Make Family Nurse Practitioner Review Easy (Precise and Concise) First Edition

Dr. Mohammad Ishaq Ibrahim Al Lahham
Dr. Abdiqani Qasim
Ms. Mawahib Samatar

ACKNOWLEDGEMENT

The completion of this book would not have been possible without the invaluable support and contributions of many individuals and institutions.

First and foremost, I thank **God** for guiding me through every challenge and blessing me with the strength and perseverance to complete this work.

I sincerely thank the dedicated Family Nurse Practitioners and healthcare professionals whose clinical insights and real-world experiences have significantly informed the content and practical approach presented herein. Their commitment to excellence in patient care continues to inspire me.

Special thanks are due to **Dr. Abdiqani Qasim,** co-author of this book, and **Mrs. Mawahib. H Samatar**, CEO of Nursing at the Ministry of Defence Health Services (MODHS). Their unwavering support and valuable contributions were instrumental throughout the development of this work.

Deep thanks go to the authors, researchers, and organizations whose evidence-based guidelines and clinical research underpin the principles outlined in this book. Their foundational work has helped shape a comprehensive and current resource for Family Nurse Practitioners.

I am equally grateful to the technical and editorial teams whose dedication, from manuscript preparation to final production, has significantly enhanced the quality and accessibility of this book.

Above all, I offer my heartfelt thanks to my family. To my parents, **Ishaq Daoud Al-Lahham** and **Massara Abdulnabi**, for their enduring love, guidance, and example. To my beloved **wife, Asmaa Radwan**, for her endless support and encouragement. And to our five wonderful children—**Qassem, Gana, Hala, Ishaq, and Ahmad**—your presence is my greatest motivation.

I hope this book serves as a practical and empowering guide for Family Nurse Practitioners, helping them advance their clinical proficiency and provide the highest standards of care.

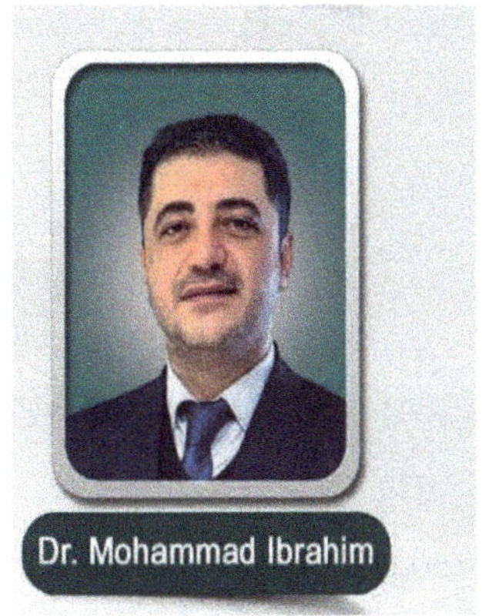

Book Author

Dr. Mohammad Ibrahim, DNP, APRN, FNP-C, MSN, CCRN, BScN

Dr. Mohammad Ibrahim is a leading authority in advanced practice nursing and healthcare research, currently serving as Director of Advanced Practice Nursing at Riyadh's Ministry of Defense Health Services (MODHS). With over two decades of clinical experience—including five years as a Family Nurse Practitioner and another fourteen as a critical care registered nurse—he brings a unique blend of expertise in primary care, critical care, and gerontology.

Dr. Ibrahim earned his Doctor of Nursing Practice from D'Youville University in Buffalo, New York, and holds nurse practitioner certifications in Ontario (Canada), New York, and Michigan (USA). His groundbreaking research, including a landmark study published in the *American Journal of Medical Science and Innovation*, compares care outcomes between nurse practitioners and primary care physicians in older patients with congestive heart failure. His work emphasizes the value of collaborative, patient-centred approaches in chronic disease management.

As the primary author of this book, Dr. Ibrahim hopes it will serve as a practical and empowering guide for Family Nurse Practitioners, helping them advance their clinical proficiency and provide the highest standards of care.

A passionate educator and visionary, Dr. Ibrahim is committed to advancing clinical practice, improving healthcare policy, and mentoring future generations of healthcare professionals. His research and leadership continue to shape innovative care models that redefine the roles of healthcare providers in the 21st century.

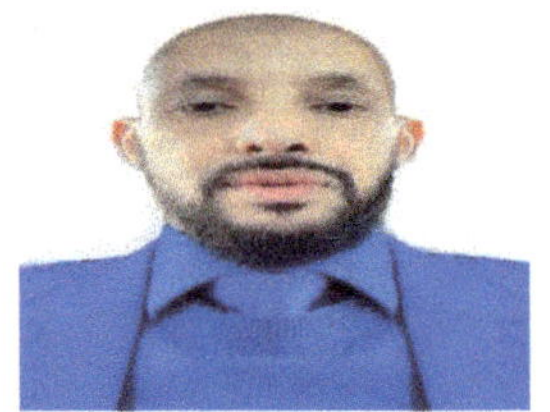

Book Coauthor

Dr. Abdiqani Qasim, DNP, MSc, FNP, ACNP(c), RN

Dr. Abdiqani Qasim is the Executive Director of Training & Continuous Professional Development at the Ministry of Defense Health Services, Nursing Administration. With over 30 years of dedicated service in healthcare, he has held influential roles, including Nursing Consultant to the Executive Nursing Administration at King Fahad Medical City (KFMC) in Riyadh.

Dr. Qasim holds a Doctor of Nursing Practice in Executive Educational Leadership and is recognized for his leadership in nursing management, advanced practice nursing, education, and hospital performance improvement. He is a certified Family and Acute Care Nurse Practitioner with active RN licenses in Canada, the United States, and Saudi Arabia.

Throughout his career, Dr. Abdiqani Qasim has led and implemented numerous transformative initiatives that have advanced nursing practice and healthcare quality. These include establishing hospital-based nursing education infrastructure, introducing advanced nursing practice at King Fahad Medical City (KFMC) and the Ministry of Defense Health Services (MODHS), and launching the first nursing shared governance models in both institutions. He has also led efforts in achieving Magnet Recognition and implementing NDNQI projects, contributed significantly to JCIA and CBAHI accreditation processes, advocated for safe nurse-to-patient ratios, and organized multiple international nursing congresses to promote knowledge exchange and professional development.

A passionate advocate for professional development, Dr. Qasim is committed to mentoring younger generations of nurses. He has published extensively, presented at national and international forums, and is a peer reviewer for the *International Journal of Africa Nursing Sciences.*

Dr. Qasim continues to shape the future of nursing through innovation, education, and strategic leadership in healthcare systems worldwide.

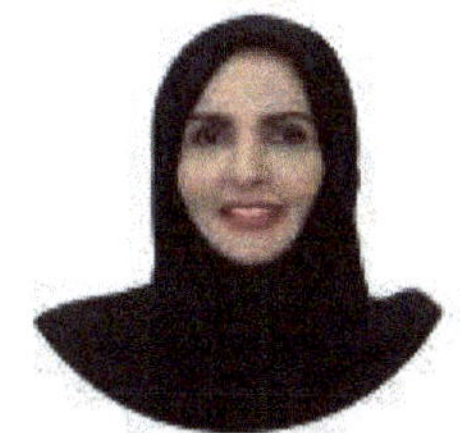

Book Coauthor

Mrs. Mawahib. H Samatar, MSN, CCRN, BScN

Mrs. Mawahib is the Executive Director of Nursing Administration at the Ministry of Defense Health Services. She graduated from Walden University in Minneapolis, Minnesota, with a Master's Degree in Healthcare Management and Leadership. Mrs. Mawahib has extensive experience in clinical and managerial areas, and her areas of expertise include critical care nursing and leadership.

Mrs. Mawahib introduced the Magnet Recognition program to the Director of Nursing in all Eastern Province Military Hospitals and served as Chairperson on the Nursing Executive Committee.

Most recently, Mrs. Mawahib has been involved with the National Transformational Program 2030 at the national level to assist with planning nursing pathways.

Mrs. Mawahib serves as the Executive Director of Nursing Administration at the Ministry of Defense Health Services in Riyadh, overseeing 25 hospitals and approximately 15,000 nurses.

Mrs. Mawahib is a dynamic and result-oriented nurse leader who sets high standards for herself and her team. A leader who prioritizes patient care while empowering and motivating nurses and physicians to reach their highest potential.

Mrs. Mawahib has also led efforts in implementing NDNQI projects, contributed significantly to JCIA and CBAHI accreditation processes, advocated for safe nurse-to-patient ratios, and organized multiple international nursing congresses to promote knowledge exchange and professional development.

SUMMARY

This book serves as a comprehensive guide for Family Nurse Practitioners (FNPs), focusing on core aspects of clinical practice, patient care, and the essential skills required in managing diverse healthcare needs. The first chapter introduces the role of an FNP, emphasizing the significance of evidence-based practice (EBP) and offering practical approaches to diagnostic and treatment principles. It also highlights the importance of system-based reviews to understand common medical conditions and disorders encountered in clinical settings. SOAP notes are discussed in detail, with an emphasis on their clinical application, helping practitioners efficiently document patient care and avoid common mistakes. Subsequent chapters dive deep into specific body systems, such as cardiovascular, respiratory, gastrointestinal, musculoskeletal, and nervous systems, detailing anatomy, physiology, and prevalent conditions. The book outlines the management of chronic diseases, such as hypertension, diabetes, and heart failure, while also addressing urgent conditions like stroke and myocardial infarction. FNPs are guided through clinical decision-making frameworks, promoting critical thinking and effective interventions. Pharmacology, including drug classifications, pharmacokinetics, and pharmacodynamics, is also thoroughly explored, providing FNPs with essential knowledge for safe prescribing and understanding drug interactions. Emphasis is placed on the importance of preventive care, health promotion, and disease management, particularly in vulnerable populations like the elderly, pregnant women, and children. Practical tips are provided for improving patient outcomes, along with tools for managing complex cases. The book also touches on legal and ethical considerations, stressing the importance of cultural competency in healthcare and addressing the challenges that FNPs face in clinical practice. Overall, the text equips Family Nurse Practitioners with the necessary tools and knowledge to excel in patient care, diagnose effectively, and stay up to date with the latest clinical practices and guidelines.

Contents

List of Tables

List of Figures

1 Chapter 1: Introduction to the Family Nurse Practitioner Role

1.1 Role of an FNP in Patient Care

1.1.1 Overview of the Family Nurse Practitioner (FNP) Role

In today's healthcare field, the **Family Nurse Practitioner (FNP)** has become an essential professional for filling the shortages and needs in primary care, chronic illness care, and preventive services. FNPs are postgraduate professional nurses with knowledge and skills that enable them to offer **patient-centred care** throughout their lifespan using both nursing and medical concepts (Berglund 2019). Their function has been gaining importance in countries with a deficit of physicians, a growing population, and heightened expectations of healthcare services (Melo et al., 2019).

They have the capacity to practice independently in a lot of areas, areas that embrace diagnosing, treating and managing of both acute and chronic illnesses. In accordance with national policies and regulations, most **FNPs practice independently**, although they may, at times, work in multi-disciplinary teams. Currently, most states and provinces have embraced the FPA allowing FNP practice without medical supervision in countries like the **United States and Canada**. On the other hand, in **France and Italy**, the autonomy of advanced practice nurses is somewhat limited; hence, they cannot prescribe medicines or undertake particular medical procedures independently without the assistance of physicians (OECD, 2024).

The role of an FNP is a highly favourable one because of the focus on preventative medicine, educating patients, and providing follow-up appointments. Compared to the conventional workforce modelled by physicians, FNPs take more time to counsel, educate and interact with patients hence **patients' satisfaction and compliance to treatment** regiments as postulated in the WHO 2024. The Netherlands remains an outstanding case of a **'best-practice'** model of FNP integration to full practice, as NPs in the Netherlands were able to produce equivalent or even better patient outcomes than their **physician counterparts**, which subsequently led to NP autonomy by means of policy changes that formally reaffirmed the clinical and legal authority of independent **FNPs** (WHO, 2024). As the healthcare system advances, FNPs are liable to be even more involved with identifying issues, enhancing the availability of care, and implementing direction and coordination of other professionals to enhance performance and value in healthcare services.

1.1.2 Responsibilities of an FNP

The FNP as a professional is a clinically oriented person who possesses varying competencies, knowledge, and skills in the disease management-promoting health literacy approach. They perform various clinical, educational, and leadership roles to make them vital in ensuring health care delivery in primary, acute, and speciality care facilities (Melo et al., 2019).

One of the most important roles of an FNP is the p**rovision of valid and precise assessments of patients** that involve taking health histories, clinical assessments, and risk assessments. These assessments allow FNPs to build what can be described as tailored care plans that are compatible with guidelines. FSN practice within this role involves ordering of diagnostic tests such as **laboratory, imaging and ECG**. It remains the most important tool for diagnosing diseases in the early stages and avoiding complications (OECD, 2024).

In addition to the assessment of the patient, another essential duty of an FNP is in the prescription and administration of the right medications. In most FPA, FNPs autonomously **prescribe and modify prescriptions,** including controlled substances, in concordance with protocols. However, in the restricted practice environment, the FNPs are allowed to prescribe some drugs but this will require them to enter into an agreement with a physician (WHO, 2024). In addition to medication, FNPs use **non-drug therapies, or non-pharmacologic treatments**, for long-term effective counseling on lifestyle changes, and dietary and mental health issues.

Scholars indicate that FNP practice focuses on patient education and health promotion, including chronic conditions such as **Diabetes, hypertension, and cardiovascular diseases**. According to the studies, the patient receiving continuous care from the FNP improves better medicine compliance, better disease management, and better satisfaction level compared to the physician's model of care (Fraze et al., 2017). Also, FNPs perform preventive care, **including immunizations, mammography, Pap smear, and family planning**, thus avoiding hospitalization and emergency department utilization.

In addition to direct patient care, FNPs act as intercessors between physicians, nurses, social workers, and other specialists involved in patient treatment. They are involved in policy-making, research, quality improvement, evidence-based practice (EBP), and the advancement of healthcare (Dotson, 2024). Since the focus of healthcare has shifted to more cost-efficient approaches, FNPs' roles in primary care, rural healthcare, and telemedicine for various populations remain a growing trend. **Following are the key 5 responsibilities of FNP:**

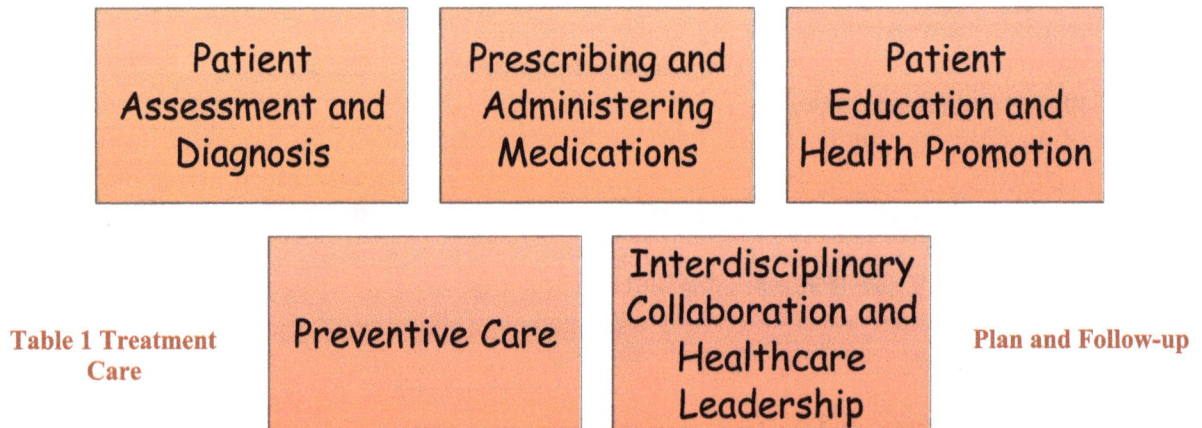

Patient Assessment and Diagnosis

Prescribing and Administering Medications

Patient Education and Health Promotion

Preventive Care

Interdisciplinary Collaboration and Healthcare Leadership

Table 1 Treatment Care Plan and Follow-up

Condition	Treatment Plan	Follow-Up Care
Hypertension	Prescribe antihypertensives, and lifestyle changes, and monitor comorbidities.	Follow-up in 4 weeks, assess BP control, adjust meds.
Diabetes Mellitus	Initiate metformin/insulin, dietary counseling, and glucose monitoring.	Follow-up in 6-8 weeks, check glucose levels and monitor complications.
Hyperlipidemia	Start statins, heart-healthy diet, and cardiovascular risk assessment.	Follow-up in 6-12 weeks, lipid panel check, annual monitoring.
Asthma	Prescribe inhaled corticosteroids/bronchodilators, develop action plan.	Follow-up in 4-6 weeks, assess symptoms and medication adherence.

COPD (Chronic Obstructive Pulmonary Disease)	Prescribe bronchodilators/corticosteroids, smoking cessation, rehab.	Follow-up in 4-6 weeks, assess symptoms, annual spirometry.
Obesity	Structured weight-loss plan, exercise, behavioral therapy.	Follow-up in 1 month, assess weight loss progress, ongoing support.
Depression/Anxiety	Start SSRIs/therapy, assess for suicidal ideation.	Follow-up in 2-4 weeks, check med tolerance, adjust therapy.
Osteoarthritis	Prescribe NSAIDs, physical therapy, consider injections.	Follow-up in 4-6 weeks, assess pain control, adjust treatment.
Hypothyroidism	Initiate levothyroxine therapy, monitor TSH levels.	Follow-up in 6-8 weeks, recheck TSH, adjust dosage.
Chronic Kidney Disease (CKD)	Control hypertension/diabetes, adjust medications, monitor kidney function.	Follow-up every 3-6 months, renal function tests, urine analysis.

1.1.3 Special Populations & Considerations

Family Nurse Practitioners are competent in dealing with the number one health issue affecting diverse populations around the world, therefore, FNPs must possess culturally sensitive tolerance and the knowledge of how to handle different issues concerning community's health. Some of the focus populations include **children and adolescents, the elderly, minorities, and populations with chronic and complicated diseases** that require special attention due to disparities in access and care outcomes.

Certainly one of the most vulnerable patient populations that FNPs work with managing is the pediatric population, in which their responsibilities go beyond simple annual physicals, screening for **developmental delays, administering immunizations, and counseling parents.** These pediatric FNPs evaluate childhood development and recommended nutritional intake; acute and chronic childhood diseases such as asthma, obesity, and behavioral health issues (WHO, 2024). Due to rising cases of **childhood obesity and type 2 diabetes,** FNPs are significant in counseling for health improvement, weight control, dietary directions, and early diagnosis in children.

Another area of practice for FNPs is the care of elderly people due to the increasing population and incidence of chronic disorders worldwide. These populations have complex medical needs, including **polypharmacy, falls, advanced care planning, and hospice referral** at the end of life. In nursing homes and assisted living facilities, FNPs manage the care of complex elderly patient populations guaranteeing that the implementation of their medical plan is in synergy with the patient's needs and preferences (Fraze et al., 2017). Research conducted in the Netherlands has established that FNP-driven geriatric programs are effective in improving **functional status, medication safety, and patient satisfaction** (WHO, 2024).

It is also important to mention that FNPs serve patients with limited access to care, especially, those in rural areas. In low-resource areas, FNPs play a role in filling the gap that is caused by shortages of physicians. This includes the treatment of long-established diseases, care of mothers and their offspring as well as preventive care. Studies from the United States and Canada show that **FNP-led clinics enhance accessibility** of care and decrease hospitalization rates in rural settings (OECD, 2024). But there is still some issues that inhibit FNPs from responding to these disparities adequately; these include scarce funds, inadequate workforce, and restrictive policies.

There is also the need to consider the care of patients with acute and stable chronic and complicated diseases such as **diabetes, cardiovascular disease of different types, mental diseases, autoimmune diseases.** To address these afflictions, FNPs need to use a **biopsychosocial**, life span approach and treat these disorders **medically, psychologically, and lifestyle-wise**. Telemedicine and remote patient monitoring have become crucial in chronic disease management since FNPs can monitor patient progress, modify treatment plans, and introduce numerous educational components without seeing the patient often (WHO, 2024).

Cultural competence and health equity initiatives are pivotal to nursing evaluation and management of ethnocultural populations, immigrants, and patients of diverse sexual orientation, and disability. Despite the intention to provide quality and culturally sensitive care, FNPs are confronted with **language barriers, disparities, and stigma** in creating equal access for all clients. According to the Pan American Health Organization (PAHO, 2022), FNP training should focus on **cultural intelligence and trauma-informed care** to address how past prejudice and disparities affect patient care and engagement.

Applying care models, advancing policies, and using technology are all challenging roles performed by FNPs to reduce health inequalities and promote improvements in vulnerable and underrepresented groups. The essence of nurses is in their ability to deliver individually tailored, holistic care solutions in various contexts, thus making them agents of fairness and access to healthcare for all.

1.2 Overview of System-Based Reviews

1.2.1 Purpose of System-Based Reviews

Integrated system assessments involve the complete process of evaluation, diagnosis and care delivery for a patient which makes it easy not to overlook any spot of a patient's status (Gubala et al., 2012). This helps the FNPs to address patient complaints systematically focus on particular organ systems and order relevant diagnostic tests based on patient clinical presentation. It also improves efficiency in clinical practices, accuracy in diagnosis, and precision in the management of patients with illnesses. This can be challenging since patients in primary care frequently come with a multiplicity of symptoms and complaints affecting various body systems, thus urging the FNPs to distinguish between **local and constitutional complaints**. It is beneficial for a patient as a system approach ensures that symptoms are evaluated systematically and hence different possibilities are not overlooked. For instance, a particular patient who complains of **fatigue and weight gain** may require an evaluation of the endocrine system, which could be caused by hypothyroidism and not depression. According to the **OECD Health System Characteristics survey** (2023), systematic bias minimizes cost issues that emanate from the health facility besides emphasizing that where such strips exist, the diagnostic tools used are often highly developed for any setting that may lack resources to afford them. In this way, using a more structured approach, FNPs avoid unnecessary and costly re-visits, provide timely and adequate care, and increase demand for healthcare facilities.

1.2.2 Key Body Systems & Common Conditions

1.2.2.1 Cardiovascular System

The cardiovascular is one of the most reviewed systems in system-based reviews because of its attendant critical diseases like heart diseases, hypertension and stroke. **Cardiovascular diseases and hypertension rank top** among the most frequent diseases affecting the global population; in primary care, people suffer from **CAD** and **CHF** (Celermajer et al., 2012). Cardiovascular diseases are closely monitored, diagnosed and prevented by FNPs in the initial stage. Hypertension also known as the **"silent killer"**, the patients should have periodic blood pressure checks (WHO, 2023). Counseling regarding changes in lifestyle should be on medication to control hypertension and reduce risks of stroke and myocardial infarction. Moreover, infections cause ECG abnormalities together with inflammation and vascular obstruction which result in severe heart complications. The **Figure 1** presents strategies for risk reduction through public health programs as well as preventive measures and diagnostic guidelines together with treatment protocols and international collaboration. To decrease infection-associated cardiac conditions healthcare professionals need to raise awareness while conducting data collection and implementing preventive measures. Components of CHF management **include control of the daily intake of fluids, maintaining compliance with prescribed medication, and educating the patient about the need to reduce salt intake and the daily self-weighing** (Kekii 2014). Thus, in patients with CAD it is critical for FNPs to discuss the issue of cholesterol, smoking cessation, and exercise as to avoid disease progression. That is why FNP–led cardiovascular risk reduction programs contribute to the enhanced patient outcomes with the help of **education, medications, and lifestyle changes** (Fraze et al., 2017). Since the prevalence of CVDs is on the rise, FNPs are crucial to provide early and comprehensive management of CVDs to decrease morbidity and mortality.

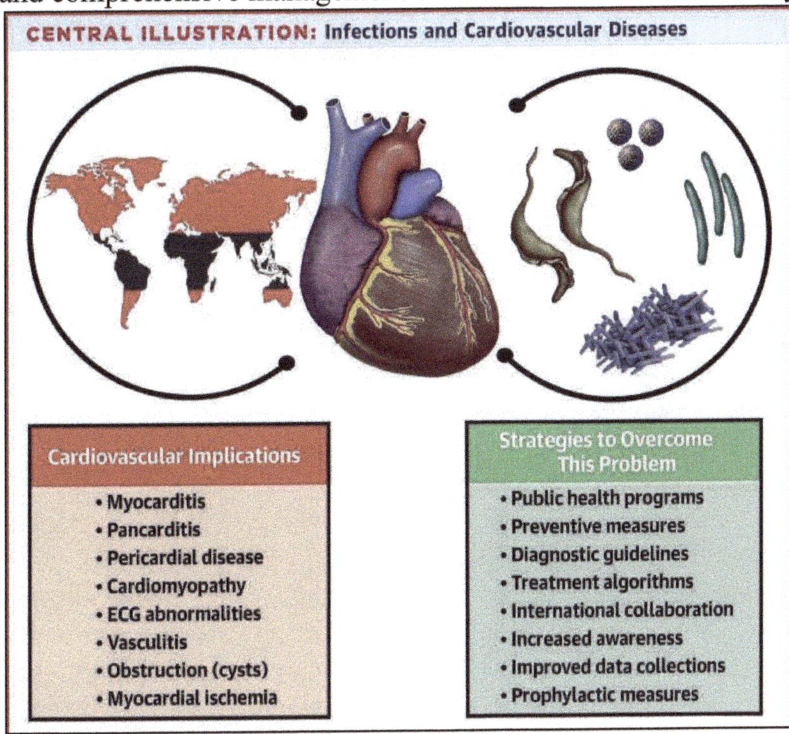

CENTRAL ILLUSTRATION: Infections and Cardiovascular Diseases
Cardiovascular Implications
• Myocarditis
• Pancarditis
• Pericardial disease
• Cardiomyopathy
• ECG abnormalities
• Vasculitis
• Obstruction (cysts)
• Myocardial ischemia
Strategies to Overcome This Problem
• Public health programs
• Preventive measures
• Diagnostic guidelines
• Treatment algorithms
• International collaboration
• Increased awareness
• Improved data collections
• Prophylactic measures

Figure 1 Impact of Infections on Cardiovascular Diseases and Strategies for Prevention

1.2.2.2 Respiratory System

Respiratory diseases are common in the outpatient clinic and this calls for the early recognition and management of conditions like asthma, COPD, pneumonia, and tuberculosis among others (Senno et al., 2022). **Dyspnea is one of the common complaints** presented to FNP and other respiratory-related symptoms such as cough, wheezing and chest pain: require that FNP conduct a structured respiratory system assessment to establish the nature and cause of the complaint. **Asthma and Chronic obstructive pulmonary disease (COPD)** are conditions that are very popular among patients with chronic diseases (Yin et al., 2017). Asthma is defined as episodic reversibility of the airflow obstruction due to bronchoconstriction with inflammation thus it needs the use of **inhalational steroids, bronchodilators as well as patient counseling on ways** of preventing triggers. COPD is primarily associated with smoking and environmental pollution with necessary **spirometry, smoking cessation and appropriate counselling**, and other **pharmacological therapy, including LABA, LAMA and ICS** (Figure 2) (Amegadzie, 2021; Prosser et al., 2017).

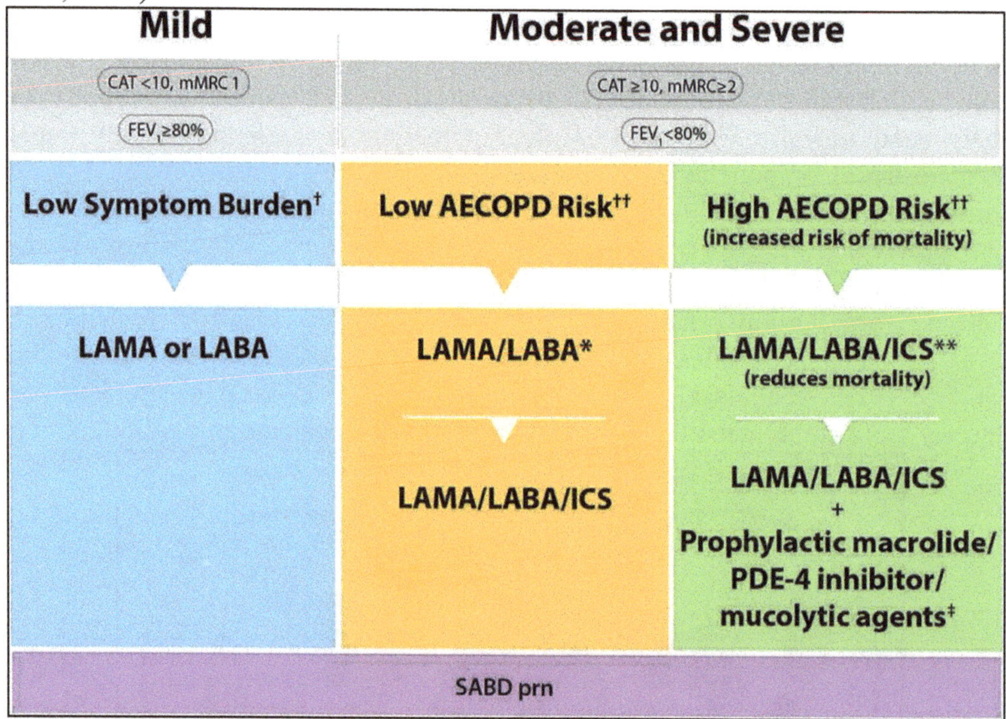

Figure 2 COPD Management Based on Severity and Risk

1.2.2.3 Endocrine System

Metabolic regulation, hormonal balance and homeostasis are key areas covered by the endocrine system, and thus, any system-based review needs to include this system. **Diabetes mellitus, thyroid disorders and adrenal insufficiency are the most common endocrine diseases** found in primary care. **Diabetes mellitus (DM)** is a common health problem and T2DM is on the rise due to the increased prevalence of obesity and a sedentary lifestyle (Zheng et al., 2018). To implement the testing and management of **DM, FNPs monitor HbA1c test results, fasting blood glucose level**, and patient education on diet, physical activity, and medication regimens. Figure 3 illustrates the **HbA1c test range for pre-diabetes,** indicating that levels between **6.0% and 6.5%** suggest an **increased risk** of developing diabetes. It emphasizes that continuous monitoring and lifestyle modifications are essential to prevent progression to type 2 diabetes. It is important to note that diabetes management cannot be solely achieved by medications, but requires nutrition education, medication and comprehensive lifestyle changes. The evaluation of energy level, changes in weight and cardiovascular system is important in the cases of hypothyroidism and hyperthyroidism. For hypothyroidism, common intervention includes supplementing with **levothyroxine while hyperthyroidism may require the use of antithyroid medications, beta-blockers or radioactive iodine treatment** (Hughes et al., 2021). Adrenal disorders are less frequent and should be distinguished from adrenal insufficiency; **fatigue, hypotension, and electrolyte abnormalities,** which may warrant hormone substitution therapy (Godshall et al., 2013). Based on the increasing rate of endocrine diseases, FNPs need to be on the lookout for signs and symptoms of diseases and promptly diagnose them for ongoing medical management.

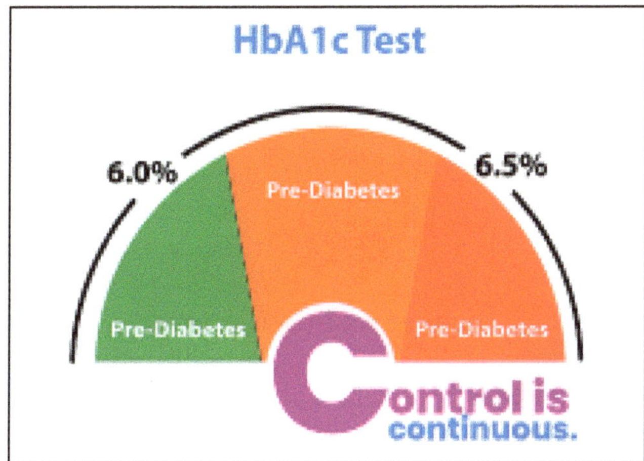

Figure 3 Identifying Pre-Diabetes Risk through HbA1c Test

1.2.2.4 Gastrointestinal System

GI problems represent one of the primary drivers for outpatient consultation; they include functional GI disorders such as **irritable bowel syndrome and organic diseases like colorectal cancer.** Among them are abdominal pains, nausea, bloating, and changes in bowel movement, which have to be distinguished between normal and serious illnesses. GERD is relatively common and should be treated through dieting, some changes in behaviours, and PPIs for relief of the symptoms (Martin et al., 2022). **Irritable bowel syndrome (IBS)** necessitates a patient-specific approach, incorporating dietary changes, stress management, and pharmacologic interventions. More severe conditions than **GERD include peptic ulcer disease (PUD)** and **inflammatory bowel disease (IBD)** that need endoscopy **H. pylori testing** and the use of **immunosuppressants** (Figure 4) (Dumic et al., 2019). They further need to assume a more proactive approach to informing clients about colorectal cancer screening, including fecal occult blood tests and colonoscopies among the targeted population.

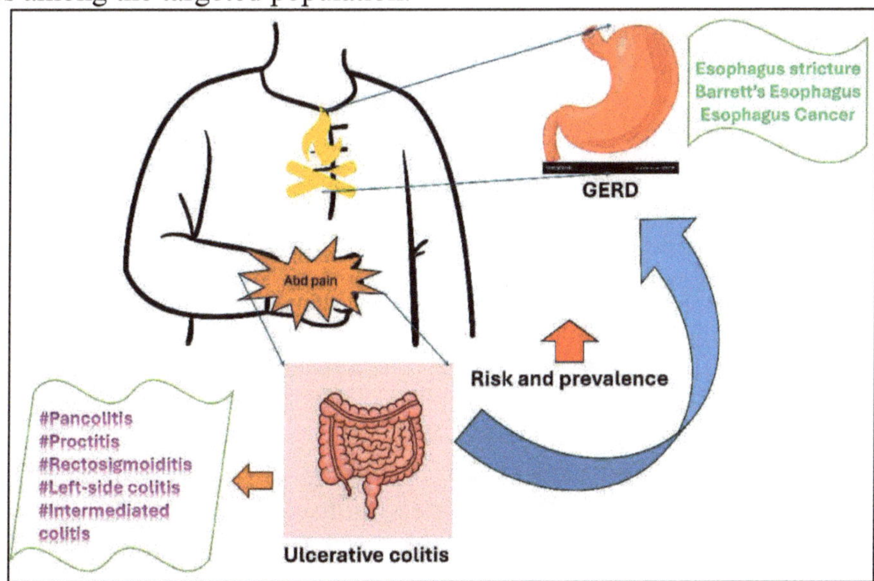

Figure 4 Enhanced Risk of Gastroesophageal Reflux Disease

1.2.2.5 Neurological System

Neurological disorders involve a multitude of symptoms which may manifest broadly across the body and have the possibility to cause disability over an extended period of time thus, it calls for a systematic assessment. Some of the most common diseases are stroke, migraines, epilepsy, and other convulsive disorders. It is important for stroke screening, especially in patients with **hypertension, atrial consulted, and diabetes.** Furthermore, FNPs must understand symptoms such as acute neurological changes, facial weakness, arm weakness, and speech abnormalities, which require an emergency response (Fenstermacher et al., 2019). Migraine and tension headache are two essential diagnoses which should be distinguished from secondary causes like **cerebral hemorrhage or meningitis.** Management of migraine deals with lifestyle changes, **pharmacological prevention (beta-blockers, triptans), and avoidance of potential triggers** (Haghdoost et al., 2022). Epilepsy requires continuous treatment with antiepileptic medications and adherence to safety measures to avoid seizure triggers. It is also crucial since FNP has to pay much attention to psychosocial treatment where a patient requires referral to counseling, support, or additional educational materials.

1.2.2.6 Musculoskeletal System

Many patients presenting with musculoskeletal disorders seek treatment in primary care, and some of the most common conditions include OA, RA, and low back pain which should be assessed systematically. **Osteoarthritis (OA)** treatment involves pain management, physical therapy, and changes in lifestyle, medication with NSAIDs and intra-articular corticosteroid injections being equally used (Nowaczyk et al., 2022). **Rheumatoid Arthritis (RA)** is an autoimmune disease that must be diagnosed as early as possible and the drug of choice is disease-modifying **antirheumatic drugs (DMARD)** (Lin et al., 2020). It is very common for people to complain of lower back pains, which may be caused by **muscle strain, a herniated disc or spinal stenosis**. Such patients present with complications such as unclear **mechanical vs inflammatory** causes, managing physical therapy, ultrasounds, and pain modality issues.

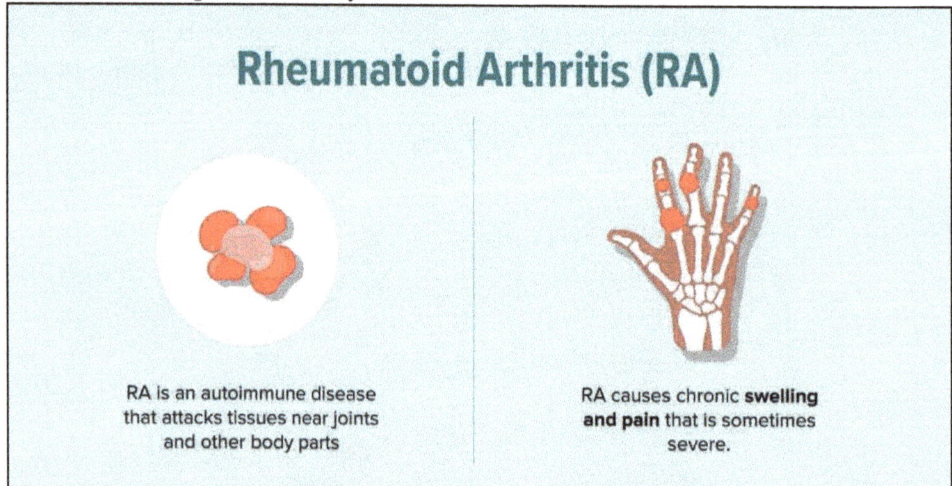

Rheumatoid Arthritis (RA)
RA is an autoimmune disease that attacks tissues near joints and other body parts
RA causes chronic swelling and pain that is sometimes severe.

Figure 5 Description of Rheumatoid Arthritis

1.2.2.7 Dermatological System

Eczema, psoriasis, and acne are examples of skin disorders that need specific treatments. Eczema takes treatment by use of moisturizers, steroids, and avoiding the triggers while psoriasis is treated with topical **agents, immunomodulators, and lifestyle changes**. The treatment of acne involves medicines that can be applied directly on the skin, such as retinoids and benzyl peroxide, oral medications such as antibiotics, and hormonal therapies. Through these system-based reviews, FNPCS enable proper diagnosis, treatment, and prevention of diseases, hence enhancing the physical fitness of patients.

1.3 SOAP Note Format & Clinical Application

1.3.1 What is a SOAP Note?

SOAP is a structured documentation tool which is frequently used by many healthcare providers, as well as FNPs, to be certain that documentation is coherent and complete. SOAP notes, created by **Dr. Lawrence Weed in the 1960s**, are a technique of reporting the patient record that enhances the organization of information, critical thinking, shared information exchange, and patient care coordination (Podder et al., 2020). There are four main elements in the SOAP note, the acronym of which is derived from the first letters of these parts: **S= Subjective, O=Objective, A=Assessment, P=Plan.**

1.3.1.1 Subjective (S)

This section encompasses the patient's own words as to what their symptoms are, what they are worried about, and other details of their medical history, such as the chief complaint (CC) and **history of present illness (HPI).** It should also contain the history of the disease, history of surgical procedures, drugs, allergies, family history and social history of the patient. The **Review of Systems (ROS),** which is a wide-spectrum symptom assessment, is also noted here. A systematic approach like the **OLDCARTS (Onset, Location, Duration, Character, Factors that Aggravate/Relieve, Radiation, Time, Severity)** framework assists in obtaining the details (Pearce et al., 2016).

1.3.1.2 Objective (O)

This section will entail information derived from commonly testable and observable findings from the patient: physical examination findings, laboratory investigations and radiological findings. Physiological observations like temperature, pulse, respiration, and language development, as well as outcomes from other examinations and tests, such as **blood tests, X-rays, and ECGs,** are recorded here (Podder et al., 2020).

1.3.1.3 Assessment (A)

Assessment refers to clinical judgmental and diagnostic evaluation of the **subjective and objective health status of a patient.** It usually begins with a differential diagnosis, i.e., a list of potential diseases accompanied by the diagnosis that the doctor considers to be the primary probable diagnosis. If the diagnosis is unclear, the assessment should specify why **further tests are needed** or if the student needs to be referred to someone else (Podder et al., 2020).

1.3.1.4 Plan (P)

This section presents treatment and management plans for the patient. These can be **medication, non-drug management, changes in personal behaviour and lifestyles, admitting a patient to other specialists,** providing information and advice to the patient, and the overall plan of action to be taken after treatment. The plan should be **realistic, supportable by data, and undertaken about the patient's condition and wishes** (Podder et al., 2020).

SOAP notes are vital in continuity as they help the different caregivers giving care to a patient to have records on the **progress of a patient, efficacy of treatment given, as well as management changes made from one visit to another**. Documenting SOAP records promotes the general efficiency of practice, decreases the likelihood of medical mistakes as well as legal claims, and complies with legal and reimbursement standards (Podder et al., 2023).

1.4 Clinical Application of SOAP Notes

1.4.1 Clinical Application of SOAP Notes

SOAP notes are especially common in primary, urgent, and chronic care, as they are conducive to directing the patient evaluation and development of the management plan effectively. In the case of a FNP, SOAP notes are important as these are used to outline the strategy of diagnosis and treatment planning while at the same time putting the provider in a legal standpoint (Donohoe, 2015). **In primary care,** FNPs are expected to come across several patients who present with ambiguous complaints that need systematic evaluation. For instance, **lethargy and weight gain** may have so many causes, which may include **hypothyroidism, anemia, depression, or diabetes**. According to the SOAP format, the **FNP gathers subjective information** (symptom history – onset, duration, accompanying features); **objective information** (physical assessment findings and laboratory results like TSH and CBC); **develops an assessment** (differential diagnosis); and **establishes a plan** (additional testing, prescribed medication and lifestyle changes) (Lin et al., 2013).

SOAP notes are also used in follow-up visits for chronic diseases to maintain order. For example, a patient with **hypertension (HTN)** is a chronic disease that needs continuous surveillance and medication changes. SOAP format helps the FNP to document **BP trends, medication compliance, side effect findings, and behavior changes**, making it easier to assess the effectiveness of the treatment plan and make necessary modifications (Podder et al., 2023). When it comes to the acute care context, including the evaluation of a patient's healthcare status, the SOAP note is an indispensable tool. Further, a patient who has **acute chest pain** must be assessed through the establishment of an acute SOAP chart based on the type of pain (sharp/dull), area affiliation, factors that worsen/magnify the pain, and physical examination findings such as **pulse rate, blood pressure, ECG, and cardiac enzymes** to rule out myocardial infarction, angina, or musculoskeletal pain and to determine a definitive referral to the **cardiology department, administration of aspirin, or further cardiac tests.**

SOAP notes also enable smooth communication between different professionals in the field of healthcare. **Medical practitioners, doctors, specialists, and other caregivers** commonly use SOAP notes as a way of comprehending the patient's progress and individual medical treatment and management plan. In a hospital context, SOAP notes help in the handover process, hence minimizing mistakes and thereby enhancing patient care outcomes (Podder et al., 2023). Besides, the SOAP notes meet legal and billing requirements. **Standard documentation** helps in avoiding cases of complicated malpractice suits since there will be a record of the events that took place in the presence of the patient, their assessment, and the overall treatment plan. SOAP notes are critical to providing insurers and healthcare payers **adequate documentation** of the services to be reimbursed, as well as adhering to regulatory policies. Thus, it is quite apparent that SOAP notes have not lost their significance in modern healthcare practice as they help to standardize documentation, increase the accuracy rate of diagnoses, and balance patient management.

1.4.2 Example SOAP Notes & Common Mistakes

Table 2 Example SOAP Note – Hypertension Follow-up

Category	Main Details	Additional Information	Notes
Subjective (S)	A 55-year-old male presents for a follow-up on hypertension.	Reports occasional headaches and mild dizziness. Denies chest pain, dyspnea, or palpitations. Admits non-adherence to prescribed low-sodium diet but takes medications regularly.	Patients should be encouraged to adhere to a low-sodium diet to help manage hypertension.
Objective (O)	BP: 148/92 mmHg, HR: 78	No signs of edema or jugular venous distension. Normal heart	Monitor BP regularly and

	bpm, RR: 16, BMI: 30 kg/m^2.	sounds, no murmurs. Lab results: Serum creatinine normal, LDL cholesterol 160 mg/dL.	encourage physical activity to aid in weight management.
Assessment (A)	Primary Hypertension - Uncontrolled due to poor dietary adherence.	Hyperlipidemia - Elevated LDL cholesterol requiring intervention.	Consider statin therapy if LDL remains elevated after lifestyle interventions.
Plan (P)	Increase antihypertensive dosage.	Initiate dietary counseling for salt restriction. Lipid panel re-evaluation in 3 months. Patient education on medication adherence and lifestyle modifications. Follow-up in 4 weeks to assess BP response.	Emphasize importance of adherence to both medication and lifestyle changes to improve outcomes.

1.5 Diagnostic & Treatment Principles

1.5.1 Diagnostic Approach

The diagnostic approach in clinical practice comprises of a model used by FNPs for the assessment of diseases that enables them to eliminate differential diagnoses and treatment plans. Diagnosis is a vital and complex process that involves critical thinking, evidence-based analysis, and patient-centered care.

1.5.1.1 Step 1: Comprehensive History-Taking

One of the most important procedures in diagnosing a disease is taking a history of a patient since some of the observations made by the patient may be crucial in identifying the conditions affecting him/ her. Based on the case scenario mentioned above, the FNP follows a **standardized technique** such as the mnemonic **OLDRACTS** to elicit appropriate information.

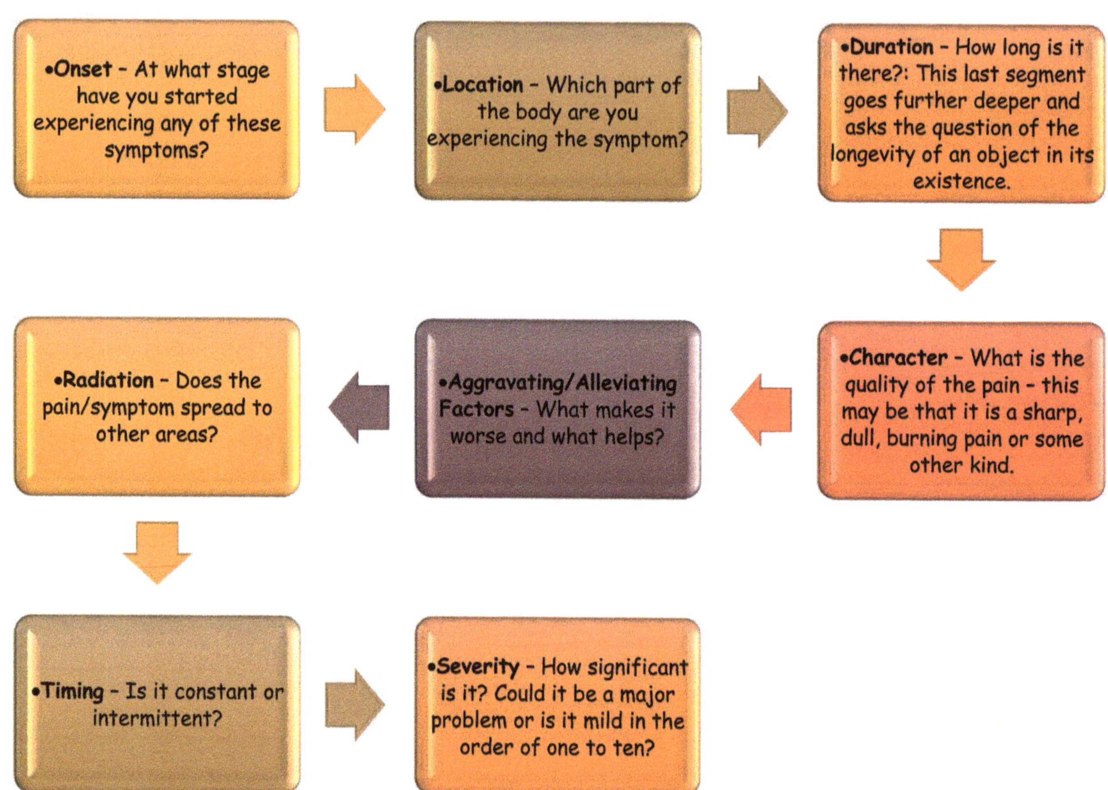

•Onset - At what stage have you started experiencing any of these symptoms?
•Location - Which part of the body are you experiencing the symptom?
•Duration - How long is it there?: This last segment goes further deeper and asks the question of the longevity of an object in its existence.
•Character - What is the quality of the pain - this may be that it is a sharp, dull, burning pain or some other kind.
•Aggravating/Alleviating Factors - What makes it worse and what helps?
•Radiation - Does the pain/symptom spread to other areas?
•Timing - Is it constant or intermittent?
•Severity - How significant is it? Could it be a major problem or is it mild in the order of one to ten?

For instance, when the patient complains of chest pain, history-taking to differentiate it as cardiac **(angina, myocardial infarction), musculoskeletal (costochondritis), gastrointestinal (GERD), or psychological (panic attack)** has to be done. Also, there is a need to gather the following information by FNPs:

Table 3 Important Information to Gather

Findings	Description
Past medical history	Existing conditions (e.g., hypertension, diabetes).
Drugs	having prescribed, purchased and used medicines - prescription drugs, non-prescribed drugs, supplements, vitamins that one takes regularly.
Family history	Genetic predisposition (e.g., cancer, cardiovascular disease).
Survey data based of social habits	Smoking, alcohol, drug use, occupation and stressors.

1.5.1.2 Step 2: Physical Examination

The physical examination is also done once history has been taken with an aim of identifying objective findings. This includes:

Table 4 Key Details for Physical Examination

Physical Observation	Findings
Vital signs	Blood pressure, heart rate, respiratory rate, temperature, oxygen saturation.
Physical condition	Improper posture, anxious, difficulty breathing or is pale, has a blue tinge on her skin or is yellowish.

Organ based assessment	It involves inspection, palpation, percussion, and auscultation based on the body organ affected.

For example, in a patient presented with pneumonia, FNP examines for crackles or decreased breath sound, coarse tactile feathery friable sign, and dull percussion note.

1.5.1.3 Step 3: Diagnostic Testing & Imaging

If physical examination does not give adequate results in diagnosing them, then diagnostic tests help to confirm with absolute certainty. Common investigations include:

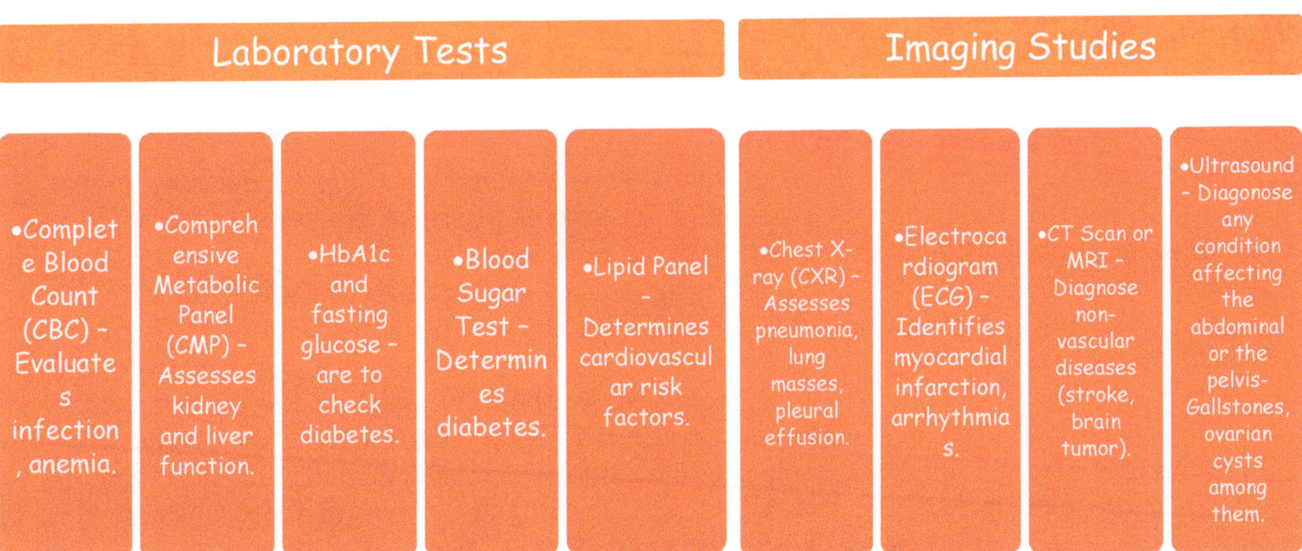
Investigation
Laboratory Tests
Imaging Studies
•Complete Blood Count (CBC) - Evaluates infection, anemia.
•Comprehensive Metabolic Panel (CMP) - Assesses kidney and liver function.
•HbA1c and fasting glucose - are to check diabetes.
•Blood Sugar Test - Determines diabetes.
•Lipid Panel - Determines cardiovascular risk factors.
•Chest X-ray (CXR) - Assesses pneumonia, lung masses, pleural effusion.
•Electrocardiogram (ECG) - Identifies myocardial infarction, arrhythmias.
•CT Scan or MRI - Diagnose non-vascular diseases (stroke, brain tumor).
•Ultrasound - Diagonose any condition affecting the abdominal or the pelvis- Gallstones, ovarian cysts among them.

Figure 6 Steps in Diagnosis and Imaging Approaches

From these determinations, the differential diagnoses and related clinical decisions would be made: After history taking, **physical examination and investigations** have been done, FNPs apply differential diagnosis to come up with the potential conditions. The following structured approach may be considered, and one of the examples is the **VINDICATE mnemonic**:

Table 5 Mnemonic for FNPs

VINDICATE Mnemonic	Examples
Vascular	Stroke, deep vein thrombosis.
Inflammatory	Rheumatoid arthritis, lupus.
Neoplastic	Cancer, tumors
Degenerative	Osteoarthritis, Alzheimer's disease
Infections	pneumonia, urinary system infection (UTI).
Congenital	Genetic disorders, birth defects.
Auto-Immune	Multiple sclerosis, type 1 diabetes
Traumatic	Fractures, concussions

Endocrine	Hypothyroidism, diabetes.

While assessing symptoms, lab results, and patient risks, FNPs come up with the final diagnostic analysis that is the basis of the management plan.

1.5.2 Treatment Guidelines

In management, treatment planning also subscribes to the set clinical guidelines as the management strategies developed post-diagnosis are comprehensive and evidence-based. The current national bodies that issue standard protocols on the management of patients include The **Centers for Disease Control and Prevention (CDC)**, the **American Association of Nurse Practitioners (AANP)**, and **United States Preventive Services Task Force (USPSTF).** Medications are a very important part of the treatment plan, and drug choices are made on the basis of effectiveness, side effects, and the patient's ability to take the medications as prescribed. Hypertension management involves **ACE inhibitors like lisinopril, calcium channel blockers like amlodipine, and diuretics like hydrochlorothiazide**. Diabetic or renal-identified patients may need special considerations in terms of medication choice, for instance, the use of **ARBs** to protect the kidneys.

In T2DM, the pharmacologic treatment starts with metformin because it enhances insulin sensitivity and reduces hepatic glucose output. In case of persistent dysglycemia, second-line medications including **GLP-1 receptor agonists (semaglutide) or SGLT2 inhibitors (empagliflozin)** can be used (Wilcox et al., 2020). These newer medications have proven to be better as they present extra cardiovascular and renal shields to patients with heart or kidney conditions. **Asthma and Chronic obstructive pulmonary disease (COPD)** illnesses, in particular, are diseases that are responsive to the severity of the illness and the level of their control (Holtzman, 2012). **Albuterol** is considered a rescue medication for an acute asthmatic attack while the long-term management is achieved using fluticasone and salmeterol. Other drugs that can be used to treat COPD include **phosphodiesterase-4 inhibitors and drugs** to assist smoker to quit smoking since smoking accelerates the disease progression (Chipps et al., 2021).

One of the most important cornerstones of pharmacologic care is, thus, trying to avoid developing **resistance to antimicrobial agents**. For instance, common **upper respiratory tract infections (URTIs)** are caused by viruses and do not call for antibiotic treatment, but a streptococcal pharyngitis requires **penicillin or amoxicillin**. For example, the management of uncomplicated UTIs involves using **nitrofurantoin or trimethoprim/sulfamethoxazole**, while complicated UTIs may involve the use of **fluoroquinolone (ciprofloxacin)** (Porreca et al., 2021). In addition to pharmacologic treatment, non-pharmacologic measures are significant in handling out chronic diseases and avoiding their consequences. They are part of the recommended internal medicine treatment for chronicity as they entail reduced i**ntake of sugars, frequent exercise, manageable stress, and cessation of smoking**. The recommended diet for patients with cardiovascular disease or hypertension is low in sodium and high in **vegetables, lean protein, and healthy fats** following the **Mediterranean-style diet.** Weight loss is more advisable in patients who have obesity-associated diseases such as metabolic syndrome, diabetes and osteoarthritis.

Exercise therapy is the other proven approach for handling different health issues. OA patients as well as those with **lower back pain need physical therapy**, **and programmed and exercises** in order to restore movement and relieve pain respectively (Baldania et al., 2024). Likewise, people with mental disorders, including depression and anxiety benefit greatly from aerobics and **Cognitive Behavioral Therapy (CBT)** (Gilbert et al., 2021). Currently, early interventions and knowledge enhancement procedures should be considered the landmarks of effective disease treatment. FNPs are crucial in increasing patients' knowledge about disease prevention, lifestyle transitions, medication regimens, and signs of complications. These vaccinations such as the annual **influenza vaccines, pneumococcal vaccines for older adults**, and **HPV** for the youth control contagious diseases and lower the incidences of illnesses.

Preventive approaches in healthcare include recommendations for screening for various chronic ailments or cancers. For instance, **colonoscopy screening for colorectal cancer** is done at fifty years with a repeat in ten years while mammography for breast cancer screening is done after two years in women aged between fifty and seventy-four (Sung et al., 2021). **Pap smears** should be conducted every three years for women 21-65 years, while co-testing, which includes HPV, should also be done but at longer intervals (Cooper et al., 2018). Other strategies of care planning are also encompassed in patient-centred care, where an FNP takes into consideration the patient's views, **cultural practices, economic significance, and literacy levels.** The use of shared decision-making is more productive and can also lead to better health since the patient feels he or she has a say in the management of the condition. Through the use of risk management strategies, medication reconciliation, wellness promotion, and health promotion, FNPs are uniquely positioned to address this need and play a positive, active role in disease prevention and healthcare optimization among various patient populations. Employing guidelines and patient centered care guarantees the provision of high quality and sustainable health care services.

Table 6 Treatment Guidelines Summary

Condition	Pharmacologic Treatment	Non-Pharmacologic Treatment
Hypertension	ACE inhibitors (lisinopril), calcium channel blockers (amlodipine), diuretics (hydrochlorothiazide). ARBs for diabetic/renal patients.	Dietary sodium restriction, weight loss, exercise.
Type 2 Diabetes Mellitus (T2DM)	Metformin (first-line), GLP-1 receptor agonists (semaglutide), and SGLT2 inhibitors (empagliflozin) for added cardiovascular and renal protection.	Lifestyle modifications, dietary control, exercise.
Asthma	Albuterol (rescue medication), fluticasone, and salmeterol (long-term management).	Trigger avoidance, breathing exercises.
Chronic Obstructive Pulmonary Disease (COPD)	LAMA, LABA, ICS; phosphodiesterase-4 inhibitors, smoking cessation medications.	Smoking cessation, pulmonary rehabilitation.
Upper Respiratory Tract Infections (URTIs)	No antibiotics are needed for viral infections; streptococcal pharyngitis is treated with penicillin or amoxicillin.	Symptomatic treatment with fluids and rest.
Uncomplicated Urinary Tract Infections (UTIs)	Nitrofurantoin or trimethoprim/sulfamethoxazole.	Hydration, hygiene practices.
Complicated UTIs	Fluoroquinolone (ciprofloxacin).	Hydration, avoidance of risk factors.
Cardiovascular Disease/Hypertension	Low-sodium, Mediterranean-style diet with vegetables, lean protein, and healthy fats.	Exercise, stress management.
Obesity-Associated Diseases	Weight loss recommended for metabolic syndrome, diabetes, osteoarthritis.	Dietary modification, regular physical activity.
Mental Disorders (Depression, Anxiety)	Cognitive Behavioral Therapy (CBT), aerobic exercise.	Stress management, psychotherapy.

Osteoarthritis (OA) & Lower Back Pain	Physical therapy and exercise programs.	Weight-bearing exercises, posture correction.
Vaccination	Annual influenza, pneumococcal (for older adults), HPV (youth).	Health education, disease prevention awareness.
Cancer Screening	Colonoscopy (every 10 years from age 50), mammography (every 2 years for women 50-74), Pap smear (every 3 years for women 21-65).	Early detection and awareness campaigns.
Patient-Centered Care	Shared decision-making, risk management, medication reconciliation, wellness promotion.	Holistic approach considering patient's preferences, culture, and literacy levels.

1.6 Importance of Evidence-Based Practice (EBP)

1.6.1 Definition of EBP & Why It Matters

Evidence based practice mainly involves the practical application of clinical experts, evidence available from research findings, as well as the patient preferences for healthcare decisions. EBP is derived from EBM which **Sackett et al. (1998)** defined as the process of integrating up to date best research evidence with clinical expertise and patient preferences in individual clinical practice. EBP is now regarded as one of the best practices in healthcare as it is founded on sound evidence, best practice, and theories instead of relying on **historical practices and myths**.

For FNPs, EBP is critical as it helps in determining the best practices inpatient care, promote patient safety and overall betterment of the healthcare system (Connor et al., 2023). By integrating EBP into their practice, these FNP's are guaranteed that they are sticking with the latest evidence and best practices, thus providing better recovery rates among their clients, fewer mistakes, and efficient healthcare delivery at a lower fee. For instance, in the treatment of hypertension, according to EBP, pharmacologic therapy should include **ACE inhibitors, calcium channel blockers, or thiazide diuretics as first-line therapy** due to the effectiveness noted from RCTs on reducing cardiovascular risk factors.

EBP also help in the development of critical thinking and professional standards. In contrast to other approaches, FNPs use peer-reviewed **medical studies, evidence-based clinical protocols, and systematic literature reviews** to support their treatment choices. This is especially useful where there is either new knowledge, techniques or diseases that a practitioner needs to update their knowledge with because the knowledge as per distance learned may prove to be obsolete. EBP was particularly evident during the **COVID-19 pandemic**, as practices and policies in infection control, treatment, and vaccination programs changed frequently due to new research findings (Olalekan et al., 2021).

1.6.2 Reliable Sources for FNPs

In order to be able to practice EBC, FNPs must use reputable sources that include scholarly articles, peer reviewed articles and scientifically researched publications in decision making. Medical databases such as **CINAHL**, clinical guidelines, and peer-reviewed articles as well as professional organizations offer the most credible data.

Among such resources, **PubMed** is one of the most common, free, and developed by the **National Library of Medicine (NLM).** Google Scholar is highly useful in obtaining a larger number of articles, whereas PubMed covers millions of medical studies, systematic reviews and clinical trials, so with help of these FNP could find information on the disease management, treatment effectiveness, trends in medicine etc. Like in the case of **Pubmed**, **Cochrane Library** provides research articles that include systematic reviews and meta-analysis, which presents the best evidence of clinical effectiveness of the treatment by following a strict methodological approach.

Healthcare associations and societies also produce clinical reference tools that present research-backed best practices in management of patients. Both the **American Association of Nurse Practitioners (AANP)** and the **American Academy of Family Physicians (AAFP)** offer current clinical practice guidelines that are specific for primary care providers. Moreover, governmental and academic institutions such as the **Centers for Disease Control and Prevention (CDC)** and the World Health Organization (WHO) disseminate public health recommendations such as recommendation of vaccines, as well as epidemic reports that are imperative in the fight against infectious diseases and other population health issues.

In addition, FNP can also use the resources such as **UpToDate, DynaMed and Medscape** that provide summarized evidence, treatment guideline and point of care decision support tools. These platforms combine experience with current medical information to make effective clinical decisions that can lead to quicker diagnoses. Conversely, periodicals like the **Journal for Nurse Practitioners, BMJ, NEJM, The Lancet** are professional, peer-reviewed journals that provide the most up-to-date information, research, and treatments empowering FNPs with the latest developments in the field. With these resources, FNPs can be confident that their clinical judgments are evidence-based, current, and compliant with the standards of the profession.

1.6.3 Barriers to EBP and Solutions

There are some major challenges that pose significant impediments to the implementation of **evidence-based practice (EBP)** in clinical practice. The most frequently reported difficulties are known time, inadequate literature in databases, organizational reluctance to change, and weak institutional backing. To overcome these barriers and enhance the implementation of EBP, **particular solutions** need to be applied that **facilitate its adoption in everyday practice** (Solomons et al., 2011). Another challenge is the time within which one is supposed to accomplish his/her activities, missions, and objectives. Most FNPs practice in facilities where they are inundated with patients and have **minimal opportunities for research and tracking of literature** critically. To overcome these issues, more healthcare institutions have to introduce EBP training and digital decision-support tools into practice. Information sources like **UpToDate and DynaMed** provide access to point of care resources that saves the time providers spend on searching for the evidence within their clinical practice.

Another challenge is the inability to obtain research materials of quality and this information is vital in developing good policies. Subscription to many peer-reviewed journals and databases is extremely expensive, something that makes it hard for FNPs practicing in low resource setting to access current body of evidence. **One solution** is to engage with the support of universities and medical institutions that offer access to medical databases, trials, and training at little or no cost. Also, **PLOS Medicine and BMC Nursing and** other similar journals provide free, reviewed medical papers and widen the sources for the healthcare workers globally. Another challenge is resistance to change and this can be attributed to the fact that most of the clinicians who are resisting the use of the technology are seasoned ones used to practicing in a traditional way. Some of the practitioners do not follow new guidelines because they feel uncomfortable with change, or they are not convinced that the research evidence can be applied in the clinical setting. To address this, there is need for constant EBP training, workshops, and mentorship to enable the FNPs to build confidence when it comes to the interpretation of evidence as well as applying evidential knowledge into practice.

1.7 Moh Golden Points & 10 Summary Questions and Answers

1.7.1 Moh Golden Points

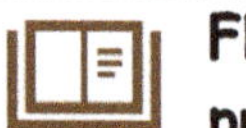	FNPs provide primary healthcare across the lifespan with a focus on health promotion and disease prevention.
	System-based reviews help streamline patient evaluations and aid in organ system management.
	SOAP notes are crucial for clinical decisions, legal issues, and patient advocacy.
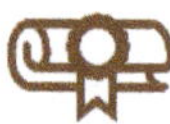	A detailed history, physical examination, and investigations help in diagnosis and exclusion of fatal illnesses
	Differential diagnosis is essential; mnemonics like VINDICATE assist in identifying possible conditions.
	Diabetes management includes diet, exercise, and medications like metformin, GLP-1 receptor agonists, and SGLT2 inhibitors.
	Musculoskeletal disorders like OA and RA are treated with physiotherapy, NSAIDs, and DMARDs in severe cases.
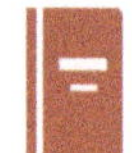	Stroke care follows the FAST approach: Facial droop, Arm weakness, Speech difficulty, Time to call an ambulance.
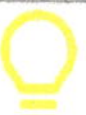	Preventive care includes screenings (mammography, Pap smear, colonoscopy) and vaccinations (influenza, pneumococcal, HPV), plus lifestyle counseling.

1.7.2 Ten Summary Questions & Answers

1. **What are the four components of a SOAP note?**
   a) Beta-blockers (e.g., metoprolol)
   b) Loop diuretics (e.g., furosemide)
   c) ACE inhibitors (e.g., lisinopril) or calcium channel blockers (e.g., amlodipine)
   d) Alpha-blockers (e.g., prazosin)
2. **What is the first-line treatment for hypertension in most patients?**
   a) Beta-blockers (e.g., metoprolol)
   b) Loop diuretics (e.g., furosemide)
   c) ACE inhibitors (e.g., lisinopril) or calcium channel blockers (e.g., amlodipine)
   d) Alpha-blockers (e.g., prazosin)
3. **Why is Evidence-Based Practice (EBP) important in FNP practice?**
   a) It reduces patient autonomy in healthcare decisions
   b) It ensures clinical decisions are based on the best available scientific evidence
   c) It relies primarily on anecdotal experiences of providers
   d) It replaces clinical judgment and expertise
4. **How do FNPs differentiate between bacterial and viral infections when prescribing antibiotics?**
   a) Prescribe antibiotics for all infections to avoid complications
   b) Use clinical judgment and diagnostic testing such as rapid strep tests
   c) Treat viral infections with antibiotics only if symptoms persist for more than 10 days
   d) Assume all fevers above 100°F indicate bacterial infections
5. **What is the recommended screening schedule for colorectal cancer?**
6. **What are the key differences between osteoarthritis (OA) and rheumatoid arthritis (RA)?**
   a) OA is an autoimmune disease, while RA is degenerative
   b) OA affects multiple joints symmetrically, while RA is typically unilateral
   c) OA is managed with NSAIDs and physical therapy, while RA requires DMARDs
   d) RA affects weight-bearing joints, while OA primarily affects smaller joints
7. **What are the first-line pharmacologic treatments for asthma?**
   a) Short-acting beta-agonists (SABAs) like albuterol
   b) Inhaled corticosteroids (ICS) like fluticasone
   c) Oral antihistamines like loratadine
   d) Systemic corticosteroids for all patients
8. **What mnemonic is used to assess stroke symptoms?**
   a) Fatigue, Arrhythmia, Slurred Speech, Thirst
   b) Facial drooping, Arm weakness, Speech difficulty, Time to call 911
   c) Fever, Anemia, Seizures, Tremors
   d) Foot drop, Asymmetry, Slurred speech, Tachycardia
9. **How can FNPs ensure effective antibiotic stewardship?**
   a) Prescribe broad-spectrum antibiotics for all infections
   b) Encourage patients to stop antibiotics as soon as they feel better
   c) Select narrow-spectrum antibiotics when appropriate and educate patients on adherence
   d) Always prescribe a 10-day course, regardless of the condition
10. **What are the best resources for FNPs to stay updated with EBP guidelines?**

a) UpToDate
b) Cochrane Library
c) Social media blogs
d) CDC and WHO guidelines

1.7.3 Rationales

1. **Answer: b) Subjective, Objective, Assessment, Plan (SOAP)**

Rationale: SOAP notes provide a structured way of documenting patient encounters, ensuring clear communication among healthcare providers.

2. **Answer: c) ACE inhibitors (e.g., lisinopril) or calcium channel blockers (e.g., amlodipine)**

Rationale: These medications are first-line treatments for hypertension because they have proven efficacy in lowering blood pressure and reducing cardiovascular risks.

3. **Answer: b) It ensures clinical decisions are based on the best available scientific evidence**

Rationale: Evidence-Based Practice (EBP) ensures that clinical decisions rely on current research, expert consensus, and patient values rather than outdated methods or personal opinions.

4. **Answer: b) Use clinical judgment and diagnostic testing such as rapid strep tests**

Rationale: Differentiating bacterial from viral infections helps prevent unnecessary antibiotic prescriptions, reducing the risk of antimicrobial resistance.

5. **Answer: a) Colonoscopy every 10 years starting at age 50**

Rationale: The USPSTF recommends colonoscopy every 10 years for adults aged 50-75 to detect colorectal cancer early and improve outcomes.

6. **Answer: c) OA is managed with NSAIDs and physical therapy, while RA requires DMARDs**

Rationale: OA is a degenerative joint disease treated with pain relief and physical therapy, while RA is an autoimmune condition requiring DMARDs to slow disease progression.

7. **Answer: b) Inhaled corticosteroids (ICS) like fluticasone**

Rationale: Inhaled corticosteroids are the cornerstone of long-term asthma management as they reduce airway inflammation and prevent exacerbations.

8. **Answer: b) Facial drooping, Arm weakness, Speech difficulty, Time to call 911**

Rationale: The FAST mnemonic helps quickly identify stroke symptoms, promoting early intervention and reducing the risk of permanent disability.

9. **Answer: c) Select narrow-spectrum antibiotics when appropriate and educate patients on adherence**

Rationale: Using the most specific antibiotic and ensuring adherence helps reduce antimicrobial resistance and improve treatment efficacy.

10. **Answer: a) UpToDate, b) Cochrane Library, d) CDC and WHO guidelines**

Rationale: These sources provide reliable, peer-reviewed, and regularly updated clinical guidelines essential for evidence-based practice.

2 Chapter 2: Cardiovascular System

2.1 Anatomy & Physiology of the Cardiovascular System

The cardiovascular system plays an essential role in transporting oxygen and nutrients with waste products across the entire body. The cardiovascular system integrates the heart with blood vessels along with blood to preserve **hemodynamic stability**. The heart positions within the mediastinum as a muscular organ contains four chambers including the right atrium and right ventricle along with the left atrium and left ventricle. **Blood flows** from the body into the **right atrium** through the **superior and inferior vena cava** before entering the **right ventricle** to travel through the **pulmonary artery to the lungs for oxygenation**. **Oxygenated blood** reaches the left atrium through pulmonary veins before traveling to the left ventricle which pumps it forward through the aorta for systemic **blood distribution (Figure 8)**. **Figure 9** shows an anatomical view of the human heart with both **internal and external elements** that maintain blood circulation. Blood distribution in the **human heart** occurs through **four chambers**: the **right atrium** and **right ventricle** handle deoxygenated blood and the **left atrium** along with the **left ventricle** operate for pumping oxygenated blood. The **tricuspid valve** exists between the **right atrial and ventricular spaces** while the **mitral valve** enables blood circulation between **left ventricles and atria**. The **aortic and pulmonary semilunar valves** serve to maintain normal blood circulation by preventing bloodstream reversal into the **ventricles**. Deoxygenated blood from the **superior and inferior vena cava** enters the **right atrium** before flowing through **pulmonary arteries** to the **lungs for oxygenation** and later reentering the heart through **left atrium**. Blood which has become oxygenated from the lungs enters the **left atrium through pulmonary veins** before being transported by the aorta to reach the tissue of the **systemic circulation**. The figure 2 displays the **papillary muscles** together with **chordae tendineae** that help valves work efficiently while presenting all heart wall layers starting from **endocardium** through **myocardium** finishing with epicardium that enables heart **contractions and defense processes**.

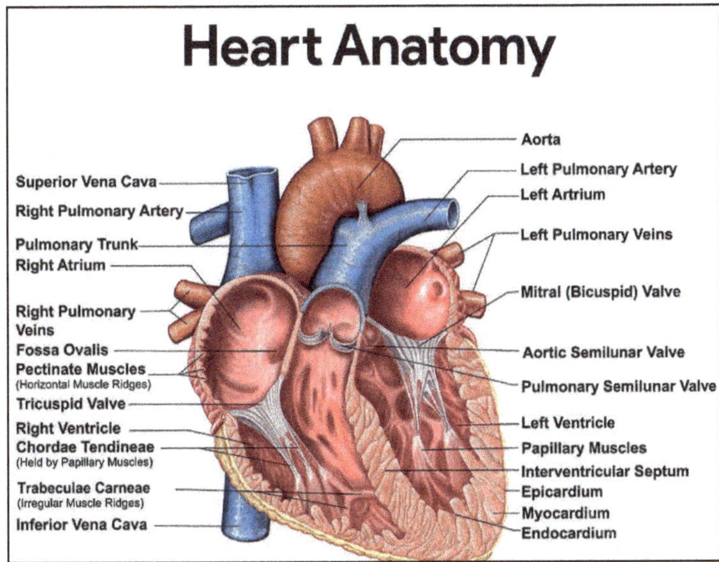

Figure 7 Anatomy of Heart

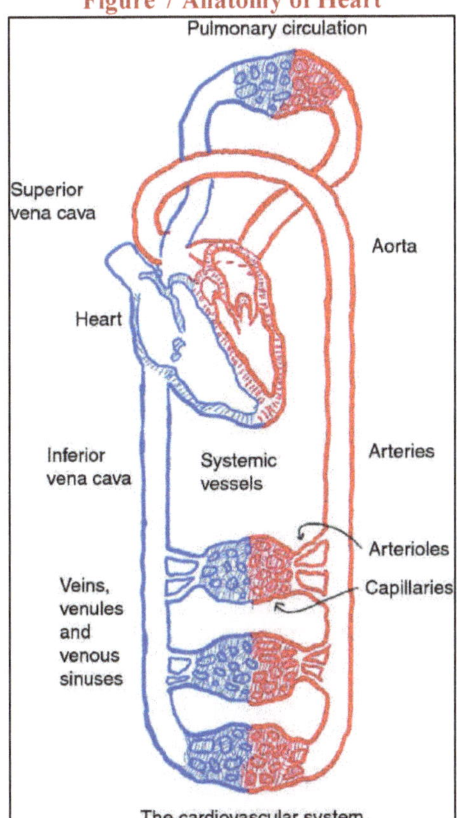

Figure 8 Physiology of Cardiovascular System

An electrical conduction system regulates heart function to maintain coherent movement between the different chambers. The natural pacemaker function of the **sinoatrial (SA) node** generates electrical impulses that proceed through the **atrioventricular (AV) node** to the **bundle of His** and then to the **Purkinje fibers** to synchronize ventricular activity. The circulatory system consists of interconnected blood pathways between **arteries, veins, and capillaries**. Blood transport begins through arteries that transport oxygenated blood from the heart and continues through veins that bring **deoxygenated blood back to the heart**. At the tissue level gas exchange occurs through minuscule blood vessels known as capillaries. Cardiovascular function relies on appropriate **cardiac output and blood pressure management** along with intact vascular structures for proper performance. Figure 9 illustrates the **cardiovascular system,** depicting the **systemic and pulmonary circulation** through the heart. **Oxygenated blood (red)** flows from the **heart through the aorta and arteries to systemic capillaries**, while **deoxygenated blood (blue) returns via veins**, the superior and inferior vena cava, and enters the **pulmonary circulation for oxygenation.**

2.2 Common Cardiovascular Conditions

The table below summarizes the common CVD conditions, highlighting their **causes, key symptoms, diagnostic tools, and treatment options**, providing a concise reference for understanding and managing cardiovascular diseases. To memorize **common cardiovascular diseases**, remember **VIN MH2V—Valve disorders, Infections, Neurotransmitters, Myocardial infarction with angina, Hypertension, Heart failure, and Vascular diseases**—which cover key conditions affecting heart function, circulation, and vascular integrity.

Table 7 Most prevalent CVD conditions

VIN MH2V—Valve disorders, Infections, Neurotransmitters, Myocardial infarction with angina, Hypertension, Heart failure, and Vascular diseases				
Condition	**Description**	**Key Symptoms**	**Diagnostic Tools**	**Treatment Options**
Valve Disorders	Murmurs are caused by conditions like mitral regurgitation, aortic stenosis, and tricuspid regurgitation.	Heart murmur, breathlessness, fatigue	Echocardiogram, auscultation	Valve replacement, medications (diuretics, beta-blockers)
Myocardial Infarction (MI) with Angina	MI occurs due to coronary artery blockage leading to myocardial necrosis; angina results from transient ischemia without tissue death.	Chest pain, shortness of breath, ECG changes	ECG, cardiac biomarkers, angiography	Aspirin, beta-blockers, statins, PCI (angioplasty)
Hypertension	Elevated blood pressure; treatment varies by ethnicity and includes ACE inhibitors, calcium channel blockers, diuretics, and lifestyle changes.	Headache, vision problems, stroke risk	BP measurement, ambulatory BP monitor	Lifestyle changes, ACE inhibitors, calcium channel blockers

Heart Failure	Types include systolic (reduced ejection fraction) and diastolic (preserved ejection fraction); classified by NYHA Class I-IV.	Edema, fatigue, shortness of breath	Echocardiogram, BNP levels, NYHA classification	Diuretics, ACE inhibitors, beta-blockers, ARNI
Vascular Disease	Includes arterial diseases (CAD, PAD) and venous diseases (DVT, varicose veins); assessed by ABI, pulse examination, and capillary refill.	Leg pain, swelling, skin discoloration	Doppler ultrasound, ABI, venography	Compression therapy, anticoagulants, bypass surgery
Infections	Includes endocarditis (heart lining infection), myocarditis (heart muscle inflammation), and pericarditis (pericardium inflammation).	Fever, chest pain, heart failure symptoms	Blood cultures, echocardiogram	Antibiotics (endocarditis), NSAIDs/steroids (pericarditis)

2.3 Major Medical Issues in Cardiovascular Health

The cardiovascular system plays an essential role in sustaining **whole-body circulation** as well as oxygen distribution across the body. Various significant cardiovascular ailments have direct effects **on heart operation**, vascular health, and **blood pressure management**.

2.3.1 Valve Disorders

Irregular blood flow causes heart valve diseases including **mitral regurgitation** together with **aortic stenosis and tricuspid regurgitation** to **produce murmurs.** These cardiovascular conditions produce symptoms of respiratory **distress as well as tiredness** alongside **heart failure signs.** The diagnosis process includes **echocardiography** and **auscultation** testing and leads to treatment options that extend from medicine drugs like **diuretics and beta-blockers up to surgical valve replacement.** The presented image shows heart valve disease by presenting four different valves **(pulmonary, tricuspid, aortic, and mitral)** and their possible pathological states. The illustration shows a comparison **between normal and stenotic aortic valves** as well as **displaying mitral valve prolapse** with an improperly **bulging leaflet** that leads to potential **regurgitation.**

2.3.1.1 Valve Disorders: Heart Murmurs

Irregular blood flow through the heart valves leads to heart murmurs which indicate conditions like **mitral regurgitation (MR), aortic stenosis (AS), tricuspid regurgitation** or other valve diseases cause these murmurs. **Heart murmurs become detectable through** auscultation tests therefore indicating potential cardiovascular conditions. The symptoms of heart valve diseases lead to **respiratory distress** combined with **fatigue and specific indications** of heart failure.

Heart murmur classification (Figure 9) occurs through the Image into systolic and diastolic categories which include three intensity patterns: **crescendo-decrescendo, holosystolic, and decrescendo**. A **crescendo-decrescendo systolic murmur** points to either left-sided aortic stenosis, hypertrophic obstructive cardiomyopathy, or right-sided pulmonic stenosis conditions. Medical professionals link **holosystolic murmurs** with stable tones to three right-sided cardiovascular conditions as well as **three left-sided cardiovascular conditions**. The combination of decrescendo pattern and **decrescendo-crescendo** pattern helps **diagnose aortic regurgitation** of the left side and pulmonic regurgitation of the right side together with left-sided mitral stenosis and **Austin-Flint murmur and right-sided tricuspid stenosis**. Healthcare providers use this system to identify heart conditions because it evaluates the type of murmurs alongside pitch changes during **systole and diastole**.

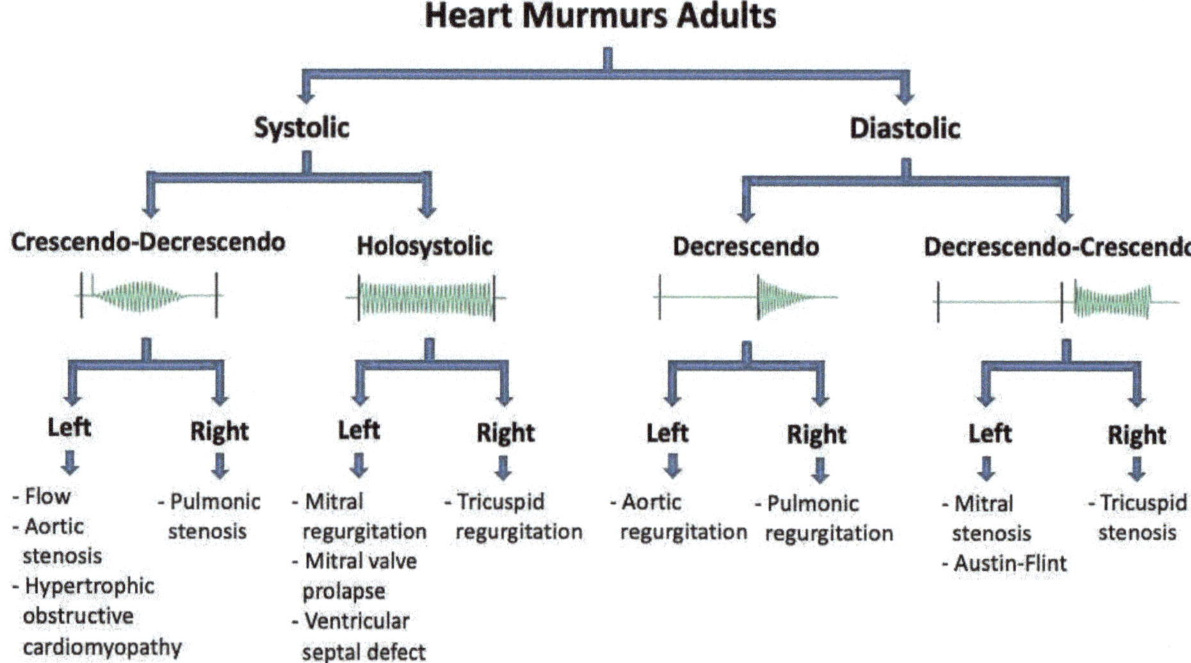

Figure 9 Classification of Heart Murmurs

Shown below is the grading of systolic murmurs which is divided by the loudness or the volume of the sound. **Grade I/VI** is feeble and can hardly be heard even when using a stethoscope and the surroundings are very serene. **Grade II/VI** is just apprising softly but also audible with the help of the standard stethoscope. **Grade III/VI** is heard without leaning close to the chest and using a regular stethoscope as a **Grade IV/VI** has an audible vibrant thrill. **Grade V/VI is** very loud, and pulsating, a thrill that can still be palpated and can be heard even when tapping on the chest lightly using the stethoscope. **Grade VI/VI** is the loudest and is accompanied by the thrill and can be heard even when the stethoscope is removed from the chest. It is very useful in assessing the loudness of the murmur and essentially in diagnosing the heart diseases that are causing them.

Grading systolic murmurs

Intensity	Description
Grade I/VI	Barely audible
Grade II/VI	Audible, but soft
Grade III/VI	Easily audible
Grade IV/VI	Easily audible and associated with a thrill
Grade V/VI	Easily audible, associated with a thrill, and still heard with the stethoscope only lightly on the chest
Grade VI/VI	Easily audible, associated with a thrill, and still heard with the stethoscope off of the chest

Figure 10 Grading of Systolic Murmurs

This image divides the **top four heart murmurs; these include; Mitral Stenosis; Mitral Regurgitation; Aortic Stenosis; and Aortic Regurgitation. Mitral Stenosis** causes a mid systolic rumbling murmur which is heard loudest at the Apex and best heard during expiration with patient in left lateral position. **Exertional dyspnea, haemoptysis, and palpitations** are some symptoms of the condition while **malar flush, atrial fibrillation, and tapping apex beat** are among the signs of the disease. This is mostly associated with rheumatic heart illness. Mitral **Regurgitation has pansystolic murmur best heard over the left sternal area, and patient complains of palpitations, fatigue and exertional dyspnoea, displacement of apex beater and atrial fibrillation** may be observed. Some of the reasons include; Mitral regurgitation and rheumatic heart disease. **Aortic Stenosis** causes ejection systolic murmur to the carotids and apex as well focusing on the symptoms like syncope and angina. They include a sharp peak and narrow pulse pressure which are mostly attributed by **senile calcification or congenital bicuspid valves.** Aortic Regurgitation results to an early diastolic murmur which is best heard on expiration while the patient is sitting forward and exhibit **palpitations and dyspnoea.** Its manifestations are indicated by water hammer pulse and widened pulse pressure and might be due to acute aortic dissection or **chronic connective tissue disorders.** This sort identifies the murmurs, the symptoms that accompany each murmur and the signs which are useful in clinical diagnosis and patient management.

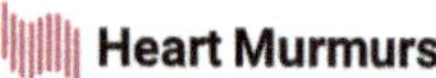

	Murmur	Symptoms	Signs	Causes
Mitral Stenosis	Rumbling mid-diastolic murmur with opening snap (best heard on expiration and patient lying on left side)	• Exertional dyspnoea • Haemoptysis (due to pulmonary oedema) • Palpitations (AF) • Chest pain	• Malar flush • Atrial fibrillation • Tapping apex beat • Low volume pulse • Loud S1	• Rheumatic heart disease (most common) • Annular calcification • Congenital • Mucopolysaccharidosis
Mitral Regurgitation	Pansystolic murmur radiating to left axilla	• Palpitations • Exertional dyspnoea • Fatigue • Weakness	• Atrial fibrillation • Displaced, thrusting apex • Soft/absent S1	• Papillary muscle rupture/ dysfunction (e.g. post-MI) • Mitral valve prolapse • Rheumatic heart disease • Infective endocarditis • Connective tissue disorders
Aortic Stenosis	Ejection systolic murmur radiating to carotids and apex	Triad of • Syncope • Angina • Dyspnoea	• Sustained, heaving apex • Slow rising pulse • Narrow pulse pressure • Soft S2 if severe	• Senile calcification of valve • Congenital bicuspid valve • Rheumatic heart disease
Aortic Regurgitation	Early diastolic murmur (best heard on expiration with patient sat forward)	• Palpitations • Angina • Dyspnoea	• Water hammer pulse • Wide pulse pressure • Displaced apex • Eponymous signs: *Corrigan's (carotid pulsation), De Musset's (head nodding with heartbeat), Quincke's (capillary pulsation in nail bed)*	**Acute** • Aortic dissection • Infective endocarditis **Chronic** • Connective tissue disorders • Rheumatic heart disease • RA, AS, Takayasu's

GRAM PROJECT

Figure 11 Classification of Heart Murmurs

2.3.1.2 Cardiac Valvular Disorders: Systolic and Diastolic Phases

During the cardiac cycle the heart operates through two essential phases known as systolic and diastolic. These phases involve blood pumping followed by **heart relaxation for refilling. Abnormal blood flow** develops from heart valve disorders which results in several health conditions affecting the patient.

Medical conditions with the name **Systolic (AS, MR Systolic) (Mr. Systolic)** appear during heart contractive periods known as systole. The narrowing of the aortic valve that controls the left ventricle to the aorta blood passage qualifies as **Aortic Stenosis (AS).** The narrowed passageway **blocks blood movement** and presses the **left ventricle** to generate more effort which results in symptoms including **chest pain and fatigue** alongside fainting episodes. The mitral valve lacks proper closure between the left atrium and left ventricle structure during **MR (Mitral Regurgitation).** A backward **blood flow (regurgitation)** enters the **left atrium** when the **left ventricle** contracts in systole thus causing shortness of **breath and fatigue** because of inadequate blood circulation.

During heart relaxation and blood filling time known as **diastole AR and MS Diastolic (Ms. Diastolic)** develop. During diastole, the **aortic valve** of people with **Aortic Regurgitation** cannot close properly which causes blood to leak continuously into the **left ventricle. Heart failure** becomes likely when the ventricle suffers from volume **overload due to the condition.** MS develops because the mitral **valve thickens** and stiffens to create an obstruction for blood moving from the left atrium to the left ventricle during the diastolic phase. The **elevated pressure** in the left atrium produces symptoms of breathlessness and exhaustion due to the condition. When dealing with **AR and MS** improper management leads to important medical issues.

Table 8 Systolic and Diastolic Murmurs – Normal and Abnormal Conditions

Phase	Condition	Normal Situation	Abnormal Situation (Pathogenic Murmur)

Systolic	Aortic Stenosis (AS)	Innocent Systolic Murmur: Soft, localized murmur in healthy individuals, usually in children or young adults, caused by increased blood flow through normal heart valves.	Harsh, crescendo-decrescendo murmur heard at the right upper sternal border; often associated with symptoms like chest pain, syncope, and shortness of breath.
Systolic	Mitral Regurgitation (MR)	Innocent Systolic Murmur: Typically soft, often due to normal physiological variations.	High-pitched, holosystolic murmur heard at the apex, radiating to the axilla; commonly associated with fatigue, shortness of breath, and fluid retention.
Diastolic	Aortic Regurgitation (AR)	Innocent Diastolic Murmur: Rare, soft murmur, can occur in some young individuals.	Diastolic decrescendo murmur heard along the left sternal border; can lead to fatigue, palpitations, and heart failure in severe cases.
Diastolic	Mitral Stenosis (MS)	Innocent Diastolic Murmur: Rare, soft murmur, may occur due to slight variations in normal valve motion.	Low-pitched, diastolic rumbling murmur was heard at the apex with the patient in the left lateral decubitus position; symptoms may include dyspnea, fatigue, and hemoptysis.

2.3.1.3 Types of Valvular Heart Disorders

The figure 12 displays **six different valvular heart diseases** which separate the conditions into **stenosis and regurgitation (insufficiency)** between the valves of the **aortic, mitral and tricuspid sections.** Blood leakage from **improper valve closure appears** as red marks corresponding to **regurgitation** while the **narrowing of heart valves** shows as blue marks that indicate **stenosis**.

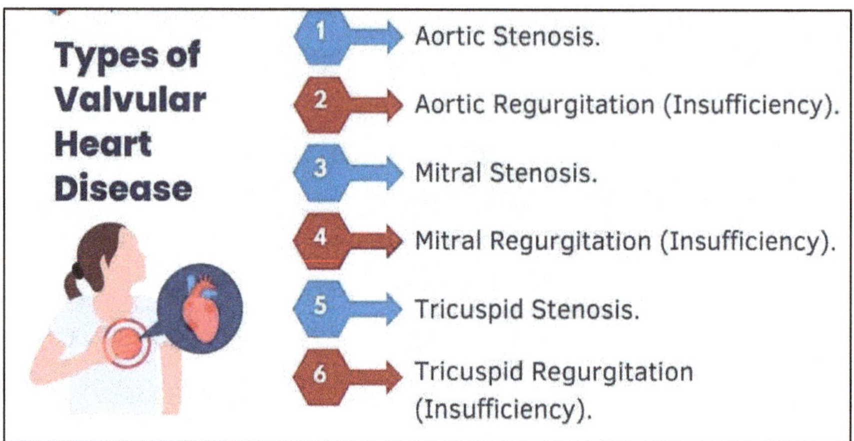

Figure 12 Classification of Valve Disorders

2.3.1.4 Possibilities of Normal and Pathological Cardiac Sounds in Valve Disorders

Figure 13 depicts **normal and pathological cardiac sounds as phonocardiograms** that display how various diseases of the heart valves create different patterns of sound waves. **Normal heart sounds** consist of **separate first and second heart sounds** accompanied by minimal **background noise (A)** but patients with **aortic stenosis** show **excessive vibrations** after their **first heart sound (B) that reveal a turbulent bloodstream**. The pathological disruptions that affect normal heart valve function lead to specific **wave abnormalities** in conditions like **mitral regurgitation (C), aortic regurgitation (D), and mitral stenosis (E).**

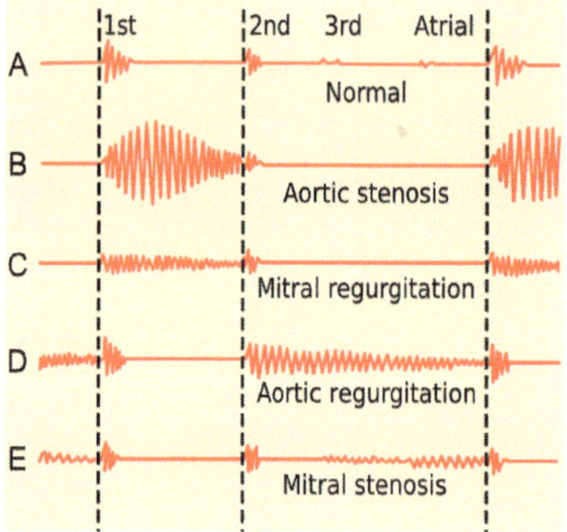

Figure 13 Phonocardiogram of normal and abnormal heartbeats.

2.3.1.5 Possible Pharmacological Treatments for Valve Disorders

Figure 14 includes medical classes for **heart conditions** and demonstrates their intended **therapeutic outcomes**. **ACE**

inhibitors enable **blood pressure reduction** to slow down **heart failure progression** while **antiarrhythmic drugs** normalize **heart rhythms.** Patients with heart conditions require **antibiotics** to prevent **infections** while **anticoagulants** reduce **thromboembolism risk, beta-blockers, and vasodilators** lower **cardiac workload,** and diuretics aid in **edema management** and **cardiac strain reduction**.

Medication Category	Goal of Therapy
ACE inhibitors	Reduce blood pressure and slow progression of heart failure
Antiarrhythmics	Restore normal rhythm
Antibiotics	Prevent infections
Anticoagulants	Reduce risk of thromboembolism, which can lead to stroke
Beta-blockers	Reduce cardiac workload via reduction in heart rate; reduce palpitations
Diuretics	Reduce edema and cardiac workload
Vasodilators	Reduce cardiac workload; reduce valvular leakage

Figure 14 Medical Categories for Heart Conditions

2.3.1.6 SOAP Notes for Valve Disorder

Table 9 SOAP Notes for Valve Disorder

Component	Details
Subjective (S)	The patient presents with progressive shortness of breath, fatigue, and heart palpitations. Reports worsening exertional dyspnea and swelling in the lower extremities.
Objective (O)	Vitals: BP 130/85 mmHg, HR 88 bpm, RR 20 bpm. Cardiac exam: Auscultation reveals systolic murmur (mitral regurgitation) and diastolic murmur (aortic stenosis). Signs of pulmonary congestion and mild peripheral edema were noted.
Assessment (A)	Differential Diagnoses: 1. Mitral Regurgitation 2. Aortic Stenosis 3. Tricuspid Regurgitation.
Plan (P)	Investigations: Echocardiogram, cardiac catheterization, BNP levels. Pharmacological Treatment: Diuretics (furosemide), beta-blockers, ACE inhibitors for heart failure prevention (See algorithms and figures below). Non-Pharmacological Treatment: Salt restriction, fluid management, and cardiac rehabilitation. Education: Explain disease progression, medication adherence, and signs requiring urgent care. Referral: Cardiologist evaluation for possible valve replacement surgery. Follow-up: Reassess symptoms and echocardiographic findings in 3-6 months.

Table 10 Algorithm for Pharmacological Treatment of Valve Disorder

Medications are not a cure for heart valve disease, but in some cases it can be successful in the treatment of symptoms caused by heart valve disease.			
Medication Management Algorithm for Heart Valve Disorders			
Step 1: Initial Assessment and Diagnosis	**Identify the type of heart valve disorder**: (e.g., aortic stenosis, mitral regurgitation, etc.) **Evaluate symptoms**: Fatigue, shortness of breath, chest pain, palpitations, etc. **Assess hemodynamic impact**: Presence of heart failure, arrhythmias, or other complications. **Comorbid conditions**: Hypertension, diabetes, heart failure, arrhythmias.		
Step 2: Medications to Control Heart Rate and Rhythm	**Beta-blockers**: • **Indication**: Used to control heart rate and prevent arrhythmias in heart valve disorders. • **Common drugs**: Metoprolol, Atenolol. • **Mechanism**: Reduces heart rate and myocardial oxygen demand, helps with arrhythmias. • **Monitoring**: Heart rate, blood pressure, risk of bradycardia.	**Digoxin**: • **Indication**: For rate control in atrial fibrillation, especially in patients with heart valve disease and heart failure. • **Mechanism**: Increases myocardial contractility and slows the heart rate. • **Monitoring**: Digoxin levels, renal function, potassium levels.	**Calcium Channel Blockers**: • **Indication**: For rate control, especially if beta-blockers are contraindicated. • **Common drugs**: Diltiazem, Verapamil. • **Mechanism**: Slows AV node conduction and heart rate. • **Monitoring**: Heart rate, blood pressure, risk of bradycardia.

Step 3: Medications to Control Blood Pressure	**Diuretics**: • **Indication**: For fluid retention, especially in heart failure associated with valve disease. • **Common drugs**: Furosemide, Hydrochlorothiazide. • **Mechanism**: Reduces fluid volume and venous pressure, easing the workload on the heart. • **Monitoring**: Electrolytes, renal function, fluid status, blood pressure. **Vasodilators**: • **Indication**: To reduce afterload, helping the heart pump more effectively, particularly in aortic valve disease. • **Common drugs**: ACE inhibitors (e.g., Enalapril, Lisinopril), ARBs (e.g., Losartan), Hydralazine. • **Mechanism**: Relaxes blood vessels, decreasing the force against which the heart pumps. • **Monitoring**: Blood pressure, renal function, electrolytes.
Step 4: Symptom Management and Supportive Medications	**Anticoagulants** (if atrial fibrillation or thromboembolism risk exists): • **Indication**: To prevent thromboembolism in patients with atrial fibrillation or mechanical heart valves. • **Common drugs**: Warfarin, Apixaban, Dabigatran. • **Monitoring**: INR for Warfarin, renal function, bleeding risk
Step 5: Considerations for Advanced Disease	**Advanced disease management**: In severe heart valve disorders, medications may alleviate symptoms but may not halt disease progression. **Consider valve repair/replacement**: If symptoms are severe or if heart failure or other complications arise.
Step 6: Monitoring and Follow-up	**Routine monitoring**: Regular echocardiograms, ECGs, and blood pressure checks. **Adjust medications**: Based on symptom control, disease progression, and any side effects.

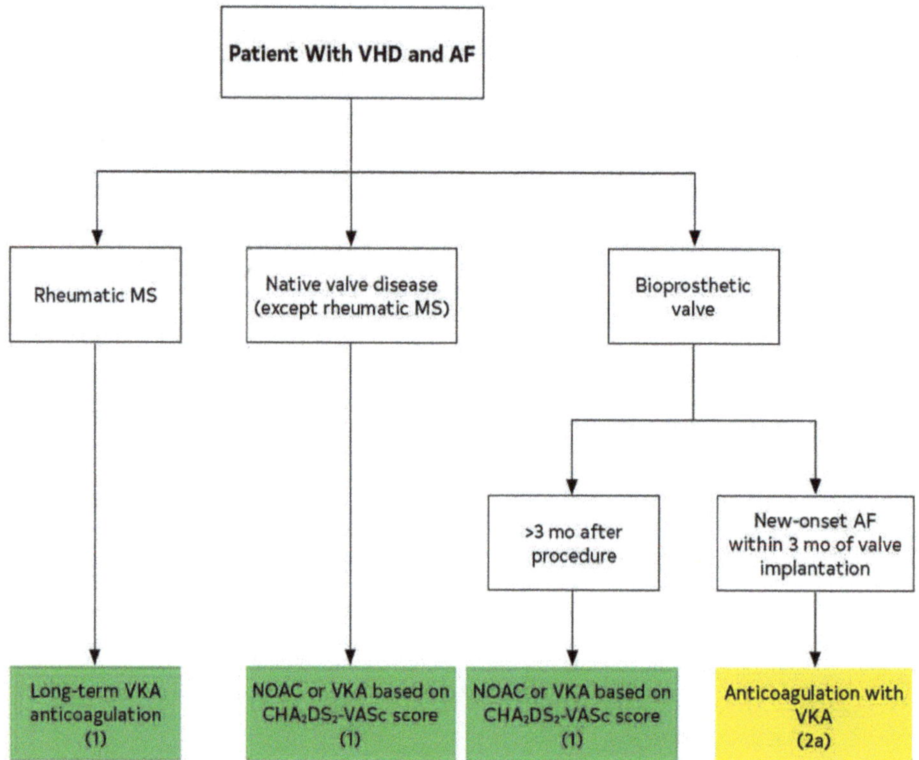

Figure 16 Treatment Approaches for Patient with VHD and AF

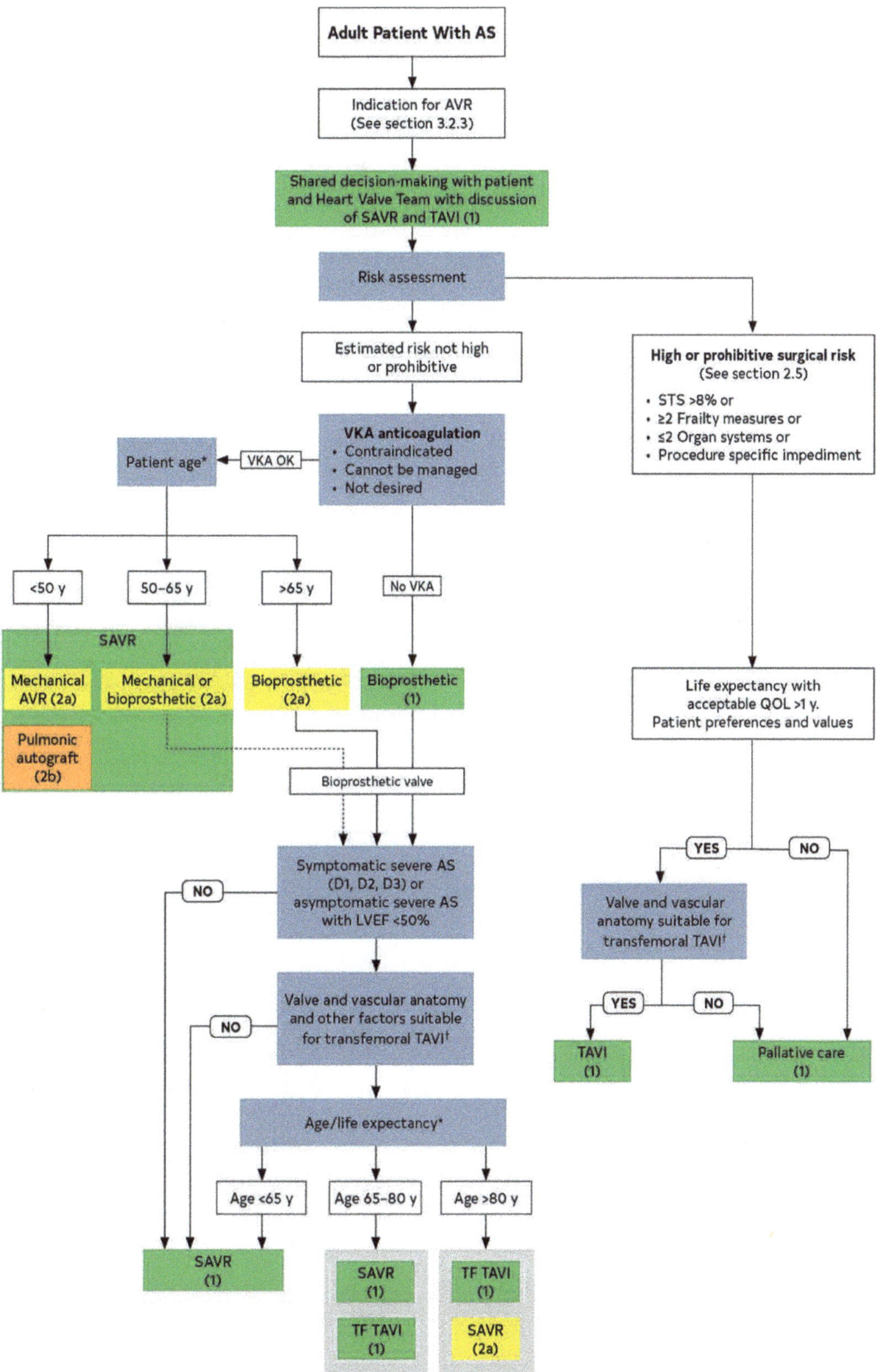

Figure 17 Treatment Approaches for the Patient with AS

2.3.2 Heart Block

Heart block is a **medical condition** that **blocks or delays heart electrical signals** therefore disrupting normal heart rhythm. The conduction system that manages heartbeat regulation fails **because of an impairment. Signal transmission** delays in heart block progress from the least severe **first-degree through intermediate second-degree** to the most dangerous **third-degree block** that separates atrial from **ventricular heartbeats**. A heart block often causes decreased heart rate along with dizziness and faintness that may need pacemaker therapy. The illustration reveals multiple heart block patterns that appear in **electrocardiogram (ECG)** results. In 1st Degree Heart Block, the **PR interval is prolonged (>0.2 ms)** but remains constant, with every P-wave followed by a QRS complex, indicating delayed but normal conduction. 2nd **Degree Heart Block (Mobitz I)** is characterized by a progressively lengthening PR interval until a **QRS complex** is dropped, reflecting a delay in impulse conduction that eventually leads to a block. 2nd Degree **Heart Block (Mobitz II) shows a fixed PR interval** with some **P-waves not followed by QRS** complexes, indicating a block in the His-Purkinje system, which can be more dangerous than Mobitz I. **3rd Degree Heart Block (Complete Block)** results in independent atria and ventricle beating since their intervals remain unrelated pointing to a serious blockage that commonly needs **pacemaker installation.** These blocks enable proper medical diagnosis through their ability to evaluate the extent of heart conduction failures for determining specific therapy options.

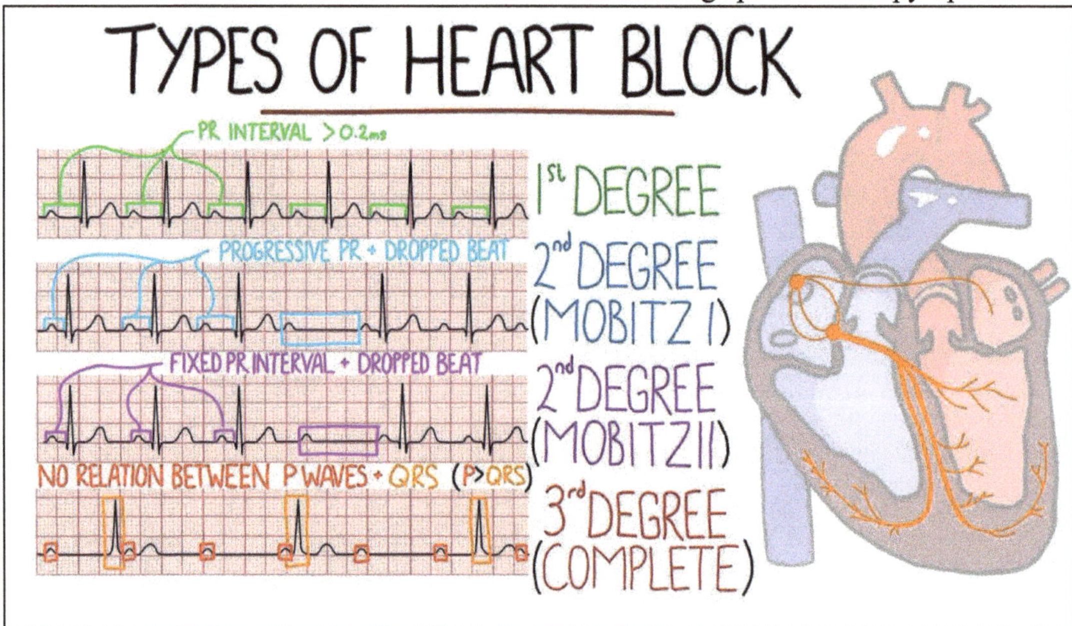

Figure 18 Classification of Heart Block

2.3.2.1 SOAP Notes for Heart Block

Table 11 SOAP Notes for Heart Block

Component	Details
Subjective (S)	The patient presents with dizziness, lightheadedness, and intermittent episodes of syncope. Reports feeling fatigued over the past few days and describes an unusual "slow" heartbeat sensation. Denies chest pain, shortness of breath, or palpitations. The patient has a history of hypertension and diabetes mellitus. No recent trauma or fever.

Objective (O)	BP: 130/85 mmHg, HR: 40 bpm (irregular), RR: 18 bpm, Oxygen Saturation: 98% on room air. ECG: Evidence of second-degree heart block (Mobitz type I) with progressively lengthening PR interval followed by a dropped beat. Cardiac biomarkers: Within normal limits. Physical Examination: No signs of acute distress, but patient is bradycardic with irregular rhythm.
Assessment (A)	Differential Diagnoses: 1. Second-degree AV block (Mobitz type I), 2. Sinus bradycardia, 3. Hypothyroidism, 4. Medications (e.g., beta-blockers) causing heart rate suppression
Plan (P)	**Investigations:** Repeat ECG in 24-48 hours, Holter monitor for continuous rhythm assessment, Thyroid function tests, and Electrophysiological study if indicated. **Pharmacological Treatment:** Adjust current medications (e.g., reduce beta-blockers if applicable). Consider Atropine if symptomatic bradycardia persists (See the algorithm below). **Non-Pharmacological Treatment:** Monitor heart rate and rhythm closely, especially during episodes of dizziness or syncope. **Education:** Educate patient on recognizing symptoms of heart block, such as dizziness and syncope, and the importance of seeking medical care if symptoms worsen. **Referral:** Cardiology referral for further evaluation, including possible pacemaker implantation if heart block worsens. Follow-up: Re-evaluate in 1 week for further monitoring of symptoms and adjustments to treatment plan.

Table 12 Algorithm for the Management of AV Block

Algorithm for the Management of AV Block		
Step 1: Initial Diagnosis and Assessment	**Confirm AV Block type** via ECG: • **First-degree AV block**: PR interval > 300 ms. • **Mobitz type I (Wenckebach)**: Progressive PR interval prolongation until a beat is dropped.	**Evaluate patient status**: • **Symptomatic**: Hypotension, syncope, dizziness, bradycardia. • **Asymptomatic**: Routine ECG surveillance may be sufficient.

	• **Mobitz type II**: Fixed PR interval with occasional dropped beats. • **Third-degree AV block**: Complete dissociation between atrial and ventricular activity.	

Step 2: Management of First-Degree AV Block	**Treatment**:
	• **No treatment required** for the majority of cases.
	• **Surveillance**: Monitor with routine ECGs for progression.
	• **Indications for treatment** (rare):
	    ○ **Symptomatic** (PR interval > 0.30 seconds).
	    ○ **Coexisting neuromuscular disease** or prolonged QRS interval.
	    ○ **Consider pacemaker placement** if symptomatic or progression.	

Step 3: Management of Mobitz Type I (Wenckebach)	**Initial Approach**: • **No treatment required** for most cases unless symptomatic. • **Symptomatic**: If bradycardia leads to hypotension, administer **Atropine**. • **If unresponsive to Atropine**: ○ **Pacing** (transcutaneous or transvenous) should be initiated. • **Medication adjustment**: Reduce or discontinue **beta blockers, calcium channel blockers, or digoxin.** • **Monitoring**: Admit and monitor for progression.	
Step 4: Management of Mobitz Type II	**Immediate Action**: • **Pacing required**: Initiate **transvenous pacing** as soon as identified.	

	• **Risk of deterioration**: Type II block may progress to **complete heart block**, requiring urgent pacing. • **Hypotension/bradycardia**: Atropine **unlikely to be effective**. • **Further Action**: ○ **Consult electrophysiology** for possible permanent pacemaker placement. • **Monitoring**: Admit for continuous monitoring. • **Medication adjustment**: Consider reducing medications that may exacerbate AV block.	

Step 5: Management of Third-Degree AV Block	**Immediate Action**:
	• **Atropine**: Often ineffective due to AV node dysfunction.
	• **Temporary pacing**:
	  ○ **Transcutaneous pacing** is first-line for immediate stabilization.
	  ○ **Transvenous pacing** if transcutaneous pacing fails.
	  ○ **Dopamine or epinephrine** can be used as temporary measures for symptomatic bradycardia.
		Long-term treatment:
		• **Permanent pacemaker** implantation is often required once stabilization is achieved.
		 Underlying causes: Treat underlying conditions (e.g., myocardial infarction, drug toxicity).

Step 6: Special Considerations in Heart Block due to Myocardial Infarction	**For acute myocardial infarction (MI)**: • **Inferior MI (Right Coronary Artery occlusion)**: Often improves with reperfusion; **temporary pacing** may be considered until recovery.	

	• **Anterior MI**: High likelihood of requiring **permanent pacemaker**. • **Management**: Prioritize **restoration of myocardial perfusion** (cardiac catheterization) to restore native rhythm. • **Monitor closely**: Continue monitoring post-MI patients with heart block for progression. • **Temporary pacing**: Only if required for hemodynamic support until perfusion is restored.
Step 7: Permanent Pacemaker Consideration	▯ **Indications for permanent pacemaker:** • Mobitz type II or high-degree AV block with symptoms. • Third-degree AV block requiring stabilization. • Failure to respond to temporary pacing or recurrent symptomatic AV block. • Persistent bifascicular block with associated high-grade AV block. ▯ Timing: Implantation should be performed once stabilization is achieved.

Step 8: Management of Complications with Temporary Pacemaker	• **Complications to monitor for:**
	    o Device malfunction (e.g., failure to capture, lead displacement).
	    o Infection risk.
	    o Thromboembolism.
	    o Cardiac perforation.
	• Minimize duration: Keep temporary pacing duration as short as possible to avoid complications.
	• Careful consideration: Weigh the risk-benefit ratio of continuing temporary pacing versus transitioning to permanent pacemaker.

Summary	• ***First-degree AV block:*** Generally requires no treatment beyond surveillance unless symptomatic or associated with significant comorbidities. • ***Mobitz type I (Wenckebach):*** Atropine for symptomatic cases, pacing if unresponsive.

	• ***Mobitz type II:*** Requires immediate pacing due to risk of progression to third-degree block. • ***Third-degree AV block:*** Pacing is required immediately, either transcutaneous or transvenous. Long-term management involves permanent pacemaker placement. • ***Heart block due to MI:*** Temporary pacing may be required until perfusion is restored; anterior MI often leads to need for a permanent pacemaker.

2.3.3 Myocardial Infarction (MI) with Angina

A heart attack develops when coronary artery **blockages trigger myocardial tissue** destruction but **angina** appears as brief cardiac interruptions without resulting myocardial death. The symptoms of these patients include **chest pain** and **shortness of breath** combined with **ECG abnormalities**. Medical staff diagnose MI with angina via **ECG results, cardiac biomarkers, and angiographic tests** before managing patients with **aspirin followed by beta-blockers, statins, and PCI procedures**. The Figure 19 differentiates acute myocardial infarction (MI) between Type 1 and Type 2 by determining acute coronary obstruction status. The first subtype of **Type 1 MI** develops from acute **coronary artery blockage** and includes **four distinct subcategories**: plaque rupture combined with **thrombus formation (Type 1A)** and spontaneous coronary artery dissection cases **(Type 1B)** and coronary embolism cases **(Type 1C)** and patients experiencing **vasospasm or microvascular dysfunction (Type 1D).** Patients with **Type 2 MI develop shortages between oxygen supply and demand** which include two subtypes: **Type 2A** with existing **obstructive coronary artery disease** and **Type 2B** with no obstructive coronary artery disease.

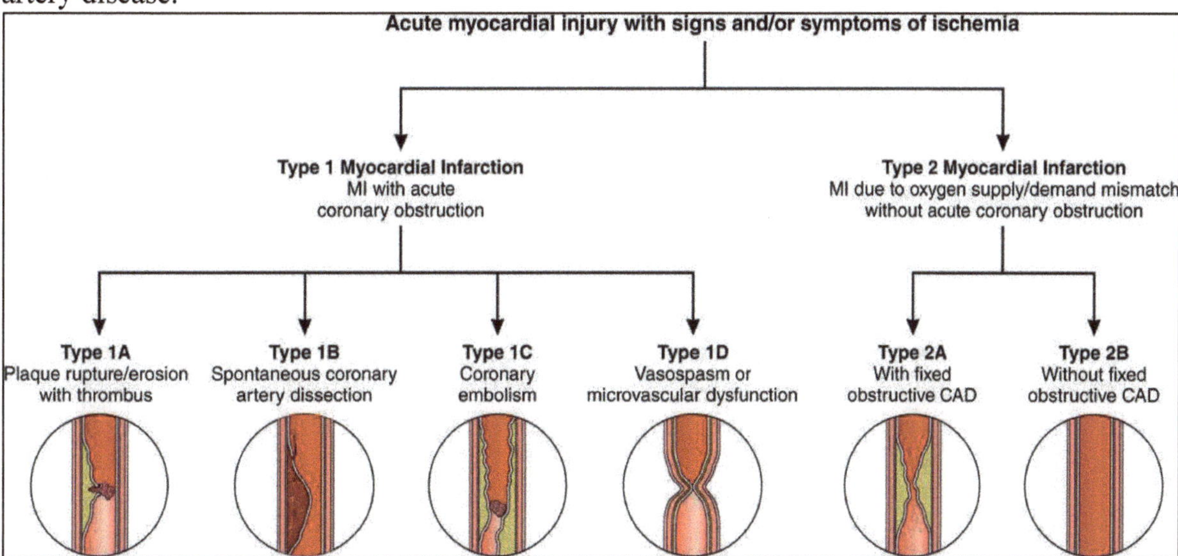

Figure 19 Classification of Acute MI

2.3.3.1 Types of MI and Their ECG

1. Type #1: Anterior ST Segment Elevation MI

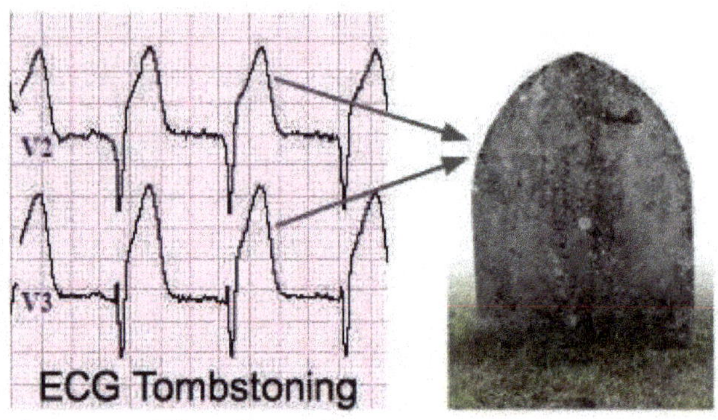

2. Type #2: Inferior ST Segment Elevation MI

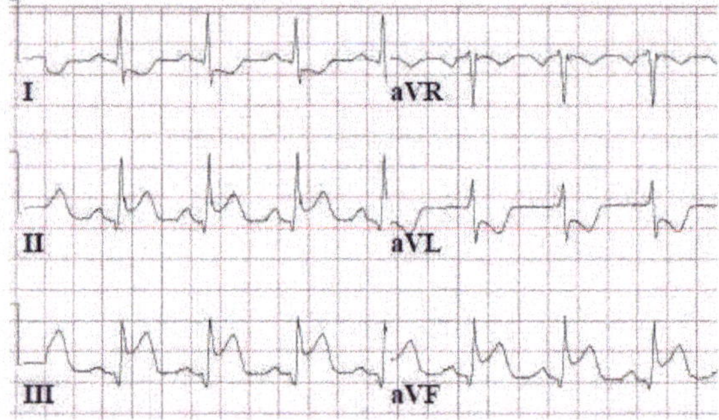

3. Type #3: Posterior ST Segment Elevation MI

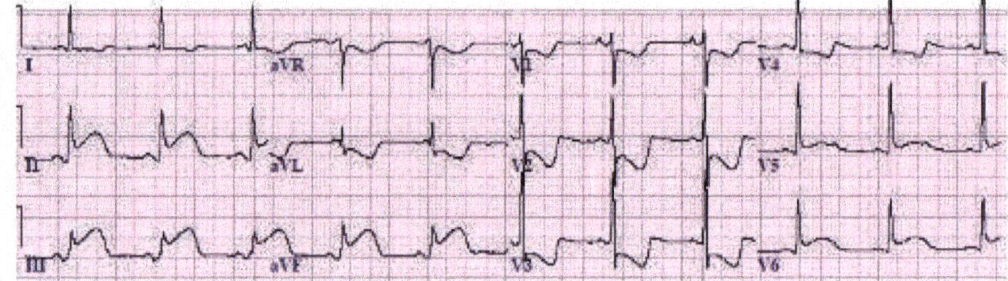

4. Type #4: Acute MI with a Right Bundle Branch Block

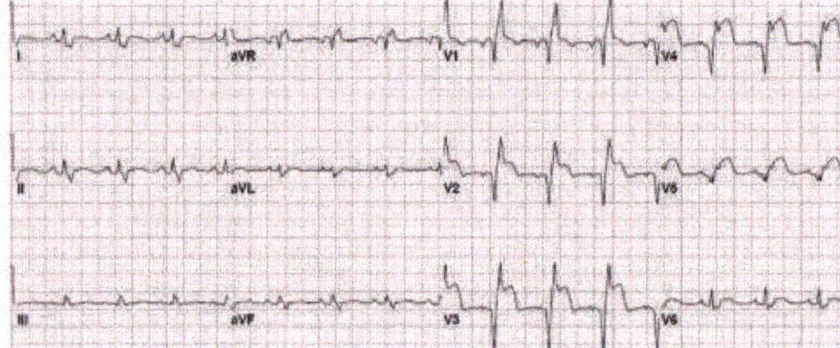

5. Type #5: A New Left Bundle Branch Block – Equivalent to a STEMI

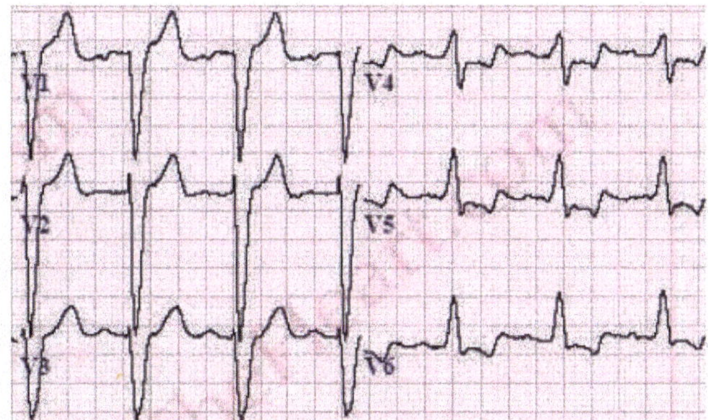

2.3.3.2 SOAP Notes for MI and Angina

Table 13 SOAP Notes for MI and Angina

Component	Details
Subjective (S)	Patient presents with severe chest pain, radiating to the left arm and jaw, associated with shortness of breath and diaphoresis. Reports a history of hypertension and hyperlipidemia. No recent trauma or fever.
Objective (O)	BP: 160/100 mmHg, HR: 95 bpm, RR: 20 bpm, Oxygen Saturation: 94% on room air. ECG: ST-segment elevation in leads II, III, aVF. Cardiac biomarkers: Troponin I elevated.
Assessment (A)	Differential Diagnoses: 1. Acute ST-Elevation Myocardial Infarction (STEMI) 2. Unstable Angina 3. Pulmonary Embolism
Plan (P)	Investigations: Serial ECG, Troponin I levels, Echocardiogram, Coronary Angiography. Pharmacological Treatment: Administer Aspirin 325 mg, Clopidogrel 75 mg, Heparin IV, and Nitroglycerin sublingual (See the following algorithm). Non-Pharmacological Treatment: Oxygen therapy (if SpO2 < 90%), lifestyle modifications (low-fat diet, exercise). Education: Educate the patient about MI warning signs and the importance of early intervention. Referral: Urgent referral for PCI or thrombolytic therapy. Follow-up: Re-evaluate within 48-72 hours post-procedure, monitor cardiac function.

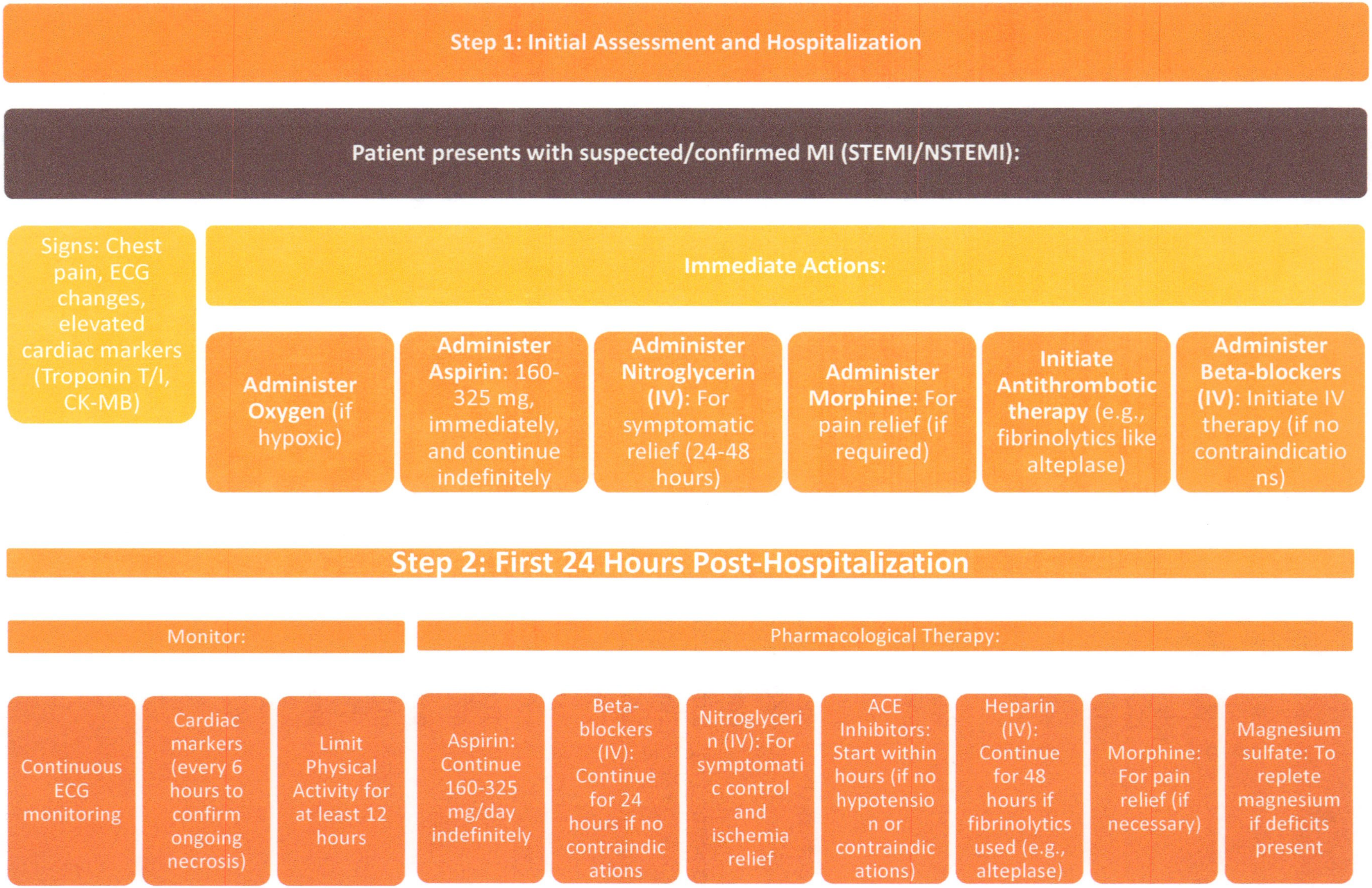

Step 1: Initial Assessment and Hospitalization

Patient presents with suspected/confirmed MI (STEMI/NSTEMI):

Signs: Chest pain, ECG changes, elevated cardiac markers (Troponin T/I, CK-MB)

Immediate Actions:

- **Administer Oxygen** (if hypoxic)
- **Administer Aspirin**: 160-325 mg, immediately, and continue indefinitely
- **Administer Nitroglycerin (IV)**: For symptomatic relief (24-48 hours)
- **Administer Morphine**: For pain relief (if required)
- **Initiate Antithrombotic therapy** (e.g., fibrinolytics like alteplase)
- **Administer Beta-blockers (IV)**: Initiate IV therapy (if no contraindications)

Step 2: First 24 Hours Post-Hospitalization

Monitor:

- Continuous ECG monitoring
- Cardiac markers (every 6 hours to confirm ongoing necrosis)
- Limit Physical Activity for at least 12 hours

Pharmacological Therapy:

- Aspirin: Continue 160-325 mg/day indefinitely
- Beta-blockers (IV): Continue for 24 hours if no contraindications
- Nitroglycerin (IV): For symptomatic control and ischemia relief
- ACE Inhibitors: Start within hours (if no hypotension or contraindications)
- Heparin (IV): Continue for 48 hours if fibrinolytics used (e.g., alteplase)
- Morphine: For pain relief (if necessary)
- Magnesium sulfate: To replete magnesium if deficits present

Step 3: After 24 Hours - Ongoing Management

Continue Pharmacotherapy:

- **Aspirin**: 160-325 mg/day indefinitely
- **Beta-blockers**: Continue orally after IV therapy (if no contraindications)
- **ACE Inhibitors**: Continue for at least 6 weeks, or indefinitely if LV dysfunction or CHF
- **Nitroglycerin (IV)**: Continue for 24-48 hours, or use oral long-term if necessary
- **Heparin**: Continue for 48 hours if alteplase (TPA) was administered
- **Statins**: Start lipid-lowering therapy based on lipid profile

Additional Therapy Based on Patient Status:

For high-risk patients (e.g., large anterior MI, LV mural thrombus):

- Administer **Intravenous heparin** to reduce embolic stroke risk
- **Consider coronary angiography** and **PCI** if needed

For bradycardia or AV block:

- **Atropine** or **Temporary pacing** if needed

For atrial fibrillation or ventricular arrhythmias:

- **Rate control** with **beta-blockers** or **digitalis** (for atrial fibrillation)
- **DC cardioversion** for hemodynamically unstable arrhythmias
- **Lidocaine or amiodarone** for ventricular arrhythmias

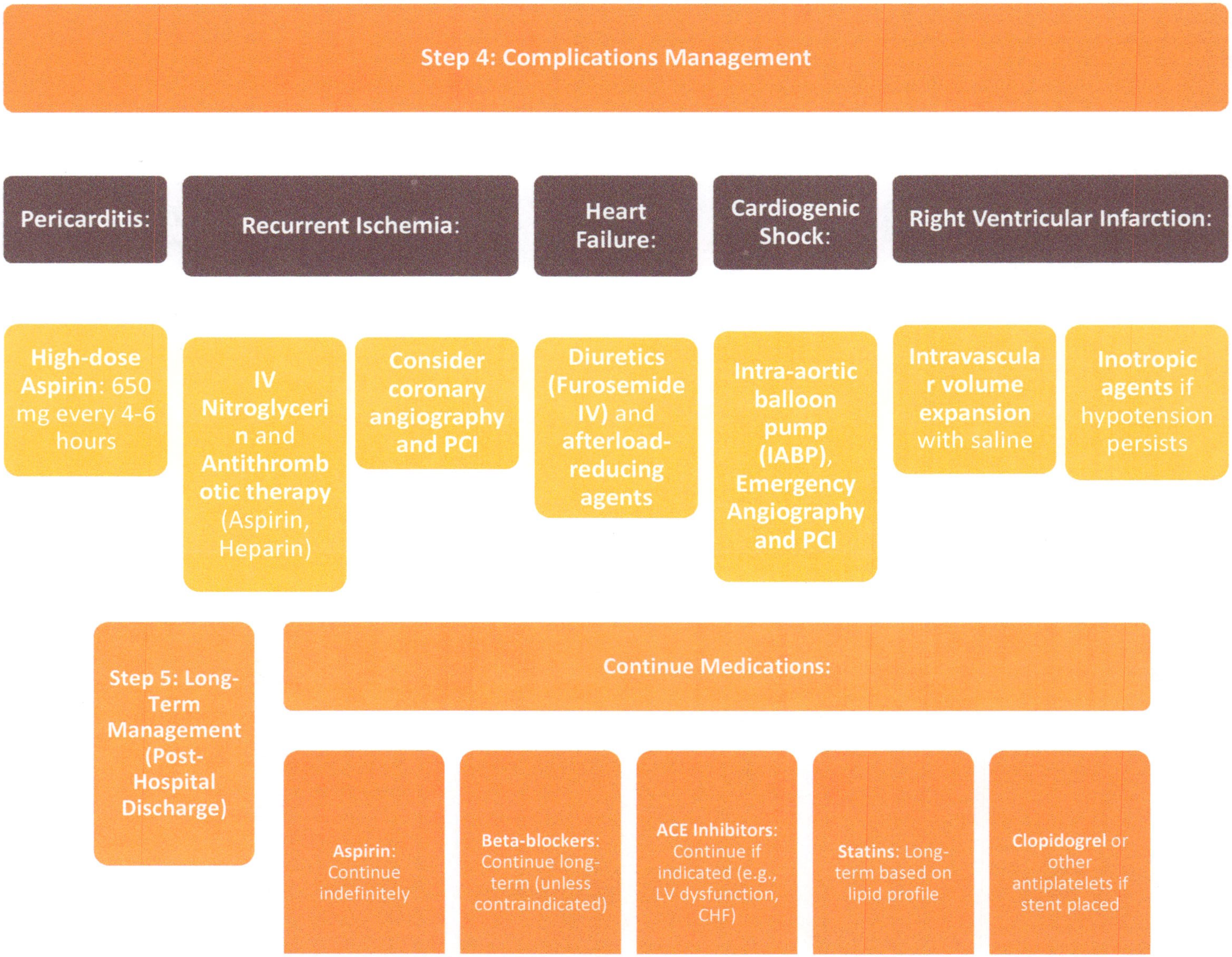

Step 4: Complications Management

Pericarditis:
- **High-dose Aspirin**: 650 mg every 4-6 hours

Recurrent Ischemia:
- **IV Nitroglycerin and Antithrombotic therapy** (Aspirin, Heparin)
- **Consider coronary angiography and PCI**

Heart Failure:
- **Diuretics (Furosemide IV)** and **afterload-reducing agents**

Cardiogenic Shock:
- **Intra-aortic balloon pump (IABP), Emergency Angiography and PCI**

Right Ventricular Infarction:
- **Intravascular volume expansion** with saline
- **Inotropic agents** if hypotension persists

Step 5: Long-Term Management (Post-Hospital Discharge)

Continue Medications:
- **Aspirin**: Continue indefinitely
- **Beta-blockers**: Continue long-term (unless contraindicated)
- **ACE Inhibitors**: Continue if indicated (e.g., LV dysfunction, CHF)
- **Statins**: Long-term based on lipid profile
- **Clopidogrel** or other antiplatelets if stent placed

Figure 20 Treatment Approaches for MI

2.3.4 Hypertension (HTN)

Stroke with **heart failure and kidney disease** develop primarily from persistent hypertension. The condition produces **three distinct symptoms** which include **severe headaches together with vision problems and an elevated propensity to suffer a stroke**. Medical staff diagnoses patients using blood pressure measurements before selecting individual treatments for different ethnic groups between **ACE inhibitors and calcium channel blockers** together with **lifestyle change programs.** The Figure 15 demonstrates the **REASOH hypertensive classification** system which divides hypertension into **six distinct categories** regarding their **root causes and therapeutic approaches.** Each letter represents a different form: ***Renin-dependent hypertension (R)*** linked to high plasma renin activity and treated with ARNI, ACEIs, or ARBs; ***Elderly Arteriosclerosis-based hypertension (E)*** diagnosed through pulse wave velocity and treated with calcium channel blockers (CCB); ***Sympathetic-Active hypertension (A)*** associated with high heart rate and stress, managed using beta-blockers and renal denervation; ***Secondary hypertension (S)*** requiring identification of primary causes for targeted treatment; ***Salt-sensitive hypertension (O)*** diagnosed via sodium levels and managed with a low-salt diet and diuretics; and ***Hyperhomocysteinemia hypertension (H)*** linked to elevated homocysteine, treatable with folic acid and enalapril. Specific pathophysiological factors help physicians create individualized hypertension treatment plans through this classification system.

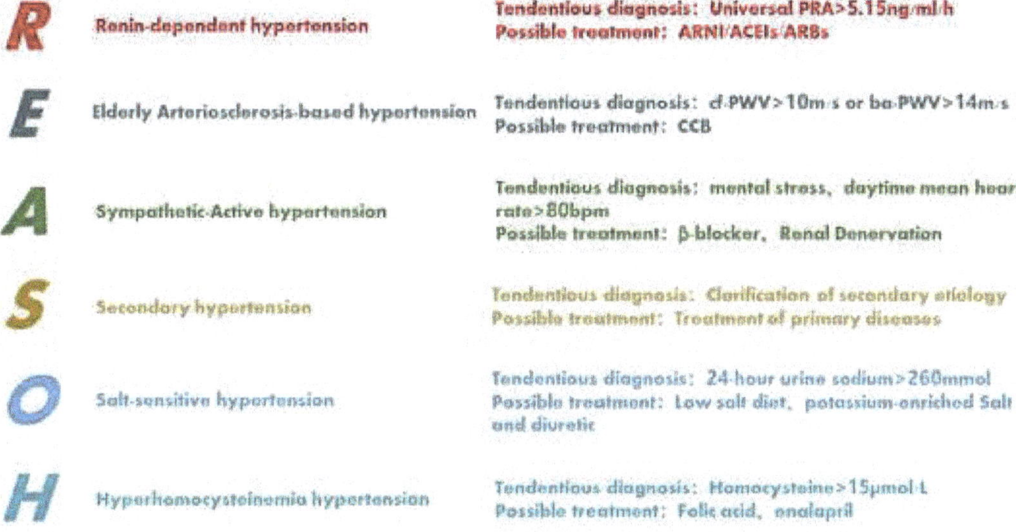

R
Renin-dependent hypertension
Tendentious diagnosis: Universal PRA>5.15ng/ml/h
Possible treatment: ARNI/ACEIs/ARBs
E
Elderly Arteriosclerosis-based hypertension
Tendentious diagnosis: cf-PWV>10m/s or ba-PWV>14m/s
Possible treatment: CCB
A
Sympathetic-Active hypertension
Tendentious diagnosis: mental stress, daytime mean heart rate>80bpm
Possible treatment: β-blocker, Renal Denervation
S
Secondary hypertension
Tendentious diagnosis: Clarification of secondary etiology
Possible treatment: Treatment of primary diseases
O
Salt-sensitive hypertension
Tendentious diagnosis: 24-hour urine sodium>260mmol
Possible treatment: Low salt diet, potassium-enriched Salt and diuretic
H
Hyperhomocysteinemia hypertension
Tendentious diagnosis: Homocysteine>15μmol/L
Possible treatment: Folic acid, enalapril

Figure 21 REASOH Classification of Hypertension

2.3.4.1 Analytical Framework of Hypertension Management

The figure 23 provides an approach for managing hypertension by addressing essential **clinical questions** that specify medication **initiation and enhancement procedures**. Adults with **diagnosed HTN** who made **lifestyle changes** enter the framework before moving onto medication **start times and test requirements** and risk evaluations. The model analyzes **hypertension treatment approaches** by **comparing single medications with multiple medications** while it assesses both **blood pressure results and hypertension management** rates as intermediate outcomes. The system also evaluates end health results including **cardiovascular mortality and**

myocardial infarction (MI) and stroke and heart failure while taking into account adverse effects alongside management approaches between **physician and non-physician providers**.

2.3.4.2 Classification of Hypertensive Drugs

Figure 24 organizes **antihypertensive drug** classes along with their respective drug names and examples as well as mechanisms of action for each class and their effects on blood pressure measurements. Different classes of antihypertensive drugs include **ACE inhibitors (lisinopril and**

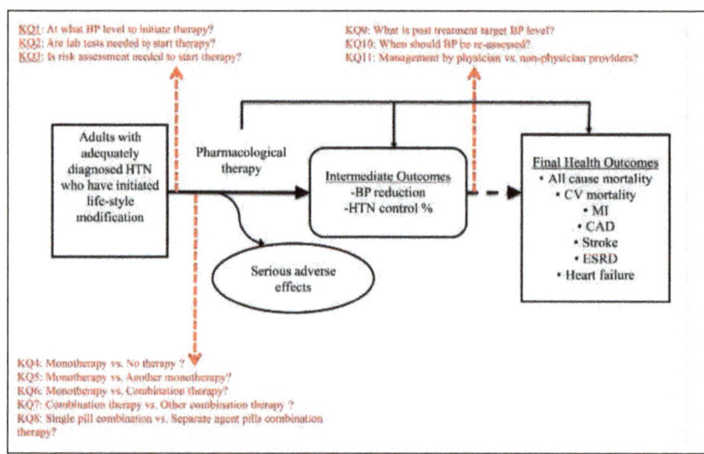

Figure 22 Analytical Framework for HTN Management

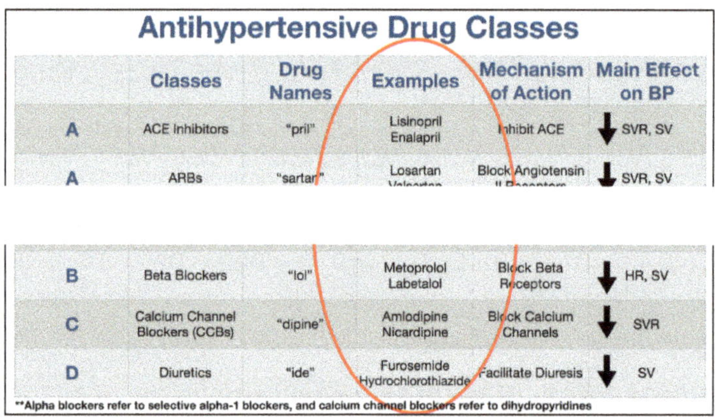

Antihypertensive Drug Classes

	Classes	Drug Names	Examples	Mechanism of Action	Main Effect on BP
A	ACE Inhibitors	"pril"	Lisinopril Enalapril	Inhibit ACE	↓ SVR, SV
A	ARBs	"sartan"	Losartan	Block Angiotensin	↓ SVR, SV
B	Beta Blockers	"lol"	Metoprolol Labetalol	Block Beta Receptors	↓ HR, SV
C	Calcium Channel Blockers (CCBs)	"dipine"	Amlodipine Nicardipine	Block Calcium Channels	↓ SVR
D	Diuretics	"ide"	Furosemide Hydrochlorothiazide	Facilitate Diuresis	↓ SV

**Alpha blockers refer to selective alpha-1 blockers, and calcium channel blockers refer to dihydropyridines

Figure 23 Classification of Antihypertensive Drugs

enalapril) alongside **ARBs (losartan and valsartan)** and **alpha-blockers (doxazosin and terazosin)** as well as **beta-blockers (metoprolol and labetalol)** and **calcium channel blockers (CCBs) (amlodipine and nicardipine)** and **diuretics (furosemide and hydrochlorothiazide).** Different BP-lowering pathways exist within each class that either block angiotensin II or alpha/beta receptors, inhibit **ACE or blockade calcium channels,** or **trigger diuretic** effects that decrease **systemic vascular resistance (SVR), stroke volume (SV), and heart rate (HR).**

2.3.4.3 SOAP Notes for Hypertension

Table 14 SOAP Notes for HTN

Component	Details
Subjective (S)	Patient presents with headaches, dizziness, and occasional blurred vision. Reports fatigue, shortness of breath on exertion, and chest discomfort. Family history of hypertension and cardiovascular disease noted. Lifestyle factors include high salt intake, sedentary lifestyle, and stress. No history of smoking, but moderate alcohol consumption.
Objective (O)	**Vitals:** BP 150/95 mmHg (elevated), HR 82 bpm, RR 18 bpm, BMI 29 (overweight). **Physical Exam:** No jugular venous distention (JVD), normal heart sounds, mild peripheral edema noted. **Investigations:** ECG: Normal sinus rhythm; Echocardiogram: Mild left ventricular hypertrophy (if applicable); Blood Tests: Elevated LDL cholesterol, normal kidney function.
Assessment (A)	**Differential Diagnoses:** 1. Primary (Essential) Hypertension 2. Secondary Hypertension (due to renal dysfunction, endocrine disorders, or medication use) 3. White Coat Hypertension. **Risk Factors Identified:** Family history, obesity, high salt intake, stress.
Plan (P)	**Investigations:** 24-hour ambulatory BP monitoring, renal function tests, lipid profile, fasting glucose, and urine analysis for proteinuria. **Pharmacological Treatment:** Initiation of antihypertensive therapy (ACE inhibitors, ARBs, calcium channel blockers, or diuretics based on patient profile) (See Figure and algorithm below). **Non-Pharmacological Treatment:** Low-sodium DASH diet, weight management, regular physical activity, stress reduction techniques. **Education:** Counseling on lifestyle modifications, the importance of medication adherence, and BP self-monitoring. **Referral:** Nephrology or endocrinology consultation if secondary hypertension is suspected. **Follow-up:** Reassess in 4-6 weeks to monitor BP control and medication response.

The management strategy for hypertension patients follows a decision flowchart that accounts for blood pressure intensity and patient risk attributes as well as drug accessibility for treatment. The first step of care for all patients diagnosed with hypertension includes receiving lifestyle recommendation advice. The healthcare industry divides hypertension into two categories: **Grade 1 (BP 140–159/90–99 mmHg) along with Grade 2 (BP ≥160/100 mmHg)**. Picking drug therapy stands as the vital and most effective treatment method for every patient with Stage 2 hypertension. Drug treatment receives essential and optimal status right away for **Grade 1 hypertensive patients who face higher risk including those with CVD, CKD, DM or HMOD**. Doctor-prescribed drugs should only be recommended to uncontrolled blood pressure patients who fall into the low to moderate-risk category following **their participation in 3–6 months of lifestyle intervention** period.

Medical treatment initiation depends on whether effective medications are available to patients. The management of lower-risk individuals should start with lifestyle changes for a **period of 3–6 months** while medication access remains limited in their settings. Treatment through medication should be started for patients **between 50–80 years** who have uncontrolled blood pressure. When medication access is not a limitation the healthcare team should start treating patients with low to moderate risk after the initial lifestyle intervention period. This flowchart applies a risk-based structure for **hypertension management** to deliver prompt **pharmacological care** for high-risk patients while patients at lower risk can make lifestyle adjustments before starting drug treatment.

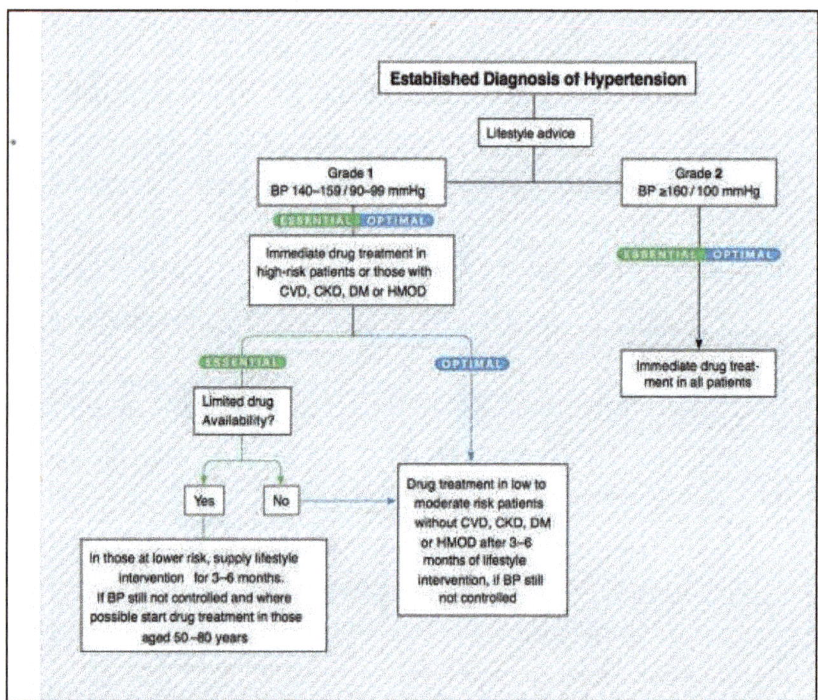

Figure 24 The management strategy for hypertension patients

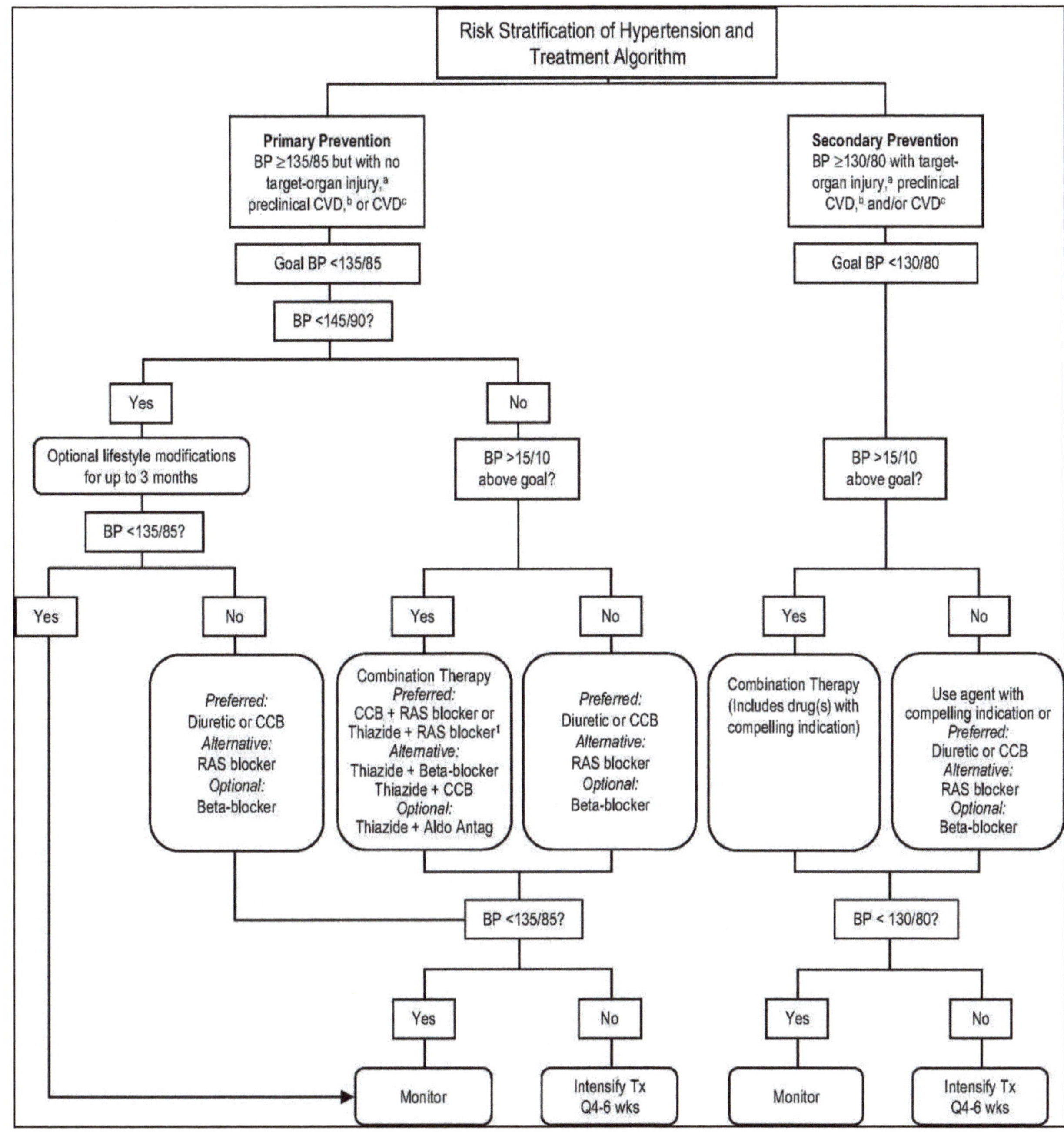

Figure 25 Algorithm of Hypertension Management in Black

Table 15 Algorithm for HTN Management

Section	Subsection	Condition	Recommended Drugs	Recommendation
1. First-Line Pharmacological Treatment		Nondiabetic hypertensive patients	ACE Inhibitors (e.g., Enalapril), ARBs (e.g., Losartan), CCBs (e.g., Amlodipine), Thiazide Diuretics (e.g., Hydrochlorothiazide)	Start with one of the following classes based on individual tolerance and comorbidities. (A)
	General Population	SBP 140-159 mmHg or DBP 90-99 mmHg	ACE Inhibitors (e.g., Ramipril), ARBs (e.g., Irbesartan), CCBs (e.g., Lercanidipine), Diuretics (e.g., Indapamide)	Monotherapy is appropriate for mild hypertension (A)
	Mild Hypertension	SBP 140-159 mmHg or DBP 90-99 mmHg	ACE Inhibitors (e.g., Ramipril), ARBs (e.g., Irbesartan), CCBs (e.g., Amlodipine), Diuretics (e.g., Indapamide)	Monotherapy is appropriate for mild hypertension (A)
2. Second-Line Treatment		Hypertension not controlled with one drug	ACE Inhibitor + Calcium Channel Blocker / ARB + Thiazide Diuretic	Most patients with resistant hypertension need a combination of drugs to achieve goal BP (C)
	Resistant Hypertension	Hypertension not controlled with one drug	ACE Inhibitor + Calcium Channel Blocker / ARB + Thiazide Diuretic	Combination therapy with different classes is required for better control (C)
3. Specific Populations		Diabetic patients with hypertension	ACE Inhibitors (e.g., Lisinopril), ARBs (e.g., Valsartan), Calcium Channel Blockers (e.g., Diltiazem), Thiazide Diuretics (e.g., Chlorthalidone)	ACE inhibitors or ARBs preferred due to renal protection (B)
	Diabetes Mellitus	Diabetic patients with hypertension	ACE Inhibitors (e.g., Lisinopril), ARBs (e.g., Valsartan), Calcium Channel Blockers (e.g., Diltiazem), Thiazide Diuretics (e.g., Chlorthalidone)	ACE inhibitors or ARBs preferred due to renal protection (B)

	Chronic Kidney Disease (CKD)	CKD patients with hypertension	ACE Inhibitors (e.g., Enalapril), ARBs (e.g., Losartan), Calcium Channel Blockers (e.g., Amlodipine)	First-line choice to prevent progression of kidney disease (A)
	Elderly	Elderly patients with hypertension	Calcium Channel Blockers (e.g., Amlodipine), Thiazide Diuretics (e.g., Chlorthalidone), ACE Inhibitors (e.g., Ramipril)	Lower starting doses and gradual titration to avoid side effects (C)
4. Combination Therapy		Hypertensive patients requiring more than one drug	ACE Inhibitors + Calcium Channel Blocker (e.g., Amlodipine), ARB + Diuretic (e.g., Hydrochlorothiazide)	Combine drugs from different classes for effective BP control (A)
	Dual Therapy	Hypertensive patients requiring more than one drug	ACE Inhibitors + Calcium Channel Blocker + Diuretic	Triple therapy is effective when dual therapy is insufficient (C)
	Triple Therapy	Patients requiring three drugs to control BP	Methyldopa, Labetalol	Avoid ACE Inhibitors, ARBs, and diuretics due to fetal risk. Methyldopa and labetalol are safe alternatives (A)
5. Other Considerations		Pregnant women with hypertension	ACE Inhibitors (e.g., Lisinopril), ARBs (e.g., Valsartan), Beta-Blockers (e.g., Bisoprolol), Statins (e.g., Atorvastatin)	ACE inhibitors and ARBs are preferred to reduce the risk of recurrent CVD events (A)

2.3.4.4 Racial Differences in Antihypertensive Medication Use and Blood Pressure Management

The researchers (Stamm et al., 2022) evaluated medication usage patterns of antihypertensive medications between **Black and White participants across two-time frames (2003–2007 and 2013–2016).** The research discovered that **Black participants took more antihypertensive**

medications than White participants when examining both stroke-free subjects and patients who had suffered strokes. Provided data showed that **ACE inhibitors and diuretics** distribution rates among **Black participants exceeded those of White participants**. During the second visit **ACE inhibitor usage rates between ethnic groups became closer though Black patients continued using higher levels of diuretics.** The initial preference for calcium channel blockers among Black patients diminished over time as White patients also started using CCBs more often. Throughout both study visits Black participants demonstrated elevated blood pressure readings than **White participants in both systolic and diastolic measures**. Adjusting for demographic socioeconomic and medical factors the research used mixed-effects logistic regression models to examine racial discrepancies. The research findings demonstrate that **racial discrepancies existed in hypertension management** as well as **medication adherence from one time period to the next**. Similarly, race affects how people of different ethnic backgrounds respond to individual **antihypertensive medicines.** According to Sehgal (2004), the contrasting responses between **white and black patients** become prominent features in review documents that establish clinical recommendations. The magnitude of blood pressure adjustments from drugs remains substantially diverse throughout all racial groups. An analysis of fifteen studies involved a combined total **of 9307 white participants together with 2902 black participants.** The average difference between white and black blood pressure responses to drugs reached between **0.6 and 3.0 mm Hg** yet the measurement variability within each racial group varied from 5.0 to 10.1 mm Hg. The data showed that diuretics, β**-blockers, calcium channel blockers, and angiotensin-converting enzyme inhibitors** had comparable drug-associated changes in diastolic blood pressure between whites and blacks at levels of **90% (95% confidence interval: 81 to 99) and 90% (95% CI: 83 to 97) and 95% (95% CI: 92 to 98) and 81% (95% CI: 76 to 86),** respectively. Research studies indicated that between 83% to 93% of participants from both white and black groups displayed identical pressure changes measured in systolic blood pressure. The majority of blacks and whites show comparable reactions to antihypertensive drugs which are frequently used in medical treatment. The selection of medication in clinical practice is determined by other essential factors which include the individual treatment response and the strain evidence together with financial considerations.

The selection of medications for hypertension treatment depends critically on the **patient renal function and racial background**. The clinical team needs to use CCBs and diuretics instead of **ACE inhibitors along with ARBs** for individuals with kidney disease since these choices protect kidney function more effectively. Black patients demonstrate improved responses to calcium channel blockers and diuretics than **ACE inhibitors and ARBs because their natural renin baseline levels are lower**. **ACE inhibitors and ARBs** produce greater effectiveness in White patients than in any other group so they represent the most appropriate initial hypertension medications while also serving as excellent kidney protective agents.

2.3.5 Vascular Diseases

Arterial conditions like **coronary artery disease (CAD)** and **peripheral artery disease (PAD)** fall under this category while venous diseases such as **deep vein thrombosis (DVT)** and **varicose veins** also belong there. Treatment of these conditions requires **Doppler ultrasound** and **ABI measurements** to identify symptoms which include **leg pain** together with **swelling** and **skin discoloration.** The treatment options include **compression therapy and anticoagulants with bypass surgery as an alternative.**

2.3.5.1 Classification of Vascular Diseases

The displayed classification division in Figure 26 groups **vascular diseases** based on **three categories** which include **venous** along with **arterial** and **lymphatic disorders**. **Nonatherosclerotic occlusive disorders** exist as venous diseases that impact multiple circulatory regions including the **coronary arteries, cerebral blood vessels, peripheral arteries, kidneys, and mesenteric bloodstream.** The **systemic atherosclerosis** group belongs to arterial diseases alongside **aneurysms** that target the **aorta and aortic branches and peripheral arteries**. **The lymphatic system** serves as a **vascular disease** component yet remains unclassified in the presented diagram.

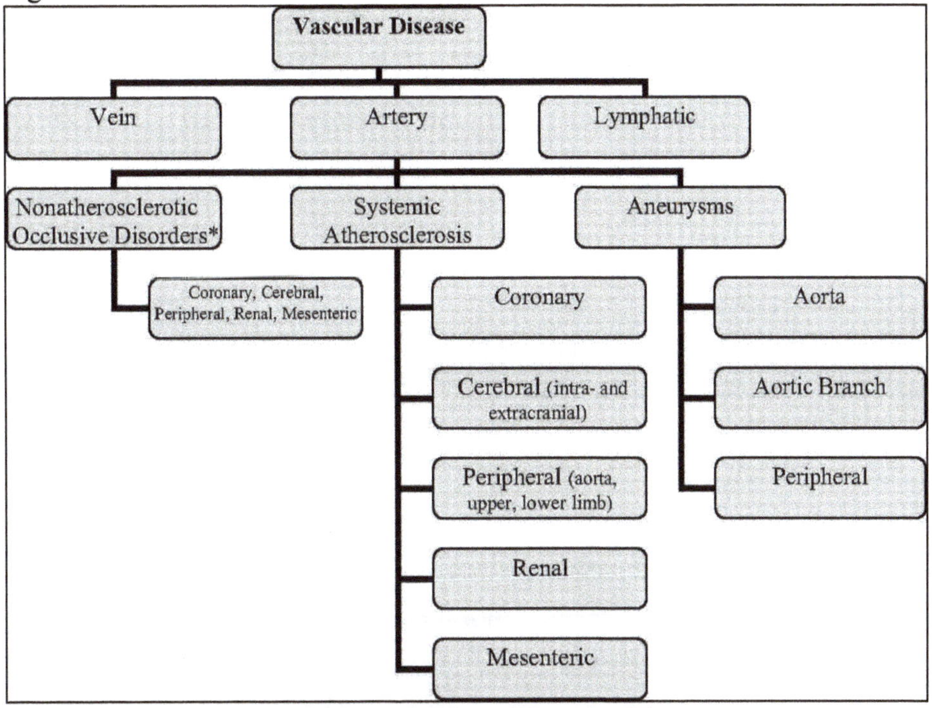

Figure 26 Classification of Vascular Diseases

2.3.5.2 SOAP Notes for Vascular Disease

Table 16 SOAP Notes for MI with Angina

Component	Details
Subjective (S)	Patient presents with unilateral leg swelling, pain, and redness that developed over the past few days. Reports a feeling of heaviness and warmth in the affected limb. History of prolonged immobility (e.g., recent long flight, surgery, or bed rest), oral contraceptive use, or family history of clotting disorders. No significant trauma to the limb.
Objective (O)	**Vitals:** BP 130/85 mmHg, HR 95 bpm, RR 18 bpm, Temp 37.2°C. **Physical Exam:** Unilateral lower extremity swelling, erythema, tenderness along the deep veins, positive **Homan's sign** (pain with dorsiflexion of foot, though not specific for DVT). **Investigations:** Doppler ultrasound (showing thrombus in deep veins), **D-dimer test** (elevated, if used for screening), CBC, coagulation profile, and renal function tests for anticoagulation planning.
Assessment (A)	**Differential Diagnoses:** 1. Deep Vein Thrombosis (DVT) 2. Cellulitis 3. Chronic Venous Insufficiency 4. Baker's Cyst 5. Compartment Syndrome.
Plan (P)	**Investigations:** Confirm diagnosis with **compression ultrasound**, assess for risk factors, and consider thrombophilia screening if indicated. **Pharmacological Treatment:** Initiate anticoagulation therapy (e.g., Apixaban, Rivaroxaban, LMWH bridging to Warfarin, or IV Heparin in high-risk cases). Consider thrombolysis in massive DVT with phlegmasia cerulea dolens (See figures 20-22 below and the algorithm table). **Non-Pharmacological Treatment:** Leg elevation, compression stockings, and early ambulation if appropriate. **Education:** Counsel patient on signs of pulmonary embolism (PE) (e.g., sudden shortness of breath, chest pain), the importance of medication adherence, and risk factor modification (hydration, avoiding prolonged immobility). **Referral:** Hematology for hypercoagulability workup if recurrent or unprovoked DVT. **Follow-up:** Reassess in 3-6 months to determine the need for continued anticoagulation based on risk factors.

Figure 27 demonstrates how to manage **antithrombotic treatment for PAD** patients who fall into **asymptomatic and symptomatic categories** as well as those undergoing **revascularization procedures.** The treatment plan for **asymptomatic PAD** patients should include aspirin administration particularly when **PAD is additionally present** in a different **vascular area**. The therapy for symptomatic patients includes **aspirin or clopidogrel alone or aspirin with rivaroxaban** due to their effectiveness in reducing **limb and cardiovascular complications** even **though rivaroxaban** causes increased bleeding. Individuals who received a coronary stent recently or have **acute coronary syndrome necessitate dual antiplatelet therapy (DAPT)** to determine their long-term risk between **ischemic events and bleeding complications**. After both surgical and endovascular **revascularization procedures** patients should undergo treatment with **dual antiplatelet therapy for one to six months.** Patients with elevated limb complications require either **aspirin or clopidogrel medications** or a **combined treatment of aspirin alongside rivaroxaban.**

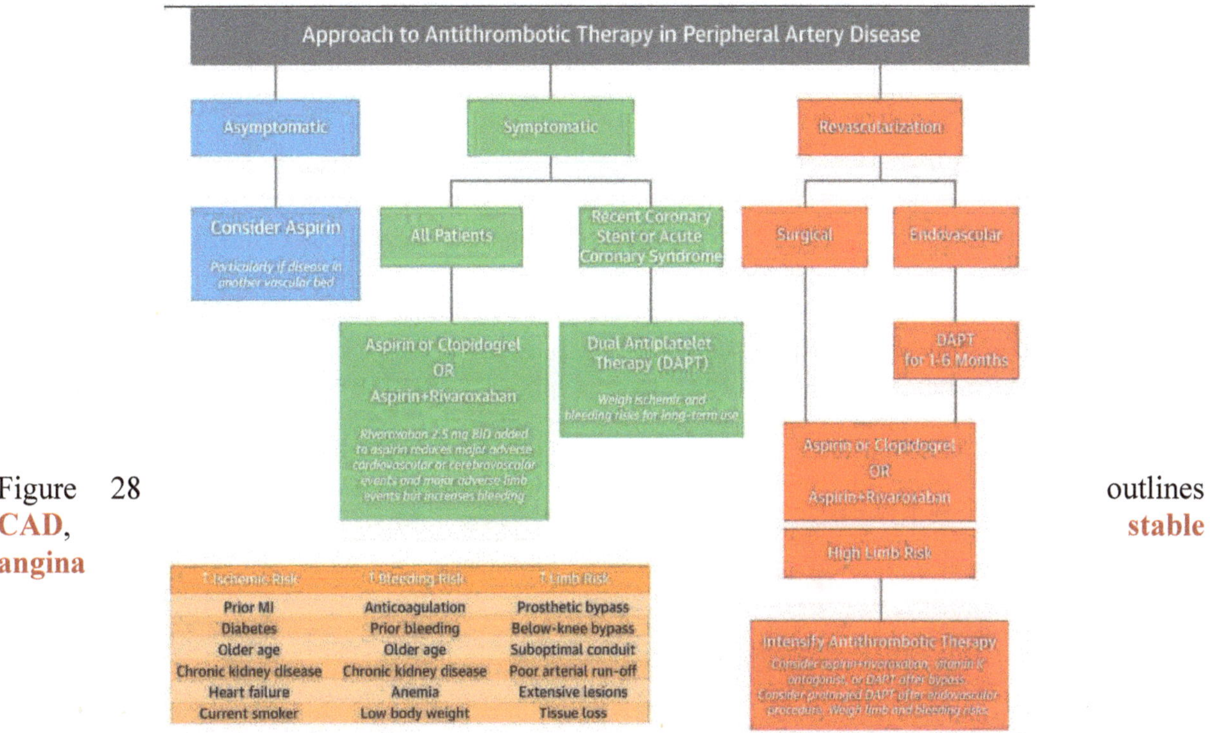

Figure 27 Classification of PAD Pharmacological Treatment

Figure 28 outlines **CAD**, **stable angina** management through **sequential strategies** for treating angina attacks and preventing future events. Patients can start drugs from **the first or second treatment line including nitrates, beta-blockers, and CCBs for angina relief** before progressing to **ivabradine, long-acting nitrates, nicorandil, or ranolazine** and possibly requiring **angiography and PCI or CABG intervention.** Risk factor control along with patient education and aspirin as well as **statins**, **ACE inhibitors, and ARBs** forms the basis of event prevention strategies.

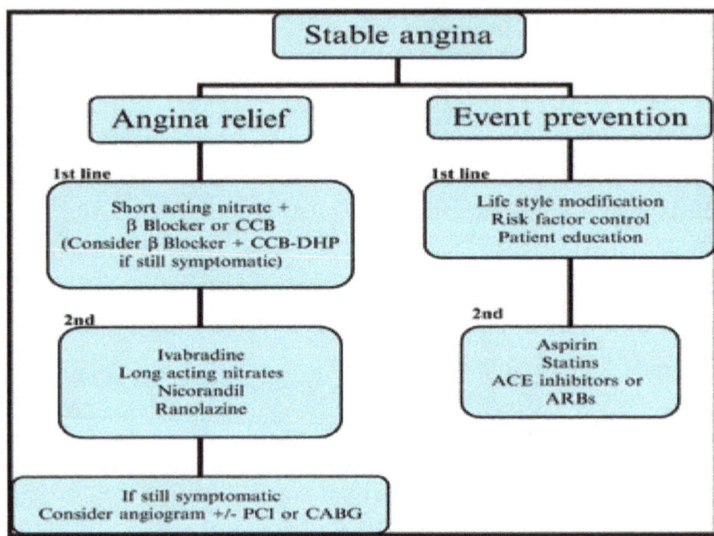

Figure 28 Medical Management of CAD

Figure 29 presents a structured **anticoagulation treatment plan for DVT** divided into three phases: **Initial (5-21 days), Long-term (first 3 months), and Extended (>3 months)**. Different anticoagulants, including **Apixaban, Dabigatran, Edoxaban, Rivaroxaban, and Vitamin K Antagonists (VKA)**, are prescribed based on duration and clinical considerations such as renal function and concurrent medications. The extended phase allows dose reductions for some drugs (e.g., **Apixaban 2.5 mg bid or Rivaroxaban 10 mg od beyond 6 months**) to balance efficacy and bleeding risks.

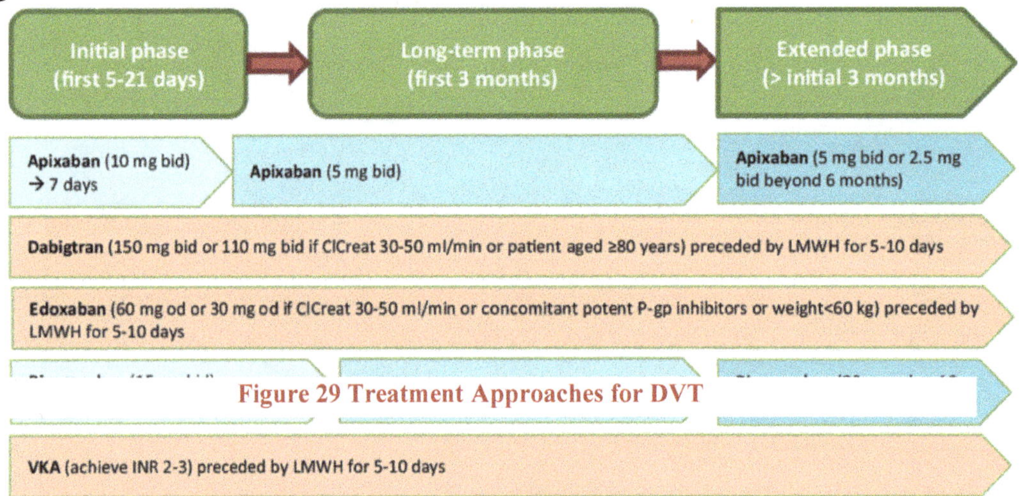

Figure 29 Treatment Approaches for DVT

Table 17 Algorithm for PAD

Antithrombotic Therapy Algorithm for PAD			
Initial Assessment	**Confirm diagnosis of PAD**: ABI ≤ 0.90 (for symptomatic PAD) or ABI 0.91 - 0.99 (asymptomatic with risk factors). **Evaluate cardiovascular risk**: Determine presence of comorbidities (hypertension, diabetes, hyperlipidemia, previous MI, stroke, or TIA). **Assess bleeding risk**: History of major bleeding, coagulopathies, or previous stroke/TIA.		
Step 1: Antiplatelet Therapy (First-line)	For Symptomatic PAD (ABI ≤ 0.85): • **Aspirin 75–150 mg daily** or **Clopidogrel 75 mg daily** (either as monotherapy). • **Indication**: To reduce the risk of MI, stroke, and vascular death.	Dual Antiplatelet Therapy (DAPT): • **Aspirin + Clopidogrel**: ○ Consider in **high-risk patients** with multiple atherothrombotic risk factors (e.g., history of MI, stroke). ○ **Monitor for bleeding risk**. ○ **Evidence**: CHARISMA trial showed some benefit in PAD subgroup.	**For Asymptomatic PAD (ABI between 0.91 and 0.99):** • Role of antiplatelet therapy is less well-established. • Consider based on individual cardiovascular risk factors.
Step 2: Add-on Therapy (Optional)	**Vorapaxar** (PAR-1 antagonist): • **Indication**: For **patients without history of stroke/TIA** who have symptomatic PAD. • **Efficacy**: Reduces cardiovascular events when combined with aspirin or clopidogrel.		

	• **Risk**: Increased bleeding risk, especially moderate bleeding. • **Caution**: Not recommended for patients with a history of stroke or TIA due to the risk of intracranial hemorrhage.	
Step 3: Avoid Anticoagulants (Unless Another Indication Exists)	**Warfarin**: • **Not recommended** as an alternative to antiplatelet therapy unless another indication (e.g., atrial fibrillation, mechanical heart valve). • **Risk**: Increased bleeding risk without additional cardiovascular benefit compared to antiplatelet therapy.	**Vitamin K Antagonists (e.g., Warfarin)**: • **Efficacy**: No significant reduction in cardiovascular events in PAD (Warfarin Antiplatelet Vascular Evaluation trial). • **Bleeding Risk**: Significantly increased compared to antiplatelet therapy.

Step 4: Ongoing Monitoring & Risk Management	**Regular follow-up** for:
	• **Bleeding complications** (monitor gastrointestinal or intracranial hemorrhage risks, especially with dual antiplatelet therapy).
		• **Continue or adjust** antiplatelet therapy based on:
		  ○ Symptom progression.
		  ○ New cardiovascular events.
		  ○ Tolerability of medications.

	• **Cardiovascular event monitoring** (e.g., MI, stroke, revascularization events). • **Adjustments in therapy** based on risk-benefit analysis.	
Summary	**First-line**: Monotherapy with **Aspirin** or **Clopidogrel** (preferred for symptomatic PAD). **Dual antiplatelet therapy** may be considered for **high-risk patients** but requires careful monitoring due to the increased bleeding risk. **Vorapaxar** offers additional benefit in patients without a history of stroke/TIA but should be used cautiously. **Anticoagulation** with warfarin is not recommended in PAD patients unless there is a concurrent indication (e.g., atrial fibrillation).	

2.3.6 Heart Failure (HF)

The **classification of heart failure** consists of systolic HF with reduced ejection fraction and diastolic HF with preserved ejection fraction and **NYHA** categories extend from I to IV. The **diagnosis of heart failure** is based on echocardiography results and **BNP** measurements while the primary symptoms are fatigue as well as edema and shortness of breath. The combination of diuretics together with ACE inhibitors beta-blockers and ARNI represents the main course of treatment. The **Universal Definition and Classification of Heart Failure (HF)** describes it as a **syndrome producing symptoms** resulting from **heart structural or functional issues** that cause **reduced cardiac output.** The assessment includes two primary subsections which are Stages and Classification by **Ejection Fraction (EF).** Heart function deterioration becomes more apparent during different HF stages from **At-risk HF** through **to Advanced HF**. There are three EF-based classification groups according to clinical classifications including **HFpEF and HFrEF as well as HFimpEF.**

2.3.6.1 Classification of Heart Failure

The image presents a **heart failure stage model** which uses both **disease severity and symptom appearance** as classification criteria. The initial phase includes people with high heart failure risk despite having a healthy heart at this time. Different risk elements that lead to heart failure consist of hypertension along with diabetes and valve abnormalities and exposure to cardiotoxic chemotherapy drugs. **During Stage B** patients experience **asymptomatic structural heart disease** that shows early indications of **cardiotoxicity through LVEF below 55% and GLS impairments** along with diastolic dysfunction. **Stage C heart disease** displays symptomatic structural heart disease because patients experience **declining LVEF levels** together with deteriorating heart toxic effects. **Stage D heart failure** constitutes the most advanced condition because it represents treatment-resistant failure alongside severe toxic effects on the heart. The development of the disease demonstrates growing severity and advancing negative cardiac effects.

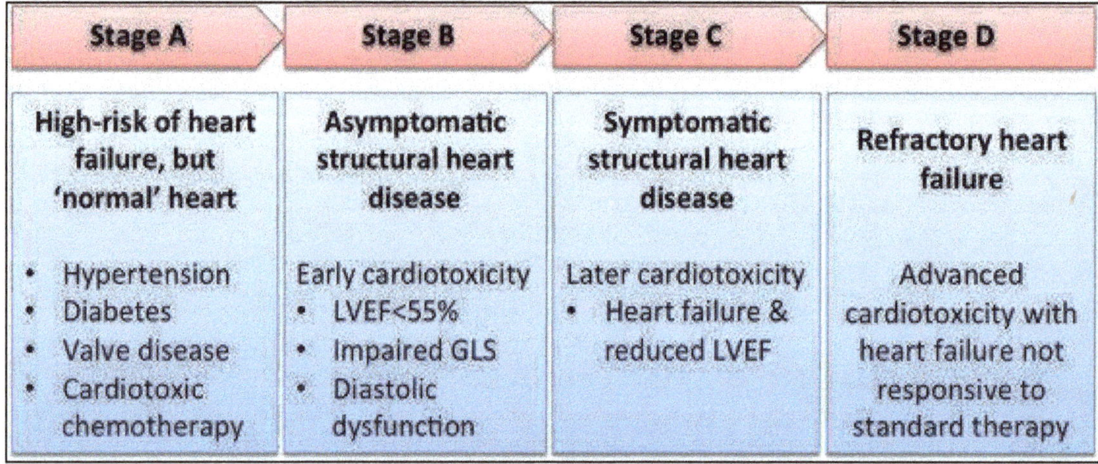

Stage A
Stage B
Stage C
Stage D
High-risk of heart failure, but 'normal' heart
• Hypertension
• Diabetes
• Valve disease
• Cardiotoxic chemotherapy
Asymptomatic structural heart disease
Early cardiotoxicity
• LVEF<55%
• Impaired GLS
• Diastolic dysfunction
Symptomatic structural heart disease
Later cardiotoxicity
• Heart failure & reduced LVEF
Refractory heart failure
Advanced cardiotoxicity with heart failure not responsive to standard therapy

Figure 30 Stages of Heart Failure

2.3.7 SOAP Notes for Heart Failure

Table 18 SOAP Notes for Heart Failure

Component	Details
Subjective (S)	The patient presenting with increasing shortness of breath, fatigue, and leg swelling over the past month. He reports difficulty lying flat due to orthopnea and waking up at night feeling short of breath (paroxysmal nocturnal dyspnea). He has a history of hypertension, diabetes, and coronary artery disease.
Objective (O)	BP: 145/90 mmHg, HR: 88 bpm, RR: 20 bpm, Oxygen Saturation: 94%. Physical exam reveals an S3 gallop, elevated JVP, bibasilar rales, and bilateral pitting edema. ECG shows sinus rhythm. Echocardiogram: LVEF 35%, dilated left ventricle, moderate mitral regurgitation. BNP elevated at 400 pg/mL.
Assessment (A)	**Differential Diagnoses:** Chronic heart failure with reduced ejection fraction (HFrEF), exacerbated by uncontrolled hypertension and diabetes. Differential diagnoses include an acute exacerbation of heart failure.
Plan (P)	Investigations: Repeat echocardiogram in 6 months to assess progression of heart failure. Monitor renal function and electrolytes regularly. **Pharmacological Treatment:** Initiate ACE inhibitor (Lisinopril 20 mg daily) for afterload reduction. Start Beta-blocker (Carvedilol 12.5 mg twice daily) for heart rate control and symptom relief. Diuretic (Furosemide 40 mg daily) to manage fluid overload and improve symptoms. Aldosterone antagonist (Spironolactone 25 mg daily) to reduce hospitalizations and mortality (See the algorithm below). **Non-Pharmacological Treatment:** Recommend a low-sodium diet and fluid restriction. Educate the patient about daily weight monitoring and symptom tracking (orthopnea, edema), Encourage moderate physical activity as tolerated **Referral:** Refer to cardiology for long-term management and possible evaluation for implantable cardioverter-defibrillator (ICD) or heart failure device therapy if needed. **Follow-up:** Re-assess within 1 week for symptom monitoring and medication adjustment. Follow-up with cardiology in 1 month for further evaluation of heart failure management

Table 19 Algorithm for the Management of Heart Failure

<table>
<tr><th colspan="4">Medication Management Algorithm for Heart Failure</th></tr>
<tr><td>Step 1: Initial Assessment</td><td colspan="3">Diagnose heart failure type: Assess if the patient has HFrEF (Heart Failure with reduced Ejection Fraction) or HFpEF (Heart Failure with preserved Ejection Fraction).
Evaluate symptom severity: Assess for common symptoms such as shortness of breath, fatigue, edema, and reduced exercise tolerance.</td></tr>
<tr><td>Step 2: Initiate First-Line Medications</td><td>ACE Inhibitors:
• Indication: For all patients with HFrEF, helps relax blood vessels and reduce blood pressure.
• Examples: Ramipril, Lisinopril, Enalapril.
• Common side effect: Dry cough (switch to ARB if persistent).</td><td>Angiotensin II Receptor Blockers (ARBs):
• Indication: Alternative for patients who can't tolerate ACE inhibitors.
• Examples: Losartan, Candesartan.
• Side effects: Low blood pressure, high potassium levels.</td><td>Beta-Blockers:
• Indication: Slows heart rate, reduces workload on the heart, and improves outcomes in heart failure.
• Examples: Bisoprolol, Carvedilol, Nebivolol.
• Side effects: Dizziness, tiredness, blurred vision.</td></tr>
<tr><td>Step 3: Add-on Therapy for Symptom Control</td><td>Mineralocorticoid Receptor Antagonists (MRAs):
• Indication: Reduces fluid retention and</td><td colspan="2">Diuretics (Water pills):
• Indication: Relieves fluid retention, swelling, and breathlessness.
• Examples: Furosemide, Bumetanide.</td></tr>
</table>

	helps manage blood pressure. • **Examples**: Spironolactone, Eplerenone. • **Side effects**: High potassium levels, gynecomastia (Spironolactone), dizziness (Eplerenone).	• **Side effects**: Dehydration, electrolyte imbalances.	
Step 4: Consider Additional Medications if Necessary	**Ivabradine**: • **Indication**: Slows heart rate, useful when beta-blockers are insufficient or poorly tolerated. • **Side effects**: Headaches, dizziness, blurred vision.	**Sacubitril Valsartan**: • **Indication**: For more severe heart failure, combining ARB and neprilysin inhibitor. • **Side effects**: Low blood pressure, kidney problems, high potassium levels.	**Hydralazine with Nitrate**: • **Indication**: For patients who can't take ACE inhibitors or ARBs. • **Side effects**: Headaches, palpitations, fast heartbeat
Step 5: Add-on Medications for Symptom Relief	**Digoxin**: 1. **Indication**: For patients with persistent symptoms	**SGLT2 Inhibitors**: • **Indication**: Used as an add-on therapy to improve heart failure symptoms and lower blood sugar levels.	

	despite other treatments. 2. **Side effects**: Dizziness, nausea, blurred vision, irregular heartbeat.	• **Examples**: Empagliflozin, Dapagliflozin. **Side effects**: Increased urination, thrush, back pain.
Step 6: Ongoing Monitoring	• Monitor kidney function, electrolyte levels, and blood pressure regularly. • Adjust medications based on symptom control, side effects, and lab results. • Periodic follow-up with echocardiograms and heart function assessments.	
Summary	First-line therapies: ACE inhibitors or ARBs, beta-blockers, and diuretics. Add-on therapies: Ivabradine, sacubitril valsartan, hydralazine with nitrate, and digoxin. SGLT2 inhibitors are increasingly included as an adjunct in the treatment of heart failure with reduced ejection fraction.	

2.3.8 Neurotransmitter Dysfunctions in Cardiac Regulation

Heart rate becomes elevated due to **Beta-1 receptors** interaction with **norepinephrine but parasympathetic muscarinic receptors** control it down with acetylcholine delivery. **Pathway disorders** create **heart rhythm** problems and **high or low blood pressure** along with impaired **autonomic responses** that need either **adrenergic or cholinergic medical procedures** . The illustration depicts the **Nervous System** through a hierarchical structure that separates it into Central and Peripheral parts. The **Peripheral Nervous System** includes two divisions that encompass **Sensory functions while its Motor functions split into Somatic control and Autonomic (ANS).** Autonomic control comprises **SNS and PNS.** The Autonomic Nervous System contains two separate subdivisions called Sympathetic Nervous System (SNS) with **Alpha (1,2) and Beta (1,2) receptors and Parasympathetic Nervous System (PNS) with Nicotinic and Muscarinic receptors.**

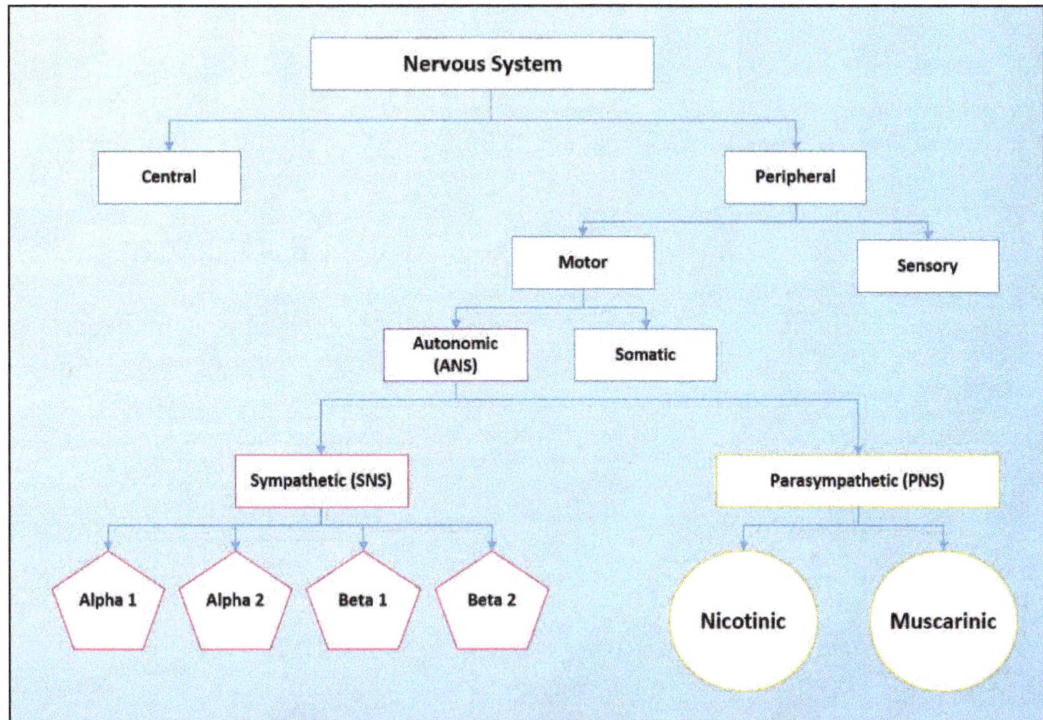

Figure 31 A hierarchical overview of the Nervous System, illustrating its major divisions and receptor classifications within the Autonomic Nervous System

A graphical comparison in figure shows how the parasympathetic and sympathetic systems influence different organs through their autonomic nervous system divisions. The **parasympathetic** system functions through **green pathways to control rest and digest operations** that slow heart rate and promote digestion but the sympathetic system operates through **orange pathways** to trigger **fight or flight responses** through **heart rate acceleration** along with **pupil dilation and delayed digestion**. The mapping illustrates the neural pathways which lead **nerve signals** through brain and spinal cord channels to all major body organs.

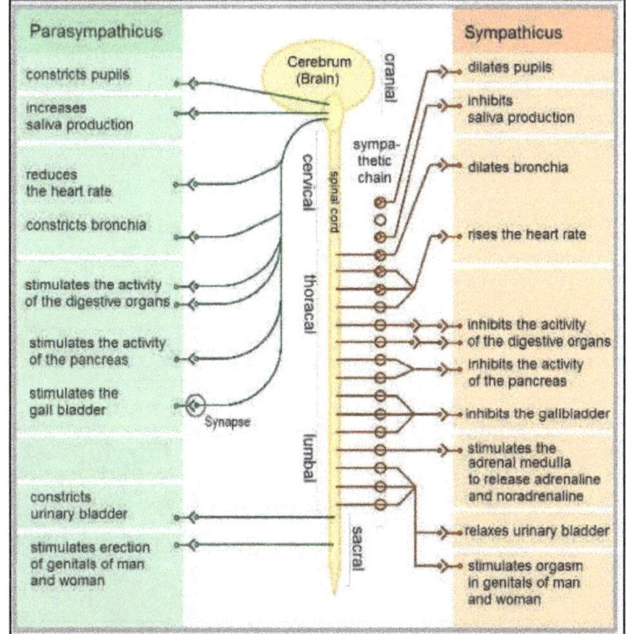

Figure 32 Classification of sympathetic and parasympathetic NS

2.3.8.1 Key Functions of Neurotransmitter

Figure 34 displays **neurotransmitter functionality** by grouping them according to their **functions involving pleasure, mood, learning, stress response, and relaxation behaviors**. **Dopamine** plays a key role in **pleasure responses** alongside its functions **to regulate cognition and decision-making skills** but also **controls serotonin concentrations** which influence **mood state regulation alongside** appetite control **and social behavior responses. Norepinephrine** and epinephrine serve as **"flight or fight" neurotransmitters** that amplify heart rate together with blood flow while improving physical capabilities yet **GABA operates** as a relaxing **neurotransmitter** to limit stress while fostering a state of calm. The neurotransmitter **acetylcholine (Ach)** stands out due to its essential contribution to **learning and memory** as well as concentration processes in the brain.

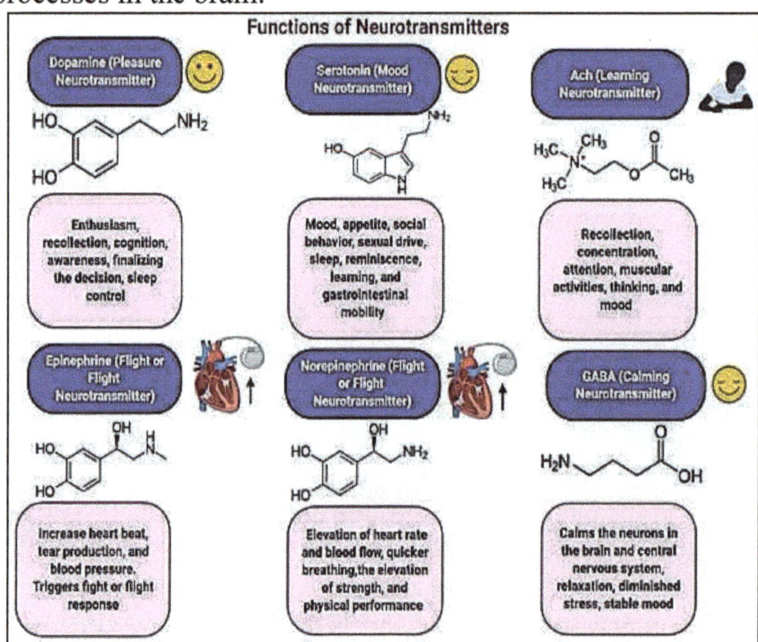

Figure 33 Functions of Neurotransmitter

2.3.8.2 SOAP Notes for Neurological Dysfunction

Table 20 SOAP Notes for Neurological Dysfunction

Component	Details
Subjective (S)	Patient reports episodes of palpitations, dizziness, and fluctuating blood pressure. Complains of sudden increases in heart rate, especially during stress or exertion, along with occasional fainting spells. Reports fatigue and exercise intolerance.
Objective (O)	Vitals: BP 145/90 mmHg (hypertensive episodes), HR 102 bpm (tachycardia) at rest, RR 18 bpm. Cardiac exam: Irregular heart rate with occasional ectopic beats. Neurological exam: No focal deficits, but autonomic instability is suspected. ECG: Shows sinus tachycardia with intermittent premature ventricular contractions (PVCs).

Assessment (A)	Differential Diagnoses: 1. Dysautonomia (Autonomic Nervous System Dysfunction) 2. Adrenergic Overactivity (Excess Norepinephrine) 3. Cholinergic Dysfunction (Impaired Acetylcholine Regulation) 4. Neurocardiogenic Syncope.
Plan (P)	**Investigations:** Holter monitoring, autonomic function testing, tilt table test, catecholamine levels, and cardiac MRI (if structural concerns arise). **Pharmacological Treatment:** Beta-blockers (e.g., metoprolol) to control excessive sympathetic activation, alpha-blockers (if necessary), and potential cholinergic modulation (e.g., pyridostigmine). **Non-Pharmacological Treatment:** Hydration, high-salt diet for dysautonomia, avoiding triggers such as stress or rapid postural changes, and vagal maneuvers for heart rate control. **Education:** Patient advised on lifestyle modifications, warning signs of severe dysautonomia, and medication adherence (See table and figure below). **Referral:** Neurologist and cardiologist consultation for further autonomic evaluation and management. **Follow-up:** Reassessment in 4-6 weeks with a repeat ECG, blood pressure monitoring, and symptom evaluation.

Table 21 Treatment Approaches for Cholinergic dysfunction

Indication	Medication/Agent	Rationale/Notes
Myasthenia gravis	Pyridostigmine (first-line), Neostigmine	Used as anticholinesterase therapy to improve neuromuscular transmission.
Dementia	Rivastigmine, Donepezil, Galantamine	Cholinesterase inhibitors improve cognition in Alzheimer's and other dementias.
Ophthalmology	Pilocarpine, Carbachol	Pilocarpine and Carbachol reduce intraocular pressure in open-angle glaucoma.
Reversal of nondepolarizing neuromuscular blockade after surgery	Neostigmine preceded by atropine	Neostigmine reverses neuromuscular blockade after surgery with atropine to counteract muscarinic effects.
Postoperative urinary retention	Neostigmine, Bethanechol	Neostigmine prevents and treats urinary retention; Bethanechol is used for non-obstructive urinary retention.
Neurogenic bladder	Bethanechol	Bethanechol helps in complete bladder emptying for those with hypotonic bladder.
Acute colonic pseudo-obstruction	Neostigmine (off-label)	Neostigmine is used off-label for acute colonic pseudo-obstruction.
Xerostomia	Cevimeline	Cevimeline is used in patients with dry mouth due to Sjogren's syndrome or post-radiation.
Anticholinergic overdose	Physostigmine	Physostigmine is used as an antidote for life-threatening anticholinergic toxicity.
Tensilon test	Edrophonium (discontinued)	Edrophonium was previously used for diagnosing myasthenia gravis but has been discontinued.

Snakebite	Neostigmine	Neostigmine helps with neurotoxic snakebites when antivenom is unavailable or ineffective.

2.3.9 Infections

The cardiovascular system becomes vulnerable to infections that produce severe consequences on heart functioning and total health status. **The inner heart lining** suffers an infection known as **endocarditis** which primarily **affects heart valve structures. Bacteria entry through the bloodstream triggers** this condition which leads to heart failure symptoms among other cardiac manifestations and also **generates fever with chest pain**. Physicians validate **endocarditis through the analysis of blood cultures and echocardiograms.** Prolonged antibiotic treatment serves as the main therapeutic approach for the elimination of heart infections.

Heart muscle inflammation known as myocarditis arises from viral infection as well as autoimmune diseases or bacterial causes. Such an illness leads to **extreme tiredness as well as heart damage and irregular heart rhythms**. The identification of the condition depends on clinical signs combined with blood tests and imaging methods. Healthy treatment of this condition requires anti-inflammatory medication and symptom management medicine.

Medical experts identify pericarditis as the inflammation which affects the pericardium that envelops the heart. This infection emerges due to viral or autoimmune illnesses and leads to chest pain together with fever symptoms. **NSAIDs and steroids** serve as treatments to minimize inflammation in patients. Stepwise detection paired with prompt medical care plays a vital role in averting heart failure among patients.

The diagnostic pathway for **Infective Endocarditis (IE)** (Figure 34) depends on low or high patient risk along with clinical suspicion according to the flowchart design. When patients display low initial risk along with low suspicion an echocardiography TTE becomes the initial diagnostic procedure. A **Transesophageal Echocardiogram (TEE)** becomes necessary to check for complications when patient suspicion develops throughout their clinical treatment. The initiation of treatment takes place simultaneously with the need for additional **TEE to monitor post-treatment complications** when **high-risk echo abnormalities appear.** The patient does not need extra imaging tests since high-risk features are absent yet retesting may occur for deteriorating clinical conditions. High-risk patients requiring **confirmatory echo tests** receive a **TEE** at first assessment and later require another one in case their suspicions remain elevated. The healthcare provider will redirect their attention to other possible symptom sources if suspicion subsides or another medical condition confirms the diagnosis. Reassessment imaging must be completed based on clinical requirements to evaluate vegetation and **treatment response as well as complications.** A structured diagnostic management process helps doctors determine infective endocarditis properly while delivering it in a timely manner.

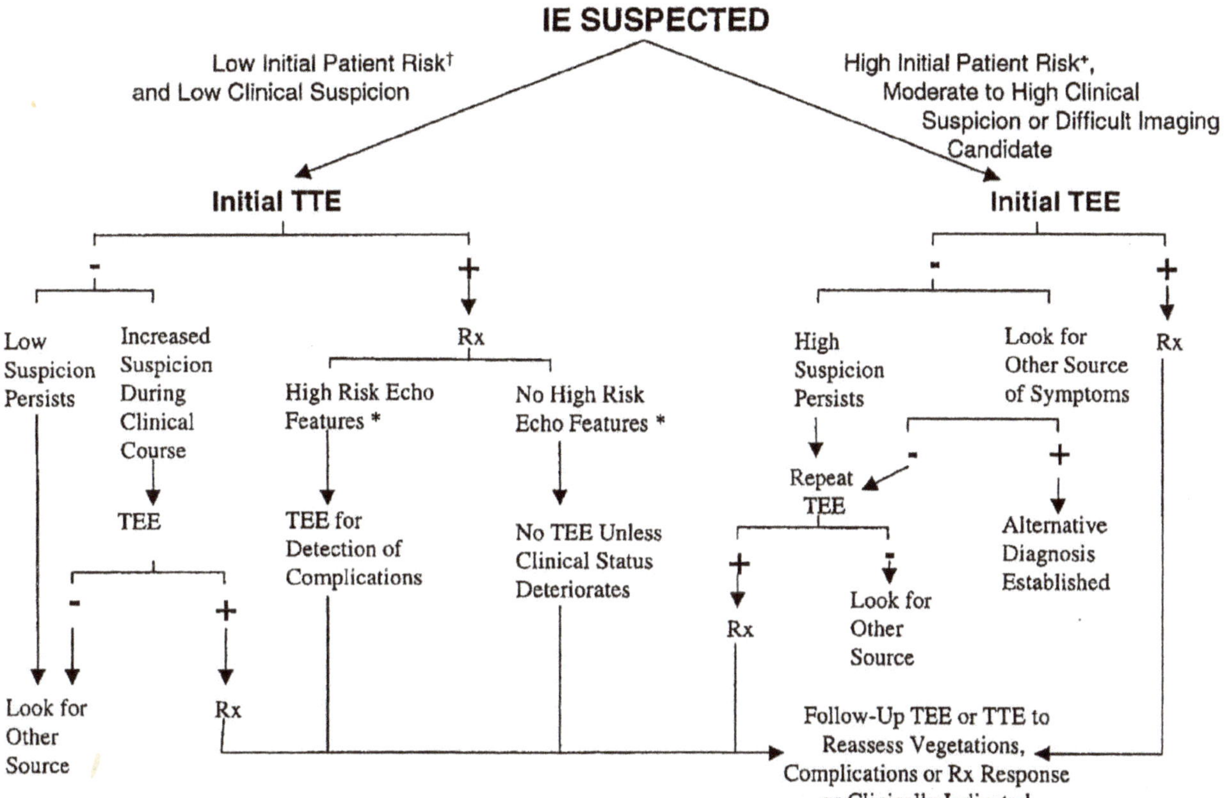

Figure 34 Flowchart of Infected Endocarditis

Figure 36 shows how viral heart disease together with **myocarditis advance** while showing different possible end results. **Antiviral cytokines** are produced upon a viral infection to fight against the virus **causing tissue inflammation**. Success in eliminating the virus allows inflammation to disappear yet the possible outcomes remain different. The **heart heals** itself from myocarditis when there is no **myocardial dysfunction** thus avoiding the need for particular medical treatment. A disorder of myocardial function will result in dilated cardiomyopathy and the subsequent deterioration of heart muscle performance. **The infection will progress to chronic myocarditis** or **inflammatory cardiomyopathy** when **myocardial inflammation continues** thereby leading to heart failure. People with these long-term illnesses might require medications to suppress their immune system as well as procedures to take out **inflammatory cells to reduce swelling.** Antiviral medications become necessary to treat viral heart disease when it occurs after a **chronic viral infection with or without inflammation**. The diagram illustrates that viral infections together with inflammatory responses and selected treatment approaches guide the development of myocarditis and viral heart disease.

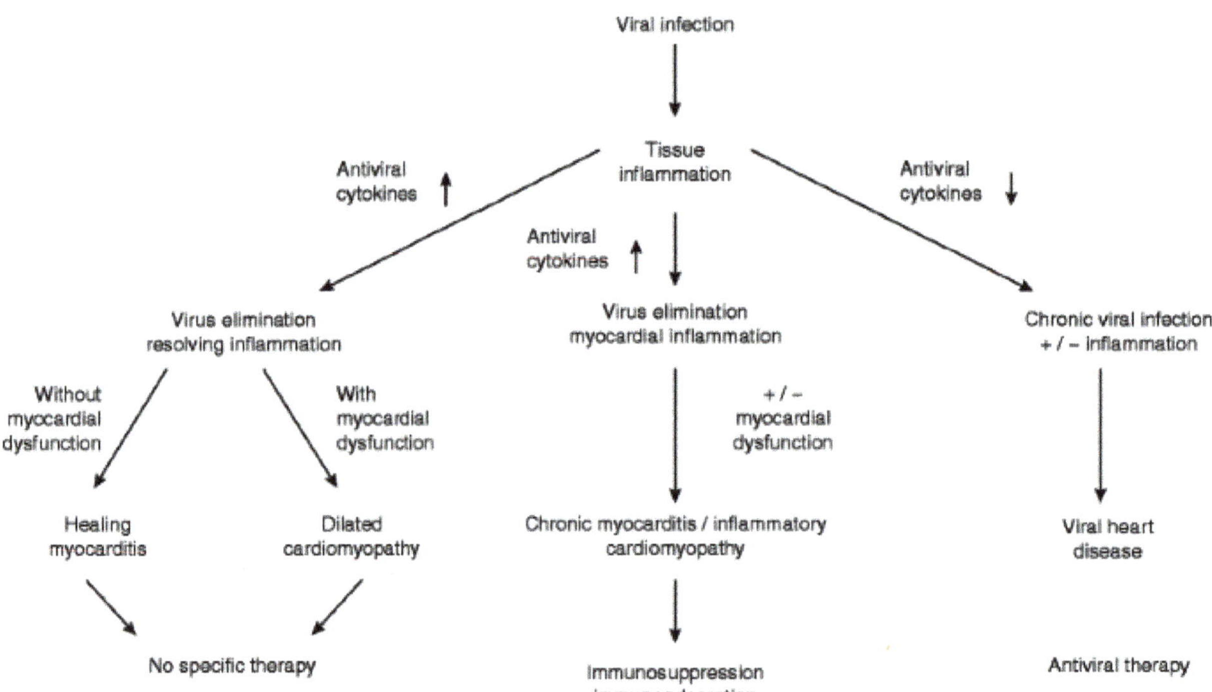

Figure 35 Flowchart of Viral Infection Progression in Myocarditis and Viral Heart Disease

Acute Pericarditis patients (Figure 36) with excessive effusion **above 20mm may need pericardiocentesis or pericardial biopsy** to investigate the condition. A **lower than 20mm effusion** usually requires **NSAID therapy** as treatment with either positive or negative clinical outcomes for recovery. When patients fail to recover the situation demands additional procedures including pericardiocentesis and biopsy. When there is effusion in **Constrictive Pericarditis** the clinical **workflow demands pericardiocentesis** combined with pericardial biopsy followed by microbiological testing or histopathology investigations to reach a full diagnosis. The surgical **removal of the pericardium** becomes the necessary therapeutic option when there is no presence of effusion. **Cytology** analysis and molecular testing specifically **PCR** and special staining along with other specific examination methods are strongly recommended for determining the cause of the disease. A defined strategy enables health professionals to deliver suitable medical interventions according to the extent of the effusion alongside medical signs. The illustration depicts the **multiple origins of pericarditis** which describes **an inflammatory situation** that affects the **heart-wrapping pericardium**. **Post-Cardiac Injury Syndrome** stands as one of the **leading causes of pericarditis** because it happens after cardiac surgeries and pacemaker insertions together with other cardiac interventions. **Idiopathic pericarditis** refers to a **pericardial inflammation** situation without detected origins. **Pericardium inflammation** arises mainly due to infection either from viruses or bacteria or fungi. Pericarditis develops partially due to **Cancer and Cancer Therapies** since specific tumors together with therapeutic agents like immune checkpoint inhibitors produce the condition. **Pericarditis** develops as a side effect of autoimmune diseases along with hypothyroidism due to their inflammatory effects on the body. The various **causes of pericarditis** demonstrate how the condition can manifest through medical operations and diseases as well as infectious agents and constant health conditions.

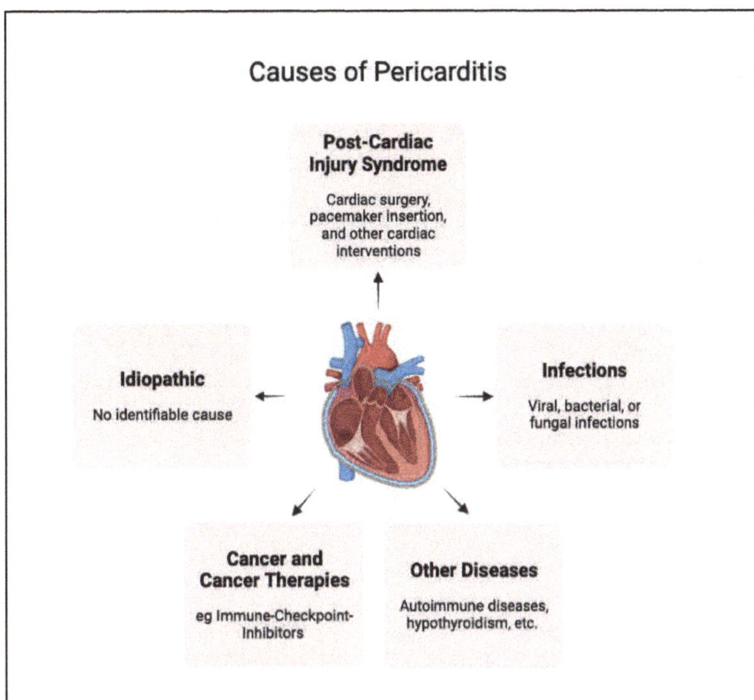

Figure 36 Causes of Pericarditis

2.3.9.1 SOAP Notes for Infections

Table 22 SOAP Notes for the Cardiovascular Infections

Component	Details
Subjective (S)	Patient reports recent episodes of fever, fatigue, and shortness of breath. Complains of chest pain that worsens with deep breathing. History of recent dental surgery and intravenous drug use. Denies recent travel or contact with sick individuals. The patient reports no prior heart conditions but mentions occasional palpitations and swelling in the legs. The patient is concerned about possible complications due to recent illness and risk factors.
Objective (O)	Vitals: BP 130/85 mmHg, HR 110 bpm (tachycardia), RR 20 bpm, Temp 38.2°C (febrile). Cardiac exam: Heart sounds are distant, with a systolic murmur heard at the apex, which radiates to the axilla. Neurological exam: No focal deficits observed. ECG: Shows sinus tachycardia and non-specific ST changes. Blood tests: Elevated WBC (14,000/µL), elevated CRP, and positive blood cultures for **Streptococcus viridans**. Chest X-ray: No significant findings. Echocardiogram: Shows vegetations on the mitral valve, suggestive of **infective endocarditis**.

Assessment (A)	Differential Diagnoses: 1. **Infective Endocarditis** - Likely due to bacteremia following dental surgery and potential intravenous drug use. 2. **Myocarditis** - Considered due to fever, chest pain, and tachycardia, though less likely based on presentation. 3. **Pericarditis** - Symptoms of chest pain and fever align but are less consistent with pericardial friction rub. 4. **Septicemia** - Given fever, positive blood cultures, and systemic symptoms, further investigation required to rule out generalized infection.
Plan (P)	Investigations: Blood cultures (repeat if needed), Transesophageal echocardiogram (TEE), CT chest if suspicion of embolic events. Pharmacological Treatment: Start **IV antibiotics** (vancomycin and ceftriaxone) based on blood culture results. Consider antifungal therapy if fungi are suspected (See algorithms below). Non-Pharmacological Treatment: Bed rest, hydration, and nutrition. Education: Educate the patient on infective endocarditis, the importance of completing the full course of antibiotics, and preventive measures (e.g., prophylactic antibiotics for future dental procedures). Referral: Referral to cardiologist for further evaluation and possible valve surgery if needed. Referral to infectious disease specialist for targeted therapy and management. Follow-up: Reassess in 1-2 weeks for symptom resolution and repeat echocardiogram to assess valve function and vegetations. Schedule follow-up blood cultures and clinical assessment for the next 6 months to ensure full resolution of infection.

Table 23 Algorithm for the Endocarditis Management

Category	Recommendation	Class/Level of Evidence	Details
Antibiotic Therapy	Routine use of rifampin for staphylococcal NVE	Class III; Level of Evidence B	Not recommended for routine use due to limited evidence of benefit in the treatment of staphylococcal NVE.
	Management of IE caused by vancomycin-resistant staphylococci	Class I; Level of Evidence C	Should be managed in conjunction with an infectious diseases consultant.
	Empirical antimicrobial therapy for undefined febrile illnesses	Class III; Level of Evidence C	Should be avoided unless the patient's condition (e.g., sepsis) warrants it.
	Initiation of antimicrobial therapy	Class I; Level of Evidence C	Antimicrobial therapy should be started promptly for infective endocarditis, usually with a combination of broad-spectrum antibiotics like vancomycin or ceftriaxone until specific organisms are identified.
	Targeted antimicrobial therapy	Class I; Level of Evidence C	Once the causative organism is identified, therapy should be adjusted accordingly (e.g., penicillin, ceftriaxone, or nafcillin for specific pathogens).
	Antimicrobial therapy for long-term treatment	Class IIb; Level of Evidence C	For patients receiving long-term aminoglycosides, serial audiograms may be considered due to the risk of ototoxicity.
	Antifungal therapy	Class I; Level of Evidence C	Consider if fungal infections are suspected or identified, particularly in immunocompromised patients or those with prosthetic heart valves.

	Removal of intravenous catheters	Class I; Level of Evidence *C*	All indwelling intravenous catheters used for antimicrobial treatment should be removed promptly at the end of therapy to reduce the risk of infection.
Surgical Considerations	Surgical intervention	Class I; Level of Evidence B	Valve replacement or repair may be necessary in cases of severe valve damage, persistent bacteremia, or heart failure despite adequate antimicrobial therapy.
Prevention & Monitoring	Ongoing observation for recurrent infection and valve dysfunction after treatment	Class I; Level of Evidence *C*	Ongoing monitoring for recurrence of infection and evaluation of valve function (e.g., echocardiography).
	Prophylaxis before dental/surgical procedures	Class I; Level of Evidence *C*	Prophylactic antibiotics should be administered before dental, surgical, or invasive procedures to prevent recurrent infections.
	Echocardiography before or at completion of antimicrobial therapy	Class IIa; Level of Evidence *C*	Echocardiography should be done to establish a new baseline and evaluate the heart valves at the end of antimicrobial therapy.
Follow-up Care	Serial audiograms for aminoglycoside therapy	Class IIb; Level of Evidence *C*	For patients receiving long-term aminoglycosides, particularly those with underlying renal or otic disorders, serial audiograms may be considered during therapy.
	Blood cultures and echocardiography after completing antimicrobial therapy	Class III; Level of Evidence *C*	Routine blood cultures are not recommended after the completion of antimicrobial therapy unless there is clinical suspicion of relapse.

	Monitoring for complications like IE relapse and heart failure	Class I; Level of Evidence C	Patients should be monitored for the development of IE relapse, heart failure, and other complications in the short-term follow-up.
	Immediate medical evaluation for symptoms of relapse	Class I; Level of Evidence C	New onset of fever, chills, or systemic toxicity should prompt immediate evaluation, including blood cultures and echocardiogram.
	Removal of intravenous catheters	Class I; Level of Evidence C	All indwelling intravenous catheters used to infuse antimicrobial treatment should be removed promptly at the end of therapy.
Patient Education	Avoidance of empirical antimicrobial therapy for undefined febrile illnesses	Class III; Level of Evidence C	Empirical antimicrobial therapy should not be initiated for undefined febrile illnesses unless the patient's clinical condition (e.g., sepsis) warrants it.
	Patient education on endocarditis signs and symptoms	Class I; Level of Evidence C	Educate patients about the signs of endocarditis, the importance of medication adherence, and the need for prophylactic antibiotics before certain procedures.
	Referral for drug use cessation in IDUs	Class I; Level of Evidence C	Referral to a program to assist in the cessation of drug use should be made for intravenous drug users (IDUs) to prevent recurrence of IE.
	Heart failure monitoring	Class I; Level of Evidence C	Monitor for signs of heart failure, as it is a common complication after IE. If heart failure develops or worsens, evaluate immediately for cardiac surgery.
Post-Treatment Care	Antibiotic toxicity monitoring	Class I; Level of Evidence C	Monitor for antibiotic-related toxicity, including ototoxicity (with aminoglycosides) and gastrointestinal complications like Clostridium difficile infections.

A Figure 37 shows **high-risk factors (red boxes) intermediate-risk factors (yellow boxes) and low-risk factors (green boxes)** based on **BP levels and AHF progression severity** and **LVEF** measurements from first echocardiograms and **ECG** readings which include **VT and VF or AVB**. Additional information explains how these risk factors guide the decision to send patients to specialized centers for potential cardiac support treatment including **t-MCS** and whether EMB or **CMRI** should occur with possible steroid prescription. The tag sign indicates recommended actions. **No symbol indicates not recommended**. The therapy involves immune suppression through intravenous steroid administration for patients with fulminant myocarditis even though no

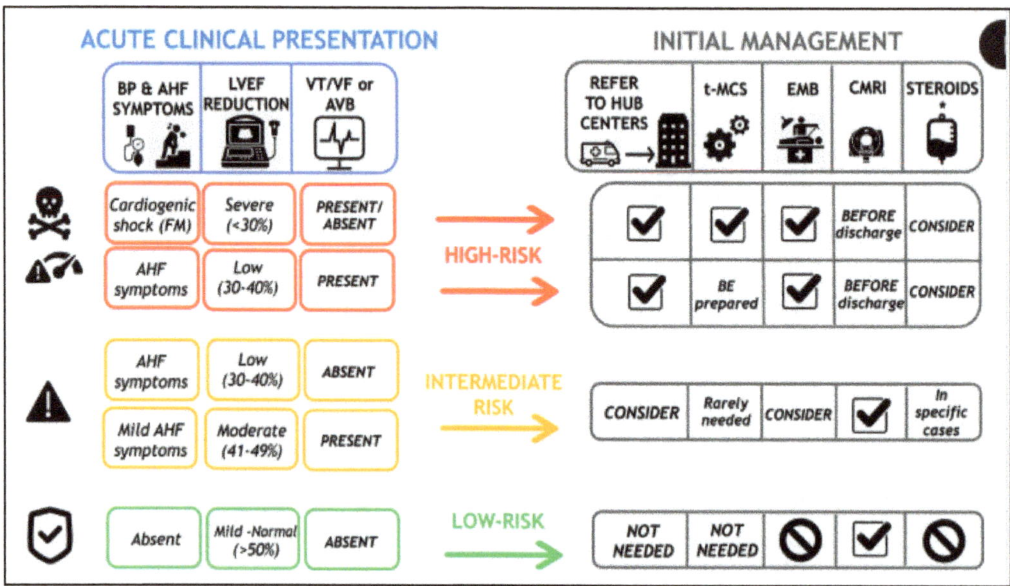

clinical research proves its effectiveness.

Figure 37 Proposed risk-based approach to acute myocarditis

Table 24 Algorithm for the Myocarditis Treatment Approaches

Type of Myocarditis	First-Line Treatment	Second-Line Treatment	Treatment Details	Notes
Lymphocytic Fulminant Myocarditis (FM)	Intravenous (i.v.) methylprednisolone (7-14 mg/kg for 3 days, then 1 mg·kg−1·day−1 with tapering)	IVIG (2 g/kg), plasmapheresis (3-5 sessions over 5-10 days)	Steroids are commonly used. IVIG and plasmapheresis are options for refractory cases.	Lymphocytic FM is often treated with high-dose corticosteroids. IVIG and plasmapheresis are considered for refractory cases or those with severe symptoms.
Immune Checkpoint Inhibitor (ICI)-Associated Myocarditis	Withdraw ICI therapy, high-dose intravenous corticosteroids	Anti-CD52 antibody (alemtuzumab), Anti-CD3 antibody (antithymocyte globulin), CTLA-4 agonist (abatacept)	ICI therapy withdrawal and high-dose corticosteroids are first-line. Secondary options include immunosuppressive agents.	ICI-Associated Myocarditis results from immune checkpoint inhibitors and requires immediate withdrawal and immunosuppression. Other immunosuppressive treatments are considered if the patient does not respond to steroids.
Eosinophilic Myocarditis (EM)	Corticosteroids, immediate withdrawal of offending drug (hypersensitivity reactions)	Cyclophosphamide, azathioprine, methotrexate, albendazole for parasitic infections	Steroids are crucial, and additional treatments depend on the underlying cause (e.g., parasitic infections).	EM is associated with hypersensitivity reactions, parasitic infections, and autoimmune conditions like EGPA. Treatment focuses on addressing the

				underlying cause.
Giant Cell Myocarditis (GCM)	Anti-T-lymphocyte therapy (e.g., antithymocyte globulin), high-dose corticosteroids	Cyclosporine, azathioprine, rituximab	Immediate corticosteroid therapy with immunosuppressive agents, and in case of FM, use anti-T-lymphocyte therapy.	GCM is a rapidly progressing myocarditis with poor prognosis. It requires high-dose corticosteroids and immunosuppressive therapies to control inflammation.
Sarcoidotic Myocarditis (CS)	Corticosteroids	Methotrexate, azathioprine, cyclophosphamide, infliximab, rarely rituximab	Corticosteroids are the primary treatment, often with methotrexate for refractory cases. Other immunosuppressives may be used for long-term management.	CS is associated with granulomatous inflammation in the myocardium. Corticosteroids are the first-line treatment, but methotrexate and other immunosuppressives may be needed for refractory cases.

Table 25 Algorithm for the Pericarditis Treatment Approaches

Condition	First-Line Treatment	Second-Line Treatment	Treatment Details	Notes
Acute Pericarditis	Aspirin or NSAIDs (e.g., ibuprofen)	Colchicine	Aspirin/NSAIDs for 1-2 weeks for pain and	Aspirin or NSAIDs are first-line for managing acute

			inflammation control, colchicine as adjunct for 3 months	pericarditis. Colchicine is added to prevent recurrences.
Incessant and Recurrent Pericarditis	Aspirin or NSAIDs (e.g., ibuprofen)	Corticosteroids (low-to-moderate doses)	Triple therapy with aspirin/NSAIDs, colchicine, and low-dose corticosteroids if needed	Corticosteroids should only be added after failure of aspirin/NSAIDs and colchicine.
Myopericarditis	Aspirin (1,500-3,000 mg/day) or NSAIDs (e.g., ibuprofen 1,200-2,400 mg/day)	Corticosteroids	Symptomatic treatment with NSAIDs, corticosteroids used if needed for intolerances or failure	NSAIDs are used to control chest pain; corticosteroids are considered for failure of other treatments.
Acute Viral Pericarditis	NSAIDs	Colchicine	Short course of NSAIDs, colchicine for recurrence prevention	Corticosteroids are not recommended due to their potential to reactivate viral infections.
Bacterial Pericarditis (e.g., Tuberculous Pericarditis)	Anti-TB therapy (if applicable)	Corticosteroids (for HIV-negative TB)	Anti-TB chemotherapy for exudative pericardial effusion in endemic areas, adjunctive steroids in non-HIV cases	Corticosteroids may be used in HIV-negative TB pericarditis, but not in HIV-associated TB.

Purulent Pericardial Effusion	Surgical drainage	Pericardiectomy	Surgical drainage to manage loculated or purulent effusions, consider intra-pericardial streptokinase	Early surgical drainage is key to prevent constriction; intra-pericardial streptokinase may be used in select cases.
Pericarditis in Autoimmune Disorders	Aspirin/NSAIDs with colchicine	Immunosuppressive agents (e.g., anti-IL, anti-TNF agents)	Target treatment of systemic autoimmune disease, often requiring adjunctive immunosuppression	Colchicine may be ineffective, and immunosuppressive agents like anti-TNF may be needed for management.
Radiation Pericarditis	NSAIDs	Pericardiotomy	Radiation therapy methods to reduce cardiac irradiation dose, pericardiotomy if needed	Pericardiotomy may be needed for constrictive pericarditis after radiation.
Drug-Induced Acute Pericarditis	Discontinue the causative drug	Symptomatic treatment	Discontinue offending agent, manage with NSAIDs or other supportive treatments	Symptomatic treatment is necessary once the causative agent is stopped.
Corticosteroid Use in Acute Pericarditis	Not recommended as first-line	N/A	Should be avoided in most cases; used when NSAIDs and colchicine	Corticosteroids can lead to recurrences and should be

			fail, but with caution	used only when necessary.
Exercise Restrictions	Exercise restriction until symptom resolution	N/A	Limit physical activity for non-athletes until CRP, ECG, and echocardiogram are normal	Exercise restrictions are recommended until the resolution of symptoms, especially for athletes.

2.4 Moh Golden Points and Summary Question Answers

2.4.1 Moh Golden Points

Heart block involves delayed or impaired conduction of electrical signals, and treatment varies from surveillance to pacemaker implantation depending on the severity and type of block.

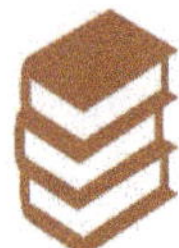

Heart valve disorders like mitral regurgitation and aortic stenosis cause murmurs, shortness of breath, and fatigue, and are treated with medications such as diuretics and beta-blockers or surgical valve replacement.

Vascular diseases, including arterial and venous conditions such as CAD, PAD, and DVT, are diagnosed using tools like Doppler ultrasound and ABI, and treated with anticoagulants, compression therapy, or surgery depending on severity.

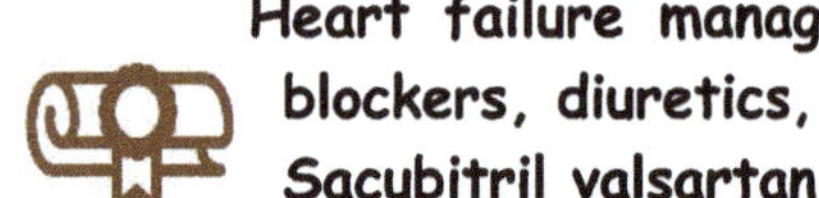

Heart failure management involves a combination of ACE inhibitors, beta-blockers, diuretics, and mineralocorticoid receptor antagonists (MRAs), with Sacubitril valsartan and SGLT2 inhibitors for more severe cases.

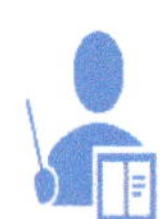

Myocardial infarction (MI) with angina is diagnosed using ECG, cardiac biomarkers, and angiography, and is treated with aspirin, beta-blockers, statins, and PCI procedures.

Hypertension is managed with antihypertensive medications like ACE inhibitors, ARBs, CCBs, and diuretics, alongside lifestyle changes including a low-sodium diet and weight management.

2.4.2 Summary Questions & Answers

1. **Which of the following is the most appropriate treatment for a patient with deep vein thrombosis (DVT)?**
   A. Compression therapy alone
   B. Anticoagulation therapy (e.g., Apixaban or Warfarin)
   C. High-dose aspirin
   D. Statins

2. **Which of the following is a key first-line medication for a patient with heart failure and reduced ejection fraction (HFrEF)?**

A. Ivabradine
B. Sacubitril valsartan
C. ACE inhibitor (e.g., Lisinopril)
D. Digoxin

3. **Which of the following is the most appropriate pharmacological treatment for a patient with acute ST-segment elevation myocardial infarction (STEMI)?**

A. Beta-blockers alone
B. Aspirin, clopidogrel, heparin, and nitroglycerin
C. ACE inhibitors
D. Diuretics

4. **Which of the following is the first-line treatment for primary hypertension in a patient with no other significant comorbidities?**

A. Beta-blockers
B. ACE inhibitors
C. Diuretics
D. Calcium channel blockers

5. **Which of the following is the most appropriate treatment for a patient with aortic stenosis and worsening heart failure symptoms?**

A. Diuretics
B. Beta-blockers
C. Valve replacement surgery
D. Anticoagulants

6. **Which of the following is the most appropriate treatment for a patient with symptomatic Mobitz Type II heart block?**

A. Observation
B. Atropine
C. Temporary pacing
D. Long-term beta-blockers

7. **Which heart murmur is typically associated with a "pansystolic murmur radiating to the left axilla" and can be caused by mitral valve prolapse or papillary muscle dysfunction?**

A) Aortic Stenosis
B) Mitral Stenosis
C) Mitral Regurgitation
D) Aortic Regurgitation

8. Which of the following murmurs is most commonly associated with a rumbling mid-diastolic sound, best heard on expiration with the patient lying on their left side?

A) Mitral Regurgitation
B) Mitral Stenosis
C) Aortic Stenosis
D) Aortic Regurgitation

9. Which of the following cholinergic medications is primarily used as a first-line treatment for Myasthenia Gravis?

A) Rivastigmine
B) Bethanechol
C) Pyridostigmine
D) Cevimeline

10. Which of the following medications is commonly used as the first-line therapy for Myasthenia Gravis?

A) Rivastigmine
B) Pyridostigmine
C) Cevimeline
D) Neostigmine

2.4.3 Rationales

1. **Answer: B. Anticoagulation therapy (e.g., Apixaban or Warfarin**

Rationale: Anticoagulation therapy is the standard treatment for deep vein thrombosis (DVT). Medications like Apixaban or Warfarin are commonly prescribed to prevent clot formation and reduce the risk of pulmonary embolism (PE). Compression therapy may also be used in conjunction with anticoagulants, but it is not a standalone treatment. Aspirin and statins are not first-line treatments for DVT.Answer: a) Joint pain and stiffness

---

2. **Answer: C. ACE inhibitor (e.g., Lisinopril)**

Rationale: ACE inhibitors like Lisinopril are first-line treatments for HFrEF. They help relax blood vessels, reduce blood pressure, and improve heart function. Other options like Ivabradine or Sacubitril valsartan may be used for more severe cases, but ACE inhibitors are fundamental in the initial management of HFrEF. Digoxin is used for symptom relief when other treatments fail but is not first-line**.**

---

3. **Answer: B. Aspirin, clopidogrel, heparin, and nitroglycerin**

Rationale: For **STEMI**, the initial treatment involves antiplatelet therapy (Aspirin, Clopidogrel), anticoagulation (Heparin), and nitrates to relieve chest pain. These medications help reduce clot formation and prevent further complications. Beta-blockers and ACE inhibitors are also used but not as initial treatments for STEMI. Diuretics are not a primary treatment for acute MI.

.

---

4. **Answer: C. Diuretics**

Rationale: **Diuretics**, such as **hydrochlorothiazide**, are often considered first-line treatment for **primary hypertension**, especially in patients without significant comorbidities. They are effective in reducing blood pressure by promoting sodium and water excretion. ACE inhibitors, beta-blockers, and calcium channel blockers are also used but may not be the first choice in uncomplicated hypertension..

---

5. **Answer: C. Valve replacement surgery**

Rationale: In patients with severe **aortic stenosis** and symptoms such as shortness of breath and fatigue, **valve replacement surgery** is typically required if medical therapy is insufficient. While diuretics and beta-blockers may help manage symptoms, they do not address the underlying valve dysfunction. Anticoagulants are not routinely used in the absence of other indications like atrial fibrillation or embolism risk.

---

6. **Answer: C. Temporary pacing**

Rationale: **Mobitz Type II** is a more serious form of heart block that can progress to complete heart block, requiring immediate intervention with **temporary pacing**. Atropine may be ineffective in Mobitz Type II, and observation alone is insufficient. Beta-blockers may exacerbate heart block and are generally avoided in this context.

7. **Answer: C) Mitral Regurgitation**

Rationale: Mitral Regurgitation is associated with a pan systolic murmur that radiates to the left axilla. It can result from mitral valve prolapse, papillary muscle rupture or dysfunction (often following a myocardial infarction), and rheumatic heart disease. Symptoms include palpitations, exertional dyspnoea, fatigue, and weakness.

8. **Answer: B) Mitral Stenosis**

Rationale: Mitral Stenosis is characterized by a rumbling mid-diastolic murmur, which is best heard on expiration when the patient is lying on their left side. This murmur is commonly caused by rheumatic heart disease and is associated with symptoms such as exertional dyspnoea, palpitations, and hemoptysis.

9. **Answer: C) Pyridostigmine**

Rationale: Pyridostigmine is the first-line treatment for **Myasthenia Gravis**, a neuromuscular disorder. It works as an anticholinesterase medication, improving neuromuscular transmission by inhibiting the enzyme acetylcholinesterase, thereby increasing acetylcholine availability at the neuromuscular junction. Other medications listed, such as **Rivastigmine** and **Cevimeline**, are used for conditions like dementia and xerostomia, respectively, and **Bethanechol** is used for urinary retention.

10. **Answer: B) Pyridostigmine**

Rationale: Pyridostigmine is the first-line anticholinesterase medication used in the treatment of Myasthenia Gravis. It works by inhibiting the breakdown of acetylcholine, thus improving neuromuscular transmission. Neostigmine is also used for this condition, but pyridostigmine is preferred due to its longer duration of action.

3 Chapter 3: Respiratory[1] System

3.1 Anatomy and Physiology of Respiratory System

The respiratory system carries out vital **gas exchange** duties that involve passing **oxygen and carbon dioxide** between human bodies and surrounding environmental zones. The system consists of two main sections known as the **upper and lower respiratory tracts**. The upper respiratory tract filters **incoming air** while warming and moistening it through the **nose, nasal cavity, pharynx, and larynx** before it reaches the lungs. The lower respiratory tract consists of four parts: **trachea, bronchi, bronchioles, and lungs**. Air enters each lung through two main bronchi and then continues to branch into progressively smaller bronchioles. Gas exchange takes place in the tiny air sacs known as **alveoli** which are located at the end of bronchioles. The thoracic cavity protects the lungs as they function as respiration's primary organs. The breathing process requires the **diaphragm** to act as a dome-shaped muscle which **contracts and relaxes** to permit air movement through the lungs. The integrated system maintains efficient lung function along with **optimal oxygen delivery** throughout the body. The trachea together with bronchi and bronchioles with the lungs compose the lower respiratory tract system. Two main bronchi originate from the trachea to penetrate each lung space where subsequent branching forms bronchioles. The bronchioles terminate in tiny alveoli structures for gas exchange to happen. The largest organs responsible for respiration exist within the **rib cage-protected thoracic cavity**. Respiration utilizes the rounded diaphragm muscle which sits beneath the lungs to enable both breathing in and out of the respiratory system through controlled actions.

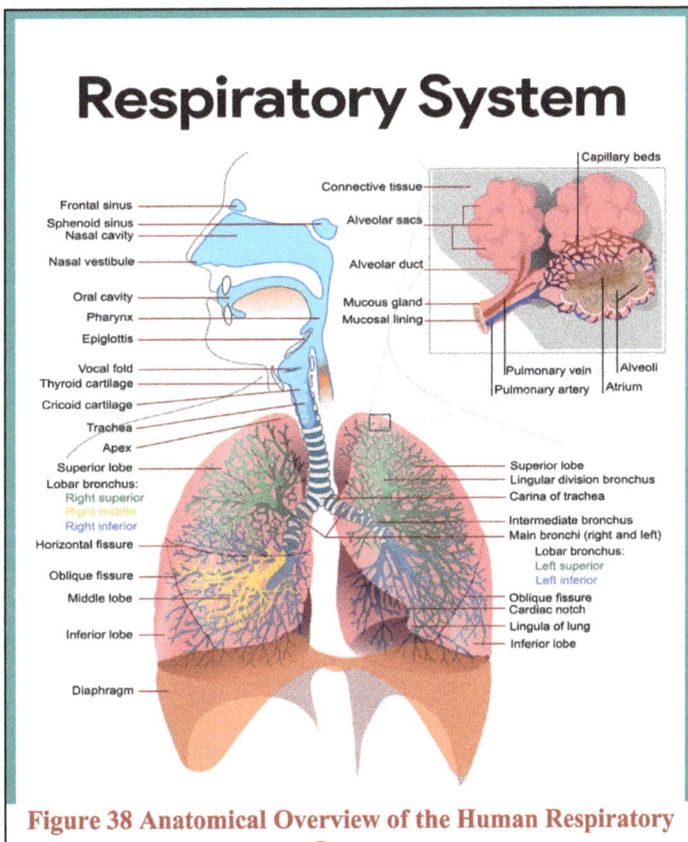

Figure 38 Anatomical Overview of the Human Respiratory System

3.2 Common Respiratory System Disorders

In order to memorize the diseases, we can remember this sentence *"A Clever Elephant Can Play Tennis, Protecting Lung Cysts".* This sentence helps to recall the conditions in a memorable way: **A** – Asthma, **C** - Chronic Obstructive Pulmonary Disease (COPD), **E** – Emphysema, **C** - Chronic Bronchitis, **P** – Pneumonia, **T** - Tuberculosis (TB), **L** - Pulmonary Embolism (PE), **C** - Lung Cancer, **C** - Cystic Fibrosis

Table 26 Common Disorders of Respiratory System

Condition	Description	Key Symptoms	Diagnostic Tools	Treatment Options
Chronic Obstructive Pulmonary Disease (COPD)	A progressive obstructive lung disease, often caused by smoking, leading to chronic bronchitis and emphysema.	Chronic cough, dyspnea, sputum production, wheezing	Spirometry (FEV1/FVC < 70%), Chest X-ray, CT scan, ABG analysis	Bronchodilators, inhaled corticosteroids, pulmonary rehabilitation, smoking cessation
Emphysema	A form of COPD characterized by the destruction of the alveoli, leading to reduced surface area for gas exchange.	Shortness of breath, chronic cough, wheezing	Chest X-ray, CT scan, Spirometry	Bronchodilators, inhaled corticosteroids, oxygen therapy, pulmonary rehabilitation
Asthma	A chronic inflammatory airway disorder causing bronchospasm, airway hyperreactivity, and reversible airflow obstruction.	Wheezing, shortness of breath, chest tightness, cough	Spirometry (FEV1/FVC), Peak Flow Measurement, Methacholine Challenge	Inhaled corticosteroids, beta-agonists (SABAs/LABAs), leukotriene inhibitors
Chronic Bronchitis	A form of COPD characterized by chronic inflammation of the bronchial	Persistent cough, sputum production, dyspnea	Chest X-ray, Spirometry, Sputum culture	Bronchodilators, inhaled corticosteroids, smoking cessation,

	tubes, leading to excess mucus production and cough.			pulmonary rehabilitation
Pneumonia	Infectious lung inflammation caused by bacteria, viruses, or fungi, resulting in alveolar consolidation.	Fever, productive cough, dyspnea, pleuritic chest pain	Chest X-ray, Sputum culture, Blood cultures, CRP, Procalcitonin	Antibiotics (bacterial pneumonia), antivirals, supportive oxygen therapy
Tuberculosis (TB)	A bacterial infection (Mycobacterium tuberculosis) that primarily affects the lungs and can become systemic.	Persistent cough, night sweats, weight loss, hemoptysis	Mantoux Tuberculin Skin Test, Sputum AFB Staining, Chest X-ray	First-line anti-TB therapy (Rifampin, Isoniazid, Ethambutol, Pyrazinamide) for 6 months
Pulmonary Embolism (PE)	A life-threatening blockage of the pulmonary artery, usually due to a blood clot, leading to ventilation-perfusion mismatch.	Sudden dyspnea, chest pain, hemoptysis, tachycardia	CT pulmonary angiography, D-dimer test, Ventilation-perfusion scan	Anticoagulation (heparin, warfarin), thrombolytics, oxygen therapy
Lung Cancer	A malignant neoplasm in lung tissue, often associated with smoking, exposure to carcinogens, or genetic mutations.	Chronic cough, hemoptysis, weight loss, fatigue	Chest CT, PET scan, Lung biopsy, Bronchoscop y	Surgical resection, chemotherapy, targeted therapy, radiation therapy
Cystic Fibrosis	A genetic disorder that affects the lungs, pancreas, and other organs,	Persistent cough, wheezing, frequent lung	Sweat test (elevated chloride levels), Genetic	Mucus-thinning drugs, bronchodilators , chest physiotherapy,

	causing thick mucus production that leads to respiratory and digestive problems.	infections, salty skin, poor growth	testing, Chest X-ray, Pulmonary function tests	antibiotics for infections, enzyme replacement therapy for digestive issues

3.3 Major Medical Issues in Respiratory System

3.3.1 Chronic Obstructive Pulmonary Disorder (COPD)

COPD stands as a persistent lung disease which **reduces lung airflow** permanently because patients spend long periods inhaling dangerous elements like **tobacco smoke**. The illness consists of two core features: **chronic bronchitis and emphysema**. The airways show persistent inflammation along with **mucus production in chronic bronchitis patients** whereas emphysema **destroys alveoli** to decrease the space available for gas exchange. **Shortness of breath, chronic cough and wheezing as well as sputum** production are included in COPD symptoms. Respiratory failure and restricted daily performance become probable consequences of the disease as it progresses. The confirmation of **COPD** diagnosis **requires spirometry testing** to assess lung capacity combined with **X-ray imaging and CT scans**. The medical approach for COPD involves two elements that work to decrease symptoms and slow disease progression although the condition is untreatable. Doctors offer patients **bronchodilators** and **inhaled corticosteroids** with **pulmonary rehabilitation** and assistance to stop smoking as their treatment options. It is essential to diagnose and treat COPD early because such actions improve patient quality of life and help avoid complications occurring.

3.3.1.1 COPD Assessment Framework

Figure 39 defines methods to evaluate **COPD severity** based on these three essential elements. The **Modified Medical Research Council Questionnaire (mMRC)** consists of five questions which help evaluate patients' breathlessness intensity. **A scoring system** offers a range from **zero to four** where higher scores show patients face severe respiratory issues and their symptoms become worse. **The 8-item CAT (COPD Assessment Test)** evaluates the entire health condition of individuals with COPD through its questionnaire format. The test produces scores that range from **zero to forty** where elevated scores indicate **worse quality of life along with greater medical effects of the disease.** The assessment model primarily relies on the **Frequency of Exacerbations per Year factor** since this metric tracks exacerbations that represent critical symptom deterioration in COPD progression. The assessment includes **Spirometric Evaluation together with FEV1 (% predicted)** for measuring lung function status. The FEV1 metric measures lung capacity during a forced breathing action whereas **the % predicted** scale reflects how a patient's lung capacity compares to that of healthy participants matched by age demographics and sex along with body dimensions. These evaluation methods assist in determining COPD severity levels to support correct medical choices.

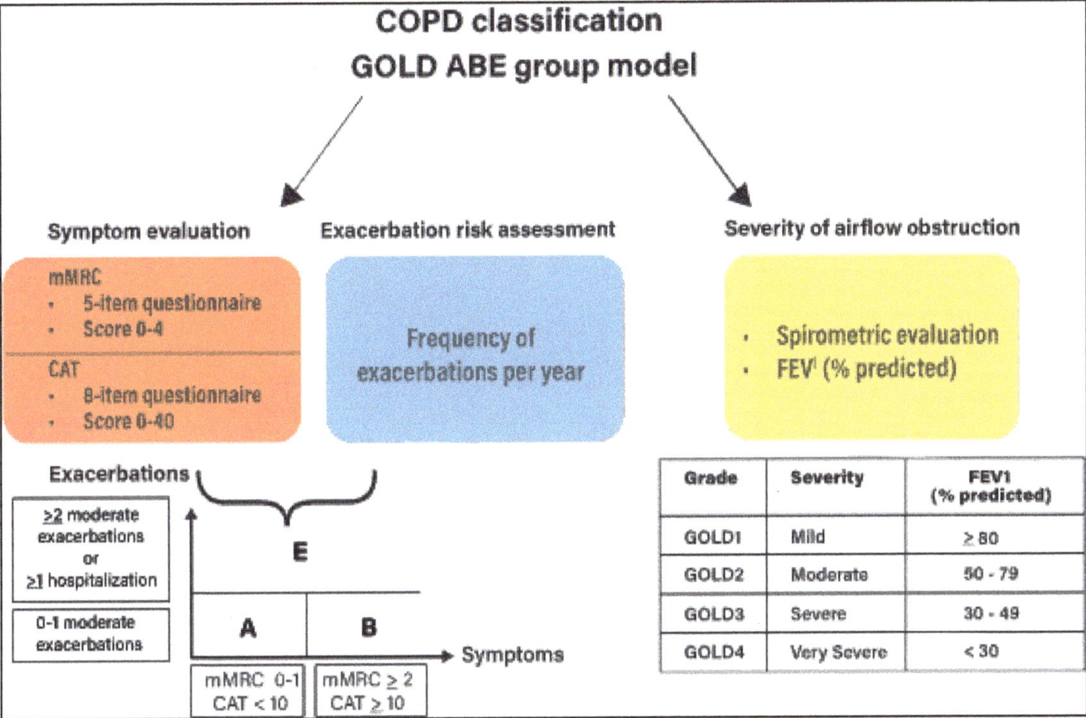

Figure 39 COPD Severity Assessment Model

3.3.1.2 Classification of COPD

GOLD established the COPD classification framework through two vital criteria which combine airflow limitation measurement by **post-bronchodilator FEV1 along with symptoms/risk of exacerbations.** The progression of airflow limitation exists in four separate categories. **At the mild (GOLD Stage I) level FEV1** values remain above 80% of the predicted value and most people experience few symptoms. **In GOLD Stage II** the predicted FEV1 value falls within 50% to 80% with escalating symptoms that cause shortness of breath. The lung function and daily activities of patients become severely restricted because **Severe (GOLD Stage III)** presents with FEV1 levels between 30% and 50% of the predicted value. When FEV1 decreases to values below 30% of predicted the condition is classified **as Very Severe (GOLD Stage IV)** because it causes major limitations which could lead to respiratory failure. COPD is classified through its symptoms and disease exacerbation risk patterns alongside **airway obstruction measures**. Individuals who display low symptoms and single or no exacerbation history fall under GOLD Category A which represents the beginning stage of COPD. **In GOLD Category C individuals** present with low symptom burden together with either frequent or severe exacerbations although no consistent diagnosis exists. **GOLD Category D** patients have both greater symptoms along with frequent or severe exacerbations needing detailed management. Medical professionals use this system to evaluate COPD patients' disease levels so they can create personalized treatment approaches.

Table 27 Classification of COPD as Defined by Global Initiative for Chronic Obstructive Lung Disease (GOLD

	COPD Classification	Definition
Classification of airflow limitation (post-BD FEV_1)	Mild GOLD Stage I	$FEV_1 \geq 80\%$ predicted
	Moderate GOLD Stage II	$FEV_1 \geq 50\%$ predicted but <80% predicted
	Severe GOLD Stage III	$FEV_1 \geq 30\%$ predicted but <50% predicted
	Very severe GOLD Stage IV	FEV_1 <30% predicted
Classification of symptoms/risk of exacerbation	GOLD category A	mMRC 0-1 or CAT <10 (low symptom burden) History of 0 or 1 moderate or severe exacerbations (not leading to hospital admission)
	GOLD category B	mMRC ≥ 2 or CAT ≥10 (higher symptom burden) History of 0 or 1 moderate or severe exacerbations (not leading to hospital admission)
	GOLD category C	mMRC 0-1 or CAT <10 (low symptom burden) History of ≥2 moderate/severe exacerbations or ≥1 exacerbation (leading to hospital admission)
	GOLD category D	mMRC ≥ 2 or CAT ≥10 (higher symptom burden) History of ≥2 moderate/severe exacerbations or ≥1 exacerbation (leading to hospital admission)

3.3.1.3 SOAP Notes for COPD

Table 28 SOAP Notes for COPD Management

Component	Details
Subjective (S)	The patient reports chronic cough, shortness of breath, and frequent sputum production, particularly in the mornings. Complaints of worsening dyspnea with exertion and difficulty completing daily

	activities. Experiences fatigue and occasional wheezing. Denies chest pain but has a history of smoking for 20 years.
Objective (O)	Vitals: BP 130/85 mmHg, HR 88 bpm (tachycardia), RR 20 bpm. Cardiac exam: Normal heart sounds, no murmurs. Respiratory exam: Decreased breath sounds, wheezing, and prolonged expiration. Chest X-ray: Hyperinflated lungs with flattened diaphragms. Spirometry: FEV1/FVC ratio < 70%, FEV1 55% predicted.
Assessment (A)	Differential Diagnoses: 1. Chronic Obstructive Pulmonary Disease (COPD) 2. Asthma (less likely given age of onset and smoking history) 3. Bronchiectasis (given sputum production and wheezing) 4. Interstitial lung disease (less likely given clinical presentation).
Plan (P)	Investigations: Chest CT scan to assess for emphysema, repeat spirometry to monitor disease progression, and alpha-1 antitrypsin testing (if family history of COPD). Pharmacological Treatment: Inhaled corticosteroids (ICS), long-acting beta-agonists (LABAs), and long-acting muscarinic antagonists (LAMAs) for symptom control. Short-acting bronchodilators (SABAs) for rescue use (See he figures below). Non-Pharmacological Treatment: Smoking cessation program, pulmonary rehabilitation, and oxygen therapy if required based on oxygen saturation levels. Education: Medication adherence, lifestyle modifications, and recognizing exacerbation symptoms. Referral: Pulmonologist consultation for further management and potential enrollment in pulmonary rehab. Follow-up: Reassess in 4-6 weeks, including repeat spirometry and symptom evaluation.

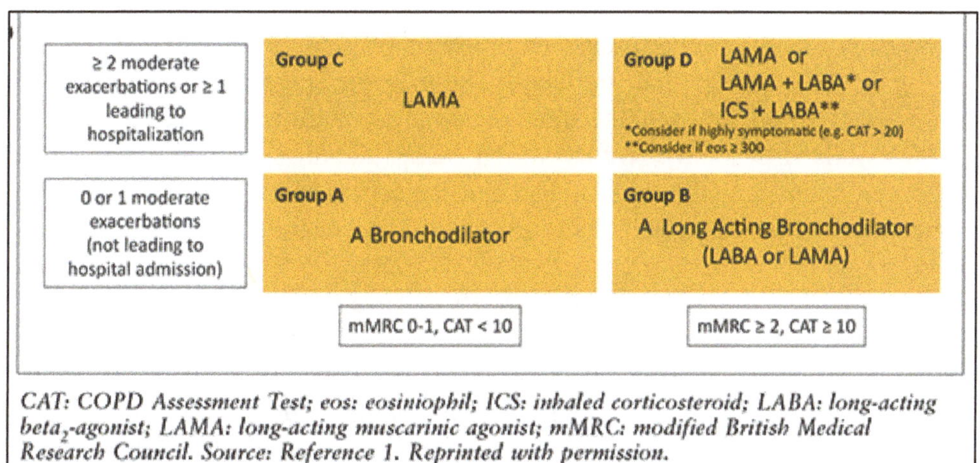

CAT: COPD Assessment Test; eos: eosiniophil; ICS: inhaled corticosteroid; LABA: long-acting beta$_2$-agonist; LAMA: long-acting muscarinic agonist; mMRC: modified British Medical Research Council. Source: Reference 1. Reprinted with permission.

Figure 40 Initial treatment approaches for COPD

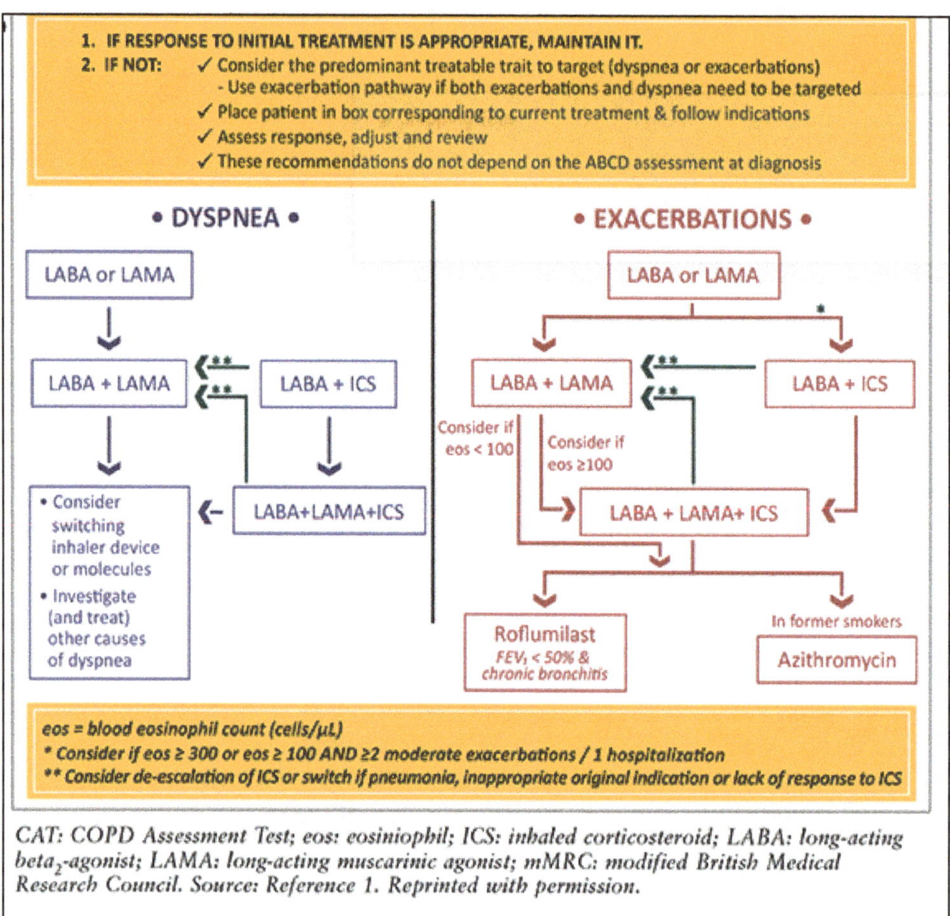

CAT: COPD Assessment Test; eos: eosiniophil; ICS: inhaled corticosteroid; LABA: long-acting beta$_2$-agonist; LAMA: long-acting muscarinic agonist; mMRC: modified British Medical Research Council. Source: Reference 1. Reprinted with permission.

Figure 41 Follow-up pharmacological treatment of COPD

3.3.2 Emphysema

The main cause of progressive lung disease emphysema originates from **persistent contact with harmful airborne substances** that frequently stem from cigarette smoking. **Emphysema** damages **both alveoli** which represent the small air sacs responsible for gas exchange. The damage to alveoli creates walls with **less flexibility** which causes the air spaces to expand and decreases the area for oxygen exchange (Figure 43). The disease causes **breathing problems** that become more pronounced when the individual tries to exercise. Three main emphysema symptoms consist of **continuous coughing, breathing trouble, and wheezing sounds.** Speedy diagnosis happens through spirometry by showing **low forced expiratory volume (FEV1)** and additional tests such as **chest X-rays or CT scans** provide imaging results. Treatment seeks to control emphysema symptoms alongside attempts to reduce its progression even though a cure is unavailable for this condition. People with emphysema receive medical treatment using **bronchodilators, inhaled corticosteroids, oxygen therapy**, and **programs to stop smoking**. Along with pulmonary rehabilitation patients need to follow lifestyle modifications that include staying away from respiratory irritants to manage their condition effectively.

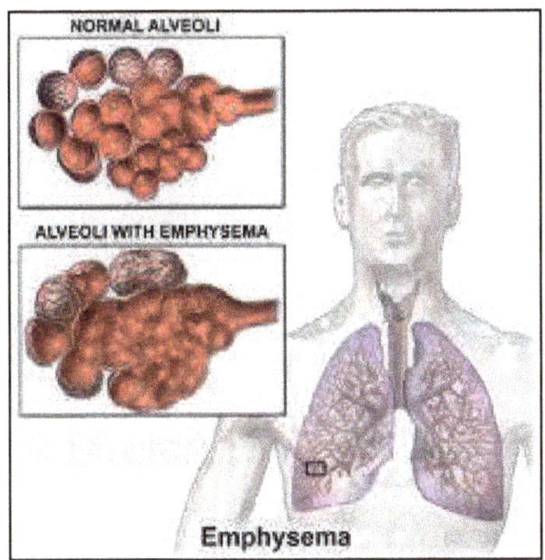

Figure 42 Visual representation of emphysema

3.3.2.1 Classification of Emphysema

Figure 44 displays categorizations of emphysema depending on where the disease affects the **pulmonary lobule.** The classification system identifies four distinct types of emphysema which include **irregular emphysema, paraseptal, panacinar and centrilobular emphysema**. The respiratory bronchioles occupy the central regions of the lobule as the main target area during **centrilobular emphysema** progression but the alveolar sacs remain untouched. The smoking-related form of **emphysema destroys bronchioles** and adjacent **alveolar structures** which induces serious airflow blockage as its main effect. Panacinar emphysema destroys every portion of the lobule by affecting both its inner and outer sections. Patients with **alpha-1 antitrypsin deficiency** tend to develop major lung function disability from the broad destruction of alveolar walls. The paraseptal form of emphysema targets the **sacs of alveoli** which are located near **interlobular septa** found in the distal parts of the lobule. The development of **bullae, large air-filled lung spaces** is a rare occurrence of this type of damage. Within irregular emphysema, there is no standardized pattern within the lobule which allows the condition to appear anywhere in the affected area. The condition typically presents from **scarring tissue** following **prior lung injuries** along with **prior infections** although it might not necessarily cause serious **airflow blockage**. The clinical understanding of lung damage dispersion becomes possible through these classification methods along with their capability to direct proper treatment for **emphysema patients**.

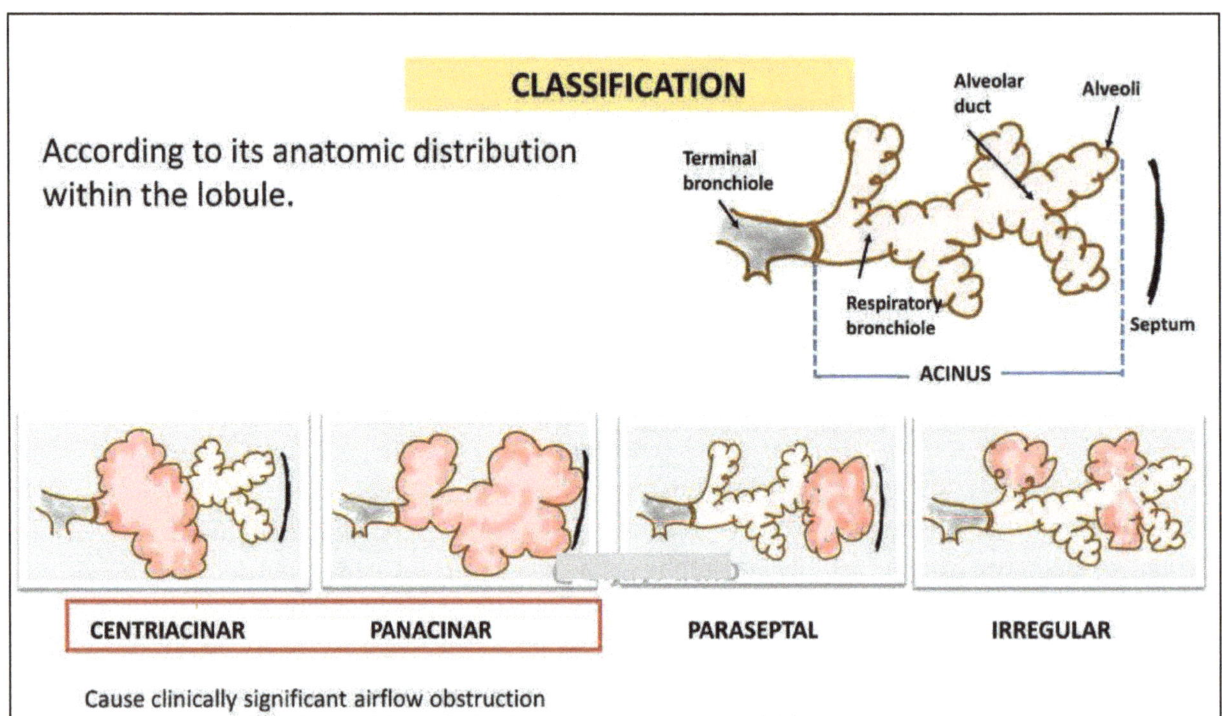

Figure 43 Classification of Emphysema

3.3.2.2 SOAP Notes for Emphysema

Table 29 SOAP Notes for Emphysema

Component	Details
Subjective (S)	Patient reports chronic shortness of breath, especially with exertion. Complains of a persistent cough, primarily in the mornings, with occasional sputum production. States that symptoms have worsened over the past few months, with increasing difficulty performing daily activities. Has a 30-year smoking history. Denies chest pain but experiences fatigue and frequent wheezing.
Objective (O)	Vitals: BP 128/84 mmHg, HR 95 bpm, RR 18 bpm. Cardiac exam: Normal heart sounds, no murmurs. Respiratory exam: Decreased breath sounds, wheezing, prolonged expiration. Chest X-ray: Hyperinflation with flattened diaphragms. Spirometry: FEV1/FVC ratio < 70%, FEV1 55% predicted, indicative of obstructive lung disease.
Assessment (A)	Differential Diagnoses: 1. Emphysema (COPD) 2. Chronic Bronchitis 3. Asthma (less likely given the history of smoking) 4. Pulmonary fibrosis (unlikely given clinical presentation). Based on spirometry and patient history, a diagnosis of emphysema is most likely.
Plan (P)	Investigations: Repeat spirometry for monitoring progression, chest CT scan to assess for emphysema, and alpha-1 antitrypsin testing if family history of COPD. Pharmacological Treatment: Inhaled corticosteroids (ICS), long-acting beta-agonists (LABAs), long-acting muscarinic antagonists (LAMAs) for maintenance, short-acting bronchodilators (SABAs) for symptom relief (See algorithm below). Non-

	Pharmacological Treatment: Smoking cessation program, pulmonary rehabilitation, oxygen therapy if required, and a high-salt diet for managing symptoms. Education: Patient advised on the importance of smoking cessation, inhaler techniques, recognizing exacerbation symptoms, and avoiding respiratory irritants. Referral: Pulmonologist consultation for further management and potential enrollment in pulmonary rehabilitation. Follow-up: Reassess in 4-6 weeks, including repeat spirometry, chest X-ray, and symptom evaluation.

Table 30 Algorithm for pharmacological management of emphysema

Medication Type	Purpose	Examples	Potential Side Effects	Notes
Bronchodilators	Relax smooth muscle in the airways to improve airflow	Beta2-agonists (SABA & LABA): albuterol, levosalbutamol, salmeterol, formoterol Antimuscarinics (SAMA & LAMA): ipratropium, tiotropium	Headaches, nervous tension, trembling, muscle cramps, heart palpitations	Used to relieve symptoms and improve airflow.
Inhaled Corticosteroids	Reduce inflammation in the airways	budesonide (Pulmicort), flunisolide, ciclesonide (Alvesco)	Cough, sore mouth/throat, nosebleeds, hoarseness, oral thrush	Often combined with LABAs for better symptom control.
Systemic Glucocorticoids	Reduce inflammation during acute flare-ups	prednisone, methylprednisolone	Increased blood glucose, weight gain, muscle breakdown, infections, osteoporosis	Not recommended for long-term use due to serious side effects.
Phosphodiesterase-4 Inhibitors	Reduce inflammation and prevent flare-ups	roflumilast (Daliresp)	Nausea, vomiting, gastrointestinal issues	Prescribed for severe emphysema to reduce exacerbations.

Antibiotics	Reduce frequency of flare-ups caused by infections	azithromycin (Zithromax)	Gastrointestinal issues, hearing impairment, prolonged QT interval	Prescribed for people with frequent flare-ups or infections.
Methylxanthines	Relax smooth muscle of the airways	theophylline (Elixophyllin), dyphylline (Lufyllin)	Headaches, nausea, insomnia, tremors, palpitations, gastrointestinal issues	Less commonly used but may be considered in specific cases.

3.3.3 Asthma

Asthma is a long-term airway **inflammatory condition** which **triggers breathing problems, nighttime coughs, as well as daytime wheezing and chest tightness**. Inflammation creates air passages which become narrower so that air cannot pass through the lungs easily. Various possible asthmatic triggers exist that include **allergens, exercise, respiratory infections, exposure to cold air and irritants from smoke and pollutants.** Asthma symptoms differ between people with some individuals experiencing occasional mild attacks as well as others needing to manage severe regular attacks. Medical researchers have determined that the full explanation for asthma origins remains unclear but **heredity, external triggers, and improper immune system functions** contribute to its development. Patients with asthma usually need **inhaled bronchodilators and inhaled corticosteroids** to treat their condition and reduce airway muscle tightness along with inflammation. The control of asthma symptoms and prevention of worsening conditions requires patients to both avoid their triggers and follow medicine instructions while obtaining regular monitoring tests.

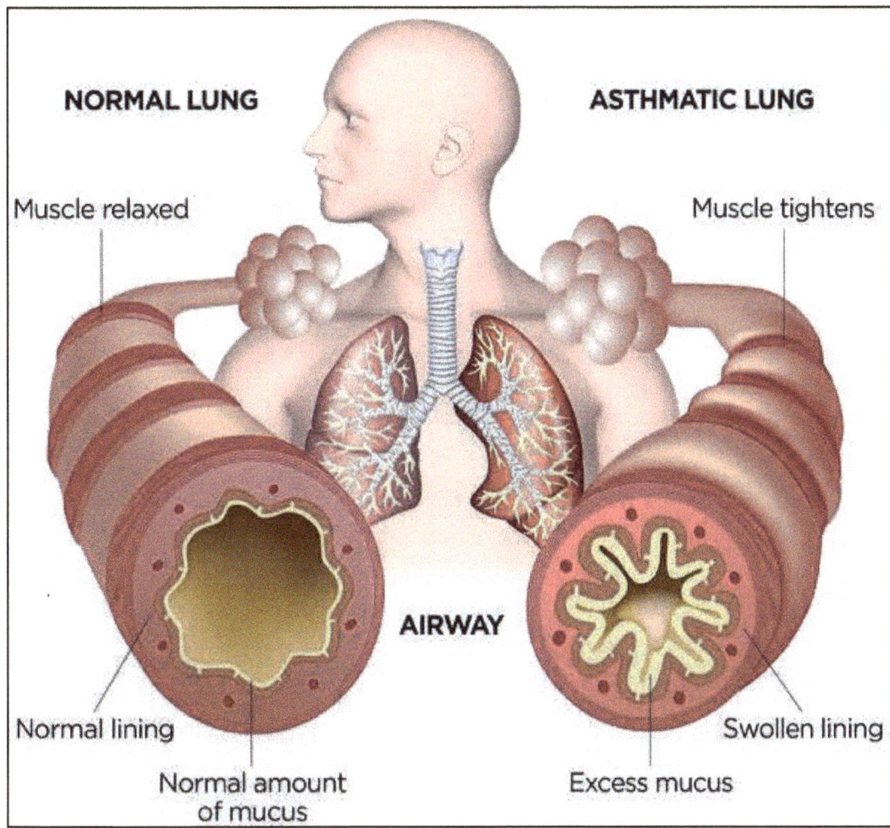

Figure 44 Comparison of Normal and Asthmatic Lungs

Figure 44 demonstrates the distinction between healthy lung airways and asthma-induced changes. A healthy lung contains wide open airways and their linings exist in **normal conditions while mucus maintains equilibrium.** Relaxed smooth muscle in the airways permits free air movement to promote **adequate breathing** and **gas exchange functions**. An asthmatic lung results in restricted airways because of smooth **muscle tightness**, **both lining inflammation** and **excessive mucus production**. The pathway becomes harder to breathe through because airways narrow down because of these changes and produces symptoms including wheezing together with shortness of breath along with coughing.

3.3.3.1 Types of Asthma

There are different categories of asthma which physicians use to distinguish different types of asthma according to their triggers or fundamental origins. **Environmental substances** such as pollen dust mites and pet dander serve as the main precipitating factors for **extrinsic asthma**. The **immune system** reacts harshly to **non-harmful substances** which leads to **allergic reactions**. **Intrinsic asthma** operates based on **environmental elements and infections** together with irritants like smoke alongside air pollution which do not result in **allergic reactions**. The individual in manufacturing businesses or agricultural settings develops **occupational asthma** when they encounter **work-based natural allergens** such as dust, chemicals or fumes during their shifts. The combination of asthma symptoms triggered by **aspirin and other nonsteroidal anti-inflammatory drugs (NSAIDs)** leads to **Aspirin-Induced Asthma** which is usually connected to **aspirin-exacerbated respiratory disease (AERD).** The condition known as asthma of infancy emerges in infants because of their exposure to allergens and viruses during early life and it may persist throughout their later developmental stages (Figure 45).

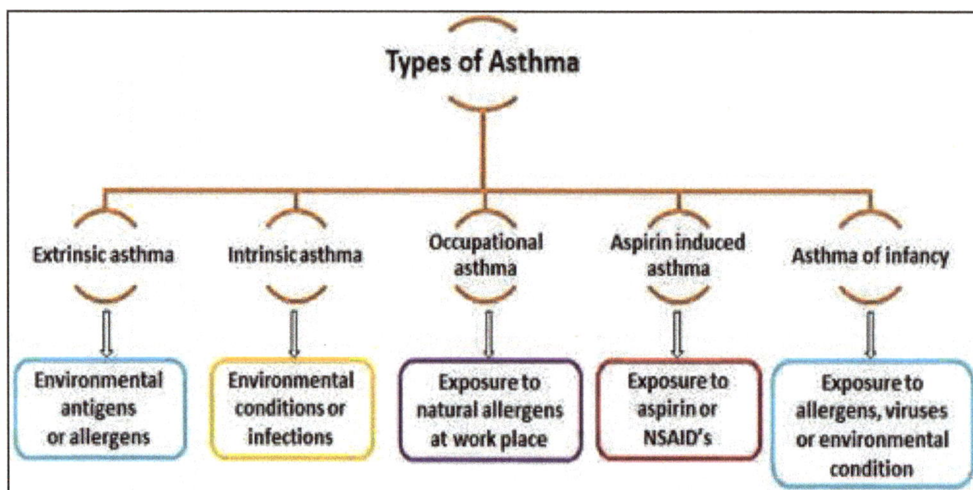

Figure 45 Types of Asthma

3.3.3.2 Classification of Asthma

A clinical asthma severity determination system exists to classify asthma severity levels in individuals who are at least 12 years old according to the **frequency of their symptoms, nighttime symptoms, their lung function, and short-acting beta-agonist (SABA) consumption (Table 31)**. Permanent asthma characterizes symptoms that appear **no more than twice weekly** combined with **two or fewer night-time symptoms** in a monthly period. **The %FEV1 measurement exceeds 80% while maintaining lower than 20% variability** and patients need to use **SABAs** for no more than two days during a week. People with **Mild Persistent asthma** experience symptoms more than twice per week although they avoid daily occurrences which are accompanied by **3-4 nocturnal symptoms monthly.** The patients exhibit **FEV1 levels that meet 80%** of the predicted value and **FEV1 variable at 20-30% levels** while using SABA medication more than two days per week. One defining characteristic of **Moderate Persistent asthma** includes daily symptoms as well as more than one night-time symptom each week and FEV1 levels between **60–80% alongside FEV1 variability above 30% and daily SABA usage**. Patients with Severe Persistent asthma show non-stop symptom frequency lasting throughout all seven days of the week together with FEV1 values below **60% and exceeding 30% in FEV1 variations.** SABA use is **≥twice a day**. These clinical parameters allow practitioners to determine the asthma severity through the classification system which promotes effective treatment options.

Table 31 Clinical Classification of Asthma (for ≥ 12 years old)

Severity	Symptom frequency	Night-time symptoms	%FEV$_1$ of predicted	FEV$_1$ variability	SABA use
Intermittent	≤2/week	≤2/month	≥80%	<20%	≤2 days/week
Mild persistent	>2/week	3–4/month	≥80%	20–30%	>2 days/week
Moderate persistent	Daily	>1/week	60–80%	>30%	daily
Severe persistent	Continuously	Frequent (7/week)	<60%	>30%	≥twice/day

Table 32 presents a four-level classification system which ranges from **Near-fatal to Life-threatening to Acute severe and ends with Moderate asthma exacerbations.** A near-fatal exacerbation manifests as **high $PaCO_2$** levels or requires mechanical ventilation of the patient. The near-fatal condition shows **changes to patient consciousness** along with **exhaustion and arrhythmias** followed by **low blood pressure and cyanosis** resulting in a **silent chest with poor breathing effort.** Key measurements in this condition present both peak flow values less than one-third of predicted amounts and oxygen saturation readings **under 92% combined with PaO_2 levels below 8 kPa.** A life-threatening exacerbation arises when patients manifest one of the defined clinical signs together with **peak flow levels within 33% to 50% and PaO_2 lower than 8 kPa.** Acute severe exacerbations show themselves through rapid breathing above 25 times per minute combined with **heart rates beyond 110 beats per minute** while making patients unable to finish multiple sentences during one breath cycle when **peak flow falls within 33% to 50%.** The key indicators of moderate exacerbations include predicted **peak flow readings between 50% and 80%** with **deteriorating asthma symptoms** yet without signs of acute severe asthma. A comprehensive classification framework enables healthcare providers to evaluate asthma attacks by their clinical signals and objective measurements in order to select proper medical interventions.

Table 32 Severity of an acute exacerbation of Asthma

Near-fatal	High $PaCO_2$, or requiring mechanical ventilation, or both	
Life-threatening (any one of)	**Clinical signs**	**Measurements**
	Altered level of consciousness	Peak flow < 33%
	Exhaustion	Oxygen saturation < 92%
	Arrhythmia	PaO_2 < 8 kPa
	Low blood pressure	"Normal" $PaCO_2$
	Cyanosis	
	Silent chest	
	Poor respiratory effort	
Acute severe (any one of)	Peak flow 33–50%	
	Respiratory rate ≥ 25 breaths per minute	
	Heart rate ≥ 110 beats per minute	
	Unable to complete sentences in one breath	
Moderate	Worsening symptoms	
	Peak flow 50–80% best or predicted	
	No features of acute severe asthma	

3.3.3.3 SOAP Notes for Asthma

Table 33 SOAP Notes for Asthma

Component	Details
Subjective (S)	Patient reports frequent episodes of wheezing, shortness of breath, and coughing, particularly at night and early in the morning. Symptoms worsen with exposure to allergens, exercise, and cold air. Denies chest pain, but has a history of seasonal allergies and frequent respiratory infections. Uses a rescue inhaler (SABA) up to 3 times a week for relief.
Objective (O)	Vitals: BP 120/80 mmHg, HR 92 bpm, RR 20 bpm. Respiratory exam: Mild wheezing on expiration, prolonged expiration phase, no use of accessory muscles. Peak flow: 70% of predicted value. Oxygen saturation: 96%. Chest X-ray: Normal. Spirometry: FEV1/FVC ratio < 70%, FEV1 65% predicted, indicating moderate obstructive pattern.

Assessment (A)	Differential Diagnosis: 1. Asthma (based on symptoms, spirometry results, and wheezing). 2. Chronic obstructive pulmonary disease (COPD) (unlikely based on age and smoking history). 3. Upper respiratory infection (less likely due to chronicity and recurring symptoms). The diagnosis of asthma is confirmed, given the chronic symptoms, response to SABA, and spirometry results.
Plan (P)	Investigations: Repeat spirometry in 6 months for monitoring, and consider allergy testing if triggers are unclear. Pharmacological Treatment: Start inhaled corticosteroid (ICS) (e.g., fluticasone) daily, continue short-acting beta-agonist (SABA) as needed, and add long-acting beta-agonist (LABA) (e.g., salmeterol) if control is not achieved with ICS alone (See the figure below). Non-Pharmacological Treatment: Avoid known triggers, use an air purifier, and recommend regular physical activity. Education: Teach proper inhaler technique, reinforce adherence to daily medication, and advise on the use of a peak flow meter. Referral: Consider referral to an allergist for further evaluation if environmental or allergic triggers are suspected. Follow-up: Reassess in 4 weeks to evaluate symptom control, inhaler technique, and adjust medications if necessary.

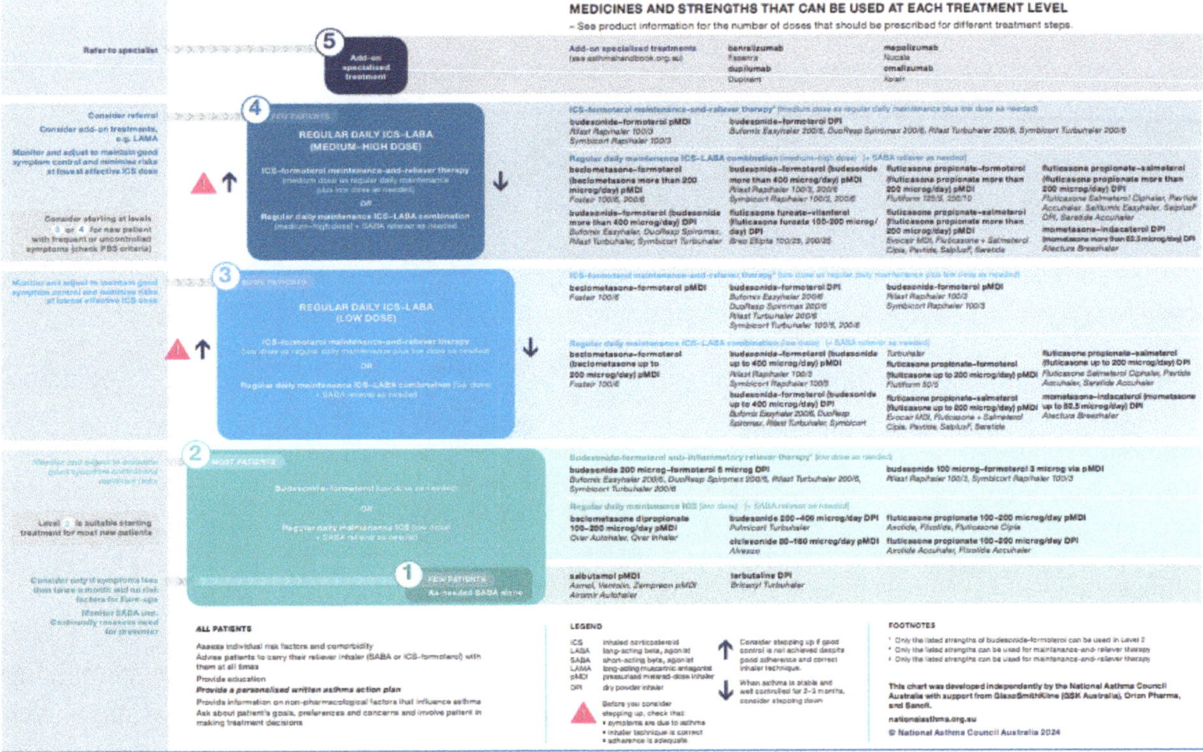

Figure 46 Asthma Management

3.3.4 Chronic Bronchitis

Chronic bronchitis functions as one form of COPD because it continuously **inflames bronchial tubes responsible for air transportation to the lungs**. Prolonged interaction with **tobacco smoke together with air pollution and dust** mainly produces this condition. The inflammatory response triggers **mucus production** exceeding normal levels thus **causing continuous coughing** along with **wheezing and limited breathing capability**. The illness causes patients to develop a continuous cough with productive secretions for at least three months within two successive years. **The airway blockage in chronic bronchitis** wedges the airways to narrow down so that both lung oxygen exchange and respiratory passage function decrease. **Shortness of breath with fatigue and regular respiratory infections** appear as results of the condition. Ongoing **injuries to airways** ultimately result in serious lung complications that cause permanent destruction of lung tissue. The main objective of **chronic bronchitis** treatment is symptom relief and improved lung function together with disease progression reduction. Doctors typically treat this condition with **bronchodilators together with corticosteroids** in combination with **respiratory infection antibiotics**. Preventing **additional harm from smoking** requires a person to stop using cigarettes while **pulmonary rehabilitation** creates useful health benefits for daily living. The therapy **requires oxygen** as a treatment method for severe cases. Patients with **chronic bronchitis** require treatment through medicine combined with other approaches and routine assessment to stop disease progression and complication development.

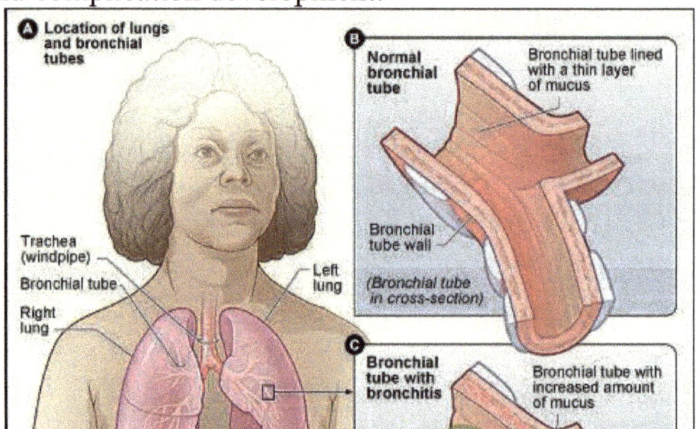

Figure 47 Chronic Bronchitis

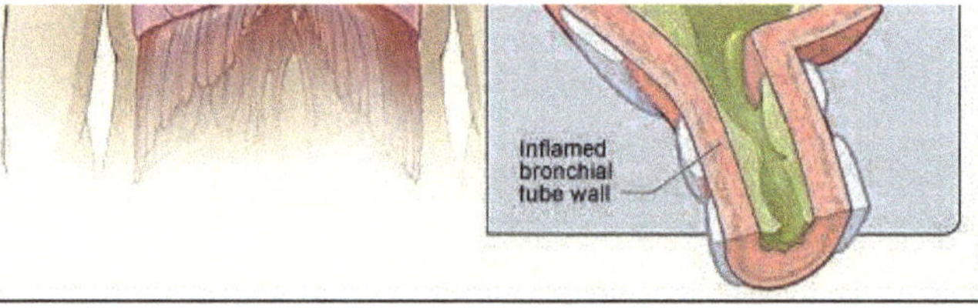

Figure 47 compares and contrasts healthy bronchial tubes with bronchitic ones to display airway structural transformations. **Panel A** shows the general **location of the lungs and bronchial tubes** in the body, with **labels for the trachea (windpipe), bronchial tubes, and both the right and left lungs.** The bronchial tube wall includes a thin mucus layer according to the illustrated cross-sectional view in **Panel B**. Air enters the respiratory **system through respiratory tubes** containing mucus that functions as a trap for airborne elements without obstructing air passages. The bronchitis state shown in **Panel C** displays bronchial tubes with bronchitis condition which **produces inflammation and thickness of the bronchial wall with abnormally high mucous production.** The inflated bronchial passages compress due to excessive mucus buildup and subsequent swelling therefore air moves more slowly causing bronchitis symptoms including

persistent coughing along with wheezing and trouble breathing. The depicted image shows bronchitis creates breathing difficulties through its blockage of regular airflow.

3.3.4.1 Risk Factors Associated with Chronic Bronchitis

Table 34 displays the relationship between risk factors of chronic bronchitis and their specific impact levels. The major contributing factor leading to chronic bronchitis appears in **cigarette smoking** because this habit creates the most significant association with its development. Various **occupational conditions** that expose workers to harmful substances demonstrate **a moderate relationship with chronic bronchitis development**. The risk factors come from **coal miners' substance exposure as well as hard-rock miners' exposure, tunnel workers' exposure, exposure to concrete manufacturers, and livestock farmers**. A variety of moderate-risk factors that cause chronic bronchitis exist in relation to agricultural pesticide exposure and both domestic solid fuel use and electronic cigarette consumption. The development of chronic bronchitis is **weakly affected by marijuana smoking and air pollution exposure**. Environmental and lifestyle triggers have a minor influence on forming chronic bronchitis while increasing its intensity. This table demonstrates the range of effects multiple risk factors generate when it comes to both initiating chronic bronchitis and its advancement.

Table 34 Risk Factors Associated with Chronic Bronchitis

Risk Factor	Association
Cigarette Smoking	Strong
Occupational Exposures:	Moderate
1. Coal miners	
2. Hard-rock miners	
3. Tunnel workers	
4. Concrete manufacturers	
5. Livestock farming	
Exposure to Agricultural Pesticides	Moderate
Use of Domestic Solid Fuels	Moderate
Electronic Cigarettes	Weak
Marijuana Smoking	Weak
Air Pollution	Weak

3.3.4.2 Management of Chronic Bronchitis

The flowchart presents an extensive method to handle patients suffering from chronic respiratory diseases including **chronic bronchitis and COPD** which covers diagnostic assessment combined with therapeutic interventions as well as **prolonged care management**. The diagnostic and symptomatic evaluation begins the process before patients receive recommendations **for exercise therapy, healthy lifestyle habits, and necessary vaccinations.** When a patient persists in smoking behavior the healthcare provider needs to implement active smoking cessation programs. Medical professionals diagnose **airway obstruction** before prescribing suitable drugs for treatment and teaching patients about medication use. **Post-treatment evaluation** includes a check for **hypoxemia** and the patient gets started **on oxygen therapy with proper educational instructions about usage.** The healthcare provider assesses how well the patient responds to treatment specifically in situations with frequent hospital visits combined with severe symptoms. The nurse sends the patient to **a multidisciplinary rehabilitation program** when this intervention proves necessary. Monitoring of patient condition occurs through periodic assessments in order to provide

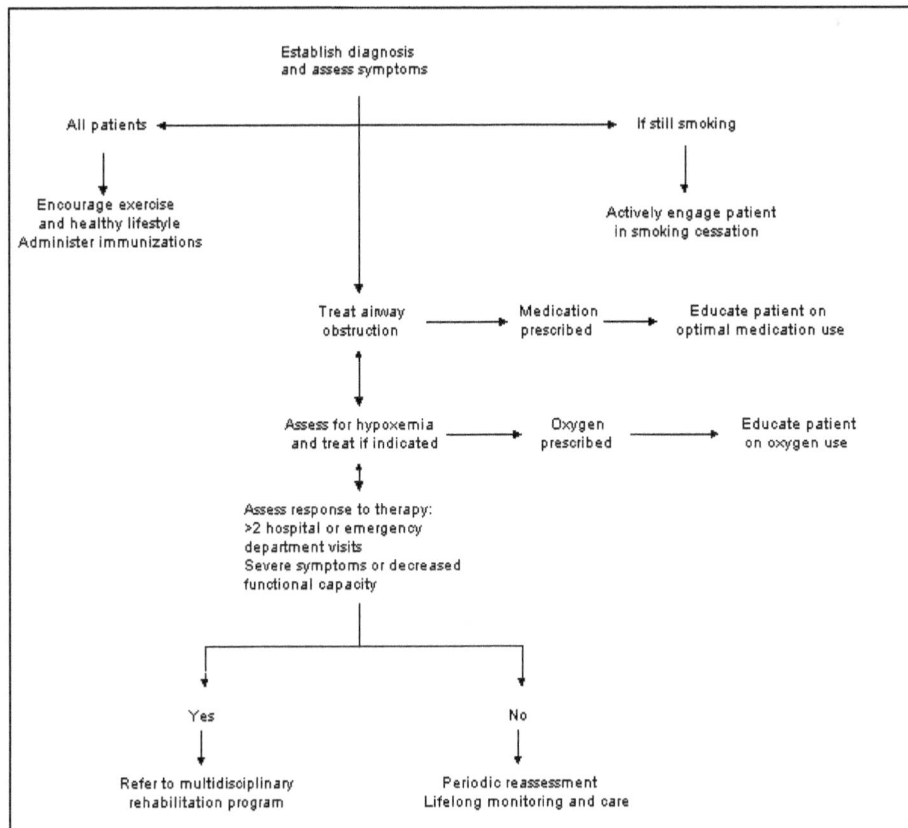

continuous care and management throughout their lifetime.

3.3.4.3 SOAP Notes for Chronic Bronchitis

Figure 48 Flowchart for the Chronic Bronchitis Management

Component	Details
Subjective (S)	Patient reports a persistent cough with clear to yellowish sputum production, especially in the mornings. Complains of shortness of breath that worsens with exertion and during colder months. History of smoking for 25 years and regular exposure to dust in the workplace as a construction worker. Denies chest pain but feels fatigued and experiences occasional wheezing. Symptoms have been ongoing for over 3 months.
Objective (O)	Vitals: BP 130/85 mmHg, HR 98 bpm, RR 18 bpm. Respiratory exam: Mild wheezing on expiration, decreased breath sounds, and prolonged expiration. Chest X-ray: Hyperinflated lungs, no evidence of consolidation or masses. Spirometry: FEV1/FVC ratio < 70%, FEV1 55% predicted, indicating moderate obstructive pattern. Oxygen saturation: 95%.
Assessment (A)	Differential Diagnosis: 1. Chronic Bronchitis (most likely given symptoms, smoking history, and spirometry results). 2. Asthma (unlikely due to the absence of a history of allergy or childhood asthma). 3. COPD (considered due to smoking history but less likely with current exam findings). Chronic bronchitis is confirmed based on the persistent cough, sputum production, and obstructive spirometry findings.
Plan (P)	Investigations: Repeat spirometry in 6 months to monitor disease progression. Consider alpha-1 antitrypsin testing if a family history of lung disease is present. Pharmacological Treatment: Start inhaled corticosteroid (ICS) for reducing inflammation, long-acting bronchodilator (LABA), and short-acting bronchodilator (SABA) for symptom relief. Consider antibiotics for any acute exacerbations (See algorithm below). Non-Pharmacological Treatment: Smoking cessation program, pulmonary rehabilitation, avoiding exposure to dust, use of a face mask, and improving indoor air quality. Education: Teach proper inhaler technique, reinforce the importance of smoking cessation, and educate on avoiding triggers such as dust or cold air. Referral: Refer to a pulmonologist for further management and possible evaluation for pulmonary rehabilitation. Follow-up: Reassess in 4-6 weeks for symptom control, and inhaler technique, and adjust medications if necessary.

Table 35 Algorithm for Pharmacological Management of Chronic Bronchitis

Treatment/Management Area	Description	Specific Recommendations
Primary Objectives	The main goals are to reduce excessive mucus production, decrease mucus hypersecretion, enhance ciliary transport, lower mucus viscosity, and support effective cough mechanisms. Smoking cessation is crucial.	Quit smoking, minimize exposure to environmental irritants.

Smoking Cessation	Quitting smoking and avoiding secondhand smoke significantly improve mucociliary function, reduce airway damage, and decrease goblet cell hyperplasia.	A 30-year study found 42% incidence in smokers, 26% in ex-smokers, and 22% in non-smokers.
Mucolytics	There is debate over mucolytics like N-acetylcysteine, carbocysteine, and erdosteine. GOLD recommends their use for reducing exacerbation frequency, while the American Academy of Chest Physicians advises against them.	GOLD recommends mucolytics for a modest reduction in exacerbations and improvement in quality of life.
Bronchodilators for Acute Exacerbations	Short-acting bronchodilators like albuterol are used to treat acute exacerbations. Nebulizers or MDIs can be used with a combination of albuterol and ipratropium.	Use every 20 minutes for 2-3 doses, then every 2-4 hours as needed. Combine with ipratropium for more severe cases.
Systemic Steroids for Acute Exacerbations	Systemic steroids (e.g., prednisone) are given for 5 days for moderate to severe symptoms of acute exacerbations.	40 mg of prednisone daily for 5 days.
Antibiotic Therapy	Antibiotics are prescribed when there are increased dyspnea, sputum volume, or sputum purulence. The choice of antibiotic depends on risk factors and local resistance patterns.	Macrolides, second/third-generation cephalosporins, or respiratory quinolones for patients at risk. For high-risk, consider amoxicillin-clavulanic acid or quinolones like levofloxacin.
PDE-4 Inhibitors	PDE-4 inhibitors like roflumilast can reduce exacerbations in patients with severe COPD and chronic bronchitis by decreasing inflammation and promoting airway smooth muscle relaxation.	Consider adding roflumilast in severe COPD with FEV1 < 50% and history of exacerbations or hospitalizations.
Pulmonary Rehabilitation	Pulmonary rehabilitation for at least 6 weeks is essential, which includes supervised exercise, self-management education, and psychosocial support to improve overall health and reduce hospitalizations.	Undergo at least 6 weeks of supervised exercise, self-management, and psychosocial support.

3.3.5 Pneumonia

Pneumonia involves **lung infection** that triggers **air sac inflammation** with potential accumulation of **fluid or pus** which produces **coughing, fever, chills and respiratory distress symptoms.** Multiple pathogens such as **bacteria, viruses, fungi or parasites** contribute to developing this condition. The treatment of bacterial pneumonia requires antibiotics whereas viral pneumonia mostly heals independently yet specific cases might require antiviral medications. Pneumonia risks are higher for both young and old individuals as well as those with impaired **immune systems, asthma, diabetes, and tobacco users**. Medical diagnosis of pneumonia occurs through **physical examination combined with chest X-rays and lab tests.** Pneumonia varies from mild to dangerous for susceptible groups and calls for **hospital-based treatment** of extreme cases. Preventing pneumonia relies on **vaccinations** alongside practicing **hygiene and refraining from smoking activities.** The specific treatment approach relies on several factors including infection type and its severity level. This image presents a thorough analysis of healthy and pneumonic lung conditions. This presentation displays the lungs from an anatomical perspective where **lobar pneumonia** impacts the left lung section while showing airway positions through its presentation of bacterial ***Streptococcus pneumoniae***. The small **air sacs (alveoli)** for **gas exchange** appear regular in structure as shown in Panel B. The alveoli have an open configuration which enables free air movement bringing oxygen into the body. In Panel C the pneumonia infection is shown as it affects the alveoli. This image shows that **alveolar wall inflammation** causes **fluid, pus, and blood cells** to build up until **normal gas exchange becomes impossible**. Fluid and inflammatory cells that accumulate in alveolar spaces during pneumonia cause physical obstruction that results in respiratory distress with subsequent oxygen depletion among patients.

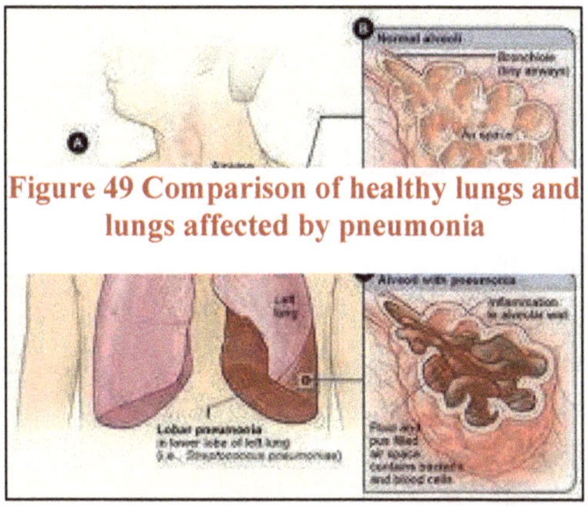

Figure 49 Comparison of healthy lungs and lungs affected by pneumonia

3.3.5.1 Types of Pneumonia

As shown in the figure, there are **different kinds of pneumonia** that stem from **different origins**. The main classifications of pneumonia include **bacterial, viral, atypical, fungal, and exposure-related types**. The different forms of bacterial pneumonia are **community-acquired, hospital-acquired pneumonia, and flu-related pneumonia** each possesses its own specific causes and risk elements. Bacterial pneumonia patients outside hospitals acquire their infection through **community settings** whereas the same infection presents in hospital patients **as hospital-acquired pneumonia** against **antibiotic-resistant bacteria**. The complication of influenza leads to the development of **flu-related pneumonia.** There are two categories of viral pneumonia including **common respiratory virus infections** from influenza, **respiratory syncytial virus,** and pandemic **SARS-Type virus infections that include SARS-CoV.** The bacteria that cause atypical pneumonia lead to symptoms known as **walking pneumonia and generate milder illness**

manifestations. The presence of fungal pneumonia primarily occurs within people with compromised immune function while pneumonia arising from **environmental exposure** develops from **inhaling toxic substances** in the environment. The classification system emphasizes the multiple pathogens responsible for pneumonia due to its varied nature thus requiring specific therapeutic strategies.

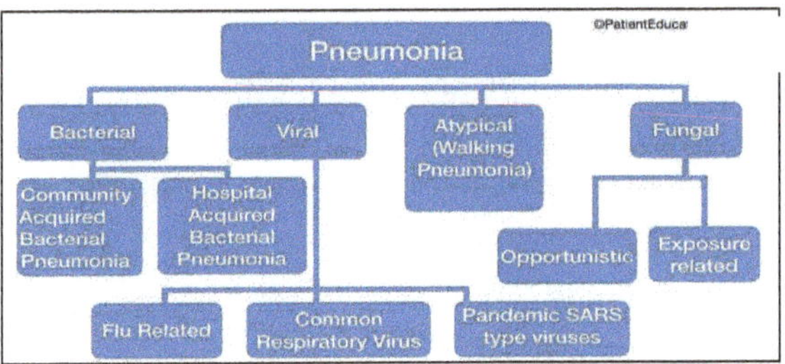

Figure 50 Classification of Pneumonia

The table outlines the different types of pneumonia based on the setting in which they are acquired and their key characteristics.

Table 36 Summary of Types of Pneumonia

Type of Pneumonia	Description	Key Characteristics
Community-Acquired Pneumonia (CAP)	Acquired outside healthcare settings.	Less likely to involve multidrug-resistant bacteria; may involve typical pathogens like *Streptococcus pneumoniae.*
Healthcare-Associated Pneumonia (HCAP)	Infection is linked to recent exposure to healthcare settings such as hospitals, outpatient clinics, etc.	A higher risk for multidrug-resistant pathogens; often involves individuals with pre-existing medical conditions.
Hospital-Acquired Pneumonia (HAP)	Pneumonia that develops at least 48 hours after hospital admission.	More likely to involve resistant bacteria and more severe cases due to patients' compromised health conditions.
Ventilator-Associated Pneumonia (VAP)	Pneumonia occurs more than 48 to 72 hours after endotracheal intubation in patients using mechanical ventilation.	Often caused by multidrug-resistant bacteria; associated with extended use of ventilation.
Aspiration Pneumonia	Pneumonia is caused by the inhalation of food, liquid, or vomit into the lungs.	Often caused by anaerobic bacteria; can lead to lung abscesses or other complications.

3.3.5.2 Pneumonia Management

The presented table displays the **CURB-65 scoring system** that functions as a clinical assessment model to evaluate **pneumonia intensity for decision-making** regarding patient care. Each point in the CURB 65 scoring system **represents one criterion** including **confusion or altered mental state along with SBP lower than 90 mmHg and DBP lower than 60 mmHg before age 65**. The medical provider can gauge infection severity **through the total score**. The severity of pneumonia gets stronger as the score increases thereby requiring hospital admission or advanced intervention. The results of this test indicate whether hospital admission is necessary for treatment. The **CURB-65 tool** serves as a vital tool in patient management because it helps practitioners decide between hospital admission and **home-based treatment** regarding pneumonia care.

Table 37 CURB Score for Pneumonia Management

CURB-65	
Symptom	**Points**
Confusion	1
Urea>7 mmol/L	1
Respiratory rate>30	1
SBP<90mmHg, D**B**P<60mmHg	1
Age>=**65**	1

3.3.5.3 SOAP Notes for Pneumonia

Table 38 SOAP Notes for Pneumonia

Component	Details
Subjective (S)	Patient presents with a 5-day history of fever, chills, productive cough with greenish sputum, and shortness of breath. Reports fatigue and general malaise. Denies chest pain but has been experiencing pleuritic pain on deep breathing. No history of recent travel, sick contacts, or hospitalizations. History of smoking for 15 years but quit 3 years ago. Symptoms have worsened over the past 24 hours.
Objective (O)	Vitals: BP 128/76 mmHg, HR 102 bpm, RR 22 bpm, Temp 39°C (102.2°F). Respiratory exam: Decreased breath sounds on the right lower lobe, crackles on auscultation, and dullness to percussion in the same area. Chest X-ray: Consolidation in the right lower lobe consistent with bacterial pneumonia. Oxygen saturation: 92% on room air. Lab results: Elevated white blood cell count (WBC 15,000/mm^3), positive sputum culture for *Streptococcus pneumoniae*.
Assessment (A)	Diagnosis: Community-acquired pneumonia (CAP) most likely caused by *Streptococcus pneumoniae* based on clinical presentation and positive sputum culture. Differential Diagnosis: 1. Viral pneumonia (less likely due to the

	bacterial culture and localized consolidation on X-ray). 2. Aspiration pneumonia (unlikely due to the absence of risk factors such as recent aspiration events).
Plan (P)	Investigations: Blood cultures to assess for bacteremia, repeat chest X-ray in 1 week to monitor response to treatment. Pharmacological Treatment: Start on intravenous (IV) antibiotics—ceftriaxone and azithromycin to cover common bacterial pathogens (including *Streptococcus pneumoniae*). Switch to oral antibiotics if the patient improves (See Tables below). Non-Pharmacological Treatment: Encourage hydration, rest, and the use of a humidifier for respiratory comfort. Oxygen therapy if saturation drops below 92%. Education: Educate the patient on the importance of completing the full course of antibiotics, signs of worsening symptoms (such as increased difficulty breathing), and the need for follow-up care. Referral: Refer to pulmonology if no improvement within 48-72 hours or if complications arise (e.g., pleural effusion). Follow-up: Reassess in 3-5 days for symptom improvement and response to treatment. If symptoms persist or worsen, consider hospitalization or further investigation for complications.

Table 39 Treatment Approaches for Pneumonia

Category	Treatment/Management Component	Details
Initial Assessment	Risk Assessment	Determines whether the patient should receive outpatient or inpatient care. Immediate initiation of therapy is essential in severe bacterial pneumonia to prevent sepsis.
	Empirical Antibiotic Therapy	Empirical antibiotics depend on local pathogens; options include benzylpenicillin, third-generation cephalosporins, macrolides, carbapenems, and fluoroquinolones.
	Adjust Treatment Based on Culture	Once a culture result is positive, treatment should be adjusted based on susceptibility to the specific pathogen.
Antibiotic Therapy	Combination Therapy for Severe Cases	Combination therapy may enhance survival in severe bacterial pneumonia, particularly in patients with shock.
	Outpatient Management	For patients without comorbidities, options include penicillin, macrolides, or tetracyclines. For those with comorbidities, respiratory fluoroquinolones or amoxicillin/clavulanate with macrolides are recommended.
	Inpatient Management	Inpatients should undergo microbiological testing (sputum/blood cultures) to guide

		treatment. Empirical antibiotics may be adjusted based on results.
Outpatient Management	Antipyretic Therapy	Antipyretics should be given to reduce fever and alleviate symptoms.
	Non-invasive Ventilation	For bacterial pneumonia cases without respiratory failure, non-invasive ventilation is debated, especially for patients with COPD.
Inpatient Management	Bronchodilators	Bronchodilator therapy may offer limited benefit in COPD patients with pneumonia, without corticosteroid use.
	Corticosteroids	Corticosteroids are used in cases of persistent hypotension with presumed adrenal insufficiency and in severe cases of CAP within 24 hours.
Supportive Care	Non-invasive Ventilation	Non-invasive ventilation is debated for bacterial pneumonia cases without respiratory failure, especially in patients with COPD.
	Bronchodilators	Bronchodilator therapy may offer limited benefit in COPD patients with pneumonia, without corticosteroid use.
Corticosteroid Use	Corticosteroids	Corticosteroids are used in cases of persistent hypotension with presumed adrenal insufficiency and in severe cases of CAP within 24 hours.
	Follow-Up	For home-based treatment, follow-up should be scheduled within 2 to 3 days to assess complications. For hospitalized patients, follow-up should occur in 7 days.
Monitoring and Follow-up	Smoking Cessation	Essential for patients with pneumonia, especially those with a history of smoking.
	Vaccination	Ensure vaccination against influenza, COVID-19, and pneumococcus to prevent future infections.
Non-Pharmacological Management	Chest Physiotherapy	The effectiveness of chest physiotherapy in pneumonia is debated, but it may reduce hospitalization duration and the need for mechanical ventilation.
	Hydration	Ensures proper hydration, which is vital in pneumonia management.
	Mechanical Support	Provides mechanical support for patients in acute respiratory distress.
	Nutrition	Adequate nutrition is essential for recovery.

Additional Measures	Early Mobilization	Encourages early mobilization, especially in hospitalized patients, to reduce complications.

Table 40 Pharmacological Management for Community-Acquired Pneumonia

Table 4. Dosage and Cost of Some IV Antibiotics for Empiric Treatment of CAP in Hospitalized Patients

Drug	Some Formulations	Usual Adult Dosage[1]	Cost[2]
Cephalosporins			
Cefotaxime – generic	1 g vials	1-2 g IV q8h	$75.50
Ceftaroline – *Teflaro* (Allergan)	400, 600 mg vials	600 mg IV q12h	2118.20
Ceftriaxone – generic	250 mg, 500 mg, 1 g, 2 g, 10 g vials; 1, 2 g/50 mL soln	1-2 g IV once/day	17.70
Fluoroquinolones			
Delafloxacin – *Baxdela* (Melinta)	300 mg vials	300 mg IV q12h	1325.00
Levofloxacin – generic	250 mg/50 mL, 500 mg/100 mL, 750 mg/150 mL soln; 25 mg/mL vials	750 mg IV once/day	40.00
Moxifloxacin – generic *Avelox IV* (Bayer)	400 mg/250 mL soln	400 mg IV once/day	225.20 255.30
Macrolides			
Azithromycin – generic *Zithromax*	500 mg vials	500 mg IV once/day	27.90 30.20
Pleuromutilins			
Lefamulin – *Xenleta* (Nabriva)	150 mg vials	150 mg IV q12h	1025.00
Penicillins			
Ampicillin/sulbactam – generic *Unasyn* (Pfizer)	1.5, 3, 15 g vials	1.5-3 g IV q6h	100.60 152.80
Tetracyclines			
Doxycycline – generic *Doxy* (Fresenius)	100 mg vials	100 mg IV q12h	204.20 210.00
Omadacycline – *Nuzyra* (Paratek)	100 mg vials	200 mg IV on day 1,[3] then 100 mg once/day	2196.10

soln = solution

1. Dosage adjustments may be needed for renal or hepatic impairment.
2. Approximate WAC for 5 days' treatment at the lowest usual adult dosage. WAC = wholesaler acquisition cost or manufacturer's published price to wholesalers; WAC represents a published catalogue or list price and may not represent an actual transactional price. Source: AnalySource® Monthly. January 5, 2021. Reprinted with permission by First Databank, Inc. All rights reserved. ©2021. www.fdbhealth.com/policies/drug-pricing-policy.
3. 200 mg loading dose is infused over 60 minutes. Alternative loading dose is 100 mg IV infused over 30 minutes twice on day 1.

Table 41 Pharmacological Management of Hospital Acquired Pneumonia

Early onset (< 5 days since admission) and no MDR risk factors	Dosing
Ceftriaxone	2 g i.v. or i.m. every 24 h
Levofloxacin	750 mg i.v. or PO every 24 h
Moxifloxacin	400 mg i.v. or PO every 24 h
Ciprofloxacin	400 mg i.v.every 8 h
Ampicillin-sulbactam	3 g i.v. or i.m. every 6 h
Ertapenem	1 g i.v. or i.m. every 24 h
Late onset (≥ 5 days since admission), with MDR risk factors	
Cefepime	2 g i.v. every 8 h
Ceftazidime	2 g i.v. every 8 h
Imipenem	500 mg i.v. every 6 h or 1 g i.v. every 8 h
Meropenem	2 g every 8 h
Piperacillin-tazobactam	4.5 g every 8 h
Vancomycin	15 mg/kg every 12 h
Linezolid	600 mg every 12 h
Ciprofloxacin	400 mg every 8 h
Levofloxacin	750 mg every 24 h
Fluconazole	800 mg every 12 h
Caspofungin	50 mg every 24 h
Voriconazole	4 mg/kg every 12 h

i.v.: Intravenous; MDR: Multidrug-resistant; PO: Per oral administration.

3.3.6 Tuberculosis (TB)

Tuberculosis (TB) functions as an infectious disease that mostly targets the lungs because of ***Mycobacterium tuberculosis*** infection. The bacteria moves by **air transmission** from the **coughs sneezes or spits of infected individuals**. Around one-quarter of the total global human population carries the tuberculosis bacteria yet only five to ten percent of them develop active **TB symptoms**. Those who have TB disease can receive treatment with antibiotics which saves their life but death becomes likely when they do not receive **antibiotics.** Patients who have **diabetes, weakened immune systems, experience malnutrition, tobacco users, and alcohol abusers** are at higher risk for developing TB. The major symptoms of TB include **coughing for an extended period together with bloody cough and chest discomfort as well as weakness, exhaustion, substantial weight loss, fever, and night sweats**. TB causes infections outside the lungs by spreading to kidney tissue and the brain as well as the spine and skin tissue. The prevention strategies focus on **early medical care, tests, and proper hygienic approaches** for high-risk groups and patients. The diagnosis process depends on molecular tests although it remains challenging to detect drug-resistant TB and TB cases in children. Figure 51 demonstrates how *Mycobacterium tuberculosis* causes **tuberculosis** which advances through different stages. After **bacterial entry into the lungs**, the pathogen creates a **primary lesion** that contains infected **macrophages, T cells, and foam giant cells.** The caseous core of the lesion serves to **protect bacteria from growth** yet it allows the bacteria to remain active within the lesion tissue. Tuberculosis spreads through the body to lymph nodes so ***Mycobacterium tuberculosis*** maintains its survival within tissues that are infected and those that show no signs of infection. The advance of the disease causes **post-primary disease** to occur when **cavitating lesions** start forming in the lungs. **The pulmonary tissue disintegrates** due to bacterial infection leading to lung cavity development. The path of infection shows that TB exists as a chronic disease that breaks down lung tissue while moving throughout the body's tissue.

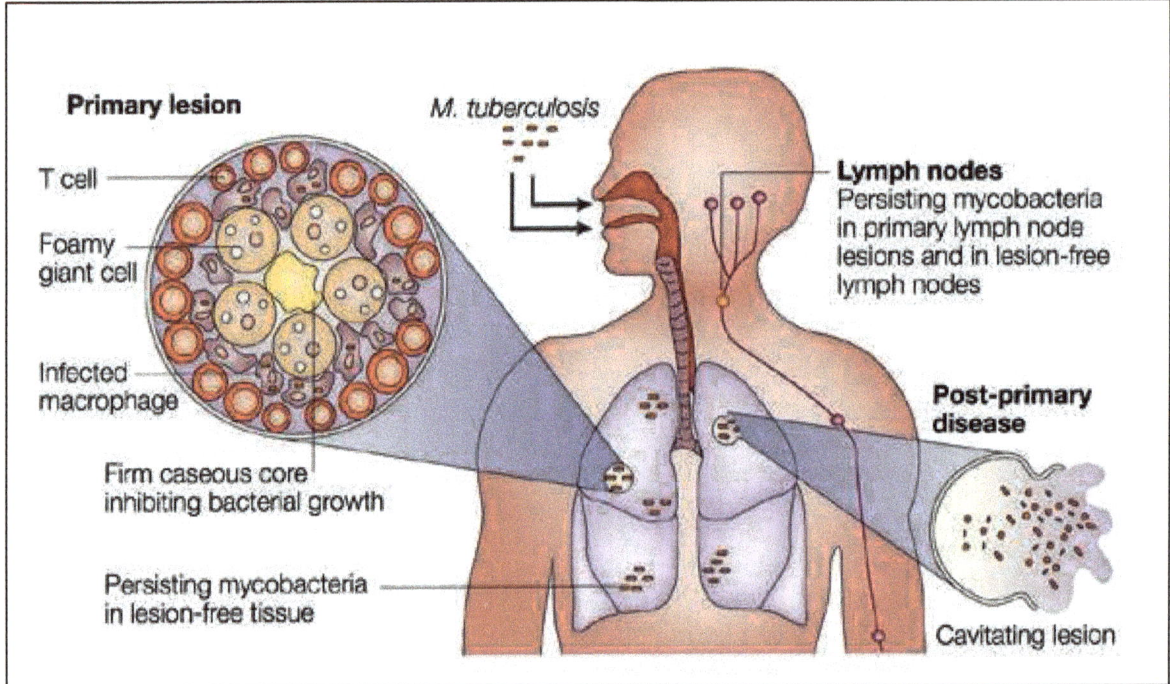

Figure 51 Progression and pathological features of tuberculosis (TB) infection

Figure 52 establishes an extensive model to understand **tuberculosis (TB)** by subdividing infection **into stages** and describing how screening and treatment measures **benefit patients** in addition to possible treatment **results within each phase**. The **five stages** covered in **panel A** discuss macroscopic pathology, transmission ability, and diagnostic signs of TB infection. During ***Mycobacterium tuberculosis*** infection persons acquire the infection **before exhibiting symptoms or turning infectious.** During **Subclinical tuberculosis, non-infectious** the infected person retains the illness without displaying its symptoms while avoiding disease transmission to others. During **Subclinical tuberculosis, infectious** individuals have no symptoms yet remain capable of spreading the infection. At the **fourth stage of Clinical tuberculosis**, **non-infectious**, the disease manifests itself while the person remains incapable of transmitting it. **Clinical tuberculosis**, infectious describes the last stage when patients have **symptoms and high contagiousness**. The diagnostic process combined with intervention can produce **five essential benefits** for individual and population health according to each stage of the diagnosis: **preventing disease, stopping**

further harm, resolving early illness, blocking symptoms' outbreak, and minimizing spread potential.

The possible TB infection developments are shown in **Panel B** through their evolution from **no symptoms to worse disease manifestations.** The human body sometimes clears infections automatically through **natural self-healing processes** among persons who have no tuberculosis disease. The proper medical intervention will lead infected individuals to either **complete recovery or long-lasting tuberculosis-related consequences**. The lack of appropriate care or mistreatment of tuberculosis infections can lead to fatal outcomes. **Early identification** of tuberculosis cases combined with proper treatments serves as crucial elements for halting disease spread and reducing tissue damage.

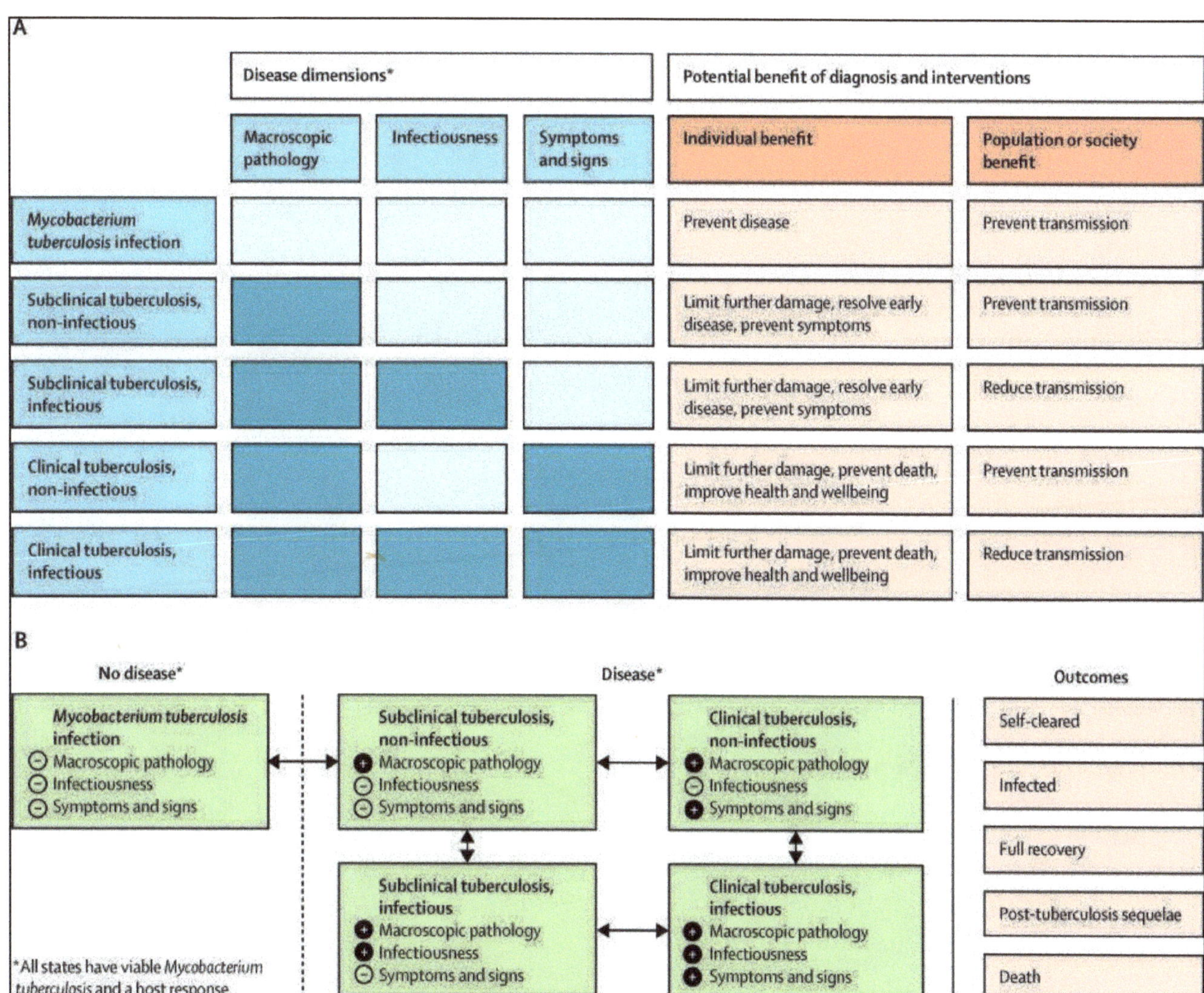

Figure 52 Classification of Early Tuberculosis State

3.3.6.1 Diagnosis of TB

The flowchart demonstrates how healthcare decisions are made about **secondary tuberculosis symptoms** and why patients may need testing or vaccination. The evaluation starts by recognizing essential risk elements that help form TB symptoms. Primary risk factors for secondary tuberculosis develop when people engage in **smoking, consume alcohol or drugs, have HIV,**

diabetes, pneumonia, kidney disease, receive cancer treatment, or contract COVID-19. The work environment itself restricts individuals to certain jobs which automatically puts them at higher risk for developing TB from exposure. The flowchart creates two distinct paths to direct people either toward **BCG vaccination and TB testing recommendations** when symptoms exist or risk factors are detected. Individuals without symptoms or risk factors for tuberculosis should not undergo testing for the condition. The diagram underscores how proper detection of TB symptoms and risk factors should determine decisions about testing and vaccine administration.

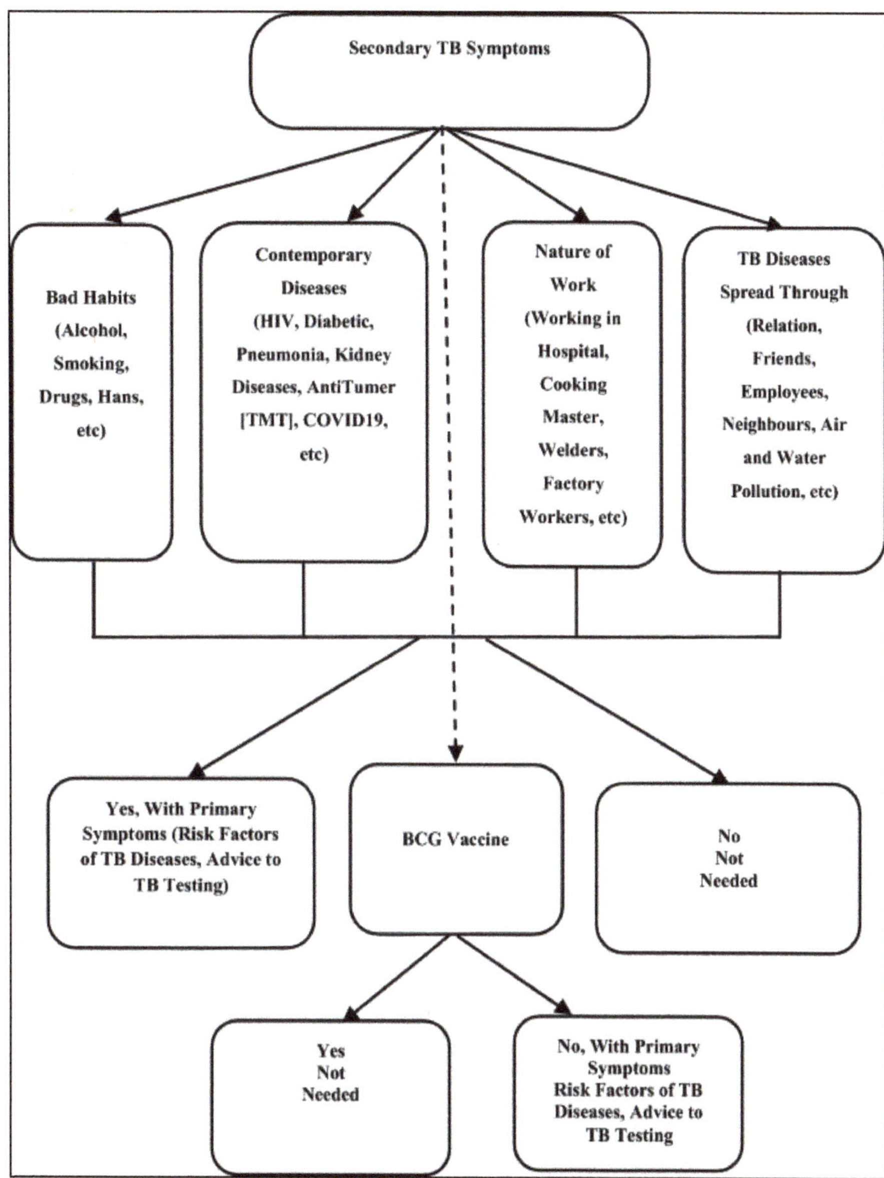

Figure 53 The decision process for TB testing and BCG vaccination based on secondary TB symptoms and risk factors.

3.3.6.2 Tuberculosis Transmission

As shown n figure 54, a person with tuberculosis spreads the disease to others by **exhaling respiratory particles** into the air during **common activities** such as **coughing, speaking, or sneezing**. Small particles among these airborne droplets are the most **endangering to others** due to their capability of **staying within the air while reaching distances up to 1–2 meters**. The size of particles matters because those that appear during **coughing or talking stay close to the ground** and do not spread as effectively **as smaller ones**. Aerosol particles of **smaller dimensions penetrate deeply into lung regions starting from the upper locations making them highly infectious**. The body absorbs these bacteria through the lungs where bacteria multiplication occurs to develop disease. Both **wearing face masks and keeping proper distance** from sick patients along with sufficient ventilation help reduce bacterial transmission through the air. In addition to the infectiousness of the individual, **environmental factors such as air circulation, humidity, and UV light** play a critical role in the viability of the **TB bacteria in the air.** An insufficient airflow within enclosed spaces allows bacteria to **stay suspended in the air** therefore increasing chances of particle transmission resulting in infection. TB transmission risks grow higher when the target population consists of individuals with **compromised immune function** including **HIV patients** along with **diabetic patients** and persons **whose lung health is compromised**. Bacteria exposure brings a greater risk of TB disease development to such individuals. TB transmission prevention requires these factors to achieve control while **good hygiene, adequate ventilation, and protective masks** remain important regarding high-risk transmission events.

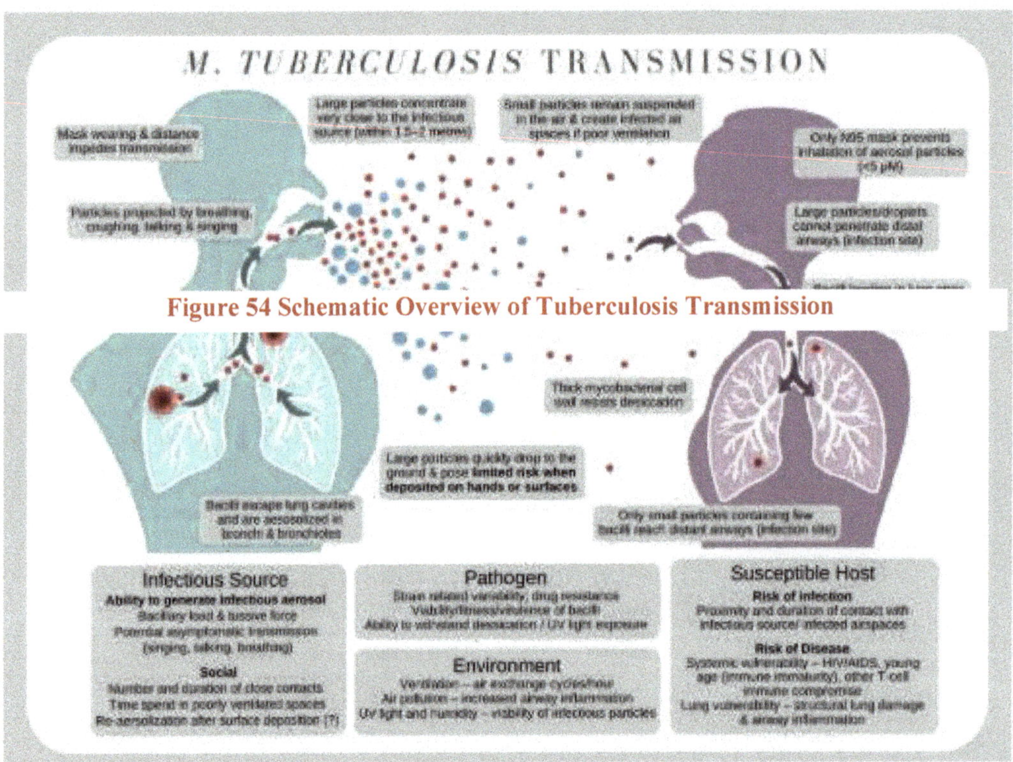

Figure 54 Schematic Overview of Tuberculosis Transmission

3.3.6.3 Modes of Transmission

TB transmission mainly occurs **through the air** when infected individuals such as Person A cough or sneeze and release ***Mycobacterium tuberculosis*** **bacteria-laden droplets.** The airborne bacteria stay suspended until **Person B breathes them** in through their **nasal passages** until they reach the respiratory system. After entering the lungs the bacteria start an infection that causes disease in the pulmonary area. TB affects the lungs the most frequently which leads to symptoms like **ongoing coughs, chest pain, shortness of breath, and intense coughing**. The bacteria that cause tuberculosis can cause **gastrointestinal infections when Person B unintentionally consumes respiratory drops** that contain the bacteria through personal **coughing or exposure to contaminated surfaces**. The infection risk for Person B becomes heightened when their immune system is weak because of HIV or imbalanced conditions so the bacteria have better chances to transform into active TB disease. The path of transmission through eating or drinking highlights the importance of focusing on prevention and monitoring those who face the highest risks of developing active TB disease.

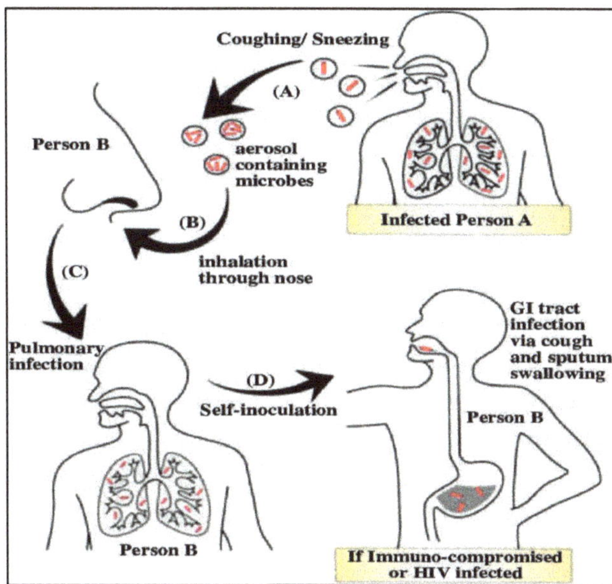

Figure 55 Transmission Routes of Tuberculosis

3.3.6.4 SOAP Notes for Tuberculosis

Table 42 SOAP Notes for Tuberculosis

Component	Details
Subjective (S)	The patient presents with a 4-week history of persistent cough, night sweats, and weight loss. The patient also reports fatigue and occasional hemoptysis (blood in sputum). They deny any recent travel, sick contacts, or hospitalizations. The patient has a history of smoking for 20 years and is currently immunocompromised (HIV positive). The symptoms have progressively worsened over the past week.
Objective (O)	The patient's vitals are BP 118/76 mmHg, HR 88 bpm, RR 18 bpm, and Temp 38.5°C (101.3°F). On respiratory examination, decreased breath sounds are noted in the upper right lung along with crackles and wheezing on auscultation. The chest X-ray shows a cavitary lesion in the upper right lung, which is indicative of active tuberculosis. The sputum smear is positive for *Mycobacterium tuberculosis*. The patient also has a positive HIV test with a CD4 count of 350 cells/mm^3.
Assessment (A)	Tuberculosis (TB) is suspected based on the patient's clinical presentation, the positive sputum smear for *Mycobacterium tuberculosis*, and the cavitary lesion visible on the chest X-ray. The differential diagnosis includes lung cancer, although the imaging findings and history make it unlikely, pneumonia (less likely given the positive sputum smear and cavitary lesion), and bronchitis (unlikely as symptoms are more severe and prolonged). The primary diagnosis is active tuberculosis.
Plan (P)	The next steps include HIV viral load testing, drug susceptibility testing for TB, and liver and kidney function tests to assess the patient's ability to

tolerate treatment. Pharmacologically, the patient will start the first-line TB regimen with Isoniazid, Rifampin, Pyrazinamide, and Ethambutol (RIPE therapy). Vitamin B6 supplementation will be prescribed to prevent peripheral neuropathy caused by Isoniazid. (See algorithms and Tables below). Non-pharmacologically, the patient is advised to stay hydrated, rest, and use a humidifier for respiratory comfort. Isolation in a well-ventilated room is recommended until the patient is no longer infectious. Education will be provided to the patient regarding the importance of completing the full course of TB treatment, recognizing signs of worsening symptoms, and the need for follow-up care. Referral to a pulmonologist will be made if the patient does not show improvement within 48-72 hours or if complications arise. Follow-up visits will be scheduled in 3-5 days to assess symptom improvement, response to treatment, and any adverse effects. If symptoms persist or worsen, hospitalization or further investigation for complications will be considered.

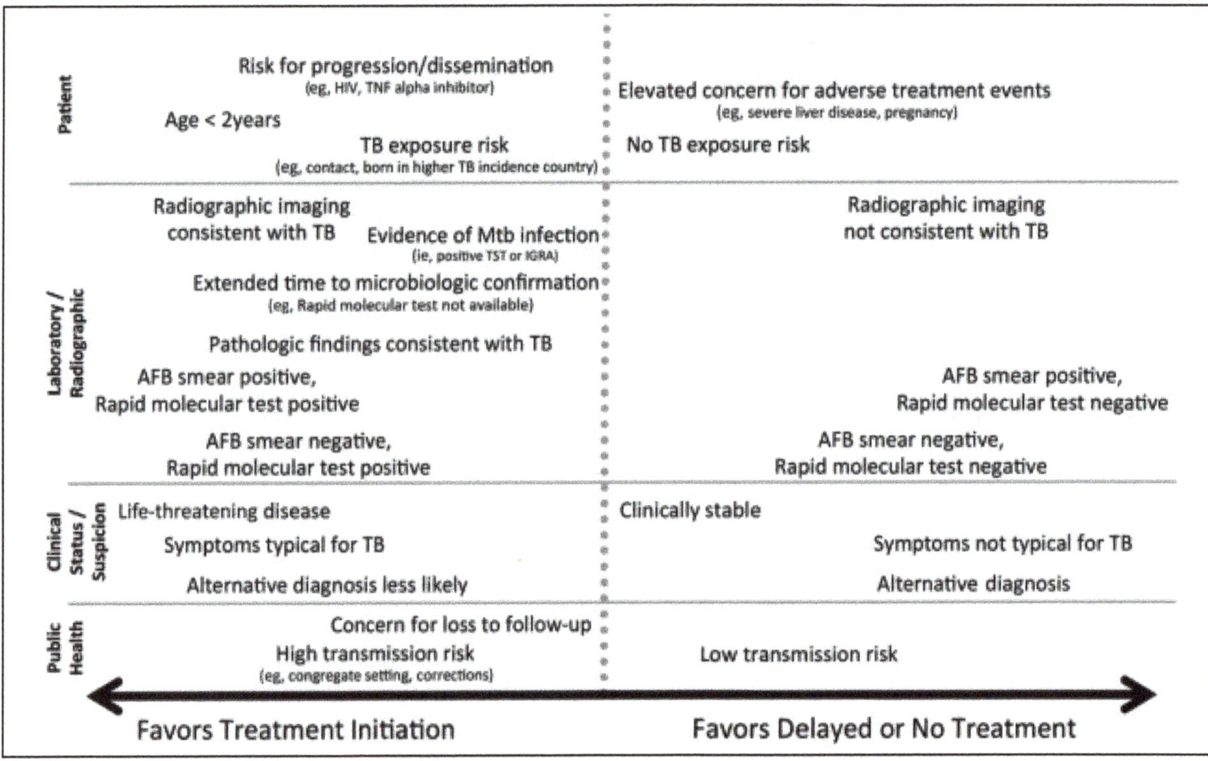

Figure 56 Algorithm/Factors to be considered in deciding to initiate treatment empirically for active tuberculosis (TB) (prior to microbiologic confirmation).

Table 43 Drug Regimens for Microbiologically Confirmed Pulmonary Tuberculosis Caused by Drug-Susceptible Organisms

	Intensive Phase		Continuation Phase				
Regimen	Drug[a]	Interval and Dose[b] (Minimum Duration)	Drugs	Interval and Dose[b, c] (Minimum Duration)	Range of Total Doses	Comments[c,d]	Regimen Effectiveness
1	INH RIF PZA EMB	7 d/wk for 56 doses (8 wk), or 5 d/wk for 40 doses (8 wk)	INH RIF	7 d/wk for 126 doses (18 wk), or 5 d/wk for 90 doses (18 wk)	182–130	This is the preferred regimen for patients with newly diagnosed pulmonary tuberculosis.	Greater
2	INH RIF PZA EMB	7 d/wk for 56 doses (8 wk), or 5 d/wk for 40 doses (8 wk)	INH RIF	3 times weekly for 54 doses (18 wk)	110–94	Preferred alternative regimen in situations in which more frequent DOT during continuation phase is difficult to achieve.	
3	INH RIF PZA EMB	3 times weekly for 24 doses (8 wk)	INH RIF	3 times weekly for 54 doses (18 wk)	78	Use regimen with caution in patients with HIV and/or cavitary disease. Missed doses can lead to treatment failure, relapse, and acquired drug resistance.	
4	INH RIF PZA EMB	7 d/wk for 14 doses then twice weekly for 12 doses[e]	INH RIF	Twice weekly for 36 doses (18 wk)	62	Do not use twice-weekly regimens in HIV-infected patients or patients with smear-positive and/or cavitary disease. If doses are missed, then therapy is equivalent to once weekly, which is inferior.	Lesser

Abbreviations: DOT, directly observed therapy; EMB, ethambutol; HIV, human immunodeficiency virus; INH, isoniazid; PZA, pyrazinamide; RIF, rifampin.

[a] Other combinations may be appropriate in certain circumstances; additional details are provided in the section "Recommended Treatment Regimens."

[b] When DOT is used, drugs may be given 5 days per week and the necessary number of doses adjusted accordingly. Although there are no studies that compare 5 with 7 daily doses, extensive experience indicates this would be an effective practice. DOT should be used when drugs are administered <7 days per week.

[c] Based on expert opinion, patients with cavitation on initial chest radiograph and positive cultures at completion of 2 months of therapy should receive a 7-month (31-week) continuation phase.

[d] Pyridoxine (vitamin B6), 25–50 mg/day, is given with INH to all persons at risk of neuropathy (eg, pregnant women; breastfeeding infants; persons with HIV; patients with diabetes, alcoholism, malnutrition, or chronic renal failure; or patients with advanced age). For patients with peripheral neuropathy, experts recommend increasing pyridoxine dose to 100 mg/day.

Table 44 Doses of Antituberculosis Drugs for Adults and Children

Drug	Preparation	Population	Daily	Once-Weekly	Twice-Weekly	Thrice-Weekly
First-line drugs						
Isoniazid	Tablets (50 mg, 100 mg, 300 mg); elixir (50 mg/5 mL); aqueous solution (100 mg/mL) for intravenous or intramuscular injection. Note: Pyridoxine (vitamin B6), 25–50 mg/day, is given with INH to all persons at risk of neuropathy (eg, pregnant women; breastfeeding infants; persons with HIV; patients with diabetes, alcoholism, malnutrition, or chronic renal failure; or patients with advanced age). For patients with peripheral neuropathy, experts recommend increasing pyridoxine dose to 100 mg/d.	Adults	5 mg/kg (typically 300 mg)	15 mg/kg (typically 900 mg)	15 mg/kg (typically 900 mg)	15 mg/kg (typically 900 mg)
		Children	10–15 mg/kg	...	20–30 mg/kg	...[b]
Rifampin	Capsule (150 mg, 300 mg). Powder may be suspended for oral administration. Aqueous solution for intravenous injection.	Adults[c]	10 mg/kg (typically 600 mg)	...	10 mg/kg (typically 600 mg)	10 mg/kg (typically 600 mg)
		Children	10–20 mg/kg	...	10–20 mg/kg	...[b]
Rifabutin	Capsule (150 mg)	Adults[d]	5 mg/kg (typically 300 mg)	...	Not recommended	Not recommended
		Children	Appropriate dosing for children is unknown. Estimated at 5 mg/kg.			
Rifapentine	Tablet (150 mg film coated)	Adults		10–20 mg/kg[e]		
		Children	Active tuberculosis: for children ≥12 y of age, same dosing as for adults, administered once weekly. Rifapentine is not FDA-approved for treatment of active tuberculosis in children <12 y of age.			
Pyrazinamide	Tablet (500 mg scored)	Adults	See Table 10	...	See Table 10	See Table 10
		Children	35 (30–40) mg/kg	...	50 mg/kg	...[b]
Ethambutol	Tablet (100 mg, 400 mg)	Adults	See Table 11	...	See Table 11	See Table 11
		Children[f]	20 (15–25) mg/kg	...	50 mg/kg	...[b]
Second-line drugs						
Cycloserine	Capsule (250 mg)	Adults[g]	10–15 mg/kg total (usually 250–500 mg once or twice daily)	There are inadequate data to support intermittent administration.		
		Children	15–20 mg/kg total (divided 1–2 times daily)			
Ethionamide	Tablet (250 mg)	Adults[h]	15–20 mg/kg total (usually 250–500 mg once or twice daily)	There are inadequate data to support intermittent administration.		
		Children	15–20 mg/kg total (divided 1–2 times daily)			
Streptomycin	Aqueous solution (1 g vials) for IM or IV administration.	Adults	15 mg/kg daily. Some clinicians prefer 25 mg/kg 3 times weekly. Patients with decreased renal function may require the 15 mg/kg dose to be given			

Table 45 Management of Treatment Interruptions

Interruption	Details of Interruption	Approach
During intensive phase	Lapse is <14 d in duration	Continue treatment to complete planned total number of doses (as long as all doses are completed within 3 mo)
	Lapse is ≥14 d in duration	Restart treatment from the beginning
During continuation phase	Received ≥80% of doses and sputum was AFB smear negative on initial testing	Further therapy may not be necessary
	Received ≥80% of doses and sputum was AFB smear positive on initial testing	Continue therapy until all doses are completed
	Received <80% of doses and accumulative lapse is <3 mo in duration	Continue therapy until all doses are completed (full course), unless consecutive lapse is >2 mo. If treatment cannot be completed within recommended time frame for regimen, restart therapy from the beginning (ie, restart intensive phase, to be followed by continuation phase)[b]
	Received <80% of doses and lapse is ≥3 mo in duration	Restart therapy from the beginning, new intensive and continuation phases (ie, restart intensive phase, to be followed by continuation phase)

Abbreviation: AFB, acid-fast bacilli.

[a] According to expert opinion, patients who are lost to follow-up (on treatment) and brought back to therapy, with interim treatment interruption, should have sputum resent for AFB smear, culture, and drug susceptibility testing.

[b] The recommended time frame for regimen, in tuberculosis control programs in the United States and in several European countries, is to administer all of the specified number of doses for the intensive phase within 3 months and those for the 4-month continuation phase within 6 months, so that the 6-month regimen is completed within 9 months.

3.3.7 Pulmonary embolism (PE)

A pulmonary embolism exists as a dangerous medical emergency **that arises from blood clots or different obstructive** materials including **fat tissue, air bubbles, or tumors blocking pulmonary arteries. Deep vein thrombosis (DVT) formation** in the lower leg veins creates the primary reason for pulmonary embolism development because **clots migrate into lung pulmonary arteries (Figure 57)**. Blood circulation becomes blocked which weakens lung tissue oxygen supply while simultaneously putting excessive strain on the heart. The extent of pulmonary embolism depends on the **dimensions of the clot along with the area of blockage in the lungs**. Pulmonary emboli of different sizes may result in either **no obvious symptoms or mild complaints** yet larger emboli obstruct substantial pulmonary arterial sections creating **severe breathing problems accompanied by lung tissue collapse** leading potentially to death. PE typically brings about sudden **breathlessness combined with severe chest pain and dizziness along with quickened heart rate and coughing episodes that may cause minor bleeding through the lungs (hemoptysis).**

Pregnancy alongside cancer represents a major **pulmonary embolism risk factor** together with prolonged immobility that develops after **surgical procedures or flights including previous occurrences of DVT or PE** and conditions such as **obesity** which increase blood coagulation potential. **Unionized individuals** and those patients who suffer from **heart disease cancer or stroke** experience increased vulnerability to pulmonary embolism. PE diagnosis depends on **clinical examination results, imaging procedures, and blood testing procedures.** Medical specialists use **D-dimer tests** to exclude clotting irregularities yet this test shows **false elevation when other health issues occur. CTPA** remains the most effective test for **PE diagnosis** since it creates precise images that reveal precise clot positions in the pulmonary arteries. Medical professionals sometimes utilize a **ventilation-perfusion (V/Q) scan because CT scans** either cannot be accessed or are unsuitable for the condition.

Treatment for pulmonary embolism targets major objectives: **minimizing clot size reduction while stopping additional complications from happening.** Most people with pulmonary embolism receive treatment with anticoagulants such as **heparin combined with warfarin** to prevent new clots and make existing emboli smaller. Patients with serious pulmonary embolism receive **clot-busting drugs for dissolving the clot**. Patients requiring life-threatening care and those who do not respond to current treatments may need either surgical treatment or catheter-directed thrombolytic therapy. It is essential to prevent PE especially among people who have a **high risk of developing the condition.** Preventing deep vein thrombosis through surgical patient activation, compression stocking wear and anticoagulant therapy for vulnerable patients diminishes pulmonary embolus development risks.

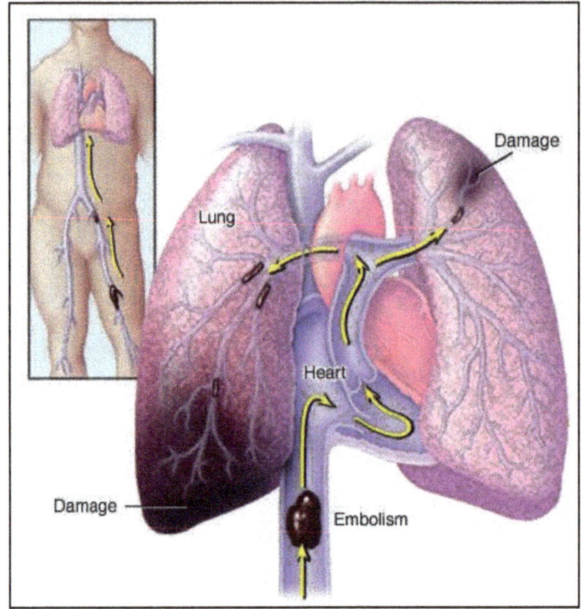

Figure 57 Pulmonary Embolism

3.3.7.1 The Pathophysiological Sequence of Pulmonary Embolism

Figure 58 shows the pathophysiological sequence of pulmonary embolism (PE) which begins with an **anatomic obstruction from embolism into pulmonary arteries**. The pulmonary artery vascular resistance becomes **higher when an obstruction occurs** which results in **increased difficulty for blood to flow through the lungs**. Heart pressure from **pulmonary embolism** causes increased right ventricular afterload that continues to strain the heart. The additional workload creates adverse effects on **right ventricle coronary perfusion** so the heart tissue becomes **ischemic because of decreased oxygen supply**. The oxygen requirements of the **right ventricle** further deteriorate during ischemia thus leading to dysfunction of the right ventricle. The right ventricle becomes **less efficient and expands to increased RV volume** that continues to stress the heart. The right ventricle's expanded volume produces **septal leftward bowing and pericardial limitation of heart motion** that **blocks normal heart expansion and contractions**. The left ventricle develops **reduced elasticity** during filling due to which blood properly enters the chamber. The decreased LV preload condition makes less blood available for **left ventricular pumping** which leads to a substantial reduction in cardiac output. The final result is severely **reduced cardiac output** because both right and **left ventricles fail** to operate correctly which diminishes body-wide oxygen delivery and might trigger organ malfunction.

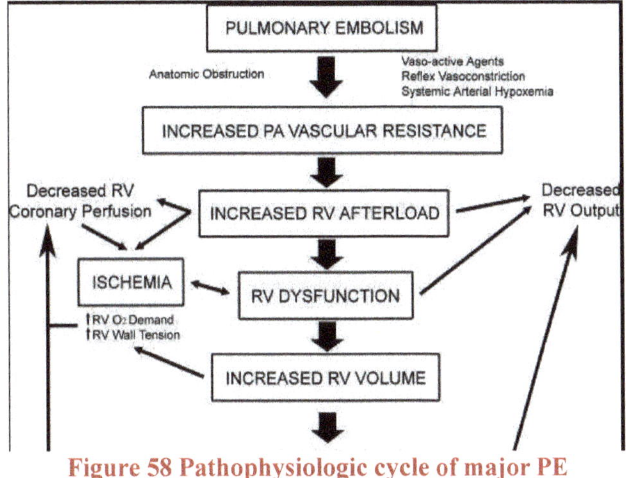

Figure 58 Pathophysiologic cycle of major PE

3.3.7.2 Types of Pulmonary Embolism

As shown in Figure 59, A pulmonary embolism from **Venous Thromboembolism (VTE)** develops when a **deep vein blood clot travels** from the body to the lungs. The passage of a **heart-derived arterial blood** clot blocks **lung blood flow** which creates an arterial embolism. **Pulmonary emboli** of this type are more severe than **VTE** because deaths may occur when prompt medical treatment is not available. A pulmonary embolism develops after **fat emboli** make their way through the bloodstream to block blood flow in **small arteries and capillaries** in the lungs thereby causing this condition. **Pulmonary embolisms occur primarily following traumatic injuries** that include long bone fractures with a breakdown of fat tissue from surrounding regions that enter blood flow. Death is a **possible outcome** when air enters circulation since air emboli form through puncture wounds or major airways such as the **trachea or bronchus** during surgical procedures.

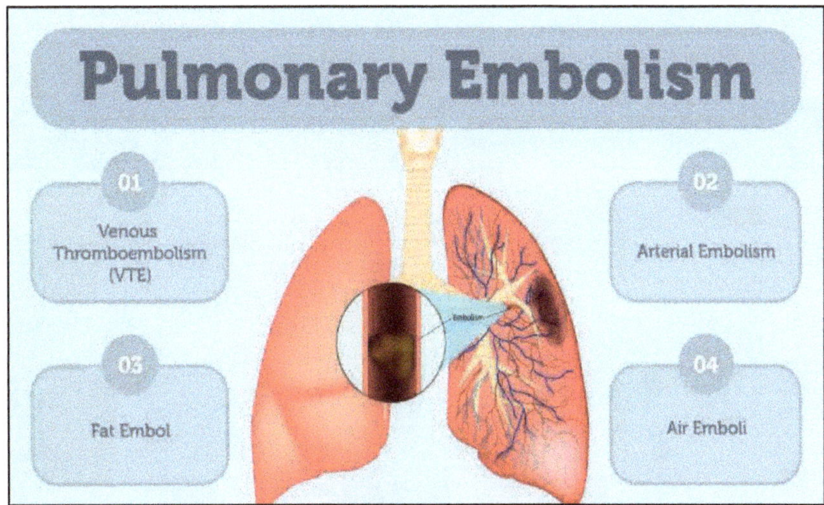

Figure 59 Types of Pulmonary Embolism

3.3.7.3 Medical Management of Pulmonary Embolism

The initial diagnostic assessments for a suspected PE begin with evaluating **whether shock or hypotension exists.** A high risk exists for severe pulmonary embolism when either **shock or hypotension is detected.** The main objective is to verify **a PE diagnosis** followed **by beginning primary reperfusion therapy** that normally utilizes **thrombolysis or surgical methods** to restore blood flow. **Patients without shock or hypotension** receive a diagnosis of **intermediate-risk PE.** Clinical risk evaluation requires the use of **PE Severity Index (PESI)** or **simplified PESI (sPESI)** scoring systems at this point. Primary management strategies depend on outcome assessments of patient clinical status. The therapeutic plan for high-risk intermediate patients who show **PESI Class III-V or sPESI** at values of one or more includes **anticoagulants and active surveillance** along with **rescue reperfusion** being an available option should the patient's condition deteriorate. Medical professionals should provide treatment by anticoagulation to patients who fall within **PESI Class I-II or have sPESI** values of 0 while **hospitalization is optional** in their care management. Patients who stay stable after treatment have the alternative of leaving the hospital early for home-based care. Resource distribution happens optimally through this method because it matches financial allocations to patient risk factors and **acute PE severity** levels leading to enhanced treatment results.

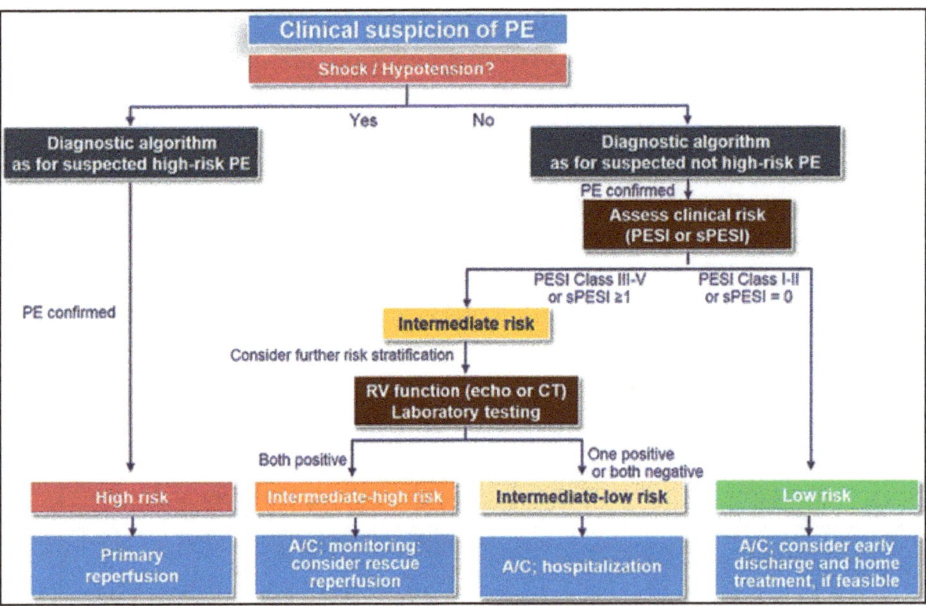

Figure 60 Flowchart/Algorithm for the Management of PE

3.3.7.4 SOAP Notes for Pulmonary Embolism

Table 46 SOAP Notes for Pulmonary Embolism

Component	Details
Subjective (S)	A 55-year-old male presents with sudden onset of shortness of breath, sharp chest pain, and dizziness that began approximately 6 hours ago after a long flight. The patient reports fatigue and has a history of deep vein thrombosis (DVT) from 3 years ago but has had no recent symptoms. He denies any recent trauma or surgery. The patient is a former smoker with a 20-year smoking history, quitting 5 years ago. He is concerned about a blood clot due to his past history of DVT and the recent long flight.
Objective (O)	Vitals show a BP of 110/70 mmHg, HR of 120 bpm, RR of 22 bpm, and a temperature of 37.8°C (100°F). The respiratory exam reveals tachypnea with decreased breath sounds on the right side and mild wheezing. Cardiovascular exam shows tachycardia but no murmurs or gallops. Chest X-ray shows no significant abnormalities, while ECG reveals sinus tachycardia with no signs of acute ischemia. Lab results show an elevated D-dimer. CT pulmonary angiography confirms a large embolus in the right pulmonary artery.
Assessment (A)	The primary diagnosis is pulmonary embolism (PE), confirmed by CT pulmonary angiography, likely originating from a previous DVT. Differential diagnoses include acute myocardial infarction (ruled out by ECG and D-dimer), pneumonia (ruled out by normal chest X-ray), and pulmonary edema (unlikely due to lack of heart failure signs).
Plan (P)	Immediate treatment includes starting IV heparin for anticoagulation and oxygen therapy to maintain oxygen saturation above 94%. Further investigations include obtaining arterial blood gases (ABG) and repeating CT pulmonary angiography in 48 hours if symptoms worsen. Pharmacologically, continue heparin until stable, then switch to oral warfarin or DOACs (See Figure and Algorithm below). Non-pharmacologically, encourage early mobilization and consider compression stockings for long-term prevention of DVT. Education on the importance of medication adherence, avoiding activities that increase bleeding risk, and follow-up with a pulmonologist for long-term anticoagulation management is provided. The patient will be closely monitored over the next 24-48 hours in the hospital.

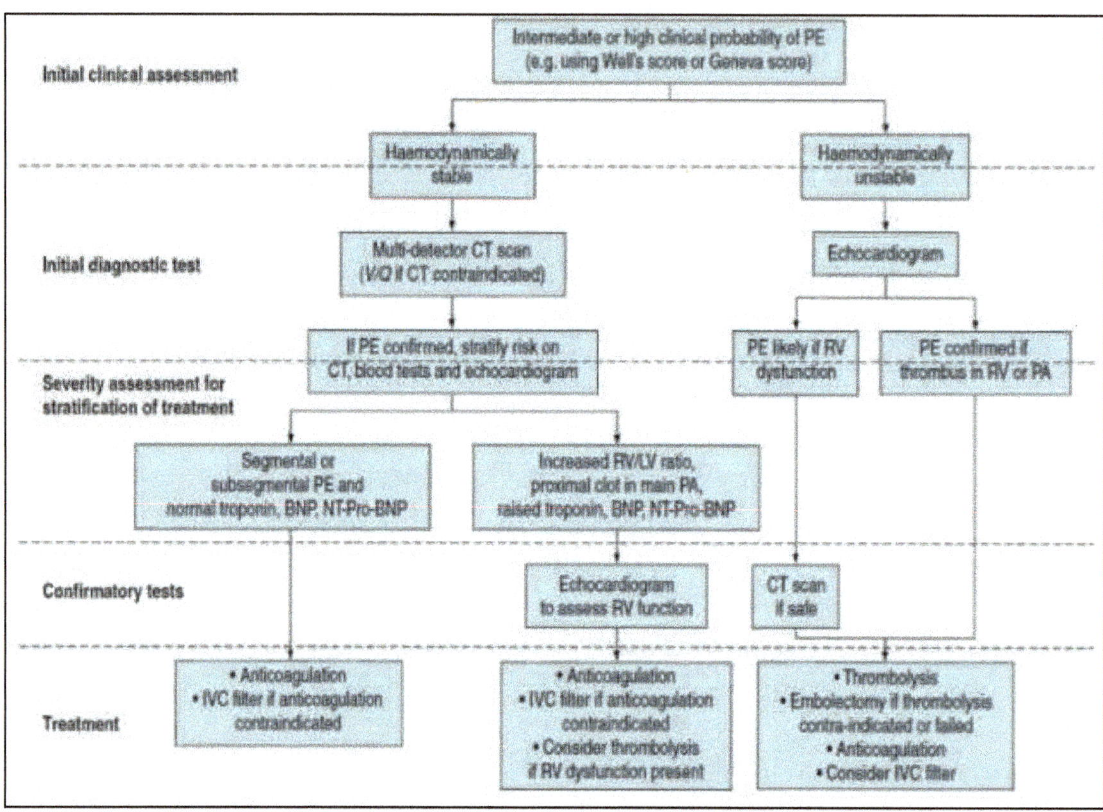

Figure 61 Algorithm for the Management of Pulmonary Embolism

Table 47 Algorithm for the Pharmacological Management of Pulmonary Embolism

Category	Phase/Treatment	Description
Management Phases	Initial Phase	The goal in the initial phase is to reduce mortality and recurrence in the first 5 to 10 days after PE presentation. Treatment options include thrombolytics, parenteral anticoagulants, oral anticoagulants, and nonpharmacologic interventions.
	Long-Term Treatment	Long-term treatment is given for at least 3 months with anticoagulants (parenteral or oral). Reevaluation at 3 months determines if extended therapy is necessary, especially for unprovoked PE or ongoing risk factors.
	Extended Anticoagulation	Extended anticoagulation therapy involves continuing anticoagulation beyond 3-6 months, particularly for patients with persistent risk factors, cancer-associated PE, or recurrent PE, regardless of bleeding risk.
Risk Classification	Massive PE (High Risk)	Massive PE is characterized by shock, sustained hypotension (SBP <90 mmHg for ≥15 minutes), or no pulse. Immediate resuscitation is required, including thrombolytics and parenteral anticoagulation. Other options like catheter-directed thrombolysis or surgical embolectomy may be considered.
	Submassive PE (Moderate Risk)	Submassive PE involves right ventricular dysfunction or myocardial necrosis but no hypotension (SBP ≥90 mmHg). Thrombolytics may be considered if clinical instability worsens, with anticoagulation as the primary treatment.
	Nonmassive PE (Low Risk)	Nonmassive PE is clinically stable, with no right ventricular dysfunction. These patients can often be treated as outpatients with anticoagulants and receive long-term therapy if necessary based on recurrence risk.
Anticoagulation Therapy	Parenteral Anticoagulation	Parenteral anticoagulants like heparin or LMWH are used in the initial phase to prevent clot extension and formation of new clots.
	Oral Anticoagulation	After the initial phase, patients transition to oral anticoagulants such as warfarin or DOACs (apixaban, rivaroxaban) to continue treatment and prevent further PE episodes.

Thrombolytic Therapy	Systemic Thrombolysis	Systemic thrombolytics such as tPA are used in high-risk patients (massive PE) to rapidly dissolve the clot. This treatment has a higher bleeding risk and is typically used in emergencies.
	Catheter-Directed Thrombolysis	Catheter-directed thrombolysis involves directly delivering clot-dissolving medication to the pulmonary arteries and is an option when systemic thrombolysis is contraindicated.
	Surgical Embolectomy	Surgical embolectomy may be performed when thrombolytics are contraindicated or ineffective, especially in high-risk patients with massive PE.
Bleeding Risk Consideration	Low Bleeding Risk	For patients with low bleeding risk, extended anticoagulation therapy can continue with regular monitoring of clotting parameters to prevent further clots.
	Moderate Bleeding Risk	Patients with moderate bleeding risk may continue anticoagulation therapy with close monitoring to manage potential bleeding complications while preventing further clots.
	High Bleeding Risk	In high bleeding risk patients, anticoagulation therapy may be limited to the initial phase, and alternative treatments or nonpharmacologic options should be considered.
Supportive Care	Oxygen Therapy	Oxygen therapy is provided to maintain oxygen saturation levels in PE patients, especially those with moderate to high risk where oxygenation can be compromised.
	IV Fluids	IV fluids are used to manage hypotension in massive PE patients and help stabilize their hemodynamic condition.
	Ventilatory Support	Ventilatory support, including mechanical ventilation, may be required in severe cases of PE to ensure adequate oxygenation and prevent respiratory failure.
Follow-up and Monitoring	Repeat Imaging	Repeat imaging, such as CT pulmonary angiography or echocardiography, is used to monitor the resolution of the embolus and evaluate right ventricular function in moderate to high-risk patients.
	Clinical Monitoring	Continuous monitoring of vital signs, oxygen saturation, and clinical signs of deterioration (e.g., worsening chest pain, and shortness of breath) is

		essential, particularly in the first few days of treatment.

3.3.8 Lung Cancer

Lung cancer stands as a form of **malignant tumor** known as **lung carcinoma** which develops in the pulmonary tissue. Airway cells obtain their **DNA damage from cigarette exposure and exposure to harmful chemicals** that ultimately create lung cancer. Tumor formation develops when **damaged airway cells** obtain unlimited **duplicating ability**. Unmanaged tumors will infect the entire lung area **while damaging its functions. Metastasizing lung tumors** progress to spread their growth through different regions in the body. The early stages of lung cancer only reveal themselves through **medical imaging** because patients usually **show no detectable symptoms**. The disease's advancement leads most patients to develop **generic respiratory complications** that include **breathlessness and chest discomfort together with coughing symptoms**. The symptoms of lung cancer depend on where the tumor has grown and its size. Medical professionals use imaging tests to identify lung cancer tumors and assess their growth range when they suspect someone has lung cancer. Medical diagnosis of lung cancer depends on **pathologists examining tumor samples** taken through **biopsy under microscopic examination**. A pathologist can identify cancerous cells through examination but also classify the tumor through its **cell type origin**. The cancer diagnosis reveals that **15% of cases are small-cell lung cancer (SCLC)** while the remaining **85% include non-small-cell lung cancers or NSCLC** which are adenocarcinomas, squamous-cell carcinomas, and large-cell carcinomas. Once the diagnosis is given medical professionals obtain additional tests to stage the cancer by determining its extent of spread. **Early-stage lung cancer** requires surgical removal of the tumor which doctors often supplement with **radiation treatment and chemotherapy** for eliminating remaining cancer cells. Radiation therapy combines with chemotherapy while drug treatments target particular cancer subtypes to handle **advanced-stage lung cancer cases**. The success rate of surviving **five years after a lung cancer** diagnosis stands at **20% despite treatment intervention.** The probability of survival increases for patients who receive **early-stage diagnosis** before reaching a young age while being female. **Tobacco smoking** is responsible for producing approximately all lung cancer incidents. The remaining cases arise from contact with hazardous substances such as asbestos and radon gas whereas spontaneous genetic mutations make up the other cases. **The prevention of lung cancer** directly promotes hazardous chemical shunning and smoking cessation among people. The habit of **smoking reduces future lung cancer** risk and yields better cancer treatment results in patients who already have the disease.

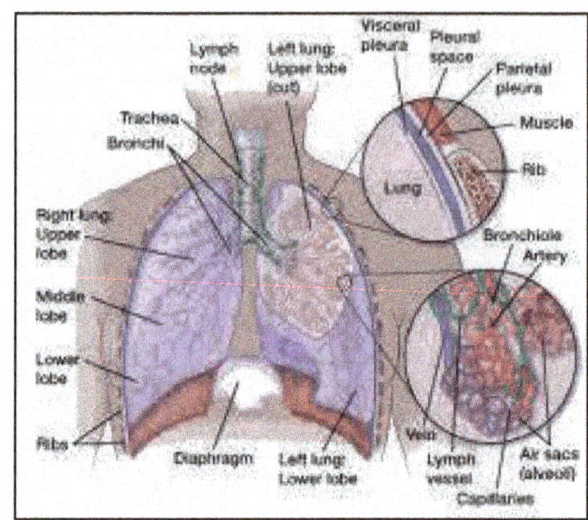

Figure 62 Anatomical Overview of Lung Cancer

3.3.8.1 Classification of Lung Cancer

Figure 63 demonstrates the WHO Classification of Lung Cancer that divides lung cancers into separate groups through c**ellular origin examinations alongside behavioral and structural classification.** Epithelial tumors form the largest category within the WHO Classification of Lung Cancer. The most prevalent lung cancer type is **adenocarcinoma** which consists of two subtypes: **minimally invasive adenocarcinoma** along with **invasive nonmucinous or mucinous adenocarcinoma**. Among epithelial tumors, several prevalent disease classes exist including **squamous cell carcinoma**, **large cell carcinoma, and adenosquamous carcinoma** together with the less common categories of **sarcomatoid carcinoma and salivary gland-type tumors.** The second essential group includes **lung neuroendocrine neoplasms** that develop from **neuroendocrine cells.** Different cancer types within the neuroendocrine category are grouped by **precursor lesions, neuroendocrine tumors, and neuroendocrine carcinoma** with specific biological traits. Lung tissue contains tumors of **ectopic tissues** which represent unusual cancers made by cells normally located outside the lungs. Tumors of the **mesenchyme** which supports organs through connections fall into the category of rare types because they **include fibrosarcomas alongside liposarcomas** and other diseases in this group. The lungs can develop lymphomas together with other hematolymphoid tumors that emerge from blood or lymphatic tissue systems. The classification scheme enables doctors and nurses to properly d**iagnose lung cancer** which enables them to choose treatment methods while determining how the disease will progress based on cancer features.

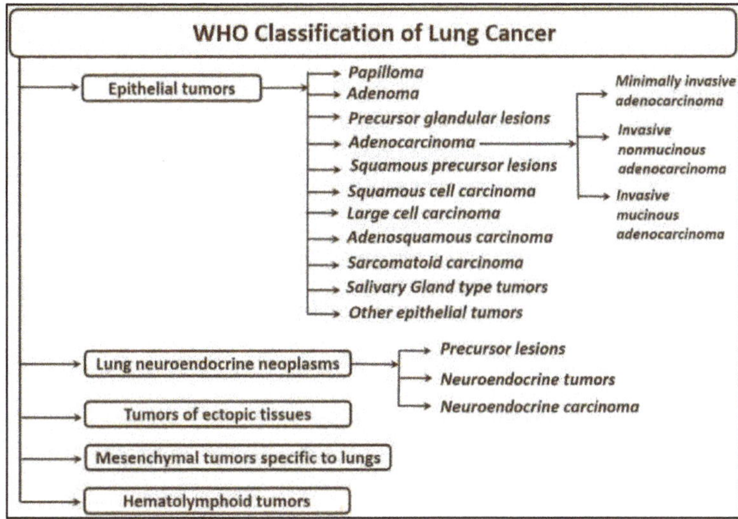

Figure 63 Flowchart for the Classification of Lung Cancer

3.3.8.2 Types of Lung Cancer

Lung cancer exists between two major cell-based classifications namely **small-cell lung cancer (SCLC) alongside non-small cell lung cancer (NSCLC) (Figure 64).** Neuroendocrine cells start SCLC which emerges as the less common version of **lung cancer at only 15% of total cases**. The fast-growth characteristics along with early spreading capabilities make this cancer type one of the most dangerous. Lung cancer cases make up 85% of all diagnoses **with NSCLC while SCLC remains at 15%.** The NSCLC subtype contains three fundamental subtypes yet each shows unique traits. The prevalent NSCLC subtype belongs to **Lung Adenocarcinoma (LUAD).** The cell type develops in **alveolar type II epithelial cells** and medical professionals mostly identify it within **nonsmoking individuals alongside adults under thirty-five years old and female patients.** The outer regions of the lungs serve as the typical starting point for **adenocarcinoma growth** since this type of lung cancer expands at a slower pace than other variants. The **bronchial basal epithelial cells** serve as the origin for **Lung Squamous Cell Carcinoma (LUSC)** as one of its subtypes of NSCLC. The risk factors of **smoking link directly to LUSC** development while this type of cancer mainly affects the central regions of the lungs. Despite its slower development rate, it possesses attributes of aggressive behavior. **LCC** stands as one of the three lung cancer subtypes resulting from the transformation of multiple types of epithelial cells present in the lungs. The **rapid nature and aggressive development of LCC** make this cancer subtype harder to treat than other NSCLC subtypes. The classification system assists medical practitioners in determining suitable therapeutic approaches alongside **predicting patient survival outcomes** and **planning effective treatment strategies for lung cancer**. The knowledge of particular cancer subtypes allows doctors to create personalized therapy plans that match the unique features of the cancer tissue for better treatment outcomes.

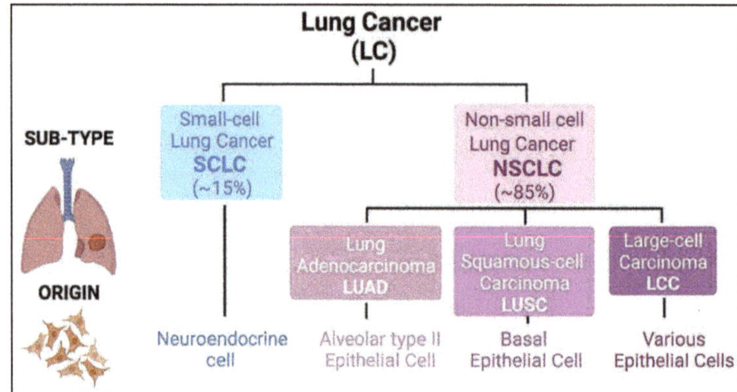

Figure 64 Broader classification of lung cancer based on its cellular origin

Figure 65 explains the classification types of non-small cell lung cancer (NSCLC) since it represents 85% of all lung cancer cases. **NSCLC includes three main classification categories**. Lung cancer takes the form of adenocarcinoma most frequently in patients who do not smoke alongside young adults and women. The first step of this cancer development occurs inside the **small glands** found in the outer parts of the lungs known as alveoli. Non-small cell lung cancer with this phenotype progresses at a moderate pace which makes it among the less hazardous NSCLC varieties. **Squamous Cell Carcinoma** ranks as the **second typical lung cancer** variety since it generally manifests in smokers. The squamous cells of the bronchi generate this cancer type in the central lung areas. **Slowness** characterizes the growth pattern of **squamous cell carcinoma** in the same way it does for adenocarcinoma. NSCLC patients rarely develop Large Cell Carcinoma though it remains the least prevalent NSCLC subtype. The condition shows itself through big cells that have **irregular shapes** while it affects the lungs from every position but mostly affects the external regions. Large cell carcinoma progresses faster than its two associated lung cancer variants since it demonstrates heightened aggressiveness.

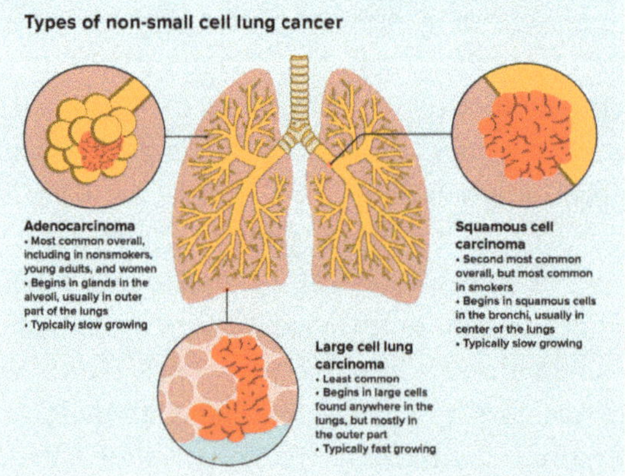

Figure 65 Types of Non-small Cell Lung Cancer

3.3.8.3 Stages of Lung Cancer

Lung cancer staging relies on the **TNM system** to determine tumor diameter and location details according to **size specifications, lymph node, and distant organ metastasis progression**. The TNM staging separates lung cancer into **T (explaining tumor dimensions and placement), N**

(illustrating local lymph node concerns), and M (providing information about metastasis progress to other body regions). Medicating doctors determine cancer severity by using numerical scales from **zero to four** which evaluate dimensions and growth patterns of the tumor and higher numbers represent more advanced cancer stages. The presence of unquantifiable tumors leads to their assessment with an X.

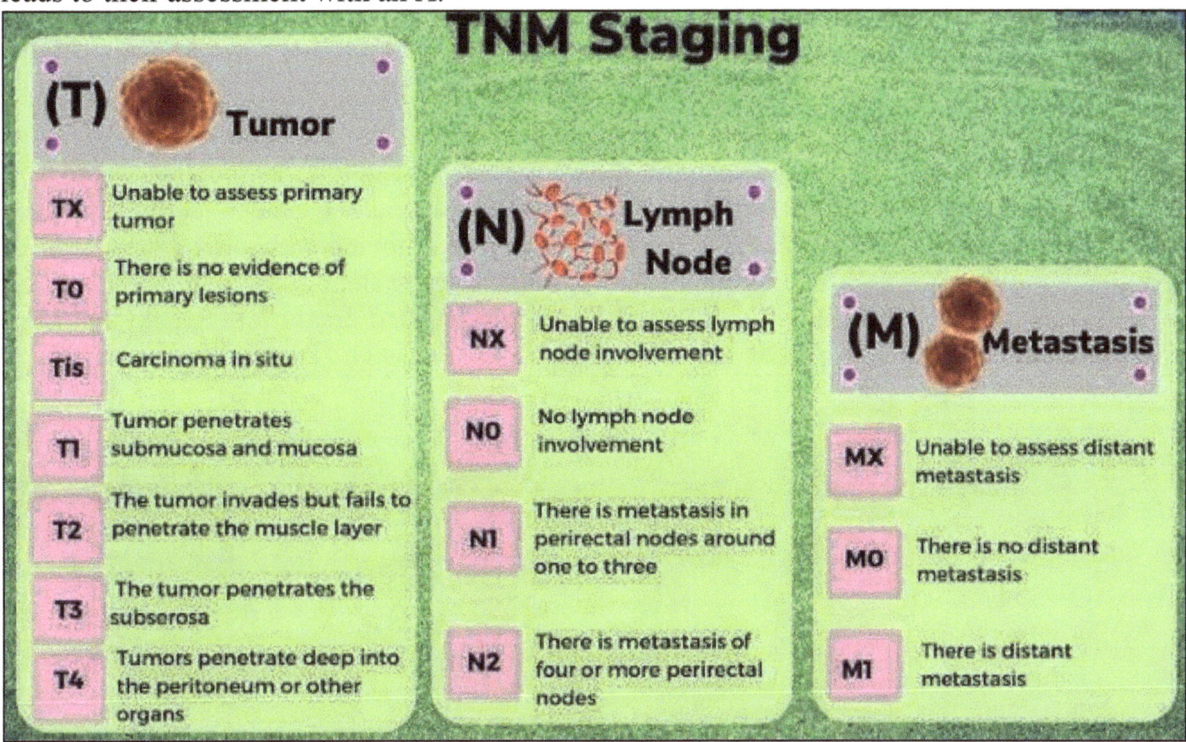

Figure 66 TNM Staging

Small-cell lung Cancer patients only receive two distinctive staging categories that classify tumors as either **limited stage or extensive stage.** The cancer stays within one area of a single lung and adjacent lymph nodes but has not moved beyond the first lung or other body organs defined limited stage. Patients with **extensive-stage tumors** show cancer growth beyond one lung that may spread to brain tissue or pleural tissue that lines the lungs. **NSCLC staging** requires a combination of **clinical and pathological examinations** to reach the final diagnosis. The clinical stage is determined through **imaging tests** but the **pathologic stage requires surgery or biopsy to assess its status**. The TNM system for NSCLC staging uses numbers from X (not measurable) to 4 to **define tumor size, location, and status of lymph node and organ metastasis.** The broader staging system for NSCLC contains multiple categories besides TNM staging. NSCLC detection requires examining mucus secretions from the lungs because this stage leaves no signs to appear in imaging results (Table 49).

Table 48 Stage (0-4) of Lung Cancer

Stage	Description
Occult Stage	The cancer is not visible in imaging scans, and it can only be detected in the mucus coughed up from the lungs.
Stage 0	This is a very early stage where the tumor is small and confined to the surface layer of the lung tissues, with no spread to deeper tissues or outside the lungs.
Stage I	The tumor is localized within the lung tissues, and there is no involvement of nearby lymph nodes.

Stage II	Cancer has spread to nearby lymph nodes within the lungs or around the chest area.
Stage III	The cancer has spread more extensively to the lymph nodes and structures in the middle of the chest, indicating a more advanced stage.
Stage IV	This stage represents the most advanced form of lung cancer, where the disease has spread widely to distant parts of the body, including the brain, bones, or liver.

Each progression level demonstrates essential consequences that guide treatment decisions and affect the predicted patient results (Table 67). The stage of 0 and I cancer requires surgical intervention but stage III and IV cancer needs chemotherapy combined with radiation or targeted therapy according to specific tumor details. Through the TNM system along with these staging categories, oncologists establish optimal treatment approaches and create foreseeable treatment success predictions.

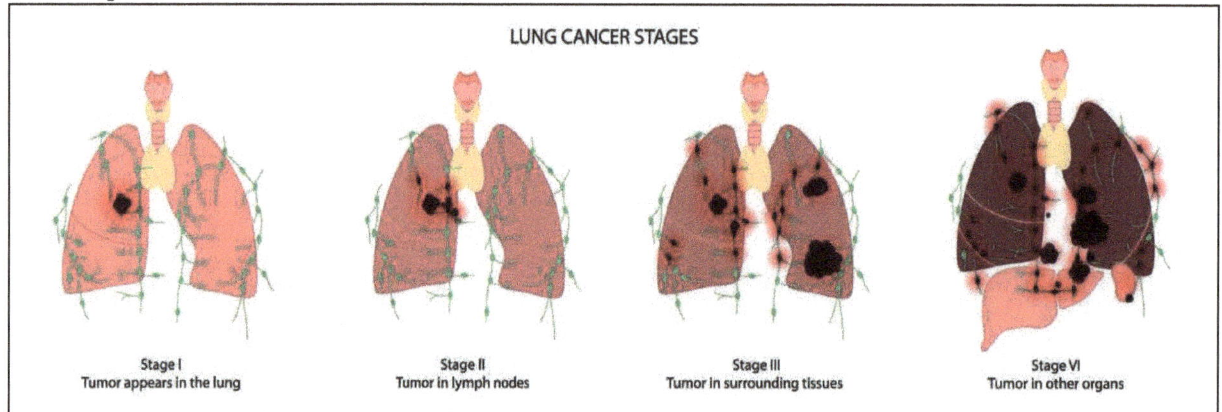

Figure 67 Lung Cancer Stages

3.3.8.4 SOAP Notes for Lung Cancer

Component	Details
Subjective (S)	The patient is a 65-year-old male with a 30-year history of smoking who presents with a 2-month history of persistent cough, weight loss, and fatigue. He reports coughing up blood-tinged sputum and experiencing occasional shortness of breath, especially with exertion. He denies any chest pain, fever, or night sweats. The patient has lost approximately 10 pounds in the last month and is concerned that these symptoms might indicate lung cancer, especially since his father had been diagnosed with lung cancer at the age of 70.
Objective (O)	On physical examination, the patient's vital signs are stable, with a blood pressure of 125/80 mmHg, heart rate of 88 bpm, and respiratory rate of 18 bpm. His temperature is 37.4°C (99.3°F). His respiratory exam reveals diminished breath sounds in the right lung base, with mild wheezing and no rales or crackles. Cardiovascular examination is unremarkable. Imaging studies, including a chest X-ray and CT scan, show a suspicious mass in the right upper lobe, along with possible mediastinal lymph node involvement. A

	biopsy was performed during bronchoscopy, and results are pending. Laboratory tests show elevated serum calcium, but CBC and liver function tests are normal. Pulmonary function tests reveal a mild restrictive pattern with an FEV1/FVC ratio of 70%.
Assessment (A)	The working diagnosis is likely **non-small cell lung cancer (NSCLC)**, based on the patient's symptoms, smoking history, and imaging findings. The biopsy results will confirm the diagnosis, and staging will be performed using a PET scan to evaluate for metastasis. Differential diagnoses include chronic obstructive pulmonary disease (COPD), though the presence of a mass on imaging makes cancer more likely, and tuberculosis or pneumonia, which are less consistent with the patient's symptoms and imaging.
Plan (P)	The plan includes waiting for biopsy results to confirm the diagnosis of lung cancer and using the staging process to guide treatment. Pharmacologically, the patient will be started on pain management with NSAIDs, and corticosteroids will be considered if inflammation causes significant symptoms (See table below). The patient will also be referred to a smoking cessation program and offered cancer support groups. If the biopsy confirms cancer and it is localized, a thoracic surgeon will evaluate for possible surgical resection. Depending on the staging, the patient may undergo chemotherapy, radiation, or targeted therapy, and immunotherapy may be considered if the cancer is metastatic. A follow-up appointment is scheduled in one week to discuss the biopsy results and further treatment planning. Regular follow-up will be essential to monitor symptoms and treatment response.

Table 49 Newer Oral Agents for Treatment of Metastatic Lung Cancer

Drug	Dosage	Class	Indication	Common AEs	Counseling Points
Erlotinib	150 mg po qd	EGFR-TKI	First-line for advanced NSCLC	Edema, rash, diarrhea, cough, conjunctivitis	Give 1 h before or 2 h after food; report symptoms of serious GI and/or pulmonary events (i.e., cough, shortness of breath, bleeding, ulceration) immediately; report abnormal eyelash growth; avoid grapefruit or grapefruit juice; report changes in cigarette smoking (dosage adjustment needed); wear sunscreen or avoid sunlight; use alcohol-free emollient cream
Afatinib	40 mg po qd until disease progression or development of intolerance	EGFR-TKI (exon 19 deletion or exon 21 substitution)	First-line for advanced NSCLC	Acneiform drug eruption, dry skin, rash, diarrhea, decreased appetite, stomatitis	Give 1 h before or 2 h after meal; report sores around mouth; report skin rashes; wear sunscreen or avoid sunlight; use alcohol-free emollient cream
Crizotinib	250 mg po bid until disease progression	ALK-TKI	*ALK*-positive NSCLC	Edema, diarrhea, constipation, N/V, vision disorders	Report symptoms of ILD or pneumonitis; report low HR; watch for symptoms of hepatotoxicity; avoid grapefruit or grapefruit juice; take missed dose ASAP (but if next dose is in <6 h, skip missed dose)

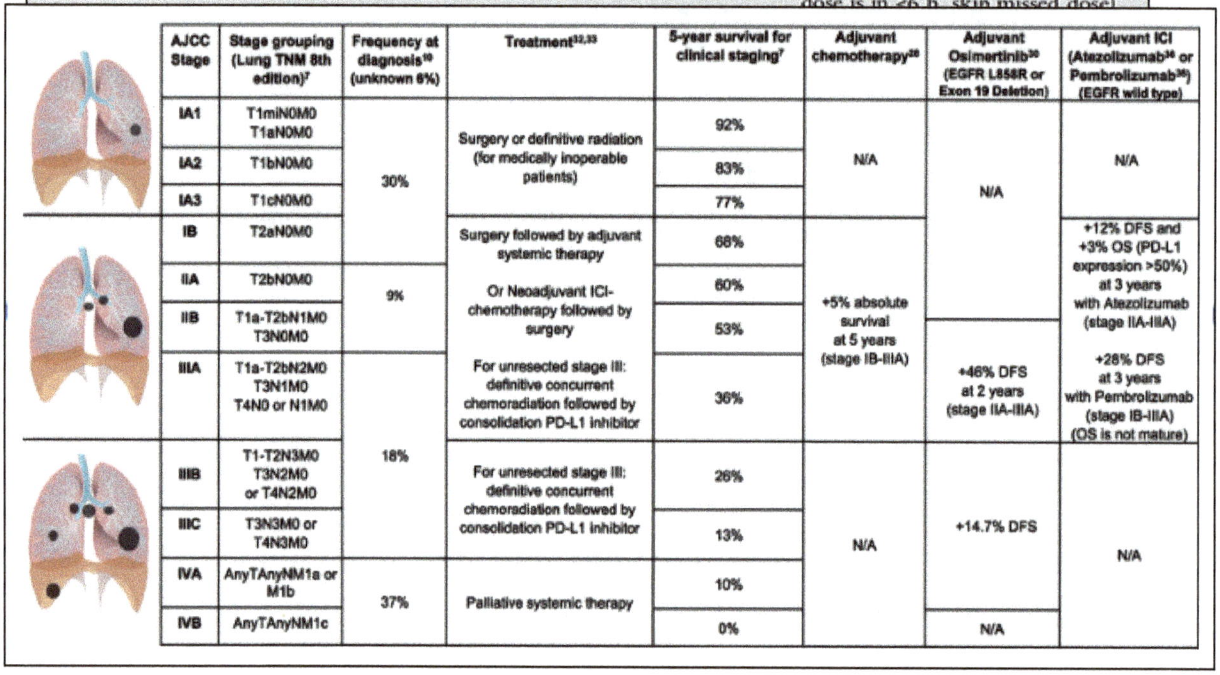

AJCC Stage	Stage grouping (Lung TNM 8th edition)[7]	Frequency at diagnosis[10] (unknown 6%)	Treatment[32,33]	5-year survival for clinical staging[7]	Adjuvant chemotherapy[28]	Adjuvant Osimertinib[30] (EGFR L858R or Exon 19 Deletion)	Adjuvant ICI (Atezolizumab[34] or Pembrolizumab[35]) (EGFR wild type)
IA1	T1miN0M0 T1aN0M0	30%	Surgery or definitive radiation (for medically inoperable patients)	92%	N/A	N/A	N/A
IA2	T1bN0M0			83%			
IA3	T1cN0M0			77%			
IB	T2aN0M0		Surgery followed by adjuvant systemic therapy Or Neoadjuvant ICI-chemotherapy followed by surgery	68%	+5% absolute survival at 5 years (stage IB-IIIA)		+12% DFS and +3% OS (PD-L1 expression >50%) at 3 years with Atezolizumab (stage IIA-IIIA) +28% DFS at 3 years with Pembrolizumab (stage IB-IIIA) (OS is not mature)
IIA	T2bN0M0	9%		60%			
IIB	T1a-T2bN1M0 T3N0M0			53%		+46% DFS at 2 years (stage IIA-IIIA)	
IIIA	T1a-T2bN2M0 T3N1M0 T4N0 or N1M0	18%	For unresected stage III: definitive concurrent chemoradiation followed by consolidation PD-L1 inhibitor	36%			
IIIB	T1-T2N3M0 T3N2M0 or T4N2M0		For unresected stage III: definitive concurrent chemoradiation followed by consolidation PD-L1 inhibitor	26%	N/A	+14.7% DFS	N/A
IIIC	T3N3M0 or T4N3M0			13%			
IVA	AnyTAnyNM1a or M1b	37%	Palliative systemic therapy	10%			
IVB	AnyTAnyNM1c			0%		N/A	

Figure 68 Stage Guided Treatment Strategy for NSCLC

3.3.9 Cystic Fibrosis

Cystic fibrosis is a hereditary condition involving the **respiratory, digestive and reproductive tracts,** in which the secretions become thick and **clog the respiratory passages** and other affected organs. Cystic fibrosis is **genetically inherited**, and it results from defects in the **CFTR gene**, which is still involved in the regulation of salt and water on the cell's membranes. Some of the **liber symptoms** include recurrent **cough with or without sputum production, shortness of breath/ breathlessness, recurrent lung infections, and diarrhoea/ poor growth and weight gain** due to malabsorption. Today, there are increased life expectancy of patients living with CF due to enhancements of their therapies in addressing issues such as **clearance of mucus, minimal risk of infections, and digestive issues**. New approaches in genetics in the form of precision medicine where a patient is treated based on specific genes have recorded positive progress in the disease. Nevertheless, the disease is chronic, so further studies are needed to enhance the treatment outcomes and identify the ways to cure the disease. The early detection and treatment of the disease as well as the required care need to be performed.

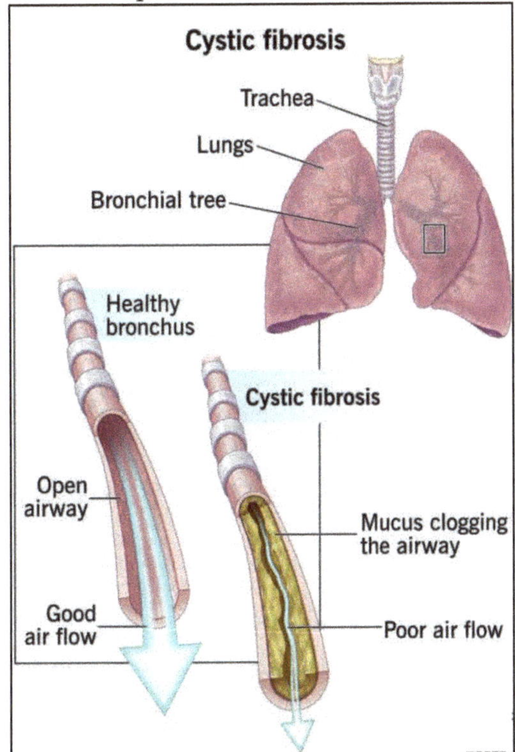

Figure 69 Cystic Fibrosis Comparison

The affected bronchus demonstrates the kind of damage caused by **cystic fibrosis (CF)** as compared to the **normal bronchus** (Figure 69). In a normal bronchus, there is no congestion and the passage is open to allow the free flow of air, thus one is able to breathe freely. However, in cystic fibrosis, **thick mucus forms in the airway and this causes obstruction**. This mucus accumulation leads to poor airflow and breathing issues due to the difficulty that it presents when breathing. This figure is designed to illustrate the effect of **CF on the bronchial tree;** more specifically, how the mucus build-up is a key characteristic of the disease and hinders breathing.

3.3.9.1 Cystic Fibrosis Transmembrane Conductance Regulator (CFTR) Mutations and Their Functional Defects

Figure 70 illustrates the six types of mutations in the CFTR gene and their defects in the function of the **CFTR protein,** which is used to transport chloride ions across the cell's membrane. In Class I, mutations such as **G542X result in the absence of CFTR** protein. Such mutations that lead to misfolding of the **CFTR protein include ΔF508** amongst others leading to failure of the protein to transport to the cell surface**. Class III mutations** including **V520F** enable the protein to get at the cell surface but it does not function well. As Class IV mutations, **R117H results in defective ion** conductance of the CFTR protein**. Class V mutation such as A455E** results in reduced biosynthesis of the CFTR protein while **Class VI mutation such as ΔF508** makes it to degradation after a short time. Some of the therapeutic strategies indicated in the table include: rescuing protein synthesis, halting the protein synthesis, repairing the structure of the protein assembled and stabilizing the normal protein structure.

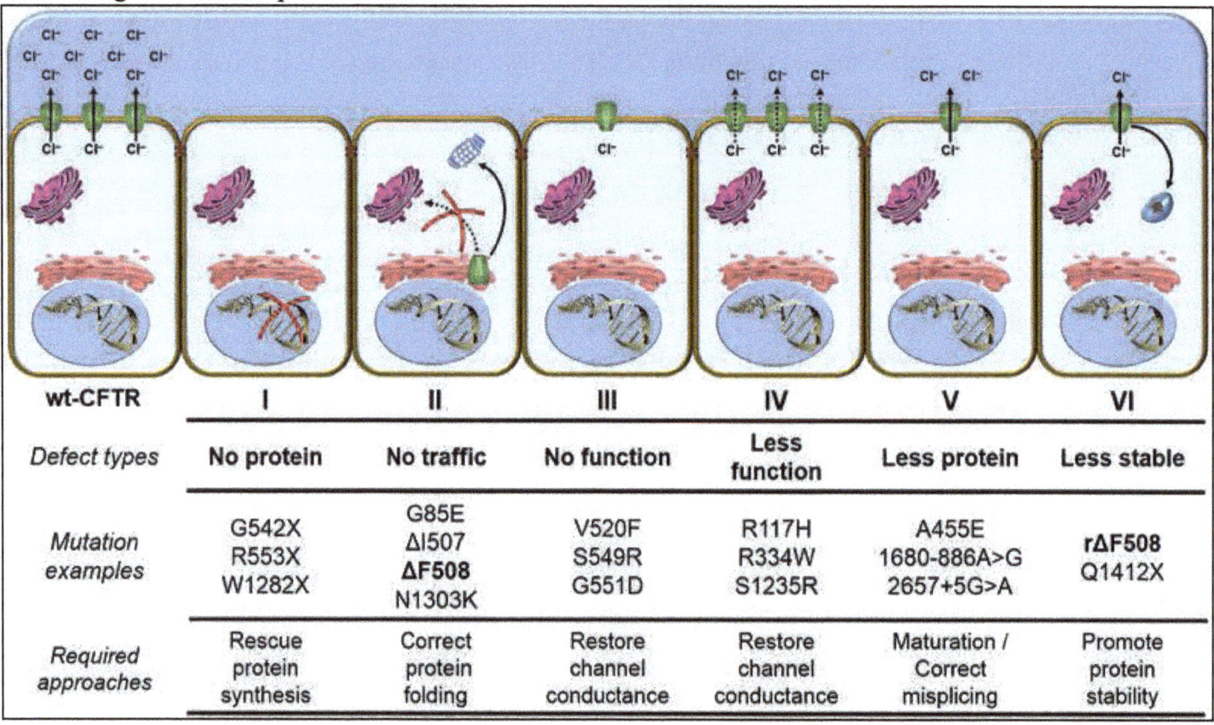

Cl⁻ Cl⁻ Cl⁻
wt-CFTR
I
II
III
IV
V
VI
Defect types
No protein
No traffic
No function
Less function
Less protein
Less stable
Mutation examples
G542X R553X W1282X
G85E ΔI507 ΔF508 N1303K
V520F S549R G551D
R117H R334W S1235R
A455E 1680-886A>G 2657+5G>A
rΔF508 Q1412X
Required approaches
Rescue protein synthesis
Correct protein folding
Restore channel conductance
Restore channel conductance
Maturation / Correct misplicing
Promote protein stability

Figure 70 CFTR Mutation Classes and Their Functional Implications

3.3.9.2 Diagnosis of Cystic Fibrosis

Cystic fibrosis is clinically identified by recurrent respiratory and digestive disorders, although there are genetic tests or sweat chloride concentration tests. There seems to be a **defect in a gene** known as the **CFTR gene, common in Chromosome 7**, which is known to be the primary cause of CF. The process of screening normally involves the measurement of immunoreactive trypsinogen in the **first few days of birth.** If positive, the next test carried out is called **the sweat test**, implemented by the use of pilocarpine to induce sweating and determination of chloride levels. High chloride levels indicate CF. For instance, diagnostic testing favours over **ninety per cent sensitivity and specificity in detecting common CFTR mutations.** Moreover, less **concentration of thiocyanate and hypothiocyanite in saliva and transepithelial potential difference** provides diagnostic significance. Nonetheless, newborn screening is employed commonly; however, the latter may present false-positive results since even carriers with normal genes for the CFTR can have increased levels of immunoreactive trypsinogen. Currently, all the states in the **United States of America and 21 countries in Europe** have enchased newborn screening programs for CF.

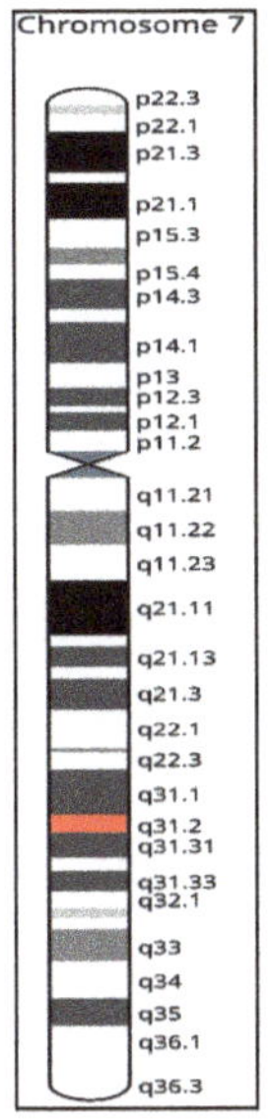

Figure 71 The location of the CFTR gene on chromosome 7

3.3.9.3 SOAP Notes for Cystic Fibrosis

Table 50 SOAP Notes for Cystic Fibrosis

Component	Details
Subjective (S)	The patient is a 28-year-old female with a history of cystic fibrosis (CF) diagnosed at age 2. She presents with a persistent cough, increased sputum production, and shortness of breath for the past month. She reports fatigue and a decrease in her exercise tolerance, stating that her usual physical activity has become more difficult. The patient has experienced a recent increase in lung infections, with more frequent antibiotic use in the past 3 months. She denies any recent weight loss, fever, or chest pain but notes that her appetite has decreased. Her family history is positive for CF, as both of her parents are carriers. She is currently adhering to her prescribed airway clearance techniques and taking pancreatic enzymes.
Objective (O)	On physical examination, the patient appears mildly distressed due to difficulty breathing. Vital signs are as follows: blood pressure 120/78 mmHg, heart rate 92 bpm, respiratory rate 20 bpm, and temperature 37.1°C (98.8°F). Respiratory examination reveals coarse crackles bilaterally, especially in the lower lobes, with occasional wheezing. There is mild clubbing of the fingers. Oxygen saturation is 94% on room air. Chest X-ray shows bilateral hyperinflation, with possible areas of consolidation in the right lower lobe. Pulmonary function tests reveal a significant decrease in forced expiratory volume (FEV1) with an FEV1/FVC ratio of 60%. The patient's serum chloride level is elevated, and her sputum culture shows growth of *Pseudomonas aeruginosa*.

Assessment (A)	The patient's symptoms, physical examination findings, and diagnostic tests are consistent with an exacerbation of cystic fibrosis. The presence of chronic lung infection, impaired pulmonary function, and elevated chloride levels support the diagnosis. The patient's condition may be worsening due to persistent bacterial colonization by *Pseudomonas aeruginosa*, which often contributes to CF exacerbations. Differential diagnoses include other chronic respiratory conditions like asthma or COPD, but these are less likely given the patient's known history of CF and the clinical presentation.
Plan (P)	The plan for the patient with cystic fibrosis will be multi-faceted, incorporating both pharmacological and non-pharmacological interventions. **Pharmacologically**, the patient will begin a course of broad-spectrum antibiotics, such as ciprofloxacin or meropenem, to target *Pseudomonas aeruginosa* and other possible respiratory pathogens, which are contributing to the current exacerbation. Additionally, inhaled bronchodilators, like albuterol, will be continued to relieve airway constriction, while corticosteroids will help reduce airway inflammation. The patient's pancreatic enzyme dosage will be adjusted if gastrointestinal symptoms or malabsorption become more pronounced, ensuring optimal digestion and nutrient absorption. **Non-pharmacologically**, the patient will be encouraged to adhere more strictly to airway clearance techniques, such as chest physiotherapy and vibrating vest therapy, to help clear mucus from the lungs and prevent further infections. Nutritional support will also be emphasized, with a focus on maintaining a high-calorie diet, and follow-up visits with a dietitian will be scheduled to monitor weight and nutritional status. If oxygen saturation drops below 92%, **oxygen therapy** will be introduced to ensure adequate oxygen levels during exertion or sleep. **Follow-up care** will include a check-up in 2 weeks to monitor progress, evaluate treatment response, and reassess lung function. The patient will also be referred to a specialized cystic fibrosis center for ongoing management and support. Finally, **genetic counseling** will be offered to discuss potential family planning, given the inherited nature of cystic fibrosis.

3.4 Moh Golden Points and Summary Question Answers

3.4.1 Moh Golden Points

Symptoms like persistent cough, weight loss, fatigue, and hemoptysis (coughing up blood) are key signs of lung cancer, especially in patients with a smoking history or occupational exposure.

NSCLC may involve surgery (for early stages), chemotherapy, radiation therapy, and increasingly, targeted therapies or immunotherapy, particularly for advanced or metastatic disease.

Lung cancer can be detected early through imaging (chest X-ray, CT scans), biopsy, and bronchoscopy, especially for patients with a smoking history or concerning symptoms like persistent cough, chest pain, or hemoptysis.

Lung cancer is primarily staged using the TNM system, which evaluates Tumor (T) size and location, Node (N) involvement, and Metastasis (M) to determine cancer extent and guide treatment.

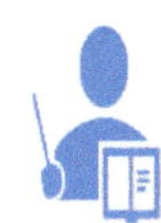

COPD is characterized by persistent airflow limitation and consists of chronic bronchitis and emphysema.

Emphysema, primarily caused by smoking, damages the alveoli and impairs gas exchange. It is classified into four types based on the location of damage within the pulmonary lobule: irregular, paraseptal, panacinar, and centrilobular.

3.4.2 Summary Questions & Answers

1. **What is the primary cause of Chronic Obstructive Pulmonary Disease (COPD)?**

A) Viral infections
B) Long-term exposure to tobacco smoke
C) Genetic factors only
D) Exposure to cold weather

2. **Which of the following is a key feature of emphysema in COPD?**

A) Persistent inflammation of airways without alveolar damage
B) Destruction of alveoli leading to reduced gas exchange
C) Increased mucus production without damage to alveoli
D) Bronchial inflammation and swelling

3. **What is the purpose of the Modified Medical Research Council Questionnaire (mMRC) in COPD assessment?**

A) To assess the patient's response to bronchodilators
B) To evaluate the intensity of the patient's breathlessness
C) To measure lung volume and airflow
D) To assess the frequency of COPD exacerbations

4. **According to the GOLD classification, which FEV1 value corresponds to Stage II COPD?**

A) FEV1 > 80%
B) FEV1 50-80% of the predicted value
C) FEV1 30-50% of the predicted value
D) FEV1 < 30% of the predicted value

5. **Which of the following conditions is the main cause of emphysema?**

A) Viral infections
B) Allergies
C) Exposure to cigarette smoke
D) Genetic disorders only

6. **In the assessment of asthma, which of the following defines Severe Persistent Asthma?**

A) Symptoms occurring less than twice a week
B) Symptoms occurring daily with FEV1 <60%
C) Symptoms occurring every other day with FEV1 >80%
D) Symptoms occurring only at night

7. **What is the first-line treatment for a moderate asthma exacerbation?**

A) Immediate intubation
B) Systemic corticosteroids
C) Short-acting bronchodilators (SABAs)
D) Long-term inhaled corticosteroids

8. **Which of the following is the primary staging system used for lung cancer?**

A) TNM Staging
B) ALTS Staging
C) BCLC Staging

D) ASA Staging

9. Which of the following is a hallmark symptom of pulmonary embolism (PE)?

A) Painless swelling of the limbs
B) Sudden onset of shortness of breath and chest pain
C) Severe headache and dizziness
D) Persistent cough with green sputum

10. What test is primarily used to confirm the diagnosis of Tuberculosis (TB)?

A) Complete blood count (CBC)
B) Sputum smear microscopy and culture
C) Chest X-ray only
D) ECG

3.4.3 Rationales

1. **Answer: B) Long-term exposure to tobacco smoke**

Rationale: COPD is primarily caused by long-term exposure to harmful substances like tobacco smoke. This leads to persistent inflammation of the airways and destruction of alveoli, which reduces lung function.

2. **Answer: B) Destruction of alveoli leading to reduced gas exchange**

Rationale: Emphysema, a key component of COPD, causes destruction of alveoli, reducing the surface area available for gas exchange, which leads to breathing difficulties.

3. **Answer: B) To evaluate the intensity of the patient's breathlessness**

Rationale: The mMRC is used to measure the severity of breathlessness in COPD patients, helping to determine the impact of the disease on their daily activities.

.

4. **Answer: B) FEV1 50-80% of the predicted value**

Rationale: GOLD Stage II COPD corresponds to moderate airflow limitation with FEV1 values ranging from 50-80% of the predicted value.

5. **Answer: C) Exposure to cigarette smoke**

Rationale: Emphysema is primarily caused by long-term exposure to harmful substances, such as cigarette smoke, which damages the alveoli and impairs gas exchange.

6. **Answer: B) Symptoms occurring daily with FEV1 <60%**

Rationale: Severe Persistent Asthma is characterized by daily symptoms, frequent nocturnal symptoms, FEV1 <60%, and significant limitations in daily activities.

7. **Answer: C) Short-acting bronchodilators (SABAs)**

Rationale: Short-acting bronchodilators (SABAs) are typically used as first-line treatment for moderate asthma exacerbations to relieve bronchospasm quickly.

8. **Answer: A) TNM Staging**

Rationale: The **TNM staging system** is the most widely used system for classifying the extent of lung cancer. It categorizes cancer based on **Tumor size**, **Node involvement**, and the presence of **Metastasis**.

9. **Answer: B) Sudden onset of shortness of breath and chest pain**

Rationale: Pulmonary embolism (PE) often presents suddenly with symptoms like shortness of breath, chest pain (often pleuritic), and sometimes hemoptysis due to blockage of pulmonary arteries.

10. **Answer: B) Sputum smear microscopy and culture**

Rationale: The diagnosis of **tuberculosis (TB)** is confirmed through **sputum smear microscopy** and **culture**, which help detect **Mycobacterium tuberculosis** bacteria. Chest X-rays are used to assess lung damage but are not definitive for TB.

4 Chapter 4: Gastrointestinal System

4.1 Anatomy and Physiology of Gastrointestinal (GIT) System

Figure 72 illustrates an **accurate representation** of the digestive anatomy of the human body and highlights the role played by various body parts in digesting the ingested food substances. Initiated in the oral cavity where the cartoon takes place and the food and **parotid, sublingual and submandibular saliva glands.** The tongue helps in shoving food to a particular backside of the mouth and the hard and soft palatal regions in mastication. It then descends through to the oropharynx and the **laryngopharynx and passes through the larynx to get to the oesophagus** where peristalsis carries it to the stomach. In the stomach, food continues to be ground or churned and crushed and further mixed with gastric juices causing the digestion of proteins to begin. The liver, gallbladder and pancreas secrete bile and digestive enzymes play a crucial role in the digestion of **fats, carbohydrates and proteins** the major site is the second part of the small intestine, also called the duodenum. The jejunum and ileum are the principal sites of absorption of nutrients such as **carbohydrates, fats, proteins, and vitamins that enter the bloodstream.** Substrate two gets into the large intestine and water with blowing and iron salts added further causes the movement of substrate two, while beneficial bacteria decompose a considerable portion of the unfermentable food. It then proceeds into the **ascending colon, transverse colon, descends in the descending colon** and finally into the **sigmoid colon prior to entering the rectum.** On the last note, the anus is also useful in the expulsion of faeces from the body. Especially, this detailed diagram presents major structures and organs participating in the digestion process, illustrating the main steps that include digestion, absorption and waste expulsion.

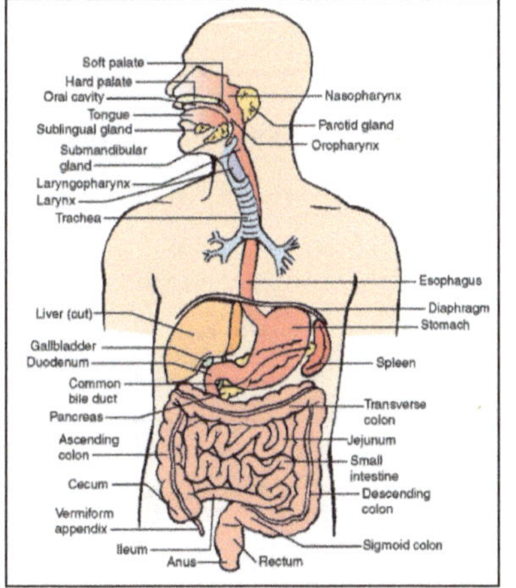

Figure 72 Anatomical Overview of GIT

The **GIT** is a physiological function which plays a significant role in the body through the process **of digestion, absorption and excretion of food substances** that people take. However, digestion starts even in the **mouth by chewing the food and enzymes** like amylase in the saliva that helps in breaking down **starchy foods.** Food is then passed onto the **oesophagus through the pharynx** and then the food is churned in the stomach through muscular contractions known as peristalsis. In the stomach, there is both **mechanical digestion** and **chemical digestion** of the food that has been taken in. **Swallowing churns** the food with stomach acids that are a combination of hydrochloric acid and an enzyme known as **pepsin that starts the digestion of protein**. It also has the role of neutralizing any pathogens that may have sneaked into the stomach through the ingested food. When the food has been **sufficiently chewed** it then moves to the small intestine where most digestion takes place as well as nutrient absorption. **Enzymes from the pancreas and bile from the liver** assist in the breakdown of fats, proteins, and carbohydrates. In digestion, through villi, the small intestine is able to absorb some nutrients including glucose, amino acids, fatty acids and vitamins. The large intestine mostly reabsorbs water and salts along with some **vitamins and pigments, and compaction of the rest forming the faeces.** There also resides good bacteria in the large intestine that aid in the digestion of certain parts of food and the **synthesis of vitamins such as K and B12.** Last but not least, the rectum holds formed faecal matter for a while until its defecation is conducted **through the anus**. During this process secretion, peristalsis, and absorption occur simultaneously so that food must be broken down, nutrients absorbed and at the same time wastes produced eliminated. The GIT also has equivalent responsibilities of defending the body against invaders such as bacteria, viruses, and toxins within its lining. Also, **the enteric nervous system, known as the second brain, controls most of these processes and controls the GIT function autonomously from the brain.**

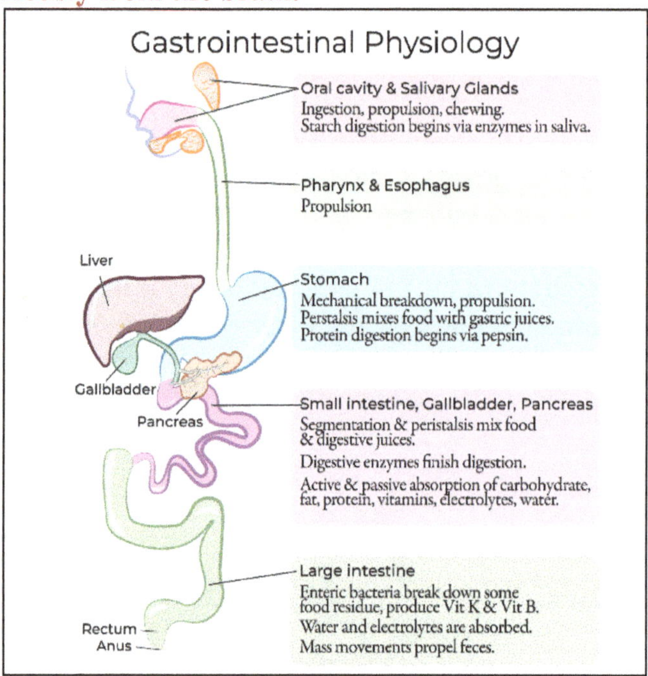

Figure 73 Physiology of GIT System

4.2 Common Gastrointestinal Tract Disorders

The mnemonic "**Good Intelligent Humans Prefer Clear Galloping, Foodful Appetites**" can be used, where each word corresponds to a different condition: **Good** stands for **Gastroesophageal Reflux Disease (GERD), Intelligent** represents **Irritable Bowel Syndrome (IBS) and Inflammatory Bowel Disease (IBD) Humans** refers to **Hepatitis**, **Prefer** helps recall **Peptic Ulcers**, **Clear** for **Celiac Disease**, **Galloping** stands for **Gallbladder Disease**, **Foodful** is for **Food Poisoning**, and **Appetites** represents **Appendicitis**. This mnemonic simplifies the process of recalling these gastrointestinal and liver disorders by linking each condition to a memorable word in the phrase.

Condition	Description	Key Symptoms	Diagnostic Tools	Treatment Options
Gastroesop hageal	A chronic digestive condition where	Heartburn, regurgitation,	Endoscopy, pH	Antacids, proton pump inhibitors

Reflux Disease (GERD)	stomach acid or bile irritates the food pipe lining.	chest pain, difficulty swallowing, cough	monitoring, Barium swallow, Esophageal manometry	(PPIs), H2-receptor antagonists, lifestyle changes, surgery (Nissen fundoplication)
Diverticulitis	Inflammation or infection of one or more diverticula in the colon, often related to low fiber diet.	Left lower abdominal pain, bloating, nausea, changes in bowel movements, fever (in severe cases)	CT scan, Colonoscopy, Abdominal X-ray, Laboratory tests (WBC count)	Antibiotics (e.g., Ciprofloxacin, Metronidazole), low-fiber diet initially, rest, in severe cases, surgery (resection or drainage)
Irritable Bowel Syndrome (IBS)	A functional gastrointestinal disorder causing abdominal discomfort, bloating, and changes in bowel habits.	Abdominal pain, bloating, diarrhea or constipation, mucus in stool	Clinical diagnosis, Rome criteria, Colonoscopy (to rule out other conditions)	Dietary changes (low FODMAP), antispasmodics, fiber supplements, probiotics, stress management
Inflammatory Bowel Disease (IBD)	Chronic inflammation of the gastrointestinal tract, including Crohn's disease and ulcerative colitis.	Abdominal pain, diarrhea, weight loss, fatigue, blood in stool	Colonoscopy, Blood tests (CRP, CBC), Stool tests (calprotectin)	Immunosuppressants (azathioprine), corticosteroids, biologics (TNF inhibitors), surgery
Hepatitis	Inflammation of the liver, often caused by viral infections (Hepatitis A, B, C) or alcohol.	Fatigue, jaundice, abdominal pain, nausea, dark urine, light-colored stool	Blood tests (liver enzymes, viral markers), Ultrasound, Liver biopsy	Antiviral medications (for Hepatitis B or C), corticosteroids (for autoimmune), lifestyle changes, liver transplant
Pancreatitis (chronic)	Inflammation of the pancreas that leads to long-term damage, often caused by alcohol abuse or gallstones.	Abdominal pain, nausea, vomiting, weight loss, fatty stools	Blood tests (amylase, lipase), CT scan, MRI, Endoscopic ultrasound	Enzyme replacement, pain management, avoiding alcohol, pancreatic surgery

Celiac disease	An autoimmune disorder where ingestion of gluten damages the small intestine lining.	Diarrhea, bloating, fatigue, weight loss, dermatitis herpetiformis, anemia	Blood tests (anti-tTG, anti-EMA), Endoscopy with biopsy	Strict lifelong gluten-free diet, nutritional support
Gallbladder disease	Includes conditions like gallstones or cholecystitis, where the gallbladder becomes inflamed or obstructed.	Abdominal pain (especially after eating fatty foods), nausea, vomiting, jaundice	Ultrasound, CT scan, HIDA scan	Gallbladder removal (cholecystectomy), medications for gallstone dissolution (ursodiol)
Gastroenteritis	Inflammation of the stomach and intestines, usually caused by viral or bacterial infections.	Diarrhea, vomiting, abdominal cramps, fever, dehydration	Stool tests (for pathogens), Blood tests, Ultrasound (in severe cases)	Hydration, antiemetics, antibiotics (for bacterial infections), probiotics
Diverticulitis				
Food poisoning	Illness caused by ingesting contaminated food, often due to bacteria, viruses, or toxins.	Nausea, vomiting, diarrhea, abdominal pain, fever	Stool culture, Blood tests (for dehydration, infection)	Hydration, rest, antibiotics (if bacterial), antidiarrheals (in some cases)
Appendicitis	Inflammation of the appendix, usually requiring surgical intervention.	Abdominal pain (starting around the navel and moving to the lower right abdomen), nausea, vomiting, fever	Physical exam, Blood tests (CBC), Ultrasound, CT scan	Appendectomy (surgical removal of the appendix)
Peptic ulcers	Sores that develop on the lining of the stomach, small intestine, or	Burning stomach pain, bloating, indigestion,	Endoscopy, Blood tests (H. pylori antibodies),	Antibiotics (for H. pylori), proton pump inhibitors (PPIs), H2-receptor

	esophagus, are often caused by H. pylori infection or prolonged NSAID use.	nausea, vomiting, blood in stool	Stool antigen test	antagonists, antacids

4.3 Major Medical Issues in Gastrointestinal Tract System

4.3.1 CHRONIC DISEASES

4.3.2 Gastroesophageal Reflux Disease (GERD)

Gastroesophageal reflux disease (GERD) is a condition that gives rise to symptoms such as **regurgitation, heartburn, chest pain, swallowing issues, sore throat, coughing, and shortness of breath** due to backflow of the stomach's content into the oesophagus. It can result in complications affecting the **oesophagus or pharynx to respiratory system**. Diagnosis of GERD is made clinically, through physical examination and with the help of tests which include **upper GI endoscopy, reflux test (wireless pH/pH impedance), oesophageal manometry and barium swallow.** Endoscopy of the upper part of the digestive tract enables the inspection of the **oesophagus, stomach, and a section of the duodenum** – the organ most significantly affected by *Helicobacter pylori* in most cases. Wearable pH monitoring continuously **tests the acid levels** for **48 hours and 24-hour impedance monitoring records** the reflux and its relation with the symptoms. Esophageal manometry entails probing the muscular tone and the function of the lower esophageal sphincter significant in surgical planning. It is useful in determining the narrowing of the **oesophagus and its motor function** by giving out a contrast material called **barium sulfate** to the patient for examination. These approaches help in the determination of the management and surgical approach to GERD.

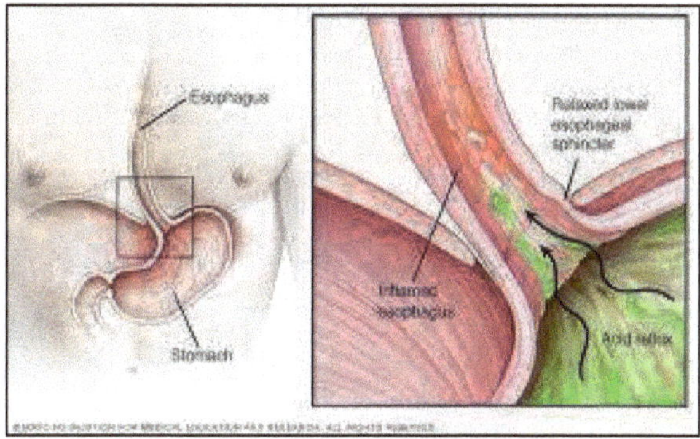

Figure 74 Overview of GERD

The picture given below highlights the problem area that is gastroesophageal reflux disease also known as GERD possibly due to its **acid peptic etiology.** On the left, there is an illustration of the **stomach and oesophagus with the area of the lower oesophagus** described where the reflux takes place. On the right, there is a view of a part of the lower oesophagus: **an inflamed oesophagus as a result of acid reflux.** The thin arrow points to a non-constricting lower **oesophagal sphincter (LES, orange colour),** which results to inflammation of the oesophagus through backward flow of stomach acid. Refluxed acid affects the lining of the oesophagus causing problems such as **heartburn, regurgitation and pain**. One of the significant causes of GERD is the relaxed LES, as it should prevent the flow of acid into the oesophagus. This image makes a considerable impact in relation to the focused topic by demonstrating the **physiological process of GRED,** whereby the reflux of acid causes inflammation and discomfort to the oesophagus.

4.3.2.1 Classification of GERD

Figure 75 helps to classify the different Esophageal Syndromes and Extraesophageal Syndromes linked to GERD. Esophageal Syndromes are classified into two forms: **the symptomatic form and the oesophagal injury form.** These are **Typical Reflux Syndrome**, which means they have the **general GERD symptoms** that include **heartburn and regurgitation, and Reflux Chest Pain Syndrome** in which chest pain is mistaken for that of heart disease due to acid reflux. **Oesophagal Injury Syndromes** are conditions resulting from exposure of the oesophagus to an acid; they include the medical conditions Reflux Esophagitis (inflammation affecting the oesophagus), Reflux Stricture (narrowing of the oesophagus which has been caused by scar tissue), **Barrett's Esophagus (pre-cancerous condition of the oesophagus) and Esophageal Adenocarcinoma**, cancer that affects the oesophagus. **Extraesophageal Syndromes** are defined as those conditions that are attributable to reflux but located outside the oesophagus and they fall under Two Classes, namely, the well-established associations where **Reflux Cough Syndrome, Reflux Laryngitis Syndrome, Reflux Asthma Syndrome, and Reflux Dental Erosion Syndrome** are contained and the yet proposed associations that include **Pharyngitis, Sinusitis, Idiopathic Pulmonary Fibrosis, and Recurrent Otitis Media** among others. This classification also shows all the symptoms and comorbidities related to GERD and its impact on both the oesophagus and other body organs.

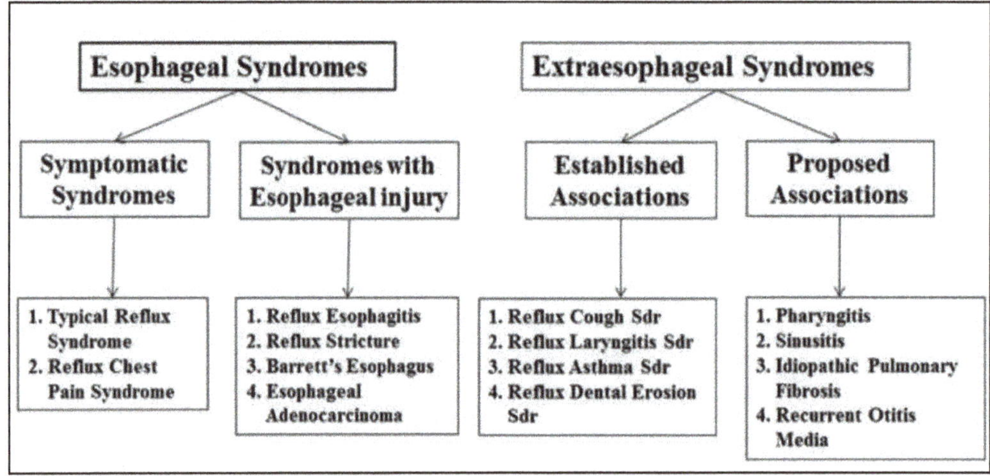

Figure 75 Classification of GERD

4.3.2.2 Comparative Analysis of Signs and Symptoms

This table shows the similarities of signs and symptoms in both adults and children suffering from GERD as well as the possible **complications, mouth symptoms, and risks such as Barrett's esophagus specific to adult patients.**

Table 51 Comparative Analysis Between Adults and Children

Category	Adults	Children/Babies
Common Symptoms	Acidic taste in the mouth, regurgitation, heartburn, pain with swallowing, sore throat, increased salivation (water brash), nausea, chest pain, coughing, globus sensation.	Repeated vomiting, effortless spitting up, coughing, respiratory issues (wheezing), crying, refusal to feed, failure to gain weight.

Less Common Symptoms	Chest pain, coughing, shortness of breath, asthma-like symptoms (wheezing), Globus sensation.	Inconsolable crying, crying for food and pulling off the bottle or breast, bad breath, burping.
Esophageal Injuries	Reflux esophagitis (inflammation, ulcers), oesophageal strictures (narrowing), Barrett's oesophagus (intestinal metaplasia), oesophageal adenocarcinoma (cancer).	N/A (though it may contribute to feeding and growth issues).
Larynx Injury	Laryngeal reflux (LPR) leads to throat problems like sore throat, and hoarseness.	N/A (however, symptoms like coughing and wheezing may occur).
Complications	Aspiration pneumonia, Barrett's oesophagus (risk of cancer).	GERD symptoms may improve by age 1 in most cases.
Mouth Symptoms	Tooth enamel erosion (breakdown), dry mouth, acid or burning sensation, bad breath, redness of the palate.	May show similar symptoms (tooth erosion) due to acid reflux into the mouth.
Barrett's Oesophagus Risk	High risk due to chronic GERD, leads to intestinal metaplasia and increases cancer risk.	N/A (Barrett's oesophagus is generally not a concern for infants).

4.3.2.3 Diagnostic Approach

Table 56 presents a **numerical rating system** that can be used to **evaluate the severity of GERD signs and symptoms.** The indicators for scoring are subdivided into **upper respiratory symptoms, local findings, gastrointestinal symptoms, comorbidity, and obesity.** Upper respiratory signs or complaints which also give an extra point when present include a **cough of more than two weeks duration, clearing the throat frequently, hoarseness, bad breath, redness of the throat lining, and vocal nodules.** Gastrointestinal symptoms consist of **nausea, gastric or epigastric pain; vomiting, and malnourishment** and any one of these adds to the score of 1. For comorbidities, asthma and in children recurrent laryngitis are assigned a point value of 1. For the obesity category, 1 point is added to the score if BMI is above the World Health Organization's growth reference median by 2 Standard deviations. The total sum refers to the GERD risk: **0-1 is a low risk, 2** represents moderate risk, and **3-4 is a high risk.** GERD is evaluated by determining the likelihood of the presence of symptoms and risk factors about the disease from the patient's case.

Table 52 Gastroesophageal reflux disease (GERD) diagnostic probability scoring tool

Upper respiratory symptoms and local findings (oropharyngoscopy and nasal fiber optic laryngoscopy)	Chronic cough Chronic throat clearing Dysphonia Halitosis Oropharyngeal redness and granulation Posterior laryngitis Vocal nodules	If present +1
Gastrointestinal symptoms	Nausea Gastric or epigastric pain Vomiting Malnourishment	If present +1
Comorbidity	Asthma Recurrent laryngitis	If present +1
Obesity	Body-mass index > 2 standard deviations above the World Health Organization growth reference median	If present +1
Score	**Low GERD risk: 0/1 points** **Moderate GERD risk: 2 points** **High GERD risk: 3-4 points**	**Total** ______

4.3.2.4 SOAP Notes for GERD

Component	Details
Subjective (S)	The patient is a 45-year-old male who presents with a 6-month history of frequent heartburn, acid regurgitation, and a sour taste in the mouth. The symptoms occur primarily after meals and are often worse when lying down. The patient also reports chronic throat clearing, occasional hoarseness, and mild chest discomfort, especially after eating spicy foods. He denies dysphagia but reports mild nausea and occasional coughing, particularly at night. The patient has a history of asthma, and symptoms sometimes exacerbate during an asthma attack. He is concerned that his condition might be linked to his chronic heartburn. He has tried over-the-counter antacids with partial relief. His family history is notable for GERD and oesophagal cancer in his father.
Objective (O)	On physical examination, the patient's vital signs are stable: blood pressure 130/80 mmHg, heart rate 82 bpm, respiratory rate 18 bpm, temperature 36.9°C (98.4°F). The patient appears generally well with no obvious distress. A thorough oropharyngeal examination reveals mild redness in the posterior pharynx but no visible lesions. There is no abnormality in the lungs upon auscultation, though slight wheezing is noted on forced exhalation. Abdominal examination is unremarkable, with no tenderness or hepatomegaly. His BMI is 30, indicating mild obesity. A review of the patient's medication history reveals he is currently taking an inhaler for asthma and occasionally uses over-the-counter antacids.

Assessment (A)	The patient's symptoms, including heartburn, acid regurgitation, and throat irritation, are consistent with gastroesophageal reflux disease (GERD). His BMI and family history increase his risk for chronic GERD and complications, such as Barrett's Oesophagus. Additionally, the patient's history of asthma may exacerbate reflux symptoms, as asthma can worsen GERD. The patient may also be experiencing mild laryngopharyngeal reflux (LPR), given his chronic throat clearing and hoarseness. Given the duration and severity of symptoms, it is important to evaluate for potential oesophagal injury.
Plan (P)	**Pharmacological**: Start a proton pump inhibitor (PPI), such as omeprazole 20 mg daily before breakfast, to reduce gastric acid production. Recommend over-the-counter H2 receptor antagonists (ranitidine) for breakthrough symptoms. Consider adding a prokinetic agent if symptoms persist despite PPI therapy (See algorithm and table below). **Lifestyle modifications**: Encourage the patient to avoid large, fatty meals and spicy foods that may trigger symptoms. Advise weight loss through a healthy diet and exercise regimen, aiming for a BMI reduction to below 25. Recommend elevating the head of the bed to reduce nighttime reflux and avoid lying down for at least 2-3 hours after meals. **Referral and follow-up**: Refer for upper endoscopy (EGD) to evaluate for potential oesophagal damage (e.g., reflux esophagitis, Barrett's oesophagus). Follow-up appointment in 4-6 weeks to assess treatment response and adjust medications as needed. Encourage regular asthma management to help control symptoms and reduce the potential for GERD exacerbations. **Patient education**: Educate the patient on the nature of GERD, potential complications, and the importance of adhering to prescribed medications and lifestyle changes to manage symptoms and prevent complications.

Table 53 Dosage Recommendations for Treatment of GERD

Medication	Recommended Daily Dose	Recommended Administration Frequency	Common Side Effects
Histamine$_2$-Receptor Antagonists (H2RAs)[a,b]			
Ranitidine	150 mg 300 mg	Twice daily At bedtime	Headache, diarrhea, thrombocytopenia
Famotidine	20 mg	Twice daily × 6 wk	
Cimetidine	400 mg 800 mg	4 times daily × 12 wk Twice daily × 12 wk	
Nizatidine	150 mg	Twice daily	
Proton Pump Inhibitors (PPIs)			
Pantoprazole Lansoprazole[b] Esomeprazole[b] Omeprazole[b] Rabeprazole Dexlansoprazole	20-40 mg 15-30 mg 20-40 mg 20-40 mg 20 mg 30-60 mg	All agents are given once daily up to 8 wk Recurrence may require an additional 4-8 wk Max dose of PPIs can be given twice daily	Pneumonia, electrolyte disturbances (e.g., magnesium), infections, *Clostridium difficile*-associated diarrhea, bone fractures, renal impairment, dementia, rebound gastritis
Miscellaneous Agents			
Metoclopramide	10-15 mg	2-4 times a day (single doses of 20 mg have been used as an alternative)	Drowsiness, agitation, irritability, depression, dystonic reactions, tardive dyskinesia
Baclofen	5-20 mg	3 times daily	Dizziness, somnolence, constipation
Melatonin[b]	3-6 mg	Daily at bedtime	Somnolence

[a] Requires renal adjustment. [b] Available OTC.
GERD: gastroesophageal reflux disease; max: maximum. Source: References 5, 7, 8.

Table 54 Algorithm for the Treatment of GERD

Category	Subcategory	Details
Pharmacologic Treatment	Antacids	Used for intermittent heartburn; effective for mild symptoms.
	H2-Blockers	Drugs like cimetidine, ranitidine, etc., used for 6-week trials in patients with mild to moderate esophagitis.
	Prokinetic Agents	Metoclopramide, cisapride; used if H2-blockers are ineffective; not recommended for long-term use due to safety and cost.
	Omeprazole (PPI)	First-line for severe erosive esophagitis; 20-40 mg daily for 8 weeks; highly effective in healing.
	Long-Term Omeprazole	For refractory or relapsing cases; may require higher doses for up to 12 weeks; potential long-term safety concerns.
Non-Pharmacologic Techniques	Eliminate Acid-Increasing Agents	Avoid coffee, fatty foods, and narcotics.

	Lifestyle Modifications	Weight loss, elevation of the head of the bed, avoid eating before bedtime.
	Avoid Drugs Worsening GERD	Discontinue anticholinergic drugs, antispasmodics, tricyclic antidepressants, and other medications that lower LES pressure.
Treatment for Severe Cases	Omeprazole for Severe Esophagitis	Omeprazole is effective in severe erosive esophagitis with an 80% healing rate.
	High Dose Omeprazole for Refractory Cases	Refractory patients may require doses up to 12 weeks for complete healing.
Concerns and Risks of Long-Term Use	Chronic Hypochlorhydria	Risks include gastric bacterial overgrowth, vitamin B12 deficiency, and benign gastric polyps.
	Genetic Factors	Some individuals (5% of Caucasians, and 20% of Orientals) may have higher plasma concentrations, increasing risks.

4.3.3 Inflammatory Bowel Disease (IBD)

IBD stands for **Inflammatory Bowel Disease** and is a group of diseases that cause inflammation in the GI tract which may lead to symptoms including **stomach pains, frequent bowel movements, fatigue, and weight loss**. Patients diagnosed with IBD are regarded to have an **abnormal response to stimuli** in their environment that causes inflammation. These include diet, smoking and infections since they are known causes of the diseases. The signs of **IBD vary from mild and severe** depending on the type and they include; **Diarrhoea with blood, and occasionally mucus in UC, abdominal pain and cramping, extreme fatigue and unwarranted weight loss**. In severe cases, possible complications may include **malnutrition and bowel perforation,** as well as an increased risk of developing **colorectal cancer** if the person has a long-standing history of **Crohn's disease**. A physical examination and medical history assessment together with blood tests that include **faecal calprotectin, endoscopic procedures, which may include colonoscopy or flexible sigmoidoscopy** to assess the disease location and severity and biopsy, CT scans, and MRIs in some cases may be used to diagnose IBD. Treatment of IBD is based on **anti-inflammatory therapy,** therapy of the exacerbations, and prevention of mucosal relapses. There are several medicines that patients use to treat the disease; some of them are **aminosalicylates, corticosteroids, and immunosuppressive agents**, while biological therapies including **TNF inhibitors like infliximab and adalimumab** are given to patients with moderate to severe UC. Other cases could warrant surgery for instance in situations where the patient fails to respond to drugs and may develop complications such as bowel perforation and obstruction. Palliation also involves the provision of adequate nutrition in order to prevent the development of malnutrition, **especially in children or those patients with weight loss**. IBD is a chronic disease for which **constant vigil** should be developed and in its complications such as colorectal cancer. As of today, there is no known cure for IBD, however, with the help of new therapies, especially biologic medications, a great many of the patients with this disease can live quite comfortably.

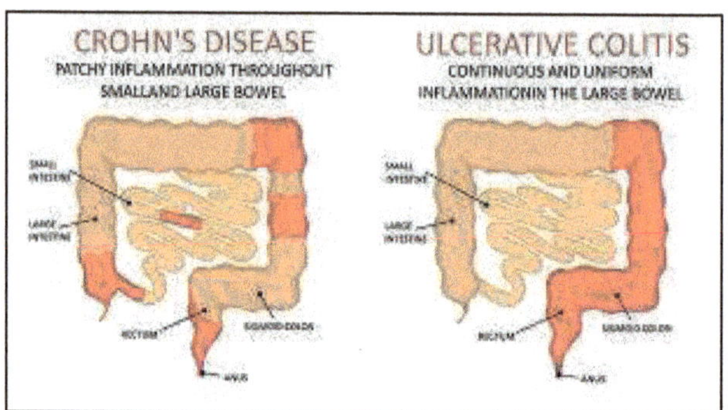

Figure 76 Inflammatory Bowel Disorder

4.3.3.1 Types of IBD

The two main classifications of IBD are **Crohn's disease and ulcerative colitis**. Crohn's disease affects any part of the gastrointestinal tract and the most typical with localization in the small intestine and the colon and with inflammation of all the layers of the bowel wall. This also results in **transmural inflammation** which means that bacteria penetrates through all the layers of the bowel wall and this brings complications such as structuring, fistulation and formation of abscesses. In contrast to Crohn's disease, **Ulcerative colitis** commonly occurs in the colon and rectum whereby the colon's inner lining realizes inflammation and ulceration. The specific origin of IBD is still not clear; however, it involves both **genetic and immunologic susceptibility** to the bowel disease. Figure 76 contrasts IBD, which are **Crohn's disease and ulcerative colitis** whereby the former affects any section of the GI tract in a transmural pattern while the latter affects the colon and ileum only in a superficial manner. Crohn's disease may occur in any section of the gastrointestinal tract with symptoms producing **transmural inflammation** affecting the layer of the bowel wall. Depending on the site this variant is specifically referred to as IBS, which is the abbreviation for **'ileal brake'**; this type of IBD is most often observed in the small intestine and sections of the large intestine. The current image intends to explain that Crohn's disease may lead to such complications as strictures and fistulas. On the other hand, **UC is limited to the colon and rectum** in which there is continuous **inflammation and ulceration of the mucosa**. Such characteristics are also identifiable in terms of categories as shown by the diagram that highlights areas of ulcerations and inflamed tissue expected of ulcerative colitis. Although both conditions develop into chronic ones, it is necessary to understand that there are some differences, which mainly refer to the way the **inflamed tissues** are affected.

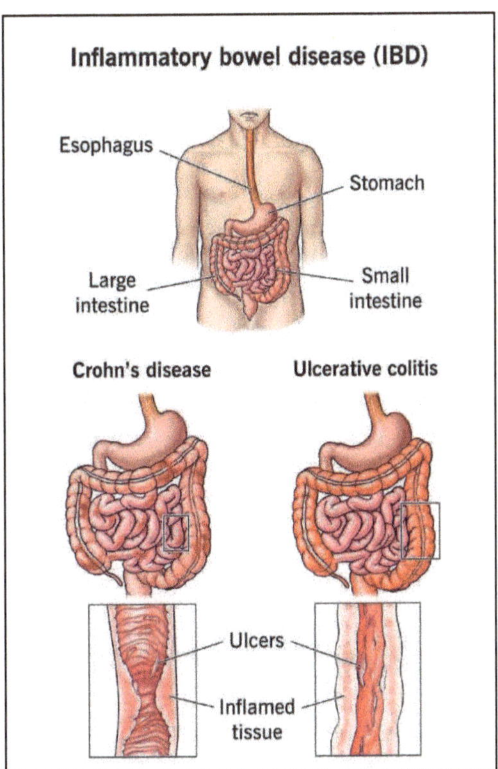

Figure 77 Comparison Between Crohn's Disease and Ulcerative Colitis

4.3.3.2 Classification of Crohn's Disease

The figure highlights the form and types of Crohn's Disease, along with diagnostic markers and pathologic manifestations. The classification of Crohn's disease based on the **site of involvement includes terminal ileal form**, which typically affects the **terminal part of the small intestine** that is referred to as ileum and the cecum, **small bowel types** like ileitis and jejunoileitis, colonic Crohn's colitis affecting the colon only**, gastroduodenal type** where the disease affects the stomach and the duodenum, perianal type that affects the region around the anus and the oral **Crohn's disease type** that has manifestations in the oral cavity in form of lesions or ulcers. The clinical manifestations of Crohn's disease include **rectal bleeding, diarrhea, abdominal pain, tenesmus, mouth ulcers, anemia, and weight loss.** Mucosal characteristics involves disappearance of **normal mucosal vessels, erythema, cobblestoning due to ulcers or erosions, spontaneous bleeding, and mucosal friability**. Pathological factors include **Crypt distortion, Crypt abscesses, shortening of crypts, infiltration of leukocytes in the lamina propria, Fistulas, and perianal changes.** These combine aspects are important tools for diagnosing this illness from other illnesses affecting the gastrointestinal tract.

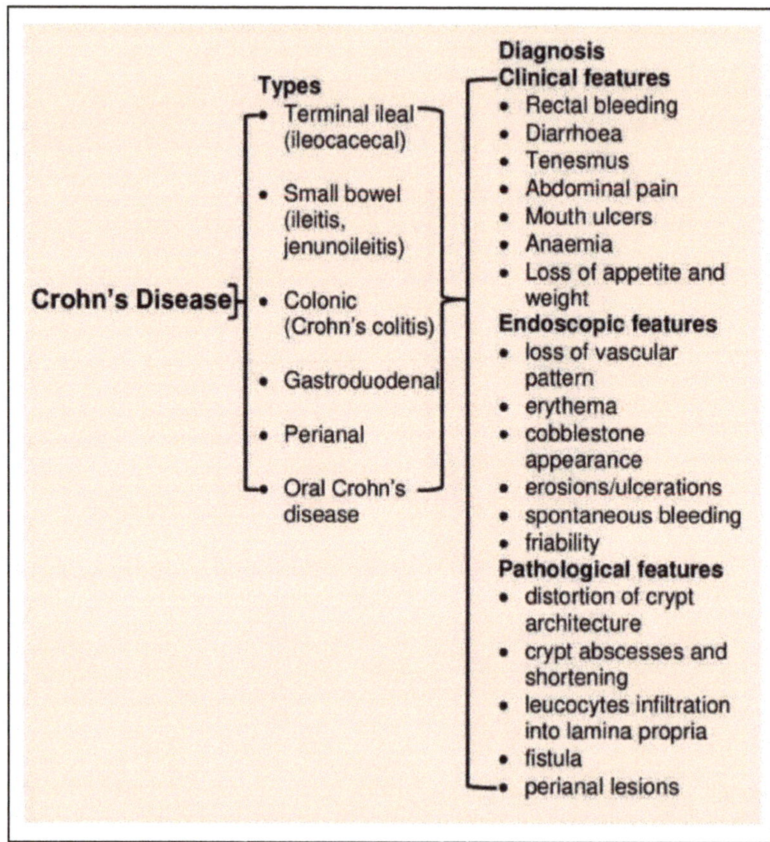

Figure 78 Classification of Crohn's Disease

4.3.3.3 Classification of Ulcerative Colitis

Figure 78 systematically outlines **Ulcerative Colitis, including types, clinical features, endoscopy, and pathology**. Ulcerative colitis can be divided into three groups; **proctitis** which affects only the rectum; **left-sided or distal colitis** which affects the left side of the colon inclusive of the descending and sigmoid; **and total colitis**, pancolitis or extensive colitis which affects the whole colon extending from the rectum to the cecum. It is achieved by several signs and symptoms which include **rectal bleeding, urgency, diarrhoea, tenesmus, abdominal cramps, fever, loss of appetite and weight loss**. Some of the endoscopic signs include changes in colouration (erythema), loss of normal mucus membrane vascular pattern, change in the surface texture (granularity), erosions or ulcers and spontaneous haemorrhage. These include **crypt architectural disruption, presence of crypt abscesses and shortening, infiltration of leukocytes to the lamina propria, secretive mucus depletion, presence of lymphoid aggregates, and ulcerations/erosions.** These along with clinical, endoscopic, and pathological features facilitate the exclusion of other diseases and to make a diagnosis of UC.

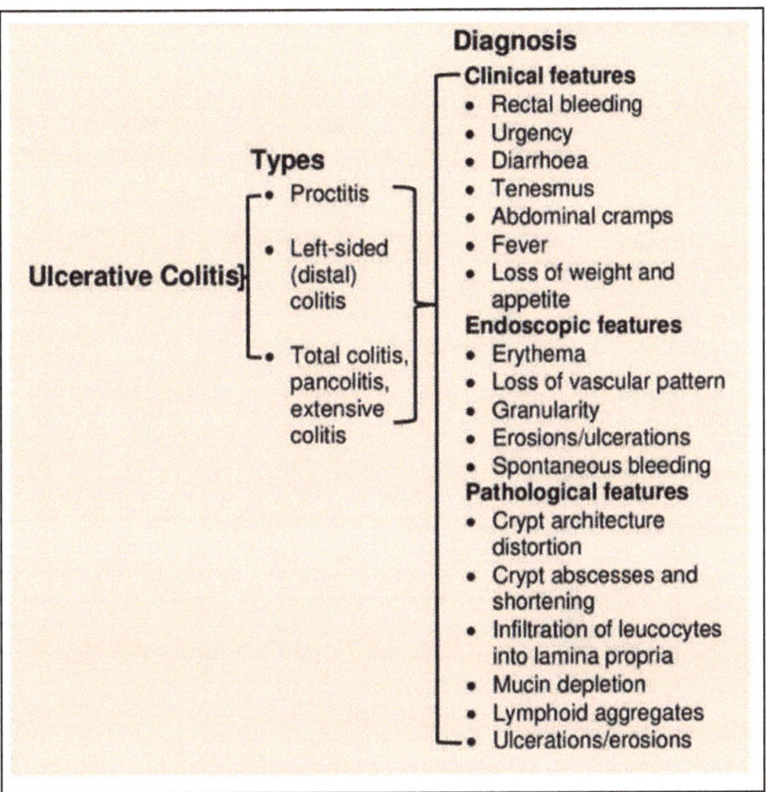

Figure 79 Classification of Ulcerative Colitis

4.3.3.4 SOAP Notes for IBD

Table 55 SOAP Notes for IBD

Component	Details
Subjective (S)	The patient is a 35-year-old male presenting with a 2-month history of persistent diarrhea, abdominal pain, and fatigue. He reports experiencing crampy abdominal pain, particularly in the lower abdomen, which is relieved after bowel movements. He has noticed blood in his stool over the past week, accompanied by mucus. The patient has unintentionally lost 5 kg in the past month and feels generally fatigued. His symptoms have been affecting his daily activities, and he is concerned about a possible underlying gastrointestinal condition. The patient has no history of recent infections or travel. His family history includes a father with a history of colorectal cancer and an uncle diagnosed with Crohn's disease. He denies fever, nausea, or vomiting.
Objective (O)	On physical examination, the patient appears mildly fatigued but is in no acute distress. Vital signs are stable: blood pressure 125/80 mmHg, heart rate 88 bpm, respiratory rate 16 bpm, and temperature 37.0°C (98.6°F). Abdominal examination reveals mild tenderness in the lower quadrants, particularly on the left side, with no guarding or rebound tenderness. Bowel sounds are hyperactive. Rectal examination reveals no abnormalities, but the patient reports discomfort with the exam. A stool sample is positive for blood and mucus. Laboratory tests show mild anemia (hemoglobin 11.2 g/dL) and

	elevated C-reactive protein (CRP), suggesting inflammation. Stool studies rule out infectious causes.
Assessment (A)	The patient's symptoms, including intermittent abdominal pain, bloating, alternating diarrhoea and constipation, are consistent with **Irritable Bowel Syndrome (IBS)**. The absence of alarming signs such as blood in the stool, weight loss, or anaemia supports this diagnosis. The patient's symptoms are likely exacerbated by stress, as is common with IBS. There is no indication of organic disease, and the normal laboratory and physical findings help rule out other gastrointestinal conditions. The diagnosis is based on the Rome IV criteria for IBS, which focuses on recurrent abdominal pain and altered bowel habits.
Plan (P)	**Diagnostic Workup**: **Colonoscopy** to assess the extent of colonic involvement and obtain biopsies for histopathological confirmation of ulcerative colitis or Crohn's disease. Stool cultures to rule out infectious causes, though this has already been done. Blood tests to monitor for anaemia, liver function, and markers of inflammation (e.g., CRP, ESR). **Pharmacological Treatment**: Start aminosalicylates (e.g., mesalamine) for anti-inflammatory effects in the colon. Corticosteroids (e.g., prednisone) may be prescribed for short-term flare management, depending on the colonoscopy results. If diagnosed with ulcerative colitis or Crohn's disease, consider immunosuppressive agents (e.g., azathioprine) for long-term control (See algorithms below). **Nutritional Support**: Refer to a dietitian for nutrition counselling, especially if malnutrition is a concern. Advise a low-residue diet during flare-ups to reduce bowel irritation. Follow-up: Schedule a follow-up visit in 1-2 weeks to review colonoscopy results, adjust medication, and assess response to treatment. Monitor for complications such as malnutrition, dehydration, or signs of infection. **Patient Education**: Educate the patient about IBD, emphasizing the importance of medication adherence to control inflammation and prevent flare-ups. Discuss lifestyle modifications, including stress management techniques, and the importance of avoiding triggers like certain foods (e.g., spicy or fatty foods). Inform the patient about the chronic nature of the disease and the need for ongoing follow-up and monitoring to manage symptoms and prevent complications.

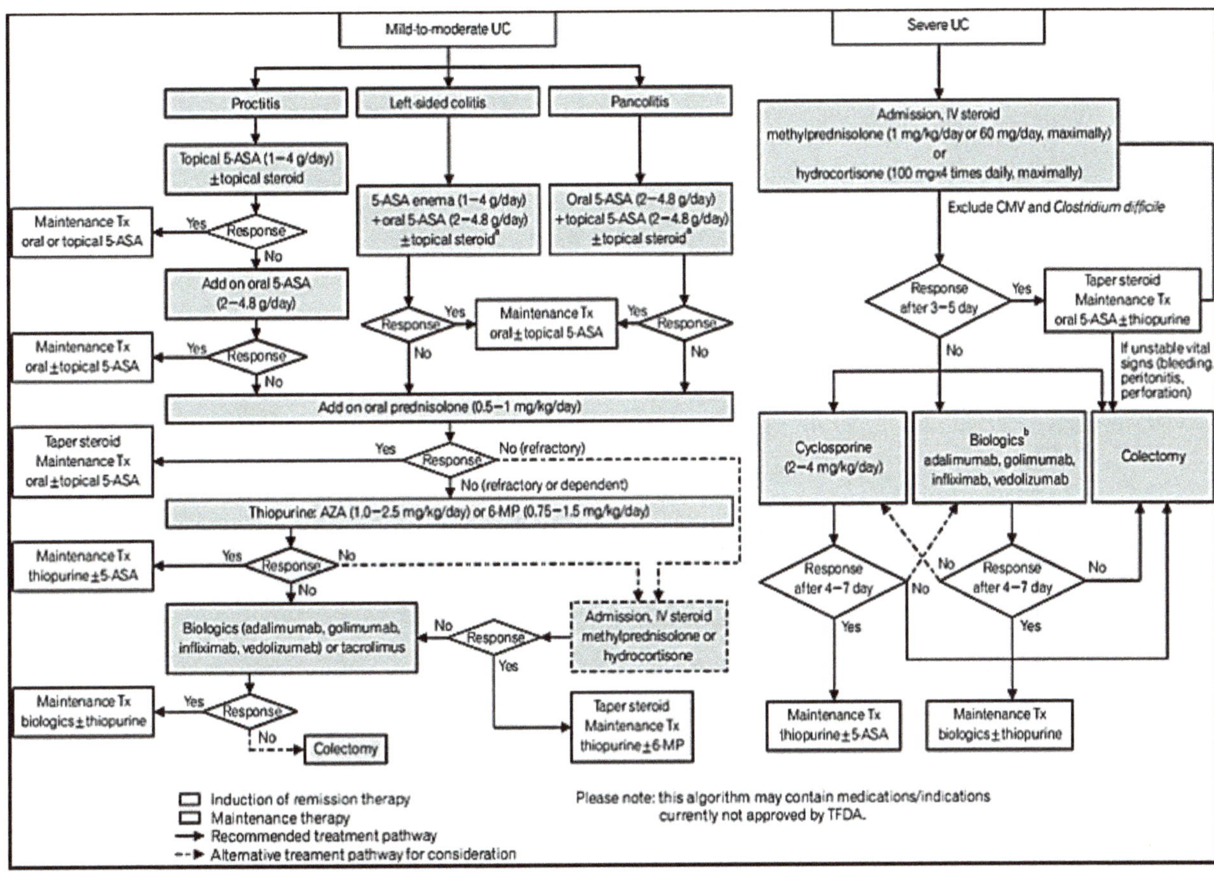
Mild-to-moderate UC
Severe UC
Proctitis
Left-sided colitis
Pancolitis
Topical 5-ASA (1–4 g/day) ±topical steroid
5-ASA enema (1–4 g/day) +oral 5-ASA (2–4.8 g/day) ±topical steroid[a]
Oral 5-ASA (2–4.8 g/day) +topical 5-ASA (2–4.8 g/day) ±topical steroid[a]
Admission, IV steroid methylprednisolone (1 mg/kg/day or 60 mg/day, maximally) or hydrocortisone (100 mgx4 times daily, maximally)
Exclude CMV and Clostridium difficile
Maintenance Tx oral or topical 5-ASA
Response
Yes
No
Add on oral 5-ASA (2–4.8 g/day)
Maintenance Tx oral ± topical 5-ASA
Response after 3–5 day
Taper steroid Maintenance Tx oral 5-ASA ± thiopurine
If unstable vital signs (bleeding, peritonitis, perforation)
Add on oral prednisolone (0.5–1 mg/kg/day)
Taper steroid Maintenance Tx oral ± topical 5-ASA
No (refractory)
No (refractory or dependent)
Thiopurine: AZA (1.0–2.5 mg/kg/day) or 6-MP (0.75–1.5 mg/kg/day)
Cyclosporine (2–4 mg/kg/day)
Biologics[b] adalimumab, golimumab, infliximab, vedolizumab
Colectomy
Maintenance Tx thiopurine ± 5-ASA
Response after 4–7 day
Biologics (adalimumab, golimumab, infliximab, vedolizumab) or tacrolimus
Admission, IV steroid methylprednisolone or hydrocortisone
Maintenance Tx biologics ± thiopurine
Taper steroid Maintenance Tx thiopurine ± 6-MP
Colectomy
Maintenance Tx thiopurine ± 5-ASA
Maintenance Tx biologics ± thiopurine
Induction of remission therapy
Maintenance therapy
Recommended treatment pathway
Alternative treament pathway for consideration
Please note: this algorithm may contain medications/indications currently not approved by TFDA.

Figure 80 Algorithm for the Management of Ulcerative Colitis

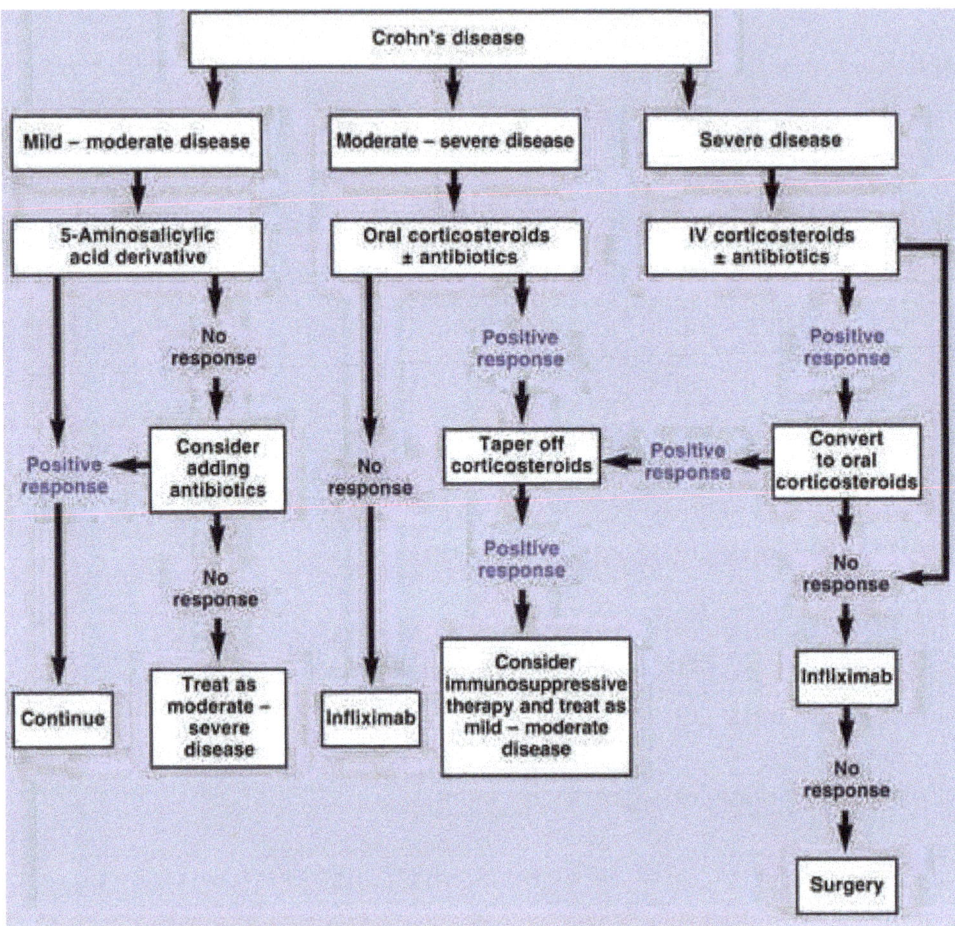

Figure 81 Algorithm for the Treatment of Crohn's Disease

4.3.4 Irritable Bowel Syndrome (IBS)

Irritable bowel Syndrome (IBS) is a type of digestive system disease that presents symptoms like **abdominal pain and discomfort with the change of bowel habits**, which may include **diarrhoea, constipation or both.** It has not been determined what causes IBS, but there is an understanding that it may involve factors like; **muscle contractions, hypersensitivity to pain, and the signals** which originate from the **gastrointestinal tract and are transmitted to the brain** and vice versa. Stress and some types of foods also trigger the symptoms of this condition in some men. Some of the signs and manifestations of IBS include **abdominal swelling, stomach aches or pains, excessive belching, and a feeling that the bowels have not been emptied properly**. More so, the diagnosis of IBS is mostly done by ruling out other probable gastrointestinal conditions because of the absence of an actual test. Treatment of IBS includes an alteration of diet, including a low **FODMAP diet, stress reduction, and pharmacological therapy** including **antispastic agents, laxatives or Diarrheal** depending on the subtype of IBS. IBS is a long-term condition but effects such as **stomach ache, bloating and diarrhoea** can be controlled through changes in diet and using medication.

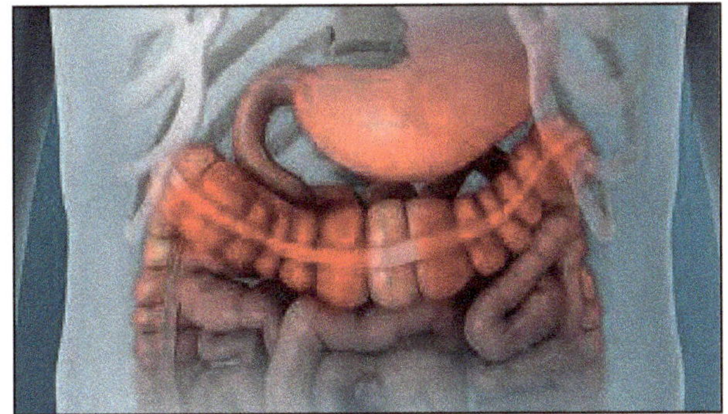

Figure 82 Irritable Bowel Syndrome

4.3.4.1 Subtypes of IBS

Figure 76 describes a classification system for IBS by using the **Bristol Stool Form Scale,** which points out the **degree of consistency of bowel movements**. The figure represents the ratio of the number of people who had hard or lumpy stools alongside those who had loose or watery stools. On the vertical axis, the scale of hard or lumpy stool is measured in percentage and so is the scale of loose or watery stool on the horizontal axis. **IBS-C (Constipation predominantly)** indicates a condition where constipation is dominant, the patient scores more than 25% of bowel movements **hard or lumpy (Briscoe type 1 and 2). IBS-D (Diarrhea predominant)** can be described by the percentage of bowel movements which is greater than 25% of loose and watery stools in the **Bristol types 6 and 7. IBS-M (Mixed) is** the consistency where the irregular bowel movements are both lumpy and watery at different times. **IBS-U (Unclassified)** occurs when there is an inability of the stool forms to conform to any of the above-mentioned categories. The 25% percentage is used in establishing the dominant stool form to categorise the subtypes of IBS.

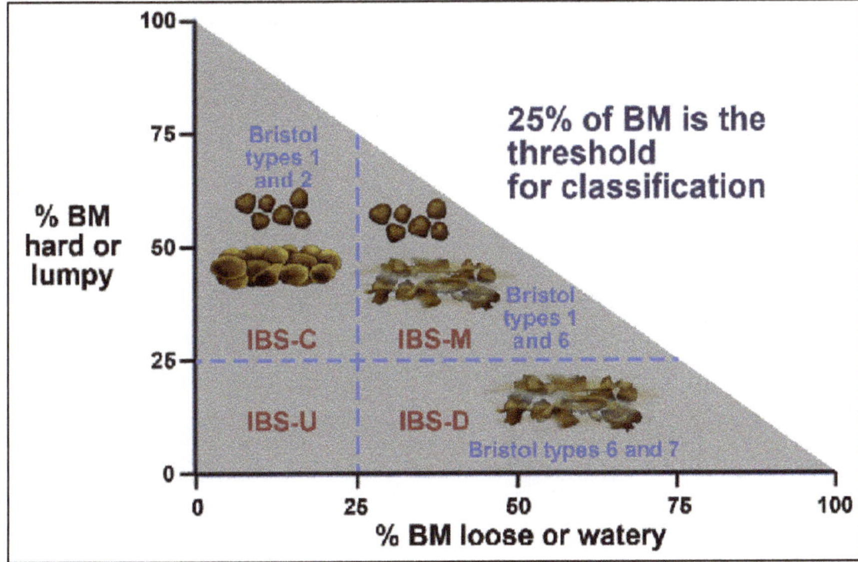

Figure 83 Sub Types of IBS

4.3.4.2 Difference Between IBS and IBD

Specifically, the image illustrates an overlapping of some features between IBD and IBS, although, the two can be different diseases. **IBD involves diseases that bring about inflammation in the gastrointestinal tracts** and therefore result in **structural changes, alterations in nutrient absorption and the likelihood of one developing colorectal cancer.** It may be inherited, though most likely, it will necessitate medical intervention throughout the life of the affected people. While IBD refers to **Inflammatory bowel disease which affects the lining of the**

gastrointestinal tract, IBS is a form of **functional bowel disorder (FBD)** which does not have an impact on the structure of the tissues. It is actually more common than IBD and is more involved with the role of nutrition. IBS does not have any specific pathological tests that would be used in the diagnosis of IBS and its treatment is more or less a management of the symptoms experienced by the patient. IBS and IBD have **overlapping features** of **symptoms, which include diarrhoea, pain, and bloating, and both disorders** affect the quality of life. Both entail a process that takes time and it requires a multidisciplinary team. This diagram elaborates on the difference between IBD and IBS in terms of their causes, symptoms and their treatment.

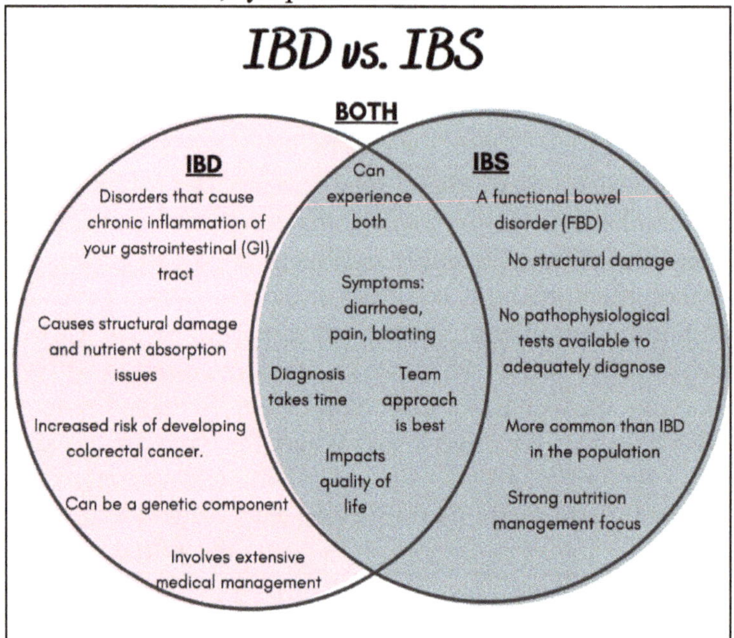
IBD vs. IBS
BOTH
IBD
Disorders that cause chronic inflammation of your gastrointestinal (GI) tract
Causes structural damage and nutrient absorption issues
Increased risk of developing colorectal cancer.
Can be a genetic component
Involves extensive medical management
Can experience both
Symptoms: diarrhoea, pain, bloating
Diagnosis takes time
Team approach is best
Impacts quality of life
IBS
A functional bowel disorder (FBD)
No structural damage
No pathophysiological tests available to adequately diagnose
More common than IBD in the population
Strong nutrition management focus

Figure 84 Difference Between IBD and IBS

4.3.4.3 SOAP Notes for IBS

Table 56 SOAP Notes for IBS

Component	Details
Subjective (S)	The patient is a 32-year-old female presenting with a 6-month history of intermittent abdominal pain, bloating, and changes in bowel habits. She reports episodes of diarrhoea alternating with constipation, often triggered by stress or after eating certain foods like dairy and fatty meals. The patient experiences relief after bowel movements but the discomfort returns as the day progresses. She denies any blood in the stool or weight loss. She also reports a sensation of incomplete bowel movements. The patient has a family history of IBS, and she has tried over-the-counter fibre supplements, which provide some relief, but her symptoms persist. She is concerned about the impact of these symptoms on her daily activities.
Objective (O)	On physical examination, the patient appears well and is in no acute distress. Vital signs are stable: blood pressure 118/76 mmHg, heart rate 74 bpm, respiratory rate 16 bpm, and temperature 36.7°C (98.1°F). Abdominal examination reveals mild tenderness in the lower abdomen, particularly in the left lower quadrant, with no guarding or rebound tenderness. Bowel sounds

	are normal, and no masses are palpated. Rectal exam is unremarkable with no evidence of blood. Laboratory tests (CBC, liver function tests, stool studies) are all normal, and no signs of anaemia or infection are present.
Assessment (A)	The patient's symptoms, including intermittent abdominal pain, bloating, alternating diarrhoea and constipation, are consistent with **Irritable Bowel Syndrome (IBS)**. The absence of alarming signs such as blood in the stool, weight loss, or anaemia supports this diagnosis. The patient's symptoms are likely exacerbated by stress, as is common with IBS. There is no indication of organic disease, and the normal laboratory and physical findings help rule out other gastrointestinal conditions. The diagnosis is based on the Rome IV criteria for IBS, which focuses on recurrent abdominal pain and altered bowel habits.
Plan (P)	**Pharmacologically**, the patient will be prescribed antispasmodics like hyoscine or dicyclomine to help alleviate abdominal cramping and pain. If constipation is more prominent, a laxative such as polyethene glycol or a fibre supplement like psyllium will be recommended to help regulate bowel movements. For patients experiencing diarrhoea, loperamide or low-dose tricyclic antidepressants may be used to reduce bowel urgency and frequency (See algorithm below). **Non-pharmacological:** dietary modifications are key to managing IBS symptoms. The patient will begin a low FODMAP diet to reduce bloating and discomfort associated with certain carbohydrates, alongside increasing their intake of soluble fibre, such as from oats or psyllium, to help normalize bowel function. Stress management will also be an important aspect of the plan, with recommendations for mindfulness, yoga, or cognitive-behavioural therapy (CBT) to help reduce stress-induced flare-ups. **Regular exercise** will be encouraged to improve gut motility and overall well-being. The patient will be scheduled for a follow-up appointment in 4-6 weeks to assess symptom control, and if symptoms persist or worsen, further testing, such as a colonoscopy, may be considered to rule out other gastrointestinal conditions. **Patient education** will focus on the chronic but manageable nature of IBS, with an emphasis on the importance of lifestyle changes, including diet and stress management, for long-term symptom relief.

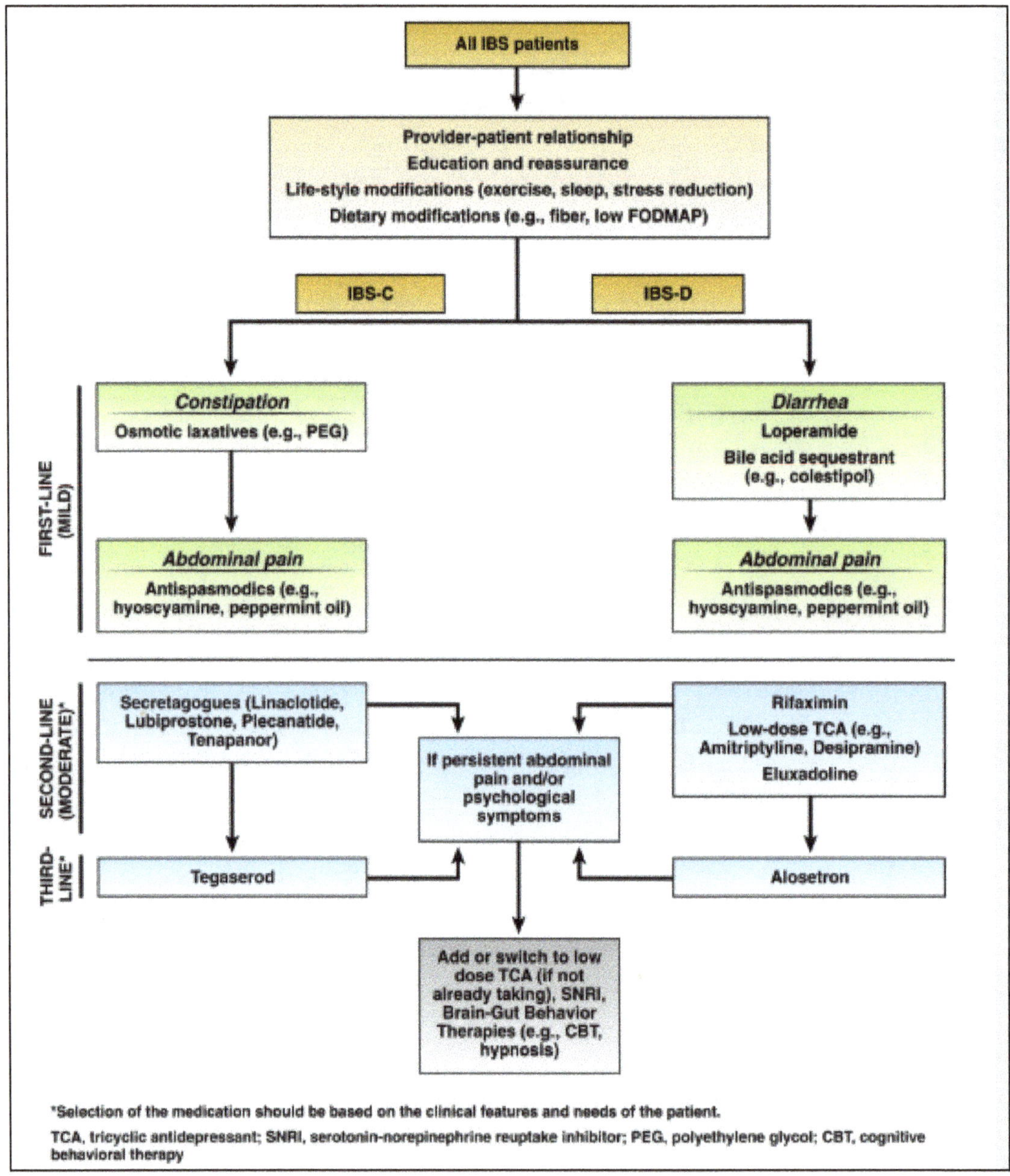

Figure 85 Clinical Decision Support Tool of IBS Management

4.3.5 Hepatitis

Hepatitis can be defined as **inflammation of the liver** and it may occur due to different factors such as **viruses, autoimmune diseases, alcohol abuse, toxic substances and certain medications** as well. In any of its types, hepatitis may cause **liver diseases, cirrhosis** and, if not well treated, liver **failure or cancer may occur**. Liver is one of the largest internal organs involved in metabolism process and has many functions such as detoxification, protein synthesis, and blood coagulation. The patients may suffer from **fatigue, vomiting, poor appetite, abdominal pain, and develop pale or yolk-colored eyes and skin, known as jaundice**. They also feel confused, have **swollen abdomen and legs, develop bruises and skin hemorrhages** due to the inability of the liver to manufacture clotting factors. **Chronic hepatitis**, if not treated eventually results in

liver damage like **cirrhosis of liver, liver failure and increased susceptibility to liver cancer**. The liver has a good capacity of regeneration but anything worsening in the liver negatively can cause damage that in the long run is irreversible. The diseases of hepatitis also establish their common blood tests which check the function of the liver as well as the presence of viral infection or any other diseases that may cause the inflammation. It is also possible to use **ultrasound or CT scans** to diagnose liver injury, though. In some occasions, a liver biopsy may be taken to determine the severity of the inflammation and fibrosis.

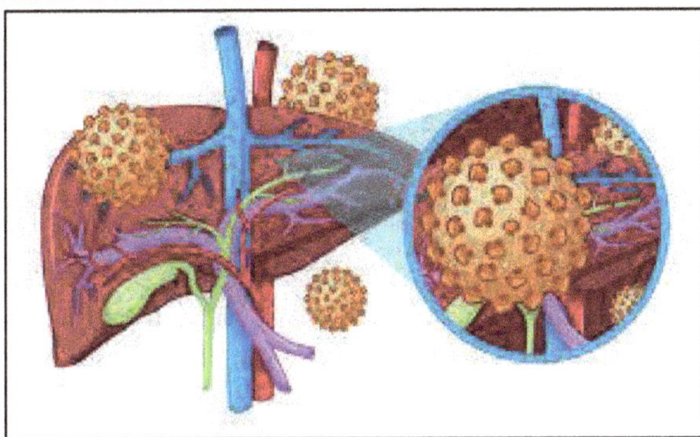

Figure 86 Pictorial Representation of Hepatitis

The treatment for hepatitis will depend on the following cause of the disorder, These include: Other types of viral **hepatitis like hepatitis B and C, and viral replication** itself may be treated using antiviral drugs. In **alcoholic hepatitis,** alcoholics are advised to stop drinking and require only supportive management while patients who have autoimmune hepatitis are put on immune suppressants because the **immune system has been attacking the liver**. In some extreme circumstances, if liver function is badly affected, the only possibility is a liver transplant. To decrease the likelihood of developing hepatitis or Hepatitis complications, people should take vaccines that are administered to curb the contraction of **hepatitis A and B**, follow standard practice, and be an aggregate for **Hepatitis C** screening besides avoiding alcohol and managing their weight. There is also a need to identify the early signs of liver diseases and treat the condition before worsening or producing fatal results, especially for patients with hepatitis.

4.3.5.1 Diagnostic Tests

Blood tests called **Liver Function Tests (LFTs)** let medical professionals assess liver health and identify possible damage to this organ. Tests of liver function measure the concentrations of different **enzymes together with proteins and biochemical compounds** that originate from or pass through the liver. The rise of two specific enzymes known as **Alanine aminotransferase (ALT) and Aspartate aminotransferase (AST)** signals liver cell damage. **Alkaline phosphatase (ALP)** shows higher levels in scenarios involving obstructed bile ducts or bone-related conditions. Elevated bilirubin levels in blood tests indicate possible liver dysfunction combined with bile duct issues that could cause jaundice. The liver's declining ability to synthesize albumin leads to reduced protein levels in patients suffering from chronic liver disease. **A prolonged prothrombin time measurement reveals impaired liver function** because it illustrates the organ's diminished capacity for clotting factor production. Liver Function Tests serve as **essential diagnostic tools** for detecting **hepatitis and cirrhosis** while identifying alcohol or medication-induced liver damage.

4.3.5.2 Classification of Hepatitis

1. **Infectious Hepatitis:**

Viral Hepatitis

It is a condition that is accompanied by hepatitic viruses like **Hepatitis A, Hepatitis B, Hepatitis C & Hepatitis E.** These forms are spread through ingestion of **food and water (Hepatitis A),** through contact with **contaminated blood and other bodily fluids (Hepatitis Bin and C)** and through **drinking water (Hepatitis E).** Hepatitis A manifests itself for the most part only during an acute period, whereas Hepatitis B and C if not treated cause chronic hepatitis, cirrhosis and mainly liver cancer. **Chronic Hepatitis B and C** can be treated using antiviral therapy in order to address the infection condition and the resulting complications.

Bacterial Hepatitis

It is relatively rarer than virus hepatitis and may be occasioned by bacteria **like Leptospira and Treponema pallidum of Syphilis.** These infections provoke the formation of inflammation and affect any area of the body, including the liver, accompanied by generalized manifestations. Management therefore requires the use of antibiotics that will be specific to the bacteria that has caused the infection in question.

Parasitic Hepatitis

Infective Hepatitis comes as a result of infection with parasitic beasts that target the liver. Some of the familiar parasitic diseases are **Amebiasis, Toxoplasmosis, Fascioliasis, Opistorchiasis, Schistosomiasis.** All these parasitic infections result from the intake of contaminated water or food. Inflammation of this vital body organ is commonly observed when the liver is implicated. It requires administration of drugs that are aimed at the type of parasite involved in the infection.

2. **Toxic Hepatitis**

Alcoholic Hepatitis

This type of hepatitis is a result of alcohol intake and complications that affect the **liver, most often resulting from alcohol addiction**. It ranges from simple steatosis to alcoholic hepatitis, alcoholic fibrosis and eventually **alcoholic cirrhosis.** Symptoms during the acute phase include jaundice, abdominal pain as well as nausea. The chronic effects include liver cirrhosis and other complications such as **liver cancer.** The best approach for patients with alcoholic hepatitis is withdrawal from alcohol and general support that will help the patient in the curing process.

Drug-Induced Hepatitis

The conditions that fall under this category are instances where hepatitis is a result of the use of certain **drugs or chemicals**. Some other drugs which may cause liver damage include: **Acetaminophen, Antibiotics, and Chemotherapy drugs.** Symptoms of drug-induced hepatitis may appear like **viral hepatitis** and the management includes stopping the use of the offending agent and supportive care. At times, corticosteroids or other related drugs might need to be administered in order to address inflammation.

Chemical Hepatitis

Chemical Hepatitis is contracted through contact with poisonous substances such as chemicals at the **workplace and contaminated foods**. They can cause harm to the liver cells, thereby causing inflammation of the liver tissues. These industries are primarily at a higher risk and the means of prevention is by reducing contact with the **chemical solution and protective clothing**. It's mainly centred on eliminating poisonous substances from the body and the general care of the liver.

3. **Other Hepatitis**

Radiation Hepatitis

It is usually a result of exposure to radiation such as those cancer patients who **undergo radiation therapy**. Irradiation of the liver brings about disorders which cause inflammation and development of **fibrosis in the liver parenchyma**. Some of the clinical signs may include sickness, vomiting, tiredness, and yellowish discolouration of the skin. The management of this condition presupposes addressing the symptoms and observing the state of the liver in the further course of the disease.

Autoimmune Hepatitis

Autoimmune Hepatitis is a medical condition that affects the liver and is primarily characterized by the immune system attacking the body's own liver cells. This often necessitates the use of immunosuppressive drugs like **corticosteroids or azathioprine** as a means of diminishing immune system activity and further harm to the body.

Genetic Hepatitis

Genetic Hepatitis is defined as a **liver disease that results from inherited disorders** like **Wilson's disease** which is characterized by the **accumulation of copper deposits and hemochromatosis** which is characterized by **iron deposits**. These are usually genetically inherited conditions which may be confirmed through DNA analysis and there is available treatment through drugs that lower the deposition of metals within the liver cells. These genetic diseases require constant check-ups to avoid the worsening of the liver and other complications.

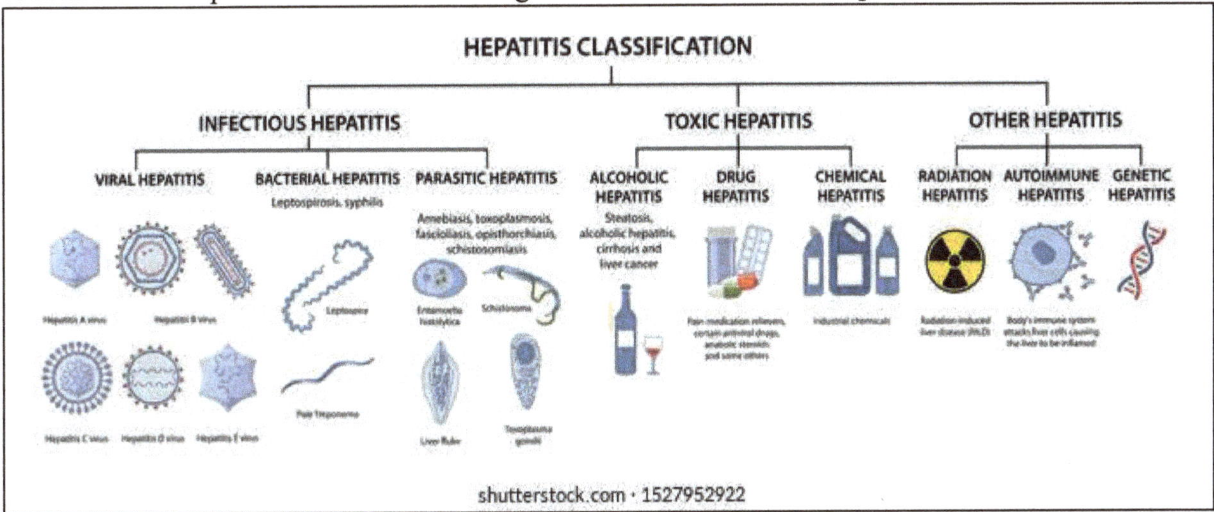

Figure 87 Classification of Hepatitis

4.3.5.3 Viruses of Hepatitis

Hepatitis A is an infectious form of hepatitis caused by the **picornavirus** which spreads chiefly through the fecal-oral route through food or water. It has a short duration of **communicability and the clinical manifestations are acute** and usually **mild or inapparent**. The fatality is however low and there is no chronic phase of infection. This means that **Hepatitis A** is not transmitted along with any other diseases with conditions such as cirrhosis or liver cancer.

Hepatitis B is the disease that is caused by hepadnavirus which is a **DNA virus** and is spread through parenteral and sexual ways. It is characterised by a slow development and a long time between the onset of symptoms and the manifestation of the disease. **Hepatitis B** can be acute or chronic, but in general, it is not **very dangerous and can be lethal** in a small percentage of cases only. It is more frequently a carrier state because hepatitis B can cause chronic illness in many people. It is related to **hepatocellular carcinoma (HCC) and cirrhosis**.

Hepatitis C is a disease that originates from an **RNA virus** known as **the flavivirus,** like Hepatitis B, the virus is spread through the parenteral and sexual conduct. It has a long-term latent period or even an asymptomatic period, then has clinical manifestations. Hepatitis C is less fatal than other types of hepatitis virus; however, the chronic infection can contribute to **cirrhosis and hepatocellular carcinoma (HCC).**

For this reason, Hepatitis D is the only **delta virus** that cannot replicate without the presence of Hepatitis B. It has also a **parenteral and sexual mode of transmission**. The incubation period is also intermediate, but it starts abruptly and the severity, according to the patients' description, is from occasional to severe. This disease has acute to fulminant hepatitis with high to very high mortality that can result in cirrhosis. It is recurrent and there is usually a carrier status frequently. Hepatitis E is an **RNA virus, in the calici group**, and spreads through the faecal-oral route like Hepatitis A. It is characterized by a short period of communicability, clinically has an acute course, which consists of discreet-objective symptoms and is severe, especially for pregnant women. **Hepatitis E is not fatal**. The seriousness of Hepatitis E risk is low but is higher **in pregnancy cases.** Interestingly HE, in contrast with other forms of the disease, does not progress to chronic carrier status, or cirrhosis.

Table 57 Overview of Viruses in Hepatitis

PROPERTY	HEPATITIS A	HEPATITIS B	HEPATITIS C	HEPATITIS D	HEPATITIS E
Common name	Infectious	Serum	Posttransfusion non-A, non-B	Delta	Enteric non-A, non-B
Virus structure (family)	Naked, RNA (picornavirus)	Envelope, DNA (hepadnavirus)	Envelope, RNA (flavivirus)	Envelope, RNA	Naked, RNA (calici-like)
Transmission	Fecal-oral	Parenteral, sexual	Parenteral, sexual	Parenteral, sexual	Fecal-oral
Incubation period	Short	Long	Long	Intermediate	Short
Usual onset*	Abrupt	Insidious	Insidious	Abrupt	Abrupt
Severity*	Mild or asymptomatic	Occasionally severe	Usually subclinical	Occasionally to often severe	Mild, but severe in pregnant women
Mortality rate*	Very low	Low	Low	High to very high	Low but high in pregnant women
Chronicity (carrier state)	No	Yes	Yes (common)	Yes	No
Other disease associations	None	HCC, cirrhosis	HCC, cirrhosis	Cirrhosis, fulminant hepatitis	None

4.3.5.4 Hepatitis A, B, and C: Antigens and Antibodies

The identification of Hepatitis A, B and C antigens and antibodies plays a vital role in determining what stage a patient is in their hepatic viral infection and immunity status. Below you will find a structure of the immune markers used as indicators:

Hepatitis A:

- **Hepatitis A Virus (HAV) Antibody (Anti-HAV IgM)** indicates recent or current infection. The presence of a positive test indicates that the patient currently experiences acute Hepatitis infection.
- **The Hepatitis A Antibody Anti-HAV IgG** shows that the person has protection because of previous infections or intentional vaccination. Meeting the criteria of positive Anti-HAV IgG and negative IgM shows that a patient currently has immune status.

Hepatitis B:

- **Hepatitis B Surface Antigen (HBsAg)** indicates active infection. Chronic carrier status will be diagnosed when Hepatitis B Surface Antigen detection exceeds six months or longer periods of time.
- **Hepatitis B Surface Antibody (Anti-HBs)** indicates immunity either from recovery or vaccination. The patient has immunity when they test positive for HBsAg and reveal no HBsAg.
- **Hepatitis B Core Antibody (Anti-HBc)** detects previous or current infection. The detection of acute infection is most likely if neither IgM nor IgG manifests in the results.

The detection of only IgG indicates exposure to Hepatitis B at some point in the past although it might represent a carrier or someone who completed infection.

- **Hepatitis B e Antigen (HBeAg)** indicates active viral replication and high infectivity. High viral DNA levels in a patient who is HBeAg-negative indicates the patient might carry the virus chronically.

Hepatitis C:

- **Testing for Hepatitis C Antibody (Anti-HCV)** shows that a person has had contact with the virus but provides no information about the infection stage. The test lacks ability to determine between newly acquired and long-term infections. The results must be verified through tests that identify HCV RNA.
- **The test for HCV RNA** evaluates the viral number in blood. The result of this test reveals a current infection status to determine between chronic infection state and infection clearance status (undetectable levels of the virus).
- Treatment decision strategies together with infection severity determination rely on **HCV Genotype and HCV RNA Quantification.**

4.3.5.5 SOAP Notes for Hepatitis

Table 58 SOAP Notes for Hepatitis

Component	Details
Subjective (S)	The patient is a 40-year-old male presenting with a 2-week history of fatigue, nausea, abdominal pain, and yellowing of the skin (jaundice). He reports that the symptoms started gradually but have worsened over the past few days. The patient also mentions dark urine and light-colored stools. He denies any significant alcohol use but has a history of unprotected sexual encounters. He has no history of recent travel or foodborne illness. The patient is concerned about his liver and is seeking medical attention due to his ongoing symptoms. He denies any weight loss, fever, or vomiting. The patient has no significant past medical history and is not currently on any medications.
Objective (O)	On physical examination, the patient appears fatigued but is in no acute distress. Vital signs: blood pressure 120/80 mmHg, heart rate 84 bpm, respiratory rate 18 bpm, and temperature 37.2°C (99°F). The patient's sclerae are mildly jaundiced, and his skin has a yellowish hue. Abdominal examination reveals mild tenderness in the right upper quadrant with hepatomegaly but no signs of ascites or palpable masses. No rebound tenderness or guarding is noted. The liver edge is palpable 2 cm below the costal margin. Laboratory results show elevated liver enzymes (AST 180 U/L, ALT 220 U/L), bilirubin 4.5 mg/dL (direct bilirubin 3.0 mg/dL), and alkaline phosphatase 150 U/L. Hepatitis A, B, and C viral markers are pending.
Assessment (A)	The patient's presentation of jaundice, elevated liver enzymes, and fatigue is suggestive of hepatitis, likely viral in origin, though the specific cause has not yet been determined. The patient's history of unprotected sexual encounters raises concern for Hepatitis B or C, and the absence of recent foodborne illness makes Hepatitis A less likely. The mild hepatomegaly and

	elevated bilirubin suggest liver involvement, but further testing (Hepatitis A, B, C, and D markers) is needed to confirm the diagnosis. Differential diagnoses include drug-induced hepatitis and alcoholic hepatitis, but the patient's lack of alcohol use makes this less likely. The severity of the disease will depend on the type of hepatitis diagnosed, and further diagnostic tests will help guide management.
Plan (P)	**Diagnostic Tests**: Order Hepatitis A, B, C, and D viral markers to identify the specific cause of hepatitis. Repeat liver function tests (including albumin, PT/INR) in 1 week to assess liver function and monitor progression. Perform an abdominal ultrasound to assess the liver for any signs of cirrhosis or other abnormalities. **Pharmacological Treatment**: If Hepatitis A is confirmed, advise supportive care and rest as it is self-limiting. If Hepatitis B or C is diagnosed, start appropriate antiviral therapy (e.g., tenofovir for Hepatitis B or direct-acting antivirals for Hepatitis C). Consider symptomatic treatment with antiemetics (e.g., ondansetron) and pain management (acetaminophen in low doses, avoiding overuse) (See Algorithms below). **Lifestyle Modifications**: Advise complete abstinence from alcohol to reduce liver strain. Recommend rest and a well-balanced diet to support liver function. Educate the patient about safe sexual practices to prevent transmission of hepatitis B and C. Follow-up: Schedule a follow-up appointment in 2 weeks to assess progress, review diagnostic results, and adjust treatment if necessary. Instruct the patient to seek immediate care if symptoms such as severe abdominal pain, bleeding, or confusion develop, as these may indicate liver failure or complications. **Patient Education**: Educate the patient on the importance of following prescribed antiviral therapy, if needed, and avoiding further liver damage through alcohol abstinence. Explain the need for regular follow-up appointments and liver function monitoring to track the progress of the disease and manage any complications.

Table 60 Algorithm for the Management of Autoimmune Hepatitis

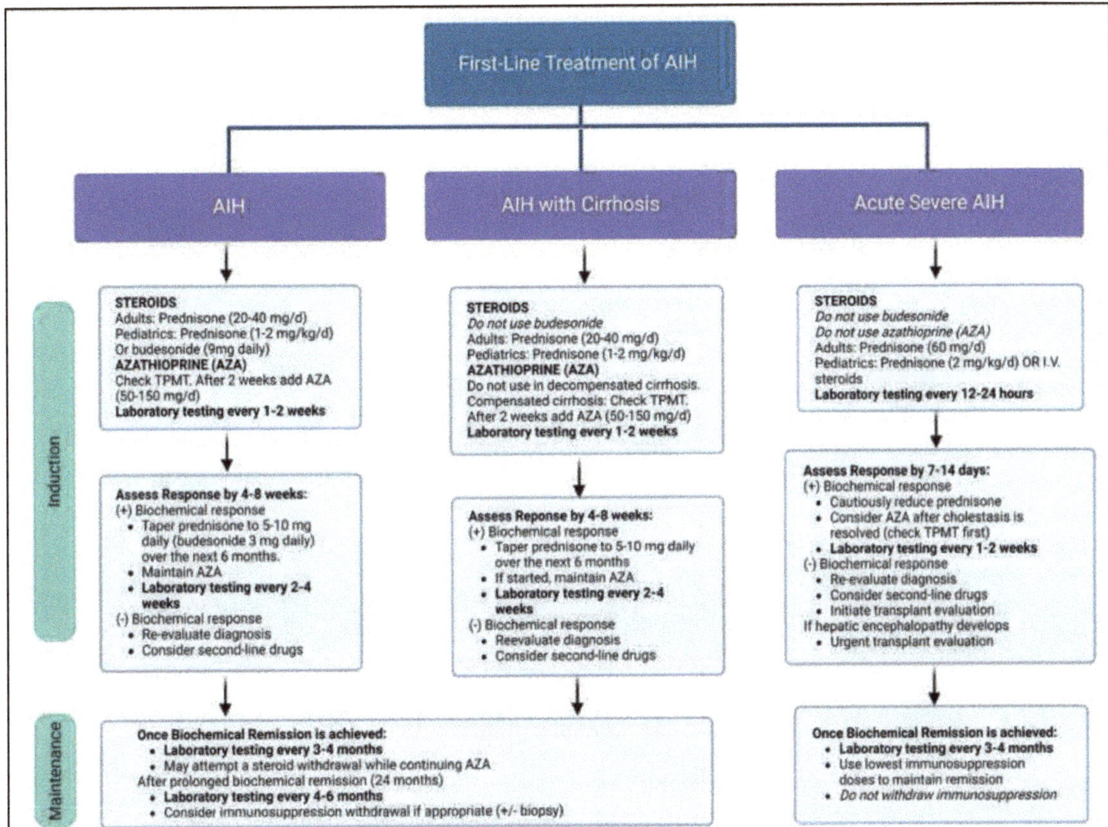

First-Line Treatment of AIH
AIH
AIH with Cirrhosis
Acute Severe AIH
Induction
Maintenance
STEROIDS
Adults: Prednisone (20-40 mg/d)
Pediatrics: Prednisone (1-2 mg/kg/d)
Or budesonide (9mg daily)
AZATHIOPRINE (AZA)
Check TPMT. After 2 weeks add AZA (50-150 mg/d)
Laboratory testing every 1-2 weeks
STEROIDS
Do not use budesonide
Adults: Prednisone (20-40 mg/d)
Pediatrics: Prednisone (1-2 mg/kg/d)
AZATHIOPRINE (AZA)
Do not use in decompensated cirrhosis.
Compensated cirrhosis: Check TPMT.
After 2 weeks add AZA (50-150 mg/d)
Laboratory testing every 1-2 weeks
STEROIDS
Do not use budesonide
Do not use azathioprine (AZA)
Adults: Prednisone (60 mg/d)
Pediatrics: Prednisone (2 mg/kg/d) OR I.V. steroids
Laboratory testing every 12-24 hours
Assess Response by 4-8 weeks:
(+) Biochemical response
• Taper prednisone to 5-10 mg daily (budesonide 3 mg daily) over the next 6 months.
• Maintain AZA
• Laboratory testing every 2-4 weeks
(-) Biochemical response
• Re-evaluate diagnosis
• Consider second-line drugs
Assess Reponse by 4-8 weeks:
(+) Biochemical response
• Taper prednisone to 5-10 mg daily over the next 6 months
• If started, maintain AZA
• Laboratory testing every 2-4 weeks
(-) Biochemical response
• Reevaluate diagnosis
• Consider second-line drugs
Assess Response by 7-14 days:
(+) Biochemical response
• Cautiously reduce prednisone
• Consider AZA after cholestasis is resolved (check TPMT first)
• Laboratory testing every 1-2 weeks
(-) Biochemical response
• Re-evaluate diagnosis
• Consider second-line drugs
• Initiate transplant evaluation
If hepatic encephalopathy develops
• Urgent transplant evaluation
Once Biochemical Remission is achieved:
• Laboratory testing every 3-4 months
• May attempt a steroid withdrawal while continuing AZA
After prolonged biochemical remission (24 months)
• Laboratory testing every 4-6 months
• Consider immunosuppression withdrawal if appropriate (+/- biopsy)
Once Biochemical Remission is achieved:
• Laboratory testing every 3-4 months
• Use lowest immunosuppression doses to maintain remission
• Do not withdraw immunosuppression

Table 59 Indications for antiviral therapy of chronic HBV infection

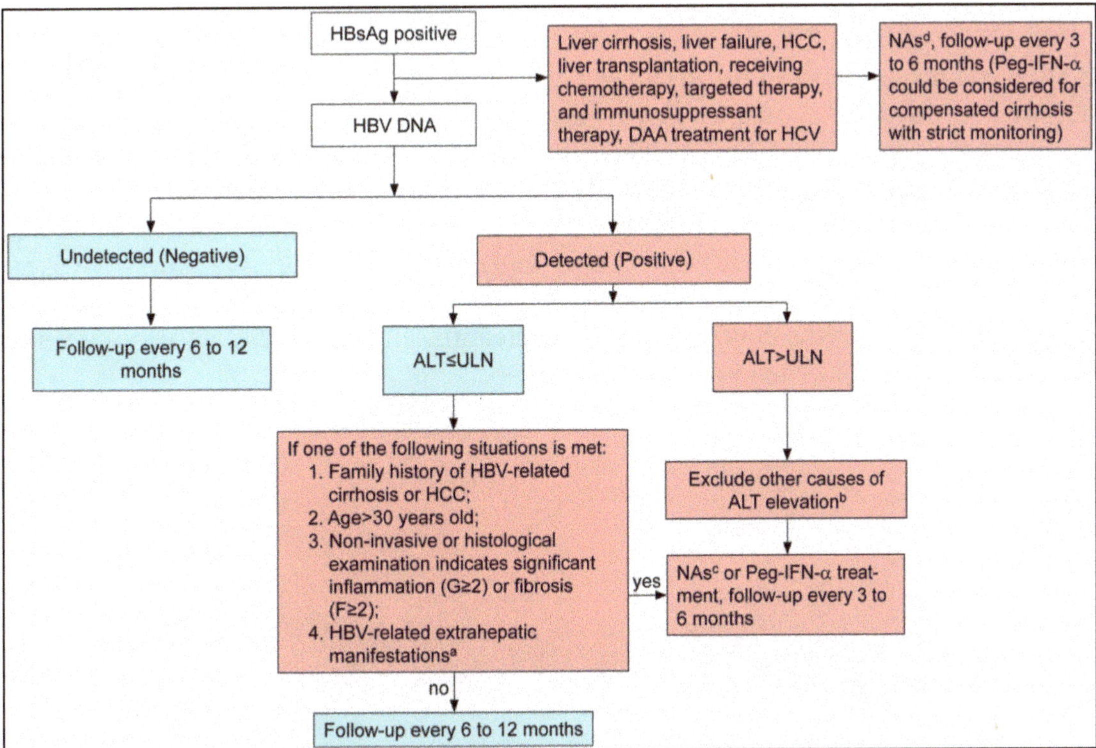

Table 61 Hepatitis C Post Exposure Management

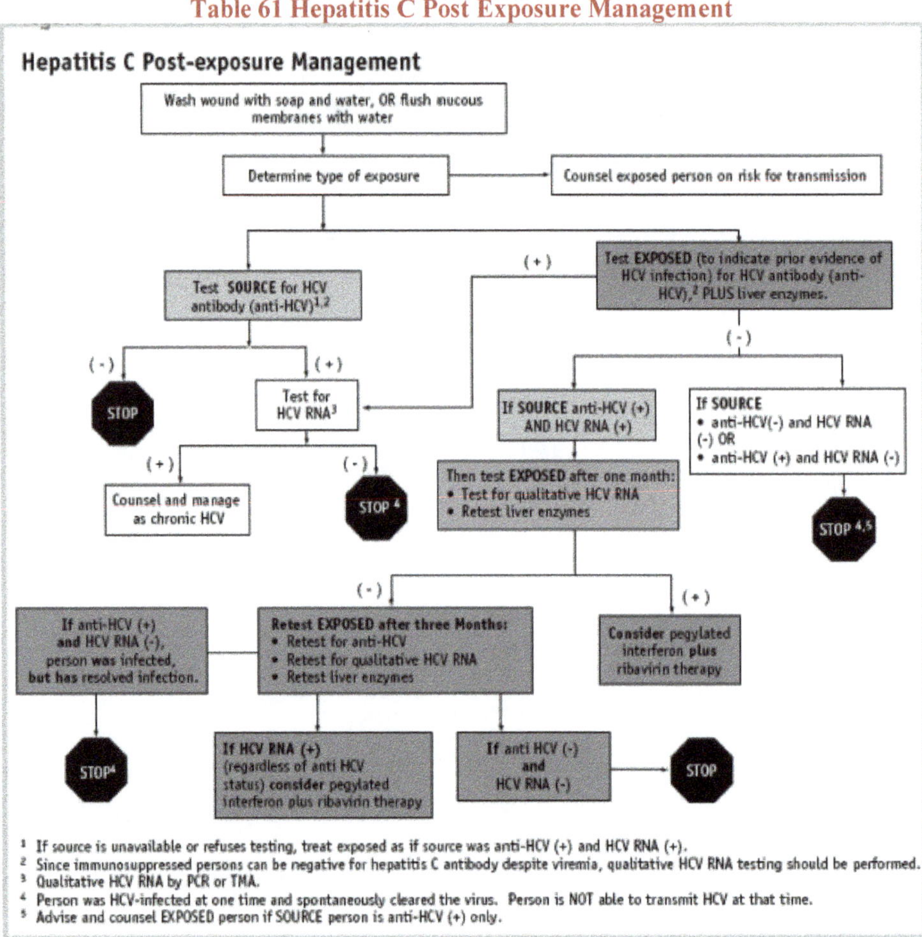

4.3.6 Pancreatitis (chronic)

Pancreatitis refers to the inflammation of the pancreas, which is a vital organ that plays a role in digestion and management of blood sugar. The cells in the pancreas secrete digestive enzymes that decomposes food and hormones that controls the **amount of glucose in the body**. That is why, in pancreatitis enzymes become activated inside the pancreas, this leads to the pancreas eating itself, inflammation and **possible destruction**. The root causes of pancreatitis are still multiple, but the two evident categories are **gallstones and alcoholism**. Other causes include being over the age limit of using the **organ, raised triglycerides, medications, pancreatic injury, viruses, and some diseases that affect the immune system**. There are certain diseases of inheritance that may lead to a predisposition to the development of pancreatitis, although these are very rare, some of them are genetic conditions and **cystic fibrosis**.

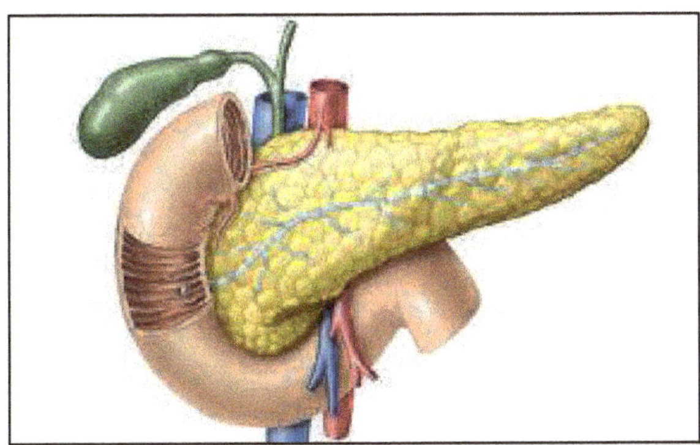

Figure 88 Acute Pancreatitis

The main and most common sign of pancreatitis is pain in the **abdominal region,** which is particularly in the upper part and may spread to the back. The symptoms manifest themselves in an increase in the intensity of pain linked to consumption of food, including fatty types of food. They include; **vomiting, nausea, fever, fatigue, jaundice** which is the condition characterized by yellowing of skin and eyes in case the inflammation impacts the bile duct. **Apathy as well as loss of appetite** and a **loss of weight** that they have not planned for may also be experienced. Thus, in severe cases, including severe **acute pancreatitis, complications may involve shock and failure of the patient's organs.**

Pancreatitis diagnosis depends on the symptoms, blood tests, and imaging examination. Blood tests also turn out to be positive for two enzymes known as amylase and lipase, which are released into the bloodstream when the pancreas is inflamed. **Vivid images** provided by **ultrasound, CT-Scans or MRI** help in making diagnostic conclusions and evaluating the extent of the injury to the pancreas. In some occasions, another procedure can be carried out endoscopically known as ERCP **(Endoscopic retrograde cholangiopancreatography)** to determine if there are blockages in the bile or pancreatic duct brought by gall stones. Pancreatitis can be managed and treated but unfortunately there is no specific cure for the ailment in equal measure. Patients are often admitted to hospitals for the purpose of controlling their conditions and guidelines against other related conditions or events. **Ongoing treatment in IV** form is used to **replenish fluids in the body** and analgesia; narcotics are used in severe cases. In the case of acute pancreatitis, the individual may be advised to fast, both the food or liquid intake is restricted for a while to give the pancreas a reprieve. In the case of gallstones, they always require their removal through surgery or even through the use of endoscopes. With regard to infection or pancreatic necrosis, antibiotics may be required and surgery might be needed as well. The other treatment for chronic pancreatitis is with the use of supplanted enzymes that help with digestion, and insulin in cases has diabetes since the pancreas is unable to produce the **correct amounts of enzymes or insulin**. Some of the most disregarded attributes include the application of a low fat diet and no alcohol consumption in the management of the condition and preventing future relapses. Pancreatitis comes with a number of complications including the **formation of pseudocysts in the pancreas, pancreatitis, organ failure and infections.** However, complications developing from acute chronic pancreatitis include pancreatic insufficiency in which the pancreas is incapable of breaking down foods and diabetes due to inactive secretion of insulin. Pancreatitis can also contribute to the formation of pancreatic cancer because chronic inflammation in the pancreas is possible. **Prevention of pancreatitis solely relies on managing the risks that help in the development of the disease.** Alcohol should be restricted, a person should follow a proper diet plan, one should regulate their blood sugar level and one should treat high cholesterol or high triglycerides. In patients with gallstones, certain follow-ups may be recommended to remove the gallbladder and ensure the prevention of pancreatitis resulting from bile duct blockage. It is recommended that early diagnosis of this disease and its management should be done so as to reduce the extent of complications as well as enhance the prognosis of the disease.

4.3.6.1 Classification of Pancreatitis

On the left, the diagram shows the normal appearance of the pancreas and the changes in the pancreas due to chronic pancreatitis. **Chronic pancreatitis,** unlike **acute, is long-term inflammation** of the pancreas which results in the **glandular tissue hardening, non-functioning or working poorly**. The picture also highlights that the pancreas is filled with ectopic tissues and ducts, chronic inflammation is evident and the pancreas may become fibrotic, a situation that will affect the production of **degradative enzymes and insulin**. Chronic pancreatitis may cause the pancreas to stop functioning as a digestive organ and the disease may also damage the cells which produce insulin hence causing diabetes. **On the right side of the picture**, the cause of acute pancreatitis by gallstones in the common bile duct and pancreatic duct is depicted. It results in inflammation of the pancreas because enzymes start working prematurely on the inside of the pancreas, digesting the organ's tissue. It is defined as **inflammation** of the pancreas rendering the organ to become **acutely swollen** with **severe abdominal pain** and could, in some cases, be life-threatening leading to pancreatic necrosis or organ failure. It underlines the reason for acute pancreatitis as obstruction of the pancreatic duct and gallstones present in the **gallbladder**.

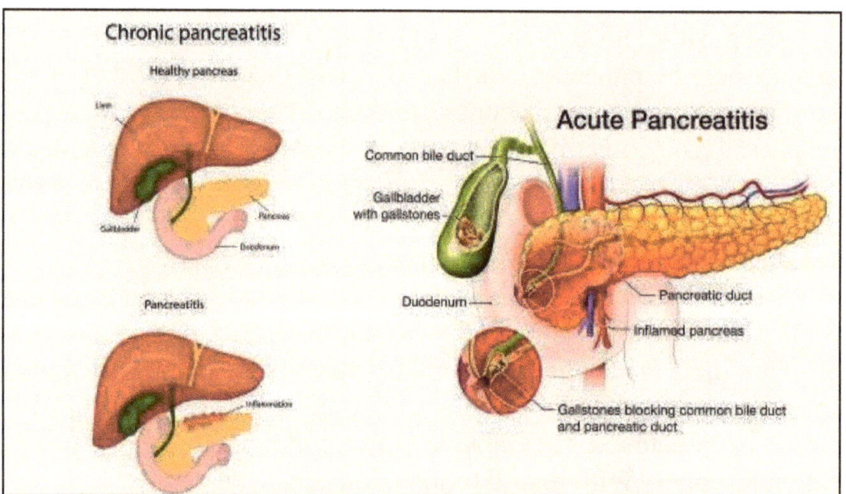

Figure 89 Classification of Pancreatitis

4.3.6.2 Types of Pancreatitis

Condition	Pathogenesis and Pathophysiology	Diagnosis	Treatment Options	Complications and Management
Acute Biliary Pancreatitis (ABP)	Inflammation of the pancreas due to bile duct obstruction, usually from gallstones. Leads to autodigestion,	At least two of the following: 1) Severe epigastric pain; 2) Serum lipase/amylase >3x normal; 3)	Supportive care (fluid resuscitation, pain management, nutritional support), early ERCP if	Severe cases: ICU management, fluid resuscitation, and pain management. Complications: Pancreatic necrosis, pseudocysts, infected necrosis (managed conservatively or with

	inflammation, and pancreatic tissue damage.	Imaging findings (US, CT, MRI).	cholangitis or obstruction is present, cholecystectomy to prevent recurrence. ERCP for bile duct drainage.	drainage), walled-off necrosis (treated with endoscopic stenting).
Acute Calculous Cholecystitis (ACC)	Obstruction of the cystic duct by gallstones leading to biliary stasis, inflammation, and ischemic necrosis. Can progress to gangrenous or purulent forms if untreated.	Diagnosis requires: 1) Local infection signs; 2) Systemic infection signs; 3) Imaging findings (US, CT, MRI).	Early laparoscopic cholecystectomy (ELC) within 7 days of hospitalization. For high-risk patients, alternative treatments include percutaneous gallbladder drainage (PGBD) or endoscopic techniques (ETGBD, EUS-GBD).	Complications: Perforation, abscess, biliary peritonitis. Management: For high-risk patients, drainage (PGBD or endoscopic techniques) before surgery. Antibiotics for complicated cases. Emergency cholecystectomy delayed in severe cases until the patient stabilizes.

4.3.6.3 SOAP Notes for Pancreatitis

Table 62 SOAP Notes for Pancreatitis

Component	Details
Subjective (S)	The patient is a 45-year-old male who presents with a 3-day history of severe upper abdominal pain that radiates to his back. The pain is described as sharp and constant, worsening after eating and improving slightly when leaning forward. The patient also reports nausea, vomiting, and loss of appetite. He denies fever but has experienced mild jaundice (yellowing of the skin). He has a history of heavy alcohol consumption (approximately 5-6 drinks per day for 15 years). The patient reports no recent trauma, infections, or surgeries. He has never been diagnosed with gallstones or had prior abdominal surgeries. He is concerned that the pain might be related to his liver or pancreas.
Objective (O)	On physical examination, the patient appears in mild distress due to abdominal pain but is alert and oriented. Vital signs are: blood pressure

	128/80 mmHg, heart rate 98 bpm, respiratory rate 18 bpm, temperature 37.4°C (99.3°F). The patient's sclerae are slightly jaundiced. Abdominal exam reveals tenderness in the upper abdomen, particularly in the epigastric and left upper quadrant regions, with no rebound tenderness or guarding. Bowel sounds are slightly decreased. The pancreatic border is palpable 2 cm below the costal margin, and the patient experiences pain on palpation. Laboratory tests show elevated serum amylase (300 U/L) and lipase (450 U/L), elevated bilirubin (2.5 mg/dL), and mild leukocytosis (WBC 12,000/µL). A CT scan of the abdomen reveals swelling of the pancreas with no evidence of pancreatic necrosis or pseudocyst formation.
Assessment (A)	The patient's clinical presentation of severe abdominal pain, nausea, vomiting, jaundice, and elevated pancreatic enzymes is consistent with acute pancreatitis, likely secondary to alcohol abuse. The mild jaundice suggests possible obstruction of the biliary or pancreatic duct, which could be due to alcohol-induced inflammation. There are no signs of severe complications such as pancreatic necrosis or infection at this point, but the patient will need careful monitoring. Differential diagnoses include gallstone pancreatitis, drug-induced pancreatitis, and pancreatic cancer, though the patient's history and imaging suggest acute inflammation rather than malignancy or infection.
Plan (P)	The pharmacological plan for managing pancreatitis involves several key treatments aimed at controlling pain, inflammation, and potential complications. Analgesics are crucial for pain relief, starting with IV acetaminophen for mild pain, and escalating to opioid analgesics like morphine for moderate to severe pain. Antiemetics such as ondansetron are prescribed to control nausea and vomiting, which are common symptoms. IV fluids, including Normal Saline or Lactated Ringer's solution, are essential for fluid resuscitation, with ongoing monitoring of electrolytes like potassium and magnesium, which may need to be replaced. If pancreatic insufficiency develops, pancreatic enzyme replacement therapy (e.g., Pancrelipase) is started once the patient is stable and able to tolerate oral intake. If hyperglycemia occurs due to pancreatic dysfunction, insulin therapy may be necessary. Antibiotics may be indicated if pancreatic necrosis or infection is suspected (See algorithm). The non-pharmacological plan includes vital lifestyle and supportive care measures to ensure recovery and prevent recurrence. Initially, the patient is kept NPO (nothing by mouth) for 24-48 hours to allow the pancreas to rest, followed by a gradual reintroduction of clear liquids and a low-fat diet. Enteral nutrition is considered for patients who cannot tolerate oral intake, using a nasogastric tube or nasoduodenal tube to reduce pancreatic stimulation. Strong advice to abstain from alcohol is essential, and a referral to an alcohol rehabilitation program is recommended for counseling and support. Bed rest is advised during the

acute phase to reduce the body's metabolic demands on the pancreas, with positioning strategies like leaning forward to relieve pain. Regular monitoring of vital signs and abdominal tenderness is crucial to detect potential complications such as necrosis or abscess formation. Educational efforts focus on the chronic nature of pancreatitis, the importance of dietary changes, and stress management to prevent further flare-ups. Finally, follow-up appointments are scheduled within 1-2 weeks to assess recovery and adjust treatment as necessary.

Table 63 Algorithm for Management of Chronic Pancreatitis

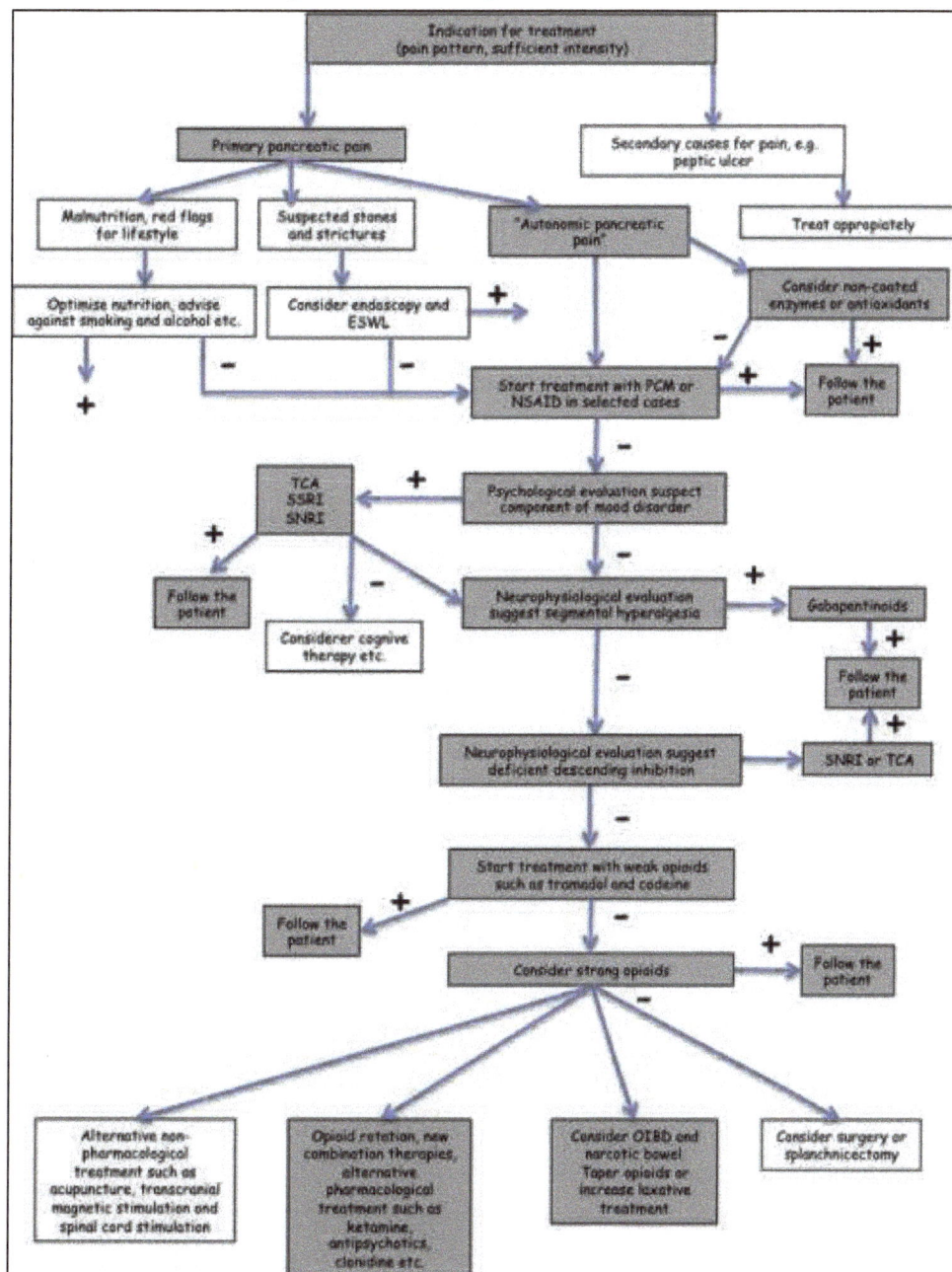

Indication for treatment (pain pattern, sufficient intensity)
Primary pancreatic pain
Secondary causes for pain, e.g. peptic ulcer
Malnutrition, red flags for lifestyle
Suspected stones and strictures
"Autonomic pancreatic pain"
Treat appropiately
Optimise nutrition, advise against smoking and alcohol etc.
Consider endoscopy and ESWL
Consider non-coated enzymes or antioxidants
Start treatment with PCM or NSAID in selected cases
Follow the patient
TCA SSRI SNRI
Psychological evaluation suspect component of mood disorder
Follow the patient
Considerer cognive therapy etc.
Neurophysiological evaluation suggest segmental hyperalgesia
Gabapentinoids
Follow the patient
Neurophysiological evaluation suggest deficient descending inhibition
SNRI or TCA
Start treatment with weak opioids such as tramadol and codeine
Follow the patient
Consider strong opioids
Follow the patient
Alternative non-pharmacological treatment such as acupuncture, transcranial magnetic stimulation and spinal cord stimulation
Opioid rotation, new combination therapies, alternative pharmacological treatment such as ketamine, antipsychotics, clonidine etc.
Consider OIBD and narcotic bowel Taper opioids or increase laxative treatment
Consider surgery or splanchnicectomy

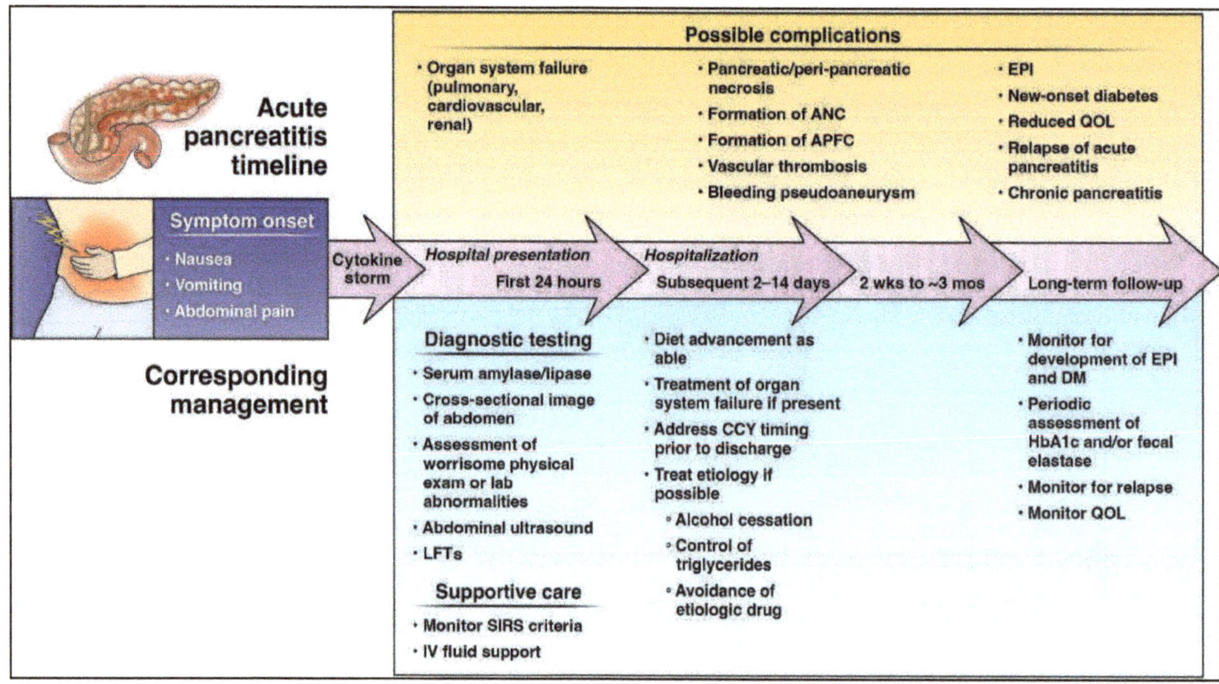

Figure 90 Management pf Acute Pancreatitis

4.3.7 Peptic Ulcer

Peptic ulcers appear as open sores which affect the **inner lining of stomach and duodenal walls and esophageal tissue** through mucosal layer breakdown. The development of **peptic ulcers** results from when protective mechanisms such as **mucus production** become unbalanced with aggressive factors including **stomach acid.** Two main triggers of **peptic ulcers** emerge from **Helicobacter pylori infection** combined with the daily usage of **nonsteroidal anti-inflammatory drugs (NSAIDs).** Peptic ulcers produce stomach burning discomfort together with abdominal enlargement along with heartburn feelings followed by nausea and vomiting which sometimes results in **blood-stained stool or vomiting**. Eating or taking antacids brings temporary relief from the pain although stomach emptying leads it to come back. Medical professionals perform endoscopy to directly examine stomach lining which confirms peptic ulcer diagnosis. Doctors also employ **H. pylori antibody blood testing** together with **urea breath testing and stool antigen testin**g to check for bacterial presence. Medical intervention primarily aims to eliminate H. pylori bacteria through antibiotic treatment while simultaneously using proton pump inhibitors for stomach acid reduction to assist in ulcer healing. **Treatment that uses H2-receptor antagonists** in combination with antacids helps decrease stomach acidity. Drugs such as **prostaglandin analogs or the complete stoppage of NSAID medications** are needed to heal ulcers. Surgery becomes necessary in uncommon situations when patients experience perforations or bleeding from their ulcers.

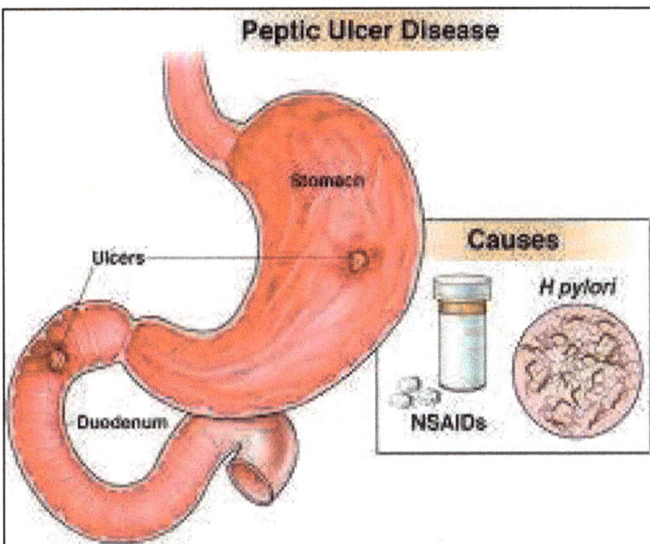

Figure 91 Peptic Ulcer

4.3.7.1 Classification of Peptic Ulcer

The illustration presents a thorough system to classify peptic ulcers as it identifies their positioning with their specific characteristics. **Gastric ulcers** appearing inside the stomach classify into acute and chronic varieties. The surface area of **acute ulcers** shows one or more erosions that remain confined above the **deeper stomach muscular layer.** Time is the determining factor that separates chronic gastric ulcers from other types since Johnson's classification defines their specific categories. **Two types of gastric ulcers exist: Type I** which appears on the lesser curve of the stomach and **Type IV** which develops proximal to the esophagogastric junction within 2 cm. The other classifications include **Type II dual ulcers and Type III prepyloric ulcers**. The two categories of duodenal ulcers include bulbar and post-bulbar ulcers depending on where they occur in the duodenal area. The cap-like duodenal segment houses duodenal cap ulcers whereas **Zollinger-Ellison Syndrome** represents an uncommon situation which stems from tumors that generate excessive stomach acid. Such classification enables medical diagnosis of peptic ulcer location and type to determine proper treatment approaches.

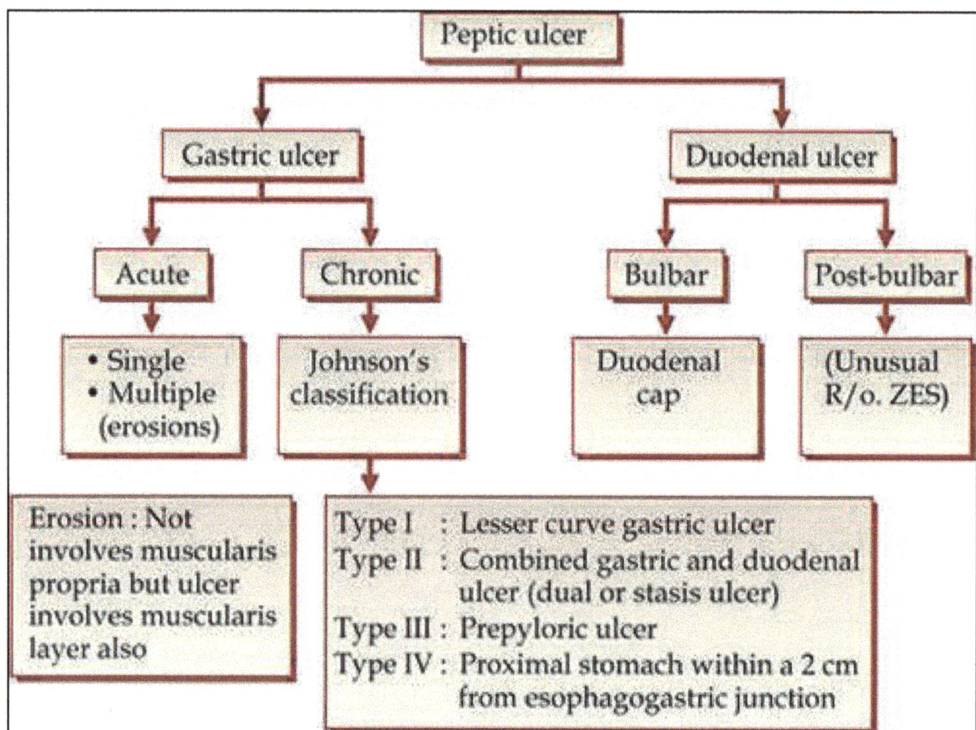

Figure 92 Classification of Peptic Ulcer

4.3.7.2 SOAP Notes for Peptic Ulcer

Component	Details
Subjective (S)	The patient is a 55-year-old male who presents with a 2-week history of recurrent burning epigastric pain, particularly after meals. The pain is described as a gnawing discomfort that improves temporarily with antacids but returns a few hours after eating. The patient reports occasional nausea and bloating but no vomiting. He has a history of frequent use of nonsteroidal anti-inflammatory drugs (NSAIDs) for chronic back pain and admits to alcohol consumption (3-4 drinks per week). He denies any recent weight loss, hematemesis, or melena. The patient is concerned about possible stomach ulcers and is seeking advice on treatment.
Objective (O)	On physical examination, the patient appears well-nourished with no signs of acute distress. Vital signs are: blood pressure 130/85 mmHg, heart rate 80 bpm, respiratory rate 16 bpm, temperature 36.9°C (98.4°F). Abdominal exam reveals tenderness on palpation of the epigastric region, but there is no rebound tenderness or guarding. Bowel sounds are normal. Laboratory tests show normal CBC, with no signs of anemia. A stool antigen test for **Helicobacter pylori** is positive, indicating active infection. An upper gastrointestinal endoscopy reveals a superficial ulcer in the duodenum and no signs of gastric malignancy.
Assessment (A)	The patient's clinical presentation of epigastric pain that improves with antacids, along with the positive **H. pylori** test, is consistent with a diagnosis of **duodenal peptic ulcer** likely caused by **H. pylori** infection. The use of

	NSAIDs may have contributed to the ulcer formation, though the primary cause appears to be infection. No signs of severe complications such as bleeding or perforation are noted at this time. The patient should be monitored for possible recurrence and complications, including gastrointestinal bleeding or obstruction. Differential diagnoses include gastroesophageal reflux disease (GERD) and functional dyspepsia, but these are less likely given the findings.
Plan (P)	The pharmacological treatment plan for this patient involves a **triple therapy** regimen for H. pylori eradication, including a proton pump inhibitor (PPI) (e.g., Omeprazole), Amoxicillin, and Clarithromycin for 14 days. This will help to both heal the ulcer and address the H. pylori infection. The patient should also be advised to avoid further NSAID use and switch to alternative pain management options, such as acetaminophen, if necessary. Additional medications may include H2-receptor antagonists (e.g., Ranitidine) or antacids to manage symptoms in the interim. If symptoms persist, endoscopic follow-up will be recommended to monitor for healing and assess for any complications. Non-pharmacological measures include dietary modifications, such as avoiding spicy, acidic, or irritating foods, and reducing alcohol consumption. The patient will be advised to follow up in 4-6 weeks to ensure successful eradication of H. pylori and monitor for symptom resolution. Education will focus on adherence to the treatment regimen and lifestyle modifications to prevent recurrence (See algorithm below).

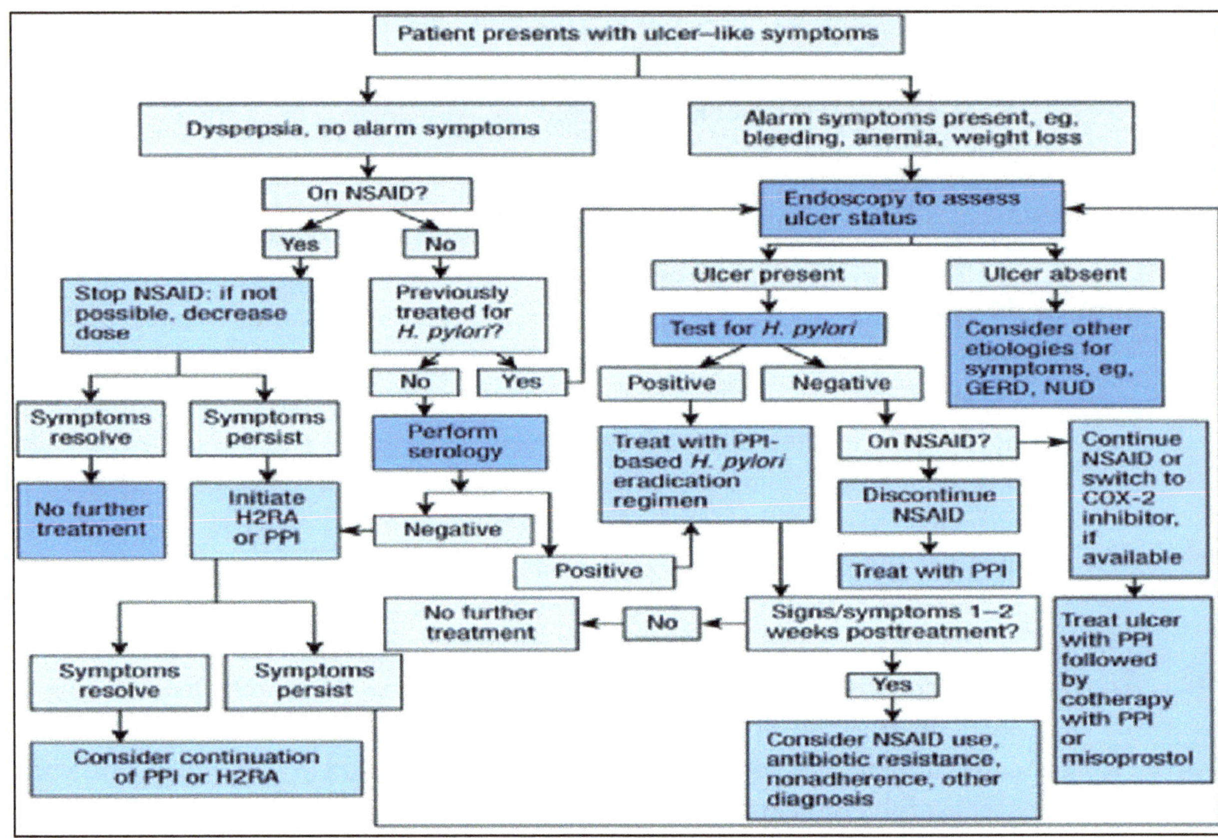

Figure 93 Algorithm for the Management for Peptic Ulcer like Symptoms

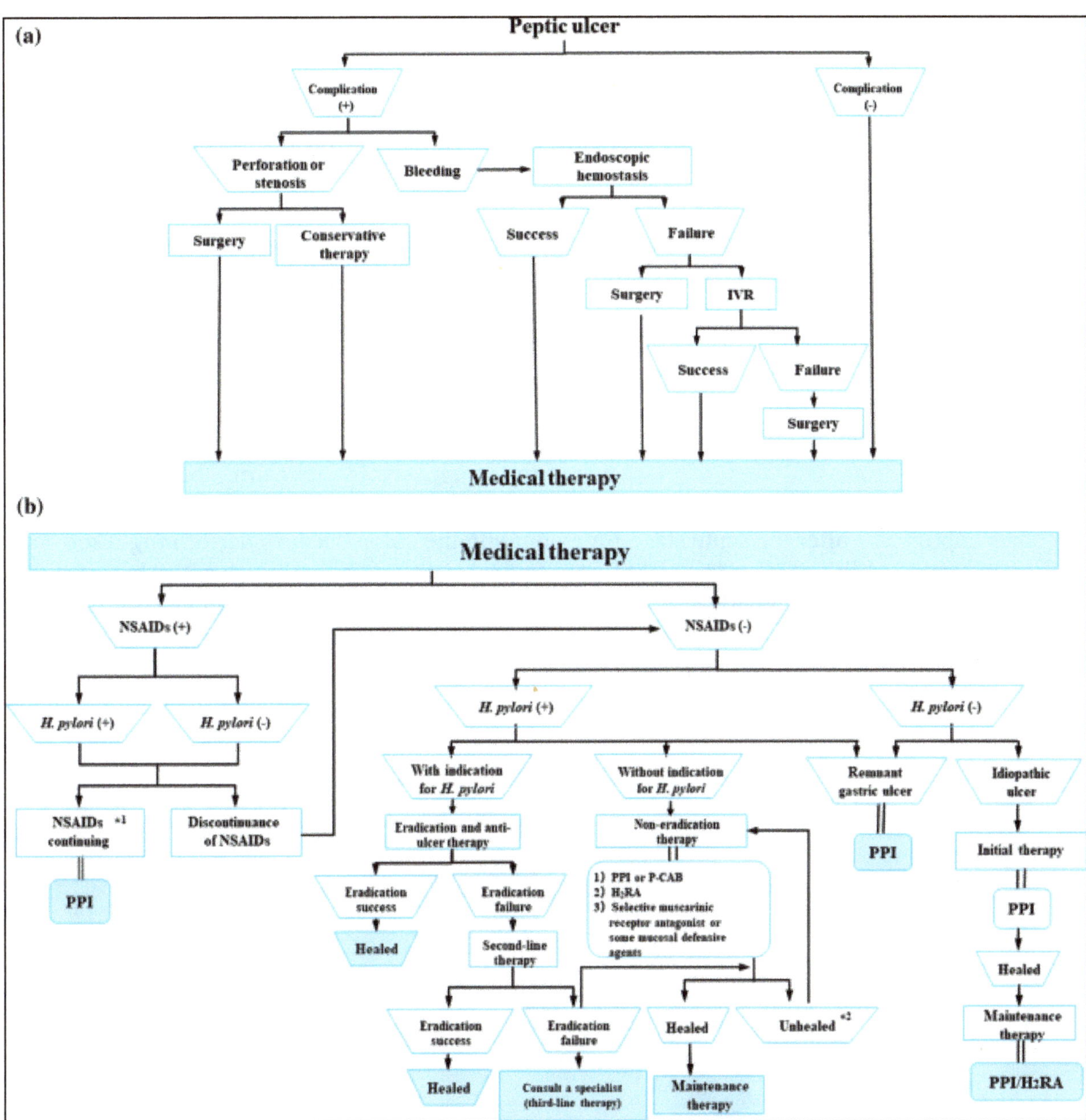

Figure 94 Algorithm for the Management of Peptic Ulcer

4.3.8 ACUTE DISEASES

4.3.9 Diverticulitis

Diverticulitis can present as either acute (sudden onset, resolves with treatment) or chronic (recurrent episodes or persistent inflammation). **Diverticulitis** occurs when infections and inflammation develop within diverticula that pop out from **colon walls** mostly in the sigmoid region. Food remains or stool trapped inside **diverticula pouches** commonly results in infections and subsequent inflammation of this condition. The development of diverticulitis represents an **inflammatory complication of diverticulosis** because **diverticulosis** refers to the pouches that form alone. The common manifestations of diverticulitis consist of pelvic or left-sided abdominal pain together with fever and nausea and possibly **constipation or diarrhea.** The condition produces worse pain levels when patients move around or when someone checks the area and they could also experience **bowel irregularities.** The development of abscesses or perforations as well as peritonitis and fistulas constitutes more severe diverticulitis complications that demand urgent medical intervention. **CT imaging confirms** the diagnosis by revealing **inflammation of diverticula** as well as abscesses together with complications of the condition. Colonoscopy becomes appropriate after the acute stage for evaluating the colon because performing it too soon carries an increased risk of **bowel perforation.** Medical treatment for **mild diverticulitis** includes both antibiotics taken by mouth and specific food restrictions like clear liquids followed by **increasing fiber intake as symptoms fade**. When severe symptoms occur with complications patients may need hospital care that includes intravenous antibiotics with surgery (for example bowel resection) becoming necessary if perforation or large abscesses develop. The risk reduction for diverticulosis becoming diverticulitis depends on **eating high-fiber food** combined with sufficient **hydration as well as performing exercise regularly**. Patients need to prevent constipation because this increases colon pressure thus promoting the growth of diverticula.

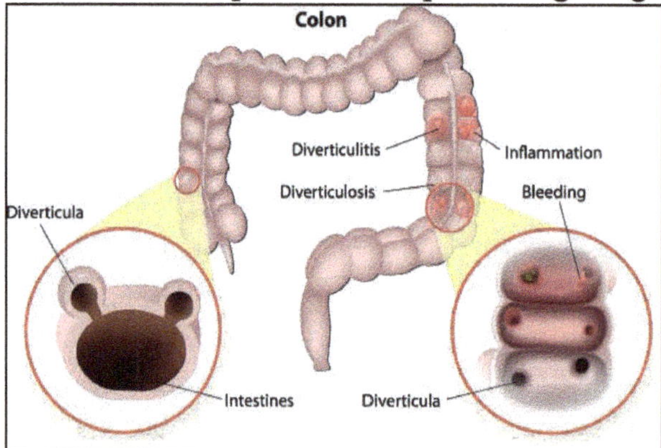

Figure 95 Diverticulitis

4.3.9.1 Stages of Diverticulitis

Modified Hinchey Classification

- **Stage 0: Mild clinical diverticulitis**—This stage refers to uncomplicated diverticulitis with mild symptoms and no significant complications.
- **Stage Ia: Confined pericolonic inflammation or phlegmon**—This stage involves localized inflammation around the colon but no abscess. It is generally considered a mild form of diverticulitis.
- **Stage Ib: Confined pericolonic abscess**—An abscess has formed, but it is still confined to the area around the colon, and there is no spread of infection.

- **Stage II**: **Pelvic, distant intra-abdominal, or retroperitoneal abscess**—The abscess has spread to other parts of the abdomen or pelvis.
- **Stage III**: **Generalized purulent peritonitis**—In this stage, infection spreads to the peritoneum, causing generalized inflammation and pus formation.
- **Stage IV**: **Generalized fecal peritonitis**—A more severe form where the infection is widespread, involving fecal matter leaking into the peritoneal cavity, often requiring urgent surgical intervention.

Ambrosetti's Classification:

- **Mild**: This stage includes findings such as **wall thickening greater than 5mm**, **pericolonic fat stranding** (indicating inflammation), and no abscess formation.
- **Severe**: This stage includes more severe findings, such as abscess formation, extramural air (which indicates perforation), and extraluminal contrast (which suggests leakage of bowel contents).

Stage	Description
Modified Hinchey classification	
0	Mild clinical diverticulitis
Ia	Confined pericolic inflammation or phlegmon
Ib	Confined pericolic abscess
II	Pelvic, distant intra-abdominal or retroperitoneal abscess
III	Generalized purulent peritonitis
IV	Generalized fecal peritonitis
Ambrosetti's classification	
Mild	-Wall thickening >5 mm
	-Pericolic fat stranding
Severe	-Abscess
	-Extraluminal air
	-Extraluminal contrast

Figure 96 Stages of Diverticulitis

4.3.9.2 SOAP Notes for Diverticulitis

Component	Details
Subjective (S)	The patient is a 60-year-old female who presents with a 3-day history of lower left abdominal pain, which is constant and sharp in nature. The pain is associated with bloating, nausea, and occasional diarrhea. The patient denies fever but has experienced mild changes in bowel movements, with some constipation alternating with loose stools. She has a history of mild diverticulosis, diagnosed during a routine colonoscopy 5 years ago, but no prior episodes of diverticulitis. She reports no recent weight loss, blood in the stool, or vomiting. The patient is concerned that her symptoms may be due to a flare-up of her diverticular disease.
Objective (O)	On physical examination, the patient appears in mild distress due to abdominal pain but is alert and oriented. Vital signs are: blood pressure 125/80 mmHg, heart rate 90 bpm, respiratory rate 18 bpm, temperature 37.2°C (99°F). Abdominal exam reveals tenderness in the lower left quadrant, with no rebound tenderness or guarding. Bowel sounds are slightly decreased.

	Laboratory tests show mild leukocytosis (WBC 10,500/µL) and normal electrolytes. A CT scan of the abdomen reveals thickening of the sigmoid colon wall and the presence of small diverticula, confirming the diagnosis of uncomplicated **diverticulitis** without any evidence of abscess formation or perforation.
Assessment (A)	The patient's clinical presentation of left lower abdominal pain, changes in bowel habits, and mild leukocytosis, along with imaging findings of diverticulitis, is consistent with acute uncomplicated diverticulitis. The absence of fever, severe leukocytosis, and complications such as perforation or abscess formation suggests that the disease is not severe at this point. Differential diagnoses include irritable bowel syndrome (IBS), gastroenteritis, and colorectal cancer, but these are less likely based on the patient's history, clinical presentation, and imaging findings.
Plan (P)	**Pharmacological Treatment**: The pharmacological approach involves oral antibiotics, such as Ciprofloxacin and Metronidazole, to target colonic bacteria. Pain management will be done with acetaminophen, avoiding NSAIDs due to their potential gastrointestinal risks. The patient will also be encouraged to ensure adequate hydration to prevent dehydration. (See algorithm below) **Non-Pharmacological Approach**: Initially, the patient is advised to follow a low-fiber diet during the acute phase, with gradual reintroduction of fiber once symptoms improve. Foods like nuts, seeds, and popcorn should be avoided to reduce irritation. The patient will be kept NPO (nothing by mouth) for 24-48 hours to allow bowel rest, followed by a gradual introduction of clear liquids and low-fiber foods. Once symptoms resolve, increasing fiber intake through fruits, vegetables, and whole grains will be encouraged. Bed rest is recommended during the acute phase to reduce abdominal strain, and physical activity should be avoided. Education will be provided on the chronic nature of diverticulitis and the importance of maintaining a fiber-rich diet and staying hydrated to prevent future flare-ups. **Follow-up**: A follow-up appointment will be scheduled in 1-2 weeks to assess symptom resolution. If symptoms do not improve or worsen, further imaging may be required to rule out complications such as abscess formation or perforation. The patient will be educated on lifestyle modifications, including increasing fiber intake and regular physical activity, to manage and prevent future episodes.

Figure 97 SOAP Notes for Divertculitis

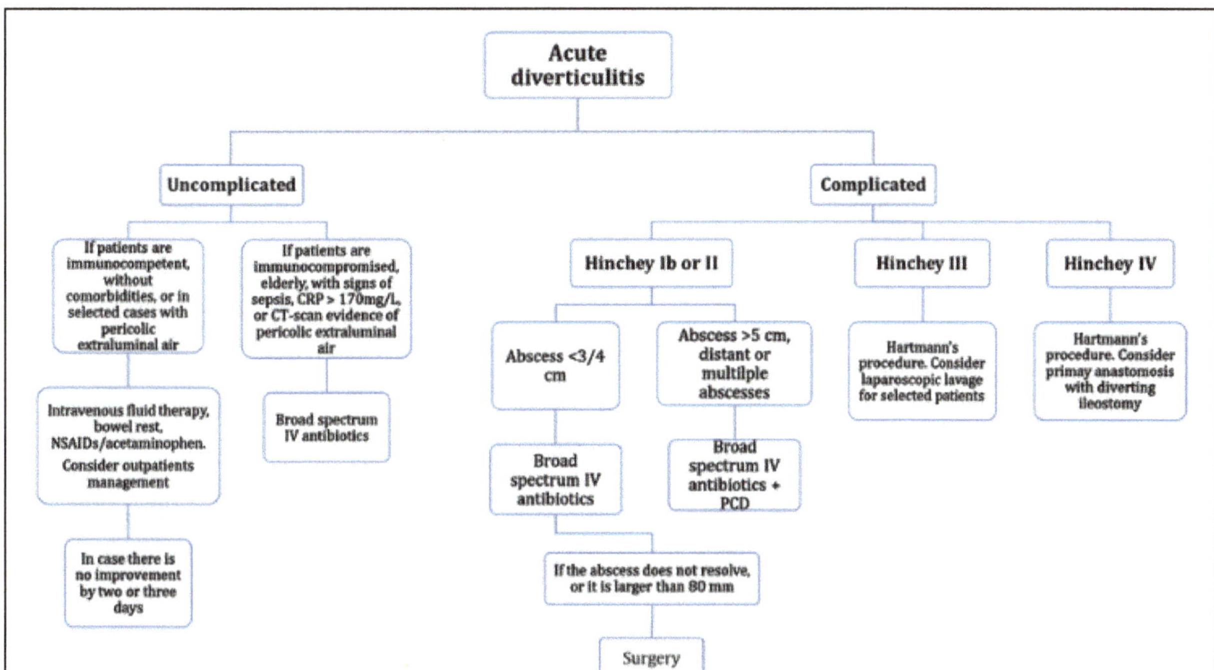

Figure 98 Management of Diverticulitis

4.3.10 *Gastroenteritis*

Gastroenteritis is an inflammation of the gut and commonly referred to as the **'stomach flu,'** which is a more accurate term because it has no relation to the influenza virus. They are usually due to **budding from viruses, bacteria or parasites**. There are two forms of **viral gastroenteritis** and the most common one is the one known commonly as the stomach flu which is usually caused by the norovirus and the rotavirus. Some of the bacteria which cause bacterial Gastroenteritis include ***Salmonella, Escherichia coli (E.coli), Campylobacter and Shigella*** and the parasitic causing ***Giardia***. There are various forms of diarrhoea which may be due to contaminated food or water, or due to contact with a carrier of the illness. Consequently, the common signs of gastroenteritis are **diarrhoea, nausea, vomiting, stomach aches or pains, and possibly fever**. These symptoms are quite common and they are manifested through sudden formation of symptoms which cause dehydration in most children and elderly people. Extreme cases of dehydration lead to dry mouth, low amounts of urine passed, dizziness and weakness. In most cases, it is **generally mild and may be cured in three to one week** and sometimes it rarely leads to complications. Treatment is mainly concerned with the administration of ORS if the patient has oral intake capacity or intravenous fluids if the conditions are severe. Some infections are due to bacteria and therefore may be treated using antibiotics, while others are a result of viruses and do not have antiviral medicine. It is therefore very essential that good hygienic practices such as **washing one's hands prevent the development of gastroenteritis.**

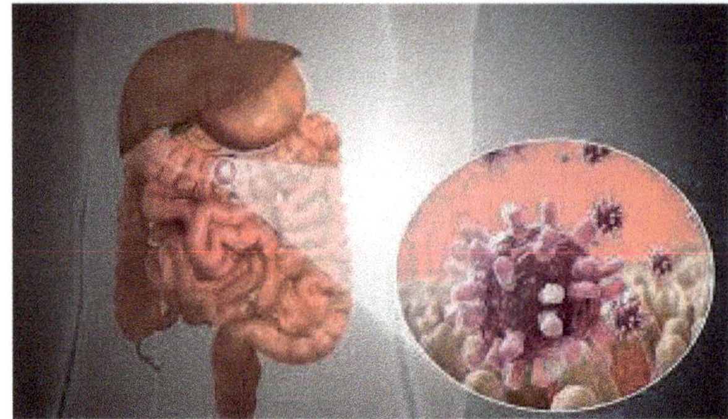

Figure 99 Gastroenteritis (Stomach Flu)

4.3.10.1 Types of Gastroenteritis

The image provides brief descriptions of three types of gastrointestinal illness different pathogens, mode of transmission, duration, and symptoms. The **travelling diarrhoea** is mainly caused by ***E.coli***, second by ***Salmonella***, third by ***Campylobacter*** and fourth by ***Shigella*** which is acquired from contaminated food or water during travelling. It is usually manifested in the first 1-5 days of incubation and the symptoms include; **Loss of appetite, abdominal pain, cramping, diarrhea, nausea, vomiting, fever, and general malaise.** The second type is the foodborne acute gastroenteritis that results from ***Clostridium difficile*** initiated from meals made from meat, ***Staphylococcus aureus*** from dairy products, eggs, and salads, ***Clostridium perfringens*** from cereals, ***Bacillus cereus*** from beans, fish, and meat, while Shigella and Salmonella are found in meat products. It is worthy of note that while ***S. aureus*** and ***B. cereus*** cause symptoms within 1-6 hours, ***C. perfringens*** within 6-48 hours; though Salmonella and Shigella have a longer duration of approximately 3-7 days. When the situation is severe food poisoning, the symptoms include severe watery diarrhoea, abdomen cramping, nausea, vomiting, and sometimes fever. Last of all, antibiotic-associated diarrhoea is the result of taking antibiotics and leads to the growth of ***Clostridium perfringens***, ***Clostridium difficile***, and ***Clostridium orbiscome***. This type is spread through the fecal-oral route and the features often appear 2- 3 weeks after the beginning of antibiotics and disappear if antibiotics are stopped. Some of the signs of cholera are tummy ache, high fever, vomiting, and severe diarrhoea resembling rice water.

Table 64 Classification of Gastroenteritis

Type	Common Pathogens	Transmission	Duration	Symptoms
Traveller's Diarrhoea	E coli followed by Salmonella, Campylobacter, Shigella	contaminated food or water	1-5 days	Malaise, anorexia, abdominal pain, cramping, watery diarrhoea nausea, vomiting and fever.
Foodborne acute gastroenteritis	Clostridium difficile, Staphylococcus aureus, Clostridium perferingens Bacillus cereus, Shigella, Salmonella etc	meat products, dairy products, eggs, salads, cereals etc.	S.aureus, B.cereus: 1-6hrs; C.perferingens: 6-48hrs; Salmonella, Shigella: 3-7 days	Severe watery diarrhoea, abdominal cramping, nausea, vomiting, fever
Antibiotic - associated diarrhoea	Increased use of antibiotics associated with risk of Clostridium difficile infection.	Faeco oral route; the continuous use of antibiotics disturbed the normal flora of the intestinal tract	symptoms seen 2-3 weeks after antibiotic usage and resolve after its stoppage	Abdominal pain fever, nausea, watery diarrhoea.

4.3.10.2 Difference between Bacterial and Viral Gastroenteritis

Gastroenteritis refers to an **inflammation of the stomach and the small intestines** as a result of a **viral or bacterial infection**. Gastric inflammation, also known as stomach influenza is a sickness that is mainly caused by **norovirus or rotavirus**. It is more usually passed through **food and water** and is not related to the consumption of meat products or travel. The array of conditions include **diarrhoea, vomiting, nausea, abdominal pain and fever.** It is normally a short illness, and blood or faecal leukocytes are not commonly identified in the faeces. This form of gastroenteritis is, in most cases, convenient and can only last for a short time; however, some potentially severe symptoms include diarrhoea, and thus causes dehydration in groups vulnerable such **as children, the elderly** and those with weak immune systems. While, bacterial diarrhoea is caused by bacteria for example **Salmonella, Shigella or Campylobacter** and food particularly meat products or contact with animals may trigger it. The bacterial infection symptoms are more severe as they include; **fever, stomach ache, vomiting, and diarrhea accompanied by blood**. Therefore, the detection of faecal leukocytes shown in this study forms a major component of bacterial gastroenteritis since it is the body's immune response to the bacteria causing the diarrhoea. This form is often **treated by antibiotics**, and it is more dangerous than other forms of gastroenteritis, which leads often to dehydration and electrolyte imbalance.

4.3.10.3 SOAP Notes for Gastroenteritis

Table 65 SOAP Notes for Gastroenteritis

Component	Details
Subjective (S)	The patient is a 28-year-old female presenting with a 2-day history of diarrhea, nausea, vomiting, and abdominal cramping. She reports that the symptoms started suddenly after returning from a family gathering, where she ate undercooked chicken and salads. She has also experienced low-grade fever and mild chills. The patient denies recent travel, blood in her stool, or previous gastrointestinal issues. She is concerned about dehydration due to her frequent vomiting. The patient has no significant medical history and takes no regular medications.
Objective (O)	On physical examination, the patient appears fatigued but is alert and oriented. Vital signs: blood pressure 110/70 mmHg, heart rate 98 bpm, respiratory rate 18 bpm, temperature 37.8°C (100°F). The patient has mild abdominal tenderness, especially in the lower quadrants, with no rebound tenderness or guarding. There are no signs of dehydration such as dry mucous membranes or low skin turgor. Bowel sounds are normal. Laboratory results show no significant abnormalities; a stool sample is negative for blood but positive for increased white blood cells, suggesting an inflammatory response.
Assessment (A)	The patient's presentation of diarrhea, vomiting, abdominal cramping, and fever, along with the recent consumption of undercooked chicken, is consistent with bacterial gastroenteritis, likely caused by Salmonella or Campylobacter. The negative stool culture for blood suggests a non-invasive bacterial infection. Although viral gastroenteritis remains a possibility, the presence of fever and recent foodborne exposure points more toward a

	bacterial cause. The patient appears to be in the early stages of dehydration, but there are no signs of severe fluid loss or shock.
Plan (P)	**Supportive Care**: Hydration: Start oral rehydration therapy (ORS) for mild dehydration. If vomiting persists or the patient is unable to tolerate oral fluids, consider IV fluids for rehydration. **Antiemetic**: Ondansetron (4 mg) for nausea and vomiting to improve fluid intake. **Antibiotics**: Antibiotic therapy is not indicated unless symptoms worsen or signs of severe infection (e.g., fever > 101°F, prolonged diarrhoea, or bloody stools) develop. If bacterial infection is confirmed, consider fluoroquinolones (e.g., ciprofloxacin) or macrolides (e.g., azithromycin) based on susceptibility. Symptom Management: Recommend anti-diarrheal medication such as loperamide for symptomatic relief, but only if no fever or blood in stools is present. Advise a BRAT diet (bananas, rice, applesauce, and toast) once vomiting subsides and progress to a bland diet as tolerated (See algorithms). **Monitoring**: Monitor for signs of severe dehydration, particularly in the next 24 hours. Follow up if symptoms persist beyond 48 hours or worsen. **Education**: Advise the patient to avoid undercooked food, especially meat and poultry, and ensure good hand hygiene to prevent future episodes. Educate on the importance of hydration and proper dietary management during recovery. Provide guidance on when to seek medical attention, such as if symptoms worsen or if severe dehydration signs occur.

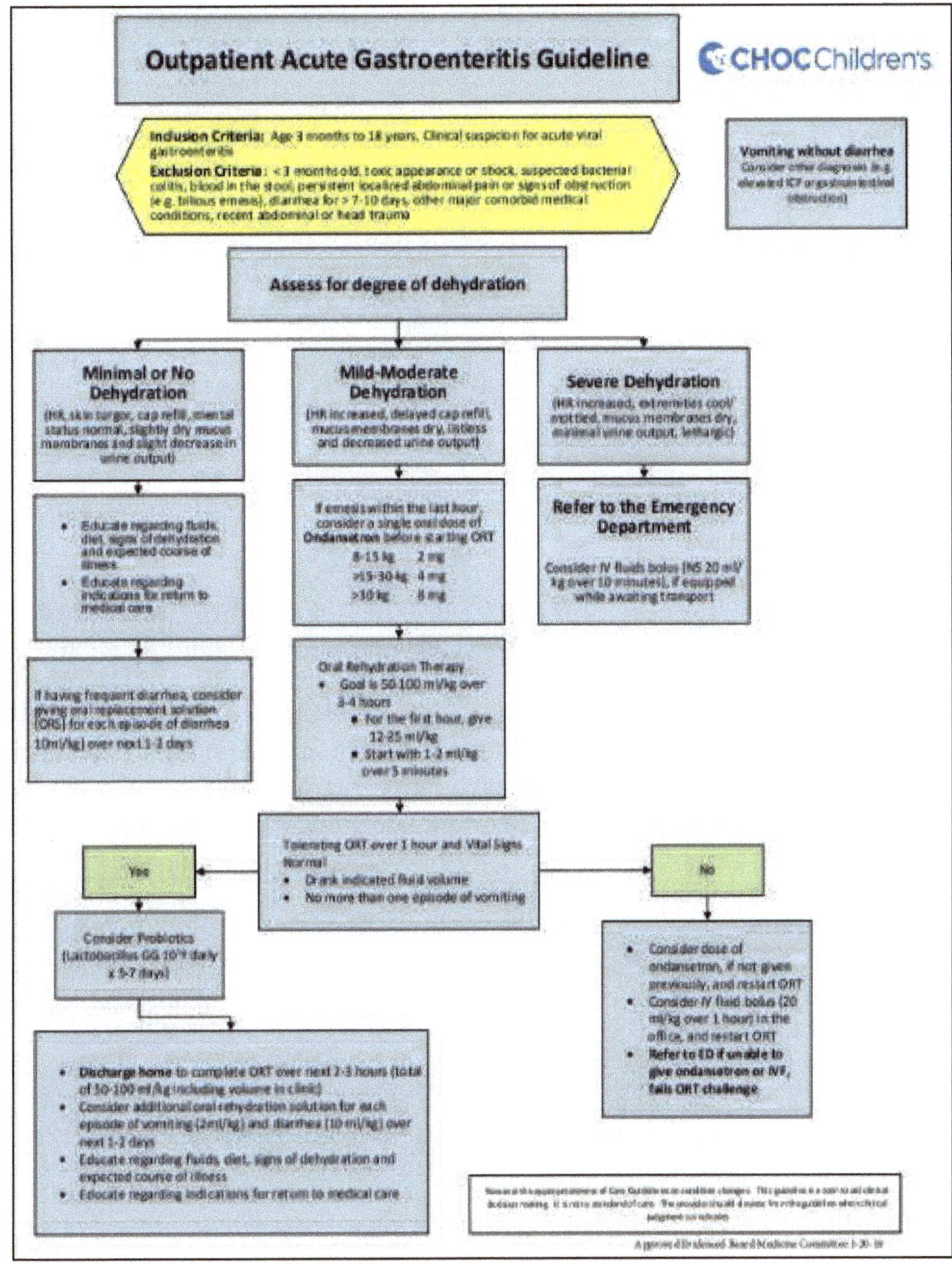

Figure 100 Algorithm for the Management of Gastroenteritis in Children

Degree of dehydration	No or minimal dehydration	Mild to moderate dehydration	Severe dehydration
Rehydration therapy	None	ORS 50–100 mL/kg body weight over 3–4 hours If vomiting is persistent, the patient (child or adult) will not take ORS and is likely to need intravenous fluids	Rehydrate with Ringer's lactate solution (100 mg/kg) intravenously within 4–6 hours Then administer ORS to maintain hydration until patient recovers
Replacement of losses	< 10 kg body weight: 50–100 mL ORS for each diarrheal stool or vomiting episode		
Nutrition	Continue breastfeeding or age-appropriate normal diet	Continue breastfeeding, or resume age-appropriate normal diet after initial hydration	

Figure 101 Management Approaches of Gastroenteritis

4.3.11 Food poisoning

Food poisoning is a common illness caused by consuming **contaminated food or beverages**, which can lead to inflammation of the stomach and intestines. This contamination may stem from **bacteria, viruses, parasitic organisms, or toxins** synthesized by these microorganisms. The primary bacteria leading to food poisoning are ***Salmonella, Escherichia coli (E. coli), Campylobacter, Listeria, Norovirus, and Clostridium botulinum.*** Also, contagious food poisoning such as Staphylococcus aureus or bacillus cereus poisoning results from the toxins secreted by bacteria before the food is ingested. Food poisoning shows different effects based on the toxin responsible for the infection, and the following are some of the effects; **Nausea, vomiting, abdominal pains, diarrhea, fever, and headaches.** Symptoms of food poisoning usually develop within **2 to 5 hours** after eating contaminated food, though some bacteria like ***Salmonella or E. coli*** have a longer onset time. Food poisoning can cause the patient to become dehydrated because of vomiting, diarrhea, and other complications which could include **kidney failure and sepsis.**

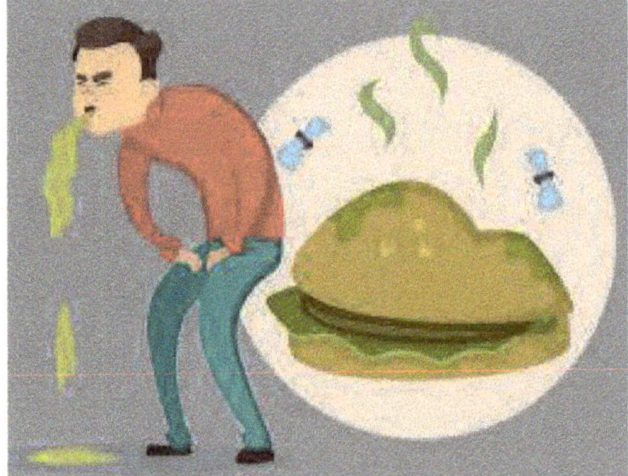

Figure 102 Food Poisoning

Management of food poisoning is mainly symptomatic, which may consist of **frequent fluid intake** to avoid dehydration, especially in children and the elderly. **Oral rehydration solutions (ORS)** are commonly advised to replace lost fluids and **electrolyte balance**. Most cases of food poisoning are mild, and the body can clear them up on its own without the use of drugs. However, antibiotics may be needed in some cases, if a bacterial infection is confirmed. If the cause is a toxin, like **botulism, then antitoxins** are given to the affected individual. Measures used in preventing food poisoning include; proper cooking of foods especially meats, **washing of hands, proper cleaning of surfaces, and right storage temperatures for the food**. Ensuring that principles of public health are upheld, including food safety by agencies like the Food and Drug Administration and the Centre for Disease Control and Prevention is thus crucial in preventing them. Washing hands and surfaces that are commonly used during food processing and handling can go a long way in preventing foodborne diseases.

4.3.11.1 Types of Food Poisoning

The flowchart shown in Figure 90 helps to classify food poisoning into two types; **Food Intoxication and Food Infection** both of which have different causative agents and different ways in which they affect the human body. Food Intoxication is one condition that results from the **consumption of toxins from foods** that have been contaminated by **microorganisms**. Some of these are botulism caused by ***Clostridium botulinum*** which results in **paralysis and respiratory failure.** Another example is staphylococcal poisoning which is caused by ***Staphylococcus aureus*** and affects individuals through **vomiting and diarrhea** after taking foods that have been contaminated by the **bacteria**. Mycotoxicosis is a condition arising from the consumption of toxic fungi like **Amanita mushrooms** that affects the liver. Phycotoxicosis or algal food poisoning is the poisonous effects of compounds produced by algae like **Gymnodinium** which commonly affects **seafood**. Furthermore, diseases such as **Polio, Hepatitis A & E, and gastroenteritis** viruses are some examples of viruses that are foodborne diseases that can be transferred through **contaminated foods or drinking water**. However, Food Infection is a disease that results from bacteria or any other pathogen invading the body through consuming any infected food. Examples include bacterial foodborne infections such as **Shigellosis (bacillary dysentery) by Shigella and *E.coli*, an acute gastrointestinal illness that can be severe, and Cholera caused by *Vibrio cholerae* that causes diarrhea** leading to severe dehydration. Other bacterial infections that can cause fever, weakness, and abdominal pain include **Brucellosis**, which is caused by Brucella bacteria. This classification shows how foodborne diseases may result from ingestion of preformed toxins or infection by pathogens entering the body.

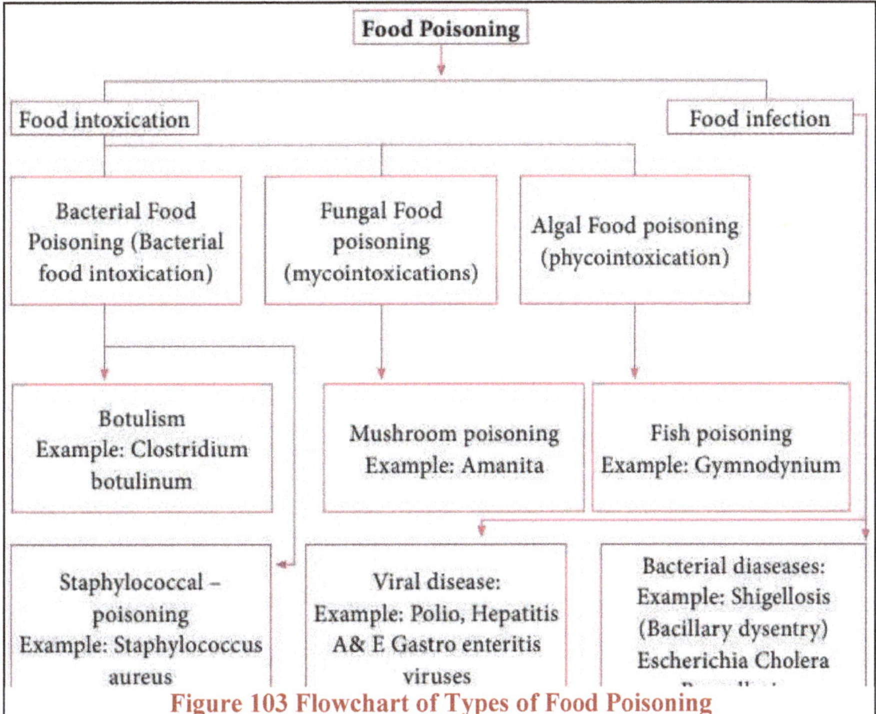

Figure 103 Flowchart of Types of Food Poisoning

4.3.11.2 Major Types of Bacterial Food Poisoning

The table below summarizes and contrasts **four common categories of bacterial food poisoning** including the type of bacteria, the time of onset, signs of the disease, foodborne, and measures taken to avoid such bacteria.

An example of a bacterial infection that's communicable is salmonellosis whose bacteria have an **incubation period of 6-48 hours.** It usually lasts for **48 to 72 hours** and the main clinical symptoms are **headache, abdominal discomfort, and gastrointestinal disorders**. It is often linked to **meats, poultry products, salads, egg custards, and other products containing protein**. Some of the measures include: washing hands to eliminate fecal contamination from food handlers and avoiding the preparation of food in an unsafe manner.

Staphylococcal poisoning, which is mainly caused by ***Staphylococcus aureus***, has the shortest **incubation period which ranges between 1-6 hours** and its duration is between **1-2 days**. Signs and symptoms of the disorder involve **stomach aches, nausea, vomiting, and diarrhea**. This condition is closely connected with foods that are cooked improperly as well as with the **cream fillings for pastries, dairy products, meat, and salads.** Precautions involve washing, proper cooking, cooling, and separation from individuals infected with food-related diseases.

Botulism, which is due to ***Clostridium botulinum***, has a longer **incubation period of 12-36 hours** and symptoms include **fatigue and headache, dizziness, visual disturbances, and difficulty in moving the tongue and swallowing**. It is commonly found in foods that are processed inadequately preserved **canned vegetables, fruits, mushrooms, fish, particularly tuna and figs**. To eliminate botulism the food must be cooked at high pressure, and temperature, and require boiling and stirring canned food for twenty minutes.

In addition, Clostridium perfringens poisoning happens between the **8th and 22nd hours** and usually takes **one day to heal**. Some of the signs include vomiting and gastrointestinal upset. This type of food poisoning stems from the consumption of foods with well-cooked textures such as **boiled, steamed, braised, or stewed meats**. Measures to reduce risk include controlling time and temperature of cooking, rapid cooling of cooked meats, and separation between raw and cooked products.

Table 66 Bacterial Food Poisoning and Prevention

Details	Salmonellosis	Staphylococcal poisoning	Botulism	Clostridium perfringens poisoning
Bacteria	Salmonella	*Staphylococcus aureus*	*Clostridium botulinum*	*Clostridium perfringens*
Incubation period	6-48 hours	1-6 hours	12-36 hours	8-22 hours
Duration of illness	2-3 days	1-2 days	Several days to a year	One day
Symptoms	Headache, abdominal pain. Plate 8.13 Symptoms	Abdominal pain, nausea, vomiting, diarrhoea.	Fatigue, headache, dizziness, visual disturbances, inability to swallow.	Abdominal pain, diarrhoea. Plate 8.14 Signs of Food Poisoning
Foods affected	Meat, meat products, poultry, salads,egg custards and other protein foods.	Improperly prepared custards, cream filled pastries,dairy products, meat poultry, salads.	Improperly processed canned foods, mushrooms, tuna, figs.	Boiled,steamed, braised, stewed meat.
Prevention	* Strict personal hygiene * Avoidance of fecal contamination from unclean food handlers. * Unsafe practices.	* Cleanliness and sanitary habits. * Proper heating and refrigeration. * Exclusion of infected food handlers.	* Pressure cooking food at high temperatures in canning. * Boiling and stirring home canned food for 20 minutes.	* Careful time and temperature control. * Quick chilling of cooked meat dishes. * Isolation of raw and cooked foods.

4.3.11.3 Comparison Between the Symptoms of Stomach Flu and Food Poisoning

Stomach flu which is also referred to as **viral gastroenteritis** has a duration of **12 to 48 hours** from the onset of exposure. The symptoms include **vomiting, diarrhea, fever, nausea, and stomach ache.** Body aches and chills are also common, but **thirst and coughing are less likely**. Stomach flu, in general, usually lasts **one to three days**. The symptoms are similar to those of stomach flu, including vomiting, diarrhea, nausea, and stomach pain. However, food poisoning tends to cause **sharp abdominal pain and is more likely to cause dehydration**. Body aches and chills are less common with food poisoning, and the symptoms can last anywhere **from 1 to 10 days**, depending on the severity and type of bacteria or toxin causing the illness..

Table 67 Stomach Flu VS. Food Poisoning

Symptoms	Stomach Flu	Food Poisoning
Onset after exposure	12 to 48 hours	Quick, 2 to 6 hours
Vomiting	Common	Common
Diarrhea	Common	Common
Fever	Common (low-grade)	Common
Nausea	Common	Common
Stomachache	Dull pain	Sharp pain
Body aches	More likely	Less likely
Sweating	Uncommon	Common
Chills	Common	Common
Confusion	Uncommon	In severe cases
Thirst	Less common	More common
Contagious	Likely yes	Likely no
Duration	Usually 1 to 3 days	Usually 1 to 10 days

4.3.11.4 SOAP Notes for Food Poisoning

Table 68 SOAP Notes for Food Poisoning

Component	Details
Subjective (S)	The patient is a 35-year-old male who presents with a 6-hour history of nausea, vomiting, abdominal cramps, and diarrhea. The patient reports that he ate undercooked chicken at a local restaurant about 6 hours before the onset of symptoms. He mentions that his symptoms began suddenly after a few hours of consuming the meal, and he has since been unable to keep any food or liquids down. He denies any fever, chills, or blood in his stool but reports feeling weak and concerned about dehydration. The patient denies any previous gastrointestinal issues or chronic conditions and is otherwise healthy. He denies recent travel or exposure to any sick individuals.
Objective (O)	The patient appears moderately dehydrated but is alert and oriented. Vital signs: blood pressure 110/70 mmHg, heart rate 96 bpm, respiratory rate 18 bpm, temperature 37.5°C (99.5°F). The abdomen is soft but tender to palpation in the epigastric area. There is no rebound tenderness or guarding. Bowel sounds are present but slightly hyperactive. The patient has dry mucous membranes, and his skin turgor is slightly reduced, indicating mild dehydration. A stool sample is negative for blood but positive for increased white blood cells, suggesting an inflammatory process. Laboratory tests show normal electrolytes, and renal function tests are within normal limits.
Assessment (A)	The patient's clinical presentation, including nausea, vomiting, abdominal cramps, and diarrhea, along with the recent consumption of undercooked chicken, is consistent with bacterial food poisoning, likely caused by Salmonella or Campylobacter. The negative stool culture for blood and the presence of fecal leukocytes suggest a bacterial cause rather than a viral infection. The patient is experiencing mild dehydration due to fluid loss, but there are no signs of severe dehydration or systemic infection at this time.

	The patient is in the early stages of recovery but requires symptomatic treatment and monitoring for complications.
Plan (P)	**Hydration:** Start oral rehydration therapy (ORS) to replace lost fluids and electrolytes. If vomiting persists or the patient is unable to tolerate oral fluids, initiate IV fluids (e.g., Normal Saline or Lactated Ringer's) for rehydration. **Symptom Management:** Antiemetics: Administer Ondansetron 4 mg IV for nausea and vomiting. Antidiarrheal: Consider Loperamide (2 mg initially, then 1 mg after each loose stool) to reduce diarrhea, but only if there is no fever or blood in stools. **Antibiotics:** Antibiotics are not routinely indicated for mild cases of food poisoning unless the infection is severe or there are signs of systemic involvement. If symptoms worsen or if a more serious bacterial infection is suspected, initiate appropriate antibiotics (e.g., ciprofloxacin for Campylobacter or Salmonella) (See algorithm below). **Monitoring:** Monitor the patient for signs of severe dehydration, such as reduced urine output, confusion, or dizziness. Regularly monitor vital signs, including blood pressure and heart rate, to assess for fluid imbalance or shock. **Patient Education:** Advise the patient to follow a BRAT diet (bananas, rice, applesauce, and toast) once vomiting subsides and to avoid dairy and high-fat foods during recovery. Educate the patient on the importance of proper food safety, including cooking meat thoroughly, washing hands, and avoiding cross-contamination to prevent future episodes. **Follow-up:** Schedule a follow-up appointment in 2-3 days if symptoms persist or worsen. If symptoms resolve, instruct the patient to monitor their condition and seek medical attention if symptoms such as fever, blood in stool, or severe abdominal pain occur.

Table 69 Algorithm for the Management of Food Poisoning

Category	Details	Additional Information	Prevention Tips
Fluids and Electrolytes	Adults: Drink water, diluted fruit juices, sports drinks, broths, and saltine crackers. For severe dehydration, older adults or immunocompromised individuals should use oral rehydration solutions like Pedialyte, Naturalyte, or CeraLyte. Children: Oral rehydration solutions like Pedialyte should be given, as directed by a doctor. Infants	Sipping small amounts of liquids like water, broths, and diluted fruit juices can prevent dehydration. If vomiting persists, IV fluids may be necessary.	Ensure proper hydration and replenishment of lost electrolytes. Use rehydration solutions for vulnerable groups, such as children and elderly.

	should continue breastfeeding or formula feeding.		
Over-the-Counter Medicines	Adults: Medicines like Loperamide (Imodium) or Bismuth subsalicylate (Pepto-Bismol, Kaopectate) can be used to treat diarrhea caused by food poisoning. These are not recommended for infants and children. Do not use these if there is bloody diarrhea or fever.	Loperamide (Imodium) and Bismuth subsalicylate (Pepto-Bismol, Kaopectate) are used for symptom management but should not be used for bacterial or parasitic infections with fever or blood in stool.	Use over-the-counter treatments for mild symptoms, but avoid them if signs of severe infection like blood in stools or fever are present. Always consult a healthcare provider if unsure.
Doctor's Treatment	Bacterial or Parasitic Infections: Doctors may prescribe antibiotics or medicines targeting parasites along with rehydration solutions. Probiotics: In some cases, probiotics may be recommended to help reduce the duration of diarrhea. Severe Cases: Hospitalization may be required for life-threatening symptoms, such as severe dehydration or complications like hemolytic uremic syndrome or paralysis.	Probiotics may help reduce the duration of diarrhea, but their use should be discussed with a doctor, particularly for vulnerable groups such as children and the elderly.	Seek medical help when symptoms persist or worsen, especially in cases of high fever or dehydration. Antibiotics and probiotics may be prescribed for specific bacterial infections.
Prevention	Safe Food Handling: Practice good hygiene by washing hands before and after handling food. Cook meats to the correct temperature, and wash fruits and vegetables before eating or cooking. Avoid Leaving Food Out: Don't eat foods that have been left out for more than 2 hours, or more than 1 hour in temperatures above 90°F (32°C).	Safe food handling practices include separating raw meats, storing food at the correct temperature, and preventing cross-contamination during meal preparation.	Follow proper food safety measures, including refrigeration, washing hands before food preparation, and cooking foods to proper temperatures. Avoid eating food that has been left

			out for extended periods.
Food Safety	Proper Storage: Keep raw meat separate from other foods, and store perishable items promptly in the refrigerator or freezer. Food Recalls: Be alert for food recalls and dispose of any recalled foods immediately.	Regularly monitor food recalls from health authorities, such as the CDC or FDA, and dispose of recalled food to prevent foodborne illnesses.	Always store food at safe temperatures, avoid cross-contamination, and practice good hygiene. Be aware of food recalls and dispose of any affected items.

4.3.12 Appendicitis

Appendicitis is the condition that is characterized by **inflammations of the appendix** which is a small fingerlike pouch located at the junction of the small intestine and the large intestine. An appendicitis is a medical condition that needs urgent attention, and this often includes **surgery that aims at removing the appendix**, commonly done through an **appendectomy**. Appendicitis is a worm-like structure connccted to the large colon that is caused by blockage of the appendix by fecal matter, foreign bodies, or infections. This results in increased pressure within the appendix, **poor blood circulation, and increased bacterial growth** within the appendix which in turn becomes very swollen.

The main sign of appendicitis is abd**ominal pain, initially around the navel, and then moving to the lower right quarter of the abdomen**. The intensity of the pain also increases and becomes localized with the progression of the disease. Other typical signs include **vomiting, gastrointestinal disturbances, lack of appetite, fever, as well as chronic constipation or diarrhea**. In addition to being localized, the pain increases with movements such as walking or coughing, and rebound tenderness is also present. Appendicitis can be diagnosed through a **physical examination, and blood tests** including white blood cell count will be conducted to observe shifts that indicate infection which will be further confirmed through ultrasound to determine the inflammation of the appendix. In some cases an examination, or observation may be warranted or a **diagnostic laparoscopy**. The conventional approach to managing appendicitis is usually through surgery, where the affected appendix is removed. This can be achieved through an open approach or through a laparoscopic approach, which is more conventional. If it has burst and **caused peritonitis (infection in the lining of the abdominal cavity),** the treatment may involve draining the peritoneum and administering antibiotics.

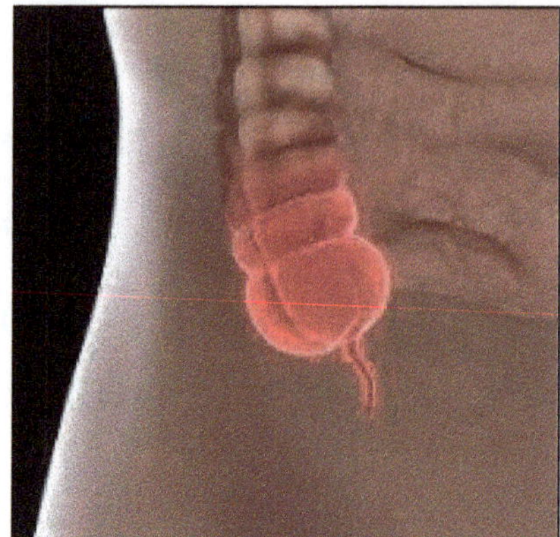

Figure 104 Appendicitis

Appendicitis, if untreated, has some of the most severe consequences possible for abdominal inflammation. In the event that these lead to appendicitis, the appendix may rupture releasing bacteria that cause peritonitis; a severe form of **infection in the abdominal cavity**. Other complications may include the formation of abscesses or even intestinal obstruction. Appropriate measures to avoid **appendicitis** cannot be taken, since the cause of the blockage is often unknown. However, **early diagnosis and subsequent treatment** should not be overlooked because they prevent the development of complications such as rupture. Today, appendicitis continues to be one of the main causes of acute abdominal pain that has to be operated on urgently.

4.3.12.1 Examination of Appendicitis

Several examination techniques in appendicitis enable healthcare providers to detect inflammation markers and peritoneal irritation. When patients experience pain at **McBurney's Point** one-third of the way from the **anterior superior iliac spine to the umbilicus the classic diagnostic indication for appendicitis is confirmed**. **The Rovsing's test** involves touching the left lower abdomen to detect pain in the opposing **right region indicating appendix inflammation**. The **Psoas Sign** assesses psoas muscle irritation by having patients attempt right hip flexion with resistance; positive results **indicate retrocecal appendicitis.** The Obturator Sign evaluates right hip joint actions through flexion and rotation to detect pelvic appendix conditions. Advanced appendicitis or possible perforation is indicated when **peritoneal inflammation** presents with **Guarding and Rebound Tenderness** signs that trigger involuntary muscle tightening and produce pain when pressure is released.

4.3.12.2 Classification of Appendicitis

For uncomplicated acute appendicitis, patients are classified further into borderline AA (type 1a) and **phlegmonous AA (type 1b).** The management of patients with a low-risk level of AA that is considered borderline entails the use of **antibiotics (AB)** to manage the risk factor, with the possible addition of ultrasound (US) to evaluate the extension of the disease. **For phlegmonous AA**, which is less severe than simple abscesses but **more severe than borderline cases**, surgical intervention is unnecessary and antibiotics can be prescribed if the condition is uncomplicated. However, for higher-risk patients, **the IV contrast should be performed** during early elective surgery within a 24-hour duration. Complicated acute appendicitis involves the following types: **PAA with obstruction and/or extraluminal fluid (type 2a), gangrenous AA (type 2b), free perforation (type 3b), PAA severe with abscess or mass (type 3a).** The management of PAA with obstruction is surgical and should ideally be done immediately within 24 hours. Perforated appendicitis involving gangrene or free perforation where there is dead tissue or a burst appendix with infection calls for surgery within 6 hours because of the fatal consequences that might occur.

Lastly, in instances where there is PAA accompanied by abscess or mass, the management is drainage of the abscess and surgery in cases with mass.

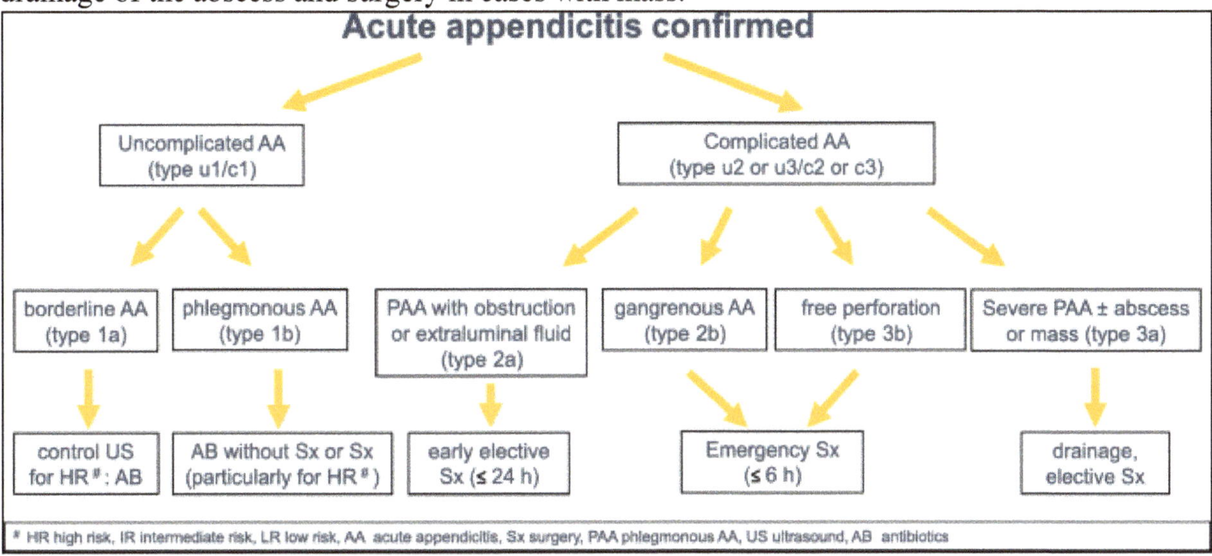

Figure 105 Classification of Acute Appendicitis

4.3.12.3 Classification of Acute Appendicitis Based on Severity

Acute appendicitis which does not involve perforation complications can be categorized into two grades. **Grade 0** describes the condition of an appendix that macroscopically exhibits no flair or injuries and if examined microscopically, there either is no pathological change or their changes are minor. **Grade I** implies appendicitis, which is hallmarked by **signs like hyperemia, edema, and at times, fibrinization. It** is also termed as mild inflammation that is not severe and does not have complications. **In complicated acute appendicitis,** the condition advances and has features of tissue ischemia and death, rupture, or abscess development. Grade II includes necrosis, or the death of tissues within the appendix, confined to a segment or extending to the base of the appendix. It takes **Grade III** which corresponds to **perforative appendicitis** when an inflammation tumor occurs. This can be with **phlegmon**, which is an extensive inflammatory process without the formation of localized suppuration, or with abscess formation, and abscesses may be small, **less than 5 cm in diameter, or large, more than 5 cm in diameter**, with the large ones, especially if they are localized in the deep tissues, additionally may require drainage or surgical intervention. Lastly, **Grade IV** is accompanied or characterized by the perforated appendix leading to diffuse peritonitis which is an infection of the whole abdominal cavity, and in such cases, surgery has to be done to treat the infection as well as prevent future complications.

Table 70 Categorization of Acute Appendicitis

Uncomplicated Acute Appendicitis	
Grade 0	Macroscopically normal/histological endoappendicitis
Grade I	Inflamed appendix (hyperemia, edema ± fibrin)
Complicated Acute Appendicitis	
Grade II	Necrosis (a) Segmental (b) Involving the base
Grade III	Perforated–inflammatory tumor (a) With phlegmon (b) With <5 cm abscess (c) With >5 cm abscess
Grade IV	Perforated with diffuse peritonitis

4.3.12.4 SOAP Notes for Appendicitis

Table 71 SOAP Notes for Appendicitis

Component	Details
Subjective (S)	The patient is a 25-year-old male who presents with a 2-day history of abdominal pain that initially started around the belly button and then shifted to the lower right side of the abdomen. He describes the pain as sharp and persistent, which worsens with movements such as walking or coughing. In addition to the abdominal pain, the patient reports nausea, loss of appetite, and a mild fever (38°C/100.4°F). He mentions no vomiting or diarrhea but states some constipation. Over the past 24 hours, the pain has intensified and become more localized to the lower right quadrant of the abdomen. The patient denies recent travel, gastrointestinal illnesses, or prior surgeries and has no known chronic medical conditions.
Objective (O)	On examination, the patient's vital signs reveal a heart rate of 98 bpm, blood pressure of 120/75 mmHg, respiratory rate of 18 bpm, and a temperature of 38°C (100.4°F), suggesting a fever likely due to an infection. Physical examination shows right lower quadrant tenderness, particularly at McBurney's point, with rebound tenderness and guarding, which are indicative of peritoneal irritation. The Rovsing's sign (pain in the right lower abdomen when palpating the left lower abdomen) is positive, further supporting the diagnosis of appendicitis. The psoas sign is also positive, indicating irritation of the iliopsoas muscle due to inflammation. Bowel sounds are slightly reduced. Laboratory findings include an elevated white blood cell count (12,000 cells/mm^3), suggesting an ongoing infection. Imaging with an abdominal ultrasound or CT scan confirms an enlarged, inflamed appendix, potentially with perforation.
Assessment (A)	The patient is diagnosed with acute appendicitis, most likely uncomplicated, but the imaging and clinical presentation suggest the possibility of perforation. The classic presentation of right lower quadrant pain, along with

	rebound tenderness and positive Rovsing's and psoas signs, strongly supports this diagnosis. The elevated white blood cell count and imaging findings confirm inflammation and possible rupture, which increases the risk of peritonitis or abscess formation. The patient is at moderate to high risk for complications if not treated promptly. Immediate surgical intervention, likely an appendectomy, is required to prevent worsening of the condition.
Plan (P)	The patient will undergo an appendectomy, the standard treatment for appendicitis. If perforation is confirmed during surgery, additional measures such as drainage and antibiotic therapy will be required to manage peritonitis. Preoperatively, the patient will be given IV fluids for hydration and IV antibiotics (e.g., Ceftriaxone and Metronidazole) to reduce the risk of infection. For pain management, the patient will receive acetaminophen or opioids as needed (See algorithm below). After surgery, the patient will be monitored closely for 24-48 hours to check for complications such as infection or abscess formation. Once the patient is stable, he will be started on oral antibiotics for 7-10 days. Postoperative care will focus on maintaining hydration, monitoring the surgical site for infection, and ensuring proper pain management. Patient education will be provided regarding wound care, signs of infection, and the importance of follow-up visits. A follow-up appointment will be scheduled within 1-2 weeks to monitor recovery and ensure no further complications arise.

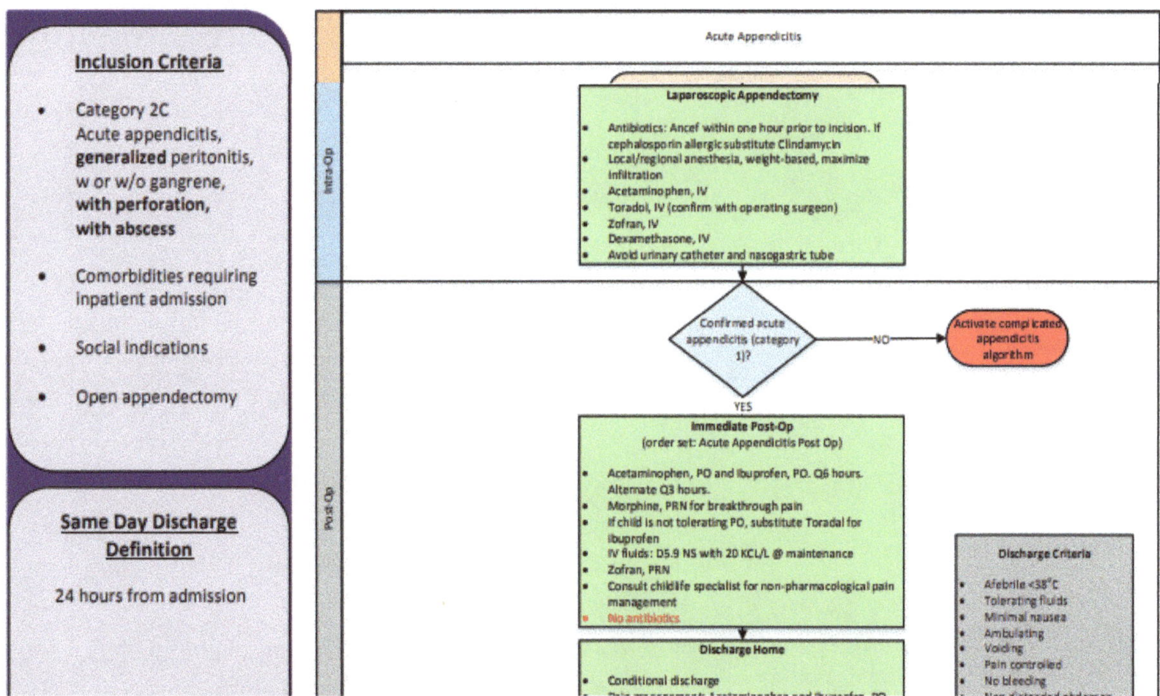

Figure 106 Algorithm for the Management and Treatment of Appendicitis in Children

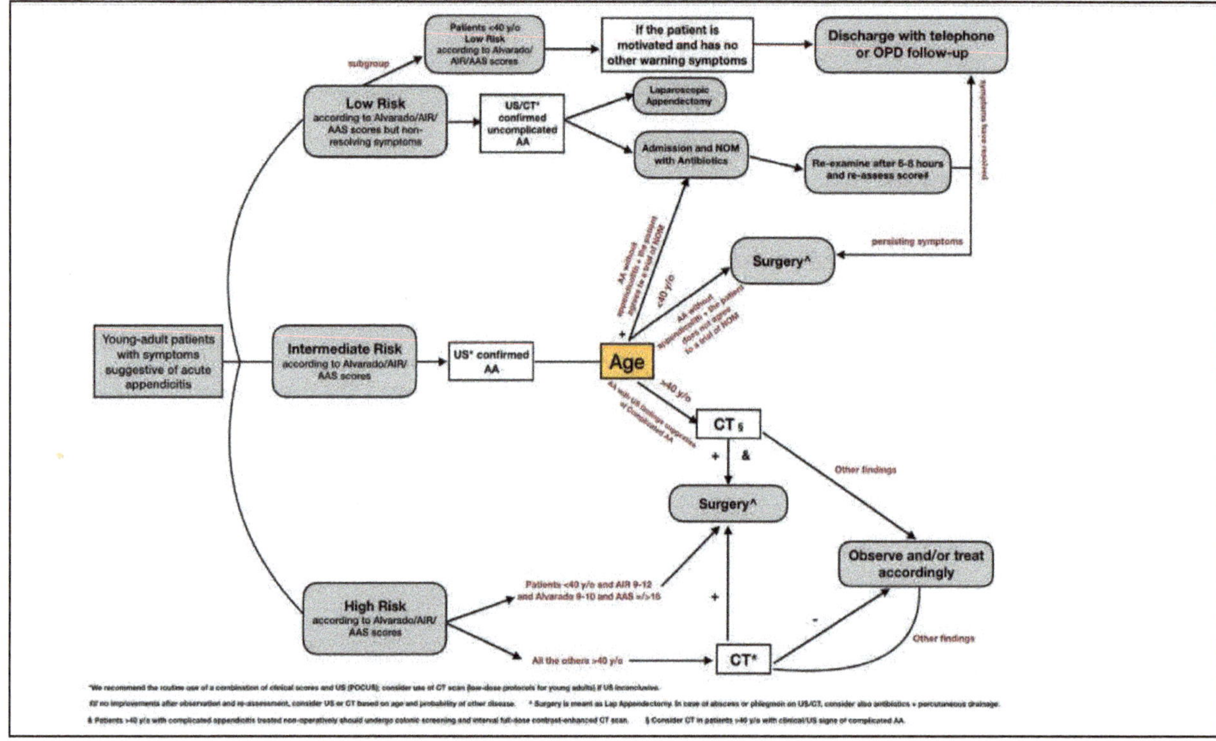

Figure 107 Management and Treatment of Appendicitis in Adults

4.4 Moh Golden Points and Summary Question Answers

4.4.1 Moh Golden Points

Viral gastroenteritis, commonly caused by norovirus or rotavirus, typically resolves on its own within a few days, while bacterial gastroenteritis may require antibiotics if caused by pathogens like Salmonella or E. coli.

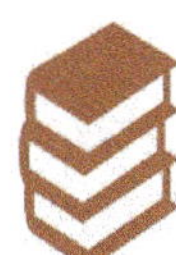

 Food poisoning can be caused by bacteria, viruses, or toxins, with symptoms such as diarrhea, vomiting, abdominal pain, and fever, and hydration is the most critical treatment to prevent dehydration.

In acute pancreatitis, the condition often presents with severe abdominal pain, nausea, vomiting, and elevated amylase and lipase levels, with treatment focusing on hydration, pain management, and IV antibiotics if infection is suspected.

Gastroesophageal reflux disease (GERD) presents with heartburn, regurgitation, and sometimes chronic cough, and management involves lifestyle modifications, antacids, and H2 blockers for symptom relief.

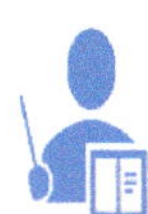

Food safety practices, such as washing hands, cooking meats thoroughly, and proper food storage, are essential in preventing foodborne illnesses like food poisoning and gastroenteritis.

Irritable Bowel Syndrome (IBS) is a functional gastrointestinal disorder characterized by abdominal pain, bloating, diarrhea, or constipation, and treatment focuses on dietary changes, stress management, and symptomatic therapy.

4.4.2 Summary Questions & Answers

1. What is the most common cause of acute gastroenteritis?
A) Salmonella
B) Norovirus
C) Clostridium botulinum
D) Shigella

2. Which of the following is a classic symptom of appendicitis?
A) Upper abdominal pain
B) Right lower quadrant pain
C) Pain in the left lower quadrant
D) Chest pain

3. In acute pancreatitis, which of the following laboratory tests is most commonly elevated?
A) AST/ALT
B) Amylase and lipase
C) Bilirubin
D) Prothrombin time

4. A patient presents with diarrhea, vomiting, fever, and right lower quadrant abdominal pain. What is the most likely diagnosis?
A) Irritable Bowel Syndrome (IBS)
B) Food poisoning
C) Appendicitis
D) Gastroesophageal reflux disease (GERD)

5. Which of the following is a common cause of bacterial gastroenteritis?
A) Rotavirus
B) E. coli
C) Norovirus
D) Influenza

6. What is the first-line treatment for uncomplicated food poisoning?
A) Antibiotics
B) Surgical intervention
C) Oral rehydration solutions (ORS)
D) Antihistamines

7. Which of the following medications is typically used to treat nausea and vomiting associated with food poisoning in adults?
A) Acetaminophen
B) Ondansetron (Zofran)
C) Amoxicillin
D) Loperamide (Imodium)

8. Which of the following is a risk factor for complicated appendicitis?
A) Older age
B) Younger age
C) Early diagnosis
D) Regular exercise

9. A 40-year-old patient with food poisoning has been vomiting and experiencing diarrhea for 24 hours. They are showing signs of dehydration. What should be the next step in management?

A) Antibiotics
B) Surgical consultation
C) IV fluid replacement
D) Antidiarrheal medication

10. What is the most common cause of viral gastroenteritis in children?

A) E. coli
B) Norovirus
C) Rotavirus
D) Campylobacter

4.4.3 Rationales

1. **Answer: B) Noravirus**

Rationale: **Norovirus** is the most common cause of viral gastroenteritis worldwide, responsible for a significant number of outbreaks, especially in settings like cruise ships and nursing homes. It is highly contagious and often causes symptoms such as vomiting and diarrhea.

2. **Answer: B) Right lower quadrant pain**

Rationale: The classic presentation of **appendicitis** involves **right lower quadrant pain**, typically starting at the **umbilicus** and later shifting to **McBurney's point** in the lower right abdomen, often accompanied by **nausea**, **vomiting**, and **fever**.

3. **Answer: B) Amylase and lipase**

Rationale: **Amylase** and **lipase** are pancreatic enzymes that are typically elevated in acute pancreatitis due to the inflammation and damage to the pancreas. These enzymes are crucial markers for diagnosing and monitoring the condition.

4. **Answer: C) Appendicitis**

Rationale: The classic symptoms of appendicitis include right lower quadrant abdominal pain, nausea, and fever. The presence of vomiting and diarrhea may also occur, although these symptoms are less common in appendicitis compared to gastroenteritis or food poisoning.

5. **Answer: B) E. coli**

Rationale: **E. coli**, especially certain strains like **E. coli O157:H7**, is a common cause of bacterial gastroenteritis, often leading to severe symptoms like **bloody diarrhea**. **Rotavirus** and **Norovirus** are viral causes, while **Influenza** causes respiratory symptoms.

6. **Answer: C) Oral rehydration solutions (ORS)**

Rationale: The primary treatment for food poisoning is the replacement of lost fluids and electrolytes to prevent dehydration. Oral rehydration solutions (ORS) are the most effective for this purpose, especially in children and the elderly.

7. **Answer: B) Ondansetron (Zofran)**

Rationale: Ondansetron (Zofran) is a commonly used antiemetic to treat **nausea** and **vomiting** associated with foodborne illnesses. **Loperamide (Imodium)** is used for diarrhea, but not for vomiting.

8. **Answer: A) Older age**

Rationale: Older age is associated with a higher risk of complications in appendicitis, including **perforation** and **abscess formation**, due to delayed presentation and differences in the immune response compared to younger patients.

9. **Answer: C) IV fluid replacement**

Rationale: The most immediate concern in a patient with food poisoning showing signs of dehydration is fluid replacement. IV fluids are indicated if the patient cannot tolerate oral hydration or if dehydration is severe.

10. **Answer: C) Rotavirus**

Rationale: Rotavirus is the leading cause of **viral gastroenteritis** in young children, responsible for a significant number of cases requiring hospitalization, especially in infants and toddlers. **Norovirus** is more common in adults.

5 Chapter 5: Musculoskeletal System

5.1 Anatomy and Physiology of Musculoskeletal System

The musculoskeletal system is a system of bones inter-connected by **muscles, tendons and ligaments** in charge of erecting the body and certain movements. As shown in the figure below, the system can be categorically divided into two broad sub-systems, which include the **skeletal system and the muscular system**. The function of some of the bones includes: supporting the structure of the body through the various bones such as the femur, humerus, and vertebrae; protecting other vital organs such as the brain and heart; the bones act as a reserve deposit of minerals such as calcium. **The bones also contain bone marrow**; blood cells are manufactured by this dark red substance. Skeletal muscles which include **deltoid, biceps, quadriceps and gastrocnemius muscles** assist in movement as a result of contraction. They contract and relax following impulses from nerves to enable walking and lifting among others.

The general muscle locations are shown in the figure, which is **pectoralis major, rectus abdominis in the upper part of the body and gluteus maximus and gastrocnemius in the lower part**. These tissues link muscles to bones, ensuring that in contracting they move the bones through the forces acting on them. Bones are connected to other bones with the help of ligaments for providing strength and flexibility to joints such as the knee and shoulder. The image displayed in this section emphasizes the main muscles and their position in the body, for example, **the pectoral muscles, including pectoralis major, and the abdominal muscles, including rectus abdominis muscles in the upper area; buttock muscles, including gluteus maximus, and the lower limb muscles, including gastrocnemius.** These muscles find attachment to bones and help in movement by pulling as a result of the contraction of the muscles. Also, tendons are covered by the skin and synovium; ligaments are the tough bands of fibres that bind bones to other bones holding several joints together like knee and shoulders.

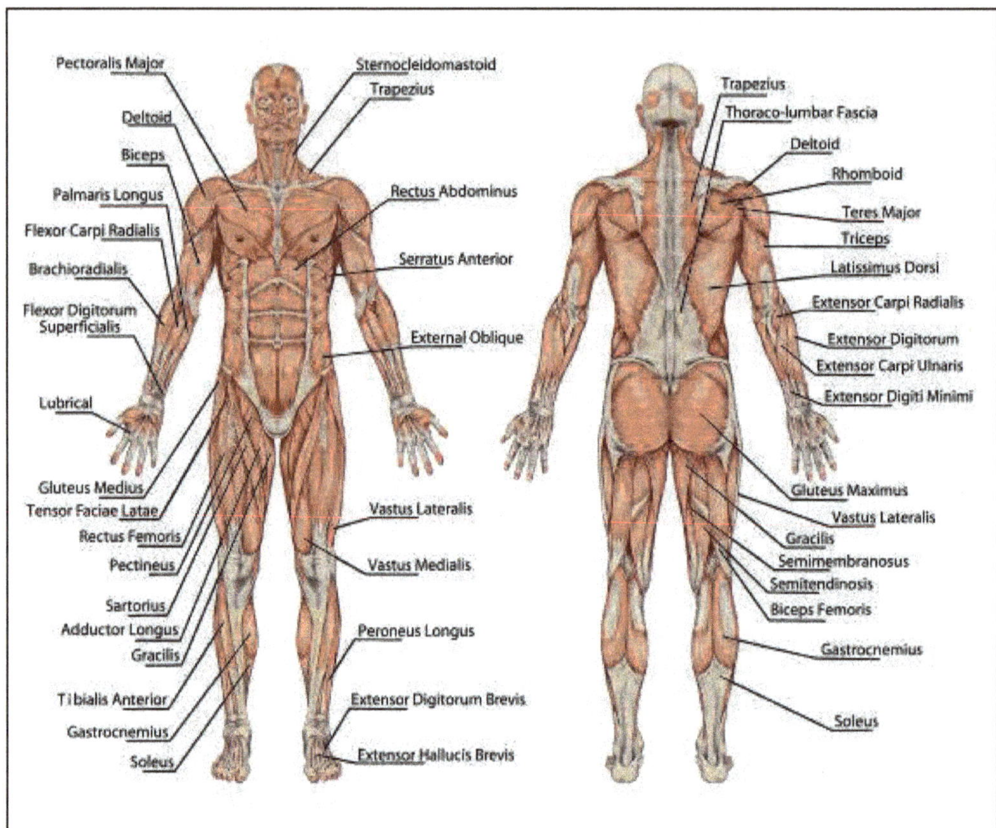

Figure 108 Anatomy and Physiology of Musculoskeletal System

5.2 Orthopaedic Manoeuvres and Their Clinical Relevance

Orthopaedic tests are also very important in **determining joint stability, ligamentous competence, and pathologic changes** in the muscles and other soft tissues in different musculoskeletal disorders. The Drawer Sign is used to assess the stability of the **anterior cruciate ligament (ACL)** and the **posterior cruciate ligament (PCL)** of the knee. The **McNeal test,** which involves the doctor pulling on the patient's knee and attempting to move their tibia too far forward or backwards beyond the femur, is a **positive test of a torn ligament.** Likewise, the **McMurray test** is usually used to detect possible meniscal injuries in the knee joint. This procedure involves bending and twisting the knee as any sound like creaking or snapping is a sign of damage to the meniscus. **Finkelstein test** is crucial in diagnosing **De Quervain's tenosynovitis** which is a medical condition that develops in the wrist region due to inflammation of tendons. It involves having the patient flex their fingers and place the thumb on the palm, and any inflammation of the tendons by the deviation of the ulnar induces pain. Finally, the **Mulder test** is used in diagnosing Morton's neuroma, which is a nerve that is **squeezed between the toes**. Confirmation of the presence of the pathology requires pain and an audible click upon applying pressure to the foot's affected region. These tests are indeed useful in providing the clinician with evidence to support his/her hypothesis or hypotheses, eliminate certain differential diagnoses, and identify the **right management plans for MSDs.**

5.3 Common Musculoskeletal Conditions

The mnemonic for major acute and chronic conditions **"ORF GIFT BOSS CAUSE DICEH"** This acronym stands for: **O**steoarthritis (OA), **R**heumatoid Arthritis (RA), **F**ibromyalgia, **G**out, **I**njuries (Sprains and Strains), **F**ractures, **T**endinitis, **B**one Metastasis, **O**steoporosis, **S**ciatica, **S**pondylitis (Ankylosing Spondylitis), **C**auda Equina Syndrome, **A**lso (for additional conditions),

Systemic Lupus Erythematosus (SLE)**, E**nvironmental (for lifestyle factors like Bursitis)**, D**isk Herniation **I**nflammation (Plantar Fasciitis)**, C**hronic Low Back Pain**, E**ndemic (referring to conditions like Carpal Tunnel Syndrome)**, and H**ip Fracture This mnemonic simplifies remembering these musculoskeletal disorders by associating each condition with a memorable word in the phrase.

Table 72 Common Disorders of Musculoskeletal System

Condition	Description	Key Symptoms	Diagnostic Tools	Treatment Options
Osteoarthritis (OA)	A degenerative joint disease causing the breakdown of cartilage, leading to pain, stiffness, and loss of joint function.	Joint pain, stiffness, decreased range of motion, swelling, crepitus (popping sounds)	X-rays, MRI, Joint aspiration, Physical exam	Pain management (acetaminophen, NSAIDs), physical therapy, joint injections (steroids, hyaluronic acid), surgery (joint replacement in severe cases)
Rheumatoid Arthritis (RA)	An autoimmune disorder causing chronic inflammation of the joints, leading to joint damage and deformities.	Joint pain, swelling, stiffness (especially in the morning), fatigue, fever, joint deformities	Blood tests (rheumatoid factor, anti-CCP antibodies), X-rays, Ultrasound	Disease-modifying antirheumatic drugs (DMARDs), biologics (TNF inhibitors), NSAIDs, corticosteroids, physical therapy
Osteoporosis	A condition characterized by weakened bones, increasing the risk of fractures, particularly in older adults.	Bone fractures (especially after minor falls), back pain, loss of height, posture changes	Bone density scan (DEXA), X-rays, Blood tests (calcium, vitamin D levels)	Bisphosphonates, calcium and vitamin D supplements, weight-bearing exercise, hormone therapy (in postmenopausal women), lifestyle changes
Fibromyalgia	A chronic condition causing widespread musculoskeletal pain, fatigue, and tenderness in specific areas of the body.	Widespread pain, fatigue, sleep disturbances, cognitive difficulties, headaches	Physical exam, Blood tests (to rule out other conditions), Tender point assessment	Pain management (NSAIDs, antidepressants, anticonvulsants), physical therapy, stress management, lifestyle changes (exercise, sleep hygiene)

Gout	A form of arthritis caused by the accumulation of uric acid crystals in the joints, leading to inflammation and severe pain.	Sudden joint pain (usually in the big toe), swelling, redness, warmth, fever	Blood tests (uric acid levels), Joint aspiration (for crystal analysis), X-rays	NSAIDs, colchicine, corticosteroids, urate-lowering medications (allopurinol), lifestyle modifications (dietary changes, weight management)
Sprains and Strains	Injuries to ligaments (sprains) or muscles/tendons (strains) often caused by overuse, stretching, or trauma.	Pain, swelling, bruising, limited movement, muscle spasms	Physical exam, X-rays (to rule out fractures), MRI	R.I.C.E. (Rest, Ice, Compression, Elevation), pain relief (NSAIDs), physical therapy, muscle relaxants, surgery (in severe cases)
Tendinitis	Inflammation of a tendon due to overuse or injury, often affecting the shoulder, elbow, wrist, knee, or ankle.	Pain and tenderness near a joint, swelling, limited range of motion, pain worsens with activity	Physical exam, Ultrasound, MRI, X-rays (to rule out other conditions)	Rest, ice, anti-inflammatory medications, physical therapy, corticosteroid injections, surgery (in severe cases)
Disk Herniation (Herniated Disc)	A condition where the inner gel-like core of a spinal disc leaks out, irritating nearby nerves and causing pain.	Lower back pain radiating to legs, numbness or tingling in extremities, muscle weakness, sciatica.	MRI, CT scan, X-rays, Physical exam	NSAIDs, Muscle relaxants, Physical therapy, Epidural steroid injections, Surgery if severe
Ankylosing Spondylitis	A chronic inflammatory disease that primarily affects the spine, leading to pain and stiffness.	Chronic lower back pain, stiffness, reduced spinal mobility, fatigue, sacroiliitis, morning stiffness.	X-rays, MRI, HLA-B27 test, Physical exam	NSAIDs, TNF inhibitors, Sulfasalazine, Physical therapy, Postural exercises, Surgery in severe cases
Plantar Fasciitis	Inflammation of the plantar fascia, often caused by	Heel pain, especially after the first steps in	Physical exam, X-rays (to rule out	Stretching exercises, Orthotics, NSAIDs, Ice,

	overuse or pressure on the heel, leading to pain.	the morning, pain in the bottom of the foot, swelling.	other conditions), Ultrasound	Corticosteroid injections, Physical therapy
Bone Metastasis	Spread of cancer from other parts of the body to the bones, leading to bone weakness and pain.	Localized pain, weight loss, fatigue, pathologic fractures, weakness, swelling at the site of metastasis.	Bone scan, X-rays, MRI, CT scan, Biopsy, PET scan	Pain management (NSAIDs, opioids), Radiation therapy, Chemotherapy, Bisphosphonates, Surgery for fractures or stabilization
Cauda Equina Syndrome	A serious condition caused by pressure on the nerve roots at the end of the spinal cord, requiring urgent treatment.	Severe lower back pain, saddle anesthesia, urinary retention, bowel incontinence, weakness in legs.	MRI, CT scan, Physical exam, Neurological assessment	Surgical decompression, Urinary catheterization, Pain management (NSAIDs, opioids), Bowel management
Osteomyelitis	Bone infection usually caused by bacteria, often due to open fractures or diabetic foot ulcers.	Pain at the infected site, swelling, fever, redness, fatigue, difficulty moving the affected limb.	Blood cultures, MRI, Bone biopsy, X-rays, CBC (elevated white count)	IV antibiotics, Oral antibiotics, Surgical debridement if needed, Pain management (NSAIDs, opioids)
Sciatica	Pain that radiates along the sciatic nerve, typically caused by compression of nerve roots in the lumbar spine.	Sharp pain radiating from the lower back to the legs, numbness or tingling in legs or feet, weakness.	MRI, X-rays, Physical exam (Straight leg raise test, Neurological examination)	NSAIDs, Muscle relaxants, Physical therapy, Epidural steroid injections, Surgery (if disc herniation is severe)
Systemic Lupus Erythematosus (SLE)	An autoimmune disease where the immune system attacks the body's tissues, causing widespread inflammation.	Joint pain, fatigue, malar (butterfly-shaped) rash, photosensitivity, fever, proteinuria,	ANA test, Anti-dsDNA, Complement levels (C3, C4), Urinalysis, Physical exam	Hydroxychloroquine, Corticosteroids, Immunosuppressants, NSAIDs, Lifestyle modifications (sun protection, diet)

		kidney involvement.		
Bursitis	Inflammation of the bursae, small fluid-filled sacs that cushion and reduce friction between bones and soft tissues.	Pain, swelling, and tenderness over the affected joint, limited range of motion, especially in the shoulders, hips, or knees.	Physical exam, Ultrasound, X-rays, MRI, Joint aspiration to rule out infection.	NSAIDs, Ice or heat therapy, Rest, Corticosteroid injections, Physical therapy, Surgery in severe cases.
Chronic Low Back Pain	A condition characterized by persistent or recurrent pain in the lower back, often due to muscle strain, poor posture, or spinal issues.	Persistent low back pain, stiffness, and difficulty with movement, radiating pain to the legs, often worsened by prolonged sitting or standing.	Physical exam, MRI, X-rays (to rule out fractures), CT scan, Blood tests to check for inflammatory markers.	NSAIDs, Muscle relaxants, Physical therapy, Chiropractic care, Heat or ice therapy, Surgery for severe cases (e.g., disc herniation).
Carpal Tunnel Syndrome	A condition caused by pressure on the median nerve in the wrist, leading to symptoms like numbness, tingling, and weakness in the hand.	Numbness, tingling, and weakness in the hand, especially in the thumb, index, and middle fingers, worsened at night.	Physical exam, Nerve conduction studies, Electromyography (EMG), Ultrasound, X-rays to rule out other conditions.	Wrist splints, NSAIDs, Corticosteroid injections, Physical therapy, Surgery (e.g., carpal tunnel release) in severe cases.
Fractures	A break or crack in a bone, often caused by trauma or excessive stress on the bone.	Pain at the site of the fracture, swelling, bruising, inability to move the affected area, deformity or abnormal positioning.	X-rays, CT scan, MRI (for complex fractures), Physical exam	Pain management (NSAIDs, opioids), Immobilization (casts, splints), Surgery (e.g., internal fixation), Physical therapy for rehabilitation.
Hip Fractures	A break or crack in the femur bone, usually due to	Severe hip pain, inability to move or bear weight,	X-rays, CT scan, MRI	Pain management (NSAIDs, opioids), surgical intervention

	trauma or falls, especially in elderly individuals with weakened bones.	bruising, swelling around the hip, pain worsening with movement		(hip replacement, internal fixation), physical therapy, rehabilitation

5.4 Major Medical Issues in Musculoskeletal System

CHRONIC CONDITIONS

5.4.1 Osteoarthritis (OA)

Osteoarthritis (OA), also known as degenerative joint disorder, is a type of joint disease in which there is a progressive loss of the articular cartilage. With time the cartilage weakens and hence causes **rubbing of bones, which results in pains, swellings and stiffness**. OA typically impacts the knee, hip or spine and can also affect the hand and fingers. The main signs of OA are pain in the joints, especially during activity, joint stiffness in the morning and after a long inactivity, and the decline of joint flexibility. The pain may become **chronic as the disease advances** and may have an impact on various aspects of life. Some of the risk factors include age, genetic factors, obesity, joint injuries, and joint overuse. The diagnosis involves clinical assessment with additional tests as **X-ray exams might reveal joint-space narrowing, bone spurs, and other evidence of cartilage degeneration.** It requires mobilization and manipulation of affected joints, medications such as Non-Steroidal Anti Inflammatory Drugs to help in pain management and acknowledging the need to alter lifestyle. In the worst-case scenario, surgical intervention may be required to fix the situation and the patient's condition in the form of joint replacement surgery.

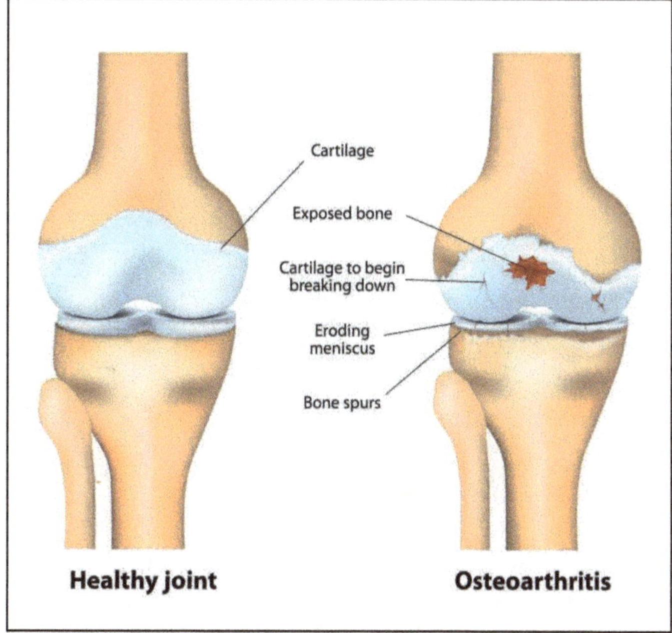

5.4.1.1 Types of Osteoarthritis (OA)

The following explains the various phases of OA according to the degree of joint space narrowing and cartilage loss. **In Stage I (Doubtful),** the joint space may narrow by up to 10%, the cartilage is almost unaffected, and the patient may not complain of any pain. **Stage II (Mild)** is where the joint space decreases and there is a very early sign of cartilage wear and tear accompanied by limited pain and stiffness. **Stage III (Moderate)** displays more joint space loss and moderate cartilage damage which causes more pain, reduced movement, and the formation of bony outgrowths called osteophytes. In **Stage IV (Severe)** joint space is narrow and there is significant cartilage erosion and large osteophytes producing severe pain leading to functional limitation and often surgical intervention may be required. These stages reflect the gradual development of OA starting from the earliest stages and up to the very development of significant disability.

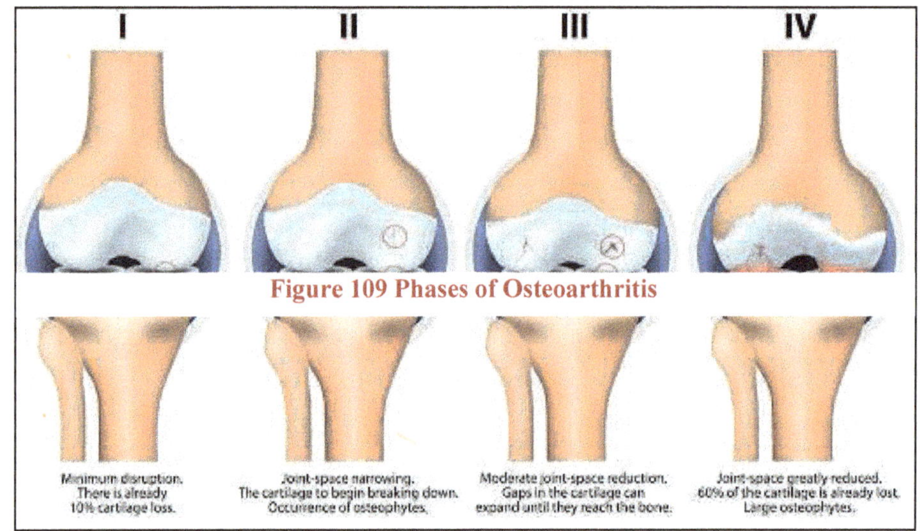

Figure 109 Phases of Osteoarthritis

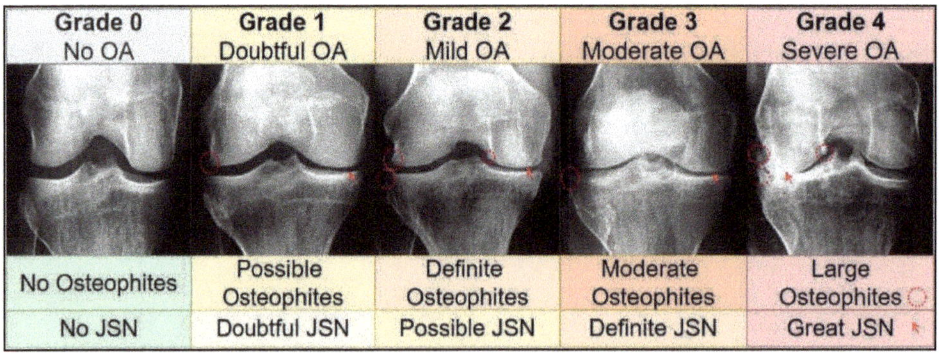

Grade 0 No OA	Grade 1 Doubtful OA	Grade 2 Mild OA	Grade 3 Moderate OA	Grade 4 Severe OA
No Osteophites	Possible Osteophites	Definite Osteophites	Moderate Osteophites	Large Osteophites
No JSN	Doubtful JSN	Possible JSN	Definite JSN	Great JSN

The image shows the radiographic grading system for osteoarthritis (OA), from Grade 0 (No OA) to Grade 4 (Severe OA). In Grade 1 (Doubtful OA), joint space narrowing (JSN) is minimal, and osteophytes may be present. As the grade progresses to Grade 2 (Mild OA), osteophytes become more pronounced, and JSN becomes more noticeable, with Grade 4 (Severe OA) showing significant joint space reduction (great JSN) and large osteophytes, reflecting advanced OA degeneration.

Figure 110 Classification of Osteoarthritis

5.4.1.2 SOAP Notes for Osteoarthritis

Table 73 SOAP Notes for Osteoporosis

Component	Details
Subjective (S)	The patient is a 68-year-old female presenting with a 6-month history of knee pain, primarily in the right knee, which has progressively worsened. The pain is described as a deep, aching sensation, occurring especially after prolonged standing or walking, and is somewhat relieved with rest and over-the-counter pain medications (acetaminophen). The patient reports stiffness in the morning, lasting about 20-30 minutes, and occasional swelling in the knee joint. She denies any recent trauma or injury but notes that the pain has affected her ability to perform daily activities, such as climbing stairs and walking long distances. She has a family history of OA and is overweight.
Objective (O)	The patient appears in mild discomfort while walking, with a slight limp on the right side. Vital signs: BP 130/85 mmHg, HR 78 bpm, Temp 36.7°C (98.1°F). On physical examination, there is tenderness over the medial joint line of the right knee, and crepitus is noted with joint movement. Range of motion is limited with pain during flexion. No signs of acute inflammation or erythema are present. X-rays show joint space narrowing and the presence of osteophytes in the right knee, consistent with mild to moderate OA. No signs of joint instability or fractures are observed.
Assessment (A)	The patient is diagnosed with osteoarthritis (OA) of the right knee, likely exacerbated by obesity and age-related degenerative changes. The symptoms of joint pain, stiffness, and crepitus, along with radiographic evidence of joint space narrowing and osteophyte formation, support the diagnosis. The condition is classified as Grade 2 (Mild OA) based on radiographic findings.
Plan (P)	Recommend acetaminophen for pain relief. If needed, NSAIDs (e.g., ibuprofen) for inflammation management. Consider corticosteroid injections if pain becomes severe or unmanageable. Initiate physical therapy focused on strengthening the quadriceps and improving knee mobility (See algorithm below). Weight management through diet and low-impact exercise (e.g., swimming, cycling) is essential to reduce stress on the joints. Schedule a follow-up visit in 6 weeks to monitor pain and functional status. If no improvement, discuss possible knee bracing or knee joint replacement options in the future. Educate the patient on lifestyle modifications, including proper weight management, the importance of regular exercise, and joint protection techniques (See algorithm below).

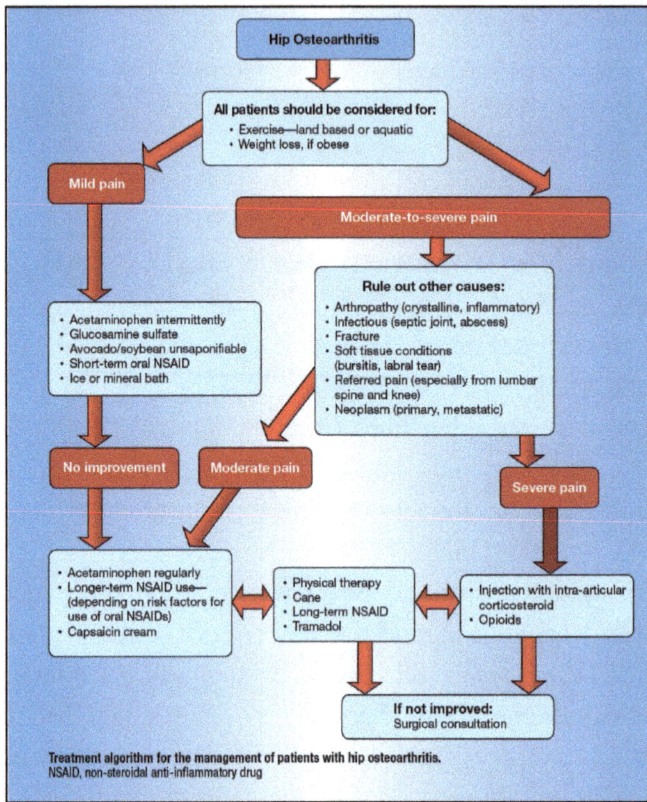

Figure 111 Algorithm for the Pharmacological Management of Osteoarthritis

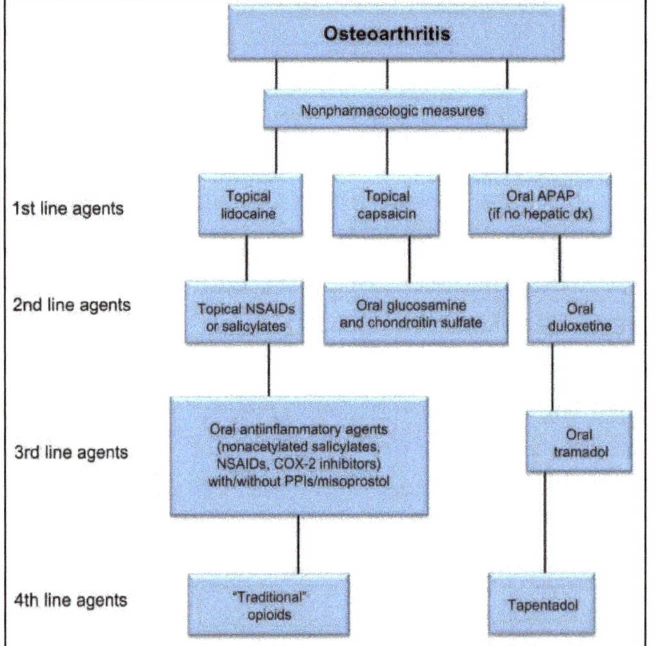

Figure 112 Algorithm for the Non-Pharmacological Management of Osteoarthritis

5.4.2 Osteoporosis

Osteoporosis is a disease that causes the bones to become **fragile**, thus posing a great risk for fractures. It is a condition that arises when bones become **less dense** as well as **qualitatively inferior** and can easily crack when one falls or is involved in a minor accident. It is mainly seen in women over the age of 45 years because of **low levels of estrogen** but it can also be seen in men with factors such as **age, low weight or long-term treatment with corticosteroids**. Some signs of osteoporosis include back pain, humps at the back, and bone fractures that happen due to a slight fall. However, osteogenesis imperfections can also be referred to as the **"silent disease"** since many patients never experience any symptoms until a fracture. The diagnosis is normally made through a **DEXA scan (dual-energy X-ray absorptiometry).** The management includes calcium and **vitamin D supplementation, bisphosphonates, and weight-bearing exercises** for strengthening the bones. Dietary modifications are an effective way of reducing the incidents of osteoporosis and these include abstaining from smoking and the use of alcohol among others.

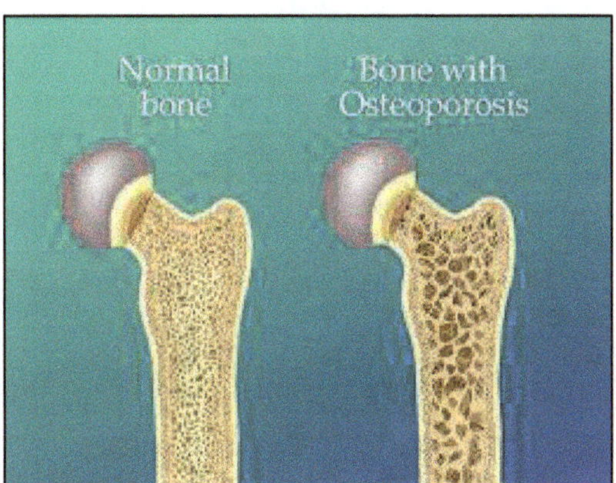

Figure 113 Comparison Between Normal and Bone with Osteoporosis

5.4.3 Types of Osteoporosis

This image illustrates that osteoporosis is categorized into two types, namely the **primary osteoporosis and the secondary osteoporosis.** Primary osteoporosis does not result from any preexisting medical condition or the use of any particular medicine. It has two subclasses: **Type 1 or Postmenopausal Osteoporosis,** where women after child bearing age are most affected due to low estrogen hormone or estrogen deficiency and the second subclass is **Type 2 or Senile Osteoporosis,** also known as age dependent osteoporosis, affecting the elderly especially those persons over 70 years of age. In contrast, **secondary osteoporosis** results from an underlying pathology or the use of certain medications for a long period of time. For example, **excessive consumption of corticosteroids or phenytoin** is a common cause of reduction in bone density resulting from treatment, increasing the fragility of bones. These classifications assist in the **diagnosis and staging of osteoporosis** since it is determined if it is age related, due to hormonal imbalance or caused by certain medication.

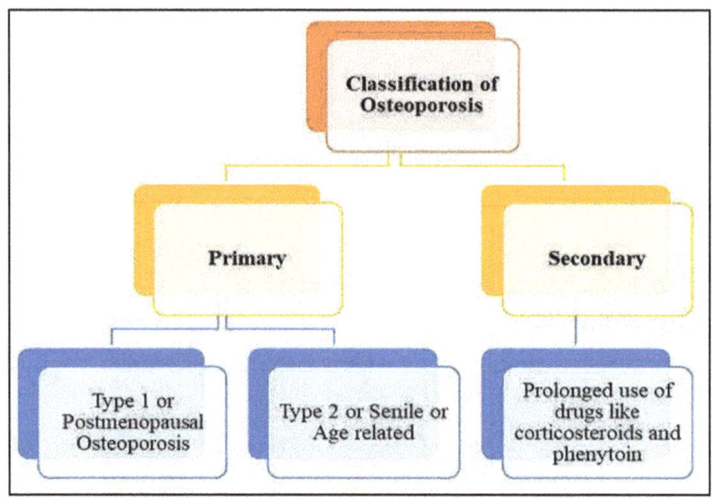

Figure 114 Classification of Osteoporosis

5.4.3.1 SOAP Notes for Osteoporosis

Table 74 SOAP Notes for Osteoporosis

Component	Details
Subjective (S)	The patient is a 67-year-old female who presents with a complaint of lower back pain that has progressively worsened over the past few months. She describes the pain as a dull ache, primarily in the lower back and hips, which becomes more pronounced with prolonged standing and walking. The patient reports that the pain improves somewhat with rest. She had a history of menopause 15 years ago and has been sedentary for the past few years. She also notes a family history of osteoporosis and fractures. The patient denies any history of trauma or significant injuries but expresses concern about her bone health. She has been taking calcium supplements for a few months but is unsure of her vitamin D intake.
Objective (O)	The patient appears well-nourished but in mild discomfort. Vital signs: BP 130/80 mmHg, HR 76 bpm, Temp 36.7°C (98.1°F). A physical exam reveals mild tenderness in the lower back, with no deformities or visible swelling. There is a slight loss of height and a stooped posture. Bone density scan (DEXA) confirms decreased bone mass with T-scores of -2.5 in the lumbar spine and hip, consistent with osteoporosis. X-rays show no acute fractures, but the patient has evidence of mild vertebral compression.
Assessment (A)	The patient is diagnosed with osteoporosis, likely exacerbated by postmenopausal hormonal changes, reduced physical activity, and a family history. The DEXA scan confirms a diagnosis of osteoporosis with a T-score of -2.5. The patient's current symptoms of chronic back pain are likely related to age-related bone density loss and vertebral compression, though no acute fractures are present. The risk of fractures in the future is elevated due to her low bone mineral density.
Plan (P)	**Pharmacological:** Start the patient on bisphosphonates (e.g., Alendronate) to reduce bone resorption and improve bone density. Recommend calcium (1200

mg daily) and vitamin D (800-1000 IU daily) supplementation. If tolerated, consider selective estrogen receptor modulators (SERMs) for additional bone protection (See algorithm below). **Non-pharmacological:** Advise weight-bearing exercises (e.g., walking, swimming) to improve bone strength and muscle mass. Encourage balance exercises to reduce the risk of falls. Recommend fall-prevention strategies and a high-protein diet to support bone health. **Follow-up: Schedule** a follow-up visit in 3 months to reassess symptoms, monitor for side effects, and evaluate bone density through a repeat DEXA scan after one year. Continue monitoring calcium and vitamin D levels. **Education:** Educate the patient on the importance of lifestyle modifications, including avoiding smoking, limiting alcohol intake, and maintaining a healthy weight to manage osteoporosis. Discuss the potential benefits of bone density testing and regular physical activity in preventing further bone loss.

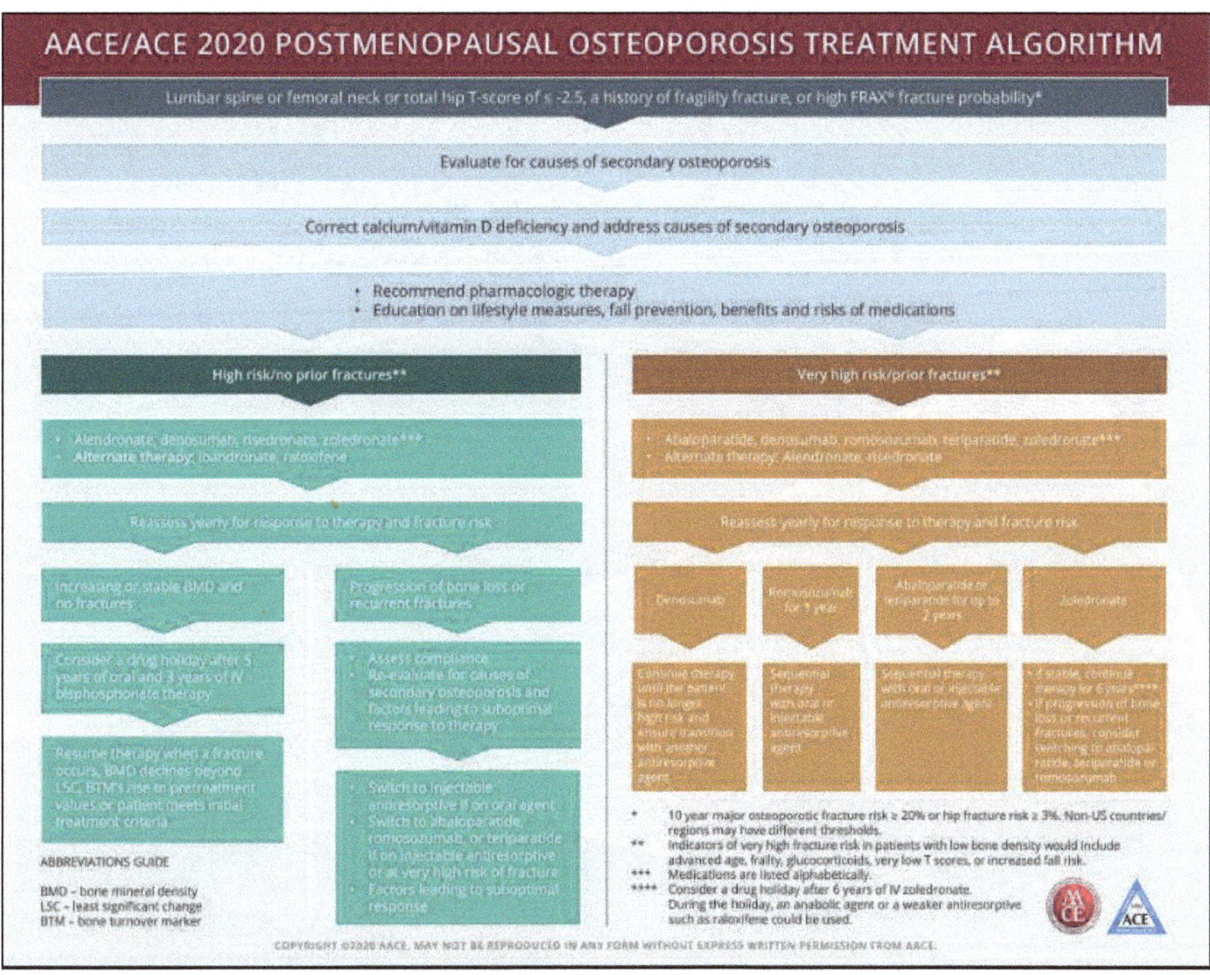

Figure 115 Algorithm for the Management of Osteoporosis

5.4.4 Rheumatoid Arthritis (RA)

Rheumatoid arthritis (RA) is a systemic autoimmune disease that mainly affects the joints with particular prevalence in the swollen and palmar side of the wrists, hands, and knees. RA, on the other hand, is a form of arthritis that results from an autoimmune disease that affects the synovium, which is the lining of the joint and therefore results in joint destruction over a period of time. It can also spread locally to affect other layers of the airway and other organs and tissues including the lungs and blood vessels and can present with **generalised systemic symptoms** which are **fatigue, fever and loss of appetite.** Some of the signs and symptoms include pains and aches in the joints, swelling, stiffness in the joints and reduced mobility, particularly in the morning hours. RA is more widespread and involves both sides of the body while osteoarthritis is commonly in **one side than the other side of the body**. Severe symptoms resolve in weeks to months however the crunchy joints often progress to joint deformity and functional impairment. **The exact cause of RA is still not clear** but it is believed to be caused by a **combination of genetics, environment, and hormones.** Rheumatoid factor and anti-CCP antibodies are blood tests used in diagnosis, whereas a physical exam, X-rays, or sonography constitutes imaging studies. Treatment is directed towards settling inflammation, minimizing pain, and minimizing the amount of joint deterioration. Specifically, treatment involves conventional synthetic **disease-modifying antirheumatic drugs (csDMARDs)** including **low-dose methotrexate and biologic DMARDs** such as **TNF inhibitors. Nonsteroidal anti-inflammatory (NSAIDs) and corticosteroids** are two forms of medication that can assist with symptom management. Therefore, identifying RA at an early stage administering medicine and correcting rheumatoid arthritis treatment is highly important in order to avoid joint destruction.

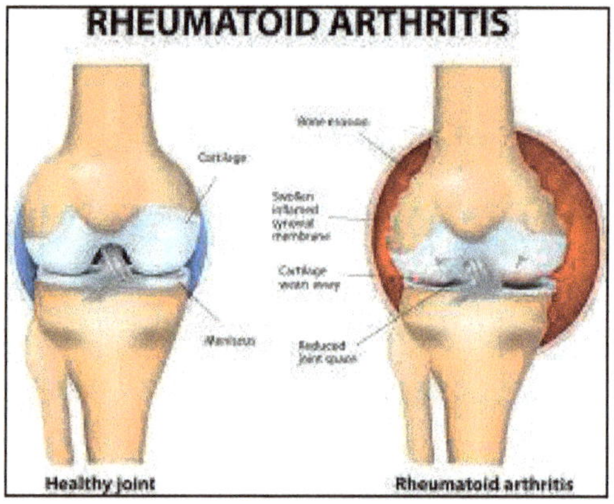

Figure 116 Comparison Between Normal and RA joint

5.4.5 Stages of Rheumatoid Arthritis

This picture demonstrates the classification of rheumatoid arthritis (RA) based on seven phases reflecting the development of joint destruction. **In Stage 1** also referred to as the Healthy Joint, the joint has not been affected and on **X-ray investigation**, there is no sign that the articular surfaces are joined. **During stage 2 (Early RA),** the changes in the affected joint are characterized by **periarticular osteoporosis and subchondral bone destruction** where some but limited joint deformities. More severe cartilage and bone destruction along with joint deformities occur in **Moderate RA or Stage 3,** which leads to some functional imitations. **In Stage 4 (Severe RA),** the joint hardens irreversibly through bony or fibrous ankylosis, leading to complete immobilization and extreme deformity that greatly reduces the functionality of the affected joint. They are useful for assessing the disease and treatment pattern in RA as a way of building a long-term plan for avoiding joint damage and disability.

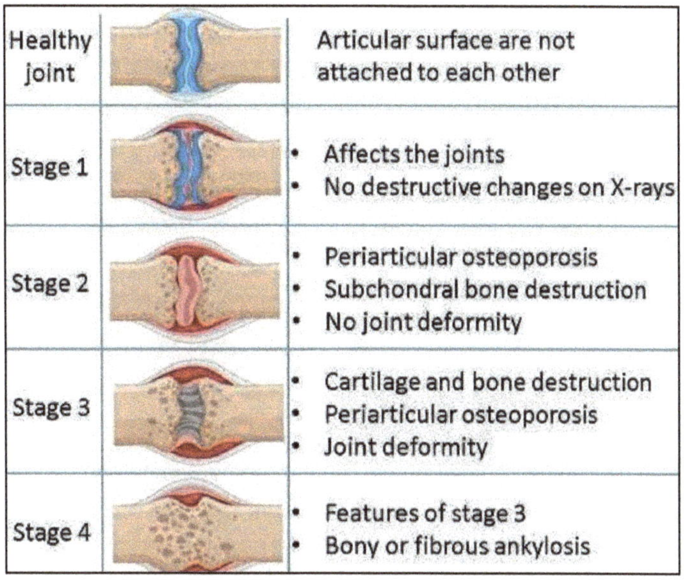

Healthy joint		Articular surface are not attached to each other
Stage 1		• Affects the joints • No destructive changes on X-rays
Stage 2		• Periarticular osteoporosis • Subchondral bone destruction • No joint deformity
Stage 3		• Cartilage and bone destruction • Periarticular osteoporosis • Joint deformity
Stage 4		• Features of stage 3 • Bony or fibrous ankylosis

Figure 117 Stages of Rheumatoid Arthritis

5.4.5.1 Targeted Therapy Strategies in Rheumatoid Arthritis

The illustration describes the processes characteristic of rheumatoid arthritis and the potential strategies that focus on certain cell types and molecular targets connected with RA. It describes, in detail, the activated cells in the RA joint and the functions they perform in the inflammatory process and joint debridement. **NK cells (a) and monocytes/macrophages (b)** thus, target therapy identifies **TNF-α and IL-6** as promising inflammation-triggering agents. **Neutrophils (c)** are involved in the inflammatory process and the therapies that involve the use of **anti-IL-6 and anti-IL-17** agents that work by depleting the neutrophils. This is true because **T and B cell activation (f, g)** plays a significant role in RA, and the therapies targeting T cells or B cells aim to control the immune cell activity. **Fibroblasts like synoviocytes (h)** are responsible for the synthesis of different pro-inflammatory cytokines, and drugs that act on the JAK pathway are used to target them. Other cells including chondrocyte (i), osteoclasts (j) and osteoblasts (k) are also involved in cartilage damage and bone resorption with a focus on RANKL, which is used to inactivate osteoclast activity. These speci c therapies consist of **TNF- α; IL-6; IL-1; IL-17; JAK; RANKL; and GM-CSF** and are equally critical to RA because they contain anti-inflammatory properties, modulate destroy joint, as well as enhance function.

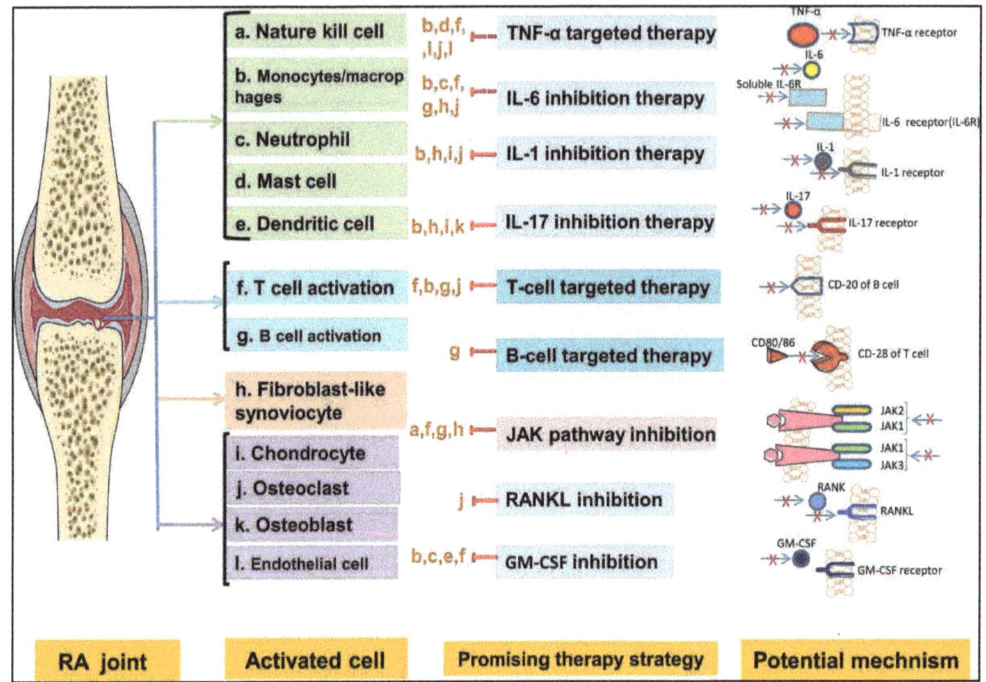

Figure 118 Rheumatoid arthritis: pathological mechanisms and modern pharmacologic therapies

5.4.5.2 SOAP Notes for Rheumatoid Arthritis

Table 75 SOAP Notes for Rheumatoid Arthritis

Component	Details
Subjective (S)	The patient is a 55-year-old female presenting with a 6-month history of symmetrical joint pain and morning stiffness that lasts for over an hour. The pain primarily affects her wrists, knees, and hands, and is accompanied by swelling and redness around the joints. She reports difficulty in performing daily activities such as gripping objects and climbing stairs. The patient mentions feeling fatigued, with occasional low-grade fever. She denies recent trauma or injuries. There is a family history of rheumatoid arthritis, and she has been experiencing these symptoms gradually. The patient is concerned about potential joint damage and long-term disability.
Objective (O)	The patient appears in mild distress due to joint pain. Vital signs: BP 125/80 mmHg, HR 80 bpm, Temp 37.2°C (99°F). Physical exam reveals bilateral joint swelling and tenderness in the proximal interphalangeal (PIP) joints, metacarpophalangeal (MCP) joints, wrists, and knees. Range of motion is limited due to pain, especially in the morning. There is no visible deformity, but joint instability is noted in the knees. Rheumatoid nodules are absent. Lab results show positive rheumatoid factor (RF) and anti-cyclic citrullinated peptide (anti-CCP) antibodies, confirming the likelihood of rheumatoid arthritis. X-rays of the hands and wrists reveal joint space narrowing, periarticular osteopenia, and the presence of osteophytes, consistent with early-stage RA.

Assessment (A)	The patient's clinical presentation, including bilateral joint pain, swelling, morning stiffness, and positive lab results (RF and anti-CCP), along with X-ray findings of early joint changes, is consistent with Rheumatoid Arthritis (RA). The condition appears to be in the early stage, and the patient is at risk for progressive joint damage if left untreated. Differential diagnoses include osteoarthritis and psoriatic arthritis, but these are less likely due to the symmetrical joint involvement and the positive serological markers for RA.
Plan (P)	**Pharmacological:** Start the patient on Methotrexate (10 mg weekly) as the first-line disease-modifying antirheumatic drug (DMARD) to reduce inflammation and prevent joint damage. NSAIDs (e.g., Ibuprofen) will be prescribed for pain relief. If symptoms persist, biological agents (e.g., TNF inhibitors) will be considered for further management (See algorithms below). **Non-pharmacological:** Refer the patient to physical therapy for joint protection exercises, strengthening, and range-of-motion exercises. Recommend regular low-impact exercises such as swimming or walking to maintain joint mobility. **Follow-up:** Schedule a follow-up in 4 weeks to assess the patient's response to Methotrexate and adjust the treatment plan as necessary. Monitor for any side effects from the medications. **Education:** Educate the patient on the chronic nature of RA, the importance of medication adherence, and the need for joint protection strategies. Discuss lifestyle modifications, including avoiding smoking, and the importance of maintaining a healthy weight to reduce stress on the joints.

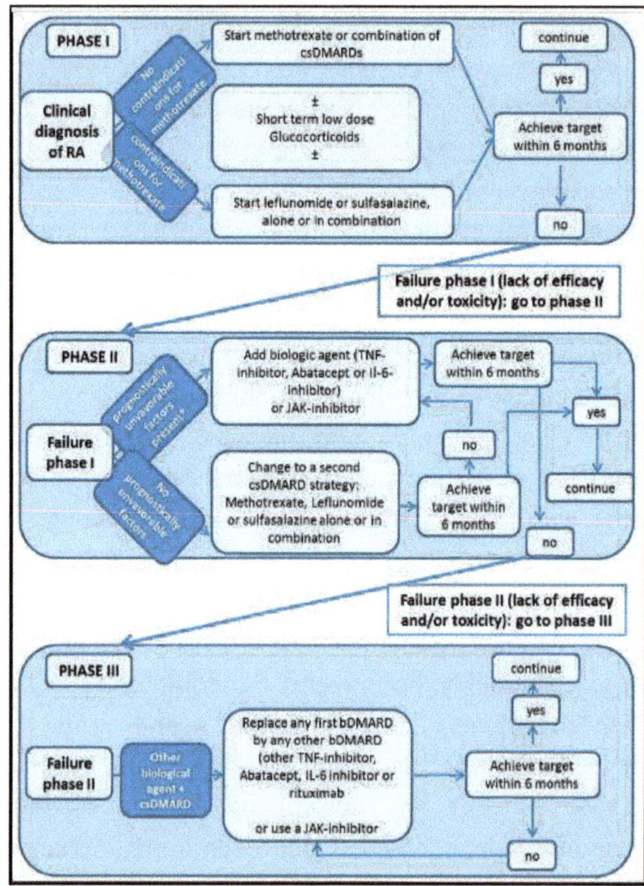

Figure 119 Algorithm for the Management of RA

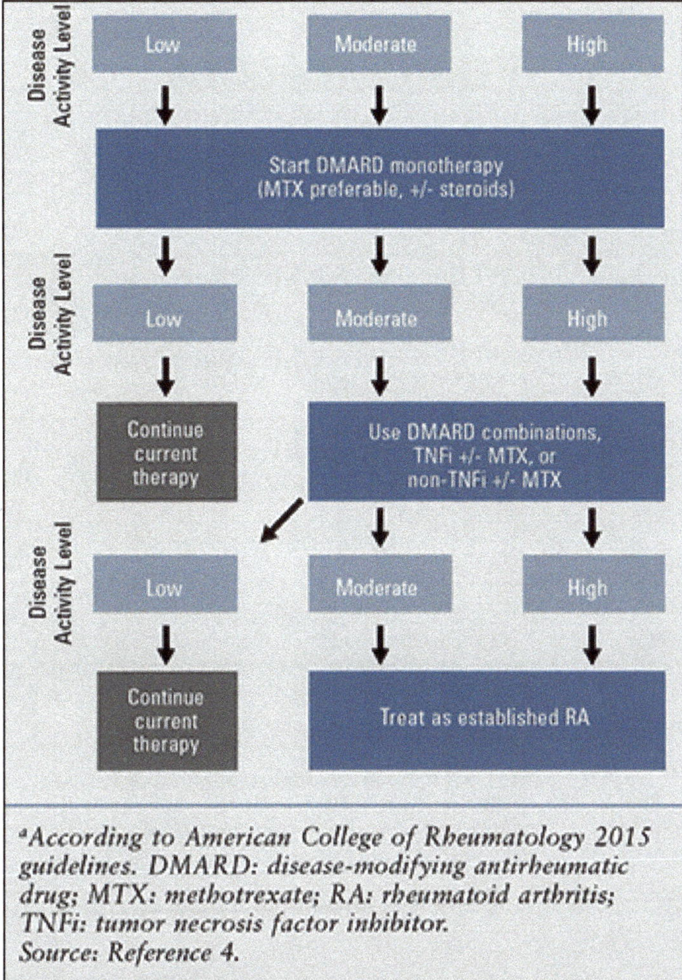

Figure 120 Abbreviated Treatment Algorithm for Early RA having symptoms <6 months

5.4.6 Fibromyalgia

Fibromyalgia is a disorder that characterizes itself in **musculoskeletal pain, fatigue and tenderness in tender points throughout the body.** Though its cause is not clearly understood, they think that it may be a result of how the **brain and nervous system process pain;** probably has to do with genetics, environment as well as psychology. Symptoms also include **sleep disturbances, memory impairment, and problems with concentration, which are collectively referred to as fibro fog.** Such an inevitable state limits one's quality of life due to possible physical and emotional stress. Unfortunately, as with **most chronic ailments**, fibromyalgia has no known cure, and the focus is on controlling manifestations to enhance quality of life. These might involve medicines including pain relievers, antidepressants, anti-seizure agents, physical therapy, and changes in one's lifestyle including **exercising and stress reduction** along with cognitive behavioural therapy. **Fibromyalgia** may be diagnosed during early stages and the efficacy of the treatment is highly dependent on the interventions the patient and the healthcare team choose to use.

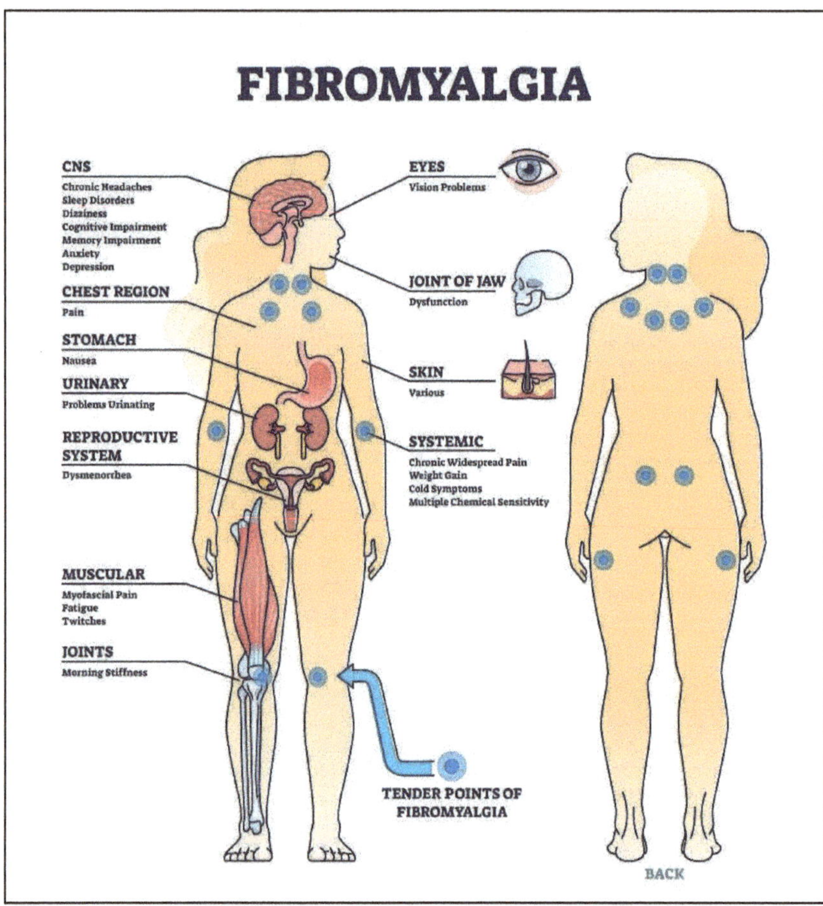

Figure 121 Overview of Fibromyalgia

This anatomical diagram shows the different systems of the human body that may be affected by fibromyalgia, **a long-term condition that results in pain throughout the body**. The diagram centres on some major areas including the **brain** which is involved in the neurological aspect since fibromyalgia is considered as an issue on the **central nervous system** and is thought to be due to abnormal processing of pain in the brain. The **muscles and arm sensitive zones** are highlighted to illustrate that musculoskeletal pain is typical for the condition, and usually occurs in the upper part of the **human body and arms.** Further, the participation of the kidneys and the bladder points to the possibility of the involvement of the other systems, as people with fibromyalgia commonly have varied symptoms related to such systems, including urinary **difficulties or autonomic nervous system disorders.** The **area C** pointed out in the figure may represent the tender facial area or TMJ which is a problem area for fibromyalgia patients.

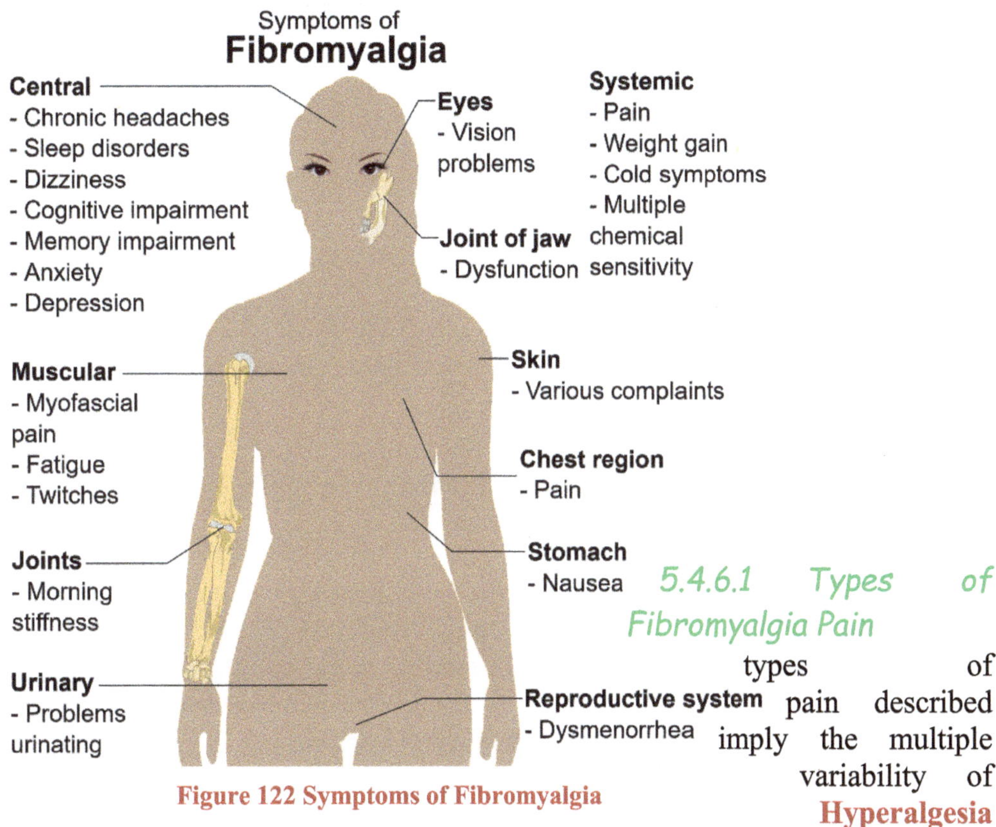

Figure 122 Symptoms of Fibromyalgia

5.4.6.1 Types of Fibromyalgia Pain

The seven types of fibromyalgia pain described in this image imply the multiple facets and variability of the illness. **Hyperalgesia** is a state in which the individual feels enhanced pain when experiencing stimuli that are usually considered painful or normal. Allodynia, in contrast to this, refers to a painful response to stimuli that under normal circumstances should not cause pain – for instance, a harmless touch. **Paresthesia** refers to the sensation that is similar to a tingling or **"pins and needles"** sensation that may manifest in the limbs and can cause pain. The **"Rattled Nerves"** pain is painted as severe and sharp, tingling shock-like pain that characterizes nerve pain. "Sparkler Burns" are stinging, burning sensations, which could be localized, similar to the sensation from a mild sparkler or burn. The **"Knife in the Voodoo Doll"** pain is defined as acute, stinging or burning, which will remind one of being pricked or stabbed. Lastly, **"Randomly Roving Pain"** refers to pain that is felt and moves randomly in an unpredictable manner throughout the body often with no form of warning. Such pains demonstrate the various and diverse characteristics of pain which are found in fibromyalgia patients.

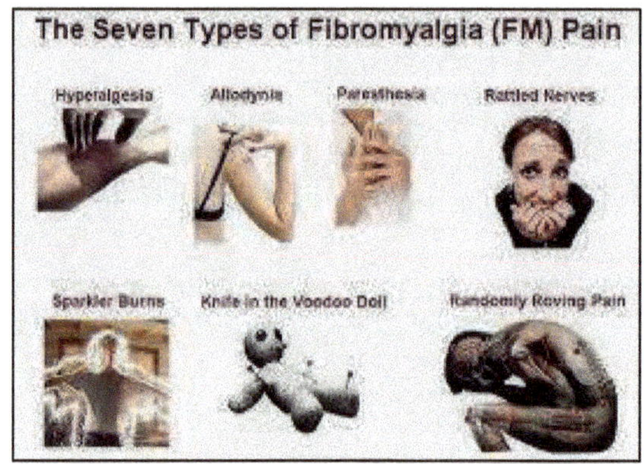

Figure 123 The Fibromyalgia Pain Chronicles

5.4.6.2 Classification of Fibromyalgia

The taxonomy of types of **fibromyalgia** here illustrates the differences in **aetiology and symptoms of the disease.** In the case of both **primary and secondary fibromyalgia**, **trauma and other conditions like osteoarthritis** create the possibility of an association making a primary fibromyalgia diagnosis one where no underlying disorder exists. Secondary fibromyalgia is a type of fibromyalgia that develops from another medical disorder, be it rh**eumatoid arthritis, osteoarthritis, hypothyroidism, polymyalgia rheumatica and the like. Mixed fibromyalgia** is similar to fibromyalgia but is accompanied by some other symptoms that are associated with other conditions including osteoarthritis or rheumatoid arthritis. **Localized fibromyalgia** for instance refers to pain that is localized and mostly attributed to strain, or some form of injury; for instance, repetitive movements which may be characteristic of some careers. It does not fit perfectly within the criteria for **fibromyalgia diagnosis** but may be a subtype of the disease. Finally, **psychogenic fibromyalgia** is when the imaged features are not physical and neuromuscular but are nonspecific, psychological, and fluctuating and are associated with an evident psychological disorder. This type does not classify into the diagnostic criteria of fibromyalgia and is actually dealing with other psychological issues.

Table 76 Classification of Fibromyalgia

Primary fibromyalgia	Characteristic features of fibromyalgia with no recognized underlying cause (eg, trauma, marked osteoarthritis)
Secondary fibromyalgia	Manifestations secondary to another cause (eg, rheumatoid arthritis, osteoarthritis, hypothyroidism, polymyalgia rheumatica)
Mixed fibromyalgia	Characteristic features of fibromyalgia, but some features attributable to concomitant condition (eg, osteoarthritis, rheumatoid arthritis)
Localized fibromyalgia	Localized pain, usually secondary to muscle strains or other trauma (eg, occupational, repetitive); similar to local or regional myofascial pain syndromes; does not satisfy accepted criteria for fibromyalgia, but may be a forme fruste or variant of more characteristic syndrome
Psychogenic fibromyalgia	Symptoms described in bizarre, vague, highly emotional, and inconsistent manner; underlying serious psychologic problem is evident; diagnosis is not fibromyalgia syndrome

5.4.6.3 Mechanism of Sensitization in Fibromyalgia

This diagram explains **Central Sensitization** which is an enhanced pain sensitivity that results from central nervous system dysfunction. The variety of related clinical syndromes is as follows: **Central Sensitivity Syndromes**. This is a broad category that comprises two main classifications of disorders – pain-centred disorders and those that have pain as a minor feature. The primary categories of central sensitivity syndromes, mainly including pain, are subdivided **into "chronic primary pain" types**.

These are chronic widespread pain which includes fibromyalgia; **Complex Regional Pain Syndromes (CRPS) type 1 and 2;** chronic primary headache or orofacial pain which may include chronic migraines or temporomandibular joint pain; and **Chronic Primary Visceral pain** which affects internal organs and it is not exclusive of irritable bowel syndrome and bladder pain syndrome. **Central sensitivity syndromes** that are less defined by chronic pain are further classified under this classification and may include **PTSD, chronic fatigue syndrome, and restless legs syndrome.** This framework thus offers an understanding of how different chronic pain conditions are diagnosed and conceptualized within the overall framework of central sensitization.

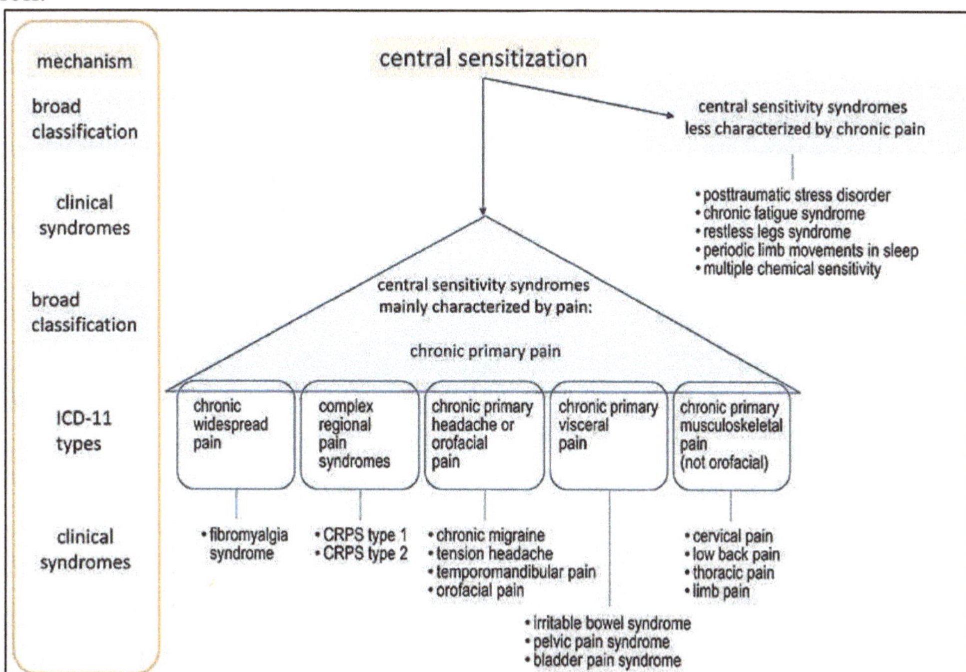

Figure 124 Cultural Sensitization

5.4.6.4 SOAP Notes for Fibromyalgia

Table 77 SOAP Notes for Fibromyalgia

Component	Details
Subjective (S)	The patient is a 45-year-old female presenting with a 9-month history of widespread musculoskeletal pain, fatigue, and sleep disturbances. The pain is described as constant, aching, and often worsens after physical activity. The pain is most intense in the shoulders, lower back, and hips, and is associated with tenderness in the joints and muscles. She reports difficulty concentrating, which she describes as "fibro fog," and experiences frequent headaches. The patient mentions feeling irritable and anxious and has trouble performing daily tasks, such as lifting objects and walking long distances. She denies any recent trauma, infections, or injuries. There is a family history of fibromyalgia. She is concerned about the impact of these symptoms on her quality of life and ability to work.
Objective (O)	The patient appears fatigued but is not in acute distress. Vital signs: BP 118/76 mmHg, HR 78 bpm, Temp 36.7°C (98°F). Physical exam shows

	tenderness on palpation of multiple trigger points, including the cervical spine, shoulders, upper chest, and knees. There is no joint swelling, redness, or deformity. Range of motion is intact, but limited by pain. Neurological exam is normal, with no signs of neuropathy. Laboratory results are within normal limits, including normal complete blood count (CBC), erythrocyte sedimentation rate (ESR), and C-reactive protein (CRP), which help exclude inflammatory or autoimmune diseases.
Assessment (A)	The patient's presentation, including widespread pain, fatigue, sleep disturbances, and cognitive difficulties, along with the absence of inflammatory markers or other underlying conditions, is consistent with fibromyalgia. The tenderness at specific trigger points further supports this diagnosis. The condition appears to be moderate in severity, significantly affecting the patient's daily functioning. Differential diagnoses include chronic fatigue syndrome, rheumatoid arthritis, and myofascial pain syndrome, but these are less likely due to the normal lab results and the specific pain pattern.
Plan (P)	**Pharmacological:** Start the patient on a low dose of Duloxetine (30 mg daily) as an antidepressant that can also help with pain management in fibromyalgia. Consider adding a low dose of Gabapentin (100 mg nightly) to help with sleep disturbances and neuropathic pain. NSAIDs (e.g., Ibuprofen) may be used for acute pain relief if needed (See algorithm below). **Non-pharmacological:** Refer the patient to physical therapy for gentle stretching exercises and strengthening. Recommend cognitive behavioural therapy (CBT) to help manage pain and stress. Encourage regular low-impact aerobic exercises, such as swimming or walking, to improve overall physical function and reduce pain. **Follow-up:** Schedule a follow-up in 4 to 6 weeks to assess the patient's response to medications and modify the treatment plan as necessary. Monitor for side effects from medications and assess any improvement in pain or sleep quality. **Education:** Educate the patient about the chronic nature of fibromyalgia, the importance of medication adherence, and the need for regular exercise and stress management. Discuss the importance of sleep hygiene, pacing of activities, and avoiding overexertion to manage flare-ups.

Table 78 Algorithm Medication Management of Fibromyalgia

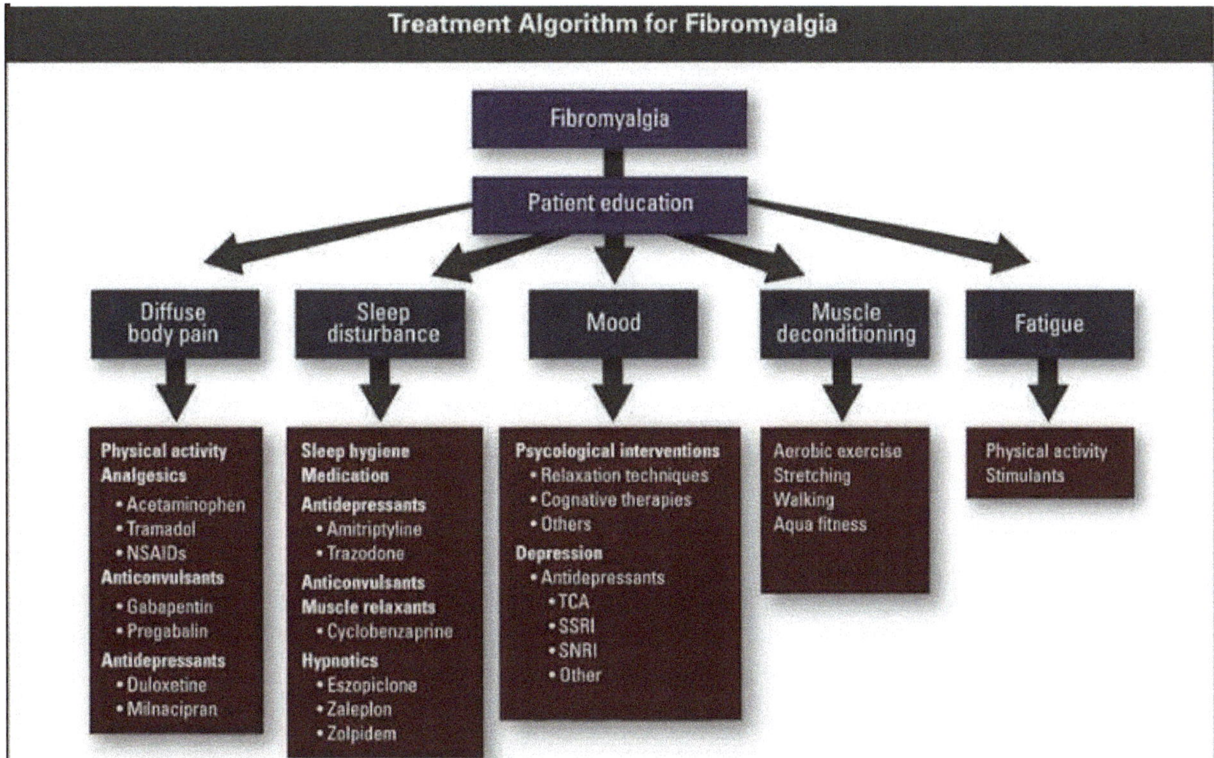

5.4.7 Bursitis

Bursitis is the **inflammation of the bursae**, which are small fluid-filled sacs that allow free gliding of the **tendons, muscles and beneath the bones** in any joint. It is common in the **shoulder, elbow, hip, and knee regions** of the body primarily because pressure and rubbing on the bursae could cause inflammatory reactions. The leading causes are **microtrauma, repeated motions, and pressure or rubbing of the bursa** for an extended period or due to other disorders like **rheumatoid arthritis or gout.** In the case of bursitis, one is likely to experience aches around the affected joint, especially in the area of the **inflamed bursa.** This pain may be severe, and increase when the joint is moved or pressure is applied on the area of the injury. They both may notice **inflammation, redness and warmth** over the affected area as well as limber confines of motion due to discomfort. At times, the joint may feel stiff or weak to some extent or it might swell or feel stiff or weak at times. For diagnosing bursitis, a doctor will perform general tests and can also request **X-rays or MRI** to exclude other conditions such as a fracture or an infection. Sometimes, it may be necessary to aspirate the joint to determine whether there are some issues with the fluids in the bursa. These consist of **nonsteroidal anti-inflammatory drugs (NSAIDs)** as an analgesic, cold or heat application, immobilization, and refraining from activities that cause discomfort to the injured area. In conditions where inflammation is **prolonged corticosteroids or in case of purulent lesions, injection of corticosteroids or surgical drainage may be expected.** This is likely to be advised in order to build up the surrounding tissues as a way of avoiding future complications of a flare-up.

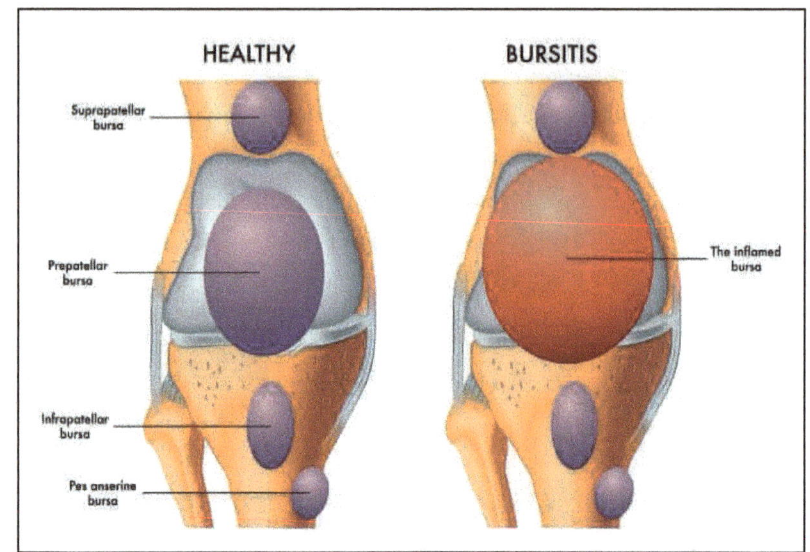

Figure 125 Bursitis Overview

5.4.7.1 Types of Bursitis

This picture illustrates the different categories of bursitis. **Shoulder bursitis** occurs as a result of overhead activities that cause abrasion to the shoulder, making it sore and with little mobility. Knee bursitis is caused mostly by **pressure or kneeling for an extended amount of time** leading to swelling and pain in the area around the kneecap. Hip bursitis is a condition that occurs in the outside of the hip in which one **feels aches while walking or squatting.** One kind of bursitis is known as 'student's elbow,' which is caused by applying pressure to the joint by leaning on it and leads to swelling and discomfort at the end of the elbow. Finally, heel bursitis develops due to pressure during activities such as running or being on your feet for most of the day as it causes pain and swelling over the back of the heel. All of these bursae cause similar symptoms which are **joint pain, swelling and stiffened movement,** while they are treated with rest, application of ice, physical therapy as well as injections of corticosteroids.

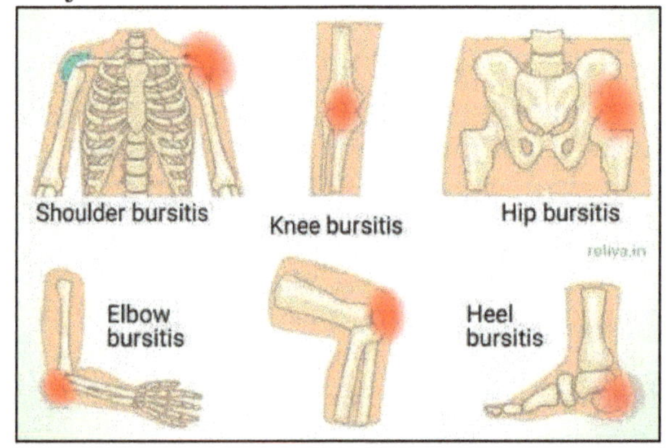

Figure 126 Types of Bursitis

5.4.7.2 SOAP Notes for Bursitis

Component	Details
Subjective (S)	The patient is a 45-year-old female presenting with a 2-week history of pain and swelling around her right shoulder. The pain started gradually after prolonged overhead work at her job as a painter. She describes the pain as a dull ache, rating it 6/10 in intensity, which worsens with reaching overhead or lifting objects. The patient also reports mild stiffness in the shoulder

	joint, especially in the morning. She denies any recent trauma or injury. The patient is concerned about the impact of the pain on her ability to work.
Objective (O)	The patient appears to be in mild discomfort but is able to move her shoulder with some difficulty. Vital signs: BP 120/78 mmHg, HR 78 bpm, Temp 36.8°C (98.2°F). Physical examination reveals tenderness over the subacromial bursa of the right shoulder. There is mild swelling and warmth around the joint. Active and passive range of motion is limited due to pain, particularly with abduction and external rotation. The Neer test and Hawkins-Kennedy test are positive, indicating possible shoulder impingement and bursitis.
Assessment (A)	The patient's clinical presentation, including pain, swelling, and limited range of motion in the shoulder, along with positive impingement tests, is consistent with subacromial bursitis of the right shoulder. The condition is likely due to repetitive overhead motions at work.
Plan (P)	**Pharmacological:** Prescribe NSAIDs (e.g., ibuprofen 400 mg every 6-8 hours) for pain relief and inflammation reduction. Consider a corticosteroid injection (e.g., methylprednisolone 40 mg) if symptoms persist despite NSAIDs (See table below). **Non-pharmacological:** Recommend R.I.C.E. (Rest, Ice, Compression, Elevation) for the first 48-72 hours. Apply ice for 20 minutes several times a day to reduce swelling. Physical therapy referral for strengthening exercises and range-of-motion exercises once the acute pain has subsided. Advise avoiding overhead activities that aggravate the pain. **Follow-up:** Schedule a follow-up in 1-2 weeks to assess symptom improvement. If symptoms persist or worsen, consider imaging studies (e.g., ultrasound or MRI) to rule out other potential causes of shoulder pain, such as rotator cuff tears. **Education:** Educate the patient on the importance of rest and avoiding activities that aggravate the condition, such as lifting or reaching overhead. Emphasize the need for physical therapy to improve shoulder strength and prevent future flare-ups. Discuss ergonomic adjustments at work to reduce strain on the shoulder.

Table 79 Management and Treatment Approaches for Bursitis

Category	Treatment/Management Option
Rest and Activity Modification	Rest the injured area and avoid activities that put pressure on the affected bursa. Ask your provider how long to rest and avoid physical activities.
At-Home Treatments	Elevation: Elevate the injured area to reduce swelling. Over-the-Counter Pain Relievers: Use ibuprofen, naproxen, or acetaminophen. Avoid using pain relievers for more than 10 days without consulting a healthcare provider. Ice: Apply a cold compress or ice pack wrapped in a towel for 15 minutes several times a day. Heat: Apply a heating pad or hot water bottle wrapped in a towel,

	alternating with ice if recommended by your provider. Splint/Sling/Brace: Use a splint, sling, or brace to support the injured area.
Additional Medical Treatments	Antibiotics: Prescribed if there is an infection causing the bursitis. Physical Therapy: To increase range of motion and improve strength. Occupational Therapy: To learn movement techniques that reduce stress on the affected area.
Invasive Treatments	Corticosteroid Injections: To reduce inflammation and pain. Surgery: If symptoms persist for six months or longer despite other treatments, surgery to remove the bursa (bursectomy) may be considered.

5.4.8 Chronic Low Back Pain

Chronic low back pain is one of the most prevalent complaints globally, and most people **experience it at least once in their lifetime.** It is described as pain that persists beyond three consecutive months and is associated with numerous health conditions like **poor posture, muscle strain, herniated disc, spinal stenosis, osteoarthritis and stress among others.** Chronic low back pain symptoms can present in different ways, manifesting as constant moderate pain or episodic severe pain. The pain intensifies during sitting, bending and lifting objects or even while standing for long durations. Other symptoms may include stiffness, restricted movements, or shooting pain down through the leg or into the legs if the sciatic nerve is pinched (sciatica). Diagnosis is usually made by asking questions about the history of contact with animals, physical examination and imaging techniques like **X-ray, MRI or CT.** These tests exclude other problems such as fractures, infections, and tumours that might also cause nerve compression. However, imaging may not always be consistent with pain, as structural changes are not always the source of the complaint. Management of **chronic pain involves a combination of interventions, both pharmacological and nonpharmacological.** Surgical treatments are not always required and patients can benefit from more conservative measures, including **physical therapy, exercise, and manual therapy.** For example, pain-killer drugs such as non-steroidal anti-inflammatory drugs, and medications for muscle contraction like muscle relaxants may be prescribed. In cases where conservative therapies for pain are not successful, epidural steroid injections or neurosurgical procedures can be administered for instance spinal fusion or disc replacement. Moreover, proper weight management, good ergonomic movement, and consistent exercise are other methods of treating and preventing it. Other interventions like **CBT, or stress, depression, and anxiety** could also go a long way in enhancing the health of patients. Chronic low back pain is often a long-term process that can be challenging to address since it must be managed over time with an individualized treatment strategy.

5.4.8.1 Types of Chronic Low Back Pain

The image depicts a taxonomy for CLBP based on the cause of the pain, which divides them into non-degenerative, degenerative, and psychogenic or unspecified origins. Non-degenerative causes include conditions such as discogenic pain which is associated with **degenerative disc disease (DDD)** predominantly isolated disc degeneration. Other related non-degenerative conditions include inflammatory DDD referred to as **MODIC 1, and DDD due to inflammation**. In addition, there is L5-S1 retrolisthesis which is caused by misalignment between the L5 and S1 vertebrae resulting in pain. The degenerative causes include a number of diseases that emanate from the regular stress that is put on the spine. This includes **facet lesions, isolated arthrosis of the facet joints and combined lesions** where the patient has both disc degeneration and facet joint disease. It also includes ligament lesions with segmental instability, which entails instability of one or several segments of the spine, and regional disorders of spinal balance, including multilevel DDD leading to the flattening of the **spine's natural curves (lordosis).** Other degenerative causes are compensatory **DDD in extension and hyperlordosis** which also refers to the inward curve of the spine. Various spinal imbalance pathologies include lumbar degenerative kyphosis that results in forward rounding of the spine and different sorts of **spinal malalignment**. Finally, the psychogenic or undetermined category involves pain that has no evident physiological cause but can be assumed to be related to **psychological aetiology** or may be related to an undiscovered pathological condition. This classification helps in determining the exact nature of CLBP, offering the most appropriate treatments concerning the cause of the condition.

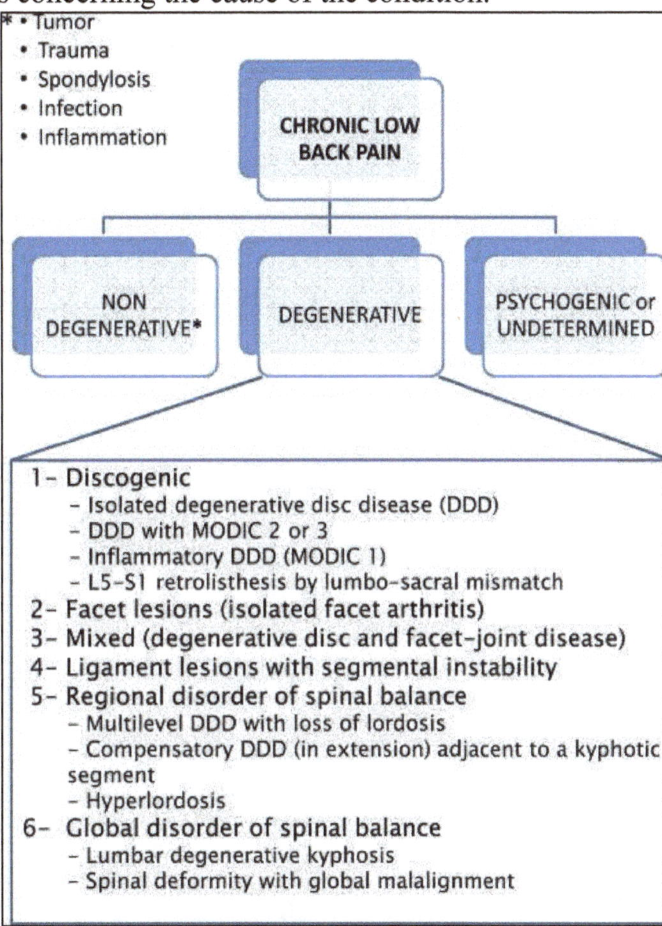

Figure 127 Types of Chronic Low Back Pain

5.4.8.2 Specific Causes of Lower Back Pain

The picture above shows **different types of causes of lower back pain** and divides them into special and transient types. Specific examples include injuries like those of sprains and strains that are caused by one or the other movement, either **sudden or repetitive,** which causes harm to muscles or ligaments in the body. Any spinal injuries or diseases like osteoporosis can lead to fractures which also cause severe pain. **Spinal disc herniation, also known as bulging discs,** are disorders where the disks compress the nerves, making it painful. Musculoskeletal and neuromuscular spinal disorders play a big role in the development of lower back pain, including scoliosis or abnormal spinal curvature for example. The major forms of arthritis are osteoarthritis and rheumatoid arthritis that cause inflammation and wear and tear in the spinal joints resulting in persistent pain. **Disease is also one of the major causes of back pain**, for instance, having a **tumor in the spinal cord.** There are also factors that lead to lower back pain, and some of them are temporary and they include menstrual cramps that make women **develop discomfort** when they are on their periods. It is a common problem because pregnancy brings about changes in posture as well as **increased weight which puts pressure on the lower back muscles.** Thirdly, back labour or the pain felt during delivery may also be a cause of low back pain. Thus, it is crucial to comprehend these predisposing factors in order to diagnose and manage the lower back pain correctly.

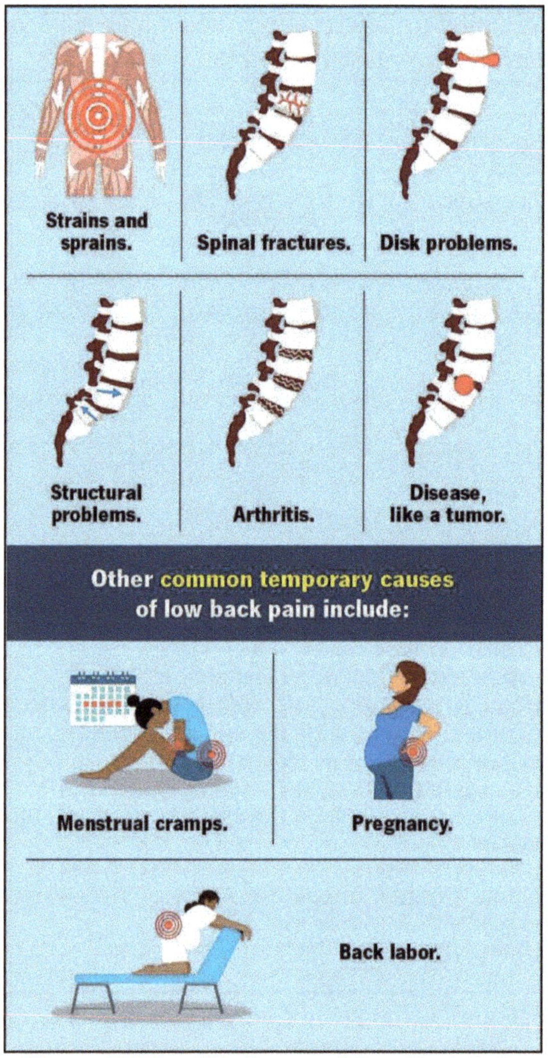

Figure 128 Specific Causes of Low Back Pain

5.4.8.3 SOAP Notes for Chronic Lower Back Pain

Table 80 SOAP Notes for Chronic Low Back Pain

Component	Details
Subjective (S)	The patient is a 50-year-old female presenting with a 6-month history of chronic lower back pain. The pain is described as a dull ache, rating 6/10 in

	intensity, with intermittent sharp episodes. It is worse after prolonged sitting or standing and improves somewhat with rest or lying down. The patient denies any trauma but reports increased discomfort after long periods of work, particularly sitting at a desk. She also experiences mild stiffness in the lower back in the morning, which improves as the day progresses. The patient has a history of poor posture and reports that the pain has gradually worsened over time. She denies numbness, tingling, or radiating pain down the legs. She is concerned about the impact on her daily activities and ability to work.
Objective (O)	The patient appears in mild discomfort but is able to move and change positions slowly. Vital signs: BP 120/78 mmHg, HR 82 bpm, Temp 36.8°C (98.2°F). Physical examination reveals tenderness over the lumbar spine and paraspinal muscles. There is reduced lumbar flexion due to pain, and the straight leg raise test is negative. X-rays of the lumbar spine show signs of degenerative disc disease and mild facet joint osteoarthritis. No signs of acute injury or structural abnormalities are noted.
Assessment (A)	The patient's chronic lower back pain, associated with degenerative changes in the lumbar spine and absence of neurological deficits, is consistent with chronic lower back pain due to degenerative disc disease and facet joint osteoarthritis. No signs of more serious conditions like tumours or fractures are present.
Plan (P)	**Pharmacological:** Initiate NSAIDs (e.g., ibuprofen 400 mg every 6-8 hours) for pain relief. If pain persists, consider muscle relaxants (e.g., cyclobenzaprine 5 mg nightly) for muscle spasms. **Non-pharmacological:** Recommend physical therapy focusing on strengthening and stretching exercises for the lumbar and core muscles to improve posture and support the spine. Advise ergonomic adjustments at work to promote better posture. Consider heat or cold therapy for acute pain relief. Encourage low-impact activities such as walking or swimming to improve overall mobility and reduce stiffness. **Follow-up:** Schedule follow-up in 4 weeks to assess the patient's progress and response to treatment. If symptoms persist or worsen, further diagnostic studies such as MRI may be considered to evaluate for any nerve impingement or herniated discs. **Education:** Educate the patient on the importance of maintaining proper posture, staying active, and engaging in low-impact exercises. Discuss the role of weight management in reducing stress on the lower back. Advise on lifestyle changes to prevent further strain and reduce symptoms.

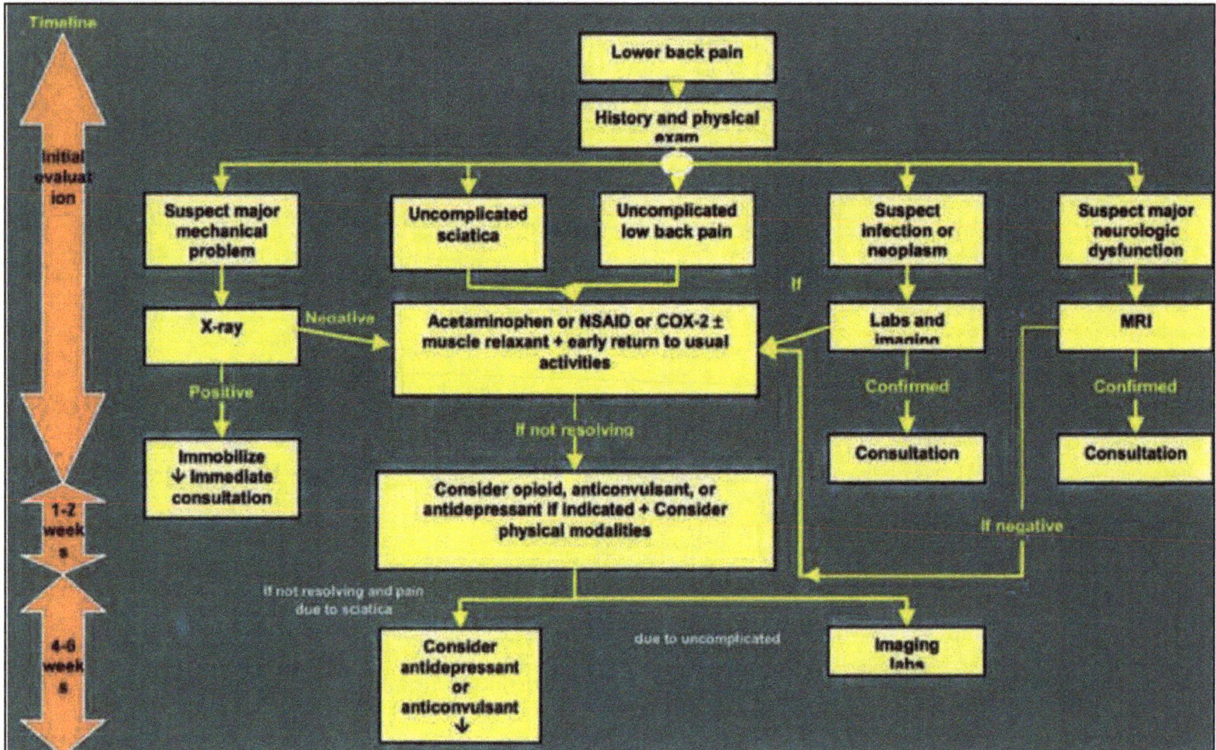

Figure 129 Algorithm for the Management of Chronic Low Back Pain

5.4.9 Carpel Tunnel Syndrome

Carpal Tunnel Syndrome (CTS) is a syndrome resulting from **compression of the median nerve in the carpal tunnel** at the wrist. The carpal tunnel is yet another vital part of the body, which is a narrow pathway made up of **bones and ligaments**, and when the tissues in this tunnel become inflamed, they can exert pressure on the said nerve and bring about several symptoms. It **controls the sensation to the palm side of the thumb, the index finger, the middle finger and half of the ring finger** plus it controls the **movements of the thumb muscles**. Some of the signs of Carpal Tunnel Syndrome include; numbness, tingling and pain that affects the palm side of the thumb, the index, middle and part of the ring fingers. This is usually **felt more at night and can even disturb the patient from sleep.** Some of the patients may also have a condition where they will develop a limp hand which cannot grasp anything properly. If neglected, there will be wasting of the **thenar muscles – the muscles in the palm at the base of the thumb.** CTS is commonly referred to with reference to hand movements that entail repeated typing, use of the mouse or any other machinery. It can also be a result of pregnancy, diabetes, rheumatoid arthritis or obesity that **puts pressure on the carpal tunnel**. The diagnosis of carpal tunnel syndrome is based on physical examination using **Tinel's sign** in which the examiner taps over the carpal tunnel to feel or elicit tingling in the fingers; **Phalen's manoeuvre** in which the wrist is flexed to simulate the symptoms of carpal tunnel syndrome. Hence, **Electromyography (EMG)** and nerve conduction studies help in ascertaining the diagnosis and exclude other potential causes. Having indicated that the manifestations of prosthetic valve endocarditis depend on the acuity of the problem, it is now pertinent to discuss the treatment options. Worn at the wrist, especially during the night to maintain the wrist in a **neutral position and pad an area** where the median nerve is compressed. These medications help in the alleviation of pain as well as inflammation and are **generically known as NSAIDs.** If the symptoms do not improve, further intervention such as supplying corticosteroid solutions may be made to decrease inflammation surrounding the nerve. It can be recommended that in more severe cases the patient has to undergo what is referred to as carpal tunnel release surgery in order to release **the pressure on the median nerve**. Carpal Tunnel Syndrome can be efficiently treated if diagnosed in its early stages and should not result in further damage to the nerve over time.

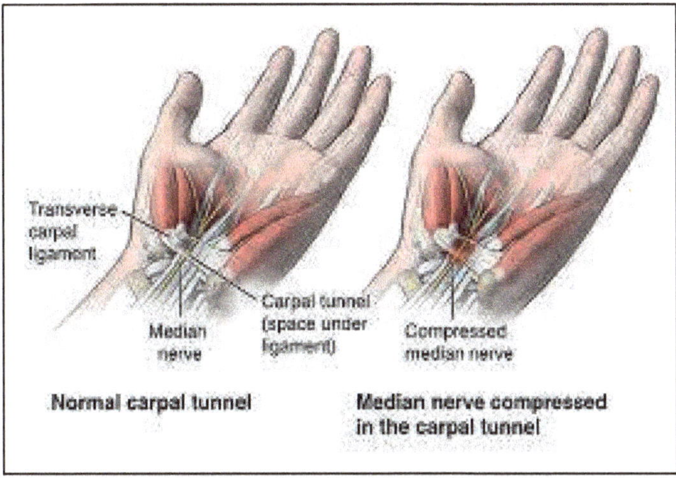

Figure 130 Carpel Tunnel Syndrome

5.4.9.1 Severity Outcomes of Carpel Tunnel Syndrome

The figure summarizes prospectively the evaluations of CTS in terms of severity and outcomes, which can be classified as subjective and objective. Subjective methods deal with techniques that incorporate patient's own observations and sensations and the effects of those sensations on their lives. These are specific health outcome measures such as the **Carpal Tunnel Syndrome Questionnaire (CTQ)** which addresses the severity and functional impact of CTS; **the Michigan Hand Outcomes Questionnaire (MHQ)** which is an assessment of hand function in the frame of CTS; the **Disabilities of the Arm, Shoulder and Hand (DASH)** score which is an upper limb outcome measure; and the SF-36 health survey, which is a comprehensive health-related quality of life measure. Disease-related assessments of CTS include the wrist flexion test also known as Phalen's test, in which the wrist is bent backwards towards the forearm to provoke symptoms, Tinel's sign which involves tapping over the carpal tunnel, Durkan's test, shooting a small flashlight directly at the palm side of the wrist and the **Katz-Stirrat Hand Diagram** in which the patient marks areas of pain or decreased sensation. Objective assessments are clinical tests such as carpal tunnel syndrome diagnosis by using **Nerve Conduction Velocity (NCV),** which determines the speed of electrical impulses along the median nerve to check for compression and **Electromyography (EMG)**, which measures electrical activity in muscles to check nerve function. They offer quantitative measures that assist the healthcare providers in establishing the severity and prognosis of the condition and develop treatment strategies.

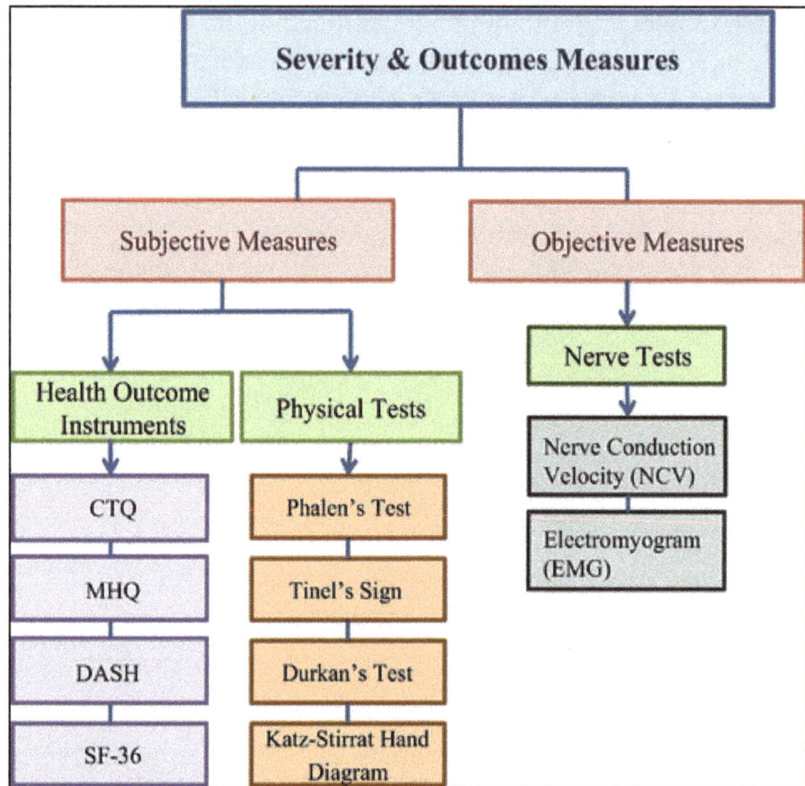

Figure 131 Severity Outcomes of Carpel Tunnel Syndrome

5.4.9.2 Grading Scale for Patients with Carpal Tunnel Syndrome

The image describes Bland's Neurophysiological Grading Scale for Carpal Tunnel Syndrome (CTS) which is grouping CTS based on nerve conduction. It begins with grade 0 where nerve conduction studies are normal and there is **no CTS to grade 6** where CTS is described as very severe. **In Grade 1 (Very Mild),** slight changes in the nerve fibres can only be demonstrated with the most sensitive of all tests and the nerve conduction velocity is slowed down in the fingers or at the wrist. **Grade 2 (Mild)** has normal terminal motor latency which suggests mild motor slowing without corresponding functional deficit. Moderate reduction in grade with changes in motor slowing, **DML of APB is less than 6.5 ms,** and sensory conduction is intact. **Grade 4 (Severe)** reveals its motor potential preservation, but **DML to APB is more than 6.5 ms,** sensory potentials are not observed. **Grade 5 (Very Severe)** applies if there are no sensory potentials and mild slowing with maximum latency of the **DML to APB above 6.5 ms.** Finally, Grade 6 (Extremely Severe) depicts the lowest impaired sensorimotor outlook with surface motor potential in the **APB being less than 0.2 mV**; it is the worst stage of CTS. The grading scale is useful to the clinicians for staging CTS and also helps in treatment planning.

Table 1. Bland's Neurophysiological Grading Scale for Patients with carpal tunnel syndrome.[17]

	Grade	Nerve Conduction Findings
0	Normal	Normal motor and sensory conduction studies
1	Very mild	CTS demonstrable only with most sensitive tests
2	Mild	Sensory nerve conduction velocity slow on finger/wrist measurement Normal terminal motor latency
3	Moderate	Sensory potential preserved Motor slowing: DML to ABP <6.5 ms
4	Severe	Sensory potentials absent Motor potential preserved: DML to APB <6.5 ms
5	Very Severe	Sensory potentials absent DML to APB >6.5 ms
6	Ext Severe	Sensory and motor potentials effectively unrecordable Surface motor potential from ABP <0.2 mV amplitude

DSL indicates distal sensory latency; DML, distal motor latency; APB, abductor pollicis brevis; and Ext, extremely.

Figure 132 Grading Scale for CTS

5.4.9.3 SOAP Notes for Carpel Tunnel Syndrome

Table 81 SOAP Notes for Carpel Tunnel Syndrome

Component	Details
Subjective (S)	The patient is a 38-year-old female presenting with a 3-month history of numbness, tingling, and pain in her right hand. The symptoms are primarily in the thumb, index, and middle fingers, with worsening at night. The patient reports that the symptoms interfere with her sleep, and she frequently shakes her hand to relieve the discomfort. She has a history of repetitive motion at her job as a data entry clerk, involving prolonged typing and using a mouse. The patient denies any trauma or injury. She is concerned about the impact of the symptoms on her ability to work.
Objective (O)	The patient appears in mild discomfort and is holding her hand in a protective posture. Vital signs: BP 120/80 mmHg, HR 75 bpm, Temp 36.9°C (98.4°F). Physical exam shows positive Tinel's sign (tingling in the fingers when tapping over the carpal tunnel) and positive Phalen's test (pain or tingling after holding the wrist in flexion for 60 seconds). There is mild atrophy in the thenar eminence. Nerve conduction studies (NCS) confirm slowed sensory conduction velocity and motor latency, consistent with Carpal Tunnel Syndrome.
Assessment (A)	The patient's clinical symptoms, positive physical tests (Tinel's and Phalen's), and nerve conduction studies confirm a diagnosis of Carpal Tunnel Syndrome (CTS). The condition is likely due to repetitive hand movements at work and is in the early stages, as there is no significant muscle weakness or advanced atrophy.
Plan (P)	**Pharmacological:** Start with NSAIDs (e.g., ibuprofen 400 mg every 6-8 hours) for pain relief and inflammation. If symptoms persist, consider a corticosteroid injection (e.g., methylprednisolone 40 mg) into the carpal tunnel (See algorithm below). **Non-pharmacological:** Recommend using a wrist splint at night to keep the wrist in a neutral position and prevent further compression of the median nerve. Advise ergonomic adjustments at

work, such as using an ergonomic keyboard and mouse, and take frequent breaks to reduce strain. Consider physical therapy to strengthen the wrist and forearm muscles and improve flexibility. **Follow-up:** Follow up in 4 weeks to assess the response to conservative treatment. If symptoms persist, further imaging (e.g., ultrasound or MRI) may be considered to evaluate the extent of nerve compression. If no improvement is noted, discuss options for surgical intervention, such as carpal tunnel release. **Education:** Educate the patient on the importance of wrist ergonomics, proper hand positioning, and the need for rest from repetitive activities. Discuss the role of splinting and physical therapy in managing symptoms and preventing long-term damage.

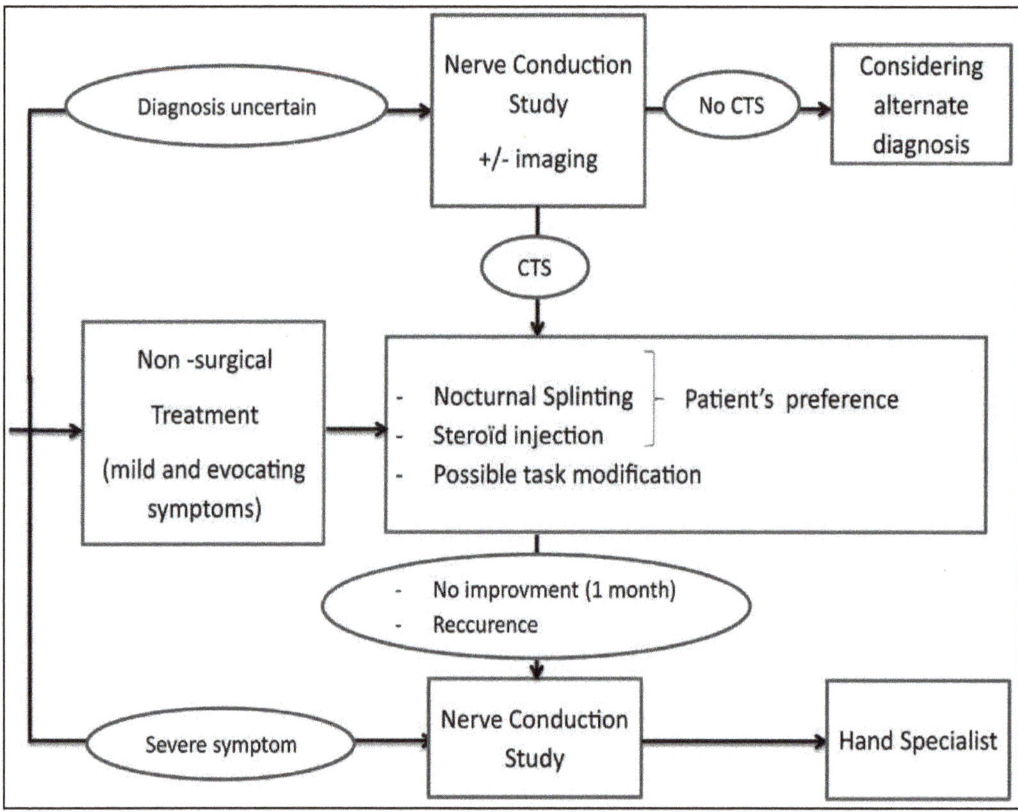

Figure 133 Primary Care Algorithm for Carpel Tunnel Syndrome

ACUTE CONDITIONS

5.4.10 Gout

Gout is said to be an **inflammatory arthritis** that is generated due to the formation of crystalline deposits of uric acid in the articulation especially because of **elevated levels of uric acid** in the blood stream. This condition is characterized by sudden severe pain, redness, and swelling over a joint, particularly the **first metatarsophalangeal joint** of the great toe. A person is likely to develop gout if they are overweight, consume too much alcohol, eat foods with high purines content such as **fatty meats and seafood** and others with medical conditions like; high blood pressure and diabetes. It is diagnosed clinically and the evidence of uric acid crystals within joint fluid. Symptomatic relief during acute gout episodes can be provided **with NSAIDs, colchicine or corticosteroids,** whereas preventive treatment entails drugs such as allopurinol to decrease serum uric acid concentrations. Lifestyle modifications, including **weight loss, a low-purine diet, and a decrease in alcohol consumption** are components of secondary prevention in the form of risk factor modification. In its advanced stage, gout can cause joint degeneration and other complications including onycholysis and gouty kidney.

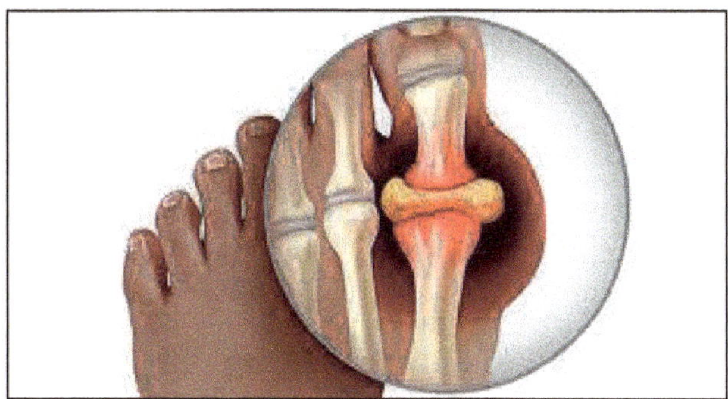

Figure 134 Gout Appearance

5.4.10.1 Stages of Gout

Gout has three stages: The first stage also referred to as **Hyperuricemia**, the second is **Gouty Arthritis,** and the third is chronic **Trapezius Gout**. **In the Asymptomatic Gout stage**, the uric acid in high amounts in the blood causes the formation of the urate in the joints without presenting any signs and symptoms. This stage can be long-lasting for years before the patient moves to an acute attack. The next stage is **Acute Intermittent Gout** which is an acute gouty attack with severe symptoms for 3-10 days. These are characterized by **pain, inflammation, redness, stiffness and tiredness,** especially in the first toe of the foot. These are commonly caused by foods high in purines such as alcohol, and in this case, the only obvious factor is dehydration. If the mentioned causes are left untreated or are **inadequately controlled**, gout may develop into **Chronic Tophaceous Gout**, in which further urate crystal deposits in the joints result in an increase in size after repeated episodes. These tophi can go on to damage the bone and cartilage as well as leading to permanent joint deformation, as well as the development of kidney disease. This point is essential to prevent the further development of this stage.

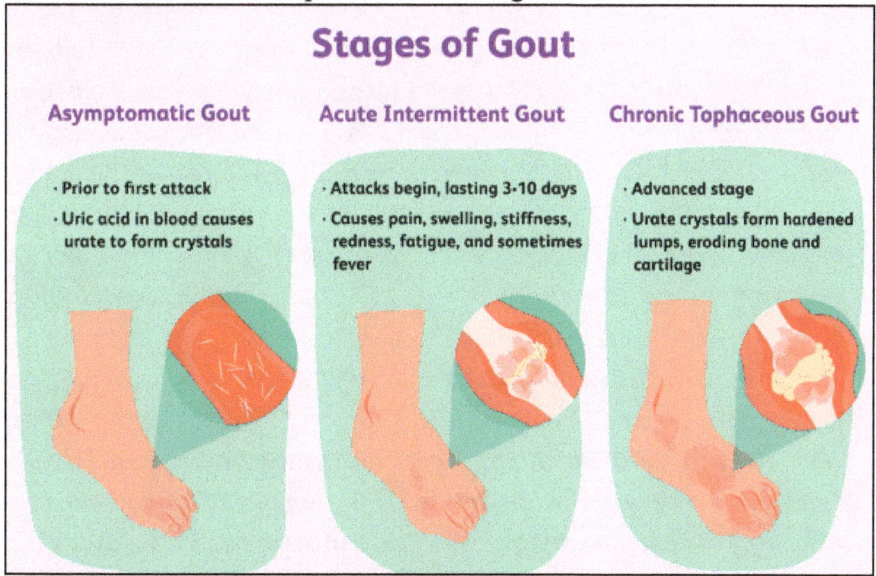

Figure 135 Stages of Gout

5.4.10.2 The Impact of Gout on Cardiovascular and Metabolic Health

Gout arises because of the **presence of excess uric acid in the blood**, hence inflammation that has adverse effects on **many systems** of the body especially cardiovascular and metabolic. **Uric acid deposits** in joints result in gout, but since uric acid is an inflammatory agent the distant organs are affected. **This inflammation** increases the risk of **coronary heart disease and atherosclerosis** which leads to heart complications. Furthermore, gout has been established to share connections with several other metabolic diseases such as **diabetes, dyslipidemia, hypertension, and metabolic syndrome.** These conditions accompany gout leading to the worsening of the risk of developing cardiovascular diseases including **heart failure.** This paper underlines the necessity of optimal gout and related inflammation and metabolic effects' management since these issues contribute to **cardiovascular** impact development.

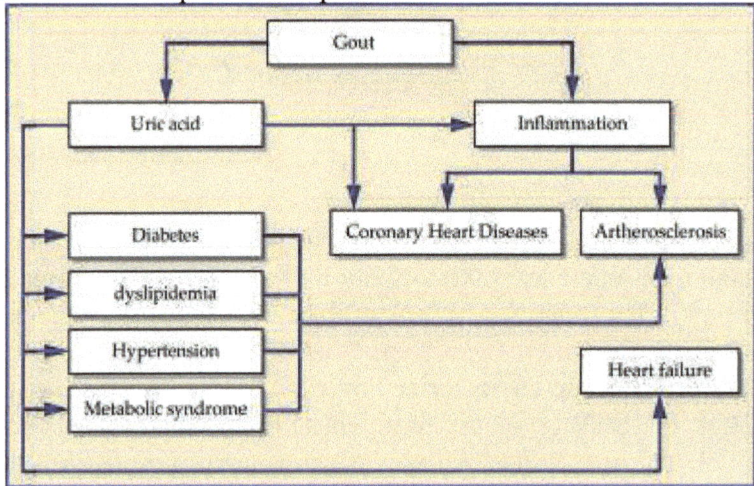

Figure 136 Flowchart of Gout Implications

5.4.10.3 SOAP Notes for Gout

Table 82 SOAP Notes for Gout

Component	Details
Subjective (S)	The patient is a 60-year-old male presenting with a 2-day history of severe pain, redness, and swelling in the big toe, which started suddenly during the night. The pain is described as sharp and excruciating, making it difficult for him to walk. The patient reports a history of occasional gout attacks, particularly after alcohol consumption or eating purine-rich foods. He denies any recent trauma, but mentions increased alcohol intake during the past weekend. He has been diagnosed with hypertension and diabetes for several years but is not on consistent medication. The patient expresses concern about frequent flare-ups and the potential for joint damage.
Objective (O)	The patient appears in moderate distress due to pain. Vital signs: BP 135/85 mmHg, HR 88 bpm, Temp 37.4°C (99.3°F). Physical exam reveals erythema, warmth, and swelling in the first metatarsophalangeal (MTP) joint of the right foot. The joint is tender to palpation, with limited range of motion due to pain. There is no deformity or skin ulceration. Laboratory results show an elevated serum uric acid level (8.2 mg/dL, normal range: 3.5-7.2 mg/dL). Joint fluid aspiration is pending for the identification of urate crystals.

Assessment (A)	The patient's presentation, including sudden onset of joint pain, erythema, swelling, and a history of recurrent gout attacks, is consistent with an acute gout flare. The elevated uric acid level further supports the diagnosis. Differential diagnoses include cellulitis and septic arthritis, but the absence of fever and the typical joint involvement make these less likely. The patient's hypertension and diabetes also increase the risk of recurrent gout attacks.
Plan (P)	**Pharmacological:** Initiate treatment with NSAIDs (e.g., ibuprofen 800 mg every 8 hours) to reduce inflammation and pain. Consider colchicine (0.6 mg twice daily) if NSAIDs are not effective or contraindicated. If symptoms persist, consider adding corticosteroids (e.g., prednisone 20 mg daily for 5 days) (See algorithm below). **Non-pharmacological:** Advise the patient to elevate the affected foot and apply ice to reduce swelling. Recommend avoiding alcohol and purine-rich foods, such as red meat, shellfish, and organ meats. **Follow-up:** Schedule a follow-up appointment in 1 week to assess the resolution of symptoms and to review the joint fluid analysis for urate crystals. If this is the patient's first severe attack, consider starting a urate-lowering therapy (e.g., allopurinol) to prevent future gout flares. **Education:** Educate the patient on gout management, including lifestyle modifications like weight loss, limiting alcohol consumption, and dietary changes to reduce uric acid levels. Discuss the importance of medication adherence for both acute and long-term gout management.

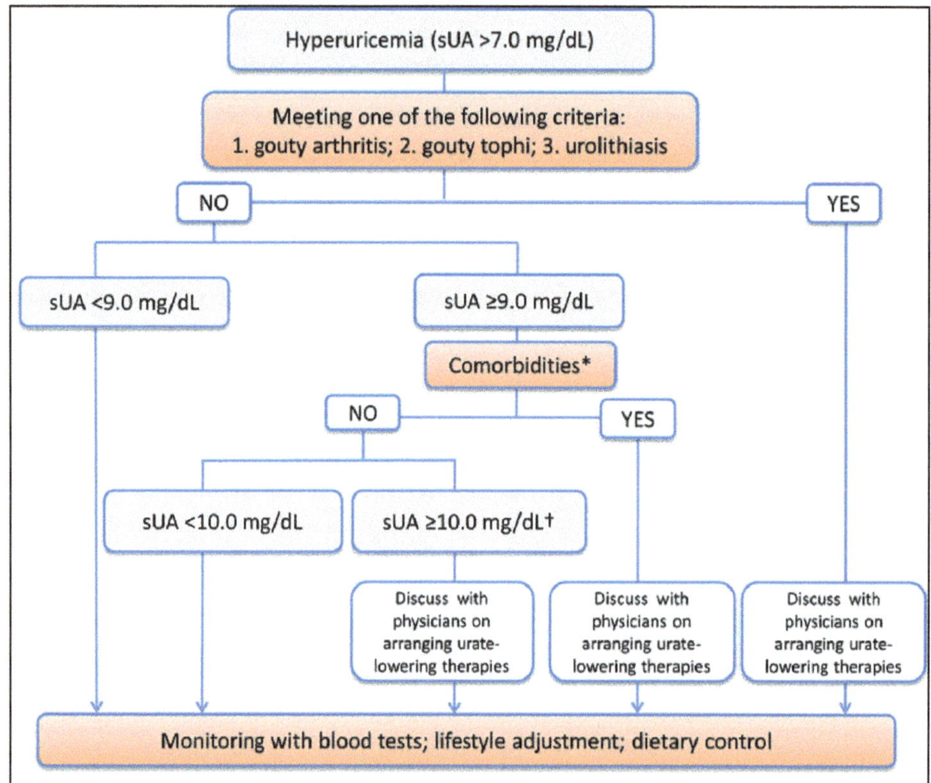

Figure 137 Algorithm for the Pharmacological Management of Gout

5.4.11 Sprains and Strains

A sprain is a **painful injury of the joint**, which results from the **stretching or tearing of ligaments** while a strain is an injury that affects **muscles or tendons in the body**. A sprain is a **ligament injury** where the tough band of tissue connecting the bones are stretched or stretched. This normally occurs as a result of somebody **stumbling or twisting his ankle, wrist or knee or** engaging in an activity that they were not prepared for physically. Some of the **inflammations contain pain, swelling, bruising and unwanted movements around the joints**. A strain, on the other hand, is a term used to describe the partial tear or break of muscles which are fibrous tissues or tendons, tissues that join muscles to bones. Strains most times are due to excessive pulling or overworking of muscles mainly during an activity that may demand a forceful pull or any repetitive use of the muscles. Some common tends to affect the **lower back, hamstrings as well as the shoulder region of the body**. Muscle pain and stiffness, contraction and twitching are also common while the joint appears less mobile than normal. Both are treated by using rest, ice, compression and elevation popularly known as **R.I.C.E and administration of anti-inflammatory pain relievers**. In severe cases, patients may require physical therapy or even surgery to have the child's bowels removed altogether.

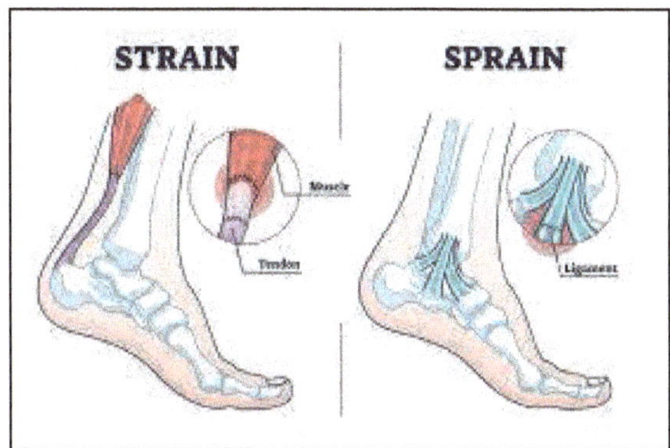

Figure 138 Strain vs. Sprain

5.4.11.1 Types of Ankle Sprain

The illustration shows distinct parts of ankle sprains **Inversion and Eversion movements.** Inversion is when the **foot turns inwards** and usually causes a sprained lateral ligament. This is a common type of sprain, often sustained **during running or any sporting activities,** which causes the foot to roll inward, straining or even rupturing the ligaments on the outer part of the ankle joint. While with eversion, there is the rolling out of the foot and one of the severest injuries that could be incurred is a **sprained medial ligament**. This type of injury is less frequent than the inversion sprains but happens when the foot rolls outside and affects **the interior ligaments of the ankle**. It also depicts the normally aligned ankle in which the foot remains in its natural position without **straining the ligaments**. Inversion and evert sprains should also be treated with rest, ice, and in some cases physical therapy.

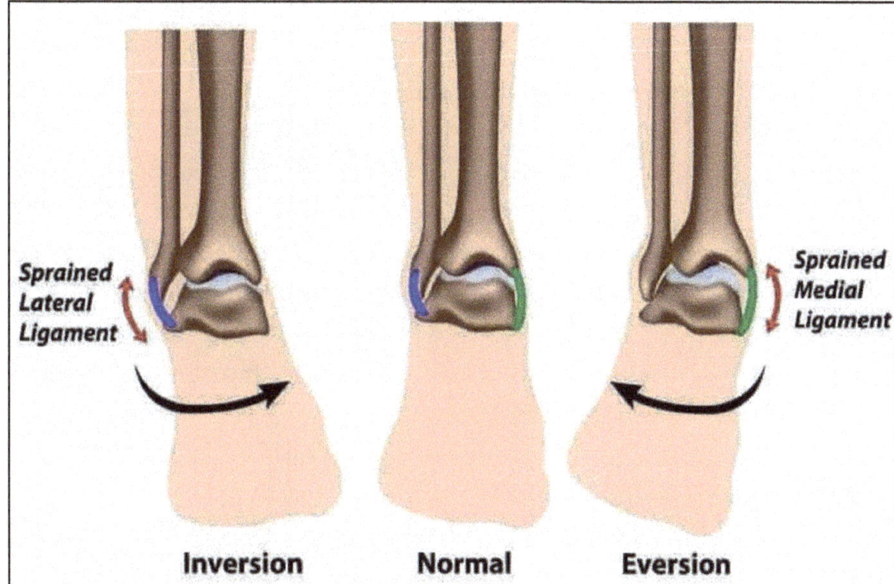

Figure 139 Types of Ankle Sprain

5.4.11.2 Classification of Muscle Strain

The image shows the classification of muscle strains based on the level of the injury as presented below; **The first-grade** strains are very non-serious because they only cause slight stretching or even tiny rips in the muscle fibres. This type produces mainly mild symptoms such as **pain and slight stiffness** but minimal strength and functional impairment. **Grade 2 strains are mild-intermediate strains** in which more number of muscle fibres are pulled. This leads to a lot of **discomfort, inflammation, as well as reduction of the capacity of the muscles,** hence it becomes hard to execute the intended force on the affected muscles. They are classified into three grades starting from **Grade 3** where the muscle is said to be torn or ruptured. This results in severe pain, inflammation, and paralysis of the muscles and on some occasions require surgery in order to be rectified. In most cases of muscle strains, **RICE (rest, ice, compression, elevation)** is used for treatment because this type of injury requires physical therapy for moderate to severe strains in terms of strength and flexibility.

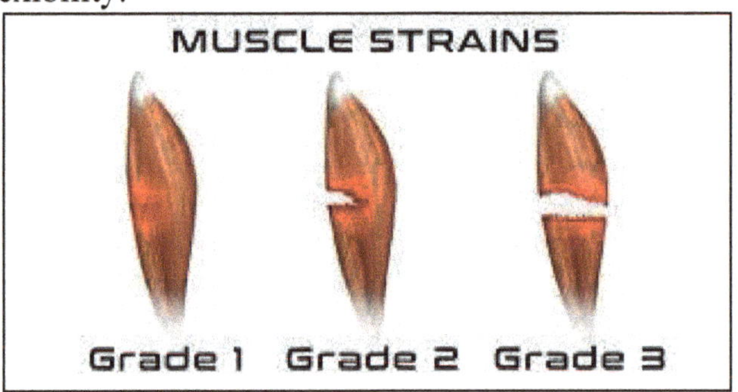

Figure 140 Classification of Muscle Strain

5.4.11.3 SOAP Notes for Sprain

Component	Details
Subjective (S)	The patient is a 35-year-old female who presents with a 1-day history of ankle pain after twisting her right ankle while jogging. The pain is described as sharp and localized around the lateral side of the ankle, with moderate swelling and bruising. The patient reports difficulty walking and bearing weight on the affected foot. She denies any previous ankle injuries but mentions occasional ankle instability during physical activities. The pain intensity is about 6/10, and the patient has been elevating and applying ice, which provides some relief.
Objective (O)	The patient appears to be in mild distress due to pain. Vital signs: BP 118/76 mmHg, HR 82 bpm, Temp 36.9°C (98.4°F). Physical exam reveals moderate swelling and bruising on the lateral aspect of the right ankle. There is tenderness over the lateral ligaments, especially when palpated along the anterior talofibular ligament. The range of motion is limited due to pain, particularly with inversion and dorsiflexion. The anterior drawer test and talar tilt test are positive, suggesting instability in the lateral ligaments. No signs of fracture are present.
Assessment (A)	The patient's symptoms, including localized pain, swelling, bruising, and positive ligament tests, are consistent with a **Grade 2 lateral ankle sprain**. This suggests a partial tear of the ligaments, specifically affecting the anterior talofibular ligament. Differential diagnoses include a fracture or tendon injury, but the absence of sharp, localized pain with palpation of bone structures and negative imaging results makes these less likely.
Plan (P)	**Pharmacological:** Prescribe NSAIDs (e.g., ibuprofen 400 mg every 6-8 hours) for pain relief and inflammation reduction. Consider a topical analgesic (e.g., diclofenac gel) for localized pain management (See algorithm below the

	table). **Non-pharmacological:** Advise the patient to follow the R.I.C.E. (Rest, Ice, Compression, Elevation) protocol for the first 48-72 hours. Recommend using an ankle brace or wrap for support and stability during walking. After 72 hours, initiate gentle range-of-motion exercises. Physical therapy referral for strengthening and proprioception training is recommended once acute pain subsides. **Follow-up:** Schedule a follow-up in 1 week to assess progress, review any swelling or bruising, and evaluate the need for further interventions. If symptoms persist or worsen, consider imaging studies (e.g., X-ray or MRI) to rule out ligament tears or fractures. **Education:** Educate the patient on the importance of following the R.I.C.E. protocol, avoiding weight-bearing activities until pain allows, and gradually increasing activity as the ankle heals. Discuss strategies for preventing future sprains, such as wearing proper footwear and incorporating ankle-strengthening exercises.

5.4.11.4 SOAP Notes for Strain

Component	Details
Subjective (S)	The patient is a 28-year-old male who presents with a 2-day history of pain in the lower back after lifting a heavy object at work. The pain started suddenly and is described as aching and sharp, worsening with movement, particularly when bending or lifting. The patient reports muscle stiffness and difficulty standing for prolonged periods. He denies any prior back injuries or weakness. No numbness or tingling in the legs. The pain intensity is about 7/10, with some relief when resting. The patient is concerned about the impact of this injury on his ability to perform daily activities and work tasks.
Objective (O)	The patient appears to be in mild discomfort but is able to move slowly. Vital signs: BP 120/80 mmHg, HR 78 bpm, Temp 36.8°C (98.2°F). Physical exam reveals tenderness over the lower back, particularly in the lumbar region. Palpation shows tightness in the muscles, with limited range of motion due to pain, especially when bending forward or rotating the trunk. No visible swelling or bruising. The neurological exam is normal, with no signs of nerve involvement. The straight leg raise test is negative, and reflexes are intact.
Assessment (A)	The patient's symptoms, including localized lower back pain, muscle tightness, and difficulty with movement after lifting, are consistent with a **muscle strain**. Given the lack of neurological signs and the history of recent lifting, this appears to be a Grade 2 strain of the lumbar muscles. Differential diagnoses include herniated discs and muscle spasms, but these are less likely due to the absence of radicular symptoms such as numbness or tingling.
Plan (P)	**Pharmacological:** Start NSAIDs (e.g., ibuprofen 400 mg every 6-8 hours) for pain relief and inflammation control. Consider a muscle relaxant (e.g., cyclobenzaprine 5 mg at night) for muscle spasms if needed (See algorithm

below). **Non-pharmacological:** Advise rest and limited activity for the next 48 hours. Apply ice to the lower back for 20 minutes, several times a day, for the first 2 days. After 48 hours, switch to heat therapy for muscle relaxation. Recommend gentle stretching and strengthening exercises after 3-5 days, once the acute pain has reduced. **Follow-up:** Schedule a follow-up in 1 week to assess recovery and adjust the treatment plan if needed. If symptoms persist or worsen, consider imaging studies (e.g., X-ray or MRI) to rule out other conditions like herniated discs or fractures. **Education:** Educate the patient on the importance of proper lifting techniques to prevent future injuries. Emphasize the need for a gradual return to normal activities, avoiding lifting heavy objects until fully healed.

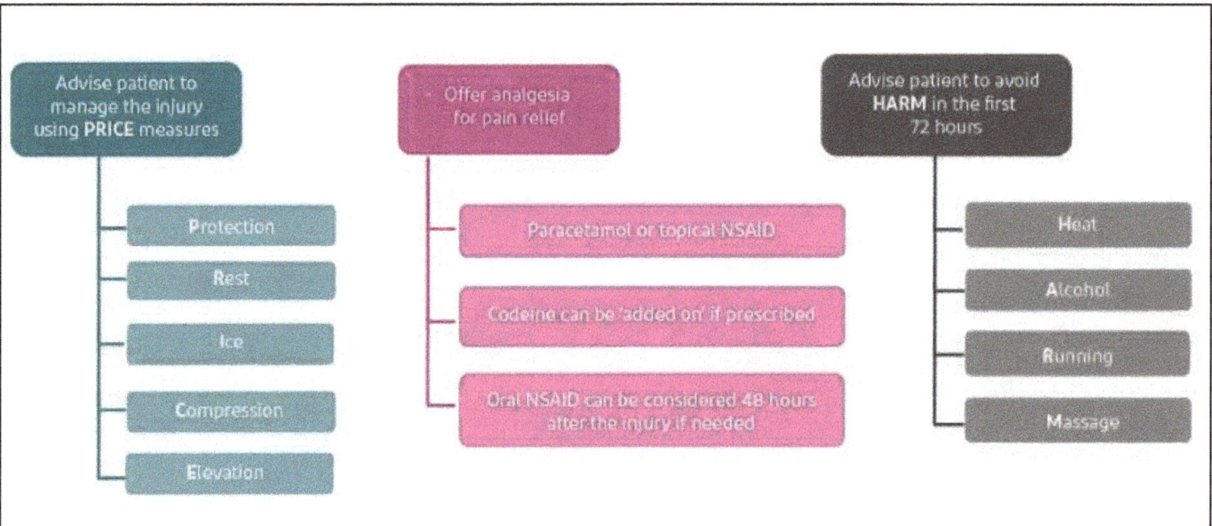

Figure 141 Management Algorithm for Sprain and Strain

5.4.12 Tendinitis

Tendinitis refers to a condition that is characterized by **inflammation or irritation of tendons**, which are the tough bands of tissue that connect muscles to bones. It is caused by **repetitive actions, overuse, or forceful activities** and also becomes common among athletes. Tendinitis is not limited to any specific tendon but is mostly located in the **shoulders, elbow (tennis elbow), wrist, knee (patellar tendinitis) and heel (Achilles tendonitis).** There's pain and inflammation where the tendon is injured and this will be worse on using the tendon. Occasionally, the tendon feels tight, and the joint can only move through a limited arc of motion. Some of the causes of tendinitis include; **ageing, poor posture, previous trauma, inadequate stretching or warm-up before activities, and repetitive movements.** The treatment of the injuries entails R.I.C.E, which stands for **rest, ice, compression, and elevation**, in addition to drugs that help to reduce inflammation and pain. For more serious conditions, potential treatments include physical therapy, injections of corticosteroids or, in some instances, surgery to help the tissue to heal. Prevention involves correct pitch, muscular strength exercises, and the non-repetition of the activity that took place before the injury.

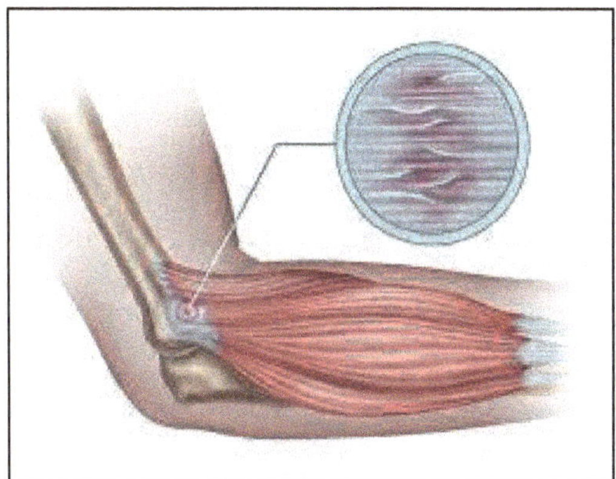

Figure 142 Tendinitis

5.4.12.1 Types of Tendinitis

This image shows various types of tendinitis, in which tendons in the body are affected differently. Tennis elbow is **lateral epicondylitis** that affects the outer aspect of the elbow where one experiences a sharp pain arising from the forearm tendons resulting from activities like gripping or swinging. **Golfer's Elbow (Medial Epicondylitis)** is the inflammation of the medial epicondyle of the humerus from the overuse of the wrist or forearm movements and can result in pain and swelling of the associated tendons. **Achilles Tendonitis** is a condition that affects the Achilles Tendon at the posterior aspect of the ankle and is caused by overuse or extreme stress during activities such as running and jumping. **Rotator Cuff Tendonitis is** a condition which affects the tendons in the shoulder by causing inflammation that leads to pains within the rotator cuff, oftentimes due to repetitive overhead movements. Lastly, **Jumper's Knee (Patellar Tendonitis)** is an injury that involves the tendon that joins the kneecap with the shin bone and is especially **common among athletes** whose activities include much jumping or those performing other activities that stress the bones heavily.

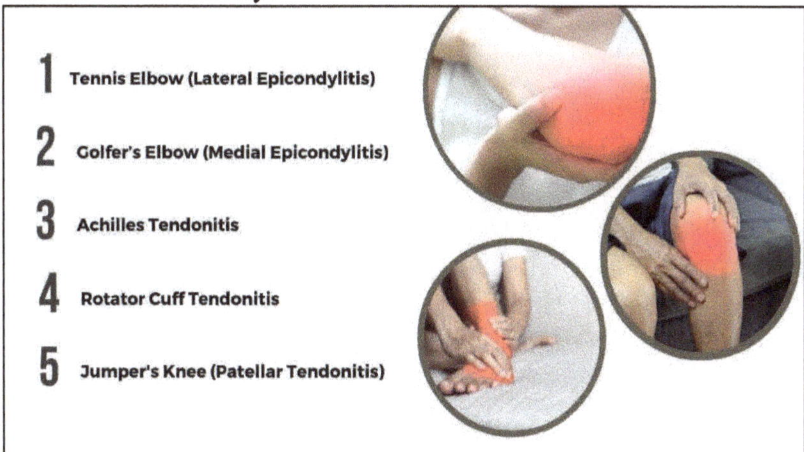

Figure 143 Tendinitis Classification

5.4.12.2 SOAP Notes for Tendinitis

Component	Details
Subjective (S)	The patient is a 40-year-old male presenting with a 1-week history of pain in the shoulder after repeated overhead movements at work. The pain is described as dull and aching, localized to the anterior shoulder and worsens with lifting or reaching overhead. The patient reports mild swelling and

	stiffness in the shoulder, with pain intensity rated as 6/10. He denies trauma but mentions that the pain has gradually worsened over the past week. The patient is concerned about the impact on his ability to work. He has no significant past medical history but engages in manual labor regularly.
Objective (O)	The patient appears in mild discomfort but is able to move his arm slowly. Vital signs: BP 118/76 mmHg, HR 80 bpm, Temp 36.9°C (98.4°F). Physical examination reveals tenderness over the anterior shoulder, particularly around the rotator cuff tendons. There is mild swelling and limited range of motion due to pain, especially with abduction and forward flexion of the arm. The Neer test and Hawkins-Kennedy test are positive for shoulder impingement. No signs of joint instability or neurological involvement.
Assessment (A)	The patient's symptoms, including pain, swelling, and limited range of motion with positive impingement tests, are consistent with **rotator cuff tendinitis**. This is likely due to repetitive overhead activities at work. The absence of trauma or neurological symptoms supports a diagnosis of tendinitis rather than a tear or fracture.
Plan (P)	**Pharmacological:** Start NSAIDs (e.g., ibuprofen 400 mg every 6-8 hours) for pain relief and inflammation. If needed, consider a short course of corticosteroids (e.g., prednisone 10 mg daily for 5 days) for more severe inflammation (See algorithms below). **Non-pharmacological:** Recommend R.I.C.E. (Rest, Ice, Compression, Elevation) for the first 48 hours. Apply ice to the shoulder for 20 minutes several times a day. Encourage the patient to rest from activities that aggravate the pain, particularly overhead movements. After 48 hours, gentle stretching and range-of-motion exercises can begin. Physical therapy referral for strengthening exercises and shoulder stabilization is recommended once the acute pain has reduced. **Follow-up:** Schedule a follow-up in 1 week to assess the response to treatment. If symptoms persist or worsen, consider imaging studies (e.g., MRI) to assess for tendon tears or other underlying conditions. **Education:** Educate the patient on avoiding aggravating activities and proper body mechanics during work to prevent further strain. Discuss the importance of stretching and strengthening exercises to promote recovery and prevent future injuries.

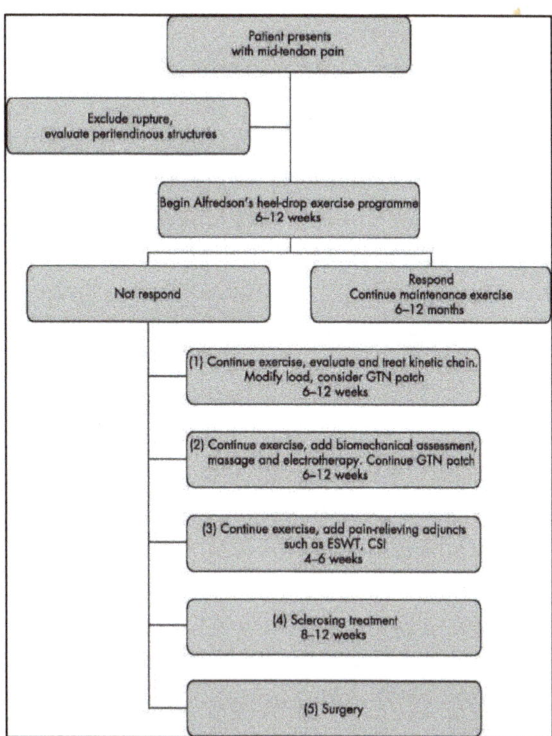

Figure 144 A Treatment Algorithm for Managing Achilles Tendinopathy

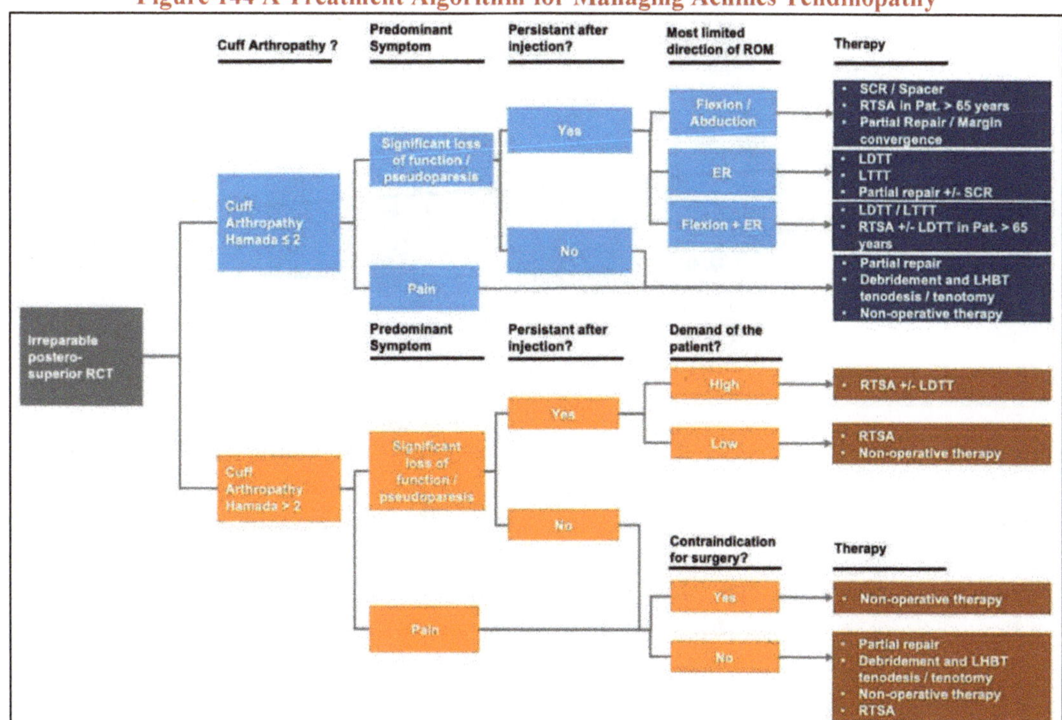

Figure 145 A treatment algorithm for Rotator Cuff Tendonitis

5.4.13 Fractures

A fracture refers to a partial or complete break in a bone that can result from **an injury, excessive force, or disease, such as osteoporosis, that dictates bone loss.** There are different types of fracture depending on the nature and site of the fracture, closed fractures, **open fractures, and comminuted fractures, among others.** Signs of a fracture include severe pain, pain, warmth, erythema, deformity in the case of **compound committed fractures, and the inability to use the affected part.** Sometimes the skin is punctured and this can reveal the bone in instances whereby the bone has fractured partly or wholly through the skin, then it is referred to as open fractures. Some degree of bruising or swelling may be expected and If the fracture is close to nerves, it may cause loss of sensation in limb or tingling. The extent of the break and its location can be established through **X-rays or computer tomographic scans.** Where necessary, an **MRI can then be carried out revealing** other damages probably to soft tissues or even nerves around the fracture region. Caring for fractures also depends on the kind of break that a person has encountered and its location. This is done in order to realign the bone and let the body fix itself naturally through the healing process. **Casts and splints** are also used a lot in the treatment of **closed fractures.** Surgery may be necessary in cases of compound fractures where particles of bone fragments and dirt have penetrated into the skin; the wound needs to be cleaned before proper alignment and fixation of the broken bone by screws, rods or plates is done. Alternatively, if needed, the doctor may **involve a bone graft in order to aid the healing process.** There may be a need for physiotherapy to help regain use, strength and flexibility in the affected part of the body after the fracture has healed. Specifically regarding the recovery period, it depends on the **location of the fracture and the extent of the damage as well.** As with any injury, certain complications might occur, for instance, in this case, infection, improper healing, malunion or non-union and nerve injury, especially in open fractures. Swift handling and proper treatment significantly contribute to the ways that would make a fracture experience to be more favourable.

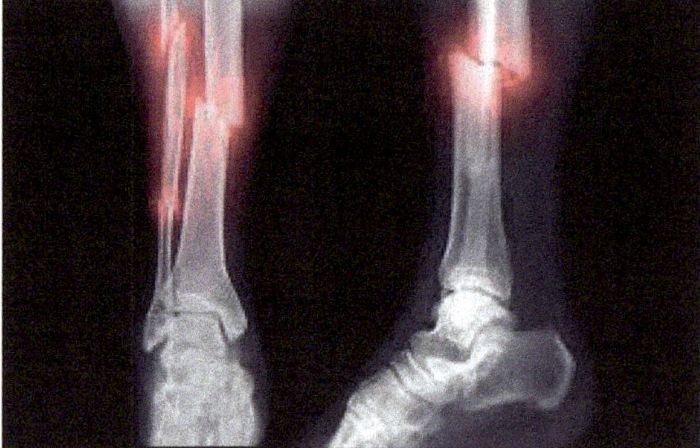

Figure 146 Fractures Representation

5.4.13.1 Types of Fractures

The picture illustrates various ways in which a bone may be broken and the classification depends on the nature of the break. The nature of bone fracture which has occurred is an important parameter in diagnosis and treatment strategy planning. In the following lines, an elaboration of the different types of fractures depicted in the image has been explained:

Transverse (Non-Displaced): This is a break that takes place perpendicular to the length of the bone and the affected part remains parallel to the other part. It is usually due to an acute injury or traumatic event or due to a physical injury or an abrupt force on the involved structure. Thus, the deformity in the case of a broken bone is temporary and the parts remain in their natural position and can be treated with keeping the bone stiff for example by casting or splinting.

Displaced – transverse: Here, too, the break is transverse, but the ends of the broken bone do not lie in the same line. This misalignment can be further precipitated by other factors or pressures that include the occurrence of forces or trauma for instance, a severe blow. In mild to severe cases, the patient may need to have the fracture put back into its proper position (reduction) by surgical means by use of rods or plates screwed to the bone.

Compound (Open) Fracture: Compound fracture is similar to a simple fracture in which in addition to the bone being cracked or shattered, the broken end of the bone emerges through the skin surface to become exposed to external influences. This type of fracture is prone to infections given that it is an open wound. Emergency response is essential and entails washing the wound and splinting the fracture as well as further involvement of surgery to treat infection in the likely event that it occurs.

Oblique Fracture: An oblique fracture is a broken bone that lies in an angled or, more precisely, a diagonal position across the shaft of the bone. This kind of a fracture is usually associated with a force that is applied from the side. Further, it can be categorised as a closed fracture in which no broken bone is protruding through the skin or an open fracture that is completely exposed. The treatment is by immobilization or surgery depending on the extent of the condition.

Comminuted Fracture: Comminuted fracture is a type of fracture in which the involved bone is divided into at least three different pieces. This type of fracture occurs usually due to extensive force, such as that which may be witnessed in car accidents or falling from a certain height. Due to the fragmentation of the bones, the process of gaining back full functionality may take a longer time, and in some cases, one needs a surgery for the relocations of these pieces to foster proper healing.

Greenstick Fracture: Greenstick is more prevalent in children comparing to adult as the bones of children are comparatively softer though slightly more rigid than those of a neonate. It is a type of fracture in which one edge of the bone is fractured while the other side flattens. It is called from the green stick of the tree which breaks but does not snap. The management of greenstick fractures entails the use of a plaster cast or an assimilation bandage in order to ensure that healing can occur effectively.

Each of the fractures deserves certain measures of management in the category of the treatment. Minor fractures heal when the area is rested and the limb is immobilized, but more severe or compound fractures which involve movements of the muscle and bones require surgery. Furthermore, those with open wound fractures or more commonly referred to as compound fractures require some form of extra caution to avoid infection and ensure proper healing. Usually, the treatment of such a wound includes the treatment of pain, physical therapy, and regular check on the progress of the same.

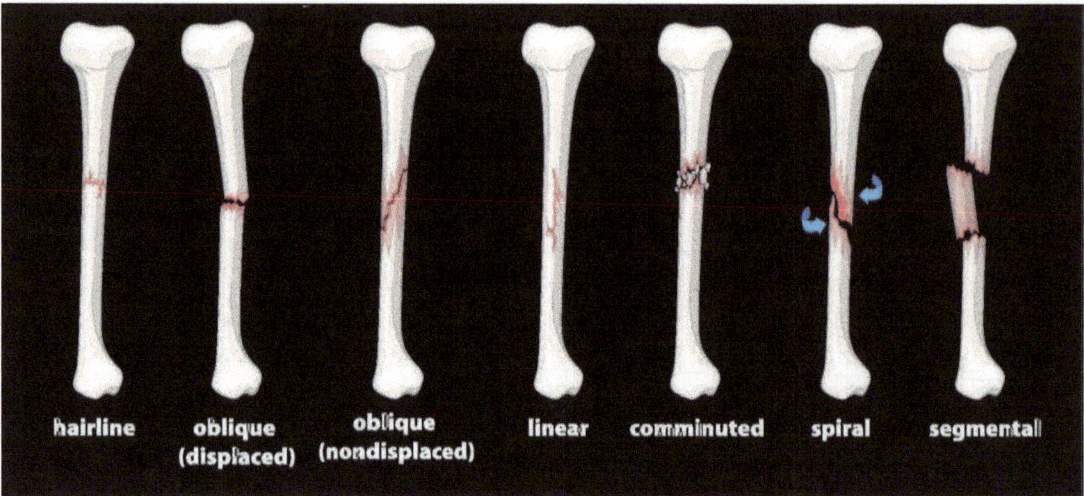

Figure 147 Types of Fractures

5.4.13.2 Classification of Fractures

Müller's classification of long bone fractures is a **certain method to classify long bone fractures** depending on the **location and pattern of fracture** to provide **accurate diagnosis and management.** The classification proposed was based on two major categories **Where? (Anatomical Region) and What? (Morphological Characteristics)**. The first lays down the type of fracture by depicting which bone is fractured, for instance, **the ulna, radius, and so on** and then the portion of the bone that is fractured, **be it the shaft, the distal, the proximal etc.**. This makes it easy to distinguish between **cervical, thoracic, lumbar or sacral breakages** and distinguish where it takes place in the middle of or towards any of the ends of the bone or at any of the joints. The second criterion evaluates the fracture type which may be **simple (AO type A), wedge (AO type B) or complex (AO type C).** Further, the fractures are classified regarding the bones that have been affected and can vary from only the ulna bones, the radius bones or even both the above without the other. For example, the **22-A3 code interprets** to simple fracture of the shaft of the forearm, and both bones of the forearm - the radius and the ulna. Thus, this classification system is valuable in **clinical management to indicate causal treatment** approaches and assess the degree of injury with a view to setting out rehabilitation procedures for various forms of long bone fractures hence providing a unified approach to handling long bone fractures.

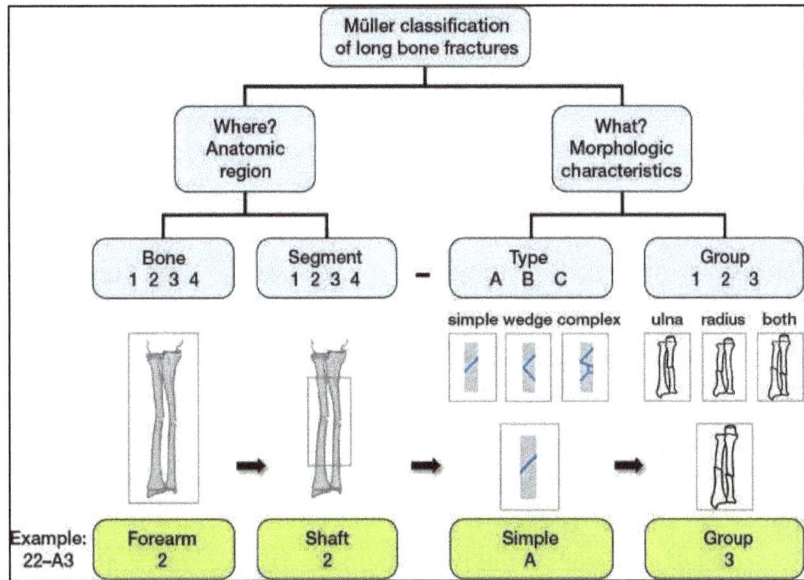

Figure 148 Muller Classification of Long Bone Fractures

This diagram shows the distribution of fractures according to the **type of bone and the segment of the body it belongs to**. Fractures are divided into different areas on **long bones;** this is important while diagnosing the fractures and the extent of treatment needed. The bone category is also more specific in that it outlines certain bones of the body such as the **humerus, radius/ulna, femur and tibia/fibular.** The segment category further subdivides the fracture location into three parts: proximal, diaphyseal, and distal. **The proximal segment refers to the area closest to the body's centre,** typically near the joints, such as the **upper end of the humerus or femur**. Diaphysis refers to the central part of the bone known as the shaft while the distal part refers to the end of the bone towards **the wrist or ankle.** This is beneficial in order to establish the specific location of the fracture, in the process of providing care to the patient, and to estimate the outcomes based on the place of the break at the human's bone.

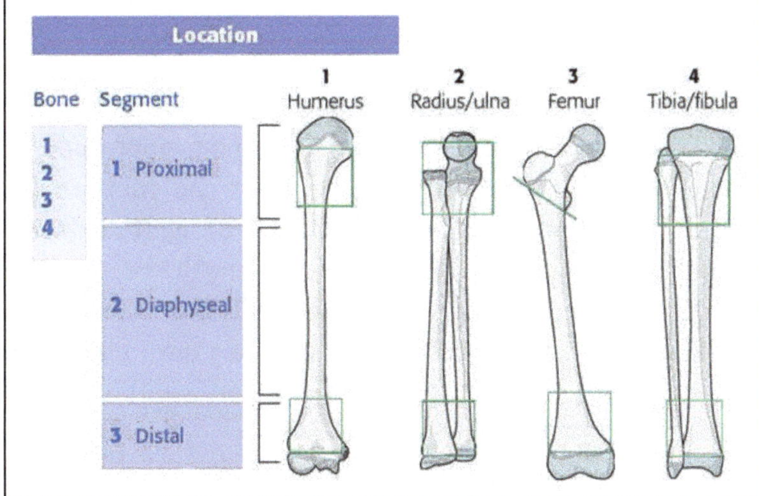

Figure 149 Classification of children's fractures

5.4.13.3 SOAP Notes for Fractures

Table 83 SOAP Notes for Fractures

Component	Details

Subjective (S)	The patient is a 40-year-old male who presents with severe pain and swelling in the right leg after falling from a ladder approximately 3 hours ago. The patient reports that he heard a popping sound at the time of injury, followed by immediate pain and difficulty bearing weight on the leg. He describes the pain as sharp, rating it 9/10 in intensity. The patient is unable to move his leg without pain and is concerned about the possibility of a broken bone. He denies any previous history of bone issues. The patient has no allergies and is generally healthy, with no prior significant medical history.
Objective (O)	The patient appears in significant distress, clutching his right leg. Vital signs: BP 130/85 mmHg, HR 92 bpm, Temp 36.8°C (98.2°F). Physical examination reveals swelling and bruising around the lower leg, specifically over the mid-shaft of the tibia. There is deformity in the shape of the leg, with an angulation at the fracture site. The patient experiences severe tenderness upon palpation, particularly along the tibia. There is an inability to bear weight on the leg. X-rays confirm a comminuted fracture of the tibia with displacement of the bone fragments. No signs of vascular or neurological compromise are noted.
Assessment (A)	The patient's symptoms, physical findings, and X-ray results are consistent with a comminuted fracture of the tibia, with bone displacement. This injury requires immediate intervention to align the bone fragments and promote healing.
Plan (P)	**Pharmacological:** Administer IV analgesics (e.g., morphine) for pain management. Initiate NSAIDs (e.g., ibuprofen) for ongoing pain relief and inflammation reduction. **Non-pharmacological:** Immobilize the leg with a splint to prevent further movement and reduce the risk of complications. Surgical intervention (e.g., internal fixation) is needed to stabilize the fracture. **Follow-up:** Arrange for immediate referral to orthopedic surgery for evaluation and surgery. Post-operative care will include monitoring for complications such as infection and ensuring proper bone healing. Schedule a follow-up in 1 week for wound assessment and further imaging. **Education:** Educate the patient on the importance of rest, immobilization, and pain management. Discuss the potential for a lengthy recovery, including the need for physical therapy after the bone has healed. Explain the importance of avoiding weight-bearing on the affected leg until cleared by the orthopedic team.

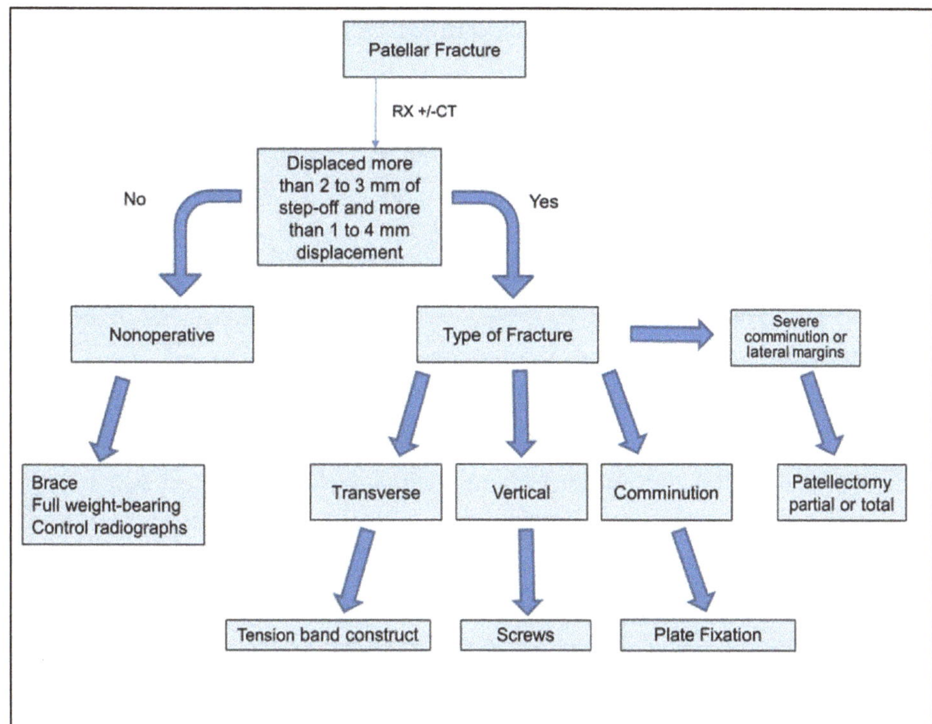

Figure 150 Algorithm for the Treatment and Management of Fractures

Other Common Conditions

5.4.14 SOAP Notes for Herniated Disc

Table 84 SOAP Notes for Herniated Disc

Component	Details
Subjective (S)	The patient is a 45-year-old male who presents with lower back pain radiating down the left leg for the past 2 weeks. The pain is sharp, described as 7/10 in intensity, and worsens with coughing, sneezing, or bending. The patient reports occasional numbness and tingling in the left leg and foot, particularly when sitting or standing for extended periods. He denies any recent trauma but mentions lifting a heavy box at work around the time the pain started. The patient expresses concern about long-term mobility issues and is unable to perform daily activities without discomfort. He has a history of mild lower back pain, but nothing as severe as this episode.
Objective (O)	The patient appears in moderate distress due to pain, especially while attempting to change positions. Vital signs: BP 125/80 mmHg, HR 82 bpm, Temp 36.8°C (98.4°F). Physical exam shows limited lumbar range of motion, particularly with flexion and extension. Positive straight leg raise test on the left at 30 degrees, suggesting sciatic nerve involvement. There is decreased sensation along the L5 dermatome. Motor strength is 5/5 in both legs, but the left ankle reflex is diminished. MRI of the lumbar spine shows a herniated disc at the L4-L5 level with compression of the left L5 nerve root.
Assessment (A)	The patient's presentation, including radicular pain, positive straight leg raise test, and MRI findings of a herniated disc at L4-L5, is consistent with lumbar

	herniated disc with sciatica. The lack of bowel or bladder incontinence and the absence of severe neurological deficits suggest no immediate need for surgical intervention but requires active management.
Plan (P)	**Pharmacological:** Prescribe NSAIDs (e.g., ibuprofen 400 mg every 6-8 hours) for pain relief and inflammation control. Consider a short course of oral corticosteroids (e.g., prednisone 10 mg daily for 5 days) to reduce inflammation around the nerve. If pain is severe, a muscle relaxant (e.g., cyclobenzaprine 5 mg nightly) may be considered. **Non-pharmacological:** Recommend rest for 2-3 days to allow the acute inflammation to subside. Initiate physical therapy once the acute pain has decreased, focusing on strengthening and stretching exercises for the lower back and legs. Ice therapy for 20 minutes several times a day during the acute phase. Avoid prolonged sitting and bending. **Follow-up:** Schedule follow-up in 2 weeks to assess progress. If symptoms persist or worsen, consider epidural steroid injections or surgical consultation. Monitor for any signs of worsening neurological deficits. **Education:** Educate the patient on proper lifting techniques, posture, and body mechanics to avoid further strain. Encourage weight loss if needed to reduce stress on the spine.

5.4.15 SOAP Notes for Plantar Fasciitis

Table 85 SOAP Notes for Plantar Fasciitis

Component	Details
Subjective (S)	The patient is a 40-year-old male who presents with heel pain, particularly during the first steps in the morning. The pain is sharp and localized to the plantar aspect of the heel, described as 6/10 in intensity. It improves slightly during the day but returns after prolonged standing or walking. The patient denies any trauma but reports increased activity recently due to his job requiring prolonged standing. He has no significant past medical history but is overweight.
Objective (O)	The patient appears to have mild discomfort when walking, especially after sitting for long periods. Vital signs: BP 118/76 mmHg, HR 80 bpm, Temp 36.9°C (98.4°F). A physical exam reveals tenderness along the plantar fascia insertion at the heel, with no visible swelling or deformity. The talar tilt test is negative.
Assessment (A)	Plantar fasciitis is confirmed based on the patient's history and physical exam findings of localized tenderness over the heel.
Plan (P)	**Pharmacological:** Recommend NSAIDs (e.g., ibuprofen 400 mg every 6-8 hours) for pain relief and inflammation control. **Non-pharmacological:** Recommend stretching exercises for the plantar fascia and Achilles tendon. Advise wearing orthotic insoles and heel cushions for added support. Ice application for 15-20 minutes several times a day to reduce swelling. **Follow-**

	up: Follow-up in 4 weeks if symptoms persist or worsen. Consider corticosteroid injections if there is no improvement. **Education:** Educate the patient on the importance of proper footwear, maintaining a healthy weight, and avoiding prolonged standing. Discuss the benefits of stretching and gentle strengthening exercises for the foot.

5.4.16 SOAP Notes for Ankylosing Spondylitis

Table 86 SOAP Notes for Ankylosing Spondylitis

Component	Details
Subjective (S)	The patient is a 30-year-old male presenting with a 6-month history of chronic lower back pain and stiffness, particularly in the mornings. The stiffness lasts for over 30 minutes and improves with activity. The pain is described as deep, and aching, and is rated 6/10 in intensity. The patient also experiences fatigue and a reduced range of motion in the lumbar spine. He reports difficulty maintaining a normal posture and has noticed progressive discomfort over the past few months. The patient has a family history of Ankylosing Spondylitis (AS) (his father was diagnosed at age 35). He denies trauma or significant physical injury.
Objective (O)	The patient appears slightly stiff, particularly when bending forward. Vital signs: BP 120/80 mmHg, HR 78 bpm, Temp 36.9°C (98.4°F). Physical examination shows reduced lumbar spine mobility with a positive Schober's test (less than 5 cm of lumbar spine flexion). There is tenderness over the sacroiliac joints. X-rays reveal sacroiliitis and early signs of bamboo spine. The HLA-B27 test is positive, confirming the likely diagnosis of Ankylosing Spondylitis.
Assessment (A)	The patient's chronic lower back pain, morning stiffness, reduced spinal mobility, and positive HLA-B27 test, along with imaging findings of sacroiliitis and bamboo spine, are consistent with Ankylosing Spondylitis (AS). The patient's family history further supports the diagnosis.
Plan (P)	**Pharmacological:** Initiate NSAIDs (e.g., naproxen 500 mg twice daily) to control inflammation and pain. If there is no improvement or if symptoms worsen, consider TNF inhibitors (e.g., etanercept) or IL-17 inhibitors (e.g., secukinumab) after referral to a rheumatologist. **Non-pharmacological:** Recommend physical therapy to improve spinal mobility and flexibility. Encourage regular low-impact aerobic exercises, such as swimming or walking, to enhance overall flexibility and reduce stiffness. **Follow-up:** Follow-up in 3 months to assess the effectiveness of NSAIDs and physical therapy. If the disease progresses, initiate biologic therapy as per the rheumatologist's advice. **Education:** Educate the patient on the chronic nature of AS and the importance of maintaining an active lifestyle to preserve mobility. Discuss

	the importance of good posture and avoiding prolonged periods of inactivity, as well as the potential complications, such as fusion of the spine.

5.4.17 SOAP Notes for Bone Metastasis

Table 87 SOAP Notes for Bone Metastasis

Component	Details
Subjective (S)	The patient is a 65-year-old male with a history of prostate cancer, presenting with persistent back pain and hip pain for the past month. The pain is described as deep and dull, rated 7/10 in intensity, and worsens with movement or pressure on the affected areas. The patient reports unintended weight loss of 8 kg over the past 2 months and generalized fatigue. He denies any recent trauma or injury. The patient is concerned about the progression of cancer and its potential effects on his mobility and quality of life.
Objective (O)	The patient appears fatigued and is in mild discomfort while sitting and standing. Vital signs: BP 125/80 mmHg, HR 80 bpm, Temp 37.2°C (99°F). On physical exam, there is tenderness over the lumbar spine and hip joints, with pain upon palpation. There is no obvious swelling or erythema, but the patient avoids certain movements due to pain. X-rays of the lumbar spine and pelvis show lytic lesions and pathological fractures in the vertebral bodies. Bone scan confirms increased uptake in the lumbar spine and hips, consistent with metastatic bone disease.
Assessment (A)	The patient's persistent pain, along with imaging findings of lytic bone lesions and a known history of prostate cancer, strongly suggest bone metastasis. The pain pattern and fatigue further support the diagnosis
Plan (P)	**Pharmacological:** Initiate pain management with NSAIDs (e.g., ibuprofen 400 mg every 6-8 hours). Consider opioids (e.g., oxycodone) for severe pain if needed. Initiate bisphosphonates (e.g., zoledronic acid) or denosumab to prevent further bone degradation and reduce fracture risk. **Non-pharmacological:** Refer to oncology for further evaluation and management, including chemotherapy or radiation therapy to treat the underlying cancer. Ensure physical therapy to maintain mobility and strengthen the surrounding muscles. **Follow-up:** Follow-up in 1-2 weeks to assess pain control and overall condition. Consider radiation therapy if the patient experiences localized pain that is not managed with medications. **Education:** Educate the patient on the chronic nature of bone metastasis, the importance of pain management, and the need for regular follow-ups with oncology. Discuss the role of physical therapy in maintaining function and preventing falls.

5.4.18 SOAP Notes for Hip Fracture

Table 88 SOAP Notes for Hip Fracture

Component	Details

Subjective (S)	The patient is a 78-year-old female with a history of osteoporosis, presenting with acute right hip pain following a fall in her bathroom two hours ago. She describes the pain as sharp, intense, and localized to the right hip, rating it 9/10 in severity. The pain worsens with any attempt to move or bear weight on the affected side. The patient is unable to stand or walk without assistance. She denies any previous hip problems but reports a history of multiple falls due to dizziness. The patient is anxious and concerned about the potential for surgery and recovery.
Objective (O)	The patient is alert and oriented but appears distressed due to pain. Vital signs: BP 130/85 mmHg, HR 92 bpm, Temp 37.4°C (99.3°F). The right hip is visibly swollen and tender to palpation, with limited range of motion. There is no open wound or visible bruising. The patient cannot perform the straight leg raise test on the right side due to severe pain. X-rays of the hip reveal a displaced femoral neck fracture. No signs of vascular compromise noted in the lower extremity. Laboratory tests show normal CBC and electrolytes.
Assessment (A)	The patient presents with a displaced femoral neck fracture, likely secondary to osteoporosis. This is consistent with the history of trauma (fall) and the physical findings (severe pain, inability to bear weight, and radiographic confirmation). The fracture is classified as high-risk due to its location and the patient's age, and surgical intervention is likely necessary.
Plan (P)	**Pharmacological:** Pain management with NSAIDs (e.g., ibuprofen 400 mg every 6 hours) for mild pain relief. Initiate opioids (e.g., oxycodone 5-10 mg every 4-6 hours) for severe pain as needed. Consider a bisphosphonate (e.g., alendronate) for osteoporosis treatment and fracture prevention, following stabilization. **Non-pharmacological:** Refer to orthopedics for evaluation of surgical options (e.g., hip replacement or internal fixation). Initiate physical therapy post-surgery to promote rehabilitation and regain mobility. Provide fall prevention education, particularly regarding environmental adjustments and balance exercises. **Follow-up:** Follow up with orthopedics in 1-2 days for surgery planning and additional imaging. Post-surgery follow-up in 1-2 weeks to assess surgical site healing and pain management. **Education:** Educate the patient on the importance of early mobilization post-surgery and the role of physical therapy in restoring function. Discuss osteoporosis management, including calcium and vitamin D supplementation, and lifestyle modifications (e.g., weight-bearing exercise). Discuss the potential risks of future fractures and strategies to prevent falls.

5.4.19 SOAP Notes for Cauda Equina Syndrome

Table 89 SOAP Notes for Cauda Equina Syndrome

Component	Details
Subjective (S)	The patient is a 50-year-old female who presents with severe lower back pain, urinary retention, and loss of sensation in the perineal area for the past

	12 hours. She reports a saddle anesthesia sensation (numbness around the genitals and anus) and difficulty urinating, despite the strong urge to do so. She also experiences bowel incontinence. The patient denies any history of trauma or injury but has been experiencing mild lower back discomfort for the past few weeks. She is concerned about the sudden onset of these symptoms and their potential long-term impact on her function.
Objective (O)	The patient appears anxious and in moderate discomfort. Vital signs: BP 130/85 mmHg, HR 88 bpm, Temp 37.0°C (98.6°F). Physical exam shows decreased sensation in the saddle region (perineal area). The straight leg raise test is negative. Reflexes are diminished at the ankles, and the anal sphincter tone is weak, indicating potential bowel involvement. MRI of the lumbar spine reveals severe compression of the cauda equina, particularly at the L4-L5 level.
Assessment (A)	The patient's presentation, including severe lower back pain, urinary retention, saddle anesthesia, and bowel incontinence, along with MRI findings of cauda equina compression, is consistent with Cauda Equina Syndrome. This is a surgical emergency requiring prompt intervention.
Plan (P)	**Pharmacological:** Start pain management with NSAIDs (e.g., ibuprofen 400 mg every 6-8 hours) for inflammation. If the pain is severe, opioid analgesics may be used until surgical intervention. **Non-pharmacological:** Urgent referral to neurosurgery for surgical decompression of the cauda equina. Catheterization should be performed immediately to relieve urinary retention. **Follow-up:** Follow-up in 24-48 hours post-surgery to assess neurological recovery and function. **Education:** Educate the patient on the seriousness of the condition and the need for immediate surgical intervention to avoid permanent damage. Discuss the potential for recovery following surgery and the importance of timely treatment to preserve function and prevent irreversible neurological deficits.

5.4.20 SOAP Notes for Osteomyelitis

Component	Details
Subjective (S)	The patient is a 60-year-old diabetic male presenting with a 2-week history of worsening pain, redness, and swelling in the left foot following a recent ulceration. The pain is described as throbbing and constant, rated 8/10 in intensity. The patient reports fever of 101°F (38.3°C) and difficulty walking due to the pain. He has had a longstanding history of diabetic neuropathy and poor wound healing. The patient is concerned about the spread of the infection and potential loss of function in his foot.
Objective (O)	The patient appears febrile and in mild discomfort. Vital signs: BP 130/85 mmHg, HR 95 bpm, Temp 38.3°C (101°F). Physical examination reveals

	erythema, swelling, and warmth over the left foot, particularly around the ulceration. There is tenderness to palpation, and the patient avoids weight-bearing on the affected foot. Blood cultures are positive for Staphylococcus aureus. MRI of the left foot reveals osteomyelitis, with bone involvement in the first metatarsal.
Assessment (A)	The patient's clinical presentation, history of diabetes, and imaging findings of bone infection are consistent with osteomyelitis of the left foot, likely secondary to the diabetic ulceration and poor blood circulation.
Plan (P)	**Pharmacological:** Start IV antibiotics (e.g., nafcillin 2 g every 4 hours) based on blood culture results. Transition to oral antibiotics once the patient is stable. Consider long-term oral antibiotics (e.g., cephalexin 500 mg 4 times daily) for 4-6 weeks. **Non-pharmacological:** Refer for surgical debridement of the necrotic tissue if necessary. Perform wound care to ensure proper healing of the ulcer. **Follow-up:** Follow-up in 1 week to assess wound healing and response to antibiotics. If the patient develops worsening pain or signs of systemic infection, further surgical intervention may be required. **Education:** Educate the patient on diabetic foot care, the importance of glucose control, and the need for regular foot inspections to prevent further infections.

5.4.21 SOAP Notes for Sciatica

Table 90 SOAP Notes for Sciatica

Component	Details
Subjective (S)	The patient is a 35-year-old male presenting with a 1-week history of sharp, shooting pain radiating from his lower back down the left leg. The pain began suddenly after lifting a heavy object. The patient reports numbness and tingling in the left foot and calf. He rates the pain 7/10 in intensity, with episodes of worsening pain when sitting or bending. The patient is concerned about the impact of the pain on his ability to work.
Objective (O)	The patient appears to be in moderate distress. Vital signs: BP 120/80 mmHg, HR 78 bpm, Temp 36.9°C (98.4°F). Physical examination shows limited lumbar range of motion due to pain. Positive straight leg raise test at 45 degrees on the left, indicating nerve root irritation. Reflexes in the left lower extremity are diminished at the ankle. MRI reveals a herniated disc at L4-L5, with compression of the left L5 nerve root.
Assessment (A)	The patient's symptoms, positive straight leg raise test, and MRI findings of a herniated disc with nerve compression are consistent with sciatica due to lumbar disc herniation.
Plan (P)	**Pharmacological:** Prescribe NSAIDs (e.g., ibuprofen 400 mg every 6-8 hours) for pain relief. If needed, initiate muscle relaxants (e.g., cyclobenzaprine 5 mg nightly) for muscle spasms. **Non-pharmacological:** Recommend rest and

	avoiding heavy lifting or prolonged sitting. Consider physical therapy to improve lumbar strength and mobility. **Follow-up:** Follow-up in 1 week to assess progress. If symptoms persist, consider epidural steroid injections or referral to neurosurgery for further evaluation. **Education:** Educate the patient on proper lifting techniques, the importance of avoiding heavy loads, and the role of exercise in strengthening the back. Discuss the potential for improvement with conservative treatment, though surgery may be required for persistent or severe cases.

5.4.22 SOAP Notes for Systemic Lupus Erythematosus (SLE)

Table 91 SOAP Notes for SLE

Component	Details
Subjective (S)	The patient is a 28-year-old female presenting with joint pain, fatigue, and a butterfly-shaped rash across her cheeks and nose. She reports feeling fatigued, especially in the afternoon, and notices pain and swelling in her wrists, elbows, and knees. She also experiences photosensitivity and occasional low-grade fever. The patient denies any history of trauma or recent infections but is concerned about the possibility of autoimmune disease due to her family history (mother with lupus).
Objective (O)	The patient appears tired but is not in acute distress. Vital signs: BP 118/76 mmHg, HR 80 bpm, Temp 37.1°C (98.8°F). Physical exam reveals a malar rash (butterfly rash) over the face and erythema in the knuckles. There is mild swelling and tenderness over the wrists and knees. ANA is positive with elevated anti-dsDNA levels, and low C3 and C4 complement levels are noted. Urinalysis shows proteinuria, indicating possible kidney involvement.
Assessment (A)	The patient's presentation, including malar rash, joint pain, positive ANA and anti-dsDNA, and low complement levels, is consistent with Systemic Lupus Erythematosus (SLE). The presence of proteinuria raises concerns for potential lupus nephritis.
Plan (P)	**Pharmacological:** Start hydroxychloroquine (200 mg daily) for disease control and to reduce inflammation. Consider low-dose corticosteroids (e.g., prednisone 10 mg daily) for flare-ups of joint pain and rash. If kidney involvement worsens, consider immunosuppressants (e.g., mycophenolate mofetil). **Non-pharmacological:** Advise the patient on sun protection to prevent photosensitivity flares. Recommend low-impact exercise to manage joint pain and fatigue. **Follow-up:** Follow-up in 1 month for monitoring response to medications, kidney function (serum creatinine, urinalysis), and potential side effects of hydroxychloroquine. **Education:** Educate the patient about the chronic nature of SLE, the importance of medication adherence, and the need for regular follow-ups to monitor disease activity.

Emphasize sun protection and avoiding environmental triggers that may worsen symptoms.

5.5 Moh Golden Points and Summary Question Answers

5.5.1 Moh Golden Points

Osteoporosis is characterized by weakened bones, making them more susceptible to fractures. This condition often develops silently, without symptoms, until a fracture occurs.

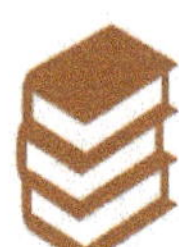
Rheumatoid arthritis (RA) is a systemic autoimmune disease that mainly affects the joints with particular prevalence in the swollen and palmar side of the wrists, hands, and knees.

Gout is associated with increased risks of cardiovascular diseases, including coronary heart disease and atherosclerosis. The inflammation caused by elevated uric acid also contributes to metabolic conditions such as diabetes and hypertension, further complicating the patient's health.

Physical therapy focusing on core and lumbar strengthening is essential for managing and preventing flare-ups.

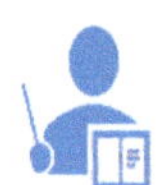
Major risk factors include age (with postmenopausal women being particularly vulnerable), family history, low body weight, smoking, excessive alcohol consumption, lack of physical activity, and low calcium or vitamin D intake.

The dual-energy X-ray absorptiometry (DEXA) scan is the standard tool for diagnosing osteoporosis. A T-score of -2.5 or lower at the spine, hip, or forearm indicates osteoporosis.

The nature of bone fracture which has occurred is an important parameter in diagnosis and treatment strategy planning.

5.5.2 Summary Questions & Answers

1. What is the most common symptom of Carpal Tunnel Syndrome (CTS)?
A) Numbness and tingling in the fingers, especially at night
B) Sharp, radiating pain in the lower back
C) Pain in the shoulder joint
D) Difficulty moving the knee joint

2. Which of the following is NOT typically used to treat Chronic Low Back Pain (CLBP)?
A) Physical therapy
B) Surgery as the first line of treatment
C) NSAIDs (Nonsteroidal Anti-inflammatory Drugs)
D) Manual therapy

3. What is the primary risk factor for Bursitis?
A) Age over 50
B) Repetitive motions or pressure on joints
C) Smoking
D) Excessive alcohol consumption

4. Which diagnostic test is commonly used to confirm Carpal Tunnel Syndrome (CTS)?
A) X-ray
B) MRI
C) Nerve conduction studies (NCS)
D) Blood test

5. What is the most common cause of Fractures in adults?
A) Osteoporosis
B) Tumors
C) Genetic disorders
D) Infections

6. **In Osteomyelitis, what is the primary treatment for the infection?**
A) Surgery to remove necrotic bone tissue
B) Rest and physical therapy
C) Topical antibiotics
D) Oral pain relievers

7. **What is a hallmark symptom of Systemic Lupus Erythematosus (SLE)**?
A) Malar (butterfly-shaped) rash
B) Nausea and vomiting
C) Joint stiffness in the morning
D) Persistent back pain

8. Which type of fracture involves the bone breaking into multiple pieces?
A) Greenstick fracture
B) Simple fracture
C) Comminuted fracture
D) Transverse fracture

9. What is the first-line treatment for Sciatica caused by a herniated disc?
A) Surgery
B) NSAIDs and physical therapy

C) Rest for more than two weeks
D) Steroid injections immediately

10. In Ankylosing Spondylitis, which of the following medications is often used to reduce inflammation and pain?

A) NSAIDs
B) Antidepressants
C) Insulin
D) Beta-blockers

5.5.3 Rationales

1. **Answer: A) Numbness and tingling in the fingers, especially at night**

Rationale: **The hallmark symptoms of CTS are numbness, tingling, and pain in the thumb, index, and middle fingers, which are typically worse at night due to pressure on the median nerve.**

---

2. **Answer: B) Surgery as the first line of treatment**

Rationale: **CLBP** is typically managed conservatively with **NSAIDs**, **physical therapy**, and **manual therapy**. Surgery is only considered in severe cases, often after other treatments have failed.

---

3. **Answer: B) Repetitive motions or pressure on joints**

Rationale: **Bursitis is most commonly caused by repetitive movements or pressure on the bursae, particularly in areas such as the shoulders, elbows, hips, or knees.**

---

4. **Answer: C) Nerve conduction studies (NCS)**

Rationale: **Nerve conduction studies (NCS) assess the function of the median nerve, which is often affected in CTS. This test measures the speed and strength of electrical signals through the nerve.**

---

5. **Answer: A) Osteoporosis**

Rationale: **Osteoporosis leads to weakened bones, making them more prone to fractures, especially in older adults**.

---

6. **Answer: A) Surgery to remove necrotic bone tissue**

Rationale: **Osteomyelitis often requires surgical intervention to remove necrotic bone tissue in addition to IV antibiotics to treat the infection.**

---

7. **Answer: C) Comminuted fracture**

Rationale: A **malar rash**, often referred to as a butterfly-shaped rash across the cheeks and nose, is a hallmark symptom of **SLE**, alongside fatigue and joint pain.

---

8. **Answer: A) Older age**

Rationale: A comminuted fracture occurs when the bone breaks into multiple fragments, often due to high-impact trauma, requiring surgical stabilization.

---

9. **Answer: B) NSAIDs and physical therapy**

Rationale: Sciatica is commonly treated with NSAIDs for pain relief and physical therapy to strengthen muscles and alleviate pressure on the sciatic nerve. Surgery is considered only for severe, unrelieved cases.

---

10. **Answer: A) NSAIDs**

Rationale: NSAIDs are often the first line of treatment for Ankylosing Spondylitis to reduce inflammation, pain, and stiffness in the spine and joints. In more severe cases, TNF inhibitors may be prescribed.

6 Chapter 6: Nervous System

6.1 Anatomy and Physiology of Nervous System

The nervous system is an extensive structure which is designed to **control and coordinate body processes.** It is divided into two broad categories namely **the central nervous system (CNS) and the peripheral nervous system (PNS).** The nervous system exclusive of the brain as well as the **spinal cord** notably coordinates the sensory input and the motor movements. The brain is the **larger part of the body that contains the ability to think, feel, learn, and perceive the environment** through the senses The spinal cord on the other hand is a **canal-like structure** that connects the brain with the rest of the body. It links the CNS to limbs and organs that would be in the body as **extremities and internal systems respectively**. It is further subdivided into two which are the **somatic division and the autonomic division**. Those are the divisions of the autonomic systems which help **control specific functions of the body like the rate of beating of the heart, digestion of food and respiratory rate among others.** There is sympathetic division and parasympathetic division of the autonomic system that function in an inverse manner to regulate the body functions. **Neurons** are the elementary structures of the nervous system which conduct electronic signals called action potentials. These signals are manifested through synapses by means of special chemical substances called neurotransmitters which ensure connection between neurons. **Astrocytes, oligodendrocytes** as well as microglial cells which are neurons' supporting type of cells help maintain homeostasis, supplying neurons with nutrients and removing waste products of their function. The specific function of the nervous system is to quickly process the information needed for the adequate functioning of the body including **reflexes, perceptions, and complex behaviours**. This system is also used in the regulation of homeostasis where the body is provided with requirements in spite of changing conditions on the outside.

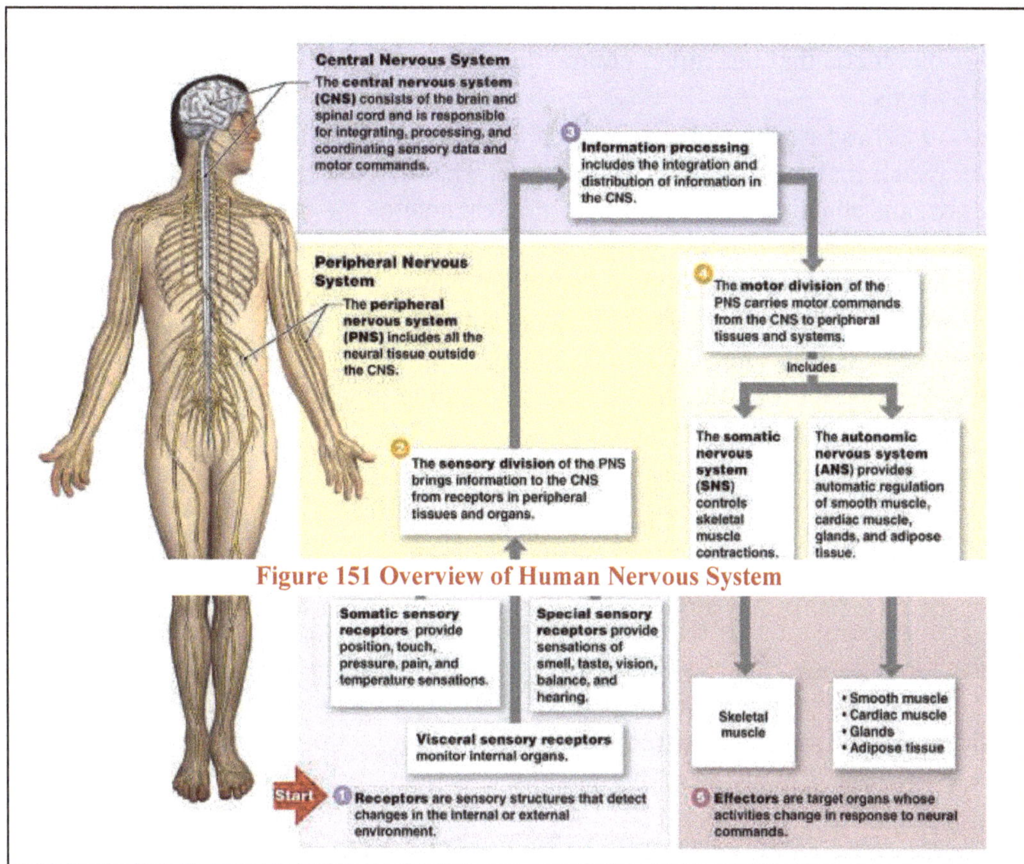

Figure 151 Overview of Human Nervous System

The following figure presents an overview of the major sub-systems of the nervous system and their functions, clearly distinguishing between the CNS and the PNS subdivisions. the following sections put into focus the components involved:

- **Receptors:** These are specialized structures that in a given stimulus, either from the external or internal environment for example **touch receptors, light receptors, sound receptors or temperature receptors, and receptors of blood pressure among others.** These are receptors that transmit information to the CNS for processing.
- **Sensory division of PNS:** This division is concerned with carrying sensory impulses from different receptors that are surrounded by the **body tissue and internal organs into the CNS**. This is further classified into general somatic receptors that differentiate touch pressure, pain, and temperature and visceral receptors that are responsible for internal organ sensations.
- **Information Processing:** Once the data enters the organism's system, the central nervous system **(comprising the brain and spinal cord)** processes the data. This entails codification and subsequent analysis of the information that is being received which is vital in decision-making and therefore formulation of responses.
- **Somatic motor division of the PNS:** This subdivision sends motor signals from the CNS to the muscles of the skin and their appendages. It includes:
- **Somatic Nervous System (SNS):** Controls voluntary muscle movements, specifically skeletal muscles.
- **Autonomic Nervous System:** ANS is the part of the peripheral nervous system that controls the automatic functions of smooth muscles, cardiac muscles, glands and fats. The

autonomic system can be divided into two groups namely the sympathetic and parasympathetic that has direct contrasting effects on the body's activities so as to help in homeostasis.

- **Effector:** These are the body parts that are targeted/affected by the signals from the nervous system such that they implement the same. The effector could be muscles, glands or any other organs which carry out the physiological change the **neural impulses have signalled for (such as muscle contraction, secretion or metabolism).**

From this structure, it is possible to understand the way the specific nervous system works and how it is able to **perceive and process** the internal stimuli as well as the external stimuli to respond to the environment appropriately. It highlights the animate role of the **CNS and PNS to co-ordinate** in providing appropriate patterns for responding to balance the entire human body and to perform any particular activity as required.

6.2 Neurologic Tests

6.2.1 Mental Status Examination

The MSE is used to guide psychiatrists or physicians in evaluating a patient's general mental state and various neurological functioning **characteristics such as memory, orientation, and behaviour**. It starts with an assessment of the individual's orientation where one has to recognize the time, place and person. This is followed by memory tests, **where patients are required to recall occurrences such as events that happened recently, names, or places**. Similarly, attention is tested by having the patient repeat simple instructions such as counting backwards sequentially from a specific number. In assessing language, **the two widely used methodologies are conversation and providing the patient with tasks** that would involve carrying out instructions or answering questions. Problem area involves skills that require sophisticated thinking and include the **evaluation of judgment, problem-solving, and abstraction. Alteration of mental status includes changes in cognition, mood, or behaviour** and is the first step of assessment when diagnosing conditions like **dementia, delirium, or psychiatric issues.**

6.2.2 Cerebellar Examination

The **Cerebellar Examination** aims at testing the patient's ability to coordinate their movements and maintain balance since these are parts of the bodily functions that are controlled by the cerebellum. The cerebellum is involved in the coordination of **movements, muscle tonus and other voluntary reflexes.** Some of these assessments include the finger-nose coordination test also known as the **heel-to-shin test** which tends to check on the ability of the patient to make fine motor movements.

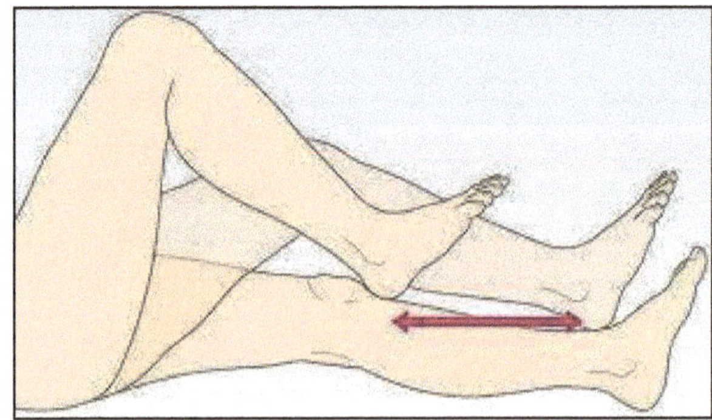

Figure 152 Heel-to-Shin Test

The difficulty in performing any of these tasks or the presence of tremors may indicate cerebellar ataxia or other disorders of the cerebellum. The next component of the cerebellar assessment is the

Romberg Test in which the patient is asked to close their eyes and stand with their legs side by side. A positive result is one where the patient shows **signs of balance loss or swaying,** which suggests proprioceptive or cerebellar disorders. Similarly, the **gait test, characterized by patient walking and especially tandem gait,** is useful to evaluate the balance and coordination of the patient; important in diagnosing multiple sclerosis or stroke, for instance.

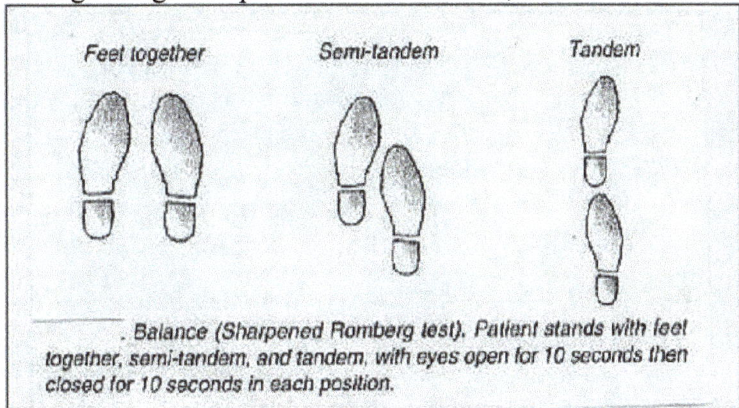

Figure 153 Romberg Test

6.2.3 Proprioception Testing

It is the technique by which the body, its parts or sense organs are aware of their location in reference to each other and the surrounding environment thus facilitating **balance and coordination during movement.** Sensory examination should include proprioception where the patient's ability to differentiate changes in joint position or to feel vibratory stimuli is tested. Another is **holding the patient's fingers or toes and trying to slide it up or down** and then telling the patient about it as the patient has their eyes closed. This is done to **check position sense** which is important in coordination. The feeling of vibration is tested by placing the tuning fork over the wrists or ankles and the patient is usually asked if they can feel the vibration. Sensory examination measures the efficiency of the Sensory tracts, especially in cases that involve **peripheral neuropathy multiple sclerosis or spinal cord injuries** where the sensory nerves are affected.

6.2.4 Cranial Nerve Examination

Cranial nerve examination is a part of the clinical examination that tests the **functionality of twelve cranial nerves** which control some of the most vital senses associated with **the head and neck region.** In addition to sensing, each cranial nerve is subjected to a motor function test. For instance, CN I (olfactory) can be considered with the help of tests of the sense of smell, and CN II (optic) includes tests of vision acuity and visual fields. **III CN VI and CN IV** can be considered significant indicators of eye movement and pupil reactions to analyze the brainstem and autonomic systems' improved status. **CN V** is tested for the sensation of the face and strength of the jaw to clench while **CN VII, facial nerve,** is tested by having the patient smile or blow air which checks for facial movement. **CN VIII** is the auditory nerve which can be tested using a tuning fork, **CN IX and X** involve swallowing tests and movement of uvula respectively. For **CN XI** – the patient is asked to shrug the shoulders and turn the head, the tongue movement test is conducted for **CN XII.** Abnormal may also reflect stroke, multiple sclerosis or even, facial nerve palsy.

The movements described in relation to the image mainly demonstrate abnormalities involving palsies of the **third (oculomoter), fourth (trochlear) and sixth (abducent) cranial nerves**. Each of these nerves is related to one of the muscles of the eye and when the nerves are impacted, then this results to different eye movements. Currently, if one is affected by schizophrenia, diagnosis of right third cranial nerve palsy will make it difficult for her/him to move the affected eye upward, downward or inwards. This is because the third cranial nerve is mostly involved in the eye movements that include upward, downward and medially directed movements. Furthermore, there may be **ptosis (drooping of the eyelids) and mydriasis (enlarged pupils)** as well. Superior oblique muscle is affected by right fourth cranial nerve palsy or trochlear nerve injury; it is involved in downward or lateral movement of the eyeballs. Therefore patients feel discomfort in looking down particularly when doing so in order to read or while going down the staircase. This **results to double vision (diplopia)** when so doing the movements. Right VI nerve palsy leads to left medial rectus paralysis that is responsible for the **adduction of the eyeball (moving it medially).** This makes the eye to turn inwards which is called esotropia, and cannot be looked outwards if one tries to do so. In conclusion, each cranial nerve palsy brings limitation in certain type of eye movement resulting into different type of vision problem or symptoms such as squinting and double vision.

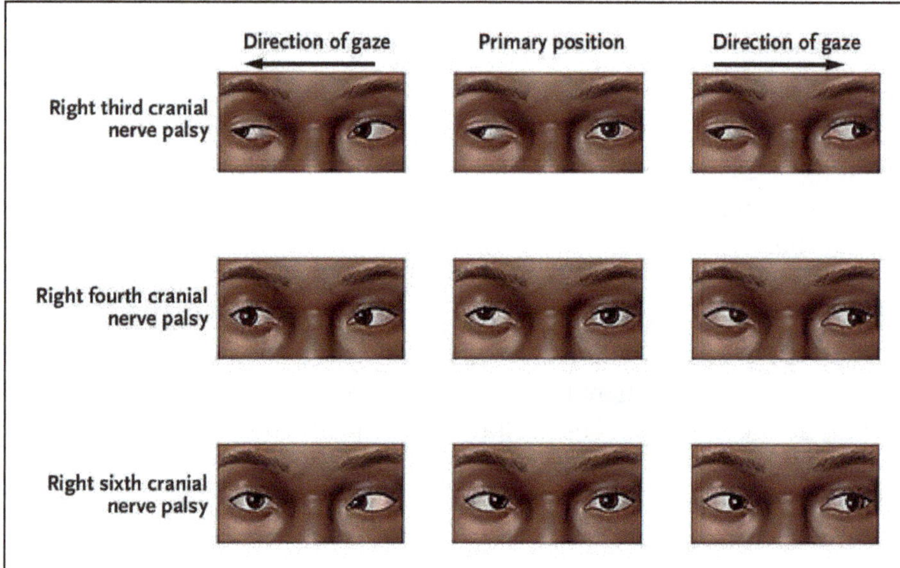

Figure 154 The effects of right-sided third, fourth, and sixth cranial nerve palsies on eye movement in different gaze directions

6.2.5 Sensory Examination

The Sensory Examination checks the patient's capacity to feel different **types of stimuli,** telling about the coordination of the **peripheral and central divisions** of the nervous system. Sensory assessment includes testing the areas of light touch, pain, temperature, vibration, as well as proprioception. **Light touch is done** by using a **cotton wisp** and the patient is required to point to the skin area being touched. **The Pinprick test** is the one that examines the ability to feel a pinprick while temperature sensation is a test that involves the use of warm and cold items on the skin. This examines vibratory perception by placing a tuning fork on various bony structures and it is taken **when the patient is no longer able to feel the vibrations.** Two-point discrimination measures the ability to perceive differences in two points applied on the skin. **Lack of sensation** in any of these areas may be due to nerve damage or dysfunction in the **sensory tracts, such as diabetic neuropathy, stroke, or peripheral neuropathies.**

6.2.6 Motor Examination

There are Four parts in the **Motor Examination** which assess **muscle strength, tone and coordination.** This is particularly important when it comes to observing disturbance of the motor function that may be a result of diseases of the central or the peripheral nervous system. This clinical assessment entails **muscle strength whereby the patient is asked to push or pull** against an examiner's hand, and muscle strength can range from 0 (zero = no power) to 5 (hood = normal). **Muscle tone** can be best described as resistance **felt during passive movement of the limbs,** increased is described as spasticity and on the other hand, decreased muscle tone is described as flaccidity. Another assessment involves testing of reflexes that stem from deep tendon reflexes like the **patellar reflex or the Achilles reflex.** Abnormality of the reflexes such as hyperreflexia means increased reflexes while hyporeflexia means decreased reflexes may show **CNS or PNS lesions. The motor exam also comprises coordinating tests, for instance, finger-nose** coordination test or heel shin tests where the physician tests a patient's advanced coordination ability to comprehend the ability of the cerebellum or other neurological disorders.

6.3 Neurologic Maneuvers: Kernig's Sign, Brudzinski's Sign, and Nuchal Rigidity

Neurologic manoeuvres are a form of physical examination test that helps to ascertain the presence of **meningeal irritation or meningitis, an inflammation of the meninges, which are the coverings over the brain and spinal cord.** These manoeuvres could come in handy in cases like bacterial or viral meningitis, subarachnoid haemorrhage, or other neurological diseases. The three neurologic signs Kernig's sign, Brudzinski's sign and Nuchal rigidity are explained below.

6.3.1 Kernig's Sign

Kernig's sign is one of the clinical tests which is used to check the presence of irritation of meninges, **especially in case of meningitis.** Standards for performing the test include having the patient in a supine position with hips and knees bent. The examiner then tries to flex **the patient's attended leg at the knee joint while the hip joint remains flexed.** Kernig's sign is positive if there is **pain and resistance to flexion** of the knee in the patient, at the lower back or posterior thigh when the knee is being extended; this may be an indication that the meninges are inflamed or the spinal nerves are irritated. This is attributed to the **patient's involuntary reflex to bend the knee** since the stimulation of the spinal meninges leads to pain in the patient. Despite the fact that the Kernig sign is sharply pathological, it is not very specific and may be present in such conditions as a hernia of the intervertebral disk.

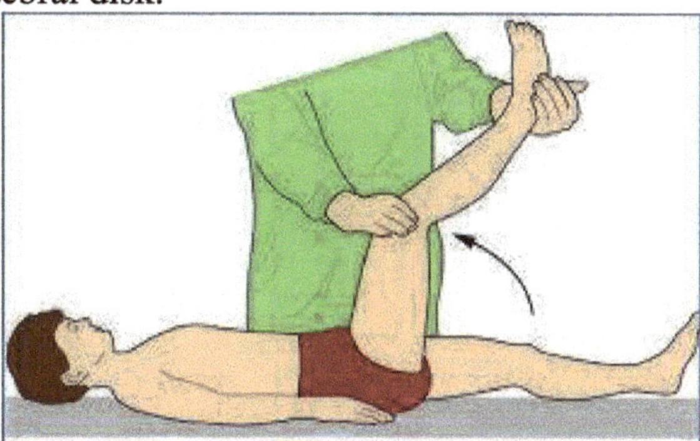

Figure 155 Kernig's Sign

6.3.2 Brudzinski's Sign

The other test for meningeal irritation is Brudzinski's sign which is usually accompanied by Kernig's sign. This is done by placing the **patient flat on the back and then, with one hand, the examiner lifts the head of the patient** without causing harm to the patient. Brudzinski's sign is performed by flexing the neck of the patient and a positive sign is evident when the patient flexes the hips and knees simultaneously. This reaction implies **meningeal irritation** as the pain and discomfort caused by the stretching of meninges make the legs flex involuntarily. A positive **Brudzinski's sign** is observed in conditions such as meningitis because the irritant of the meninges causes this reflex to take place. It is actually a better sign of meningitis as compared to Kernig's sign though this sign is also not very conclusive.

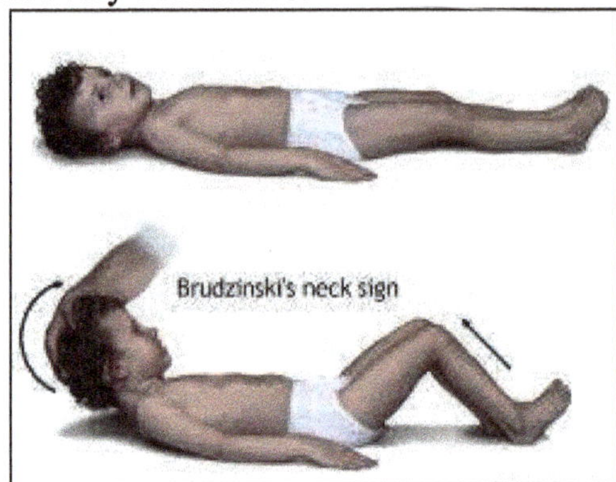

Figure 156 Budzinski's neck sign

6.3.3 Nuchal Rigidity

This can be described as the measure of the amount by which the neck cannot be easily bent backwards as it is a sign of meningeal inflammation. **Neck stiffness is performed by placing the hand on the patient's forehead to feel resistance** or attempting to flex the neck forward while the patient is lying flat. This movement, if being resisted or if the patient complained of pain during the manoeuvre, will be way positive. As already mentioned, nuchal rigidity can be seen in meningitis, but it can occur in other disorders such as **Subarachnoid haemorrhage or Cervical Spondylosis.** It is a clinical sign that is used when evaluating the patient for meningeal irritation because the meninges are irritated and the patient pulls his neck muscles to protect the spinal cord and the brain.

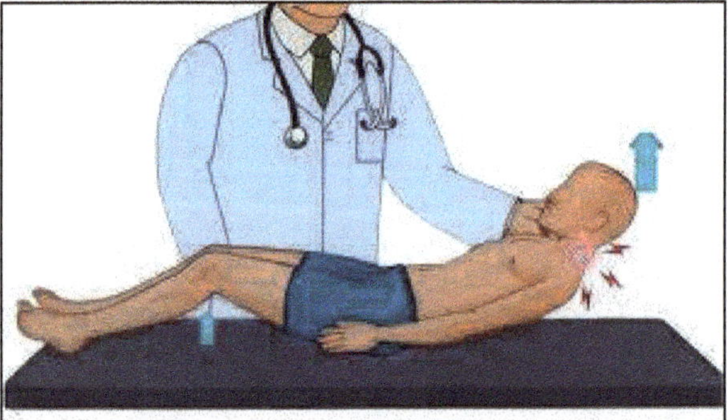

Figure 157 Nuchal Rigidity

6.4 Pathways of Sensory and Motor Neurons in the Spinal Cord

The picture shows the two major **spinocerebellar tracts which are concerned with sensory conduction and motor conduction in the body.** The ascending pathway delivers the sensation from the body to the brain and consists of the following three kinds of neurons: the first kind – **blue bullet,** which transfers the signals from the body to the spinal cord; the second kind **– pink bullet**, which transfers the signals to the brainstem or the thalamus, and the third kind – the **purple bullet**, which transfers the signal from the thalamus to the sensory cortex of the brain. They include those for processing touch, pain and temperature thus enabling the brain to interpret information received from the senses. The descending pathway on the other hand is involved in the transmission of motor signals in the body part from the brain to muscles. It starts with the upper **motor neuron (green) which is located in the motor cortex of the brain** and is communicated to the spinal cord. **The lower motor neuron (brown)** then picks the motor command from the upper motor neuron and passes it to the muscles in order to create movement. **Interneurons (orange) of the spinal cord** are also essential branches in transmitting messages between the upper and lower motor neurons, especially for instance in reflexes and movement coordination. These father and mother pathways combine in the management of the general sensory input and coordination of voluntary as well as involuntary movements. Any damage to these areas will lead to either sensory or motor dysfunction hence showing how these pathways are essential in the daily existence of human beings.

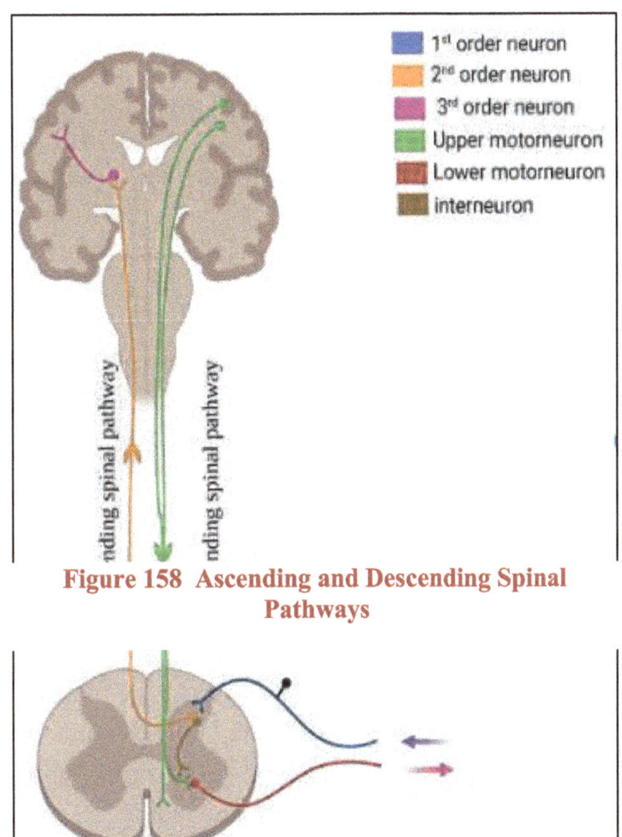

Figure 158 Ascending and Descending Spinal Pathways

6.5 Neurotransmitter and Its Types

Neurotransmitters are **chemical messengers** that transmit impulses across the synapse or the gaps between the neurons in the nervous system. Neurons are vital for the proper functioning of the brain and the rest of the body: they are responsible for **modulating mood, behaviour, muscle contractions, and even cognition**. Neurotransmitters are chemical substances that are released from the body of the presynaptic neuron and are accepted by specific receptors located on the postsynaptic neuron and set off certain **physiological responses**. By the receptors and functions, neurotransmitters can be divided into several groups. Here is a brief description of the major neurotransmitters and their functions:

The figure highlights some of the basic neurotransmitters which perform distinct activities that are essential in the overall function of any human body and brain. These chemicals facilitate the transmission of impulses between neurons and play a role in various physiological and psychological procedures.

1. **Epinephrine (Adrenaline)** is well known as the **"Fight and Flight"** hormone. It is very significant in building up the body's capacity to face stress-related factors such as increased rates of heartbeat, high blood pressure and high energy levels. This helps the body to be in a state of readiness to answer times of caution or actual physical situations that may involve fleeing from danger or physical challenges.
2. Many people are familiar with **Noradrenaline or Norepinephrine** since it is similar to adrenaline, however, its impact is more associated with increased concentration. It assists in controlling moods and focusing hence, suitable to cause alertness and concentration during a task. It also has functions of fighting stress and is involved in certain diseases such as attention-getting hyperactivity disorder and depression.
3. **Dopamine** is well-known under the name of the pleasure hormone. It is related to the evaluation of rewards, motivation, as well as positive emotions like pleasure that is felt in response to for instance **feeding or pursuing some** sort of enjoyable experience. Fair levels of dopamine are also important in those kinds of movements, and absence leads to diseases like Parkinson's disease which involves motor malfunctioning. It has an influence on conditioning which in one way or another influences addiction.
4. **Serotonin** which is associated with mood, appetite, and sleep is a chemical that helps to create an individual's feeling of contentment. It is also good to balance oneself and is associated with feelings of **satisfaction and emotional balance**. Serotonin is also another neurotransmitter chemical that affects moods and when there is unequal distribution of the drug the effects may be mood swings, especially depression and anxiety.
5. **GABA (Gamma Apartment (Aminobutyric Acid)** is one of the inhibitory neurotransmitters in the brain. It also has a sedative action having the potential to decrease neuronal excitability. Since GABA acts as an inhibitory neurotransmitter, it's critical for interrupting high activity levels in neurons which causes relaxation, reduction in anxiety, and other forms of overstimulation within the nervous system. It also acts as a muscle relaxant and is used in the treatment of anxiety and epilepsy.
6. **Acetylcholine** is a neurotransmitter that is essential for the processes linked to learning, and memory, including muscle contraction. This substance is used as a neurotransmitter in the peripheral as well as the central nervous system of the human body. Acetylcholine is also known to have its presence in the areas of the brain that deal with **memory and cognition**. It also works as a mediator of the nervous system and muscles where it controls the contraction of muscles. An imbalance of acetylcholine is associated with some disorders of cognitive type like **Alzheimer's disease**.
7. The excitatory neurotransmitter **glutamate** is the most predominant one in the brain and is directly associated with memory and learning. It is also associated with synaptic plasticity, that is, how the brain changes the efficiency of synapses based on the activity level that is necessary for learning and memorizing. Glutamate is important for synaptic transmission in the brain, however, excessive release of it which causes toxicity affects conditions such as **Alzheimer's illnesses and epilepsy**.

8. Endorphins are substances, often classified as the body's natural painkillers that are let loose in the circulation in response to exercise, stress or pain. They are involved in the dose-dependent behaviour that is experienced by athletes during vigorous physical activities; they are involved in feelings of well-being and satisfaction.

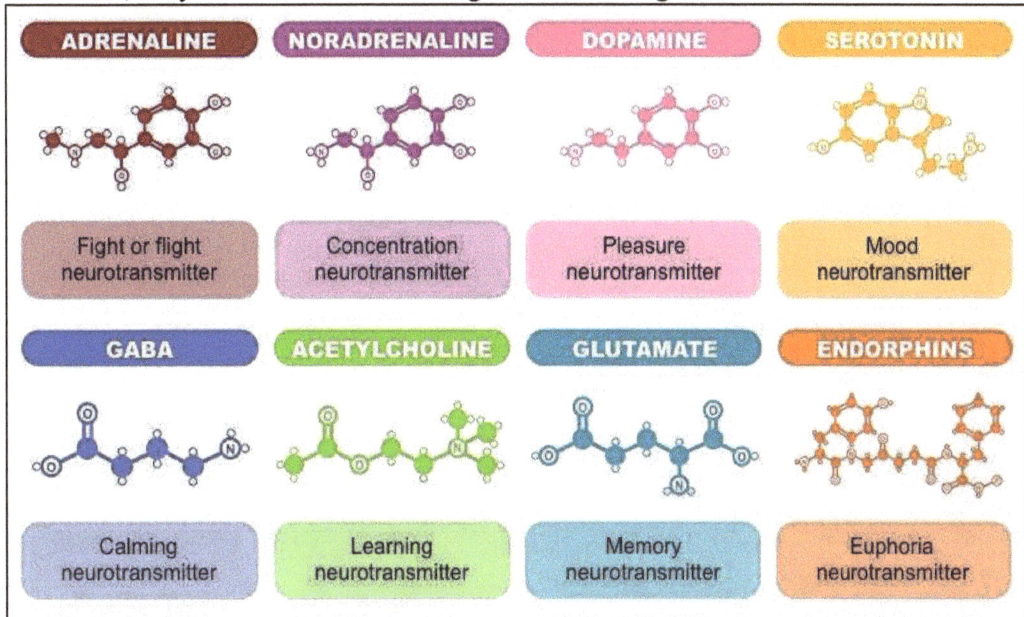

Figure 159Types of Neurotransmitters

6.6 Common Neurological Disorders

"Doctors See Great Symptoms, Consistently Treating Most Ailments, Always Hoping To Trim Brain Symptoms": **D** = Dangerous headaches, **S** = Subarachnoid hemorrhage, **G** = Giant arthritis, **S** = Subdural hematoma, **C** = Carpal Tunnel Syndrome, **T** = Traumatic Brain Injuries, **M** = Multiple Sclerosis, **A** = Amyotrophic Lateral Sclerosis, **A** = Acute bacterial Meningitis, **H** = Headaches (migraine with aura, tension, cluster), **T** = Trigeminal neuralgia (Tic), **T** = Bell's Palsy, **B** = Stroke and CVA, and **S** = Transient Ischemic Attack (TIA)

Table 92 Common Neurological Disorders

Condition	Description	Key Symptoms	Diagnostic Tools	Treatment Options
Dangerous headaches	A mass or growth of abnormal cells in the brain that can cause a variety of neurological symptoms depending on its location and size. Symptoms may include headaches,	Persistent or worsening headache, nausea, vomiting, blurred vision, seizures, personality or cognitive changes, weakness or	CT scan, MRI, physical exam.	Treatment depends on tumor type, location, and size, and may include surgery, radiation therapy, chemotherapy, or targeted therapy. Pain management and seizure control

	seizures, cognitive changes, or motor deficits.	numbness, difficulty speaking or understanding speech.		medications are also used.
Subarachnoid hemorrhage	A type of hemorrhagic stroke that occurs when there is bleeding in the space between the brain and the surrounding membrane.	Sudden severe headache, nausea, vomiting, stiff neck, loss of consciousness.	CT scan, MRI, lumbar puncture (CSF analysis).	Emergency surgery, blood pressure management, pain relief.
Giant arthritis	An autoimmune disease causing chronic inflammation and pain in the joints, often affecting the hands and wrists.	Joint pain, swelling, redness, stiffness, warmth.	Physical exam, blood tests, X-ray, MRI.	NSAIDs, DMARDs (disease-modifying antirheumatic drugs), physical therapy, joint replacement.
Subdural hematoma	A collection of blood between the brain and the dura mater, usually due to head trauma.	Headache, dizziness, nausea, confusion, loss of consciousness.	CT scan, MRI, physical exam.	Surgical removal of blood clot, monitoring in ICU, pain relief.
Carpal Tunnel Syndrome	Compression of the median nerve in the wrist, leading to pain, numbness, and tingling in the hand.	Pain, tingling, numbness, and weakness in the hand and wrist.	Nerve conduction studies, physical exam.	Wrist splinting, anti-inflammatory medications, surgery (in severe cases).
Traumatic Brain Injuries	Injuries to the brain caused by external forces, leading to brain	Headache, confusion, loss of consciousness, memory	CT scan, MRI, physical exam.	Rest, medication (acetaminophen, opioids), rehabilitation therapy, surgery.

	function impairment.	problems, dizziness.		
Multiple Sclerosis	A chronic disease where the immune system attacks the protective sheath of nerve fibers in the central nervous system.	Fatigue, muscle weakness, numbness, blurred vision, difficulty walking.	MRI, lumbar puncture (CSF analysis), blood tests.	Corticosteroids, immunosuppressive drugs, physical therapy.
Amyotrophic Lateral Sclerosis	A progressive neurodegenerative disease affecting the motor neurons, leading to muscle weakness and paralysis.	Muscle weakness, twitching, difficulty speaking, difficulty swallowing.	Electromyography (EMG), MRI, physical exam.	Riluzole, respiratory support, physical therapy, speech therapy.
Acute bacterial Meningitis	An infection of the protective membranes surrounding the brain and spinal cord, caused by bacteria.	Fever, stiff neck, headache, sensitivity to light, confusion.	Blood cultures, lumbar puncture (CSF analysis), MRI, physical exam.	Antibiotics, corticosteroids, pain management.
Headaches (migraine with aura and without, Tension, and Cluster)	A group of headache disorders that include migraines with and without aura, tension headaches, and cluster headaches.	Severe headache, nausea, vomiting, aura (visual disturbances), photophobia.	CT scan, MRI, headache diary.	Abortive treatments (NSAIDs, triptans), preventive treatments (beta-blockers, anticonvulsants), and lifestyle changes.
Trigeminal neuralgia (Tic)	A painful condition affecting the trigeminal nerve, characterized by sharp, stabbing pain in the face.	Sharp, stabbing pain in the face, usually triggered by touch or movements.	MRI, physical exam.	Carbamazepine, surgery (in severe cases), nerve blocks.

Bell's Palsy	A condition involving sudden weakness or paralysis of one side of the face, usually due to nerve inflammation.	Facial drooping, inability to close the eye, drooping mouth corner, loss of taste.	CT scan, MRI, physical exam.	Corticosteroids, physical therapy, surgery.
Transient Ischemic Attack (TIA)	A brief episode of neurological dysfunction due to temporary blockage of blood flow to the brain, is often a precursor to a stroke.	Sudden loss of speech, weakness, vision problems, dizziness, confusion.	MRI, CT scan, physical exam.	Antiplatelet drugs, surgery (if necessary), physical therapy.

6.7 Major Medical Issues in Nervous System

CHRONIC CONDITIONS

6.7.1 Traumatic Brain Injuries

Traumatic Brain Injuries (TBI) are those that are caused by some form of external force that acts on the brain and can be due to accidents like **falls, vehicle accidents, sports** and physical violence among others. TBIs can be as mild as concussion which is a mere head knock to severe allow that has lifelong influences on cognition, physical abilities and emotional processes of the injured individual. **The severity of the TBI** is determined with the help of scales that reflect the level of consciousness, the degree of memory loss and the condition of the affected tissues and cells after the injury. **Symptoms of mild TBI** include confusion and loss of consciousness that may be temporary and do not affect the body's functioning. Severe and moderate TBI results in permanent complications affecting the nervous system, which may include paralysis, memory impairment, changed personality, and inability to control muscles. TBI may also be characterized by symptoms such as headache, dizziness, confusion, nausea, blurred vision, severe neck or back pain, and unconsciousness. To diagnose **TBI, physical examination, imaging studies (CT, MRI) and cognitive status** are used. Symptoms depend on the degree of injury and may require pain-**relief medication, rest, exercise and physical and cognitive therapy,** sometimes, surgery is an option to remove the blood or to reconstruct damaged brain tissues. Some of the long-term effects of TBI are **hearing, sight, language, thinking, memory, and swaying problems** and thus, definitive care may include physical therapy, psychological guidance, and administration of care for cognitive issues, there is the need to focus on early intercession and rehabilitation.

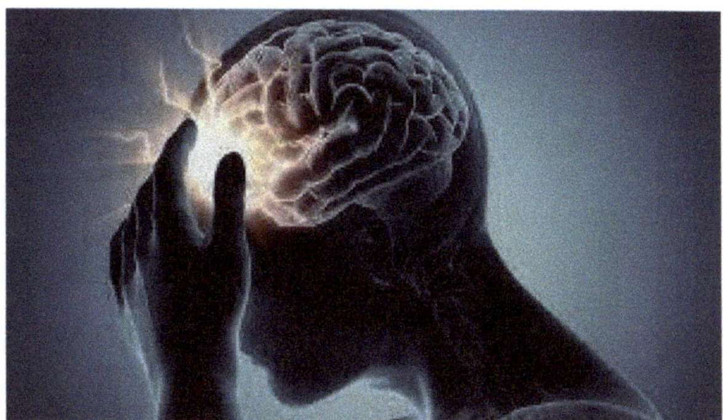

Figure 160 Traumatic Brain Injuries

6.7.1.1 Classification of Traumatic Brain Injury

The illustrated diagram displays TBI and divides it into two classes – diffuse and focal injuries In each of these classes there are subcategories as well. Diffuse injuries affect more or less all the brain tissue and occur as a result of force that impacts the whole brain. These are diffuse axonal injuries; this is where, through a **jerk or a blow on the head, forces of acceleration and deceleration** are applied to the brain which leads tearing of axons rendering communication between the brain areas impossible. A TBI's other type is the concussion which happens when the head is shaken forcefully but causes temporary cognitive or consciousness alterations which may also have a limited duration. Brain injury caused by pressure **waves from blasts**, more specifically affecting **military officers and men**, is evident as pressure waves from explosions have become rampant. **Shaken-baby syndrome or abusive head trauma is an umbrella term** for a diffuse head injury that results from the jerking of an infant. Focal injuries affect a particular region of the brain and may occur due to a direct blow or penetration. They include contusions that are bruises in the brain influenced by head shocks that cause localized inflammation accompanied by haemorrhages. The **penetrating injury** is distinguished when the head is pierced by an object, commonly a bullet, which directly affects the brain. Hematomas are pools of blood found within the brain and are usually occasioned by an injury. These can be arranged based on the layer in which they occur: epidural, which occurs between the **skull and the dura mater; subarachnoid, which is bleeding between the brain and the covering tissues; subdural, which happens between the dura mater and the brain; and intraventricular and intracerebral hematomas, which occur within the brain's ventricles and within the brain mass respectively**. It is important to note that each of these types of brain injuries calls for a distinct strategy of handling in order to ensure that the patient gets the right treatment.

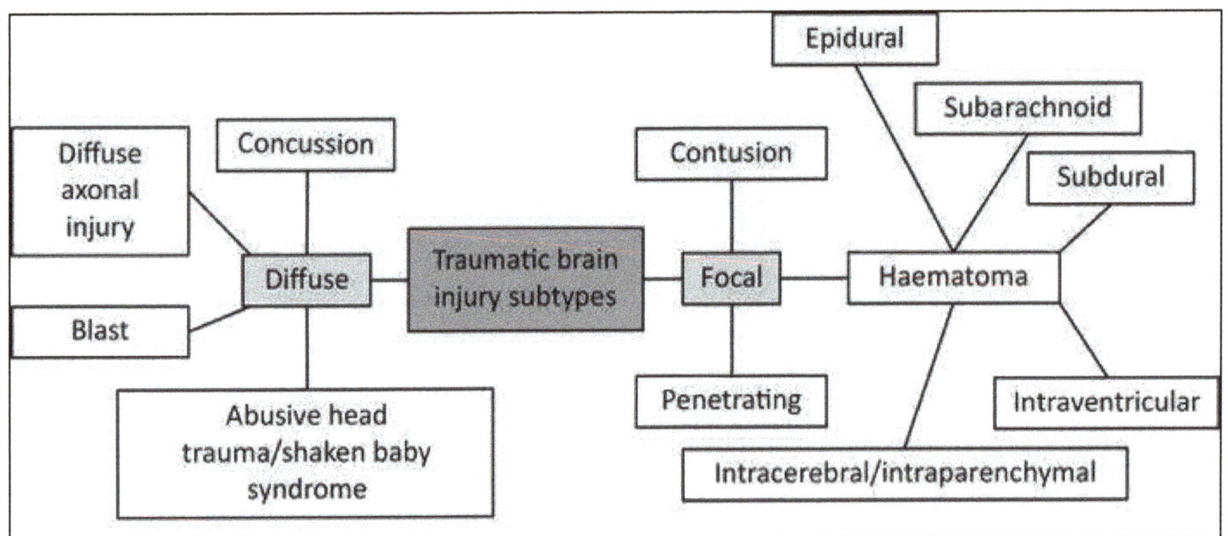

Figure 161 Classification of Traumatic Brain Injury

6.7.1.2 SOAP Notes for Traumatic Brain Injury

Table 93 SOAP Notes for Traumatic Brain Injury

Component	Details
Subjective (S)	The patient is a 32-year-old male who presents with a history of head trauma following a motor vehicle accident two days ago. He reports feeling dizzy, experiencing intermittent headaches, and has difficulty concentrating. The patient complains of nausea without vomiting, light sensitivity, and difficulty sleeping. He also mentions a mild ringing in the ears and a feeling of imbalance when standing. There is no loss of consciousness, but he does recall the incident causing a brief moment of confusion. He denies any history of previous head injuries and is concerned about potential long-term effects. No other significant medical history is reported.
Objective (O)	The patient appears alert but slightly drowsy. Vital signs: BP 120/78 mmHg, HR 72 bpm, Temp 36.8°C (98.2°F). Physical exam reveals no external signs of head trauma or scalp lacerations. Neurological examination shows normal cranial nerve function. There is mild tenderness over the frontal area of the head. Motor and sensory function are intact, but the patient exhibits mild ataxia when asked to perform heel-to-toe walking. No signs of increased intracranial pressure are noted. A CT scan of the head is ordered, which shows no fractures or acute intracranial hemorrhage. The Glasgow Coma Scale score is 15, indicating no signs of severe traumatic brain injury.
Assessment (A)	The patient's presentation, including dizziness, headache, light sensitivity, and balance issues following recent trauma, is consistent with a mild traumatic brain injury (concussion). The absence of loss of consciousness and the normal CT scan suggests no significant structural damage, but the patient's symptoms warrant close observation for possible post-concussion syndrome.

Plan (P)	**Pharmacological:** Recommend over-the-counter analgesics such as acetaminophen for headache management. Avoid NSAIDs due to the potential risk of bleeding. If symptoms persist, consider a short course of anti-nausea medication (See algorithm below). **Non-pharmacological:** Advise rest and avoid physical exertion for at least 1-2 weeks. Recommend cognitive rest, limiting screen time, and avoiding activities that may exacerbate symptoms (e.g., bright lights, loud environments). Encourage hydration and a regular sleep schedule to help with recovery. **Follow-up:** Follow-up in one week to assess symptom progression and provide further management if necessary. **Education:** Educate the patient about the signs of worsening symptoms, such as increasing headache intensity, confusion, or loss of consciousness, and instruct him to seek immediate care if these occur. Emphasize the importance of a gradual return to normal activities and stress the need to avoid further head trauma during recovery.

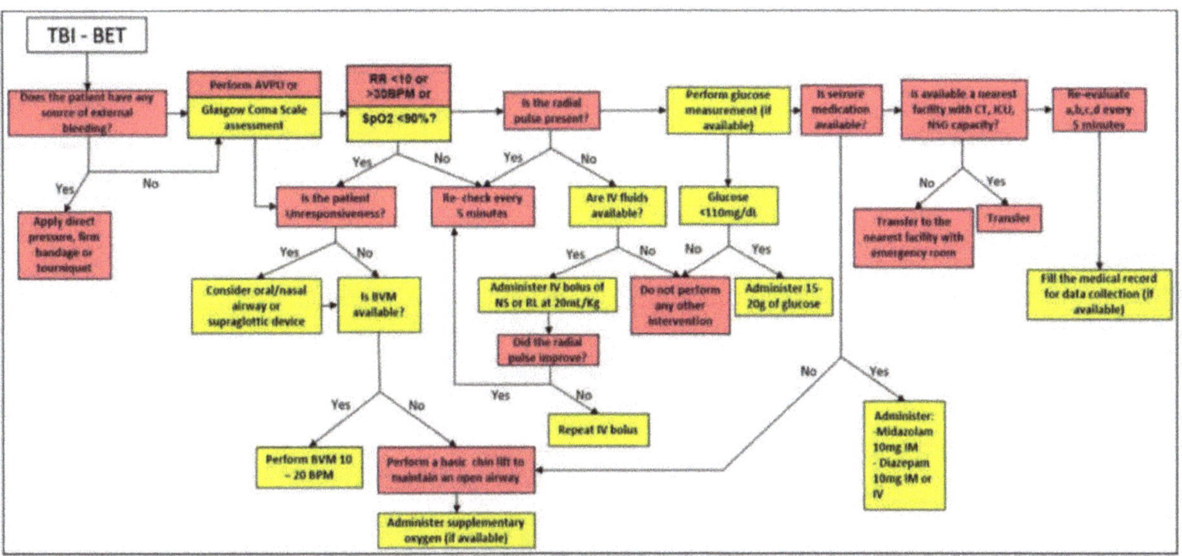

Figure 162 Algorithm for the Management of Traumatic Brain Injury

6.7.2 Multiple Sclerosis

The central nervous system (CNS) with brain and spinal cord and optic nerves becomes the target of **multiple sclerosis (MS)** which represents a **chronic autoimmune inflammatory disorder**. MS brings harm when autoimmune responses target the protective nerve fiber covering known as myelin leading to both **inflammation and myelin destruction**. The damage to the brain-body communication pathway brings about different neurological symptoms in each person with MS. Scientists have not determined the root cause of MS yet though experts believe hereditary and external elements contribute to its development. People of **northern European heritage mostly develop this condition while in the age range of 20 to 40.** People with this disease experience recurring symptom aggravations that sometimes lead to complete reductions in active symptoms. Some patients who advance in their condition do not enter remission states even though their symptoms worsen in the future. Multiple Sclerosis patients usually **experience fatigue in combination with problems walking together with numbness or tingling sensation and muscle weakness along with vision disturbances and changes in memory function**. Even though MS does not have a cure existing disease-modifying therapies known as DMT exist to help patients manage their symptoms and reduce relapse numbers while slowing disease progression. The rehabilitation efforts between physical and occupational therapy provide essential **improvements to the quality of life outcomes while preserving mobility abilities** for people affected by this condition. The best approach for managing this condition depends on early diagnosis followed by rapid intervention.

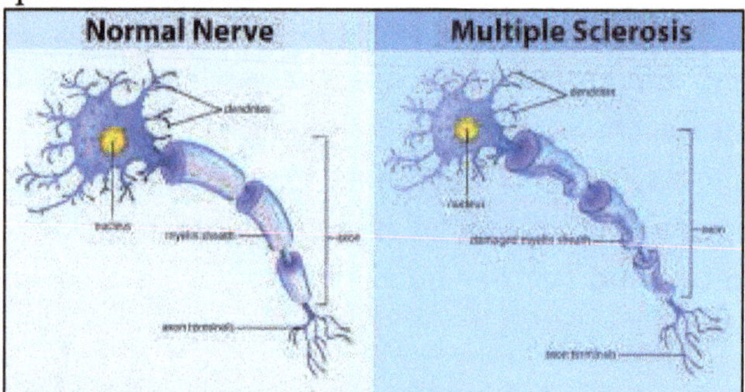

Figure 163 Comparison between Normal Nerve and Multiple Sclerosis

6.7.2.1 Types of Multiple Sclerosis

The graphic demonstrates the development of disabilities throughout the different types of Multiple Sclerosis (MS) during time periods. **Benign Multiple Sclerosis** patients experience symptom attacks that resolve during remission time which leads to no permanent disability accumulation. **The Relapsing and Remitting MS** pattern includes symptoms that worsen in relapse periods which alternates with periods of symptom recovery during remission. Patients do not develop **new disabilities during their inactive period** yet their condition may return to the same state as before attacks. The condition of **Secondary Progressive MS begins with relapsing-remitting phases** until it transitions to permanent disability growth without experiencing distinct relapses. People suffering from this form of MS exhibit a constant decrease in ability which **disregards routine relapse and remission cycles.** The disability in **Primary Progressive Multiple Sclerosis** advances continuously from the beginning and extends throughout all time periods without remission states or recurrence. Benign MS does not lead to disability accumulation as shown visually through the diagram but other types of MS cause a decline in function with Primary Progressive MS exhibiting the most consistent such patterns.

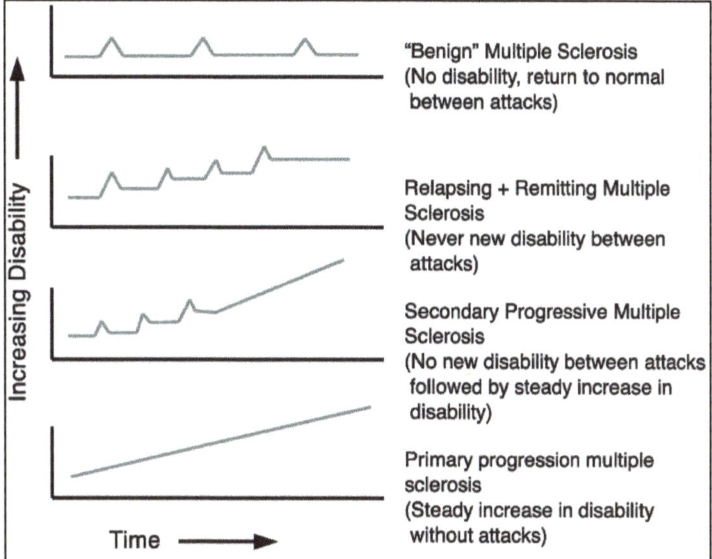

Figure 164 Different Types of Multiple Sclerosis

6.7.2.2 SOAP Notes for Multiple Sclerosis

Table 94 SOAP Notes for Multiple Sclerosis

Component	Details
Subjective (S)	The patient is a 28-year-old female who presents with a 6-month history of increasing fatigue, muscle weakness, and intermittent numbness in her legs and hands. She reports that the symptoms have gradually worsened, with occasional episodes of blurred vision and difficulty walking. The patient also experiences occasional dizziness and difficulty maintaining balance. She mentions that her symptoms tend to fluctuate, sometimes worsening after periods of stress or physical exertion. She denies any recent trauma, infections, or significant lifestyle changes. There is a family history of autoimmune diseases, including a maternal cousin with multiple sclerosis (MS), which raises concern for a potential neuroinflammatory disorder.
Objective (O)	The patient appears fatigued but is not in acute distress. Vital signs: BP 118/75 mmHg, HR 78 bpm, Temp 36.7°C (98.1°F). Neurological examination reveals decreased sensation to light touch and temperature in both lower limbs. There is slight ataxia when performing the Romberg test. Muscle strength is 4/5 in the lower limbs, with mild weakness in the hands. The patient exhibits dysmetria on finger-to-nose testing. Visual examination shows slight optic disc pallor in both eyes, and a fundoscopic exam reveals no overt retinal pathology. MRI of the brain reveals multiple areas of hyperintensity in the periventricular white matter, consistent with demyelinating lesions. CSF analysis shows mildly elevated white blood cell count with normal protein levels.
Assessment (A)	The patient's presentation, including fluctuating neurological symptoms, muscle weakness, numbness, visual changes, and MRI findings of demyelination, is highly suggestive of Multiple Sclerosis (MS). The lesions on

	MRI, combined with clinical signs of sensory disturbances and motor deficits, are indicative of a central nervous system demyelinating process. Given the family history and the typical relapsing-remitting pattern of her symptoms, MS is the most likely diagnosis. A lumbar puncture result showing mild pleocytosis further supports this diagnosis, though further confirmatory tests may be required.
Plan (P)	**Pharmacological:** Initiate disease-modifying therapy (DMT) to reduce the frequency and severity of relapses, such as interferon-beta or glatiramer acetate. Consider a short course of corticosteroids (e.g., prednisone) during flare-ups to reduce inflammation. (See algorithm below). **Non-pharmacological:** Recommend physical therapy to help manage muscle weakness and improve balance. Advise lifestyle modifications, including stress management techniques, regular low-impact exercise, and adequate rest to avoid exacerbations. **Follow-up:** Schedule a follow-up appointment in 3 months to assess response to treatment, monitor disease progression, and adjust therapy as needed. **Education:** Educate the patient about the chronic nature of MS, the importance of medication adherence, and the need for regular monitoring of symptoms and MRI imaging. Discuss strategies for managing flare-ups and emphasize the role of physical therapy in maintaining mobility.

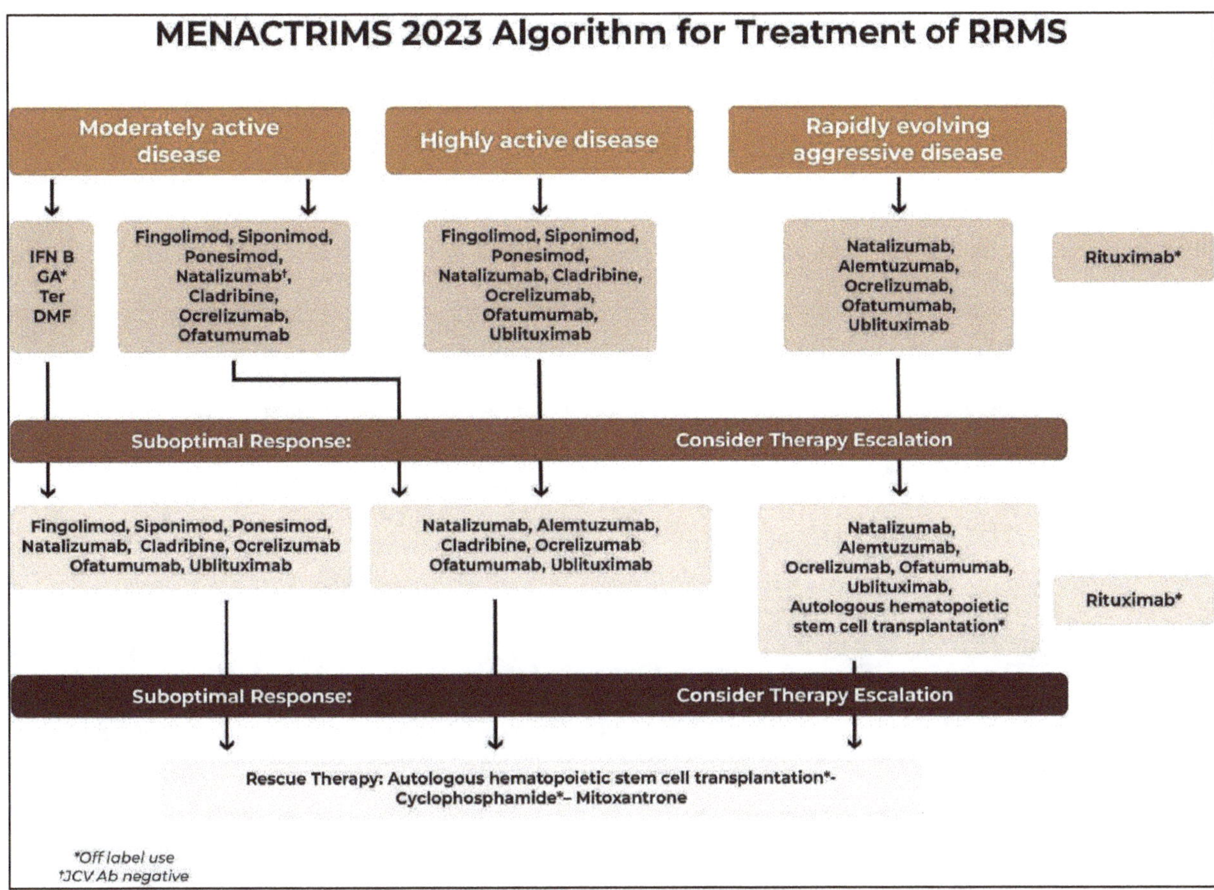

Figure 165 Consensus recommendations for diagnosis and treatment of Multiple Sclerosis

6.7.3 Amyotrophic Lateral Sclerosis

Amyotrophic Lateral Sclerosis (ALS) represents a progressive neurodegenerative condition which attacks the motor neurons that control voluntary muscle movements. People commonly refer to ALS through its alternate name **Lou Gehrig's disease**. When motor neurons in brain and spinal cord tissues progressively degenerate the patient experiences **muscle weakness as well as muscle tissue deterioration** that ultimately results in full-body paralysis. The clinical features of ALS consist of deterioration within the brain's upper motor neurons and lower motor neurons of spinal cord and brainstem. Science does not fully comprehend the root factors of ALS since this condition develops from a mixture **of inherited genetics and environmental elements and cell biology changes**. Family inheritance of ALS is responsible for 5-10% of all cases where genetic abnormalities in **C9orf72, SOD1, and TARDBP genes lead to the disease**. The majority of ALS cases occur sporadically without genetic causes although environmental factors that include exposure to toxins and heavy metals alongside trauma have shown potential links to the condition. The disease's first symptoms consist of **mild discomfort through weakness and stiffness affecting a specific area of the body such as hands, legs or mouth.** The worsening condition of the disease leads patients to develop issues with speech production and swallowing along with issues in breathing. Symptom progression in this condition causes patients to become unmanageably disabled before their death from respiratory failure occurs within a couple of years. Patients with frontotemporal dementia ALS experience cognitive decline as a less frequent yet possible development of the condition.

No cure exists for ALS but physicians can treat the condition to reduce patient discomfort and deliver better healthcare quality. The National Institute of Health has approved **riluzole as the**

only drug for ALS which extends patients' survival through its mechanism to block the excessive release of glutamate neurotransmitters. The medical community believes edaravone aids in reducing motor neuron oxidative stress and extends the lifespan of patients suffering from specific forms of ALS. The management and extension of functionality in ALS patients depend significantly on supportive treatments that combine physical exercises with respiratory therapy and occupational therapy. Scientists continue to study ALS by exploring motor neuron degeneration mechanisms and working on therapy development to target these mechanisms simultaneously with gene therapy investigation.

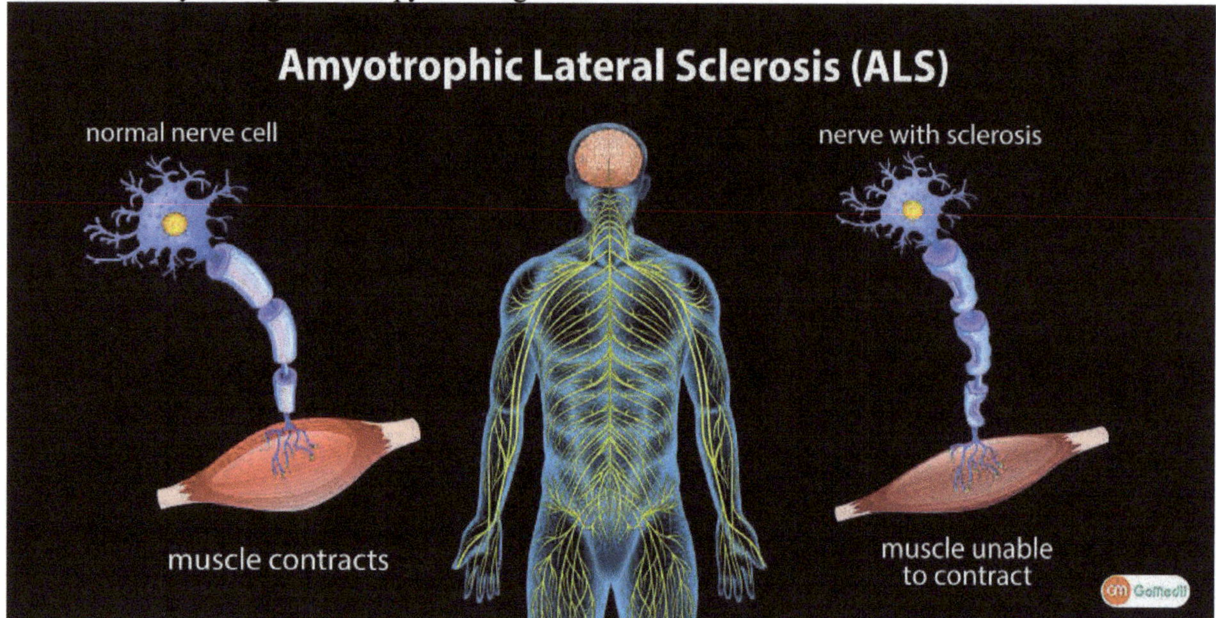

Figure 166 Comparison Between Normal and Nerves with ALS

6.7.3.1 Phenotypic Variability in ALS

The illustration shows different Amyotrophic Lateral Sclerosis (ALS) types that impact both **lower motor neuron (LMN) and upper motor neuron (UMN) nerve cells** throughout specific body areas. **Patients with Spinal Onset (a) ALS** experience degeneration of both LMN and UMN that ultimately results in limb weakness together with muscular atrophy throughout their arms and legs. **Bulbar Onset (b) ALS** specifically targets head and neck muscles leading to problems in speech and swallowing because UMN damage is severe throughout these areas. **Progressive Muscular Atrophy (c)** shows exclusively LMN dysfunction resulting in limb weakness combined with muscle degeneration throughout the body but without observable UMN damage. **Primary Lateral Sclerosis (d)** exclusively targets upper motor neurons by creating spasticity and weakness majorly affecting leg functions yet it avoids impacting lower motor neurons thus setting it apart from other variants of ALS. **Pseudopolynueritic ALS (e)** affects both LMN and UMN in the lower limbs which causes muscle weakness together with spasticity. **Hemiplegic ALS (f)** targets one side of the body by mainly affecting upper motor neurons which causes weakness and spasticity on that specific side. The condition **of Flail Arm Syndrome (g)** includes upper limb weakness and shoulder and arm muscular atrophy and **Flail Leg Syndrome (h)** specifically targets lower limbs through severe weakness and decreased muscle tone. This diagram displays motor neuron involvement through red and blue shading to illustrate the effects of ALS on different regions and motor systems.

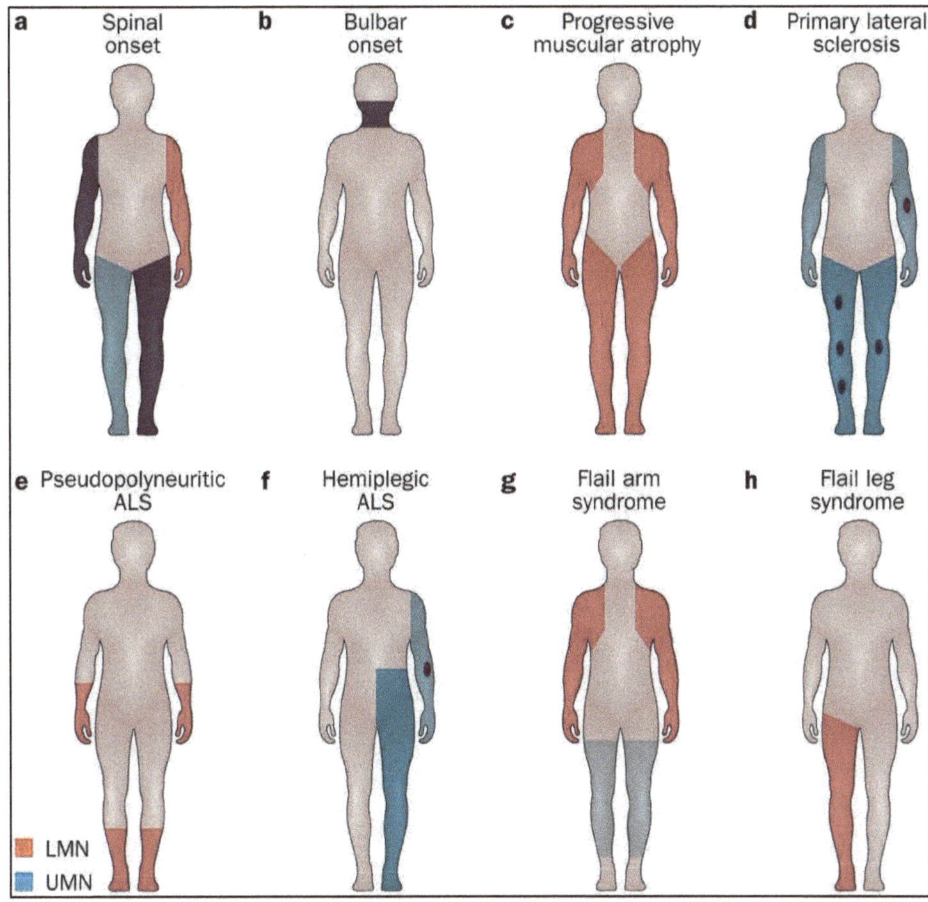

Figure 167 The phenotypic variability of amyotrophic lateral sclerosis

6.7.3.2 SOAP Notes for Amyotrophic Lateral Sclerosis

Table 95 SOAP Notes for Amyotrophic Lateral Sclerosis

Component	Details
Subjective (S)	The patient is a 55-year-old male presenting with a 6-month history of progressive muscle weakness, particularly in the arms and legs. He reports difficulty walking, clumsiness, and frequent falls. The patient also complains of muscle cramps and twitching (fasciculations) in his limbs. Over the past few months, he has noticed difficulty swallowing and occasional slurred speech. He denies any recent trauma or infections and reports no significant changes in his lifestyle. There is no family history of motor neuron diseases, but the patient is concerned about the possibility of ALS due to the gradual worsening of his symptoms.
Objective (O)	The patient appears weak and fatigued but is in no acute distress. Vital signs: BP 130/85 mmHg, HR 80 bpm, Temp 36.9°C (98.4°F). Neurological examination reveals severe muscle weakness (3/5 strength) in both upper and lower limbs, with more pronounced weakness in the distal muscles. There is noticeable muscle wasting in the arms and legs, especially in the forearms and thighs. Fasciculations are observed in the tongue and limbs. The patient exhibits dysarthria (slurred speech) and dysphagia (difficulty swallowing).

	Reflexes are hyperactive, with a positive Babinski sign. The rest of the neurological exam is otherwise unremarkable. EMG (electromyography) shows evidence of both upper and lower motor neuron degeneration, supporting a diagnosis of ALS.
Assessment (A)	The patient's clinical presentation, including progressive muscle weakness, fasciculations, dysphagia, and dysarthria, in conjunction with the EMG findings of both upper and lower motor neuron involvement, is highly suggestive of Amyotrophic Lateral Sclerosis (ALS). Given the absence of significant family history and the typical pattern of symptoms, this is likely a case of sporadic ALS. The rapid progression of symptoms, especially affecting both the limbs and bulbar region, is consistent with the clinical course of ALS.
Plan (P)	**Pharmacological:** Begin riluzole therapy (50 mg twice daily) to slow disease progression. Consider edaravone as an adjunct therapy to reduce oxidative stress, especially in patients with significant symptom progression (See algorithm below). **Non-pharmacological:** Refer the patient to a multidisciplinary ALS clinic for supportive care, including physical therapy, speech therapy, and respiratory therapy to manage muscle weakness, swallowing difficulties, and breathing issues. Recommend adaptive equipment (e.g., walking aids, communication devices) as necessary. **Follow-up:** Schedule follow-up visits every 3 months to monitor disease progression, adjust medications, and assess functional status. **Education:** Educate the patient and his family about the chronic, progressive nature of ALS and the importance of maintaining quality of life through supportive care. Discuss the role of palliative care in managing symptoms and improving comfort. Provide information on support groups and ALS resources.

Respiratory decision tree: Summary of recommendations for respiratory management in patients with amyotrophic lateral sclerosis (ALS), including ventilation (A) and airway clearance (B). Note: FVC = forced vital capacity, H_2O = water, LVR = lung volume recruitment, MIE = mechanical insufflation–exsufflation, MIP = maximal inspiratory pressure, NIV = noninvasive ventilation, PCF = peak cough flow, pCO_2 = partial pressure of carbon dioxide, SNIP = sniff nasal inspiratory pressure, SVC = slow vital capacity.

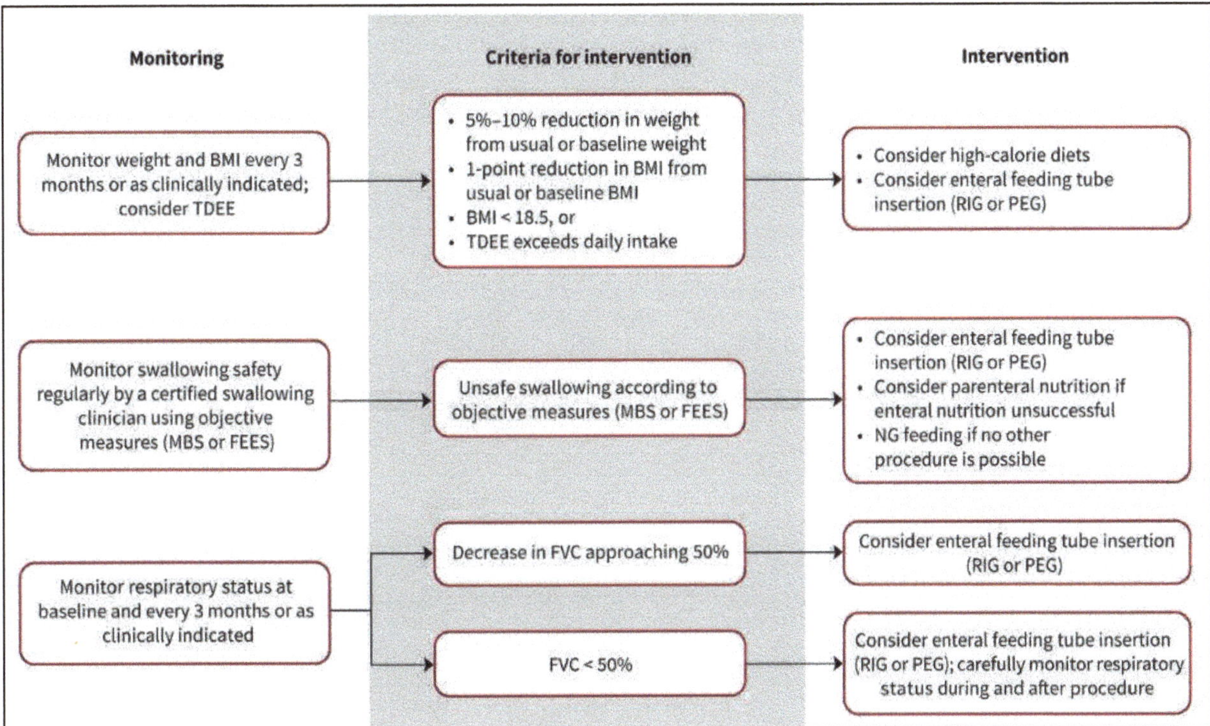

Figure 168 Management Recommendations for ALS

6.7.4 Bell's Palsy

Bell's Palsy creates sudden single-sided facial paralysis from inflammation that affects the **facial nerve (cranial nerve VII)** which manages facial muscle functions. The condition causes total or partial dysfunction of facial muscle movement on one side which emerges during short periods following hours or days. Bell's Palsy develops because of unknown factors yet medical experts believe viral infections starting with **herpes simplex virus (HSV)** lead to facial nerve swelling. When facial weakness or paralysis emerges suddenly it represents the main sign of Bell's Palsy and affects the **facial muscles on one location of the face**. It becomes challenging for a patient to close their eye on the affected side while also struggling to smile or lift their eyebrow. One can also experience jaw area pain together with ear region pain as well as front tongue taste reduction. Most Bell's Palsy cases end on their own because patients show vital improvements **between 3 to 6 months.** The timeframe for facial recovery differs across patients because some patients restore complete facial movement but some others maintain facial shortcomings.

Medical research indicates that viral infections **particularly HSV cold sore viruses** play an essential role in causing this condition although scientists have not identified the precise origin. Inflammatory viral processes linked to the infection result in facial nerve swelling which reduces nerve functioning ability. **Bell's Palsy can be set off by stress and pregnancy results and diabetic conditions and illnesses related to respiratory infections such as flu.** Standard treatment of Bell's Palsy involves both symptom reduction and recovery advancement. The most common treatment for facial nerve inflammation and swelling includes the use of the corticosteroid prednisone. The use of antiviral drugs becomes necessary when medical professionals determine a viral infection as the root cause. Patients could receive **physical therapy prescriptions** for improving both facial muscle strength and facial coordination. In unusual symptoms that continue beyond standard treatment or create complications which may cause **synkinesis (involuntary facial movements)** healthcare providers might recommend additional options such as botulinum toxin injections with potential surgical interventions. Bell's Palsy produces distress and major cosmetic difficulties yet the patient's recovery outcome tends to be positive since most people heal completely. It remains important to watch for **partial recovery symptoms because specific people** might experience prolonged facial asymmetry together with other possible enduring effects. Medical studies confirm that early medical intervention with corticosteroid administration produces better outcomes for complete recovery in patients.

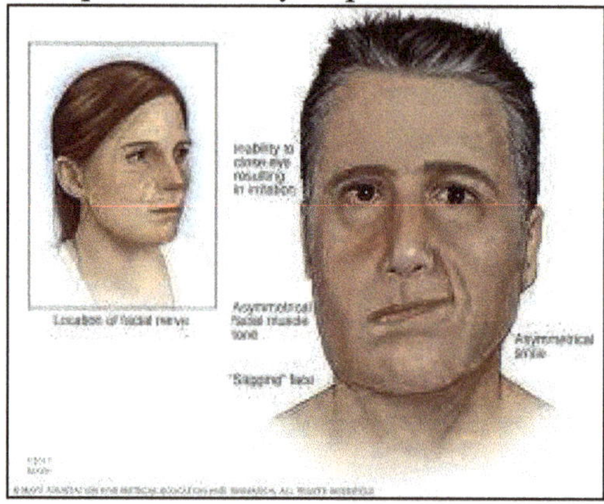

Figure 169 Bell's Palsy

6.7.4.1 SOAP Notes for Bell's Palsy

Component	Details
Subjective (S)	The patient is a 35-year-old female who presents with sudden-onset weakness and paralysis on the right side of her face, which began approximately 24 hours ago. She reports that she first noticed difficulty closing her right eye and an inability to smile on the right side of her face. The patient also mentions pain behind her right ear, which has been persistent since the onset of symptoms. She denies any recent trauma, fever, or other neurological symptoms. The patient denies any history of stroke or other neurological conditions. She is concerned about the facial asymmetry and the impact on her appearance and ability to perform routine activities such as eating and speaking.
Objective (O)	The patient appears alert and oriented but is visibly distressed by the facial weakness. Vital signs: BP 120/78 mmHg, HR 75 bpm, Temp 36.8°C (98.2°F). Neurological examination reveals asymmetric facial weakness, with the right side of the face showing drooping of the mouth and inability to close the right eyelid fully. The patient also demonstrates a diminished ability to raise the right eyebrow. Sensory examination is intact, and there is no evidence of other cranial nerve deficits. A normal examination of the rest of the neurological system, including strength and coordination, is noted. There is mild tenderness behind the right ear. No signs of recent trauma or other obvious pathologies are present. The patient does not exhibit signs of other conditions that could explain facial weakness, such as stroke.

Assessment (A)	The patient's sudden onset of unilateral facial paralysis, along with the presence of pain behind the ear, is highly suggestive of Bell's Palsy. The absence of other neurological deficits, normal sensation, and lack of recent trauma support this diagnosis. The symptoms are consistent with inflammation of the facial nerve, likely due to viral reactivation (possibly herpes simplex virus), which is a common cause of Bell's Palsy.
Plan (P)	**Pharmacological:** Start corticosteroids (prednisone 60 mg daily for 5 days) to reduce facial nerve inflammation. Consider antiviral treatment (valacyclovir 1000 mg three times daily for 7 days) if a viral aetiology is suspected (See algorithm below). **Non-pharmacological:** Advise the patient to protect the affected eye with lubricating eye drops and a patch to prevent corneal drying or injury due to incomplete eyelid closure. Recommend gentle facial exercises to improve muscle strength and coordination as part of physical therapy. **Follow-up:** Schedule a follow-up appointment in 1 week to assess response to treatment, monitor for improvement, and adjust therapy if necessary. **Education:** Educate the patient about the nature of Bell's Palsy, its self-limiting nature, and the usual recovery timeline (within 3 to 6 months). Reassure the patient that most individuals experience a full recovery, although some may have a residual weakness. Discuss the importance of eye protection and the potential need for physical therapy to aid recovery.

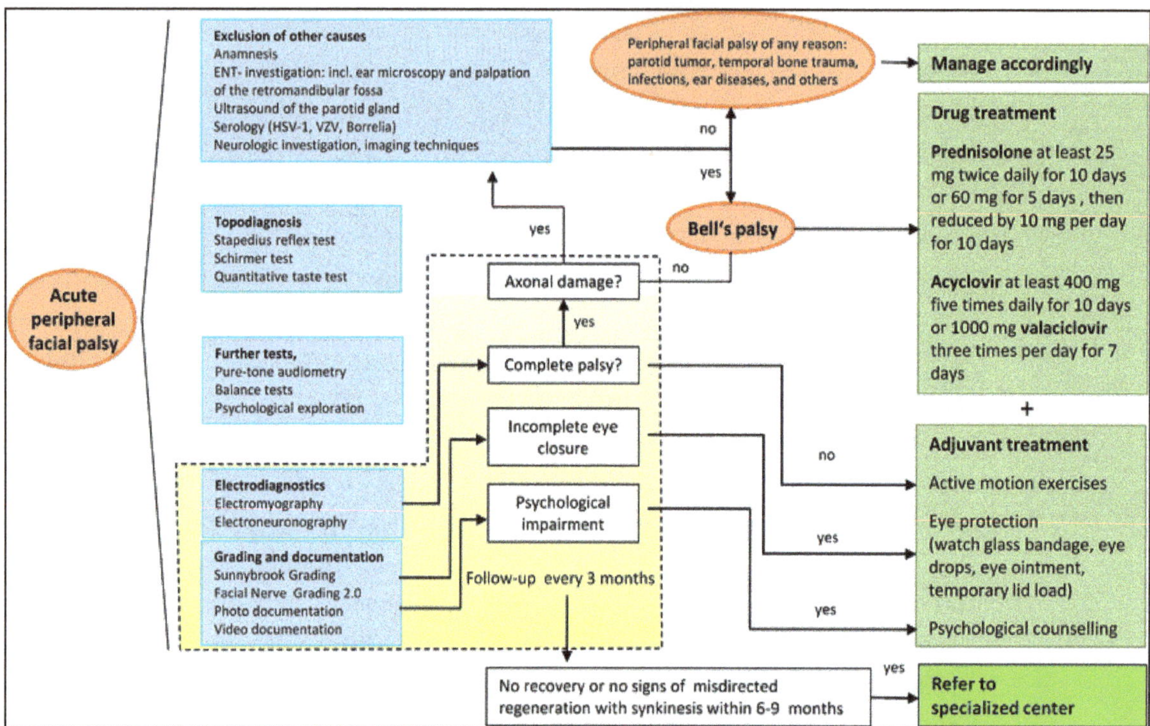

Figure 170 Management Algorithm for Bell's Palsy

ACUTE CONDITIONS

6.7.5 Acute Bacterial Meningitis

Acute bacterial meningitis represents a dangerous illness that attacks the meninges which protect the brain as well as the spinal cord. Bacteria that invade the central nervous system trigger the infection which results in meningeal inflammation and interrupt normal brain function. Medical intervention must occur right away because this condition advances quickly along with its potential to trigger fatal problems such as neurological injuries coma and mortality. **Acute bacterial meningitis frequently** develops from three main bacterial organisms which are Streptococcus pneumoniae, ***Neisseria meningitidis and Haemophilus influenzae***. Neonates usually develop meningitis from Group ***B Streptococcus or Escherichia coli*** bacteria but elderly patients with weakened systems are at risk from Listeria monocytogenes. The bacterial infection starts within the bloodstream before bacteria pass through the blood-brain barrier to reach and infect the **meninges where it starts an inflammatory process**. The resulting inflammation causes elevation of intracranial pressure alongside blood flow impairment and subsequent brain tissue damage.

The medical features of acute bacterial meningitis emerge quickly together with severe symptoms. The presentation of acute bacterial meningitis begins with severe head pain together with elevated temperature and stiff neck muscles and added manifestations of photophobia, queasiness, motion sickness and changes in mental state. Acute bacterial meningitis shows its symptoms through **irritability, lethargy, fontanelle that bulges due to increased intracranial pressure in infants and young children.** The classical indicator for meningitis diagnosis includes Kernig's sign which produces leg joint pain during flexion and extension testing of the hip or Brudzinski's sign which presents involuntary knee bending when flexing the neck. However, these signs may not always be present. The medical staff confirms the diagnosis by performing a lumbar puncture (spinal tap) to acquire **cerebrospinal fluid (CSF) samples for laboratory tests.** The CSF from acute bacterial meningitis patients presents with cloudiness along with raised pleocytosis cell counts elevated proteins and low glucose levels. Testing for the causative organism starts with Gram stain or culture of the CSF and includes the rapid identification method through PCR testing.

The medical treatment of acute bacterial meningitis requires immediate administration of antibiotics delivered through an intravenous line to eliminate the responsible bacterial infection. Labia selection depends on the **patient's age combined with immune system** status and suspected infection origin. The most frequent antibiotics used for treatment are ceftriaxone combined with cefotaxime and ampicillin while vancomycin joins other drugs that combat resistant organisms. Physicians include ampicillin in the treatment plan if ***Listeria monocytogenes*** serves as a potential infection. **Dexamethasone** serves as a corticosteroid for minimizing inflammation and preserving hearing function especially when ***Streptococcus pneumoniae*** causes the infection. The outcome of meningitis treatment depends on the patient's age and immune fitness combined with the punctuality of therapy administration and the specific organism that caused the infection. The successful treatment of bacterial meningitis does not eliminate potential lasting effects since affected patients may develop hearing loss and face cognitive defects as well as seizures and motor dysfunction. The outcome of **mortality rates and neurological complications depends greatly on the speed of diagnosis** as well as the prompt start of treatment. People with compromised immune systems as well as infants and elderly adults should receive vaccinations with Streptococcus pneumoniae, Neisseria meningitidis and ***Haemophilus influenzae*** to prevent infection. The spread of ***Neisseria meningitidis*** meningitis can be prevented by giving prophylactic antibiotics to those who had direct healthcare interactions with an infected person.

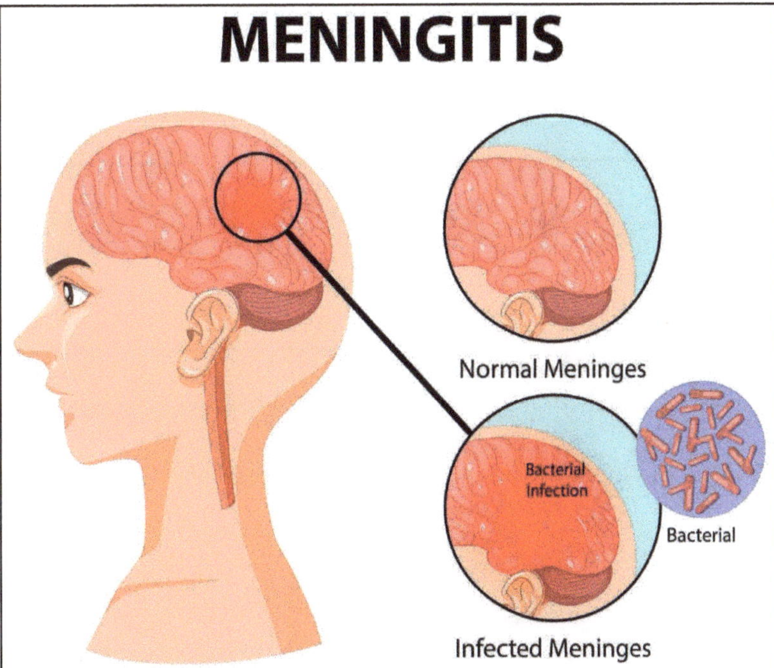

Figure 171 Acute Bacterial Meningitis

6.7.5.1 Classification of Acute Bacterial Meningitis

Bacterial meningitis exists within multiple diagnostic subtypes which differentiate infections through **bacterial behavior and progression patterns**. Bacterial infections leading to **persistent meningitis form a main category that results from partial bacterial treatment of atypical or less harmful microorganisms.** The inflammation of meninges occurs through bacterial spread from adjacent infectious sites affecting nearby parts of the brain. **Tuberculosis (TB) represents another meningitis subtype** which ***Mycobacterium tuberculosis*** causes through the development of chronic meningitis at a slow rate which mainly affects immunocompromised patients. In stage three of syphilis when caused by ***Treponema pallidum*** bacterial infection, the infection leads to neurosyphilis that produces meningitis. The infection with ***Borrelia burgdorferi*** known as Lyme disease brings about meningitis when the pathogen spreads throughout the body specifically in zones where Lyme disease prevails. Rare but important **Fungal bacterial-like meningitis** exists when ***Cryptococcus*** affects immunocompromised host, although these cases typically belong to separate classifications from classic bacterial meningitis types. Bacterial causes of meningitis come from multiple different bacterial agents which require distinctive clinical procedures for diagnosis and therapy.

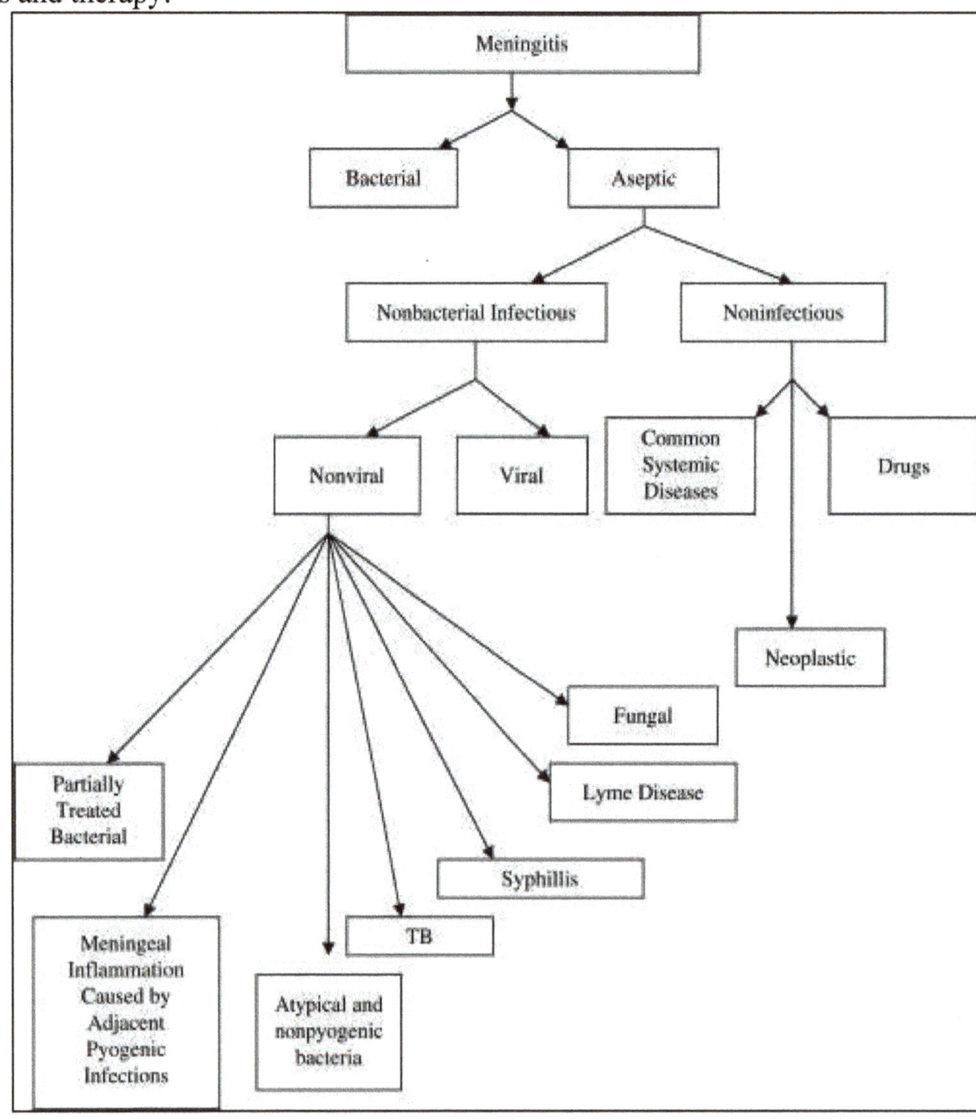

Figure 172 Classification of Acute Meningitis

6.7.5.2 SOAP Notes for Acute Bacterial Meningitis

Table 96 SOAP Notes for Acute Bacterial Meningitis

Component	Details
Subjective (S)	The patient is a 32-year-old male who presents with a 24-hour history of severe headache, fever, nausea, and vomiting. He reports that the headache is intense and located around the forehead and neck, and it is not relieved by

	over-the-counter analgesics. The patient also describes a stiff neck and increased sensitivity to light. He mentions feeling confused and having difficulty concentrating. There is no history of recent trauma, recent infections, or known exposure to any individuals with meningitis. He denies a history of chronic medical conditions but is concerned about the possibility of a serious infection due to the severity of symptoms.
Objective (O)	The patient appears ill and in moderate distress due to headache and discomfort. Vital signs: BP 130/85 mmHg, HR 110 bpm, Temp 39.2°C (102.5°F), RR 18 bpm, Oxygen saturation 98%. Physical exam reveals positive signs of meningismus (stiff neck and sensitivity to light), along with a positive Brudzinski's sign (involuntary knee flexion upon neck flexion) and a positive Kernig's sign (pain and resistance when extending the leg while the hip is flexed). Neurological examination shows confusion but no focal deficits. Cranial nerve examination is normal, and there are no signs of papilledema. A lumbar puncture is performed, revealing cerebrospinal fluid (CSF) that is cloudy with a white blood cell count of 900 cells/μL (predominantly neutrophils), low glucose levels (25 mg/dL), and elevated protein levels (150 mg/dL). Gram stain of the CSF shows gram-positive diplococci, suggesting *Streptococcus pneumoniae* as the causative pathogen.
Assessment (A)	The patient's clinical presentation, including acute onset of headache, fever, neck stiffness, photophobia, confusion, and abnormal CSF findings (elevated white blood cells, low glucose, elevated protein), is highly indicative of acute bacterial meningitis. The gram-positive diplococci observed in the CSF gram stain, along with the patient's symptoms, suggest *Streptococcus pneumoniae* as the most likely causative pathogen. This diagnosis requires immediate treatment due to the potential for rapid progression and serious complications such as neurological damage, sepsis, and death.
Plan (P)	**Pharmacological:** Start empiric intravenous antibiotics with ceftriaxone 2g IV every 12 hours and vancomycin 1g IV every 12 hours, pending final culture results. If *Streptococcus pneumoniae* is confirmed, continue ceftriaxone or cefotaxime and add dexamethasone 10 mg IV every 6 hours for the first 4 days to reduce inflammation and prevent complications such as hearing loss (See algorithm below). **Non-pharmacological:** Provide supportive care with hydration, antiemetics for nausea, and monitoring of neurological status. Ensure a quiet, dark environment to minimize discomfort from photophobia. **Follow-up:** Repeat lumbar puncture in 48-72 hours to assess CSF improvement. Schedule a follow-up visit within a week to monitor progress, neurological status, and response to treatment. **Education:** Educate the patient and family about the seriousness of bacterial meningitis and the importance of completing the full course of antibiotics. Discuss the need for isolation and the importance of notifying close contacts so they can receive prophylactic antibiotics to prevent the spread of the infection. Also, provide

information on potential complications, including hearing loss and neurological sequelae, and stress the importance of early intervention in preventing long-term damage.

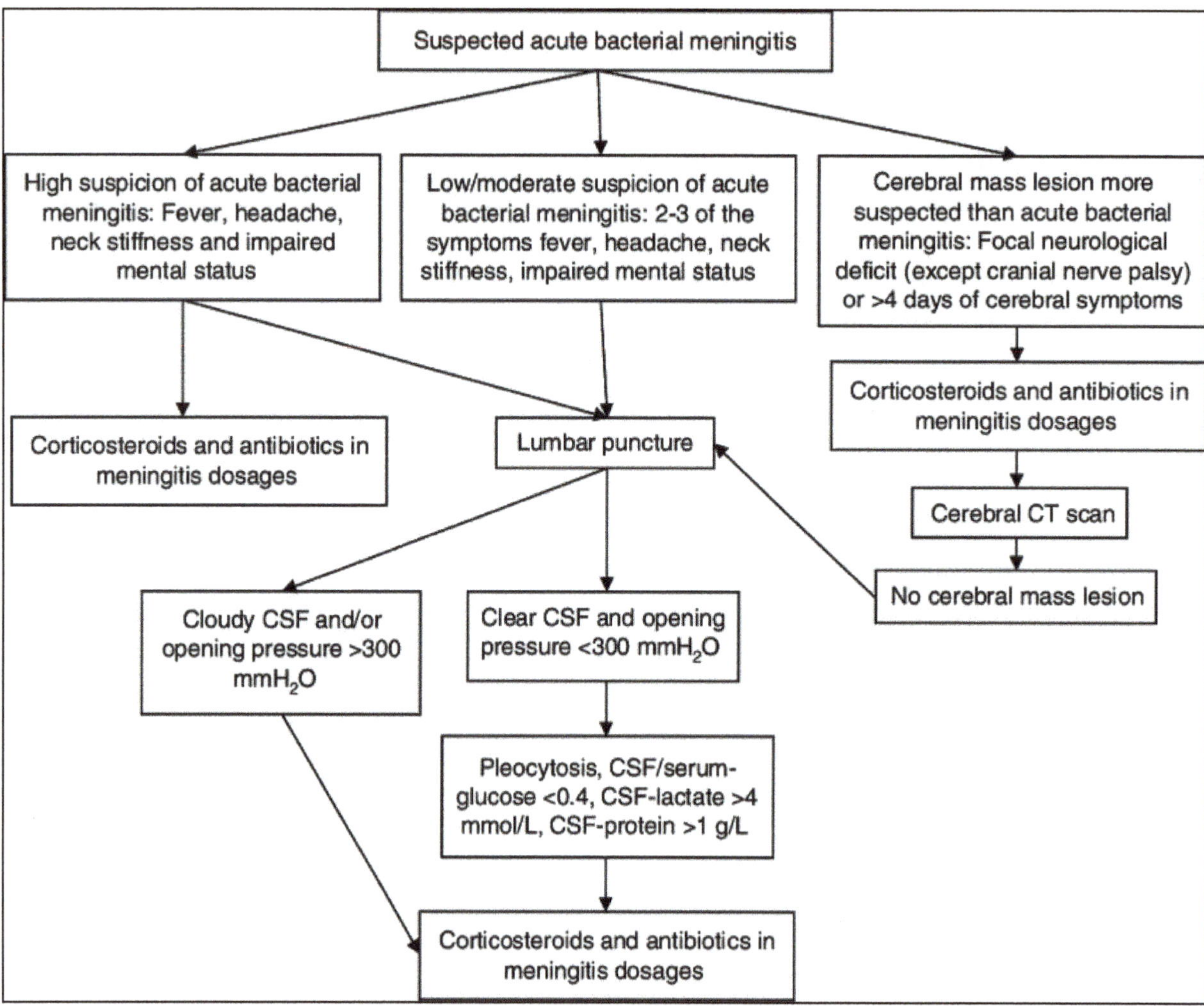

Figure 173 Algorithm for the Management of Suspected Acute Bacterial Meningitis

6.7.6 Headaches

Headaches emerge as one of the central neurological complaints which affect individuals at all stages of life from every social background. Different people experience headaches at various **levels during periods that span varying amounts of time somewhere between short and prolonged stretches** and these conditions stem from harmless medical issues through potentially dangerous medical problems. **Primary headaches exist separate** from medical conditions but most headaches fall within the primary category and secondary headaches develop because of another disorder like brain tumours or infections.

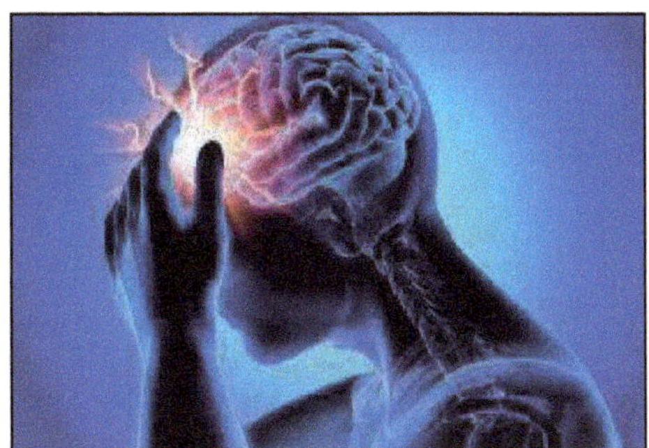

Figure 174 Headache

6.7.6.1 Types of Headache

1. **Migraine Headaches**

Most people describe migraine headaches as strong persistent headaches which develop on only one side of the head. People who experience migraines usually develop nausea along with vomiting as well as heightened **sensitivity to light sounds and smells (photophobia and phonophobia)**. Before headache onset, some sufferers experience visual symptoms that include **lightning flashes, zigzag patterns and complete vision loss.** The duration of migraine attacks ranges from four hours to seventy-two hours while keeping the patient totally disabled. Research indicates that brainstem modifications because of genetic factors combined with environmental influences generate a change in the **trigeminal nerve** while also altering brainstem activity which results in headache development in the brainstem area of the head. Strains that set off migraines occur due to **stress hormonal fluctuations, specific foods, sleep problems, environmental light conditions, and shifting weather patterns also serve as triggers.**

2. **Tension-Type Headaches**

Tension-type headaches represent the primary headache disorder which affects most people. This type of **headache produces a delayed constant pain** which creates a **band-like pressure effect across the head area.** The onset of tension headaches does not cause nausea in most cases but patients sometimes appear sensitive to environmental light or audio stimuli. The headache affects both sides of the head while existing in **different degrees of intensity from mild to moderate stages**. Current research shows that the source behind tension headaches stays unclear though the condition frequently develops due to **anxiety, body position issues, insufficient rest, neck, and shoulder muscle tightness**. These headaches present both sporadic and long-term conditions among different persons.

3. **Cluster Headaches**

People who have cluster headaches experience the most painful headaches which cause **excruciating burning or piercing pain that occurs near the eye or the side of the head.** This specific pain type stays focused in one spot as it persists from **15 minutes to 3 hours**. The headache event of cluster headaches appears in groups that cause daily attacks to continue through weeks until months at the exact same time of day. The attacks of these headaches include autonomic effects which result in tearing along with nasal congestion and drooping of eyelids on the affected side of the body.

4. **Sinus Headaches**

Frankly speaking, sinus headaches occur because of **sinus inflammation or infection** affecting the air-filled spaces named sinuses that exist both behind the eyes and in the cheeks as well as in the forehead area. The inflammatory issues of these **mucous membrane-lined cavities after sinusitis infections result in major facial discomfort, pressure, and facial pain.** The facial pain usually appears in and around the forehead together with the eye and cheek regions and intensifies when patients stoop forward or perform quick head movements.

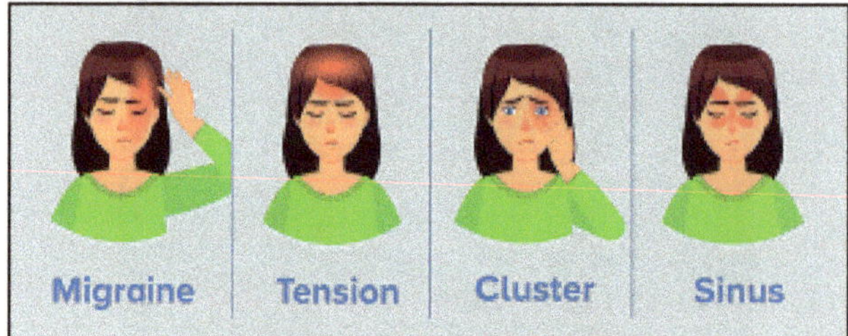

Figure 175 Types of Headaches

6.7.6.2 Classification and Treatments of Headaches

1. **Migraine with Aura (Classical Migraine)**

The main objective of abortive treatment is to start medical intervention at the initial sign of a migraine in order to stop symptoms. The abortive treatments for headaches feature **triptans (sumatriptan among them) together with NSAIDs (ibuprofen being one example) and ergotamine derivatives.** These drugs both decrease blood vessel dilation and stop pain signals from traveling from the brain area to other parts. Prophylactic treatment offers a solution to decrease both the amount and seriousness of migraine attacks that occur often. The prevention of migraine attacks is commonly achieved through **beta-blockers propranolol together with anticonvulsants topiramate and antidepressants amitriptyline.** Repeated use of triptans and NSAIDs as treatment leads to rebound headaches because patients develop a dependency on these medications. This condition results in more frequent and prolonged headaches. Medical professionals must instruct patients to restrict their intake of these medications because dependency becomes a risk. Taking too many over-the-counter pain medications leads to a higher possibility of developing medication-overuse headaches.

2. **Migraine without Aura (Common Migraine)**

For abortive management of this type of migraine, doctors prescribe **triptans, NSAIDs, and ergotamine** alongside each other. The acute migraine treatment medication known as erenumab alongside **other CGRP inhibitors** shows great potential for acute migraine treatment. The preventive measures to prevent migraine recurrence include beta-blockers together with calcium channel blockers (e.g., verapamil) along with antidepressants. **Rebound headaches will develop after excessive use of medication including triptans and NSAIDs** similar to how it happens in migraines with aura. Stretching the use of these medications must be kept minimal since this poses a threat to patient health.

3. **Tension-Type Headaches**

Patients typically benefit from managing their tension-type headaches using the pain relievers that are available without prescription such as acetaminophen and ibuprofen. The prescription of **muscle relaxants such as cyclobenzaprine or NSAIDs becomes necessary** when the headache severity demands this intervention. A prevention approach to treating chronic tension-type headaches involves giving amitriptyline which belongs to the antidepressant classification. The treatment plans for such situations may involve either **biofeedback techniques or cognitive behavioural therapy (CBT)** to treat stress and tension in the muscles. Regular consumption of painkillers including **NSAIDs or acetaminophen can trigger rebound headaches** even though patients commonly use these medications to treat their head pain. Patients need instruction about taking these medications with care that includes staying away from daily use for extended periods.

4. **Cluster Headaches**

The main abortive treatment for cluster headaches consists of oxygen therapy where patients should use **100% oxygen for 15 minutes**. For fast relief, patients can use **sumatriptan alongside an alternative medication called ergotamine.** The most effective treatment for preventing chronic cluster headaches is verapamil as a prophylactic medication. Lithium along with corticosteroids such as prednisone remain acceptable options for particular cluster headache cases. The long-term use of triptans along with ergotamine as abortive treatments often leads to medication overuse headaches. **Cluster headaches appear in short bursts** which cause healthcare providers to limit the use of these medications mainly for this reason.

6.7.6.3 SOAP Notes for Headaches

Table 97 SOAP Notes for Headaches

Component	Details
Subjective (S)	The patient is a 40-year-old female presenting with a 3-day history of recurrent headaches. The headaches are described as a dull, aching pain, predominantly located in the frontal and temporal regions. She reports that the pain is moderate in intensity (5/10 on the pain scale) and is often aggravated by stress or lack of sleep. The patient has not experienced nausea, vomiting, or visual disturbances but does report mild sensitivity to light and sound. She mentions occasional tension in her neck and shoulders, particularly after long periods of sitting at a computer. She denies any recent trauma, fever, or upper respiratory symptoms. The patient has a history of intermittent tension-type headaches, but this recent episode feels more frequent and persistent. She has been using over-the-counter ibuprofen, but it only provides temporary relief.
Objective (O)	The patient appears alert but mildly uncomfortable due to the headache. Vital signs: BP 128/80 mmHg, HR 78 bpm, Temp 36.8°C (98.2°F). Neurological examination is unremarkable with no signs of focal deficits. The patient shows no signs of papilledema or abnormal eye movement. Physical examination reveals mild muscle tightness in the neck and upper shoulders, with tenderness upon palpation. No signs of meningismus or cranial nerve abnormalities are noted. The patient's cognitive function is intact, and she does not appear confused or disoriented. There is no history of sinus congestion or any other signs suggestive of infection.
Assessment (A)	The patient's presentation of recurrent headaches, particularly with associated neck and shoulder tension, is consistent with **tension-type headaches**. The absence of nausea, vomiting, and visual changes, as well as the lack of any neurological deficits, further supports this diagnosis. While the patient has a history of intermittent headaches, the recent increase in frequency and persistence may be related to stress, poor sleep, or musculoskeletal factors (e.g., poor posture). Migraine and secondary causes, such as sinusitis or infection, are less likely given the absence of other symptoms.

Plan (P)	**Pharmacological:** Recommend NSAIDs such as ibuprofen (200-400 mg every 4-6 hours as needed, not exceeding 3,200 mg/day) for acute headache relief. If symptoms persist, consider prescribing a muscle relaxant (e.g., cyclobenzaprine) to alleviate neck and shoulder tension (See algorithm below). **Non-pharmacological:** Advise the patient on stress management techniques (e.g., deep breathing exercises, mindfulness). Recommend ergonomic adjustments to the workstation to reduce neck strain and incorporate regular breaks during prolonged computer use. Encourage regular exercise to improve posture and reduce muscle tension. **Follow-up:** Follow up in 1-2 weeks if the headaches continue or worsen to assess response to treatment and consider further investigations if secondary causes are suspected. **Education:** Educate the patient about lifestyle modifications, including improving sleep hygiene, reducing caffeine intake, and practicing relaxation techniques. Emphasize the importance of avoiding overuse of analgesics, as this could lead to rebound headaches.

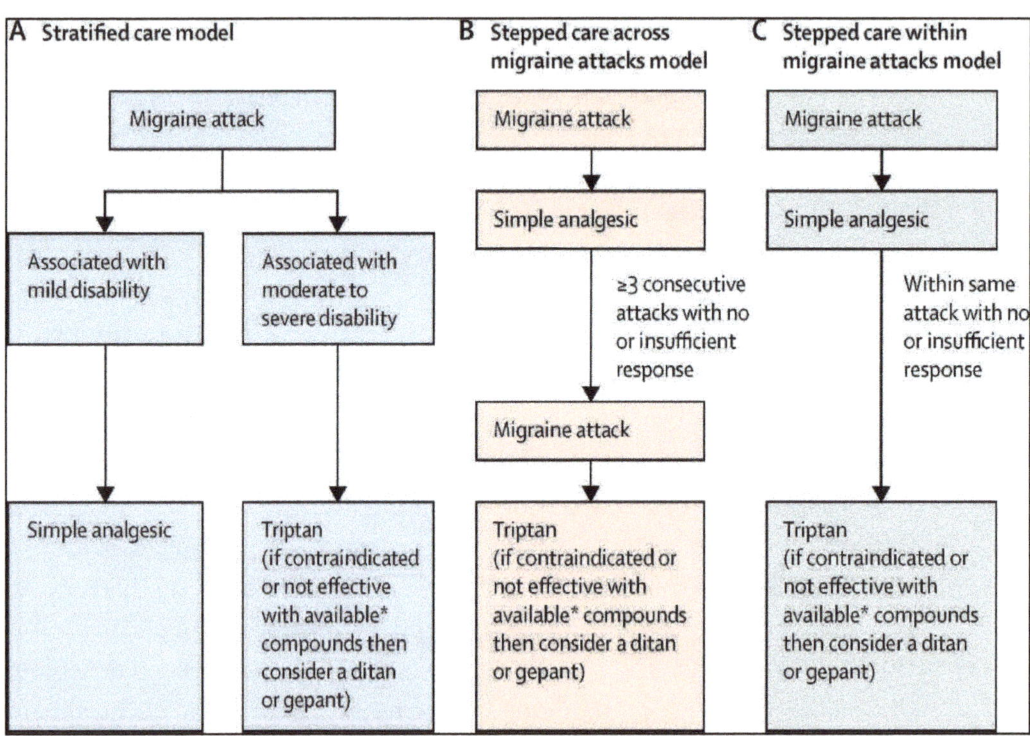

Figure 176 Management Algorithm for Headaches

6.7.7 Trigeminal neuralgia (Tic)

Trigeminal Neuralgia (Tic) commonly referred to as tic douloureux manifests as sudden intense recurring pain that targets the regions governed by the **trigeminal nerve (cranial nerve V).** Trigeminal Neuralgia pain produces **sensations of electric shock or stabbing or severe sharp pain** which occurs consistently on the patient's facial region on one side. The medical field acknowledges trigeminal neuralgia as among the most intense experiences of pain that currently exists. Vascular compression of the trigeminal nerve combined with demyelination remains the primary cause of trigeminal neuralgia although its exact origin is sometimes unclear. **Vascular**

nerve compression serves as the primary trigger for this brain disorder. The nerve firing becomes abnormal because of pressure from compression hence creating painful sensations. **Certain MS diagnoses** result in trigeminal neuralgia specifically among young patients whose trigeminal nerve demyelination stems from the disease. Three sections form the trigeminal nerve called branches.

- The V1 becomes involved by affecting both the eyeball and forehead region.
- V2 Maxillary branch of the trigeminal nerve creates pain in the cheek, upper lip and upper teeth regions.
- The lower jaw together with its teeth and portion of the tongue receives impact from the Mandibular (V3).

The pain from trigeminal neuralgia affects maximally the maxillary and mandibular regions although it might include all three nerve branches. Patients commonly experience facial pain episodes through various typical activities like eating, conversing, dental hygiene, facial contact, and windy conditions. Trigeminal neuralgia displays its primary symptom as brief yet severe facial pain which almost always appears on a single side of the face. **The facial pain emerges as brief stabbing or shooting sensations** that have durations from seconds to minutes. A person with trigeminal neuralgia experiences clusters of intense pain that can appear several times every hour or two times every day. The symptoms of this disorder present an episodic pattern because patients normally remain symptom-free between pain attacks.

The affected region shows pain corresponding to the tissue areas controlled by the **trigeminal nerve branch which has been damaged.** Some patients with this condition develop specific areas on their face which trigger **attacks when touched lightly or under movement**. Trigeminal neuralgia receives its diagnosis from patients who describe their pain experiences and properties to providers. Trigeminal neuralgia diagnosis depends heavily on face pain characteristics because these symptoms separate it from other causes involving dental issues or sinusitis. The doctor may use **MRI scanning to exclude brain tumours or microscopic abnormalities**, especially with unusual case profiles in patients aged younger than 50 years. An MRI will show vascular compression of the trigeminal nerve when used for assessment.

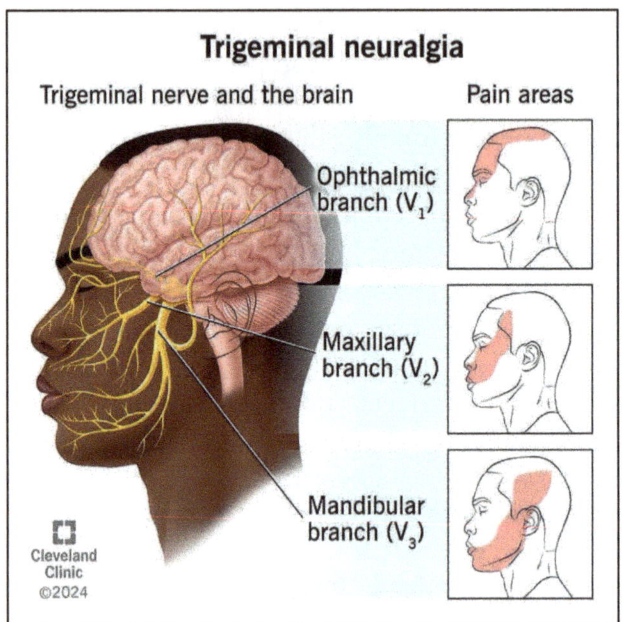

Figure 177 Trigeminal Neuralgia

6.7.7.1 Classification of Terminal Neuralgia

A diagram presents comprehensive information **regarding trigeminal neuralgia (TN) types** and their **pathophysiological characteristics** throughout different subcategories. Idiopathic trigeminal neuralgia happens to individuals with inherited susceptibilities that affect ion channels together with myelin sheaths and neurotransmitter management. Patients show a higher risk of ectopic impulse generation and epatic transmission because of their genetic vulnerability thus these basic events cause **spontaneous and evoked neuralgic pain**. The primary source of pain in classical trigeminal neuralgia occurs from neurovascular compression that involves either the superior cerebellar artery or the **trigeminal vein compressing the trigeminal nerve root entry zone resulting in axon demyelination.** Ectopic impulses along with inflammation focal arachnoiditis, central sensitization and deafferentation hypersensitivity finally produce spontaneous pain and hypersensitivity to stimuli. **Symptomatic trigeminal neuralgia** develops from other acute diseases which include herpes infections alongside **multiple sclerosis, diabetes and posterior fossa tumours or mass compressions.** The fundamental nerve damage together with trigeminal nerve atrophy and axonal loss results in central sensitization which produces continuous pain alongside the possibility of developing continuous pain. The diagram illustrates how neurovascular compression together with systemic disorders unify into pathophysiological nerve damage and **inflammatory and hypersensitivity processes which drive TN patient pain.**

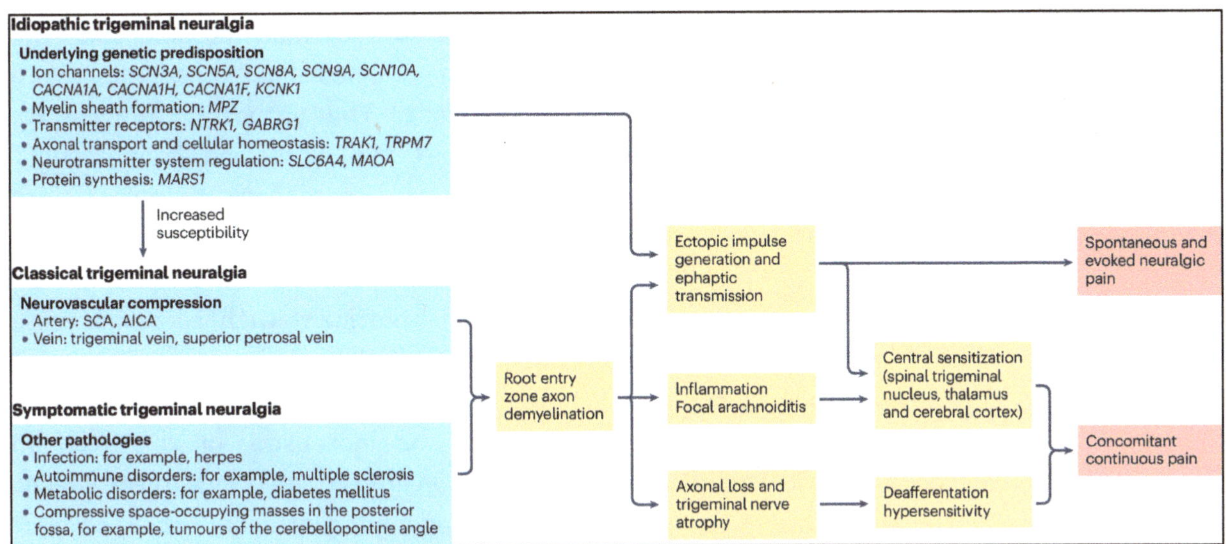

Figure 178 Classification Cascade of Trigeminal Neuralgia

6.7.7.2 SOAP Notes for Trigeminal Neuralgia

Table 98 SOAP Notes for Trigeminal Neuralgia

Component	Details
Subjective (S)	The patient is a 45-year-old female presenting with a history of trigeminal neuralgia (TN) for the past 6 months. She reports severe, sharp, stabbing pain on the right side of her face, which occurs in paroxysms lasting from a few seconds to a minute. The pain is triggered by simple activities such as chewing, brushing her teeth, or even light touch along the right cheek. She describes the pain as electric shock-like and located around the maxillary branch of the trigeminal nerve, extending to the mandibular area. The patient denies any recent trauma or systemic illness but has a history of multiple sclerosis (MS), which she believes may be related to her symptoms. She has been taking carbamazepine (200 mg twice daily) but reports partial relief, with increasing frequency and intensity of the pain over the past month. She has not experienced any other neurological deficits, such as vision changes or weakness.
Objective (O)	The patient appears in moderate distress due to facial pain but is alert and oriented. Vital signs: BP 130/85 mmHg, HR 76 bpm, Temp 36.7°C (98.1°F). Physical examination reveals right-sided facial pain upon palpation of the maxillary and mandibular branches of the trigeminal nerve. There are no signs of facial weakness, ptosis, or any other cranial nerve abnormalities. The neurological exam is otherwise normal, with no focal deficits. The patient has a history of multiple sclerosis as confirmed by previous MRI, showing demyelinating lesions in the brainstem and spinal cord. The carbamazepine is continued, but there are no signs of toxicity or side effects (e.g., ataxia or diplopia).
Assessment (A)	The patient's presentation, with sharp, paroxysmal pain localized to the right maxillary and mandibular branches of the trigeminal nerve, is consistent with

	trigeminal neuralgia. Given the patient's history of multiple sclerosis, the likely etiology is symptomatic trigeminal neuralgia, secondary to demyelination of the trigeminal nerve root. The patient's response to carbamazepine suggests partial control, but the increasing frequency of symptoms indicates potential progression of the disease or insufficient medication. Neurovascular compression is less likely in this case, given the MS history.
Plan (P)	**Pharmacological:** The patient should begin treatment with carbamazepine (200 mg twice daily) to manage trigeminal neuralgia. This medication helps reduce the frequency and intensity of pain episodes. If symptoms persist or worsen, the dose of carbamazepine may be increased, or a switch to oxcarbazepine (300 mg twice daily) can be considered, as it may offer similar benefits with fewer side effects. In cases of inadequate pain relief, adjunct therapies like gabapentin (300 mg three times a day) or baclofen (10 mg three times a day) may be introduced. The patient should be monitored for any potential side effects of carbamazepine, such as dizziness, ataxia, or rash, and adjustments should be made as needed. **Non-pharmacological:** The patient should be referred to a neurologist for further evaluation of multiple sclerosis (MS), as this could be contributing to the trigeminal neuralgia symptoms. Additionally, stress management strategies, including biofeedback and relaxation techniques like deep breathing exercises, may help reduce the frequency and severity of pain episodes. Acupuncture or physical therapy could also be considered to address any underlying musculoskeletal factors contributing to the pain, providing relief from additional discomfort. **Follow-up:** A follow-up appointment should be scheduled in 1 month to evaluate the effectiveness of the prescribed medications and assess for any potential side effects. If symptoms persist or worsen, further adjustments to the treatment plan may be required. An MRI of the brainstem should be considered to evaluate any progression of demyelinating lesions in the trigeminal nerve root, especially given the patient's history of multiple sclerosis. A follow-up assessment in 3 months is also recommended if the patient continues to experience symptoms or develops new neurological deficits. **Education:** The patient should be educated on the chronic and episodic nature of trigeminal neuralgia and the role of medications in managing symptoms. Emphasis should be placed on avoiding triggers, such as cold weather, wind, chewing, or touch, as these can exacerbate the pain.

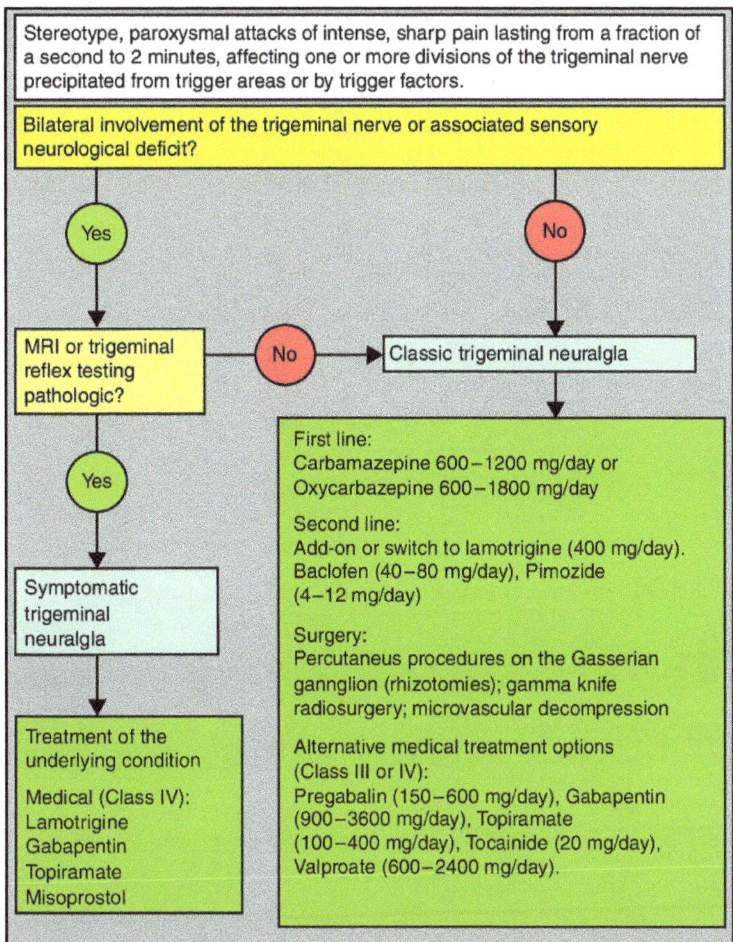
Stereotype, paroxysmal attacks of intense, sharp pain lasting from a fraction of a second to 2 minutes, affecting one or more divisions of the trigeminal nerve precipitated from trigger areas or by trigger factors.
Bilateral involvement of the trigeminal nerve or associated sensory neurological deficit?
Yes
No
MRI or trigeminal reflex testing pathologic?
No
Classic trigeminal neuralgla
Yes
Symptomatic trigeminal neuralgla
Treatment of the underlying condition
Medical (Class IV):
Lamotrigine
Gabapentin
Topiramate
Misoprostol
First line:
Carbamazepine 600–1200 mg/day or
Oxycarbazepine 600–1800 mg/day
Second line:
Add-on or switch to lamotrigine (400 mg/day).
Baclofen (40–80 mg/day), Pimozide (4–12 mg/day)
Surgery:
Percutaneus procedures on the Gasserian gannglion (rhizotomies); gamma knife radiosurgery; microvascular decompression
Alternative medical treatment options (Class III or IV):
Pregabalin (150–600 mg/day), Gabapentin (900–3600 mg/day), Topiramate (100–400 mg/day), Tocainide (20 mg/day), Valproate (600–2400 mg/day).

Figure 179 Workup and Manageent Algorithm for Trigeminal Neuralgia

6.7.8 Transient Ischemic Attack

A Transient Ischemic Attack (TIA) represents a brief moment when the **blood supply to brain tissue** stops temporarily which results in stroke-like symptoms without resulting in permanent brain tissue damage. **A TIA lasts several minutes or less than several hours** because these events never lead to lasting neurological trouble. Symptoms from a TIA present as sudden numbness or weakness on one body side and speech difficulties together with **visual problems, dizziness, and movement or balance problems.** The main reason that causes TIA is blockages from blood clots and plaque buildup which reduces blood supply through cerebral arteries. A TIA marks a brief blockage that normally dissolves but warns about an elevated stroke danger for the future since **15% of TIA patients develop a stroke within three months**. A diagnosis of transient ischemic attack requires healthcare professionals to perform clinical evaluations along with medical history gathering and imaging tests such as **CT scans or MRIs to eliminate other potential conditions**. The immediate treatment requires patients to take aspirin as **a platelet-preventing drug to stop clots** but the long-term prevention depends on managing blood pressure alongside diabetes and cholesterol levels. The passage to more serious stroke requires prompt treatment together with lifestyle adjustments as a preventive measure.

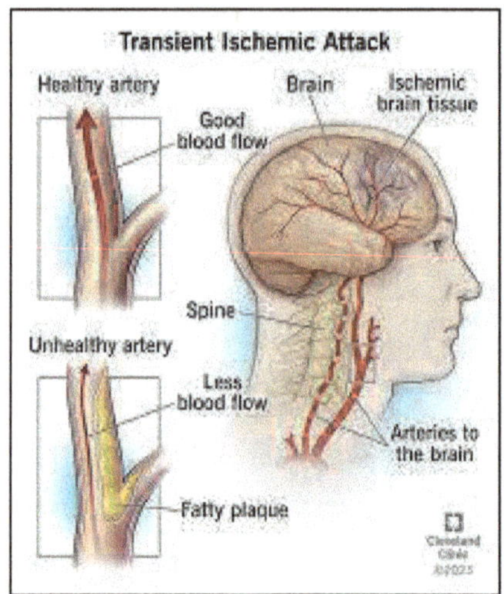

Figure 180 Schematic Diagram of Transient Ischemic Attack

6.7.8.1 SOAP Notes for Transient Ischemic Attack

Table 99 SOAP Notes for Transient Ischemic Attack

Component	Details
Subjective (S)	The patient is a 60-year-old male who presents with a sudden-onset of right-sided weakness and difficulty speaking that lasted for approximately 30 minutes earlier today. The patient describes the weakness as numbness and tingling in his right arm and leg, along with slurred speech. He reports that the symptoms completely resolved without intervention. The patient denies any headache, confusion, or loss of consciousness. He has a history of hypertension, hyperlipidemia, and type 2 diabetes, but he has not been adhering to his medications regularly. The patient is concerned because of the similarity to a stroke but is relieved that the symptoms resolved. He is seeking reassurance and guidance for preventing further episodes.
Objective (O)	The patient is alert, oriented, and in no acute distress. Vital signs: BP 145/90 mmHg, HR 78 bpm, Temp 36.7°C (98.1°F), RR 18 bpm. Neurological examination is normal with no focal deficits. Cranial nerve function is intact, and the patient demonstrates normal strength and sensation in both arms and legs without any signs of weakness or sensory abnormalities. There is no dysarthria or aphasia. No signs of fundoscopic abnormalities are observed. Based on the transient nature of symptoms and resolution, the clinical findings suggest a Transient Ischemic Attack (TIA), though further diagnostic testing is needed to rule out other causes.
Assessment (A)	The patient's history of hypertension, hyperlipidemia, and type 2 diabetes, combined with the sudden onset of right-sided weakness and slurred speech that resolved spontaneously, is consistent with a Transient Ischemic Attack (TIA). TIAs often serve as a warning sign for future strokes, and the patient's risk factors significantly increase the likelihood of a subsequent event. Immediate diagnostic testing is necessary to rule out underlying causes and assess the risk of future strokes.

Plan (P)	**Pharmacological:** Initiate aspirin 81 mg daily for antiplatelet therapy to reduce the risk of future strokes. Consider starting statins (e.g., atorvastatin 20 mg daily) to manage hyperlipidemia and reduce cardiovascular risk. Optimize blood pressure management with lisinopril (10 mg daily), targeting a goal of <130/80 mmHg. Review and adjust the patient's diabetes management plan to improve glycemic control (See algorithm below). **Non-pharmacological**: Recommend lifestyle changes, including dietary modifications, weight management, increased physical activity, and smoking cessation if applicable. Encourage stress management techniques and regular follow-up visits with his primary care physician to monitor and adjust medication as needed. **Follow-up**: Schedule follow-up in 1-2 weeks to reassess blood pressure, cholesterol, and diabetes management, and to ensure medication adherence. Consider carotid ultrasound and echocardiogram to evaluate for potential sources of embolism and assess stroke risk. Refer to a neurologist for further evaluation and consideration of advanced imaging, such as MRI or CT angiography, to confirm the diagnosis and assess risk. **Education**: Educate the patient on the nature of TIAs, their association with an increased risk of stroke, and the importance of timely intervention. Discuss lifestyle modifications to reduce risk factors, including adherence to medications, regular monitoring of blood pressure and blood sugar levels, and maintaining a heart-healthy diet. Advise the patient to seek immediate medical attention if symptoms recur or worsen.

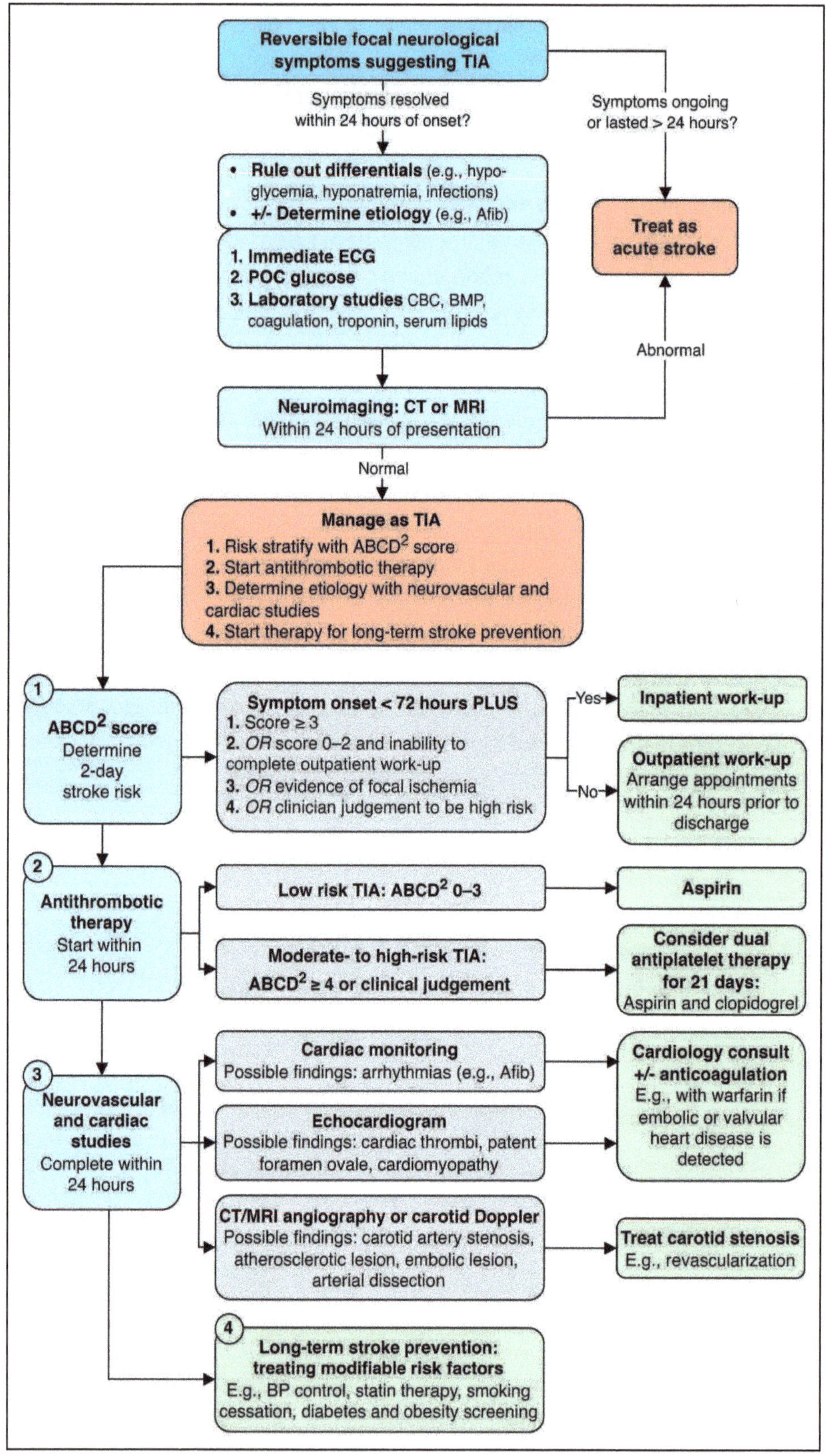

Reversible focal neurological symptoms suggesting TIA
Symptoms resolved within 24 hours of onset?
Symptoms ongoing or lasted > 24 hours?
Rule out differentials (e.g., hypoglycemia, hyponatremia, infections)
+/- Determine etiology (e.g., Afib)
Treat as acute stroke
1. Immediate ECG
2. POC glucose
3. Laboratory studies CBC, BMP, coagulation, troponin, serum lipids
Abnormal
Neuroimaging: CT or MRI
Within 24 hours of presentation
Normal
Manage as TIA
1. Risk stratify with ABCD2 score
2. Start antithrombotic therapy
3. Determine etiology with neurovascular and cardiac studies
4. Start therapy for long-term stroke prevention
1
ABCD2 score
Determine 2-day stroke risk
Symptom onset < 72 hours PLUS
1. Score ≥ 3
2. OR score 0–2 and inability to complete outpatient work-up
3. OR evidence of focal ischemia
4. OR clinician judgement to be high risk
Yes
Inpatient work-up
No
Outpatient work-up
Arrange appointments within 24 hours prior to discharge
2
Antithrombotic therapy
Start within 24 hours
Low risk TIA: ABCD2 0–3
Aspirin
Moderate- to high-risk TIA: ABCD2 ≥ 4 or clinical judgement
Consider dual antiplatelet therapy for 21 days:
Aspirin and clopidogrel
3
Neurovascular and cardiac studies
Complete within 24 hours
Cardiac monitoring
Possible findings: arrhythmias (e.g., Afib)
Echocardiogram
Possible findings: cardiac thrombi, patent foramen ovale, cardiomyopathy
Cardiology consult +/- anticoagulation
E.g., with warfarin if embolic or valvular heart disease is detected
CT/MRI angiography or carotid Doppler
Possible findings: carotid artery stenosis, atherosclerotic lesion, embolic lesion, arterial dissection
Treat carotid stenosis
E.g., revascularization
4
Long-term stroke prevention: treating modifiable risk factors
E.g., BP control, statin therapy, smoking cessation, diabetes and obesity screening

OTHER CONDITIONS

6.7.9 Dangerous headaches

Table 100 SOAP Notes for Dangerous Headaches

Component	Details
Subjective (S)	A 50-year-old male presents with a sudden-onset severe headache that started abruptly 2 hours ago, described as the "worst headache of his life." He reports associated nausea, vomiting, photophobia, and neck stiffness. The headache is concentrated in the occipital region and is not relieved by over-the-counter analgesics. He also mentions dizziness and difficulty walking. The patient has a history of hypertension, but otherwise has no significant medical history. He denies recent trauma or similar previous headaches but is concerned due to the intensity of the pain and his hypertension history.
Objective (O)	The patient appears in moderate distress due to headache and is sensitive to light. Vital signs: BP 170/100 mmHg, HR 88 bpm, Temp 37.2°C (99°F). Physical examination reveals neck rigidity and positive Brudzinski's sign and Kernig's sign. Neurological exam is notable for mild confusion but no focal deficits. CT scan of the head shows hyperdense areas in the subarachnoid space, suggestive of subarachnoid hemorrhage (SAH). The rest of the examination, including cranial nerve function and coordination, is normal.
Assessment (A)	The patient's presentation, including a severe sudden headache, neck stiffness, and positive Brudzinski's and Kernig's signs, along with CT findings, is consistent with subarachnoid hemorrhage (SAH). The hypertension and lack of prior trauma increase the suspicion of aneurysmal rupture as the cause. This is a medical emergency requiring immediate management to prevent complications like rebleeding or hydrocephalus.
Plan (P)	**Pharmacological:** Administer IV antihypertensives (e.g., labetalol) to reduce blood pressure and prevent rebleeding. Provide pain relief with acetaminophen or opioids as needed, avoiding NSAIDs due to bleeding risk. Consider anticonvulsants (e.g., levetiracetam) for seizure prophylaxis. **Non-pharmacological:** Neurosurgical consultation for assessment of potential aneurysm repair via coiling or clipping. Immediate ICU admission for monitoring and management of intracranial pressure (ICP). **Follow-up:** Schedule angiography (CT or MR angiography) to identify the source of the hemorrhage, particularly an aneurysm. Continuous monitoring for the first 24-48 hours in the ICU, with regular neurochecks for deterioration. **Education:** Educate the patient and family on the urgency of subarachnoid hemorrhage and the need for immediate intervention. Emphasize the risk of complications such as vision loss, seizures, and rebleeding.

6.7.10 Subarachnoid haemorrhage

Table 101 SOAP Notes for Subarachnoid haemorrhage

Component	Details
Subjective (S)	A 55-year-old male presents with sudden-onset severe headache described as the "worst headache of his life". He reports that the headache started abruptly while at rest and has been accompanied by nausea, vomiting, and photophobia. The patient also reports neck stiffness and light-headedness. He denies any recent head trauma but mentions a history of hypertension. He is concerned about a possible brain aneurysm since he has heard that his symptoms resemble those of a stroke.
Objective (O)	The patient appears acutely ill and in distress. Vital signs: BP 180/110 mmHg, HR 88 bpm, Temp 36.9°C (98.4°F), RR 20 bpm. Physical examination reveals neck rigidity, positive Brudzinski's sign, and Kernig's sign. The neurological exam shows alertness, but there is evidence of mild confusion. There is no focal neurological deficit. CT scan of the head shows hyperdense areas in the subarachnoid space, consistent with subarachnoid hemorrhage.
Assessment (A)	The patient's sudden onset of severe headache, associated symptoms of neck stiffness, and CT findings are highly indicative of subarachnoid hemorrhage (SAH). The patient's risk factors, including hypertension, increase the likelihood of aneurysm rupture, which is a common cause of SAH.
Plan (P)	**Pharmacological**: Administer IV antihypertensives (e.g., labetalol) to lower blood pressure to reduce the risk of rebleeding. Administer pain relief with acetaminophen or opioids, depending on severity. Anti-seizure prophylaxis with levetiracetam or phenytoin to prevent seizure activity, common in SAH. **Non-pharmacological:** Neurosurgical consult for potential clipping or coiling of the aneurysm if an aneurysm is identified. ICU admission for monitoring of neurological status, blood pressure, and possible complications such as rebleeding or hydrocephalus. **Follow-up:** Immediate CT angiography or digital subtraction angiography to identify the source of the bleeding (e.g., ruptured aneurysm). Follow-up in the ICU for 24-48 hours for monitoring. **Education:** The patient should be informed about the urgency of treatment for SAH and the potential need for surgical intervention. Emphasize blood pressure control and early detection of complications like rebleeding or hydrocephalus.

6.7.11 Giant arthritis

Table 102 SOAP Notes for Giant Arthritis

Component	Details
Subjective (S)	A 70-year-old female presents with headache, scalp tenderness, and pain in the jaw when chewing for the past week. She reports that the headache is located around the temples and is accompanied by fatigue, unexplained weight loss, and fever. She mentions that her vision has become blurry, and she is concerned that it may be related to her temporal arteries, as her

	mother had a similar condition. The patient also has a history of polymyalgia rheumatica.
Objective (O)	The patient appears fatigued but is not in acute distress. Vital signs: BP 145/90 mmHg, HR 85 bpm, Temp 37.8°C (100°F). Physical examination reveals tenderness over the temporal arteries and decreased pulse on the right side. Fundoscopic examination shows pale optic discs, and there is no papilledema. ESR is markedly elevated at 65 mm/h, and CRP is also elevated. Temporal artery biopsy is scheduled to confirm the diagnosis.
Assessment (A)	The patient's symptoms, including temporal headache, scalp tenderness, and jaw claudication, along with the elevated ESR and CRP, are highly suggestive of giant cell arteritis (GCA). The patient's history of polymyalgia rheumatica increases the likelihood of GCA, and prompt diagnosis and treatment are essential to prevent complications such as vision loss.
Plan (P)	**Pharmacological:** Start prednisone 60 mg daily for GCA to reduce inflammation and prevent complications such as vision loss. Consider a low-dose aspirin regimen (81 mg) to reduce the risk of vascular events. **Non-pharmacological:** Referral to a rheumatologist for further management and monitoring of GCA progression. **Follow-up:** Follow-up in 1 week to assess the response to steroids and adjust the dosage as needed. Consider temporal artery biopsy if not already performed to confirm the diagnosis. **Education:** The patient should be educated about the risks of untreated GCA, particularly the potential for permanent vision loss. Stress the importance of early steroid therapy and regular follow-up appointments to monitor for side effects.

6.7.12 Subdural hematoma

Table 103 SOAP Notes for Subdural Hematoma

Component	Details
Subjective (S)	A 72-year-old male presents with headache, dizziness, and confusion for the past 48 hours. The patient had a fall a week ago but did not seek medical attention at the time. He is now experiencing memory problems, difficulty concentrating, and has had difficulty walking steadily. He denies nausea, vomiting, or changes in vision but mentions feeling more fatigued than usual.
Objective (O)	The patient appears mildly confused but is oriented to person, place, and time. Vital signs: BP 130/85 mmHg, HR 78 bpm, Temp 36.6°C (97.9°F). Physical examination reveals no focal neurological deficits, but gait instability and mild dysmetria are present. CT scan of the head shows a crescent-shaped collection of blood over the right hemisphere, consistent with a subdural hematoma.
Assessment (A)	The patient's history of recent trauma, along with the onset of confusion, headache, and gait instability, is consistent with a subdural hematoma (SDH).

	The CT scan confirms the diagnosis, and the patient's age and history of falls suggest that this is likely an acute SDH.
Plan (P)	**Pharmacological:** Monitor the patient for signs of increased intracranial pressure (ICP) and manage accordingly. Consider anticonvulsant prophylaxis (e.g., levetiracetam) if the patient has a high risk of seizures. **Non-pharmacological:** Neurosurgical consult for evaluation of the hematoma. If the hematoma is significant or causing neurological deterioration, surgical intervention (e.g., craniotomy) may be required. **Follow-up:** Immediate hospital admission for monitoring and possible surgical intervention. Repeat CT scan in 24-48 hours to assess for any changes in the hematoma. **Education:** Educate the patient and family about the risks associated with subdural hematomas, including the potential for worsening symptoms and the need for prompt surgical intervention if the hematoma enlarges.

6.7.13 Carpal Tunnel Syndrome

Table 104 SOAP Notes for Carpel Tunnel Syndrome

Component	Details
Subjective (S)	A 38-year-old female presents with numbness and tingling in her right hand and wrist for the past 6 months. She describes the symptoms as worse at night and states that the tingling radiates into her thumb, index, and middle fingers. The patient works as a data entry clerk, spending long hours typing. She has tried wearing a wrist splint, but the symptoms persist. She denies any trauma or recent injury to the wrist.
Objective (O)	The patient appears in no acute distress but demonstrates mild muscle wasting in the thenar eminence of the right hand. Vital signs: BP 120/78 mmHg, HR 76 bpm, Temp 36.8°C (98.2°F). On physical examination, Tinel's sign is positive at the wrist, and Phalen's test reproduces the symptoms of tingling and numbness. Nerve conduction studies confirm median nerve compression at the level of the carpal tunnel, consistent with carpal tunnel syndrome.
Assessment (A)	The patient's symptoms, including nocturnal numbness and tingling in the distribution of the median nerve, along with positive physical exam findings and confirmation on nerve conduction studies, are consistent with carpal tunnel syndrome (CTS).
Plan (P)	**Pharmacological:** Recommend NSAIDs (e.g., ibuprofen 200-400 mg as needed) for pain relief and inflammation. Consider a short course of oral corticosteroids (e.g., prednisone) for 7-10 days if symptoms are severe or worsening. **Non-pharmacological:** Advise the patient to continue using a wrist splint at night and during activities that exacerbate the symptoms. Recommend ergonomic modifications to her workstation, including wrist positioning and breaks to reduce repetitive stress. **Follow-up:** Follow-up in 4 weeks to assess symptom improvement. If symptoms persist, consider

	corticosteroid injections or referral for surgical decompression of the carpal tunnel. **Education:** Educate the patient on the nature of CTS, including avoiding activities that exacerbate symptoms. Discuss the importance of early intervention to prevent permanent nerve damage.

6.7.14 Parkinson's Disease

Table 105 SOAP Notes for Parkinson's Disease

Component	Details
Subjective (S)	A 68-year-old male presents with a 12-month history of gradually worsening tremors in his right hand, along with stiffness and slowness of movement. The patient reports difficulty initiating movement, especially when rising from a chair or walking. He notes that the tremors worsen at rest and improve with voluntary movement. He denies any significant changes in mood or cognition. The patient has a history of hypertension and diabetes.
Objective (O)	The patient appears slightly slow in his movements but is not in acute distress. He has a resting tremor in the right hand, with a characteristic "pill-rolling" motion. On examination, there is mild rigidity in the right upper extremity (cogwheel rigidity) and bradykinesia, especially when initiating movements. Posture is slightly stooped, and there is reduced facial expressivity (masked facies). Gait is shuffling, with reduced arm swing on the right side. The Mini-Mental State Examination (MMSE) score is 28/30, indicating normal cognitive function.
Assessment (A)	The patient's symptoms of resting tremor, bradykinesia, rigidity, and postural changes, along with the clinical examination findings, are consistent with Parkinson's disease
	Pharmacological: Recommend initiating levodopa/carbidopa (e.g., Sinemet 25/100 mg three times daily) to address motor symptoms. Consider adding a dopamine agonist (e.g., pramipexole) if the response to levodopa is inadequate. **Non-pharmacological:** Refer the patient to physical therapy for gait training and balance exercises. Encourage regular exercise to maintain mobility and flexibility. Refer to speech therapy if dysphagia or vocal changes occur. **Follow-up:** Follow-up in 4-6 weeks to assess treatment efficacy and side effects. If symptoms worsen or levodopa responsiveness decreases, consider adding other medications such as MAO-B inhibitors or COMT inhibitors. **Education:** Educate the patient and family about Parkinson's disease, including the progressive nature of the disorder. Discuss the potential side effects of medications, including dyskinesia. Encourage the patient to engage in social and mental stimulation to maintain quality of life.

6.7.15 Myasthenia Gravis Diseases

Table 106 SOAP Notes for Myasthenia Gravis Disease

Component	Details
Subjective (S)	A 45-year-old female presents with a 3-month history of progressively worsening weakness in her eyelids and limbs. She reports drooping of the right eyelid, which worsens towards the end of the day, and difficulty swallowing and speaking clearly. The patient describes difficulty holding up her arms after prolonged use and increasing fatigue after activity. She denies any recent infections or trauma. Her symptoms improve with rest but worsen with sustained activity.
Objective (O)	The patient appears in no acute distress but exhibits ptosis in the right eye, which worsens with upward gaze. Muscle strength is reduced in both upper limbs, particularly with sustained abduction and flexion. There is mild dysphonia, and the patient demonstrates weakness with repetitive movements (e.g., unable to hold up arms after 1-2 minutes). Reflexes and sensation are normal. On physical examination, the weakness fluctuates with rest and activity. Ice pack test was positive for improvement of ptosis.
Assessment (A)	The patient's presentation of fluctuating muscle weakness, ptosis, dysphagia, and fatigue, along with the positive ice pack test, is consistent with Myasthenia Gravis (MG). The clinical presentation, including the involvement of ocular and bulbar muscles, raises suspicion of generalized MG.
Plan (P)	**Pharmacological:** Initiate anticholinesterase therapy (e.g., pyridostigmine 60 mg twice daily) to improve muscle strength. Consider a short course of oral corticosteroids (e.g., prednisone 30 mg daily) for exacerbation if symptoms are severe (See algorithm below). **Non-pharmacological:** Recommend frequent rest periods throughout the day to prevent fatigue and avoid prolonged activity. Advise the patient to avoid excessive heat and strenuous exercise. **Follow-up:** Follow-up in 2-4 weeks to assess medication effectiveness and side effects. If symptoms worsen or do not improve, consider initiating immune-modulating therapy such as azathioprine or intravenous immunoglobulin (IVIG). **Education:** Educate the patient and family on the chronic nature of MG, including the potential for exacerbations. Discuss the importance of medication adherence and the need for close monitoring of symptoms. Warn about the possibility of crisis situations (e.g., myasthenic crisis) and the need for emergency medical attention if respiratory symptoms worsen.

6.8 Moh Golden Points and Summary Question Answers

6.8.1 Moh Golden Points

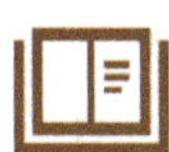
Recognizing the early signs of acute bacterial meningitis such as severe headache, fever, neck stiffness, photophobia, and confusion is critical.

Patient education about the management of medication overuse headaches and lifestyle modifications such as improving sleep hygiene and avoiding triggers

Correctly diagnosing TIA based on transient neurological symptoms like right-sided weakness, slurred speech, and the resolution of symptoms is crucial. .

Identifying multiple sclerosis early in the course of the disease is vital to providing the best management and slowing disease progression.

ALS, characterized by progressive motor neuron degeneration, requires timely initiation of pharmacological therapies.

Acute bacterial meningitis requires rapid intervention, including the administration of empiric antibiotics.

Bell's Palsy is often self-limiting but requires early medical intervention, particularly with corticosteroids like prednisone to reduce inflammation and improve recovery outcomes.

6.8.2 Summary Questions & Answers

1. What is the most common bacterial pathogen responsible for acute bacterial meningitis in adults?
a) Mycobacterium tuberculosis
b) Streptococcus pneumoniae
c) Borrelia burgdorferi
d) Treponema pallidum

2. Which of the following is a first-line treatment for acute bacterial meningitis due to *Streptococcus pneumoniae*?
a) Vancomycin and ceftriaxone
b) Azithromycin and ampicillin
c) Rifampin and acyclovir
d) Prednisone and doxycycline

3. Which of the following is the characteristic symptom of trigeminal neuralgia (tic douloureux)?
a) Dull, aching pain across the forehead
b) Sharp, electric shock-like pain along the face
c) Intense headache with photophobia
d) Nausea and vomiting associated with the headache

4. Which medication is considered the first-line treatment for acute migraine attacks with severe symptoms?
a) Acetaminophen
b) Triptans (e.g., sumatriptan)
c) Steroids
d) Calcium channel blockers

5. Which of the following is a characteristic feature of multiple sclerosis (MS)?
a) Sudden and severe onset of motor weakness
b) Progressive muscle weakness with no remissions
c) Fluctuating neurological symptoms with episodes of relapse and remission
d) Severe pain and swelling in the joints

6. What is the first-line treatment for acute bacterial meningitis caused by *Streptococcus pneumoniae*?
a) Vancomycin and ceftriaxone
b) Prednisone and acetaminophen
c) Rifampin and acyclovir
d) Amoxicillin and clindamycin

7. Which symptom is most commonly associated with amyotrophic lateral sclerosis (ALS)?
a) Unilateral facial weakness
b) Progressive muscle weakness and atrophy
c) Visual disturbances and blurred vision
d) Nausea and vomiting

8. Which of the following is a common initial symptom of Bell's Palsy?
a) Difficulty swallowing and speaking
b) Sudden-onset weakness or paralysis on one side of the face
c) Loss of vision in one eye

d) Severe headache and neck stiffness

9. What is the role of corticosteroids in the management of Bell's Palsy?

a) To prevent the spread of viral infections
b) To reduce inflammation of the facial nerve
c) To relieve pain in the affected areas
d) To improve visual symptoms

10. What diagnostic finding is most indicative of amyotrophic lateral sclerosis (ALS)?

a) Positive Brudzinski's sign
b) Evidence of both upper and lower motor neuron degeneration on EMG
c) Positive Kernig's sign
d) Elevated white blood cells in cerebrospinal fluid

6.8.3 Rationales

1. **Answer: b) *Streptococcus pneumoniae***

Rationale: ***Streptococcus pneumoniae*** **is the most common causative organism of acute bacterial meningitis in adults, as confirmed by a positive gram stain of cerebrospinal fluid (CSF) showing gram-positive diplococci, as seen in the case example.**

---

2. **Answer: a) Vancomycin and ceftriaxon**

Rationale: Empiric therapy with vancomycin and ceftriaxone is initiated to cover the most common causes of bacterial meningitis, including *Streptococcus pneumoniae*. These antibiotics provide broad coverage while awaiting final culture results..

---

3. **Answer: b) Sharp, electric shock-like pain along the face**

Rationale: Trigeminal neuralgia is characterized by sudden, sharp, electric shock-like pain in the regions governed by the trigeminal nerve (usually unilateral) and can be triggered by simple activities like chewing or brushing teeth..

---

4. **Answer: Answer: b) Triptans (e.g., sumatriptan)**

Rationale: Triptans, such as sumatriptan, are considered first-line treatment for moderate to severe migraines. They work by constricting blood vessels and inhibiting pain signals from the brain. Other medications like acetaminophen may be used for milder cases but are less effective for severe symptoms.

---

5. **Answer: c) Fluctuating neurological symptoms with episodes of relapse and remission**

Rationale: MS is known for its fluctuating neurological symptoms, which typically include episodes of relapse followed by remission. This characteristic is most commonly observed in the relapsing-remitting form of the disease.

---

6. **Answer: a) Vancomycin and ceftriaxone**

Rationale: The recommended empiric treatment for acute bacterial meningitis includes ceftriaxone and vancomycin to cover the common pathogens, including *Streptococcus pneumoniae*, until more specific information from cultures and sensitivity tests is available.

---

7. **Answer: b) Progressive muscle weakness and atrophy**

Rationale: ALS primarily affects motor neurons, leading to progressive muscle weakness, atrophy, and fasciculations. Symptoms typically involve both upper and lower motor neuron involvement and worsen over time.

---

8. **Answer: b) Sudden-onset weakness or paralysis on one side of the face**

Rationale: Bell's Palsy typically presents with sudden-onset facial weakness or paralysis, often starting with an inability to close the eye or smile on one side of the face, and may be associated with pain behind the ear..

---

9. **Answer: b) To reduce inflammation of the facial nerve**

Rationale: Corticosteroids, such as prednisone, are used to reduce the inflammation of the facial nerve in Bell's Palsy, which helps to speed up recovery and improve facial function.

---

10. **Answer: b) Evidence of both upper and lower motor neuron degeneration on EMG**

Rationale: The diagnosis of ALS is supported by electromyography (EMG) findings showing degeneration of both upper and lower motor neurons, which is characteristic of this progressive neurodegenerative disease.

7 Chapter 7: Renal System

7.1 Anatomy and Physiology of the Renal System

The renal system, also commonly called the **urinary system,** works to control volume and composition of the body fluids, to cleanse the body of **waste products, and to regulate electrolytes and acids.** The main structures of the renal system include the kidneys, which are chiefly involved in filtering blood, removing waste products and regulating ions in the body. This organ has an outer cortex and inner medulla, and consists of approximately one million nephrons, which are the working units of the kidneys. The nephron comprises the renal corpuscle and the renal tubule. **Renal corpuscle consists of the glomerulus**, a tuft of capillaries through which the blood is filtered and Bowman's capsule that receives the filtrate. The renal tubule is divided into several parts, namely, **the proximal convoluted tubule, the loop of Henle, the distal convoluted tubule, and the collecting duct.** This in turn facilitates the reabsorption of water, glucose, and electrolytes as well as the secretion of waste products like urea, creatinine and excess ions in the urine. The kidneys are also responsible **for hormone secretion as part of their functions** in the human body. They secrete erythropoietin, which is responsible for the production of the red blood cells in the bone marrow, as well as renin, which is involved in the regulation of blood pressure by the renin-angiotensin-aldosterone system. Moreover, significant roles of the kidneys are to activate vitamin D, which plays an important role in calcium absorption.

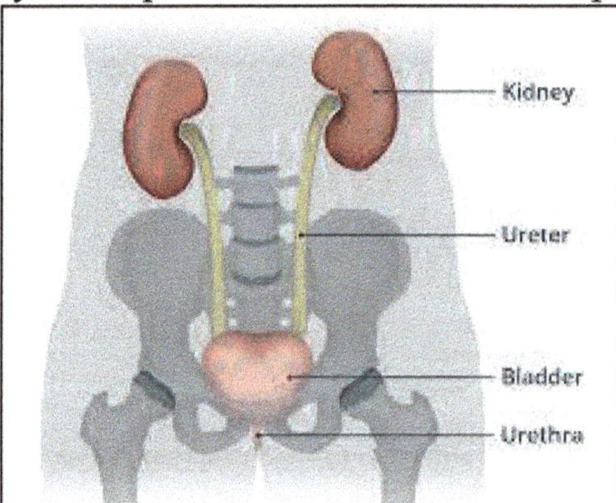

Figure 181 Overview of Renal System

7.2 ABG Buffer Systems in the Body

7.2.1 Arterial Blood Gases (ABG) and the Buffer System: A Detailed Discussion

Arterial blood gases (ABG) analysis is a critical diagnostic tool used in medicine to assess the **levels of oxygen (O_2), carbon dioxide (CO_2),** and the pH of arterial blood. It helps in diagnosing and monitoring various conditions related to acid-base balance, respiratory, and metabolic disorders. One key aspect of ABG is the role of the **buffer systems** in maintaining the body's acid-base balance. Buffer systems, particularly the **bicarbonate buffer system**, play an essential role in regulating the pH of the blood and ensuring that the body's internal environment remains stable despite fluctuations in CO_2 and H^+ concentrations.

The image illustrates the vital role of the bicarbonate buffer system in maintaining the proper pH of blood and body tissues. It highlights how the body uses two key organs, the lungs and kidneys, to regulate pH. The bicarbonate buffer system functions through a balance between **carbonic acid (H_2CO_3) and bicarbonate ions (HCO_3^-), which help to either add or remove hydrogen ions (H^+) to stabilize pH.** The **lungs** play a crucial role by adjusting the respiratory rate: when the pH drops (indicating acidosis), the lungs increase the respiratory rate to expel more CO_2, thereby decreasing acidity. Conversely, when pH rises (indicating alkalosis), the lungs decrease the respiratory rate, retaining CO_2 and reducing alkalinity. The **kidneys** assist by regulating the bicarbonate reserve, **either by reabsorbing bicarbonate ions or excreting hydrogen ions, depending on the body's pH status.** Together, these mechanisms maintain the pH of the blood and tissues within a narrow, optimal range, ensuring proper physiological function.

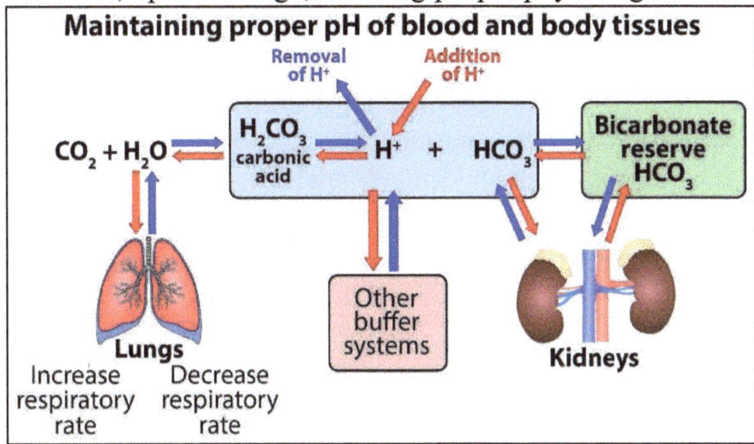

Figure 182 ABG Buffer System

7.2.1.1 Understanding Arterial Blood Gases (ABG)

ABG analysis provides a snapshot of the body's acid-base status by measuring several key parameters:

- **pH**: A measure of the acidity or alkalinity of blood, with a normal range of 7.35-7.45. Values below 7.35 indicate acidosis, while values above 7.45 indicate alkalosis.
- **Partial pressure of oxygen (PaO_2)**: Reflects the amount of oxygen in the arterial blood, normal range: 75-100 mmHg.
- **Partial pressure of carbon dioxide ($PaCO_2$)**: Represents the amount of CO_2 dissolved in the blood, normal range: 35-45 mmHg.
- **Bicarbonate (HCO_3^-)**: The primary buffer in the blood, normal range: 22-28 mEq/L.

The $PaCO_2$ and HCO_3^- levels are especially important in interpreting ABG results as they help in distinguishing between respiratory and metabolic causes of acidosis and alkalosis.

7.2.1.2 The Role of the Bicarbonate Buffer System

The **bicarbonate buffer system** is the most important buffer system in maintaining the pH of arterial blood. It functions primarily by balancing the ratio of carbonic acid (H_2CO_3) and bicarbonate ions (HCO_3^-). Carbonic acid is a weak acid that dissociates into hydrogen ions (H^+) and bicarbonate ions in a reversible reaction:

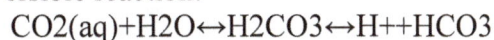

$$CO2(aq)+H2O \leftrightarrow H2CO3 \leftrightarrow H++HCO3$$

In this equilibrium:

- **CO_2 (carbon dioxide),** which is produced during metabolism, reacts with water (H_2O) in the blood to form **carbonic acid (H_2CO_3).**
- Carbonic acid dissociates into **hydrogen ions (H^+) and bicarbonate ions (HCO_3^-)**.

The concentration of CO_2 in the blood is a direct influence on the production of hydrogen ions. **$PaCO_2$** levels are tightly regulated by the respiratory system:

- When $PaCO_2$ rises (for example, due to hypoventilation), the concentration of H^+ increases, lowering the pH (leading to acidosis).

- When $PaCO_2$ decreases (for example, due to hyperventilation), the concentration of H^+ decreases, raising the pH (leading to alkalosis).

The kidneys help regulate the bicarbonate levels in the body, either by reabsorbing bicarbonate or secreting hydrogen ions into the urine, depending on the body's needs. Thus, the **bicarbonate buffer system** is the primary mechanism that prevents significant pH changes in response to fluctuations in CO_2 levels. It works in conjunction with the respiratory system, which regulates CO_2 levels, and the kidneys, which control bicarbonate levels, to maintain the blood pH within a narrow, optimal range of 7.35-7.45.

7.2.1.3 Respiratory and Metabolic Disorders in ABG

ABG analysis is essential in diagnosing and monitoring respiratory and metabolic disorders. The buffer systems play a key role in compensating for pH imbalances due to disturbances in these systems.

- **Respiratory Acidosis and Alkalosis**
- **Respiratory acidosis** occurs when the respiratory system is unable to eliminate enough CO_2, leading to an increase in $PaCO_2$. This results in an increase in hydrogen ion concentration, causing a decrease in pH (acidosis). Common causes of respiratory acidosis include chronic obstructive pulmonary disease (COPD), respiratory failure, or hypoventilation.
    - **ABG findings**: Low pH (<7.35), high $PaCO_2$ (>45 mmHg), and a compensatory increase in bicarbonate (HCO_3^-) over time as the kidneys attempt to restore pH balance.
- **Respiratory alkalosis** occurs when there is excessive CO_2 elimination, often due to hyperventilation, leading to a decrease in $PaCO_2$. This causes a reduction in hydrogen ions, increasing the pH (alkalosis). Causes include anxiety, panic attacks, and high altitudes.
    - **ABG findings**: High pH (>7.45), low $PaCO_2$ (<35 mmHg), and a compensatory decrease in bicarbonate (HCO_3^-) over time.

In both cases, the body compensates by adjusting bicarbonate levels through renal function, which may take several hours or days.

- **Metabolic Acidosis and Alkalosis**
- **Metabolic acidosis** results from an accumulation of acid in the body or a loss of bicarbonate. Causes include kidney failure, diabetic ketoacidosis, or lactic acidosis.
    - **ABG findings**: Low pH (<7.35), low HCO_3^- (<22 mEq/L), and a compensatory decrease in $PaCO_2$ as the body attempts to reduce CO_2 through hyperventilation.
- **Metabolic alkalosis** occurs when there is an excessive loss of hydrogen ions or an accumulation of bicarbonate. Causes include vomiting, excessive use of diuretics, or overuse of antacids.
    - **ABG findings**: High pH (>7.45), high HCO_3^- (>28 mEq/L), and a compensatory increase in $PaCO_2$ as the body attempts to retain CO_2 to lower the pH.

In both metabolic disorders, the **respiratory system** compensates by adjusting the $PaCO_2$ levels to counteract the pH changes. However, renal compensation is also crucial, especially in chronic conditions.

7.2.1.4 Compensation Mechanisms and ABG

Compensation refers to the body's physiological response to restore pH balance. There are two types of compensation:

- **Respiratory compensation**: The lungs can adjust the rate of CO_2 exhalation to change the pH. If the cause is metabolic acidosis (low pH), the respiratory system increases ventilation to expel more CO_2 and raise the pH. Conversely, if the cause is metabolic alkalosis (high pH), the respiratory rate decreases to retain CO_2 and lower the pH.

- **Renal compensation**: The kidneys compensate by adjusting the levels of bicarbonate in the blood. In metabolic acidosis, the kidneys increase the excretion of hydrogen ions and reabsorb bicarbonate. In metabolic alkalosis, the kidneys reduce bicarbonate reabsorption and excrete more bicarbonate to decrease the pH.

These compensatory mechanisms take time to activate, with respiratory compensation being faster (minutes to hours) and renal compensation taking longer (hours to days).

7.2.1.5 Clinical Application of ABG in Buffer Systems

ABG analysis is invaluable in clinical settings for:

- **Diagnosing acid-base disorders**: Understanding whether the cause is respiratory (due to CO_2) or metabolic (due to bicarbonate) allows clinicians to determine appropriate treatment strategies.
- **Monitoring therapy**: In critical care, ABG is used to assess the effectiveness of interventions such as mechanical ventilation or the administration of bicarbonate solutions.
- **Assessing respiratory function**: ABG analysis helps monitor oxygenation (PaO_2) and ventilation ($PaCO_2$), which are critical in diseases such as asthma, COPD, and pneumonia.

7.3 Intracellular and Extracellular Fluids: Understanding Their Role in Osmosis and Diffusion

The human body is made up of water, which constitutes a significant portion of its total mass. Water is primarily distributed between two major fluid compartments: **intracellular fluid (ICF) and extracellular fluid (ECF).** The balance between these compartments is crucial for maintaining cellular functions, homeostasis, and proper organ function. The processes that govern the movement of water and solutes between these compartments are **osmosis and diffusion. Understanding the differences between hypertonic, isotonic, and hypotonic solutions** is essential in grasping how fluids and solutes move in and out of cells, influencing their health and functioning.

7.3.1 Intracellular and Extracellular Fluid

Intracellular Fluid (ICF) refers to the fluid within the cells, making up approximately two-thirds of the total body water. This fluid is essential for maintaining the cell's internal environment, which facilitates biochemical reactions and other cellular activities. The composition of intracellular fluid includes high concentrations of **potassium ions (K^+), phosphate ions (PO_4^{3-}), and proteins, with a low concentration of sodium ions (Na^+).** The presence of these solutes is vital for maintaining the cell's osmotic balance and facilitating proper enzymatic function and cellular processes.

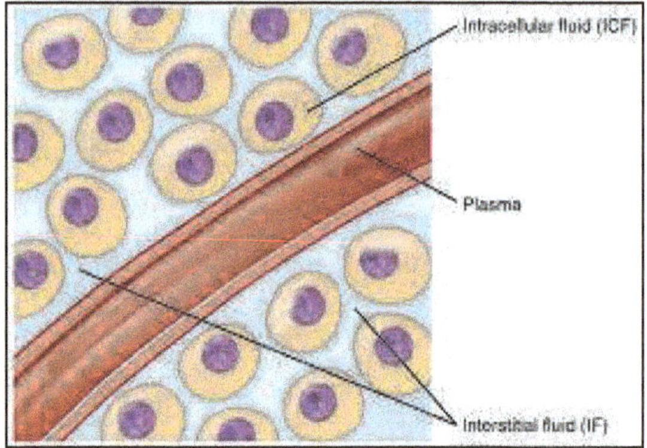

Figure 183 Understanding Intracellular Fluid

On the other hand, **extracellular fluid (ECF)** is the fluid found outside the cells, making up about one-third of the total body water. ECF is primarily composed of two parts: **interstitial fluid, which bathes the cells, and plasma**, which is the liquid component of blood. ECF contains high concentrations of **sodium ions (Na^+), chloride ions (Cl^-), and bicarbonate ions (HCO_3^-),** with relatively low concentrations of potassium and phosphate ions. The composition of ECF is crucial for maintaining blood pressure, nutrient transport, and waste removal, as well as for ensuring proper cell function by maintaining a stable environment for cells.

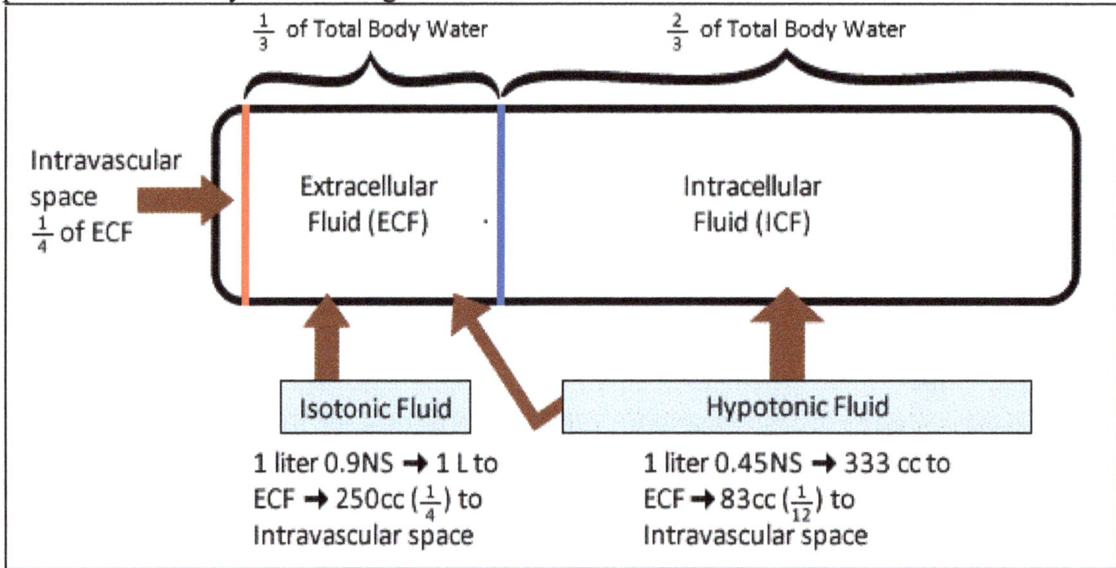

Figure 184 Understanding Extracellular Fluid

7.3.2 Osmosis and Diffusion in Fluid Movement

Osmosis is the movement of water across a semipermeable membrane, from a region of low solute concentration to a region of high solute concentration. It plays a key role in regulating the balance of water between intracellular and extracellular fluids. Osmosis occurs because water molecules move in response to **differences in the concentration of solutes across membranes, driven by the principle of osmotic pressure. Diffusion, in contrast, refers to the movement of solutes from an area of higher concentration to an area of lower concentration**. It does not require energy and occurs due to the random motion of molecules. Both osmosis and diffusion are fundamental processes that ensure proper nutrient delivery, waste removal, and fluid balance in the body.

7.3.3 The Concepts of Hypertonic, Isotonic, and Hypotonic Solutions

The terms **hypertonic, hypotonic, and isotonic** refer to the relative concentrations of solutes in solutions compared to the inside of a cell, which directly affects the movement of water and solutes.

7.3.3.1 Hypertonic Solution

A hypertonic solution has a higher concentration of solutes compared to the inside of the cell. When cells are exposed to hypertonic solutions, water moves out of the cell into the extracellular fluid to dilute the higher concentration of solutes. **This causes the cell to shrink or crenate. A common example of a hypertonic solution is seawater**. When a cell is placed in seawater, the osmotic gradient causes the cell to lose water, leading to dehydration.

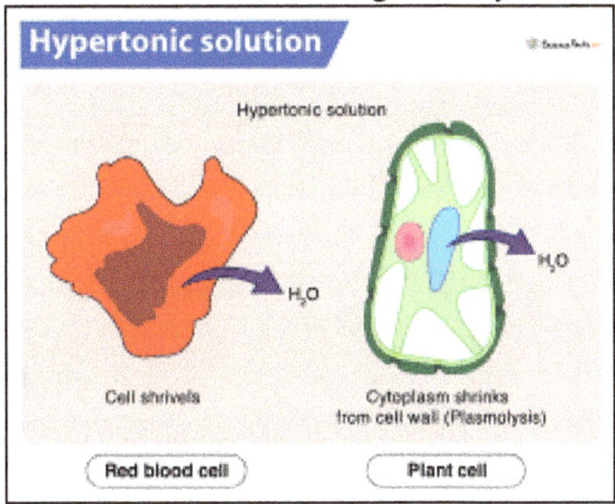

Figure 185 Hypertonic Solution

7.3.3.2 Hypotonic Solution

A hypotonic solution has a lower concentration of solutes compared to the inside of the cell. When a cell is exposed to a hypotonic solution, water moves into the cell, where the solute concentration is higher. **This influx of water causes the cell to swell and, in extreme cases, lyse (burst) if the osmotic pressure becomes too great.** An example of a hypotonic solution is pure water, which, when introduced into the body, can lead to cells absorbing excessive amounts of water.

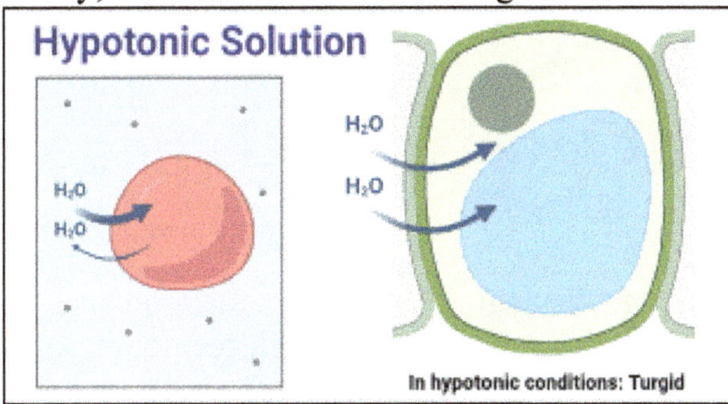

Figure 186 Hypotonic Solution

7.3.3.3 Isotonic Solution

An isotonic solution has the same concentration of solutes as the cell's interior, meaning there is no net movement of water into or out of the cell. **The cell retains its normal shape and function. An example of an isotonic solution is 0.9% saline (normal saline),** which is commonly used in medical treatments like intravenous fluids, as it maintains cellular balance.

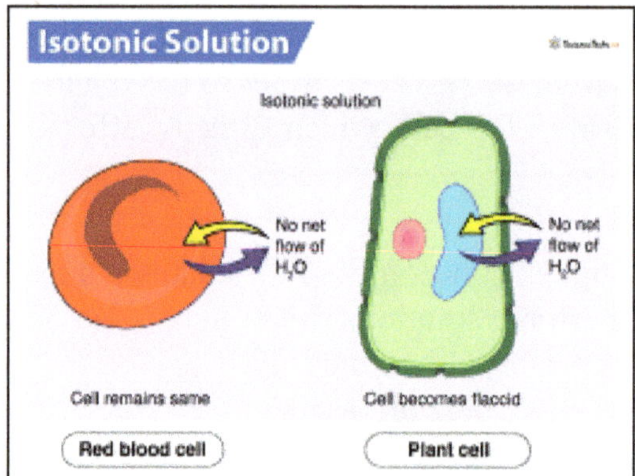

Figure 187 Isotonic Solution

7.3.4 Osmosis in Cellular Fluid Regulation

The movement of water in and out of cells is primarily governed by **osmotic pressure, which is determined by the solute concentration of the extracellular and intracellular fluids.** The **osmotic balance between the ICF and ECF** ensures that cells do not lose or gain excessive amounts of water, which could disrupt their internal environment.

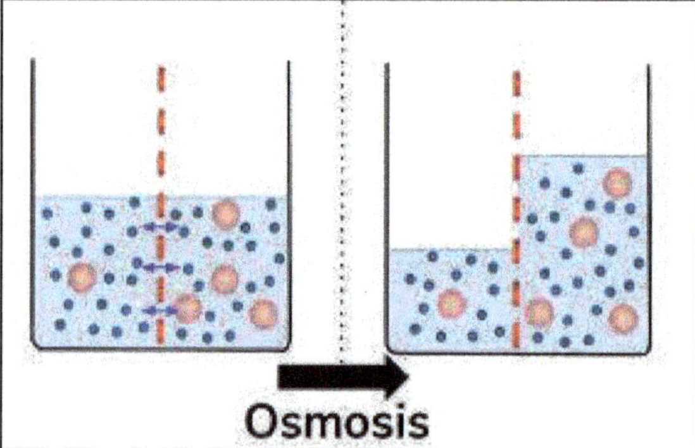

Figure 188 Osmosis Regulation

In a **hypertonic environment**, water moves out of the cells, leading to dehydration and shrinking. This can impair cellular functions and metabolic processes. For example, when red blood cells are placed in hypertonic solutions, they lose water and shrivel, impairing their ability to transport oxygen effectively. In contrast, in a **hypotonic environment**, water enters the cells, potentially causing them to swell and rupture. This can occur in certain types of kidney failure, where the kidneys are unable to properly regulate the body's fluid balance.

7.3.5 Diffusion and Its Role in Fluid Balance

While osmosis regulates water movement, **diffusion** is crucial for the movement of solutes, such as oxygen, carbon dioxide, glucose, and ions, across cell membranes. Solutes tend to move from areas of high concentration to low concentration, and this process occurs both in the extracellular and intracellular fluids. **Diffusion ensures that cells receive nutrients and oxygen and expel waste products like carbon dioxide efficiently.** The movement of gases, such as oxygen and carbon dioxide, occurs via simple diffusion across the respiratory membranes of the lungs into the bloodstream or out of the cells. For example, **in the lungs, oxygen diffuses from the alveoli (where its concentration is high) into the blood (where its concentration is low).** Similarly, carbon dioxide, which is produced as a waste product in cells, diffuses from the blood (where its concentration is high) into the alveoli to be exhaled.

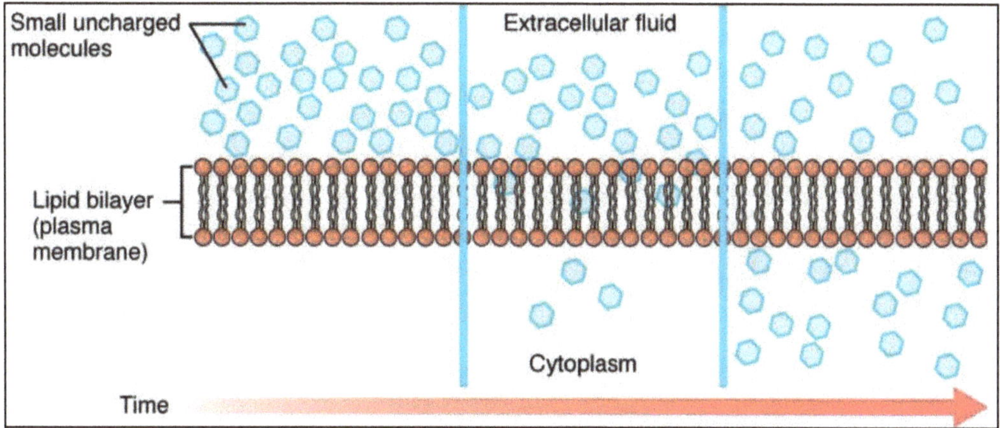

Figure 189 Difussion Transport Across Plasma Membrane

7.3.6 The Role of Membrane Proteins in Fluid and Solute Transport

Cell membranes are semipermeable and consist of lipid bilayers with embedded proteins that facilitate the movement of substances. **Aquaporins, for example, are membrane proteins that selectively allow water molecules to move in and out of cells during osmosis.** Similarly, **ion channels and transporters** are responsible for regulating the movement of specific ions and molecules. These proteins help maintain the proper concentrations of solutes and water in both intracellular and extracellular compartments. **Active transport** mechanisms, such as the **sodium-potassium pump (Na+/K+ ATPase),** also play a vital role in maintaining the balance of ions between ICF and ECF. This pump uses ATP to move sodium ions out of the cell and potassium ions into the cell, against their concentration gradients, contributing to the electrochemical gradients that drive many physiological processes, including nerve transmission and muscle contraction.

Understanding the movement of water and solutes through the processes of osmosis and diffusion is critical to maintaining fluid balance within the body. **The intracellular and extracellular fluids** must remain in a delicate equilibrium to ensure proper cellular function and overall health. By understanding the concepts of **hypertonic**, **hypotonic**, and **isotonic solutions**, as well as the role of diffusion in solute transport, it becomes clear that the body relies on highly regulated mechanisms to maintain homeostasis. These processes ensure that cells receive the nutrients and oxygen they need while efficiently removing waste products, thus enabling normal cellular and systemic functions.

7.4 Common Renal Conditions

"Aunt Patty Always Hot Pizza After Really Big Red Sauce." Here's the breakdown: Aunt = Acute and Chronic Kidney Disease, Patty = Pyelonephritis, Always = Acute Kidney Injury, Hot = Hematuria, Pizza = Proteinuria, After = Asymptomatic Bacteriuria, Really = Renal Nephrolithiasis (Kidney Stones), Big = Bladder Cancer, Red = Rhabdomyolysis, Sauce = (Remaining for clinical reminders, especially for tests and follow-ups)

Table 107 Overview of Major Clinical Conditions of Renal System

Condition	Description	Key Symptoms	Diagnostic Tools	Treatment Options
Pyelonephritis	Bacterial infection of the kidneys, usually ascending from the bladder.	Fever, flank pain, painful urination,	Urinalysis, urine culture, blood	Antibiotics, hydration, pain management

		nausea, vomiting	culture, ultrasound, CT scan	
Acute Kidney Injury (AKI)	Sudden decrease in kidney function, resulting in the buildup of waste products.	Decreased urine output, swelling, shortness of breath, confusion	Blood tests (creatinine, BUN), urine tests, ultrasound, biopsy	Fluid management, dialysis, treatment of underlying cause
Hematuria	Presence of blood in the urine, indicating a potential problem with the urinary system.	Pink or red urine, discomfort during urination	Urinalysis, urine culture, imaging (CT, ultrasound), cystoscopy	Treatment depends on the underlying cause (e.g., antibiotics, surgery)
Proteinuria	Excess protein in the urine, often indicative of kidney damage.	Frothy urine, swelling, fatigue	Urine protein test (24-hour urine collection, dipstick test)	Address underlying cause, ACE inhibitors, diuretics, lifestyle changes
Complicated and Uncomplicated UTI	Presence of bacteria in the urine without symptoms, often found in certain high-risk populations.	None	Urine culture, urinalysis	No treatment necessary unless symptomatic or at high risk of complications
Renal Nephrolithiasis (Kidney Stones)	Formation of solid crystals in the kidneys that can block the urinary tract.	Severe flank pain, hematuria, nausea, vomiting	Urinalysis, imaging (CT scan, ultrasound), X-ray	Pain management, hydration, lithotripsy, surgery (for large stones)
Bladder Cancer	Malignant growth in the bladder, often due to smoking or chemical exposure.	Hematuria, frequent urination, painful urination	Cystoscopy, urine cytology, biopsy, imaging (CT, MRI)	Surgery (resection, cystectomy), chemotherapy, immunotherapy

Rhabdomyolysis	Rapid muscle breakdown leading to the release of muscle cell contents into the bloodstream.	Muscle pain, weakness, dark urine, fatigue	Blood tests (creatinine kinase, myoglobin), urine analysis	IV fluids, addressing underlying cause, dialysis in severe cases

7.5 Major Medical Issues in the Renal System

CHRONIC CONDITIONS

7.5.1 Proteinuria

Proteinuria indicates when **proteins appear in excessive amounts in urine** and typically indicates kidney damage or dysfunction. The kidneys sustain essential proteins through their filtering process but **eliminate waste products from bloodstream during regular function**. The process of kidney filtration becomes impaired when proteins especially albumin start to leak into the urine. Proteinuria exists in two basic forms which are persistent as well as transient. The condition called **proteinuria exists only during short periods when dehydration or exercise or fever are present** before resolving when the source of these factors is corrected. Doctors analyze persistent proteinuria to diagnose serious kidney diseases among glomerulonephritis alongside diabetic nephropathy **and high blood pressure-related kidney damage**. Proteinuria does not generate major symptoms in most cases because people rarely detect its manifestation until the condition reaches advanced stages. The long-term presence of **proteinuria results in edema, fatigue along with foamy urine appearance.** Doctoral diagnosis of protein levels and kidney health involves three methods: urine **protein-to-creatinine ratio and 24-hour urine collection and urine dipstick tests.** The clinical treatment of proteinuria requires the management of fundamental causes. The prevention of kidney damage occurs when diabetes is managed alongside high blood pressure medications including **ACE inhibitors or angiotensin receptor blockers (ARBs)** which decrease protein leakage. Early detection followed by prompt intervention stands as a crucial factor which protects against the development of **chronic kidney disease (CKD).**

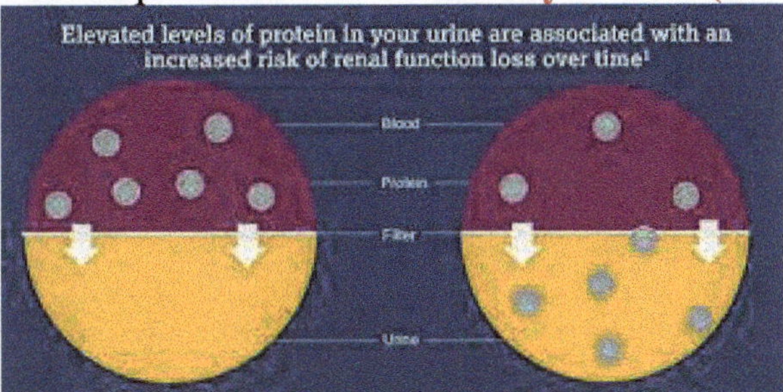

Figure 190 Proteinuria Elaboration

7.5.1.1 Classification of Proteinuria

The image displays a **proteinuria classification system that combines types with their root causes.** Transient proteinuria appears only temporarily since it develops when **fever or stress, along with dehydration or cold exposure, lead to brief periods of protein excretion**. Prolonged standing leads to orthostatic proteinuria because hidden glomerular changes and excessive changes in blood pressure create this condition. A chronic persistence of proteins in the urine implies advanced diseases like diabetes or lupus, along with other kidney disorders to indicate permanent kidney dysfunction. The urinary tract conditions, including **UTIS or kidney stones** that affect the kidneys and bring about protein leakage, account for post-renal proteinuria. The renal tubules' damage results in tubular proteinuria, which develops in Wilson's disease, cystinosis and when patients use nephrotoxic medications or experience interstitial nephritis, leading to impaired protein reabsorption. The **glomerular basement membrane** gets damaged in such cases which makes proteins (including albumin) leak into urine through the affected membrane during conditions of **IgA nephropathy or glomerulonephritis.** The kidneys become overwhelmed in their filtering capacity by excess protein production as a result of multiple myeloma and rhabdomyolysis, which leads to overflow proteinuria. The different proteinuria classifications aid both diagnosis and understanding of protein loss root causes which assists medical professionals in selecting the correct therapeutic approaches.

Table 108 Classification of Proteinuria

Proteinuria	Causes
Transient	Fever, Stress, Dehydration, Cold exposure
Orthostatic	Subtle glomerular abnormality, Exaggerated hemodynamic response
Persistent	Diabetes, Lupus, Renal disease
Post-renal	UTIs, Nephrolithiasis
Tubular	Wilson Disease, Cystinosis, Nephrotoxic medicines, interstitial nephritis, ATN
Glomerular	Glomerular basement membrane damage, Minimal change disease, IgA Nephropathy
Overflow	Multiple myeloma, Rhabdomyolysis

7.5.1.2 Types of Proteinuria

This image shows the four major types of proteinuria, which display distinct urinary protein characteristics along with their underlying causes. The main feature of glomerular proteinuria includes albumin as the **primary protein found in blood plasma.** The damage to glomerular filtration units leads to albumin leakage into urine. Medical professionals often identify glomerulonephritis along with diabetic nephropathy as conditions leading to this phenomenon. Renal tubular damage that affects how these structures absorb proteins will result in **urinary loss of small beta-2 microglobulin proteins** and other proteins with low molecular mass. The medical condition is characterised by heavy metal toxicity as well as the use of certain medication treatments, and it can also result from acute tubular necrosis. The kidneys cannot process the large amount of proteins, including **haemoglobin and Bence-Jones proteins**, and myoglobin that **results in overload proteinuria**. The appearance of proteinuria happens when the body experiences conditions such as hemolysis, as well as multiple myeloma and rhabdomyolysis. The urinary tract condition of post-renal proteinuria develops because of inflammatory processes alongside **bleeding and tumour development beneath the kidneys.** The urinary tract infection and kidney stones, together with bladder or urethral cancers, demonstrate this proteinuria condition. The different types of proteinuria serve as diagnostic tools for identifying the basis illness so doctors can select proper treatment methods.

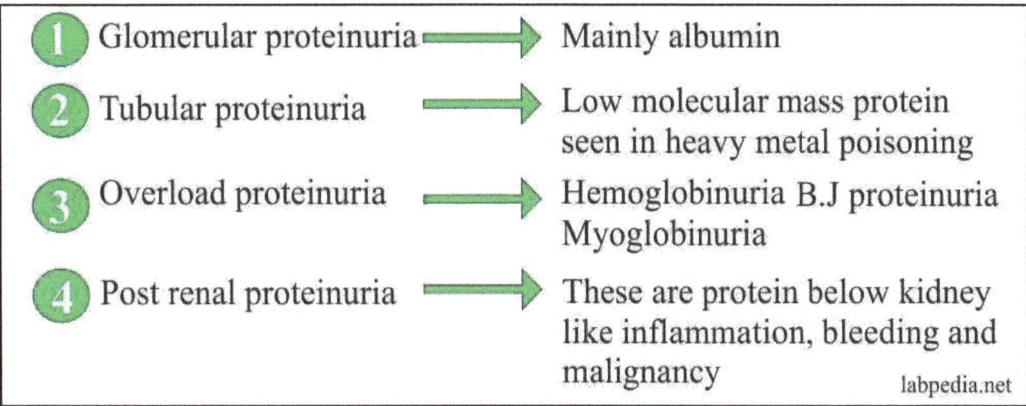

Figure 191 Types of Proteinuria

7.5.1.3 SOAP Notes for Proteinuria

Table 109 SOAP Notes for Proteinuria

Component	Details
Subjective (S)	A 52-year-old male presents with a routine health checkup where urine tests show the presence of protein in his urine. The patient denies any symptoms such as swelling, fatigue, or pain. He reports no issues with urination, no changes in frequency, and no pain while urinating. His medical history includes well-controlled hypertension and type 2 diabetes. He denies any recent infections, trauma, or strenuous physical activity. He is concerned about the findings and wants to understand their implications.
Objective (O)	The patient appears generally healthy with no signs of distress. Vital signs: BP 135/85 mmHg, HR 78 bpm, Temp 36.7°C (98.1°F). On physical examination, there is no edema or tenderness. Urinalysis shows a protein-to-creatinine ratio of 0.5 (indicating mild proteinuria). Urine dipstick test shows a trace amount of protein. The patient's blood tests reveal normal renal function with a serum creatinine level of 1.0 mg/dL and BUN of 18 mg/dL. HbA1c is 6.5%, indicating controlled diabetes. The rest of the physical exam and lab tests are unremarkable.
Assessment (A)	The patient's urinalysis and protein-to-creatinine ratio indicate mild proteinuria. Given his history of diabetes and hypertension, this is likely an early sign of kidney involvement, possibly glomerular proteinuria related to his diabetes. However, transient proteinuria due to recent physical exertion or stress cannot be ruled out. Further investigation is warranted to assess the cause, especially given the risk of diabetic nephropathy.
Plan (P)	**Pharmacological**: Continue current antihypertensive and antidiabetic medications. Consider starting an **ACE inhibitor** or **ARB** if proteinuria persists, as these medications can help reduce kidney damage (See algorithm below) **Non-pharmacological**: Advise lifestyle modifications, including weight management, increased physical activity, and reducing salt intake to control blood pressure. **Follow-up**: Schedule a follow-up visit in 3-6 months to repeat urinalysis and assess kidney function. If proteinuria

	persists or worsens, further testing, including a 24-hour urine collection, renal ultrasound, or kidney biopsy, may be needed. **Education**: Educate the patient on the significance of proteinuria as an early indicator of kidney damage, particularly in the context of diabetes and hypertension. Discuss the importance of blood pressure and blood sugar control in preventing kidney damage.

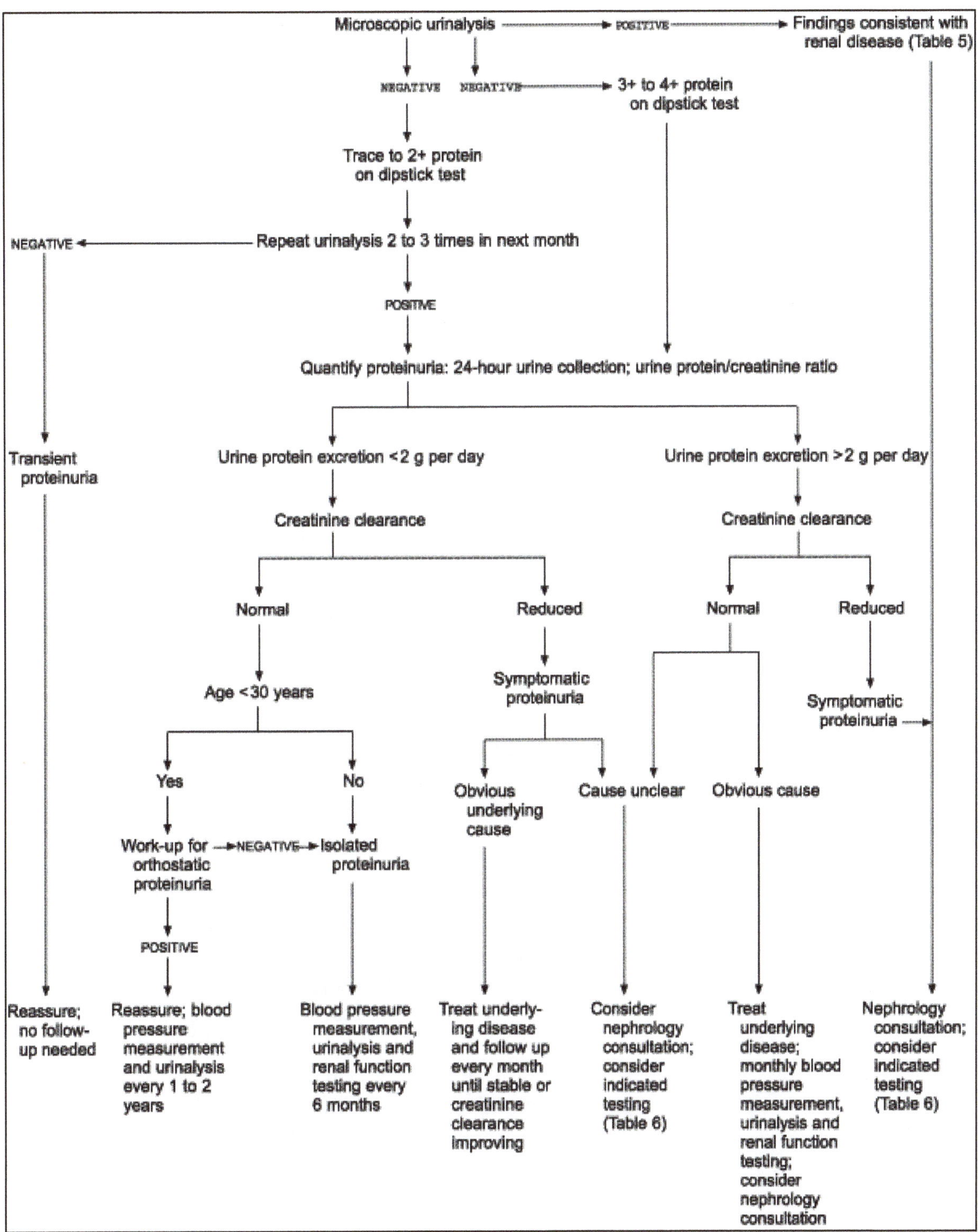

Figure 192 Management Algorithm for Proteinuria

7.5.2 Urinary Tract Infections

Asymptomatic bacteriuria refers to the presence of bacteria in the urine without any signs or symptoms of a **urinary tract infection (UTI).** Doctors typically discover this condition through standard urine testing, especially among three specific groups, including elderly patients, expectant mothers and patients with **diabetes and other ongoing medical conditions.** People who have asymptomatic bacteriuria experience no immediate symptoms, yet this situation remains dangerous for selected high-risk population groups. The absence of treatment for asymptomatic bacteria in pregnant women leads to kidney infections known as pyelonephritis, as well **as preterm labour and low birth weight for their newborns.** The condition can cause stronger infections and medical problems for people with weak immune systems and patients with invasive urinary procedures. The medical community does not require treatment of asymptomatic bacteriuria **among individuals who do not have risk factors.** Treatment initiatives for asymptomatic bacteriuria remain unnecessary unless the patient faces any of these three situations: pregnancy status, urological procedure demands or existing conditions that increase the risk of complications. A doctor uses urine culture tests to diagnose this condition through bacterial growth results while differentiating it from **UTIS by the absence of symptoms**. The standard course of action consists of antibiotic medications for certain cases, although antibiotic resistance develops when physicians prescribe antibiotics excessively to patients with **asymptomatic bacteriuria; thus, clinicians** need to follow proper treatment guidelines.

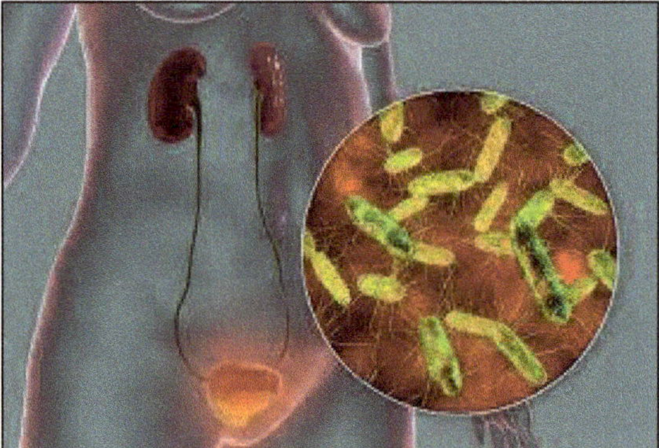

Figure 193 Overview of UTI

7.5.2.1 Classification of UTI

This image shows the progressive management of **urinary tract infections (UTIs) from asymptomatic bacteriuria (ABU)** to severe complications, which may lead **to organ failure. Asymptomatic bacteriuria (ABU)** is distinguished as a mild condition since patients display no symptoms, but medical experts confirm the diagnosis using dipstick tests and urine cultures. The infection evolves to cause dysuria together with frequency, urgency and bladder tenderness symptoms during the local symptom phase. The worsening infection causes additional symptoms of fever along with flank pain and nausea, and vomiting, which indicates both **febrile UTI along with systemic response (SIRS)** where fever and circulatory issues appear. The worst infection manifestations include circulatory failure and organ dysfunction, which can lead to complete organ failure. Medical tests become progressively more complex as the infection progresses from simple to intricate, therefore requiring blood culture testing along with renal ultrasound screening and CT scan evaluation for advanced stages. The **ORENUC framework allows health professionals to evaluate risk factors** in order to assess treatment requirements. The treatment duration for uncomplicated UTIS depends on the length of **3-5 days using one antibiotic** before progressing to two antibiotics **for seven to fourteen days**, as required for complicated UTIS. Advanced infection levels might require drainage procedures combined with surgical intervention to treat the infection effectively.

7.5.2.2 Complicated and Uncomplicated UTI

Community-acquired uncomplicated UTIs are usually observed in women, who are in a good health and with no or no **significant structural or functional abnormality of the urinary system**. They are often clinical sign because they are mostly associated with **dysuria, frequency of micturition and turbid coloured urine.** The treatment is usually with a short course of antibiotics, and the outcome is good in nearly all cases. However, **complicated UTIs are contracted by those with factors that include diabetes, anatomical structure changes, or**

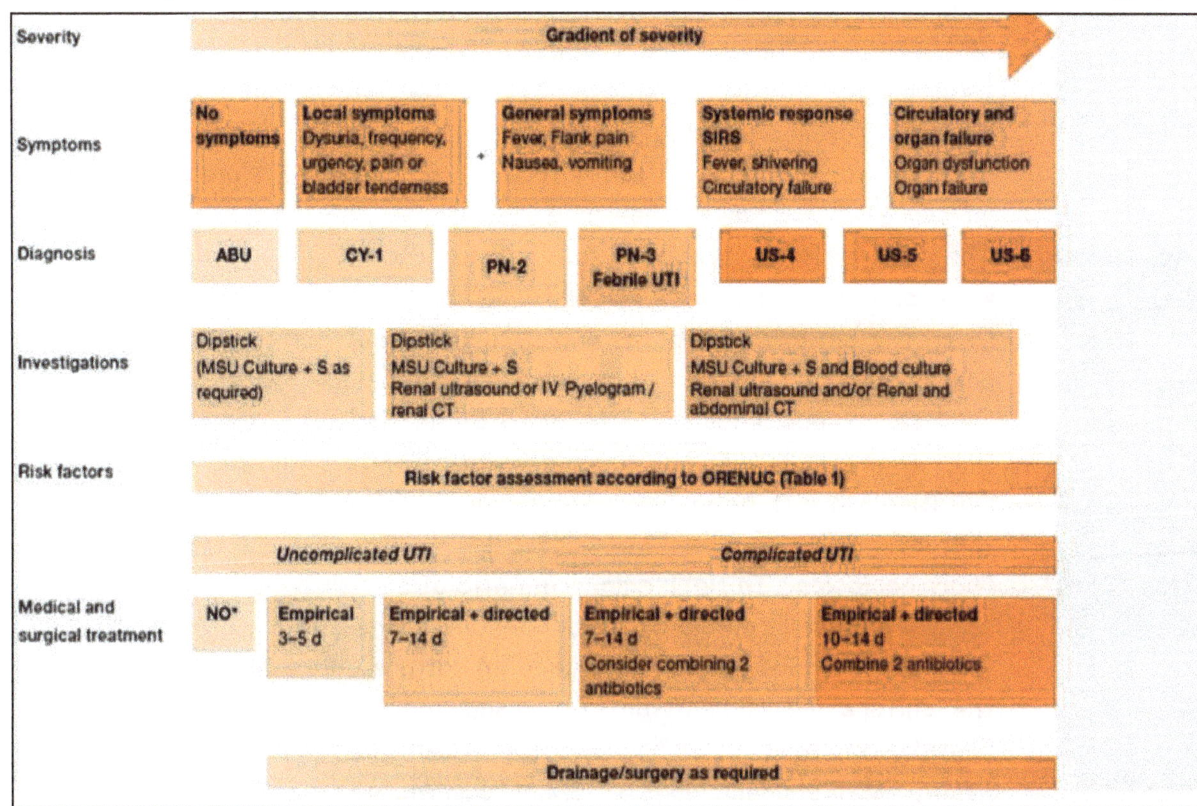

Figure 194 Classification of UTI Based on Grading of Severity

immune suppressed systems. They more frequently develop symptomatic complications; the symptoms may be more severe, for example, fever, back pains or systemic signs indicating the involvement of other body systems that require longer duration of antibiotics and more vigorous treatment. Symptomatic and asymptomatic UTIs concern the **growth of bacteria in urine, but the latter does not cause any signs or symptoms.** In this situation, the management should not be performed, unless it is imperative such as during pregnancy or in any urologic procedures, while in complicated cases, the approach depends on certain factors such as risks of renal compromise or sepsis.

7.5.2.3 SOAP Notes for UTI

Table 110 SOAP Notes for Asymptomatic Bacteriuria

Component	Details
Subjective (S)	A 65-year-old female presents with a 3-day history of dysuria, increased frequency, and urgency of urination. She reports feeling feverish and has

	experienced lower abdominal discomfort. She denies any back pain or hematuria but mentions some mild nausea. The patient has a history of recurrent UTIs but has not experienced similar symptoms recently. She is postmenopausal and has diabetes mellitus, which is poorly controlled. The patient is concerned that she may be developing another urinary infection.
Objective (O)	The patient appears slightly uncomfortable but is not in acute distress. Vital signs: BP 140/85 mmHg, HR 92 bpm, Temp 38.2°C (100.8°F). Physical exam reveals tenderness in the lower abdomen, but no costovertebral angle tenderness. Urinalysis shows leukocytes, nitrites, and a moderate amount of bacteria. Urine culture is sent for further analysis. Blood tests show elevated white blood cell count (WBC 12,000/µL) but normal kidney function (serum creatinine 0.9 mg/dL, BUN 16 mg/dL). There are no signs of dehydration, and the patient does not exhibit signs of systemic inflammatory response syndrome (SIRS).
Assessment (A)	The patient's symptoms of dysuria, fever, and increased frequency, along with positive urine culture for bacteria, are consistent with a febrile UTI. Given the patient's diabetes and recurrent UTI history, this could be a complicated UTI. Her presentation suggests local urinary tract involvement, and while her vital signs do not indicate severe infection or systemic organ failure, she is at increased risk due to her diabetes. Further investigation into her urine culture will help guide appropriate antibiotic therapy.
Plan (P)	**Pharmacological**: Initiate empirical antibiotic therapy with trimethoprim-sulfamethoxazole or ciprofloxacin pending urine culture results. Continue treatment for 7-14 days, depending on culture and sensitivity results. If the culture grows resistant organisms, adjust antibiotics accordingly. Consider starting an antipyretic for fever management (See algorithm below). **Non-pharmacological**: Encourage increased fluid intake to help flush the urinary tract. Advise the patient to rest and avoid further irritation to the urinary system. **Follow-up**: Schedule a follow-up visit in 3-5 days to assess symptoms and ensure the effectiveness of antibiotics. If symptoms persist or worsen, further imaging such as renal ultrasound may be necessary to rule out complications such as pyelonephritis or kidney stones. **Education**: Educate the patient on the importance of blood sugar control to help prevent future infections and on completing the full course of antibiotics. Discuss the potential for recurrence and the need for regular monitoring of urinary health due to her diabetes.

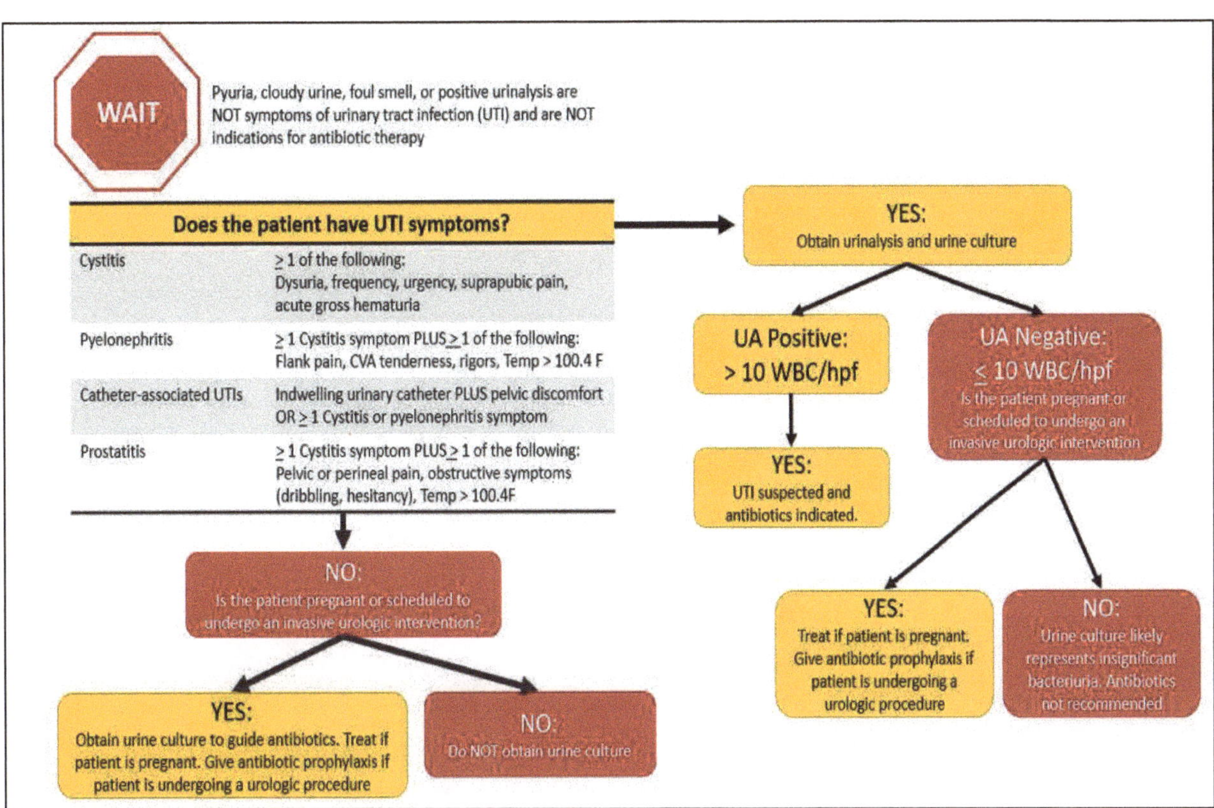

Figure 195 Management Algorithm for Urinary Tract Infections

Table 111 Management and Antibiotic Choices for Different Types of Urinary Tract Infections (UTIs)

Type of UTI	Category	First-Line Antibiotics	Second-Line Antibiotics	Other Considerations
Uncomplicated Lower UTI	Non-pregnant females	Nitrofurantoin, Trimethoprim (if low resistance risk)	Nitrofurantoin (if not used first line), Fosfomycin, Pivmecillinam, Amoxicillin	Delay antibiotics if symptoms resolve, use back-up prescriptions
	Males	Nitrofurantoin, Trimethoprim	Pyelonephritis or prostatitis management if symptoms persist	Immediate prescription, obtain urine culture before treatment
	Pregnant females	Nitrofurantoin	Amoxicillin (if susceptible), Cefalexin	Immediate treatment and culture, avoid trimethoprim and some others

Asymptomatic Bacteriuria	All groups	Amoxicillin, Cefalexin, Nitrofurantoin	-	Only treat if clinically relevant, especially during pregnancy
Recurrent UTI	Non-pregnant females (perimenopausal)	-	Vaginal estriol or estradiol, Methenamine hippurate	Prophylaxis if triggers identified, review every 6 months
	Non-pregnant females (general)	-	Single-dose antibacterial prophylaxis if identified trigger	Methenamine hippurate for prophylaxis if suitable
	Males and pregnant females	-	Methenamine hippurate if recurrent UTI not improving	Seek specialist advice for recurrent or upper UTI cases
Catheter-Associated UTI	Males and non-pregnant females	Amoxicillin (if susceptible), Nitrofurantoin, Trimethoprim (if low resistance)	Pivmecillinam Hydrochloride	Change catheter if >7 days old, culture before antibiotics
	Pregnant females	Cefalexin	-	If severely unwell, use Cefuroxime IV and consult microbiologist
Severe UTI/Upper UTI	All groups (if severely ill or unable to take oral meds)	Amikacin, Ceftriaxone, Cefuroxime, Gentamicin, Co-amoxiclav (only if combining)	Ciprofloxacin (if others inappropriate)	Intravenous treatment for severe cases, manage sepsis risk

Table 112 UTI Antibiotics Prescriptions according to American College of Clinical Pharmacy

Type of UTI	Antibiotic	Dose	Duration	Comments

Acute Uncomplicated Cystitis	Nitrofurantoin monohydrate/macrocrystal	100 mg PO BID	5 days	
	Trimethoprim/sulfamethoxazole	160/800 mg PO BID	3 days	
	Trimethoprim	100 mg PO BID	3 days	
	Fosfomycin	3 g PO once	Once	
Alternative Agents	Amoxicillin/clavulanate	500/125 mg PO q8hr	5-7 days	
	Cefpodoxime proxetil	100 mg PO BID	5-7 days	
	Cefdinir	300 mg PO BID	5-7 days	
	Cephalexin	500 mg PO BID	5-7 days	Widely used, limited data
	Ciprofloxacin	250 mg PO BID	3 days	
	Levofloxacin	250-500 mg PO daily	3 days	
Acute Uncomplicated Pyelonephritis (Outpatient)	Ciprofloxacin	500 mg PO BID	7 days	If local FQ resistance > 10%, give ceftriaxone 1 g IV once or aminoglycoside pending culture results
	Levofloxacin	750 mg PO daily	5 days	
Alternative/Definitive Therapy	Trimethoprim/sulfamethoxazole	160/800 mg PO BID	14 days	
	Cefpodoxime proxetil	200 mg PO BID	10-14 days	
	Amoxicillin/clavulanate	500 mg PO TID	10-14 days	
Inpatient (Not Severely Ill)	Ciprofloxacin	400 mg IV q12hr	7 days	May add aminoglycosi

				de pending culture results. Complete with PO antibiotics after afebrile for 48 hrs
	Levofloxacin	500 mg IV q24hr	7 days	
	Ceftriaxone	1 g IV q24hr	14 days	
	Cefepime	1-2 g IV q12hr	7-14 days	
Acute Complicated Cystitis or CA-UTI	**Ciprofloxacin**	500 mg PO BID	5-7 days	Empiric therapy based on local resistance patterns. Then streamline based on cultures.
	Levofloxacin	750 mg PO daily	5-7 days	
	Ampicillin/sulbactam	1.5-3 g IV q6hr	5-7 days	
	Ceftriaxone	1 g IV q24hr	5-7 days	
Acute Complicated Pyelonephritis or Urosepsis	**Ceftriaxone**	1 g IV q24hr	14 days	
	Ceftazidime	1-2 g IV q8hr	14 days	
	Cefepime	1 g IV q12hr	14 days	
	Piperacillin/tazobactam	3.375-4.5 g IV q6hr	14 days	
	Meropenem	1 g IV q8hr	14 days	
Antibiotic-resistant (e.g., CRE)	**Colistin**	Loading dose based on body weight	Based on look-up table	

UTIs in Pregnant Women	**Nitrofurantoin monohydrate/macrocrystals**	100 mg PO BID	5-7 days	Except during first trimester or near term
	Amoxicillin	500 mg PO TID	3-7 days	
	Amoxicillin/clavulanate	500 mg PO TID	3-7 days	
	Cephalexin	500 mg PO QID	3-7 days	
	Fosfomycin	3 g PO once	Once	
Prevention of Recurrent UTIs	**Nitrofurantoin**	50 mg PO qhs	Long-term	
	Trimethoprim/sulfamethoxazole	40/200 mg PO daily	Long-term	
UTIs in Men	**Acute Complicated Cystitis and Pyelonephritis**	See recommendations for acute complicated cystitis and pyelonephritis and treat for at least 7 days		
Acute Bacterial Prostatitis	**Ceftriaxone**	1-2 g IV q24hr	Follow with PO FQs for 2-4 weeks	
	Ciprofloxacin	400 mg IV q12hr		
	Levofloxacin	500 mg IV q24hr		
Chronic Bacterial Prostatitis	**Ciprofloxacin**	500 mg PO BID	4-6 weeks	
	Levofloxacin	500 mg PO daily	4-6 weeks	
	Trimethoprim	100 mg PO BID	4-12 weeks	

	Doxycycline	100 mg PO BID	4 weeks	

ACUTE CONDITIONS

7.5.3 Pyelonephritis

A bacterial infection known as pyelonephritis affects the kidneys, with the main infection agent being ***Escherichia coli (E. coli),*** which spreads through the lower urinary tract. Female populations are affected mostly because their urethra is shorter than males. The infection develops primarily among females because of **urinary tract obstructions and diabetes,** together with pregnancy, and in individuals who have weak immune systems. Symptoms in patients with this infection exceed those of regular urinary tract infections because they develop fever along with **flank pain and dysuria and present with nausea and vomiting, and experience general weakness.** Extremely serious situations may result in the formation of sepsis and acute kidney injury. Medical providers use clinical symptoms and urinalysis together with urine cultures, followed by imaging such as ultrasound and CT scans when necessary, to eliminate obstruction and abscesses from the diagnosis. The identification of the pathogen determines which specific antibiotics should be used, while severe situations require intravenous drug administration. Patients need proper pain control and enough hydration to enhance recovery. The prolonged absence of treatment allows pyelonephritis to inflict permanent kidney harm, up to renal failure. **The prevention of UTIS requires good personal hygiene practices together with diabetes management and antibiotic prophylaxis for people who frequently get infections.** Rapid detection of the infection combined with proper medical intervention serves as an essential components for stopping serious medical consequences and attaining complete recovery.

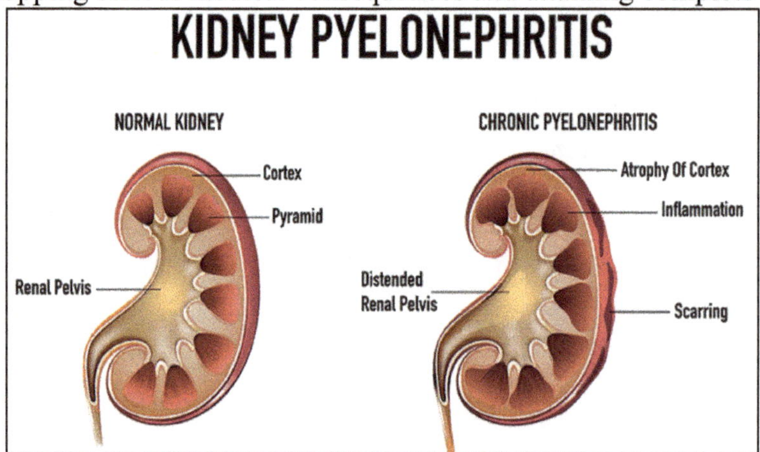

Figure 196 Schematic Overview of Kidney Pyelonephritis

7.5.3.1 Classification of Pyelonephritis

Disease classification of pyelonephritis uses three fundamental criteria to organise this condition: form, activity level and kidney function status. Primary pyelonephritis takes place without urinary tract obstructions in a condition called non-obstructive disease, while secondary pyelonephritis develops as an obstructive disease when **kidney stones or prostate enlargement block normal urine flow.** The disease presents as acute pyelonephritis for active symptomatic stages with fever and pain alongside inflammation or as chronic pyelonephritis, which manifests through noticeable symptoms or stays latent with few or no symptoms. Through different stages of the disease, patients face varying degrees of k**idney dysfunction that starts with normal renal function in**

acute phases and **evolves into functional renal disorders in chronic phases**, which impair kidney functionality. Significant permanent kidney damage develops into chronic renal insufficiency during severe cases of the condition. The classification system identifies pyelonephritis severity and tracks disease progression, which directs treatment decisions according **to organ function impairment.**

Table 113 Classification of Pyelonephritis

CLASSIFICATION OF PYELONEPHRITIS

Forms of pyelonephritis		Activity of diseases	Function of kidney
Primary *no-obstructive*	**Acute**	**Active** stage	Without functional renal disorders
Secondary *no-obstructive* *obstructive*	**Chronic** a) manifest b) latent	**Partially** clinic & labor. **remission**	With functional renal disorders
		Total clinical **remission**	Chronic renal insufficiency

7.5.3.2 SOAP Notes for Pyelonephritis

Table 114 SOAP Notes for Pyelonephritis

Component	Details
Subjective (S)	A 35-year-old female presents with a 3-day history of fever, chills, dysuria, and lower abdominal pain. She reports frequent urination with a burning sensation, and pain radiating to her back. She denies any nausea or vomiting but mentions feeling fatigued. The patient has a history of recurrent urinary tract infections (UTIs) but has not had any similar symptoms in the past year. She is sexually active and uses oral contraceptives. No known history of kidney stones or urinary tract obstructions. She is concerned due to the worsening pain and fever despite taking over-the-counter pain medications.
Objective (O)	The patient appears uncomfortable and has a temperature of 101.4°F (38.5°C). Vital signs: BP 120/78 mmHg, HR 98 bpm, Temp 101.4°F (38.5°C). On physical exam, the abdomen is tender in the lower quadrants, with mild costovertebral angle tenderness. Urine dipstick shows leukocyte esterase and nitrites. A urine culture is pending. Blood tests reveal elevated white blood cell count (WBC 14,000/µL). Kidney function tests (BUN and creatinine) are within normal limits. The rest of the physical exam, including neurological and cardiovascular, is unremarkable.
Assessment (A)	The patient's presentation, including fever, dysuria, lower abdominal pain, and costovertebral angle tenderness, is consistent with acute pyelonephritis. The positive urine dipstick for leukocyte esterase and nitrites supports this diagnosis. Her history of recurrent UTIs puts her at higher risk for pyelonephritis. The elevated WBC count indicates systemic infection. This condition is usually caused by *Escherichia coli*, but further urine culture will confirm the pathogen. Immediate treatment is necessary to prevent complications such as renal abscess or sepsis.

Plan (P)	**Pharmacological:** Start empirical antibiotics (e.g., ceftriaxone or ciprofloxacin) while awaiting urine culture results. If the culture confirms *E. coli*, adjust antibiotics based on susceptibility. Provide acetaminophen for fever and pain relief, avoiding NSAIDs due to the risk of kidney damage. Consider adding a urinary analgesic (e.g., phenazopyridine) for symptom relief (See algorithm below). **Non-pharmacological:** Encourage increased fluid intake to help flush out bacteria. **Follow-up:** Review urine culture results in 48-72 hours. If symptoms worsen or the patient develops new signs such as increased fever or chills, re-evaluate for complications like renal abscess or sepsis. Educate the patient on the importance of completing the full course of antibiotics and follow-up if symptoms persist or recur. **Education:** Explain the nature of pyelonephritis, the risk of complications, and the need to seek care promptly if symptoms worsen. Discuss preventive measures, including proper hydration and urinary hygiene practices.

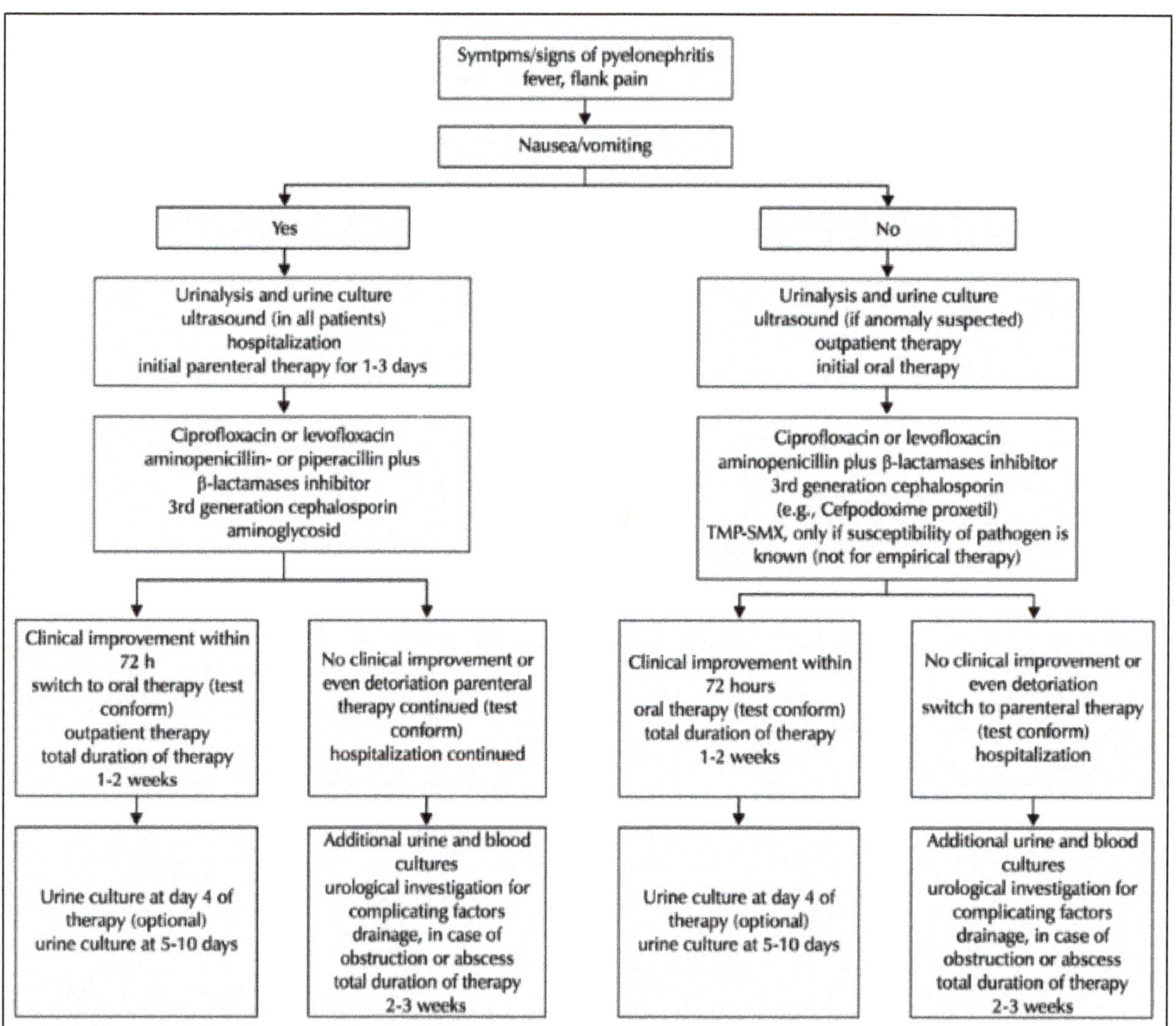

Figure 197 Algorithm for the Clinical Treatment and Management of Uncomplicated Pyelonephritis

7.5.4 Acute Kidney Injury

Acute kidney injury (AKI) represents a sudden reduction of kidney performance which develops within hours or days and triggers waste concentration throughout the body. This condition leads to both accelerated serum creatinine levels and restrained urine production. Three main categories exist for AKI causes, including prerenal issues and intrinsic damage and postrenal obstructions. The **bloodstream reduction that reaches the kidneys causes prerenal AKI** mainly because of dehydration or blood loss, or heart failure. The kidneys experience direct internal damage, leading to intrinsic AKI when people have glomerulonephritis and acute tubular necrosis (ATN) and toxic exposures. Urinary tract obstructions from kidney stones, together with prostate enlargement, result in postrenal AKI. **The main indicators of AKI are low urine output together with swelling (oedema) along with fatigue and confusion, and nausea.** The medical team uses blood tests for creatinine and BUN, along with urine tests and scanning procedures to diagnose kidney function and discover origin factors. The immediate intervention of AKI is necessary to stop irreversible damage from affecting the kidneys. The medical approach targets both the core reason for **kidney damage and fluid and electrolyte control,** and requires dialysis for extreme situations. The appropriate detection, together with prompt medical care, leads to better results and stops kidney disease from becoming long-lasting.

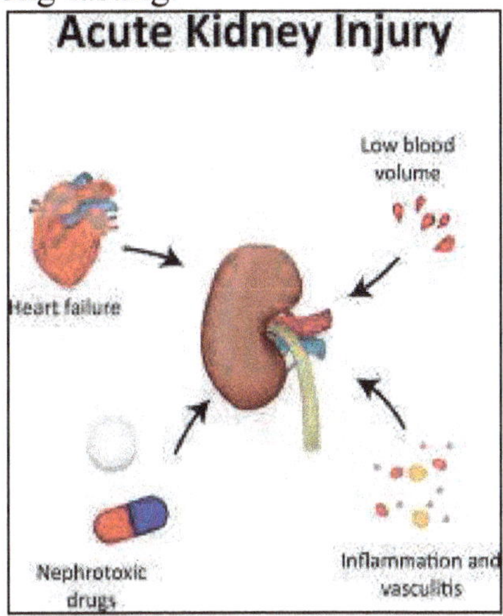

Figure 198 Acute Kidney Injury Overview

7.5.4.1 Classification of Acute Kidney Injury

A reduction in blood volume, together with blood pressure shifts, results in decreased kidney perfusion, which leads to the development of **Prerenal AKI.** Heart failure, as well as bleeding, along with burns and diarrhoea and hypovolemia, result in reduced blood flow to the kidneys, which patients experience. Multiple factors, such as **decreased blood volume together with non-steroidal anti-inflammatory drugs (NSAIDS),** severe infections or hypovolemia, contribute to AKI development. When kidney tissues suffer structural damage within the intrarenal section of the kidney, patients develop this form of AKI, especially when glomeruli or renal tubules are affected. The main kidney tissue injuries that result in this condition are **acute tubular necrosis (ATN) and glomerulonephritis.** Medical drugs, together with poisonous substances and infectious agents and inadequate blood delivery to the kidneys, can lead to this condition. The severity of this form tends to be greater because it produces actual injuries to the kidney tissues. The blockage of **normal urine flow in the urinary tract because of obstructions results in kidney damage and causes postrenal AKI.** Urinary blockages generated between renal organs and their corresponding ducts and urethra represent typical deficits in this category. Postrenal AKI develops because of kidney stones, together with tumors, an enlarged prostate, and strictures.

Table 115 Classification of Acute Kidney Injury

Category	Common abnormality	Potential causes
Pre-renal	Changes in blood volume and pressure supply to kidneys	Bleeding, fluid loss, burns, cirrhosis, recent surgery, non-steroidal anti-inflammatory drugs, impaired cardiac function, anti-hypertensive medications, sepsis
Intra-renal	Structural anomaly in the kidneys (primarily damage to blood vessels, glomeruli and tubules of nephrons)	Acute tubular necrosis, glomerulonephritis, recent surgery, nephrotoxic medications, hypertension, sepsis, severe burns or trauma, nephritis, adverse reaction to certain non-steroidal anti-inflammatory drugs and antibiotics, vasculitis
Post-renal	Urinary obstruction anywhere between kidney tubules and urethra	Kidney stones, pyelonephritis, benign prostatic hyperplasia, swollen lymph nodes (infection), transitional cell carcinoma (typically bladder, ureters or urethra), retroperitoneal fibrosis, renal papillary necrosis

Sources: Zamzami et al (2021), Kazama and Nakajima (2017), Hertzberg et al (2017), Makris and Spanou (2016).

7.5.4.2 SOAP Notes for Acute Kidney Injury

Table 116 SOAP Notes for Acute Kidney Injury

Component	Details
Subjective (S)	A 58-year-old male with a history of hypertension and type 2 diabetes mellitus presents with a 2-day history of decreased urine output and swelling in his legs. He reports feeling fatigued and experiencing nausea but denies chest pain or shortness of breath. The patient mentions that he has been feeling more thirsty than usual and has not been able to urinate much despite drinking plenty of fluids. He recently started taking an over-the-counter NSAID for mild back pain. The patient denies any recent trauma or history of kidney disease.
Objective (O)	The patient appears mildly distressed and has noticeable bilateral lower extremity edema. Vital signs: BP 160/95 mmHg, HR 92 bpm, Temp 37.5°C (99.5°F). Physical exam reveals decreased skin turgor, bilateral leg edema, and mild tenderness in the lower abdomen. The rest of the examination is unremarkable. Laboratory results show elevated serum creatinine (2.5 mg/dL), BUN (30 mg/dL), and potassium (5.3 mEq/L). Urinalysis reveals proteinuria and mild hematuria. A renal ultrasound shows normal kidney size without evidence of obstruction.
Assessment (A)	The patient's presentation, including decreased urine output, fatigue, and swelling, along with elevated serum creatinine and BUN, is consistent with acute kidney injury (AKI). Given the patient's history of hypertension and

	diabetes, the AKI is likely prerenal in origin, potentially due to dehydration or the effects of NSAIDs. The lack of obstruction on renal ultrasound supports this. Management should focus on restoring renal perfusion and correcting electrolyte imbalances.
Plan (P)	**Pharmacological:** Discontinue NSAIDs and adjust antihypertensive medications as necessary. Start intravenous (IV) fluids (e.g., normal saline) to rehydrate and improve kidney perfusion. Monitor potassium levels and consider administering IV calcium gluconate or sodium bicarbonate if hyperkalemia worsens. Adjust insulin if necessary to control blood glucose (See algorithm below). **Non-pharmacological:** Encourage the patient to avoid further NSAID use and hydrate adequately. **Follow-up:** Monitor kidney function closely with daily serum creatinine and urine output. Reassess electrolyte levels, particularly potassium. If no improvement is noted or if the condition worsens, consider further interventions such as dialysis. **Education:** Educate the patient about the importance of avoiding nephrotoxic medications, maintaining hydration, and monitoring kidney function regularly, especially in the context of diabetes and hypertension. Discuss the potential need for follow-up visits to manage the underlying risk factors.

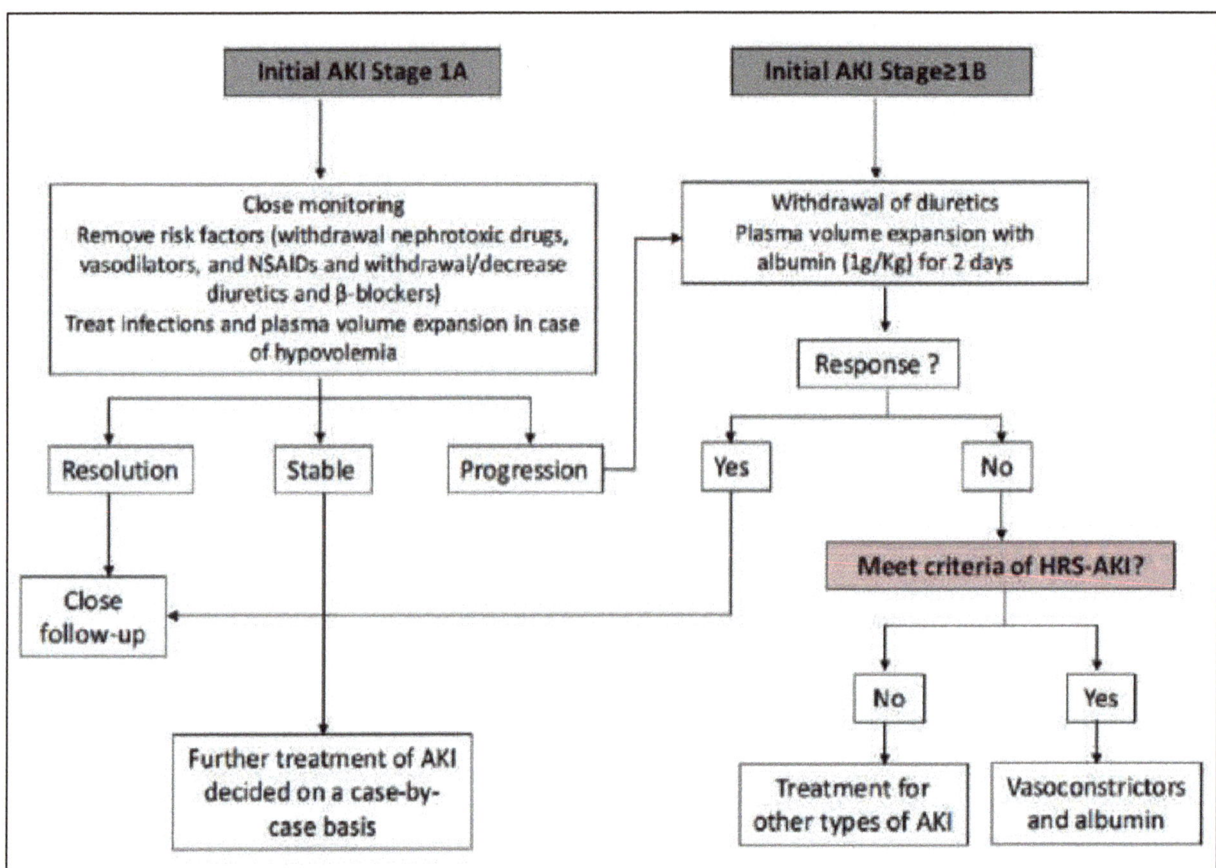

Figure 199 Management Algorithm for Acute Kidney Injury

7.5.5 Hematuria

Blood in urine leads medical professionals to diagnose various conditions affecting urinary tract organs and kidneys, together with other body parts. Two main categories exist for hematuria: microscopic hematuria requires urinary testing to **detect blood, while gross hematuria** produces visibly red or brown urine. Numerous health factors of varying severity can result in hematuria. **UTIS and kidney stones, and bladder or kidney infections (pyelonephritis),** together with urinary system traumas, represent common causes of this condition. Tumours affecting the bladder or kidneys, as well as glomerulonephritis and coagulation disorders, represent serious underlying medical conditions. **The severity of hematuria** is established based on its original source in the body. **Hematuria detected through microscopy** often occurs **without symptoms, yet testing reveals the presence, while visible amounts of blood in urine** require patients to experience pain or feel the need to urinate urgently or experience discomfort while urinating. A proper diagnosis starts with a **physical examination and history review**, and then requires urinalysis for blood detection. Medical professionals require urine cultures and imaging procedures, along with cystoscopy, to discern the root cause of the condition. **Medical professionals** provide specific treatments to resolve the root problems of urinary pathology while managing patients through antibiotics when infections exist or through surgical procedures when tumours or stones are present.

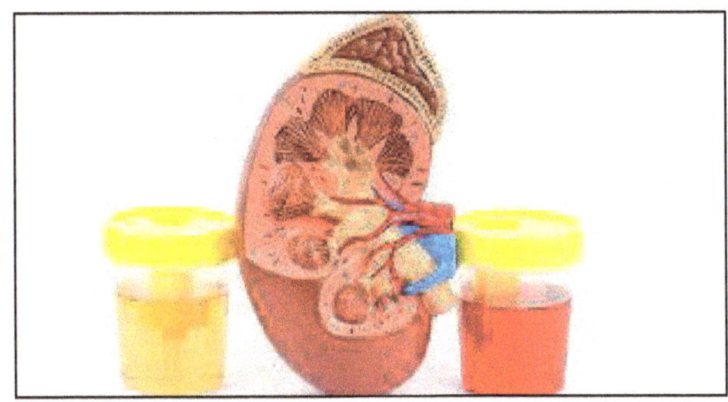

Figure 200 Difference between Normal and Hematouria Kidney

7.5.5.1 Types of Hematuria

The classification of hematuria conditions separates the presence of blood into four levels depending on blood origin and the causes that lead to bleeding. Hematuria, which affects the urinary tract, occurs as upper tract or lower tract problems inside the urinary system. The kidneys or **ureters are the body areas which produce upper tract hematuria**, and common causes include kidney stones, together with tumours and pyelonephritis infections. The urethra and bladder comprise the lower tract areas where blood appears mainly **after bladder infections or bladder cancer, or trauma.** Non-urological hematuria occurs from medical issues that exist beyond the urinary system. Medical blood disorders, such as coagulopathies and glomerulonephritis, present among the causes **which impact how the kidneys filter substances.** Within **pseudohematuria fall** all instances where urine contains substances, including haemoglobin, along with myoglobin from either **muscle injuries or hemolysis** that look like blood, even without red blood cells. A classification system supports diagnosis by identifying root causes that enable healthcare professionals to select proper treatment methods.

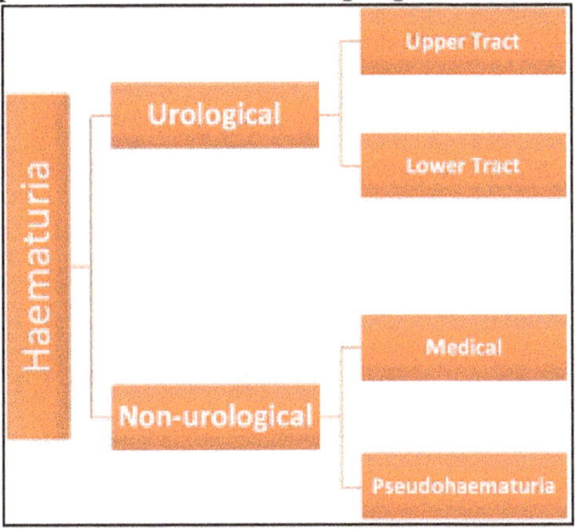

Figure 201 Hematuria Types

7.5.5.2 Classification of Hematuria

Three fundamental criteria determine the classification of hematuria as displayed in the image: **source of blood, visual characteristics and length of time for observation**. The source indicates that hematuria exists in three main forms which are glomerular, non-glomerular and extrarenal categories. **Hematuria that starts in the glomeruli affects** the kidney tissue and appears most frequently in patients. **Non-glomerular hematuria** develops in any area beyond the glomeruli of the kidneys, including the urethra or bladder or additional kidney regions, when infections or kidney stones appear. Hematuria occurring outside the kidney area is known as extrarenal hematuria, and it includes blood originating from the bladder and urethral structures. The classification of **hematuria based on visibility has two options including visible and non-**

visible conditions. Visible blood in urine manifests when red colour appears in the stream, and physicians classify these cases by initial, terminal and full stream presentation. Medical tests show blood presence in the urine, **even though the human eye cannot detect visible blood particles**. Hematuria lasts either temporarily as transient or continues as significant, which requires medical evaluation and potentially treatment. Medical classification serves as a tool to recognise root causes of hematuria because it determines which treatments become necessary.

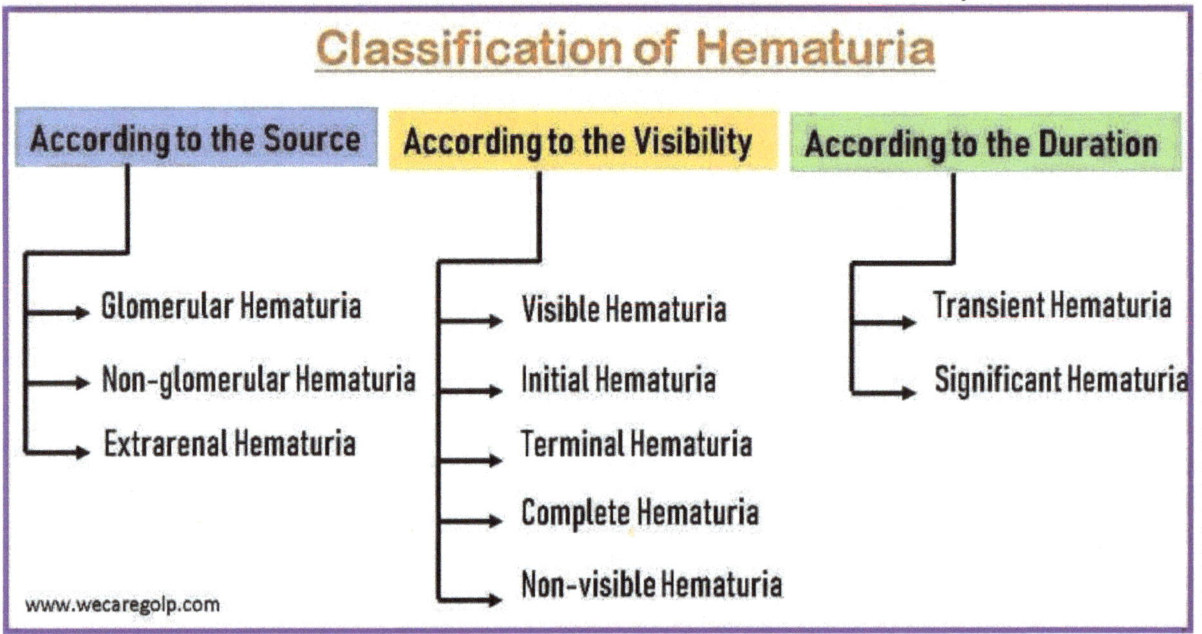

Figure 202 Classification of Hematuria

7.5.5.3 SOAP Notes for Hematuria

Table 117 SOAP Notes for Hematuria

Component	Details
Subjective (S)	A 45-year-old male presents with a 3-day history of noticeable blood in his urine. The patient reports that the urine appears red and sometimes brown, with no associated pain during urination. He denies any fever, chills, or pain in the lower abdomen or back. The patient has a history of mild hypertension and occasionally takes ibuprofen for muscle aches. He also reports increased physical activity recently, including weightlifting. He denies any recent trauma or previous history of similar symptoms. He is concerned about the cause of the blood in his urine and whether it may be a serious condition.
Objective (O)	The patient appears generally well and is in no acute distress. Vital signs: BP 130/85 mmHg, HR 82 bpm, Temp 36.8°C (98.2°F). Physical examination is unremarkable with no signs of abdominal tenderness or distension. A urine dipstick test confirms the presence of blood but no significant signs of infection (e.g., leukocytes or nitrites). Urinalysis reveals a small amount of hematuria, with no protein or glucose detected. Blood tests show normal renal function with a serum creatinine of 1.0 mg/dL and BUN of 16 mg/dL.

	A non-contrast renal ultrasound shows no signs of kidney stones or other obstructions.
Assessment (A)	The patient's presentation of visible hematuria without pain or fever, combined with a negative urine culture and normal renal ultrasound, is suggestive of non-urological hematuria. Given the patient's history of physical activity and use of ibuprofen, pseudohematuria due to muscle injury or myoglobinuria is a likely cause. However, urological causes such as bladder trauma or a mild urinary tract injury should also be considered. Further investigation is warranted to rule out any significant urological pathology.
Plan (P)	**Pharmacological**: Discontinue ibuprofen to eliminate the potential contribution to the hematuria. If muscle injury or myoglobinuria is suspected, monitor renal function closely and consider checking serum creatine kinase (CK) levels (See algorithm below). **Non-pharmacological**: Recommend the patient rest and hydrate well to prevent further kidney strain. **Follow-up**: Schedule follow-up in 3-5 days to assess any changes in symptoms and recheck urine analysis if hematuria persists. If hematuria continues or worsens, consider further imaging such as a CT scan or cystoscopy. **Education**: Advise the patient on the importance of avoiding NSAIDs, especially with increased physical exertion, and the need to monitor for any further changes in urine color. Discuss the potential causes of hematuria, including muscle injury and urological conditions, and the importance of follow-up for further evaluation.

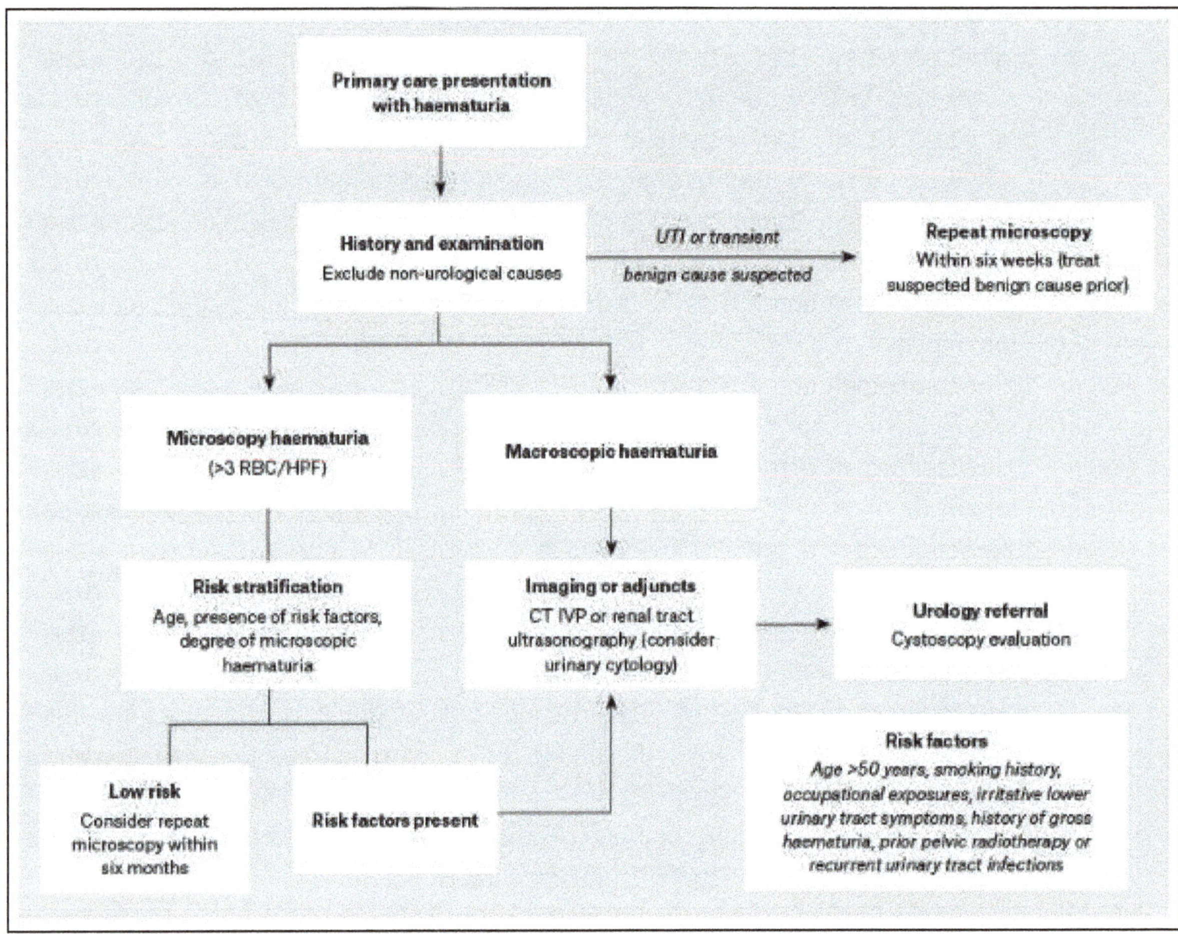

Figure 203 Algorithm for initial investigations and management of haematuria

7.5.6 Proteinuria

7.5.7 Renal Nephrolithiasis (Stones)

The formation of **hard solid crystals inside the kidneys,** which block the urinary tract, defines the medical condition known as renal nephrolithiasis, also known as kidney stones. The bodily stones consist primarily of calcium oxalate and uric acid, with struvite alongside cystine acting as **different mineralic components**. The urine becomes supersaturated with substances, such that crystals form inside your kidneys to become stones. The crystals continue to grow throughout time into renal stones with a wide range of sizes that span from minuscule masses to substantial complex formations. The main symptom of **kidney stones manifests as intense episodes of pain** which start in the lower back region and move to the flank area. These pains are often recognised as a type of colic. **Stone movement within the kidney** and its movement through the urinary tract result in **painful sensations.** The additional symptoms of kidney stone diagnosis include blood in the urine, together with nausea and vomiting and **increased need for urination**. Disclosed kidney stones might cause no symptoms, which leads to their detection only through diagnostic imaging performed for different medical reasons. People at risk of developing kidney stones include those who are dehydrated, together with those **who consume high amounts of salt** and protein and suffer from obesity or possess medical conditions such as hyperparathyroidism or gout or have an

existing family history of kidney stones. The method of treating **kidney stones** depends on both their dimensions and their position in the body. Most kidney stones will pass on their own after **fluid consumption increases and pain treatments**, yet larger stones necessitate medical procedures, including shock wave lithotripsy or ureteroscopy or surgery. Preventive steps involve drinking more fluids, together with adjusting the diet while taking treatment for managing underlying risk factors.

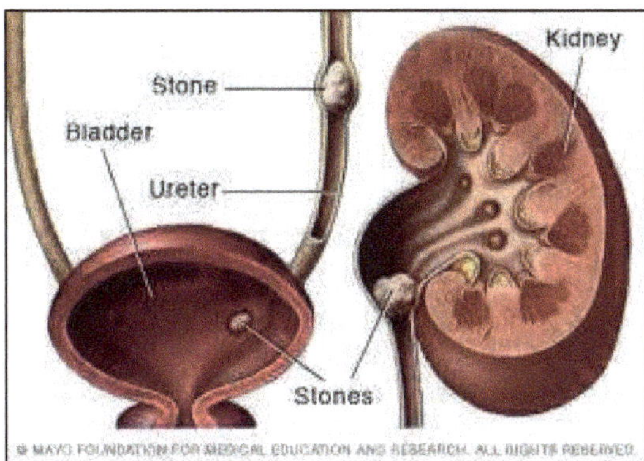

Figure 204 Kidney Stones

7.5.7.1 Types of Kidney Stones

The illustration displays the four major categories of kidney stones: calcium stones, uric acid **stones, cystine stones, and struvite stones**. Among kidney stones, calcium stones are the most typical variety, which emerge from either **calcium oxalate or calcium phosphate materials**. The formation of these stones occurs when the urine contains high levels of calcium or oxalate substances, mainly because of **dehydration or excessive dietary intake** of certain materials. The presence of excessive uric acid in urine leads to the development of uric acid stones in patients who have gout or become dehydrated. **High-protein diet consumption** and metabolic disorders have been linked to increased prevalence of these stones in people. Kidney stones that contain cystine occur rarely due to the genetic disorder cystinuria, which triggers the body to produce excessive amounts of cystine amino acid. Struvite stones form mainly due to urinary tract **infections resulting from bacteria** that create urease to elevate urine pH, thus triggering struvite crystal development. Each type of kidney stone requires various corresponding treatment methods since their causes and risk factors differ from one another, although their ability to block the urinary pathway causes **similar amounts of distress** for patients.

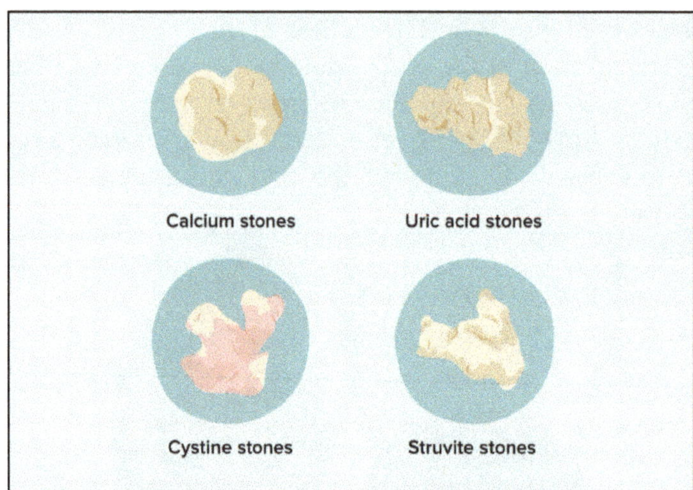

Figure 205 Types of Kidney Stones

7.5.7.2 SOAP Notes for Kidney Stones

Component	Details
Subjective (S)	A 45-year-old male presents with the sudden onset of severe, sharp pain in the lower back, radiating towards the abdomen. The pain started abruptly earlier today and has been persistent. He describes the pain as "colicky," occurring in waves. The patient also reports nausea but denies vomiting. He mentions having frequent urination and passing small amounts of urine, but no visible blood in the urine. He has no significant past medical history but reports a family history of kidney stones. The patient is concerned about the pain and suspects a kidney stone due to his family history.
Objective (O)	The patient appears in moderate distress, wincing during episodes of pain. Vital signs: BP 135/85 mmHg, HR 90 bpm, Temp 37.0°C (98.6°F). Physical exam reveals tenderness in the right lower abdomen and flank area. No signs of fever or chills. Urinalysis shows hematuria (microscopic blood in the urine), with no evidence of infection (no leukocytes or nitrites). Serum creatinine and BUN are within normal limits. A non-contrast abdominal CT scan reveals a 5mm stone in the right renal pelvis.
Assessment (A)	The patient's symptoms of severe colicky pain, hematuria, and the presence of a 5mm stone in the right renal pelvis on CT scan are consistent with renal nephrolithiasis (kidney stones). The stone is of moderate size and may be causing obstruction or irritation in the urinary tract. Given the patient's family history and symptoms, the stone is likely the cause of the acute pain.
Plan (P)	**Pharmacological**: Prescribe pain management with NSAIDS (e.g., ibuprofen) or opioids if needed for severe pain. Consider antiemetics for nausea if required (See algorithm below). **Non-pharmacological**: Advise the patient to increase fluid intake to help facilitate stone passage. Recommend rest and avoidance of strenuous physical activity. **Follow-up**: Follow up in 1 week to reassess symptoms and monitor for stone passage.

	If the stone does not pass or the pain persists, further intervention may be necessary (e.g., lithotripsy, ureteroscopy). **Education**: Educate the patient on the potential for stone recurrence and discuss lifestyle modifications, including reducing dietary sodium, oxalate, and increasing water intake. Advise the patient to monitor urine for any visible blood and seek care if symptoms worsen.

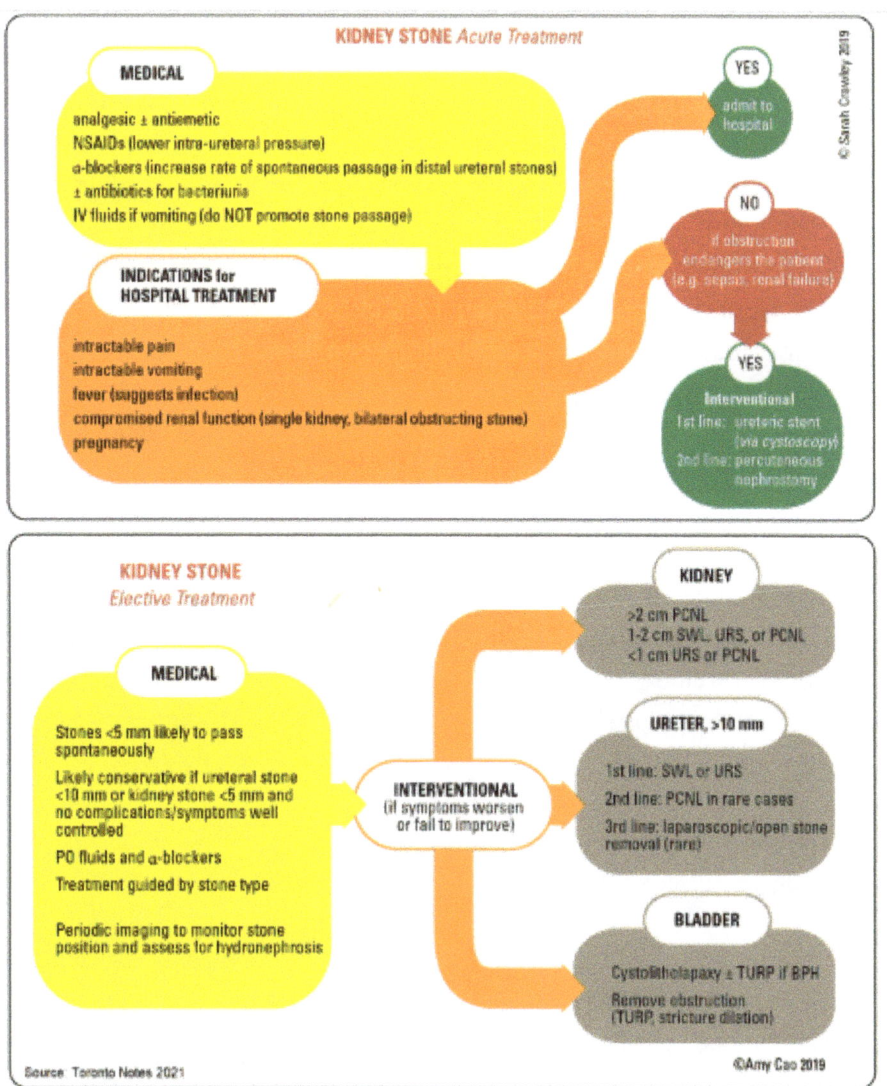

Figure 206 Treatment Approaches for Kidney Stones

OTHER CONDITIONS

7.5.8 Bladder Cancer

Table 118 SOAP Notes for Bladder Cancer

Component	Details
Subjective (S)	A 60-year-old male presents with a 2-week history of painless hematuria (blood in the urine). He has noticed the urine appearing pinkish and

	occasionally darker in color, but there is no associated pain or discomfort during urination. He reports frequent urination, especially at night, but denies any weight loss, fatigue, or pain in the lower abdomen. The patient has a significant history of smoking (30 pack-years) and has worked in chemical manufacturing for the past 25 years. He denies any history of urinary tract infections or trauma.
Objective (O)	The patient appears well, with no signs of acute distress. Vital signs: BP 130/85 mmHg, HR 80 bpm, Temp 36.8°C (98.2°F). Physical exam reveals no abdominal tenderness or palpable masses. Digital rectal exam (DRE) reveals no abnormalities. Urinalysis shows hematuria with no evidence of infection. Urine cytology is positive for atypical cells. Cystoscopy shows an irregular mass in the bladder wall. CT scan of the abdomen and pelvis reveals a lesion in the bladder.
Assessment (A)	The patient's presentation of painless hematuria and risk factors such as smoking and exposure to chemicals is highly suggestive of bladder cancer. The cystoscopy and CT scan findings confirm a bladder mass. The next step is to confirm the diagnosis with biopsy and assess for staging and potential metastasis. The patient's history and findings are consistent with transitional cell carcinoma (TCC), the most common type of bladder cancer.
Plan (P)	**Pharmacological**: Pre-operative medications include pain management and potential use of anticholinergics to control symptoms. **Non-pharmacological**: Refer to a urologist for biopsy and staging of the tumor. Discuss options for possible surgery (e.g., transurethral resection of the bladder tumor or cystectomy) and potential chemotherapy or immunotherapy post-surgery depending on the staging. **Follow-up**: Schedule follow-up in 1 week for biopsy

7.5.9 Rhabdomyolysis

Table 119 SOAP Notes for Rhabdomyolysis

Component	Details
Subjective (S)	A 30-year-old male presents with muscle pain, weakness, and dark-colored urine after an intense workout session at the gym. He reports lifting heavy weights and performing prolonged cardiovascular exercise for several hours. The next day, he noticed his urine had turned dark brown and was accompanied by generalized muscle soreness. He denies any trauma or recent illness. The patient has no significant past medical history and is otherwise healthy, although he occasionally takes over-the-counter pain medications for muscle pain.
Objective (O)	The patient appears mildly distressed and is unable to lift his arms above his head due to muscle weakness. Vital signs: BP 125/80 mmHg, HR 90 bpm, Temp 37.0°C (98.6°F). Physical examination reveals tenderness in the bilateral quadriceps and forearms with no obvious swelling or bruising.

	There is no sign of dehydration or fever. Laboratory results show elevated creatine kinase (CK) levels at 15,000 U/L (normal: 55-170 U/L), and positive myoglobin in the urine, confirming rhabdomyolysis. Renal function tests show normal creatinine and BUN levels, but urine analysis shows dark brown, tea-colored urine with no red blood cells.
Assessment (A)	The patient's clinical presentation and laboratory findings, including elevated creatine kinase and myoglobinuria, are consistent with rhabdomyolysis. The most likely cause is excessive physical exertion, particularly after a prolonged and intense workout. There are no signs of acute kidney injury (AKI) yet, but close monitoring is necessary given the potential for kidney damage from myoglobinuria.
Plan (P)	**Pharmacological**: Initiate intravenous (IV) fluids (normal saline) for hydration to help flush out the myoglobin and prevent kidney damage. Consider using bicarbonate to alkalinize the urine and reduce myoglobin-induced nephrotoxicity. Monitor electrolytes, particularly potassium, for any imbalances. **Non-pharmacological**: Rest and avoid further strenuous physical activity. **Follow-up**: Monitor renal function closely with daily serum creatinine and BUN. Recheck creatine kinase levels every 12 hours to assess for improvement. If there is evidence of kidney injury (e.g., rising creatinine or oliguria), initiate dialysis. **Education**: Educate the patient about the importance of hydration before and after exercise, avoiding overexertion, and monitoring for signs of muscle pain or weakness in future workouts to prevent recurrence. Discuss the risks of excessive physical activity and the need for proper rest and recovery.

7.6 Moh Golden Points and Summary Question Answers

7.6.1 Moh Golden Points

Proteinuria is a critical early indicator of kidney dysfunction, particularly in patients with diabetes or hypertension.

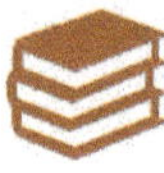

Asymptomatic bacteriuria should be treated in high-risk groups, such as pregnant women and patients undergoing urological procedures, to prevent complications like pyelonephritis and preterm labor.

Fever, flank pain, and dysuria in a patient with a history of UTIs suggest pyelonephritis, which requires prompt antibiotic treatment to prevent kidney damage or systemic infection (sepsis).

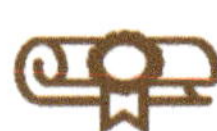

Identifying MS early is vital for managing symptoms and slowing the disease progression, offering better patient outcomes

AKI can occur due to dehydration, medications like NSAIDs, or underlying conditions like diabetes and hypertension.

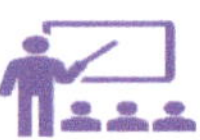

Proteinuria is a crucial early indicator of kidney damage, particularly in patients with diabetes or hypertension. .

Asymptomatic bacteriuria should be treated in high-risk populations such as pregnant women and patients with diabetes to prevent complications like pyelonephritis, preterm labor, or kidney damage.

7.6.2 Summary Questions & Answers

1. What is the first-line treatment for asymptomatic bacteriuria in pregnant women?

a) No treatment needed
b) Empirical antibiotic therapy
c) NSAIDs
d) Observation only

2. Which of the following is the most common pathogen causing pyelonephritis?

a) Escherichia coli
b) Streptococcus pneumoniae
c) Pseudomonas aeruginosa
d) Klebsiella pneumoniae

3. Which of the following is a common complication of untreated pyelonephritis?

a) Chronic kidney disease
b) Sepsis
c) Hyperkalemia
d) Hematuria

4. A patient presents with dark brown urine, muscle weakness, and pain after intense exercise. What is the likely diagnosis?

a) Acute kidney injury
b) Rhabdomyolysis
c) Urinary tract infection
d) Pyelonephritis

5. What is the first-line treatment for acute kidney injury (AKI) caused by dehydration or prerenal factors?

a) Dialysis
b) IV fluids
c) Antihypertensive medications
d) NSAIDs

6. Which of the following is a common cause of postrenal acute kidney injury (AKI)?

a) Dehydration
b) Kidney stones
c) Diabetes mellitus
d) Hypertension

7. In the management of proteinuria, what class of drugs is often prescribed to reduce kidney damage, especially in diabetic patients?

a) Diuretics
b) ACE inhibitors or ARBs
c) Calcium channel blockers
d) Beta-blockers

8. What is a typical characteristic of bladder cancer in patients presenting with hematuria?

a) Painful urination

b) Painless hematuria c) Fever and chills d) Abdominal tenderness
9. Which of the following interventions is typically used for managing a 5mm kidney stone that is causing pain but no signs of infection? a) Surgical removal b) Lithotripsy c) Pain management and increased fluid intake d) Antibiotics
10. Which of the following is a critical early sign of rhabdomyolysis that should be monitored to prevent kidney damage? a) Elevated serum creatinine b) Hematuria c) Elevated creatine kinase (CK) d) Low blood pressure

7.6.3 Rationales

1. **Answer: b) Empirical antibiotic therapy**

Rationale: ***Asymptomatic bacteriuria in pregnant women should be treated with antibiotics to prevent complications like pyelonephritis or preterm labor. This is especially important for high-risk groups.***

2. **Answer: a) Escherichia coli**

Rationale: ***Escherichia coli*** **is the most common pathogen responsible for pyelonephritis, particularly in women, due to its ability to ascend the urinary tract from the bladder to the kidneys.**

3. **Answer: b) Sepsis**

Rationale: If untreated, pyelonephritis can lead to sepsis, which is a life-threatening condition that requires immediate intervention to prevent organ failure.

4. **Answer: b) Rhabdomyolysis**

Rationale: Rhabdomyolysis is characterized by muscle pain, weakness, and dark urine (due to myoglobinuria), often triggered by intense physical activity.

5. **Answer: b) IV fluids**

Rationale: IV fluids are the primary treatment for AKI caused by dehydration or prerenal factors, as they help restore kidney perfusion and prevent further kidney damage. Dialysis is considered in severe cases when kidney function does not improve.

6. **Answer: b) Kidney stones**

Rationale: Postrenal AKI occurs due to urinary tract obstructions, such as kidney stones, which block the flow of urine and cause damage to the kidneys.

7. **Answer: b) ACE inhibitors or ARBs**

Rationale: ACE inhibitors or angiotensin receptor blockers (ARBs) are commonly prescribed to reduce proteinuria in patients with diabetes or hypertension, helping to protect the kidneys from further damage.

8. **Answer: b) Painless hematuria**

Rationale: Bladder cancer often presents with painless hematuria (blood in the urine), which is one of the hallmark signs, especially in individuals with risk factors like smoking or chemical exposure.

9. **Answer: c) Pain management and increased fluid intake**

Rationale: For small kidney stones (like a 5mm stone), the typical management involves pain management, hydration, and encouraging the stone to pass naturally, often without the need for surgery or lithotripsy.

10. **Answer: c) Elevated creatine kinase (CK)**

Rationale: Elevated creatine kinase (CK) levels are a key marker for rhabdomyolysis, indicating muscle breakdown. If untreated, myoglobin can cause kidney damage, so monitoring CK levels is essential in managing the condition.

8 Chapter 8: Genital System

8.1 Anatomy and Physiology of Genital System

Genital system or reproductive system is the system that is involved in **production, transport and nutrition of great tapetum (sperm in male and ovum in female) and support fertilization**, pregnancy and childbirth. Its structure and function in both male and female body is not similar but this system plays essential roles in the process of reproduction.

8.1.1 Male Genital System

Male reproductive system includes testes and epididymis, vas deferens, seminal vesicles and glands, prostate gland, and penis. **Testes are the male genital organs** that are responsible for male germ cell and testosterone production. Sperm generated in the testes are localized and develop in epididymis. They pass through the **vas deferens as they get joined with the seminal vesicle** and **prostate gland secretion** of sperm to form what is referred to as semen, which is ejected from the body via the penis.

8.1.2 Female Genital System

These are ovaries, fallopian tubes, uterus, vagina, and external genitalia of the woman are some parts of the Female Reproductive System. It is involved in the **production of ova (eggs)** as well as in **hormone production for female** which include **estrogen and progesterone**. A woman's ovary discharges an egg once a month to a process that is referred to as ovulation. Having reached the ovary it moves into the **fallopian tubes** to be fertilized by the sperm in case of conception. If the sperm joins with the **egg, the fertilized egg** burrows to the uterus where it forms a fetus. In the instance where there is no conception, the egg is expelled through the vagina during the next menstrual period. The processes of the male and female reproductive systems involve **intricate control by hormones signaled** from the brain and **pituitary and hypothalamus glands**. Such systems do not only regulate reproduction but are involved in other aspects of the bodies such as additional sexual characteristics and health.

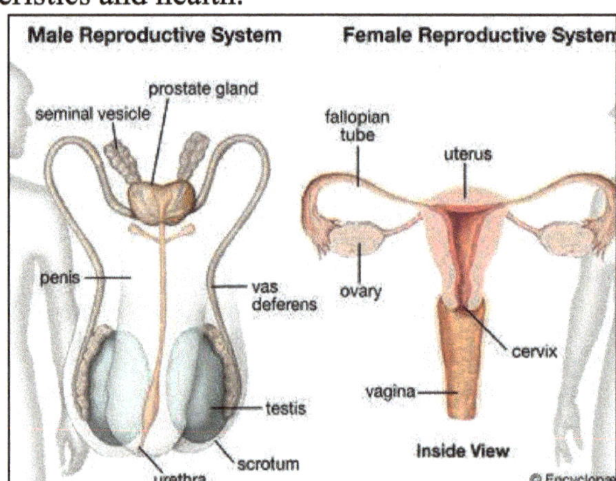

Figure 207 Anatomy and Physiology of Male and Female Reproductive System

8.2 Male Reproductive System Diagnostic Tests

8.2.1 Cryptorchidism

Cryptorchidism can be defined as one or both testes have not descended into the scrotum as they are supposed to during **fetal development or in the early stage of life.** Testes should be in the abdomen during the fetal development and the scrotum during the third trimester. In case this descent does not take place, one faces such problems as a **decreased ability for procreation, the**

possibilities of developing a tumor in the testicles and problems in the endocrine system. It is advisable to employ the administration of hormones or surgery in an operation known as orchidopexy to relocate the testes to the scrotum.

8.2.2 Testosterone

Testosterone is a steroid male sex hormone, which is synthesized in the testes and to a lesser amount in the adrenal glands. It has a very important function in the development of **male secondary sexual characteristics such as muscle mass, voice change to largo and growth of facial hair.** It also has functions that are related to sperm production and the level of sexual desire that a male is supposed to have. **Blood tests analyzing testosterone** help in diagnosing hormonal disorders that have to do with reproductive system, including hypogonadism, infertility problems and other conditions caused by androgen deficiency.

8.2.3 Spermiogenesis

Spermiogenesis is the last phase of spermatogenesis which is the process of formation of sperm cells. In spermatids, sperm production stage, the round spermatids experience **spermatogenetic transformation and change into mature spermatozoa.** This metamorphosis involves learning several significant changes such as differentiation of a tail otherwise known as the flagellum, condensation of the nucleus, **formation of the acrosome which is a cap containing enzymes** that **facilitate fertilization.** This processes takes place in the seminiferous tubules of the testes.

8.2.4 Epididymis

The epididymis is a long tube with a helical part situated on the posterior aspect of each testicle and is the place where sperm mature and are stored. They are located here after being produced in the testes **as spermatic tubule in the seminiferous tubule**. In the testes, the sperm remain immature but in the epididymis they acquire the **ability to swim and to fertilise the ovum.** The epididymis is differentiated into the head, the body and the tail, where the tail contains a storage organ for sperm.

8.2.5 Cremasteric Reflex

Cremasteric reflex is a normal phenomenon which occur due to the contraction of cremaster muscle resulting in **elevation of the testicle on the stimulated side**. This reflex is elicited by stroking the internal part of the thigh; this makes the testicle of the same side to move upward. The cremasteric reflex play a significant role in regulating the temperature of the testes because the **Cord will carry it upwards** in colder temperature and downwards if it is hot. Lack of this reflex is pathological and suggests neurologic pathology of the ilioinguinal or genitofemoral nerves.

8.2.6 Transillumination Scrotum

Scrotal transillumination is a method that involves the use of light in order to inspect the **abnormalities present in the scrotum**. This is because through a process known as transillumination where light is passed through the scrotum, a health care provider is able to identify diseases such as hydrocele where light is visible after **illuminating a fluid-filled sac** around the testes. Nonetheless, it cannot help to discover other diseases as the testicular tumors or varicocele that are **not transilluminant.** It is also typical in the physical examination to detect the enlargement of the scrotum or masses indicated by palpation apart from other diagnosis techniques such as ultrasound.

8.3 Female Reproductive Diagnostic Tests

8.3.1 Cervical Cytology

Cervical cytology may therefore be defined as the test that mainly involves **examination of cervical cells to identify abnormal cells** that could lead to cervical cancer. It entails obtaining samples from the cervix to check for dysplasia that might lead to cancer in the long run. This test can be made by the use of **PAP smear or liquid based cytology**.

8.3.2 Pap Smear

A Pap smear often termed as **Papanicolaou test** is one of the types of cervical cancer screening performed to identify precancerous as well as cancerous cells in cervix. The test is done by taking some cells from the cervix then **analyzing them using the microscope**. :For women it can help to diagnose the precancerous changes in **cervical cells, HPV infections or cervical cancer** at an early stage so that appropriate treatment can be taken. Pap smears should be started at **age 21 and then repeated every 3 years until 65** with the recommendation of the health care practitioners.

8.3.3 Table of Cervical Cancer Screening Guidelines

Counsellors have to adhere to some **certain cervical cancer screening** that is dependent on age, sexual practices and past examinations. As a result, the following are usual recommendations:

- Age 21-29: Pap smear every 3 years.
- Age 30-65: **Co-testing with both the Pap smear and HPV testing** every five years or a Pap smear alone every three years.
- Age 65 and older: The screening is not necessary if previous chest x-rays have been normal; however, further screening is necessary if previous tests have revealed some abnormalities.
- Screening for post-hysterectomy women: Women who previously **underwent hysterectomy** due to non-cancerous conditions may not require screening but their conditions depend on the evaluation of every case.

8.3.4 Bethesda System

Bethesda system is made up of a system of reporting results of **cervical cytology (Pap smear) tests**. They classify the results in order to allow clinicians make the required decisions regarding the follow-up care.

- **Negative for intraepithelial lesion or malignancy:** No signs of cancer or precancerous changes.
- **Dysplasia:** Refers to changes in the cells that are not malignant but far from being normal.
- **Low-grade squamous intraepithelial lesion (LSIL):** Refers to a mild dyskaryotic change that may be due to HPV.
- **High-grade squamous intraepithelial lesion (HSIL):** A higher degree of dyskariosis or squamous intraepithelial neoplasia, HSIL is considered precancerous.
- **Adenocarcinoma in situ (AIS):** Another type of precancerous condition of the cervical glandular cells that may cause cervical cancer.

8.3.5 Colposcopy

Colposcopy is usually done in a circumstance where the common **Pap smear test** proves to be abnormal. **A colposcope is magnifying lens** used in examining for disease of the cervix, vagina or ulcers of vulva. In case of having abnormal areas then it normally leads to a biopsy so that further assessment of the situation can be made. **Colposcopy is usually performed if a woman has an HSIL test or if she has HPV** that does not go away on its own.

8.3.6 Ablative Treatment

Ablative treatment refers to procedures that **destroy abnormal tissue in the cervix**. This kind of treatment is applicable in cases of cervical intraepithelial neoplasia diagnosed by either pap smear or colposcopy examination. Common ablative treatments include:

- Cryotherapy: Freezing of abnormal tissue.
- Photoresection : By applying laser light to the abnormal tissue to cut it.

- LEEP – A procedure where heavy growths are cut out with the electric current.

8.3.7 Potassium Hydroxide Slide

The KOH slide is used to look at the **vaginal or cervical discharge** to determine the infection like the **vaginal candidiasis.** To better analyze the results obtained through a microscope, a small portion of the discharge is added to **potassium hydroxide** solution that dissolves most cellular material and makes the fungal cells stand out. This test enables the clinician to make presumptive identification of yeasts or hyphae in the various samples obtained from a patient's body.

8.3.8 Whiff Test

Indeed, Whiff test is employed for the **diagnosis of bacterial vaginosis (BV).** A smear of the discharge is prepared from a vaginal secretion drop and it is then mixed with **10% potassium hydroxide (KOH**). The sense of a strong fishy smell is indicative of BV due to Gardnerella vaginalis or another bacteria. This is frequently employed as the first screening test for BV that is described by the alteration in the bacterial profile of the vagina.

8.3.9 Tzanck Smear

A Tzanck smear is a laboratory test that maybe employed in order to establish presence of herpes simplex virus. A small scale scraped from an ulcer or a blister of skin or mucous membranes is taken on a glass slide with a china brush and stained. Microscopically, awareness of multinucleated giant cells for identification of the **presence of HSV** is also available for both genres, that is**, HSV-1 and HSV-2.** Despite the fact that this test has been surpassed by **PCR (Polymerase Chain Reaction)** as a method that can give more precise outcomes, it is still applied to some extent.

8.4 Common Conditions of Male Genital System

"Tough Chronic Cases To Control Everything, Providing Profound Fundamentals. Going Everywhere, By Creating Practical Valuable Helpful Solutions." **T**esticular **C**ancer, **P**rostate **C**ancer, **T**esticular **T**orsion, **C**hronic and **A**cute **P**rostatitis, **E**rectile Dysfunction, **P**riapism, **P**araphimosis, **F**ournier's **G**angrene, **E**pididymitis, **B**alanitis, **C**ryptorchidism, **P**himosis, **V**aricocele, **H**ydrocele, and **S**permatocele.

Table 120 Common Conditions of Male Reproductive System

Condition	Description	Key Symptoms	Diagnostic Tools	Treatment Options
Testicular Cancer	Cancer that originates in the testicles, often affecting young men.	Painless lump in the testicle, swelling, pain, heavy feeling in scrotum.	Physical examination, ultrasound, biopsy, CT/MRI	Surgery (orchiectomy), chemotherapy, radiation therapy
Prostate Cancer	Malignant growth in the prostate gland, common in older men.	Difficulty urinating, blood in urine or semen, pelvic pain, erectile dysfunction.	Digital rectal exam, PSA test, biopsy, MRI, CT scan	Surgery (prostatectomy), radiation therapy, hormone therapy

Testicular Torsion	A condition where the spermatic cord twists, cutting off blood flow to the testicle.	Severe, sudden testicular pain, swelling, nausea, vomiting.	Physical examination, ultrasound, Doppler flow study	Surgery (orchiopexy) to untwist the spermatic cord, pain relief
Chronic Prostatitis	Long-term inflammation of the prostate, often associated with pelvic pain.	Pelvic pain, painful urination, difficulty urinating, sexual dysfunction.	Urine culture, PSA test, prostate biopsy, physical exam	Antibiotics, anti-inflammatory medications, physical therapy
Acute Prostatitis	Sudden bacterial infection causing inflammation in the prostate gland.	Fever, chills, painful urination, perineal pain, difficulty urinating.	Urine culture, blood cultures, ultrasound of the prostate	Antibiotics, analgesics, hospitalization (if severe)
Erectile Dysfunction	Inability to achieve or maintain an erection suitable for sexual intercourse.	Inability to get or keep an erection, reduced sexual desire.	Physical exam, blood tests (hormonal, lipid, glucose), penile Doppler ultrasound	Medications (Viagra, Cialis), lifestyle changes, psychotherapy
Priapism	A prolonged and often painful erection lasting more than 4 hours, not associated with sexual activity.	Painful, prolonged erection, discomfort in the penis.	Physical examination, blood gas analysis, Doppler ultrasound	Ice packs, aspiration of blood, medications (alpha-agonists), surgery (in severe cases)

Paraphimosis	A condition where the foreskin becomes stuck behind the glans penis, unable to return to normal position.	Swelling, pain, inability to reduce the foreskin, constricted blood flow.	Physical examination, ultrasound (if needed)	Manual reduction, circumcision, steroid cream (mild cases)
Fournier's Gangrene	A severe, life-threatening soft tissue infection affecting the genital area.	Severe pain, redness, swelling, fever, foul-smelling discharge.	Clinical examination, CT/MRI, blood cultures	Surgical debridement, antibiotics, supportive care
Epididymitis	Inflammation of the epididymis, often due to infection.	Scrotal pain, swelling, redness, fever, painful urination, discharge.	Physical examination, urine culture, ultrasound	Antibiotics, analgesics, rest, cold compresses
Balanitis	Inflammation of the glans penis, often due to infection, poor hygiene, or irritants.	Redness, swelling, itching, pain, discharge, sometimes a foul smell.	Physical exam, swab for culture (if infection suspected)	Topical antifungals/antibiotics, good hygiene, circumcision (in recurrent cases)
Cryptorchidism	Condition where one or both testes fail to descend into the scrotum.	No palpable testis in the scrotum, often detected in infants.	Physical exam, ultrasound, MRI (if uncertain)	Surgery (orchiopexy), hormone therapy (for minor cases)
Phimosis	A condition where the foreskin cannot be retracted	Difficulty retracting the foreskin, painful urination, swelling.	Physical examination	Topical steroids, circumcision (if severe)

	over the glans penis.			
Varicocele	Enlarged veins within the scrotum, similar to varicose veins.	Scrotal swelling, feeling of heaviness in the scrotum, infertility.	Physical exam, scrotal ultrasound	Surgery (varicocelectomy), embolization, supportive underwear
Hydrocele	Fluid-filled sac around a testicle, causing swelling in the scrotum.	Painless scrotal swelling, heaviness in the scrotum, no pain.	Physical exam, ultrasound	Surgery (hydrocelectomy), observation (if asymptomatic)
Spermatocele	A fluid-filled cyst in the epididymis, usually benign.	Painless, soft lump in the scrotum, typically near the testicle.	Physical examination, ultrasound	No treatment (if asymptomatic), surgical excision (if symptomatic)

8.5 Major Medical Issues in Male Genital System

8.5.1 Testicular Cancer

Cancer of the testicles is a type of cancer that **originates in the man's reproductive system**, in **the testis.** It is one of the frequent types of cancer affecting **young men in the age of 15 to 35 years** old, however, it can develop in any age. Little is known regarding the root causes of the disease, but a few of the predisposing factors include **family history of testicular cancer, cryptorchidism, or prior testicular cancer.** Another general sign of the disorder is a **hard, painless lump in one of the testicles** but some may **present pains in the scrotum or heaviness in the scrotum.** Cancer of the testicles is a fairly young man's disease and is easily cured if diagnosed in the early stages. Diagnosis of ovarian cancer is usually done through examination, ultrasound and **AFP and HCG blood tests.** The action taken is surgery namely orchiectomy while other options that may be used depending on the stage of the **neoplasm is chemotherapy or radiation.** It is quite a favorable one if the treatment is begun at an early stage.

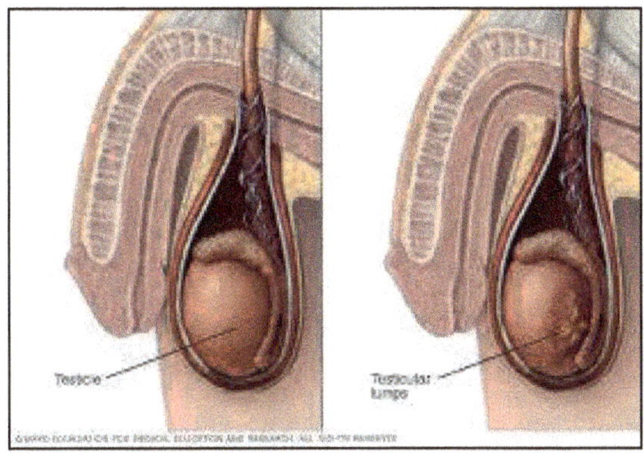

Figure 208 Testicular Cancer

8.5.1.1 Classification of Testicular Cancer

There are two major types of testicular tumor; **the germ cell tumors and non-germ cell tumors**. Testicular cancers are the male genital tract malignancies and approximately, **95% of them are germ cell tumors** which are subdivided into **seminomas and non-seminomas.** Seminoma tumors are more common than other types of **germ cell tumor with approximately 85% of all cases**. Seminomas are sub typed as classical, spermatic seminomas, and anaplastic seminomas with the latter representing **85%, 5%, and 10% respectively**. While **non seminomatous tumors** are more invasive, these are **Embryonal carcinoma, Yolk-sac tumors (endodermal sinus tumors), Teratomas and Choriocarcinomas.** These are fairly common tumors, which are somewhat more malignant as compared to seminomas and may exhibit different histopathology. Of the non-germ cell tumors accounting for about 5% of testicular tumors, there are **sex cord-stromal tumors such as Sertoli's cell tumors and Leydig's cell tumors amongst others like metastases and lymphoma**. Tumors that develop in the testicle can be classified and this classifi-cation is very important for proper diagnosis, prognosis and management of the condition.

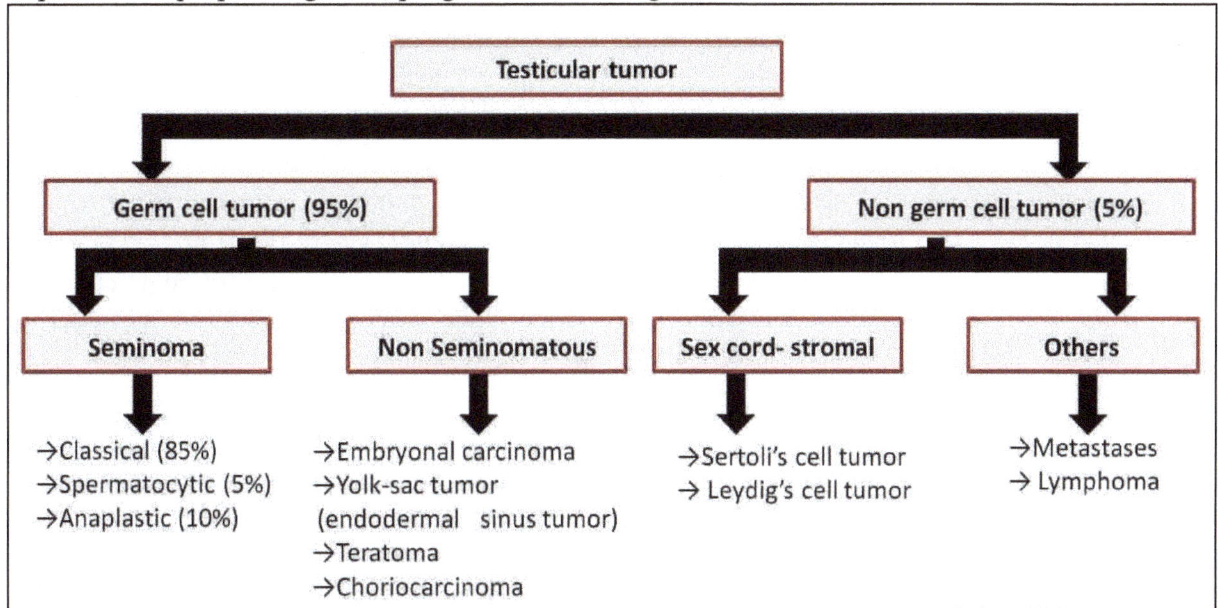

Figure 209 Classification of Testicular Cancer

8.5.1.2 SOAP Notes for Testicular Cancer

Table 121 SOAP Notes for Testicular Cancer

Component	Details

Subjective (S)	A 28-year-old male presents with a painless lump in his left testicle noticed two weeks ago. The patient reports no associated pain but feels a sensation of heaviness in the scrotum. He denies any trauma or injury to the area. There is no history of fever, weight loss, or night sweats. He mentions some mild discomfort after prolonged periods of sitting. The patient has no significant past medical history, although his father had prostate cancer. The patient is concerned because of the family history of cancer and the presence of the lump.
Objective (O)	The patient appears in no acute distress. Vital signs: BP 120/78 mmHg, HR 75 bpm, Temp 36.8°C (98.2°F). On physical examination, a firm, non-tender, irregular lump is palpated in the left testicle. No signs of scrotal edema or erythema. The right testicle is normal in size and consistency. No inguinal lymphadenopathy. Urinalysis shows no hematuria. Scrotal ultrasound reveals a solid mass in the left testicle measuring approximately 2 cm in diameter. Blood tests show elevated **alpha-fetoprotein (AFP)** and **human chorionic gonadotropin (hCG)** levels, suggesting a potential germ cell tumor.
Assessment (A)	The patient's presentation, including the painless testicular mass and elevated tumor markers (AFP and hCG), is highly suspicious for testicular cancer, likely a germ cell tumor. The scrotal ultrasound and tumor markers are consistent with a diagnosis of testicular cancer. Although there is no lymphadenopathy or signs of metastasis, further imaging and staging are needed.
Plan (P)	**Pharmacological**: No immediate pharmacological intervention is required at this stage (See algorithm below). **Diagnostic**: Refer the patient for an orchiectomy (removal of the affected testicle) for histopathological diagnosis. Schedule a CT scan of the abdomen and pelvis to assess for possible metastasis to lymph nodes or other organs. **Follow-up**: Post-surgery follow-up to assess histopathology results. If cancer is confirmed, initiate treatment with chemotherapy or radiation therapy as per staging and pathology results. **Education**: Discuss the nature of testicular cancer, the importance of early detection, and the potential for successful treatment with appropriate therapy. Provide emotional support and counseling regarding the implications of surgery on fertility and future reproductive options. Encourage the patient to monitor for any new symptoms, such as pain, swelling, or changes in bowel or urinary habits, and report them immediately.

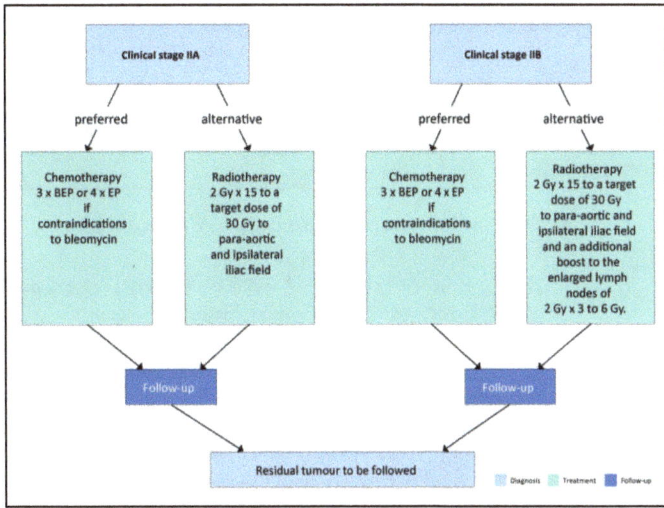

Figure 210 EAU Guidelines on Testicular Cancer

8.5.2 Prostate Cancer

Cancer of the prostate is among the commonly occurring malignancies in men especially those of over fifty years of age. Cancer of the prostate is a disease that stem from **uncontrolled growth of prostate glandular cells, which form a tumor.** However, for the initial stage of prostate cancer the patient may not experience any of the symptoms, as it progresses, one may experience painful and hard time in passing urine , find blood in the urine or in the semen and feel pains in the pelvic region. Prostate cancer risk factors **are age, family history, race (example African America men), and diet. Prostate-specific antigen test, digital rectal examination and prostate biopsy** are the usual ways of diagnosing the disease. This then calls for treatment methods that include **surgery, radiation therapy, hormonal therapy, chemotherapy, and in very rare cases, mastectomy and or hysterectomy.** In such conditions various low-risk management strategies can be applied, one of which is active surveillance. Despite this, prostate cancer is one of the most treatable forms of cancer once it is detected early enough and survival rates have risen over the years backwards **due to improvements in technology**. This policy remains pivotal in improving overall outcomes depending on the early indication received.

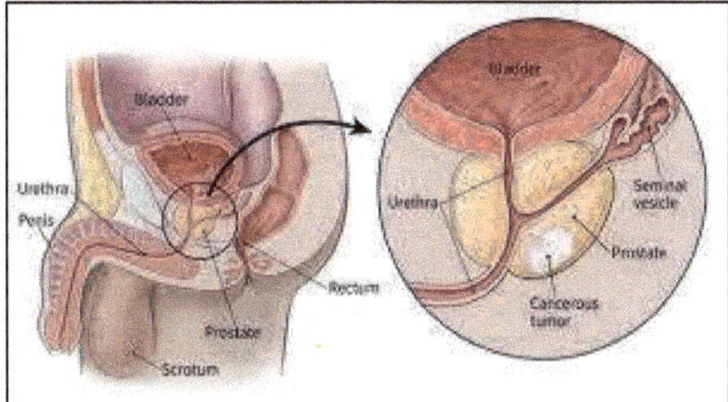

Figure 211 Prostae Cancer

8.5.2.1 Stages of Prostate Cancer

The figure depicts the various stages of prostate cancer categorized depending on the progression of cancer. **Stage I is when the cancer has not grown significantly** and can be felt only on digital rectal examination or by biopsy. **During stage II the tumour may be larger and may include both the Lobes of the prostate** but it is constrained to the gland and has not spread out. Stage III is also categorized as the **locally advanced type**; it is featured by cancer spread to the nearby structures such as lymph nodes or the seminal vesicles. The **last stage is the IV**, which advanced cancer has spread beyond the primary location to the other regions of the body like the bones, liver or lungs. Although the **cancer can spread to the bones**, persons are said to be suffering from prostate cancer and not bone cancer. They assist in reflecting on how to proceed with the patient management as well as prognosis.

Stage	Description
Stage I (Localized)	**The cancer is small and only in the prostate.**
Stage II (Localized)	**The cancer is larger and may be in both lobes of the prostate, but it is still confined to the prostate.**
Stage III (Locally Advanced)	**The cancer has spread beyond the prostate to nearby lymph glands or seminal vesicles.**
Stage IV (Metastatic/Advanced)	**The cancer has spread to other parts of the body, such as to the bones, liver, or lungs. This is referred to as metastatic or advanced prostate cancer. If prostate cancer spreads, or metastasizes, to the bone, you have prostate cancer cells in the bone—not bone cancer.**

Figure 212 Stages of Prostate Cancer

8.5.2.2 Grading of Prostate Cancer

The image also explains the **Gleason Score on how the tumor is graded** based on its microscopic appearance. **The Gleason score informs of the level of the cancer** and how active it is, or how prone it is to spread out. In the **Low/Very Low risk** group referring to the Grade Group 1, a **Gleason score of 6 or less is assigned**. This score also indicates that the tumor tissue is well differentiated – which means that it is less malignant and, it grows at a slow rate. The Intermediate risk group according to the study is the **Grade Groups 2 and 3 with Gleason scores of 3+4=7 or 4+3=7.** Some of these tumours are moderate differentiated and moderate, not too aggressive but may form new formations but are not too dangerous as to spread rapidly. Lastly, the High/Very High risk compilation is comprising of the **Grade Groups 4 and 5 with Gleason scores ranging from 8, 9 and 10**. This category of tumors lacks differentiation or is undifferentiated, and subsequently, they are very aggressive, fast-growing malignancies that are more likely to metastasize. In cases where the Gleason score is not rendered, it is signified by **Gleason 10 or referred to as Gleason X.** It is also used in calculating the prognosis of the disease as well as suggesting treatment methods of prostate cancer.

RISK GROUP	GRADE GROUP	GLEASON SCORE	DESCRIPTION
		Gleason X	Gleason score cannot be determined.
Low/Very Low	Grade Group 1	Gleason 6 (or less)	The tumor tissue is well differentiated, less aggressive, and likely to grow more slowly.
Intermediate (Favorable or Unfavorable)	Grade Group 2 Grade Group 3	Gleason 3 + 4 = 7 Gleason 4 + 3 = 7	The tumor tissue is moderately differentiated, moderately aggressive, and likely to grow but may not spread quickly.
High/Very High	Grade Group 4 Grade Group 5	Gleason 8 Gleason 9 – 10	The tumor tissue is poorly differentiated or undifferentiated, highly aggressive, and likely to grow faster and spread.

Figure 213 Grading of Prostate Cancer

8.5.2.3 SOAP Notes for Prostate Cancer

Table 122 SOAP Notes for Prostate Cancer

Component	Details
Subjective (S)	A 65-year-old male presents with difficulty urinating, weak stream, and increased frequency of urination. He reports occasional blood in the urine and mild pelvic discomfort. The patient has a family history of prostate cancer (father diagnosed at 70). He is concerned about his symptoms and potential for prostate cancer.
Objective (O)	Physical exam shows a firm, enlarged prostate on digital rectal exam (DRE). Vital signs are stable: BP 130/85 mmHg, HR 78 bpm, Temp 36.8°C (98.2°F). Urinalysis shows microscopic hematuria. PSA level is elevated at 8 ng/mL (normal range: 0-4 ng/mL). A transrectal ultrasound (TRUS) and biopsy are scheduled to assess for malignancy.
Assessment (A)	The patient's presentation, including symptoms of lower urinary tract obstruction and an elevated PSA, is suggestive of possible prostate cancer. The DRE findings and family history of prostate cancer further increase suspicion. Diagnosis needs confirmation through biopsy, and Gleason score will determine the aggressiveness of the tumor.
Plan (P)	**Pharmacological**: Consider starting a 5-alpha-reductase inhibitor (e.g., finasteride) to help manage symptoms if benign prostatic hyperplasia (BPH) is suspected (See algorithm below). **Non-pharmacological**: Proceed with a transrectal ultrasound (TRUS) and prostate biopsy to confirm diagnosis. If prostate cancer is diagnosed, staging and Gleason scoring will guide treatment options. **Follow-up**: Follow-up appointment after biopsy results for staging and discussion of treatment options (e.g., surgery, radiation, or hormone therapy). **Education**: Educate the patient about prostate cancer risk factors, the importance of biopsy for diagnosis, and treatment options.

Discuss potential side effects of treatments and the importance of regular follow-up.

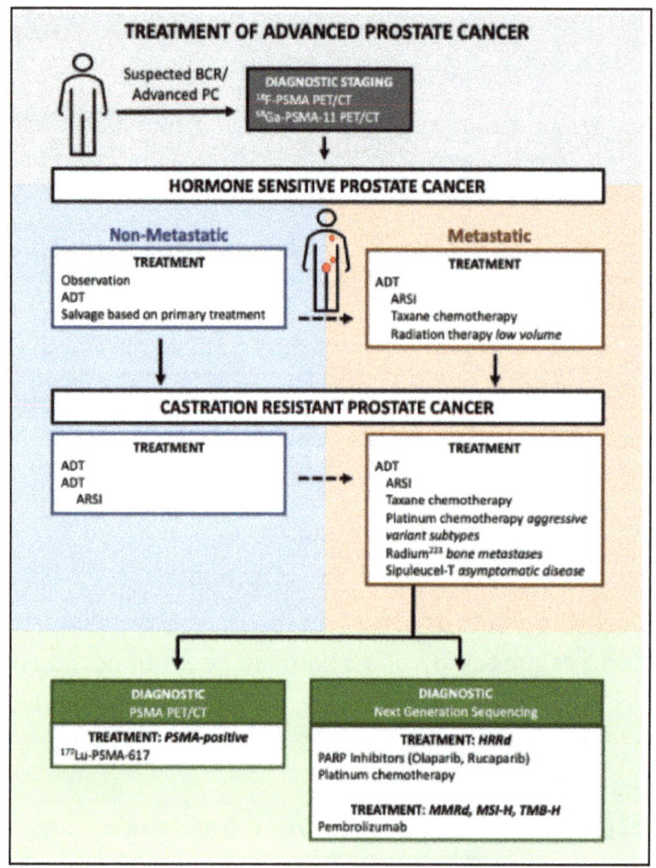

Figure 214 Treatment Algorithm for Advanced Prostate Cancer

8.5.3 Testicular Torsion

Testicular torsion is a clinical situation where the spermatic cord through which blood is supplied to the **testicle twists, and interrupts circulating blood supply.** This condition is known to affect boys in their **adolescent age of 12-18 years** but mostly manifest in any age. The main sign is pain in one of the testicles that is sharp, intense, and sudden; the **affected testicle may also be swollen**; there may also be **feelings of nausea and vomiting as well as the tummy ache**. The testicle that is affected may be located higher than the other or positioned to a position that is quite awkward. There is no certain cure for testicular torsion, but it is a surgical intervention that is triggered by either injury to the testicle or due to a **congenetic condition like the bell-clapper deformity**. In **most cases, medical attention is necessary** to avoid complications leading to loss of body functions. If the injury is not taken care of **within a span of six hours, the scrotum might become gangrenous and the testicle may have to be removed.** The common treatment plan would be to have the cord surgically untwisted to free the testicle and to anchor it.

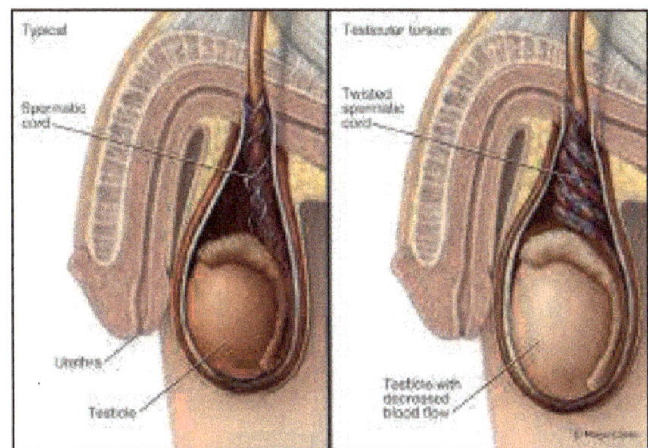

Figure 215 Testicular Torsion

8.5.3.1 Types of Testicular Torsion

The image shows **three types of testicular torsion depending on the point of attachment and structure of the spermatic cord with the testicles. Intravaginal** form represents the majority of cases, in which the testicle rotates inside the tunica vaginalis – the protective covering around it. **This chokes off the blood supply** to the testicle, leading to ischemia and possible infarction if not corrected at the soonest. it involves the torsion of the **spermatic cord and the testicle** in a spit outside the **tunica vaginalis** and is common among new born or children. This form is more comprehensive and can lead to the removal of the testicle if not treated on time. Finally, long mesorchium is a situation in which the ligament for **attaching the testicle** is longer compare to usual size and this makes the testicle more mobile. This mobility can cause torsion either intra vaginal or extra vaginal. **Surgical intervention** should be done on time, especially for all the reasons that include testicular atrophy or even infertility.

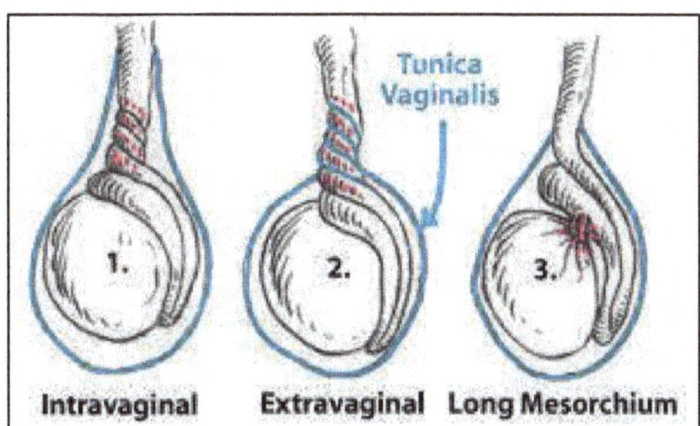

Figure 216 Types of Testicular Torsion

8.5.3.2 SOAP Notes for Testicular Torsion

Table 123 SOAP Notes for Testicular Torsion

Component	Details
Subjective (S)	A 16-year-old male presents with sudden onset of severe, unilateral scrotal pain, which began approximately 6 hours ago. He reports that the pain started spontaneously, without any known trauma or activity. He also experiences nausea and vomiting. He denies any recent history of infections or urinary problems. The patient is anxious and appears distressed due to the intense pain.
Objective (O)	The patient appears in moderate distress. On physical examination, there is significant tenderness over the right testicle, which is elevated and in a

	transverse position. The cremasteric reflex is absent on the right side. The scrotum is swollen and erythematous. Ultrasound reveals reduced blood flow to the right testicle, confirming testicular torsion.
Assessment (A)	The patient's presentation of acute scrotal pain, absent cremasteric reflex, and the findings on ultrasound suggest testicular torsion, likely intravaginal torsion. This condition is a surgical emergency, requiring prompt intervention to prevent testicular loss.
Plan (P)	**Pharmacological**: Pain management with intravenous analgesics (e.g., morphine) (See algorithm below). **Non-pharmacological**: Immediate referral to urology for emergency surgical exploration and detorsion. Consider orchiopexy on the contralateral testicle. **Follow-up**: Close monitoring post-surgery for any signs of complications such as infection or recurrence of torsion. **Education**: Educate the patient and family on the importance of early intervention for testicular torsion and the potential consequences of delayed treatment, including infertility and testicular atrophy.

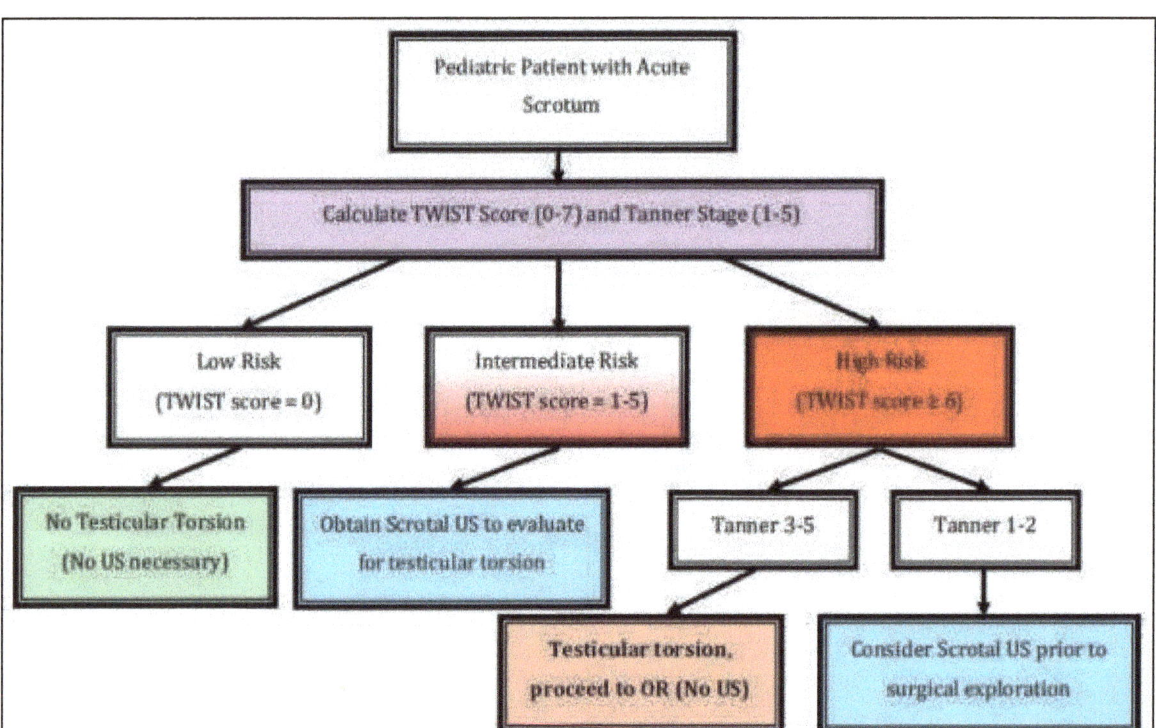

Figure 217 Management Algorithm for Testicular Torsion

8.5.4 Chronic and acute Prostatitis

Prostatitis refers to inflammation of the prostate gland, with two main types: acute and chronic. Acute prostatitis is the inflammation of the prostate due to bacterial infection in which ***E. coli*** **or any other bacteria is prevalent.** This ranges from slight to **severe manifestations, such as fever, chills, dysuria (painful urination),** lower abdomen or pelvic pain and tender quote on the prostate using the **digital rectal examination (DRE).** A challenge that the patient can experience is urinary incontinence or urinary hesitancy, that is, be able to pass urine. Acute prostatitis can be treated only medically with the use of antibiotics, including intravenous antibiotics at the initial stage and later oral antibiotics. **Hospitalization becomes necessary in such conditions**. In acute prostatitis if not treated may result in other complications like abscess formation or even sepsis.

Another pain syndrome to note is the immense one that some patients experience in the pelvic area or what is known as **Chronic Prostatitis or Chronic Pelvic Pain Syndrome**. It can be of bacterial or non-bacterial in nature, although the latter can be attributed to such issues as dysfunction of the pelvic floor and autoimmune diseases. It may be less obvious than acute prostatitis but causes considerable discomfort to a man's lifestyle. **Chronic prostatitis management still requires long-term antibiotic, anti-inflammatory drugs and pelvic floor muscles rehabilitation**. Antihypertensive medication such as alpha-blockers or other drugs could be used for the treatment of urinal symptoms. Nonbacterial prostatitis also has to be treated, and the course of therapy depends on the diagnosis made by a physician.

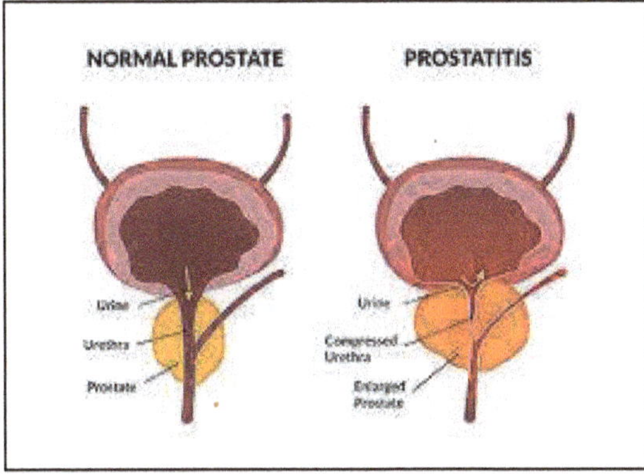

Figure 218 Prostatitis Comparison

8.5.4.1 Types of Prostatitis

The following picture gives an insight on the **types of prostatitis and the features** that may be associated with each type. Bacterial prostatitis of acute type always results from bacterial invasion and often characterised by **severe symptoms like fever, chills, pain on urination and general pelvic discomfort.** It can be treated with the help of antibiotics and one should not delay to seek medical help as the **condition can lead to sepsis**. Chronic bacterial prostatitis is a long term bacterial infection that does not clear even after repeated use of antibiotics and presents acute or chronic symptoms. This type of prostatitis may often prompt long-term antibiotics and may occasionally demand more therapy. **Chronic prostatitis is a condition that is not related to bacteria infection** but entails previous infections, immune dysfunction or stress. Delirium is not easy to manage and it poses substantial impact on a patient's daily experience. Last type of prostatitis, asymptomatic prostatitis doesn't cause symptoms and the man may experience it only if he is checked by a doctor. The cause of this type is still unidentified, and it seldom responds to **any medication unless it compromises the health of the patient.** Both types of prostatitis need management based on the cause and symptoms of each one of them.

Table 124 Types of Prostatitis

Type of Prostatitis	Cause
Acute Bacterial Prostatitis	Sudden bacterial infection
Chronic Bacterial Prostatitis	Long-term bacterial infection
Chronic Prostatitis	Not caused by bacteria; may result from a past infection, immune dysfunction, stress, or other factors
Asymptomatic Prostatitis	Unknown cause

8.5.4.2 Classification of Prostatitis

The picture depicts **NIH classification of prostatitis**, which categorizes conditions depending on their qualities. **Category I is acute bacterial prostatitis**, the inflammation of prostate gland due to bacterial infections. This category is characterized by sudden and severe symptoms including fever, chills, and pain when passing urine and demands for use of antibiotics. **As for Category II, it is chronic bacterial prostatitis** which is defined as recurrent infection of the prostate. ERP is more difficult to cure and may be treated by antibiotics in the long run. **Subcategory IIIA is inflammatory chronic pelvic pain syndrome (CPPS)** where there is Color change to Presence of white blood cells in the ejaculated semen, EPS or voided bladder urine. This type of inflammation in the prostate is not due to bacteria and is classified under infectious prostatitis. **Category IIIB is characterized as non-inflammatory CPPS**, for which there are not blood cells in semen, EPS or voided bladder urine. This type is diagnosed with the help of semen analysis and increased PSA concentration. Lastly, **the fourth category is the non-symptomatic inflammation of the prostate gland or sub-acute bacterial prostatitis** where there is no complaint from the patient, but may present some features like the elevated PSA and may be diagnosed due to incidental findings from a biopsy done on the prostate gland.

Table 125 Prostatitis Classification

NIH Classification	DEFINITION
CATEGORY I Acute Bacterial Prostatitis	Acute Infection of the Prostate Gland
CATEGORY II Chronic Bacterial Prostatitis	Recurrent infection of the Prostate
CATEGORY IIIA Inflammatory CPPS	White cells in semen/EPS/Voided Bladder Urine 3 (VB_3 or post-prostatic massage)
CATEGORY IIIB Non-inflammatory CPPS	No white cells in semen/EPS/VB_3
CATEGORY IV Asymptomatic Inflammatory Prostatitis	• Abnormal semen analysis • Elevated PSA values • Incidental findings in biopsied prostate

8.5.4.3 SOAP Notes for Prostatitis

Table 126 SOAP Notes for Prostatitis

Component	Details
Subjective (S)	A 45-year-old male presents with a 4-day history of pelvic pain, dysuria, and increased urinary frequency. He reports a low-grade fever and chills,

	but denies any back pain, hematuria, or difficulty urinating. The patient is anxious about the discomfort.
Objective (O)	Vital signs: Temperature 38°C, HR 90 bpm, BP 125/80 mmHg. Physical exam reveals tenderness on digital rectal exam (DRE) over the prostate. Urinalysis shows white blood cells and mild bacteriuria. No palpable mass or signs of abscess on physical exam.
Assessment (A)	The patient's symptoms, including pelvic pain, fever, and positive findings on DRE, are consistent with prostatitis. This could be either bacterial or non-bacterial in origin, but a bacterial etiology is more likely based on the fever and urinary symptoms. Further urine culture results will confirm the pathogen.
Plan (P)	**Pharmacological:** Initiate empirical antibiotics such as fluoroquinolones or trimethoprim-sulfamethoxazole until culture results are available (See algorithm below). **Non-pharmacological:** Increase fluid intake, encourage rest, and avoid irritants like caffeine and alcohol. **Follow-up:** Reassess in 2-3 days to monitor symptom improvement. If no improvement or worsening of symptoms, consider a change in antibiotics or further investigation.

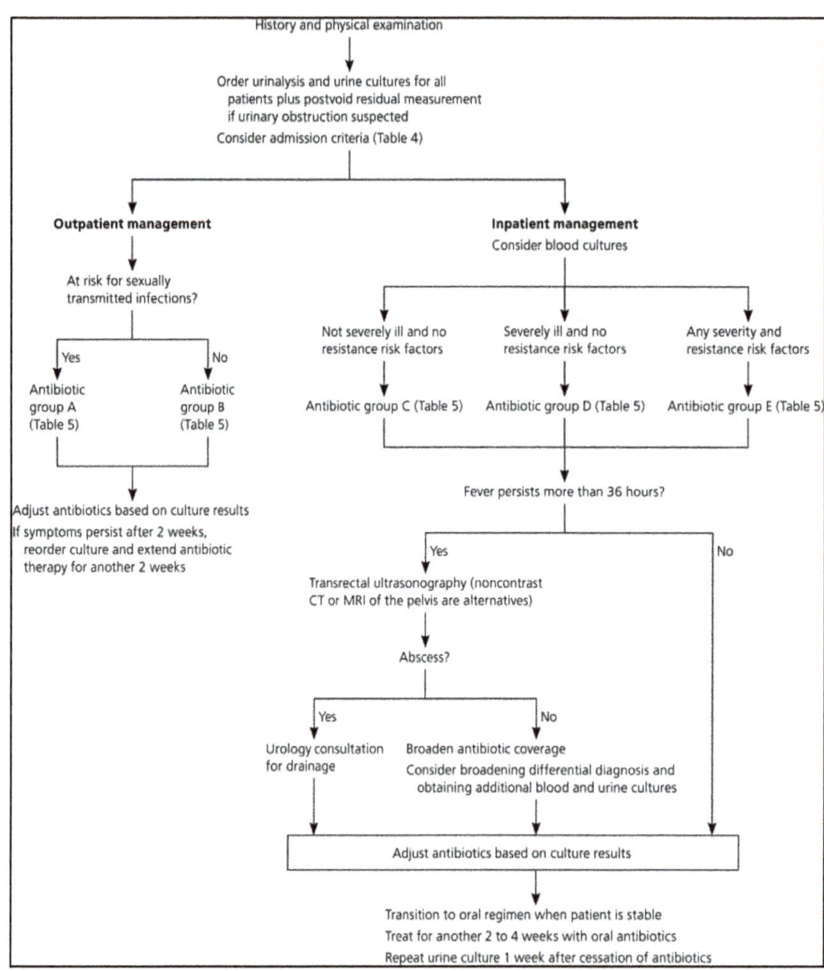

Figure 219 Management Algorithm for Prostatitis

Table 127 Admission Criteria (Table 4 mentioned in algorithm above)

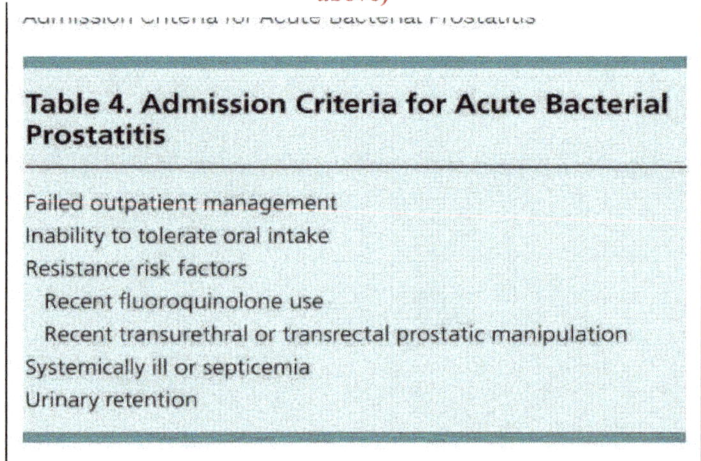

Table 4. Admission Criteria for Acute Bacterial Prostatitis

Failed outpatient management
Inability to tolerate oral intake
Resistance risk factors
  Recent fluoroquinolone use
  Recent transurethral or transrectal prostatic manipulation
Systemically ill or septicemia
Urinary retention

Table 128 Antibiotic Regimens (Table 5 mentioned in algorithm above)

Table 5. Antibiotic Regimens for Acute Bacterial Prostatitis

Group	Primary regimen	Alternative regimen	Considerations
A	Single dose of ceftriaxone (Rocephin), 250 mg intramuscularly, or single dose of cefixime (Suprax), 400 mg orally *then* Doxycycline, 100 mg orally twice daily for 10 days	—	Regimen covers *Neisseria gonorrhoeae* and *Chlamydia trachomatis* infections in addition to other common bacterial pathogens
B	Ciprofloxacin, 500 mg orally twice daily for 10 to 14 days *or* Levofloxacin (Levaquin), 500 to 750 mg orally daily for 10 to 14 days	Trimethoprim/sulfamethoxazole, 160/800 mg orally twice daily for 10 to 14 days	Extend treatment for 2 weeks if patient remains symptomatic
C	Ciprofloxacin, 400 mg IV every 12 hours *or* Levofloxacin, 500 to 750 mg IV every 24 hours	Ceftriaxone, 1 to 2 g IV every 24 hours *plus* Levofloxacin, 500 to 750 mg IV every 24 hours *or* Piperacillin/tazobactam (Zosyn), 3.375 g IV every 6 hours	Continue treatment until patient is afebrile, then transition to oral regimen (group B) for an additional 2 to 4 weeks
D	Piperacillin/tazobactam, 3.375 g IV every 6 hours *plus* aminoglycosides* *or* Cefotaxime (Claforan), 2 g IV every 4 hours *plus* aminoglycosides* *or* Ceftazidime (Fortaz), 2 g IV every 8 hours *plus* aminoglycosides*	Fluoroquinolone (group C) *plus* Aminoglycosides* *or* Ertapenem (Invanz), 1 g IV every 24 hours *or* Imipenem/cilastatin (Primaxin), 500 mg IV every 6 hours *or* Meropenem (Merrem IV), 500 mg IV every 8 hours	Continue treatment until patient is afebrile, then transition to oral regimen (group B) for an additional 2 to 4 weeks
E	**Transrectal manipulation—fluoroquinolone resistance and extended spectrum beta-lactamase–producing *Escherichia coli*** Piperacillin/tazobactam, 3.375 g IV every 6 hours *plus* aminoglycosides*	Ertapenem, 1 g IV every 24 hours *or* Imipenem/cilastatin, 500 mg IV every 6 hours	Continue treatment until patient is afebrile, then transition to oral regimen (group B) for an additional 2 to 4 weeks Carbapenems can be used if patient is unstable If patient is stable, follow primary regimen while awaiting culture results
	Transurethral manipulation—*Pseudomonas* species Piperacillin/tazobactam, 3.375 g IV every 6 hours† *or* Ceftazidime, 2 g IV every 8 hours† *or* Cefipime, 2 g IV every 12 hours†	Fluoroquinolone (group C)† *or* Imipenem/cilastatin, 500 mg IV every 6 hours *or* Meropenem, 500 mg IV every 8 hours	
	Fluoroquinolone exposure—fluoroquinolone resistance Piperacillin/tazobactam, 3.375 g IV every 6 hours† *or* Ceftazidime, 2 g IV every 8 hours† *or* Cefepime, 2 g IV every 12 hours†	Ceftriaxone, 1 g IV every 24 hours† *or* Ertapenem, 1 g IV every 24 hours	

IV = intravenously.

**—Dosing instructions: gentamicin, 7 mg per kg IV every 24 hours, peak 16 to 24 mcg per mL, trough less than 1 mcg per mL; amikacin, 15 mg per kg IV every 24 hours, peak 56 to 64 mcg per mL, trough less than 1 mcg per mL.*

†—Aminoglycosides should be added to regimen if patient is clinically unstable.

Information from references 5, 7 through 9, 15 through 17, 24, and 25.

8.5.5 Erectile dysfunction

Erectile dysfunction is a condition that is characterized by the failure to achieve and sustain an erection that is firm enough to **perform sexual intercourse.** This is something very widespread among men, regardless of the age, but it is most often **diagnosed among the elder men.** The **nonmodal causes of erectile dysfunction** include diseases of the blood vessels, diabetes, hormonal disorders and neurological disorders. Nonetheless, it is noteworthy that numerous psychological factors such as stress, anxiety, depression and problems in the partnership can also cause the **non-Commissioned Officia.** Other risk factors include education level, smoking, too much alcohol intake as well as lack of exercises. As mentioned above, the treatment for ED depends on the cause. Oral drugs include **Sildenafil also known as Viagra** that facilitates the flow of blood to the penis. In cases where medications fail to work, other treatments that are then used are the **vacuum erection devices, the injection of medications into the penis, or surgery**. Medical advice may also include psychological counseling if the client's problem has some psychological background. Other aspects include maintaining healthy habits with focusing on treatment of underlying range of conditions such as diabetes, or a possibility of improving different aspects of cardiovascular health.

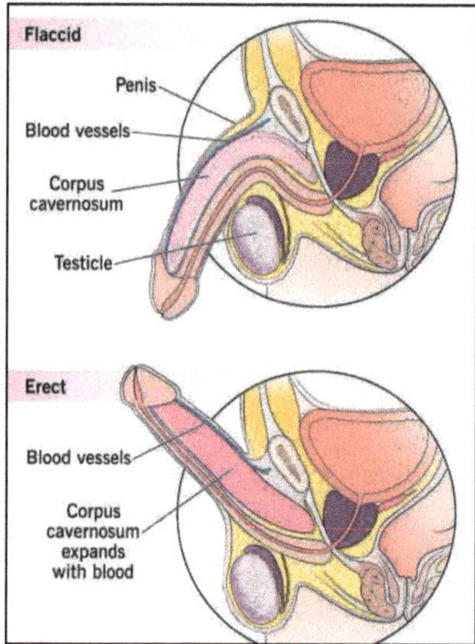

Figure 220 Erectile Dysfunction

8.5.5.1 Types of Erectile Dysfunction

Figure outlines the various classifications of **impotence (erectile dysfunction)** as comprises of primary impotence, secondary impotence with regard to rapid ejaculation, and retarded ejaculation. **Primary impotence** is defined as one that could not experience even a single erection fit for sexual intercourse at his lifetime. **This type is related most of the time to congenital or psychological disorder. Secondary impotence** is characterized as the **absence of erection ability in the man** who used to boast of this ability as a consequence of the severe diseases, including diabetes, nervous stress, or the problems with the blood circulation system. **Premature Ejaculation** is the failure of a man to delay ejaculation to the desired time during sexual activity thus resulting in unsatisfactory **sexual experience to the sexual partners**. Impaired ejaculation refers to the disability in man to ejaculate when desired to do so, or when a normal sexual stimulation is carried out, which causes **delayed orgasm and erectile dysfunction**. Every type of impotence is resulted from different causes and can be treated in particular ways.

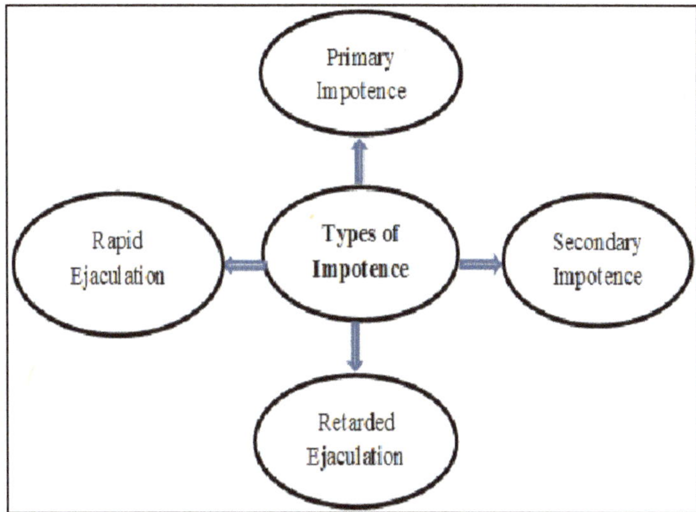

Figure 221 Types of Erectile Dysfunction

8.5.5.2 Classification of Erectile Dysfunction

The picture depicts a classification of **erectile dysfunction into two categories namely: organic and psychogenic factors.** Organic factors can be divided into vasculogenic, neurogenic, anatomic, and endocrinologic etiologies. **Vasculogenic erectile dysfunction is an arterial, cavernosal, or mixed variety,** which is associated with blood circulation. Neurogenic involves nerve issue and anatomic concerns the anatomical changes in the body that interfere with sex. According to the **psychogenic causes of the dysfunction**, there are general psychogenic dysfunction and psychogenic dysfunction related to a particular situation or event. In sexual medicine, generalized psychogenic dysfunction can be characterized by the absence of sexual show more of sexual interest or desire, which may in the **first place be congenital or developed due to aging or as a resultant of chronic illness** that does not allow for sexual activity. Situational dysfunction is then subsetted by partner related dysfunction which may include a certain degree of arousability in a certain relationship or due to c**onflict with the partner, performances arousal related arousal or any other sexual dysfunction, psychological illness or stress due to any life events**.

Organic
I. Vasculogenic
A. Arteriogenic
B. Cavernosal
C. Mixed
II. Neurogenic
III. Anatomic
IV. Endocrinologic
Psychogenic
I. Generalized type
A. Generalized unresponsiveness
1. Primary lack of sexual arousability
2. Aging-related decline in sexual arousability
B. Generalized inhibition
1. Chronic disorder of sexual intimacy
II. Situational type
A. Partner-related
1. Lack of arousability in specific relationship
2. Lack of arousability due to sexual object preference
3. High central inhibition due to partner conflict or threat
B. Performance-related
1. Associated with other sexual dysfunction/s (eg, rapid ejaculation)
2. Situational performance anxiety (eg, fear of failure)
C. Psychological distress or adjustment related
1. Associated with negative mood state (eg, depression) or major life stress (eg, death of partner)

Figure 222 Classification of Erectile Dysfunction

8.5.5.3 SOAP Notes for Erectile Dysfunction

Table 129 SOAP Notes for Erectile Dysfunction

Component	Details
Subjective (S)	A 55-year-old male presents with complaints of difficulty maintaining an erection for the past 6 months. He reports a gradual onset of erectile dysfunction and admits to experiencing occasional morning erections but struggles with sexual activity with his partner. The patient denies any pain or discomfort during erections. He has a history of hypertension and is currently taking medication for it. He also reports increased stress at work and marital concerns. The patient expresses concern about his ability to perform sexually and is seeking help.
Objective (O)	The patient appears well-groomed and in no acute distress. Vital signs: BP 130/85 mmHg, HR 75 bpm, Temp 36.9°C (98.4°F). Physical examination reveals no abnormalities in genitalia. There are no signs of penile deformities, and the testes are of normal size. Digital rectal exam (DRE) reveals a normal prostate. Laboratory results show normal testosterone levels (400 ng/dL), normal thyroid function tests, and normal lipid profile.
Assessment (A)	The patient's erectile dysfunction is likely multifactorial, involving both organic and psychogenic factors. Given the history of hypertension and the stress reported, this could be contributing to the erectile dysfunction. The absence of significant medical abnormalities and normal testosterone levels suggests a primarily functional cause, possibly related to performance anxiety or relationship stress.
Plan (P)	**Pharmacological**: Initiate treatment with oral phosphodiesterase type 5 inhibitors (e.g., sildenafil) as needed before sexual activity (See algorithm below). **Non-pharmacological**: Refer the patient to counseling for relationship stress and psychological support for performance anxiety. Recommend lifestyle modifications, including regular exercise, stress

	management techniques, and a healthy diet. Follow-up: Reassess in 1-2 months to evaluate the effectiveness of treatment and address any concerns. If symptoms persist, consider further investigations for underlying vascular or neurological causes. **Education**: Educate the patient on the role of stress and hypertension in erectile dysfunction and discuss the importance of open communication with their partner.

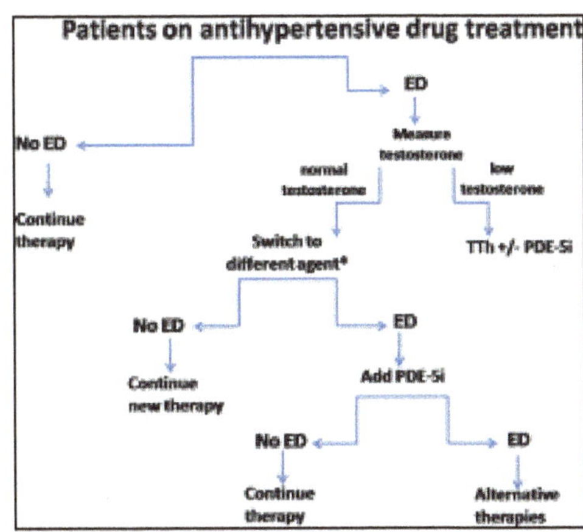

Figure 223 Management Algorithm for Erectile Dysfunction

8.5.6 Priapism

Table 130 SOAP Notes for Priapism

Component	Details
Subjective (S)	A 32-year-old male presents with a painful, persistent erection lasting over 4 hours. He reports that the erection began spontaneously without any sexual activity. He has no history of trauma or drug use, but admits to taking sildenafil earlier that evening. He is anxious about the persistent pain and is seeking immediate help.
Objective (O)	The patient is in mild distress due to pain. On physical exam, the penis is erect, and there is no tenderness on palpation of the shaft. The glans is not engorged. No signs of trauma or abnormal curvature. The patient's blood pressure is 130/85 mmHg, heart rate is 88 bpm, and temperature is 36.8°C (98.2°F).
Assessment (A)	The patient's symptoms are consistent with priapism, likely drug-induced given the use of sildenafil. This is a medical emergency that requires immediate intervention to prevent long-term damage to erectile tissue.
Plan (P)	**Pharmacological**: Administer intravenous fluids and analgesics for pain management. Consider intracavernosal injection of sympathomimetic agents (e.g., phenylephrine) if the erection persists. **Non-pharmacological**: Refer the patient to urology for

	possible aspiration of the corpora cavernosa if conservative management is ineffective. Follow-up: Monitor for resolution within 4-6 hours to avoid complications such as erectile dysfunction. **Education**: Explain the risks of priapism and encourage proper use of erectile dysfunction medications to avoid recurrence.

8.5.7 Paraphimosis

Table 131 SOAP Notes for Paraphimosis

Component	Details
Subjective (S)	A 45-year-old male presents with swelling and painful retraction of the foreskin behind the glans penis, which occurred after an attempt at cleaning the area. He reports severe discomfort, difficulty urinating, and a sense of tightness.
Objective (O)	On physical exam, the foreskin is retracted behind the glans penis and cannot be returned to its normal position. The glans is swollen and congested, and there is tenderness with palpation. No signs of infection (e.g., no discharge or fever). The patient's blood pressure is 120/75 mmHg, heart rate 78 bpm, and temperature 37.1°C (98.8°F).
Assessment (A)	The patient presents with paraphimosis, a urological emergency where the retracted foreskin causes impaired venous return, leading to swelling and ischemia.
Plan (P)	**Pharmacological**: Administer analgesics for pain relief. **Non-pharmacological**: Attempt manual reduction of the foreskin with lubrication. If unsuccessful, refer for surgical intervention (e.g., dorsal slit or circumcision). Follow-up: Monitor for complications such as tissue necrosis. **Education**: Advise on proper techniques for cleaning the genital area and the importance of not forcing the foreskin back. Discuss potential risks of recurrence.

8.5.8 Fournier's Gangrene

Table 132 SOAP Notes for Fournier's Gangrene

Component	Details
Subjective (S)	A 58-year-old male with poorly controlled diabetes presents with fever, intense pain, and swelling in the perineal area. He reports that the pain started in the scrotum and has rapidly spread to the groin. He has noticed foul-smelling discharge and increasing redness.
Objective (O)	The patient appears severely ill, with a temperature of 39.2°C (102.5°F), heart rate 110 bpm, and blood pressure of 95/60 mmHg. The scrotum is swollen, erythematous, and warm to touch, with black necrotic areas present. Crepitus is palpable in the tissue. Laboratory results show elevated white blood cells (WBC: 18,000/μL) and elevated lactate levels.

Assessment (A)	The patient's presentation is highly suggestive of Fournier's gangrene, a rapidly progressive soft tissue infection involving the perineal, genital, and abdominal areas. This is a surgical emergency requiring immediate debridement and antibiotic therapy.
Plan (P)	**Pharmacological**: Administer broad-spectrum intravenous antibiotics (e.g., piperacillin-tazobactam, vancomycin) to cover both aerobic and anaerobic organisms. **Non-pharmacological**: Emergency surgical debridement of necrotic tissue. **Follow-up**: Close monitoring in the ICU for hemodynamic stability and signs of sepsis. **Education**: Discuss the severity of the condition and the importance of controlling blood glucose to prevent recurrence.

8.5.9 Epididymitis

Table 133 SOAP Notes for Epididymitis

Component	Details
Subjective (S)	A 28-year-old male presents with a 3-day history of scrotal pain, swelling, and dysuria. He reports that the pain started in the right testicle and has progressively worsened. He admits to recent unprotected sexual activity. He denies fever or chills but reports increased urgency and frequency of urination.
Objective (O)	The patient is mildly distressed. On physical examination, the right scrotum is enlarged and tender, with a firm, swollen epididymis. There is no visible redness, and the testes are normal in appearance. The patient's vital signs are stable with a temperature of 37.5°C (99.5°F), heart rate of 85 bpm, and blood pressure of 125/80 mmHg. Urinalysis shows pyuria and positive nitrites.
Assessment (A)	The patient's presentation is consistent with epididymitis, likely due to a sexually transmitted infection (e.g., chlamydia or gonorrhea), given the sexual history and symptoms of dysuria and urethral discharge.
Plan (P)	**Pharmacological**: Start empirical antibiotic therapy with ceftriaxone and doxycycline to cover gonococcal and chlamydial infections. **Non-pharmacological**: Recommend rest, scrotal elevation, and analgesics for pain management. **Follow-up**: Reassess in 3-5 days to evaluate treatment effectiveness. If symptoms persist, consider scrotal ultrasound. **Education**: Educate the patient on the importance of completing the full course of antibiotics, practicing safe sexual practices, and informing sexual partners.

8.5.10 Balanitis

Table 134 SOAP Notes for Balanitis

Component	Details

Subjective (S)	A 40-year-old male presents with redness, swelling, and irritation of the glans penis. He reports painful urination and a discharge from the tip of his penis. He denies any history of trauma or sexually transmitted infections but admits to poor hygiene.
Objective (O)	The glans penis is erythematous, with a white, thick discharge. The foreskin is slightly swollen but can be retracted without difficulty. No signs of systemic infection (e.g., fever or chills). The patient's vital signs are stable with a temperature of 37.2°C (99°F).
Assessment (A)	The patient presents with balanitis, likely due to poor hygiene, resulting in fungal or bacterial overgrowth.
Plan (P)	**Pharmacological**: Prescribe topical antifungal or antibiotic cream depending on the cause (e.g., clotrimazole for fungal infections). **Non-pharmacological**: Advise improved genital hygiene and avoidance of irritants. **Follow-up**: Follow up in 1-2 weeks to reassess symptoms. If symptoms persist, consider further investigation for underlying conditions. **Education**: Discuss the importance of proper hygiene and safe sexual practices to prevent recurrence.

8.5.11 Cryptorchidism

Table 135 SOAP Notes for Cryptorchidism

Component	Details
Subjective (S)	A 3-month-old male is presented for a routine checkup. The parents report that they have not noticed any swelling or abnormality in the scrotum. The right testicle has not descended.
Objective (O)	On physical examination, the right scrotum is empty with no palpable testicle in the scrotum. The left testicle is normally descended. The patient's vital signs are normal (temperature 36.8°C, heart rate 120 bpm).
Assessment (A)	The patient has unilateral cryptorchidism (undescended testicle), which is likely an isolated condition but requires further investigation.
Plan (P)	**Pharmacological**: No medication is required at this stage. **Non-pharmacological**: Reassure the parents, as most cases of cryptorchidism resolve by 6 months of age. If the testicle does not descend by 6 months, referral to pediatric urology for potential surgery (orchidopexy) is warranted. **Follow-up**: Monitor for spontaneous descent and follow up at 6 months. **Education**: Explain the potential risks of undescended testicles, such as infertility and increased risk of testicular cancer, and the importance of follow-up.

8.5.12 Phimosis

Table 136 SOAP Notes for Phimosis

Component	Details

Subjective (S)	A 5-year-old male presents with difficulty retracting his foreskin during diaper changes. The parents report that the child has not shown any discomfort but expresses occasional difficulty during urination.
Objective (O)	On examination, the foreskin is tight and non-retractable over the glans penis. The glans appears normal, with no signs of infection or inflammation. The patient's vital signs are normal (temperature 36.9°C, heart rate 110 bpm).
Assessment (A)	The child presents with physiologic phimosis, which is common in younger children.
Plan (P)	**Pharmacological**: No medications are needed at this stage. **Non-pharmacological**: Advise parents to avoid forcing retraction and gently clean the area during baths. Most cases resolve by age 3 to 5. **Follow-up**: Reassess in 6 months. If the phimosis persists or causes urinary obstruction or infection, consider referral to a pediatric urologist for further management. **Education**: Provide education on the normal development of the foreskin and the risks of forced retraction.

8.5.13 *Varicocele*

Table 137 SOAP Notes for Varicocele

Component	Details
Subjective (S)	A 25-year-old male presents with a dull ache in the left scrotum that worsens with standing for long periods. He denies trauma or significant changes in urination.
Objective (O)	On examination, the left scrotum is enlarged with a "bag of worms" appearance. The varicocele is more pronounced when the patient stands and is reduced in size when the patient is lying down. The right testicle appears normal. Vital signs are stable (temperature 36.8°C, heart rate 80 bpm).
Assessment (A)	The patient presents with a left varicocele, which is likely contributing to the scrotal discomfort and could impact fertility.
Plan (P)	**Pharmacological**: Over-the-counter pain relievers for discomfort (e.g., ibuprofen). **Non-pharmacological**: Recommend wearing supportive underwear or an athletic supporter to reduce discomfort. If fertility issues are suspected or symptoms worsen, refer to urology for possible surgical intervention (e.g., varicocelectomy). **Follow-up**: Follow-up in 3-6 months to reassess symptoms and fertility status. **Education**: Educate the patient about the potential impact of varicoceles on fertility and the treatment options available.

8.5.14 *Hydrocele*

Table 138 SOAP Notes for Hydrocele

Component	Details

Subjective (S)	A 2-year-old male presents with a painless swelling in the scrotum, which is noticed primarily in the evenings. The parents report that the swelling has been present for several weeks but does not seem to cause discomfort.
Objective (O)	On physical examination, the scrotum is enlarged with a smooth, translucent swelling. Transillumination of the scrotum is positive, confirming the presence of a fluid-filled sac. Vital signs are normal.
Assessment (A)	The patient has a congenital hydrocele, which is typically benign and resolves in most cases by age 1.
Plan (P)	**Pharmacological**: No medications required. **Non-pharmacological**: Reassure the parents, as the hydrocele is likely to resolve on its own. **Follow-up**: Reassess in 6 months to monitor for spontaneous resolution. If it persists beyond 1 year or causes discomfort, consider referral to urology for possible surgical intervention. **Education**: Educate the parents on the condition, its benign nature, and the low likelihood of long-term issues.

8.5.15 Spermatocele

Table 139 SOAP Notes for Spermatocele

Component	Details
Subjective (S)	A 30-year-old male presents with a painless lump in the scrotum that he noticed during self-examination. The patient reports no associated discomfort or changes in urination.
Objective (O)	On examination, a firm, smooth, and mobile mass is palpated in the upper part of the scrotum, above the testicle. The mass is transilluminated, confirming it is cystic in nature. Vital signs are normal (temperature 36.9°C, heart rate 85 bpm).
Assessment (A)	The patient likely has a spermatocele, a benign cyst of the epididymis that contains sperm.
Plan (P)	**Pharmacological**: No medications required. **Non-pharmacological**: Advise the patient that spermatoceles are usually benign and may not require treatment unless symptomatic. If the mass increases in size or becomes painful, refer for further evaluation and possible surgical removal. **Follow-up**: Follow-up if symptoms worsen or if there are any changes in the size of the cyst. **Education**: Educate the patient about the benign nature of the condition and that surgical intervention is typically only required if the cyst causes pain or discomfort.

8.6 Essential Menstrual Cycle Explanation with all hormones

The human female body shows a natural periodic cycle which readies it for possible pregnancy. Vaginal bleeding during menstruation normally **spans 28 days yet ranges between 21 to 35 days**. A series of intricate connections between hypothalamus and pituitary gland as well as ovaries and uterus controls the cycle. The female reproductive cycle unfolds through the four different stages which include the **menstrual phase and follicular phase and ovulation and the luteal phase**. A set of hormonal changes controls every phase within the menstrual cycle.

8.6.1 Menstrual Phase (Day 1-5)

A female body starts the menstrual cycle during the menstrual phase when the **endometrium lining of the uterus sheds through menstruation**. When pregnancy fails to occur the body reduces its estrogen and progesterone hormone levels. Hormonal decreases trigger the endometrial lining to disintegrate from the body.

8.6.1.1 Key Hormones

- Estrogen and Progesterone: Low levels.
- When the body prepares for future cycles the follicle-stimulating hormone FSH starts rising.

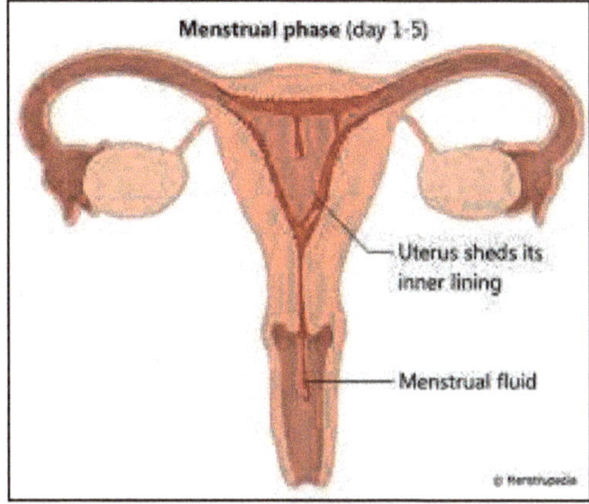

Figure 224 Menstrual Phase

8.6.2 Follicular Phase (Day 1-13)

The period beginning with menstruation extends through the period before ovulation constitutes the follicular phase. At this time the anterior pituitary **gland uses FSH to trigger the growth of ovarian follicles.** These follicles contain immature eggs. The active follicles generate estrogen to create a thick uterine lining for pregnancy potential.

8.6.2.1 Key Hormones

- **FSH (Follicle-stimulating hormone):** Stimulates the growth of ovarian follicles.
- The maturing follicles generate estrogen which builds up the uterine lining tissues.
- The hormone **Luteinizing Hormone (LH)** initiates its rise toward the conclusion of the follicular phase to initiate ovulation.

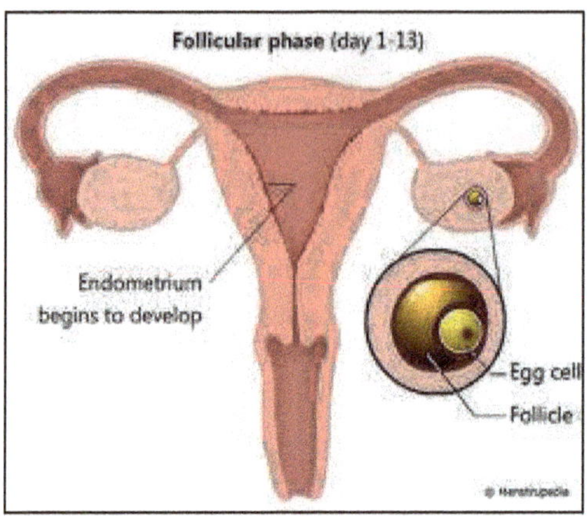

Figure 225 Follicular Phase

8.6.3 Ovulation (Day 14)

The ovary releases its mature egg as a result of ovulation from the dominant follicle. A fast influx of LH emerges after **estrogen reaches its peak point to trigger** the process of ovulation. Afteregg travels through the fallopian tube toward sperm for possible fertilization. The LH levels increase sharply while FSH decreases steeply during this period.

8.6.3.1 Key Hormones

- LH (Luteinizing Hormone): A surge in LH triggers ovulation.
- The maturation of follicles toward ovulation is supported by FSH (Follicle-stimulating hormone) hormone surge.
- Before ovulation estrogen reaches its highest point which triggers the release of LH.

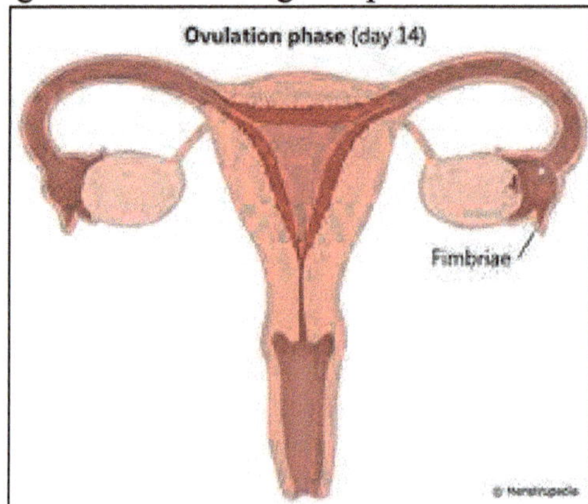

Figure 226 Ovulation Phase

8.6.4 Luteal Phase (Day 15-28)

After follicle rupture the human body transforms the remaining cavity into a structure named corpus luteum that produces **progesterone together with some estrogen**. The thickened lining of the uterus gets maintained through progesterone secretion as a pregnancy's potential formation depends on this. An egg which becomes fertilized will embed itself **within the lining for pregnancy to take place.** During the time without fertilization the corpus luteum breaks down thereby causing estrogen as well as progesterone to decrease marking the start of menstruation.

8.6.4.1 Key Hormones

- The corpus luteum produces progesterone that keeps the uterus ready for possible pregnancy by sustaining the thickened endometrium.
- Estrogen: Produced in smaller amounts by the corpus luteum.

- The secretory phase exhibits minimal activity of FSH and LH hormone production.

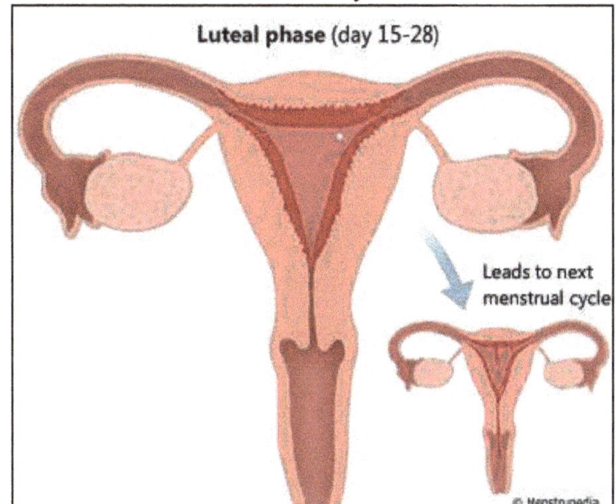

Figure 227 Luteal Phase

8.6.5 Hormonal Interactions

The hypothalamus together with the pituitary glands located in the brain function as the controllers of the menstrual cycle. **GnRH from the hypothalamus triggers** the stimulation of FSH and LH from the pituitary gland. Estrogen and progesterone production in the ovaries depends on hormone signals from these glands. The moving hormone levels between higher and lower concentrations **create various stages of the menstrual cycle**. The complex hormonal operations maintain proper functioning of the menstruation cycle as a naturally occurring method. A pregnancy-ready uterine lining requires estrogen and progesterone but **FSH and LH control both egg maturation and ovulation respectively**. A new menstrual cycle initiates after fertilization fails to happen.

8.6.6 Female Reproductive Hormonal Cycle

This diagram illustrates the hormonal fluctuations during the menstrual cycle, including the ovarian cycle, body temperature changes, and uterine cycle. The cycle starts with the **follicular phase**, where **follicle-stimulating hormone (FSH)** stimulates the growth of ovarian follicles, which produce **estradiol (estrogen)**. As the follicle matures, **luteinizing hormone (LH)** levels rise, leading to ovulation at around day 14. Following ovulation, the **luteal phase** begins, marked by the formation of the **corpus luteum**, which secretes **progesterone** to prepare the uterus for potential pregnancy. As progesterone levels rise, the uterine lining thickens in preparation for embryo implantation. If pregnancy does not occur, the corpus luteum degenerates into the **corpus albicans**, progesterone levels drop, and menstruation begins. Body temperature slightly increases after ovulation due to higher progesterone levels. This intricate hormonal interplay regulates the menstrual cycle, influencing fertility and the uterine environment.

8.7 Common Conditions of Female Genital System

"Can All People Deal Painfully, Very Violently?" **C**: Contraception, **A**: Amenorrhea, **P**: Polycystic Ovary Syndrome (PCOS), **D**: Dysmenorrhea, **P**: (All) Breast Cancer Types and Benign

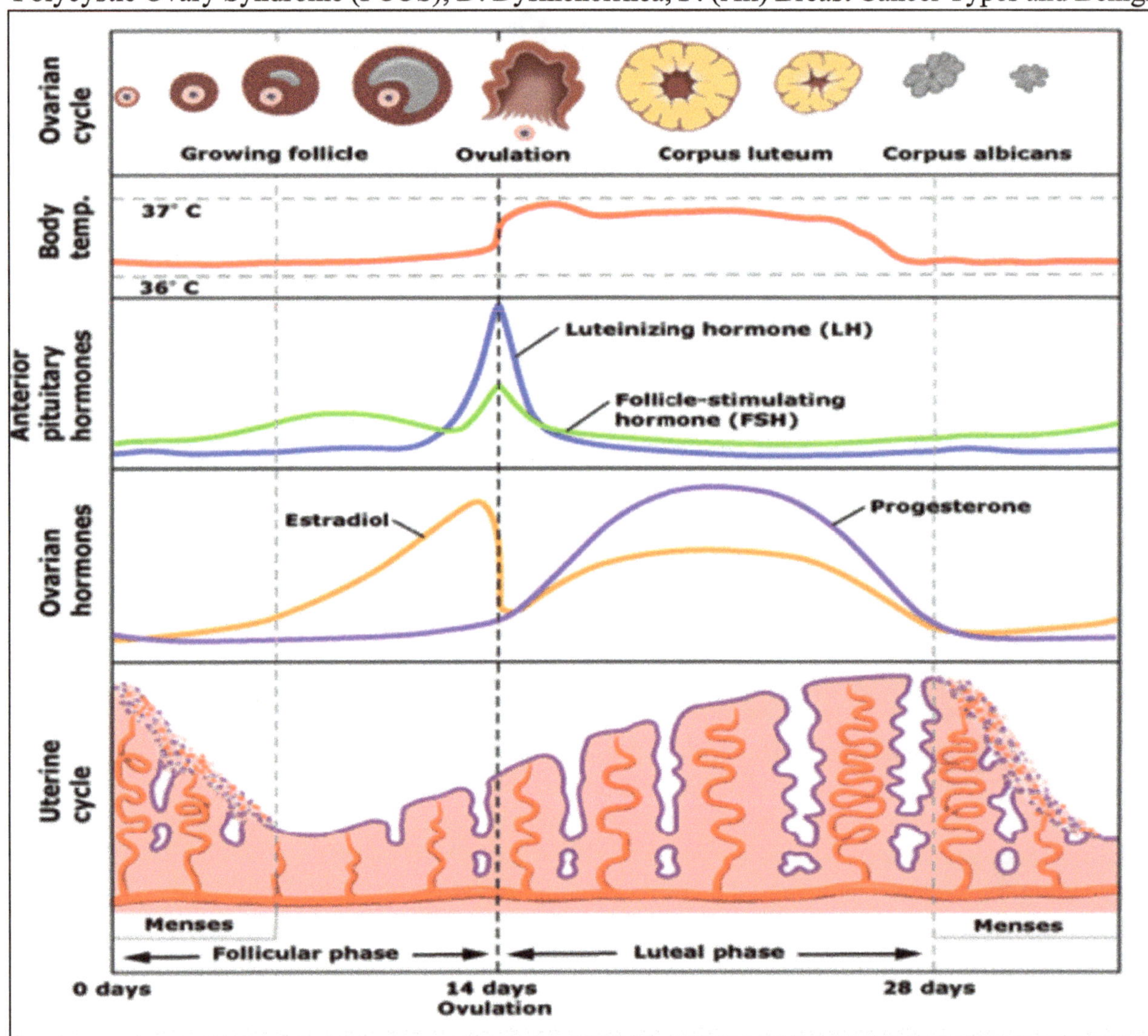

Figure 228 Hormones Trajectory in Menstrual Cycle

Masses, **V**: Vulvovaginal Infections, **V**: Atrophic Vaginitis

Table 140 Common Conditions of Female Genital System

Condition	Description	Key Symptoms	Diagnostic Tools	Treatment Options
Contraception	Methods to prevent pregnancy, including	Nausea, headaches (hormonal), or irritation	Physical exam, medical history, imaging (e.g.,	Oral contraceptives, IUD, implants,

	hormonal, barrier, permanent, and natural.	(barrier). Absence of pregnancy.	ultrasound), pregnancy test.	barrier methods, sterilization.
Amenorrhea	Absence of menstruation, can be primary or secondary.	Absence of menstrual periods, depending on age and history.	Pregnancy test, blood tests (FSH, LH, prolactin), ultrasound, MRI (for pituitary issues).	Hormonal therapy, treatment of underlying cause (e.g., weight loss, thyroid therapy).
All Breast Cancer Types and Benign Masses	Malignant tumors or non-cancerous lumps in the breast.	Painless lump, changes in breast appearance or size, nipple discharge, skin dimpling.	Mammography, ultrasound, biopsy (core needle or excisional), MRI.	Surgery (lumpectomy, mastectomy), chemotherapy, radiation, hormonal therapy.
Dysmenorrhea	Painful menstruation, either primary (no underlying condition) or secondary.	Severe cramps, pelvic pain, nausea, vomiting, fatigue.	Pelvic exam, ultrasound (for secondary causes), laparoscopy.	NSAIDs, hormonal contraceptives, laparoscopic surgery (for underlying conditions).
Polycystic Ovary Syndrome (PCOS)	A hormonal disorder causing enlarged ovaries with cysts.	Irregular periods, acne, excessive hair growth (hirsutism), obesity.	Blood tests (FSH, LH, testosterone, insulin), pelvic ultrasound.	Birth control pills, metformin, anti-androgens (e.g., spironolactone), lifestyle changes.
Vulvovaginal Infections	Infections affecting the vulva and vagina (e.g., yeast infection, bacterial vaginosis).	Itching, discharge, burning, pain during intercourse or urination.	Vaginal pH testing, wet mount microscopy, culture, PCR.	Antifungal medications, antibiotics, lifestyle changes (e.g., hygiene practices).
Atrophic Vaginitis	Thinning, drying, and inflammation of the vaginal			

	walls, usually post-men			

8.8 Major Medical Conditions of Female Reproductive System

8.8.1 Contraception

The **prevention of pregnancy exists through different methods** known as contraception. Different techniques fall under contraception including hormonal methods represented by pills and IUDs and barrier methods including **contraceptive devices**. The surgical methods which block reproduction permanently are vasectomy or tubal ligation. The practice of fertility tracking **comprises natural methods of contraception which is coupled with emergency contraception** that helps stop pregnancy after intimate contact. A person taking hormonal contraception experiences hormonal changes that stop their ovaries from releasing eggs and produce thick mucus or thin the uterus to prevent pregnancy. The barrier method stops sperm cells from reaching the egg whereas the **IUD stops pregnancy** by making the uterus unfavorable for implantation. Using contraception prevents **unintended pregnancies and controls menstrual cycles** and minimizes the risk of specific cancers as well as treating skin acne. Each person must select an appropriate birth control approach according to their reproductive goals and their overall health condition as well as their daily life needs.

8.8.2 Types of Contraception

Multiple birth control options visible in the image provide pregnancy prevention methods. Different pregnancy prevention methods sort into hormonal, barrier and permanent choices. Chosen **hormonal contraceptives** contain two components: combined **oral contraceptive pills use estrogen and progesterone** to stop ovulation and progestogen-only pills make cervical mucus thicker. The contraceptive injection together with **implant and vaginal ring** use continuous hormone release to stop pregnancy. The long-term birth control options mainly consist of hormonal **IUDs together with copper IUDs**. These devices stop conception by making the female reproductive area unfavorable for sperm. The blockage of sperm entry into the uterus is achieved through male condoms while diaphragms cover the **cervix as another barrier method**. Healthcare providers recommend consulting with individuals to help select pregnancy prevention methods since each contraceptive has its own effectiveness rating together with benefits but also potential side effects.

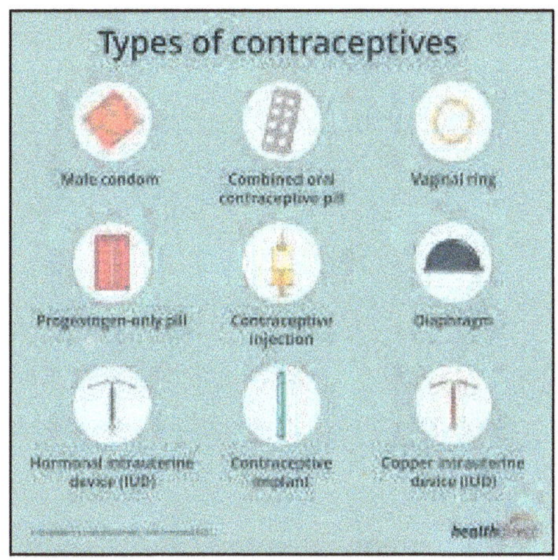

Figure 229 Types of Contraception

8.8.3 Comparison of All Contraception Methods

The first table compares the **benefits** of several contraceptive methods. It assesses factors like **pregnancy prevention**, **acne control**, and **PMS relief**, while also noting whether the method contains hormones. The implant and injection rank high for pregnancy prevention and less painful periods, while methods like condoms and fertility awareness do not rely on hormones and are often used for STI prevention. Hormonal methods (like the pill, patch, and vaginal ring) are more suitable for individuals seeking menstrual regulation, acne reduction, and PMS relief.

Table 141 Comparing all contraception methods

	Best at preventing pregnancy	Less need to remember	STI protection	For regular periods	For no periods	For less painful periods	Less acne	Less PMS	Hormones
Implant	●●●	●●●	○○○	○○○	●●○	●●●	○○○	●●○	Yes
Hormonal Coil / IUS	●●●	●●●	○○○	○○○	●●○	●●●	○○○	●●○	Low levels
Copper Coil / IUD	●●●	●●●	○○○	●●●	○○○	○○○	○○○	○○○	No
Injection	●●●	●●○	○○○	●●●	●●○	●●●	○○○	●●○	Yes
Combined Pill	●●○	○○○	○○○	●●●	●●●	●●●	●●○	●●○	Yes
Mini Pill	●●○	○○○	○○○	●○○	●○○	●●○	○○○	●○○	Yes
Patch	●●○	●○○	○○○	●●●	●●●	●●●	●●○	●●○	Yes
The Vaginal Ring	●●○	●●○	○○○	●●●	●●●	●●●	●●○	●●○	Yes
Diaphragm	●○○	○○○	●○○	●●●	○○○	○○○	○○○	○○○	No
Condoms	●○○	○○○	●●●	●●●	○○○	○○○	○○○	○○○	No
Fertility Awareness	○○○	○○○	○○○	●●●	○○○	○○○	○○○	○○○	No
Withdrawal	○○○	○○○	○○○	●●●	○○○	○○○	○○○	○○○	No

The second table compares various **contraceptive methods**, categorizing their **effectiveness**, **advantages**, and **disadvantages**. Methods such as the **contraceptive patch**, **vaginal ring**, and

combined pill are effective with perfect use (over 99% effectiveness). However, typical use shows lower effectiveness due to incorrect use. The **external condom** and **fertility awareness** methods have lower effectiveness in typical use but help prevent sexually transmitted infections (STIs).

Table 142 Contradictions of Contraceptive Methods

	Contraceptive patch	Contraceptive vaginal ring	Combined pill (COC)	Progestogen-only pill (POP)	External condom	Internal condom	Diaphragm/cap with spermicide	Fertility awareness methods
What is it?	A small patch stuck to the skin releases estrogen and progestogen.	A small, flexible, plastic ring put into the vagina releases estrogen and progestogen.	A pill containing estrogen and progestogen, taken orally.	A pill containing progestogen, taken orally.	A very thin latex (rubber) polyurethane (plastic) or synthetic sheath, put over the erect penis.	Soft, thin polyurethane sheath that loosely lines the vagina and covers the area just outside.	A flexible latex (rubber) or silicone device, used with spermicide, is put into the vagina to cover the cervix.	Fertile and infertile times of the menstrual cycle are identified by noting different fertility indicators.
PERFECT USE MEANS USING THE METHOD CORRECTLY EVERY TIME. TYPICAL USE IS WHEN YOU DON'T ALWAYS USE THE METHOD CORRECTLY.								
Effectiveness	Perfect use: over 99%. Typical use: around 91%.	Perfect use: over 99%. Typical use: around 91%.	Perfect use: over 99%. Typical use: around 91%.	Perfect use: over 99%. Typical use: around 91%.	Perfect use: 98%. Typical use: around 82%.	Perfect use: 95%. Typical use: around 79%.	Perfect use: 92–96%. Typical use: 71–88%.	Perfect use: up to 99%. Typical use: around 76%.
Advantage	Can make bleeds regular, lighter and less painful.	One ring stays in for 3 weeks – you don't have to think about contraception every day.	Often reduces bleeding and period pain, and may help with premenstrual symptoms.	Can be used if you smoke and are over 35.	Condoms are the best way to help protect yourself from sexually transmitted infections.		Can be put in any time before sex.	No physical side effects, and can be used to plan as well as prevent pregnancy.
Disadvantage	May be seen and can cause skin irritation.	You must be comfortable with inserting and removing it.	Missing pills, vomiting or severe diarrhoea can make it less effective.	Late pills, vomiting or severe diarrhoea can make it less effective.	May slip off or split if not used correctly or if wrong size or shape.	Not as widely available as male condoms.	You need to use the right size. If you have sex again extra spermicide is needed.	Need to avoid sex or use a condom at fertile times of the cycle.

8.8.3.1 SOAP Notes for Contraception

Table 143 SOAP Notes for Contraception

Component	Details
Subjective (S)	A 28-year-old female presents for a follow-up visit to discuss contraception options. She has been sexually active for the past 5 years and has no current pregnancies. She is interested in long-term contraception but is unsure of which method to choose. She reports regular menstrual cycles and no history of smoking or medical conditions that would contraindicate contraception. She is not experiencing any side effects from her current method, but she is looking for a more convenient form of birth control.
Objective (O)	The patient appears healthy with no apparent distress. Vital signs are normal: BP 118/76 mmHg, HR 72 bpm, Temp 98.6°F. There are no signs of complications or contraindications for hormonal contraceptives or IUD use.
Assessment (A)	The patient is seeking contraception for family planning and is interested in options that require minimal intervention. Given her health history and preferences, options such as a hormonal IUD or contraceptive implant may be ideal for long-term contraception. A discussion on benefits, risks, and effectiveness of various methods, including the side effects of hormonal methods, is needed.
Plan (P)	Pharmacological: Discuss hormonal methods (e.g., IUD, implant, oral contraceptives) and non-hormonal options (e.g., copper IUD). Review the pros and cons of each method with the patient. If she opts for a hormonal IUD or implant, arrange for a consultation for fitting or insertion. Non-pharmacological: Provide information on proper use and potential side effects of different methods. Follow-up: Schedule a follow-up visit after 1-3 months for evaluation and to address any side effects or concerns.

Education: Educate the patient on how different contraceptive methods work and emphasize the importance of consistent and correct use to ensure effectiveness.

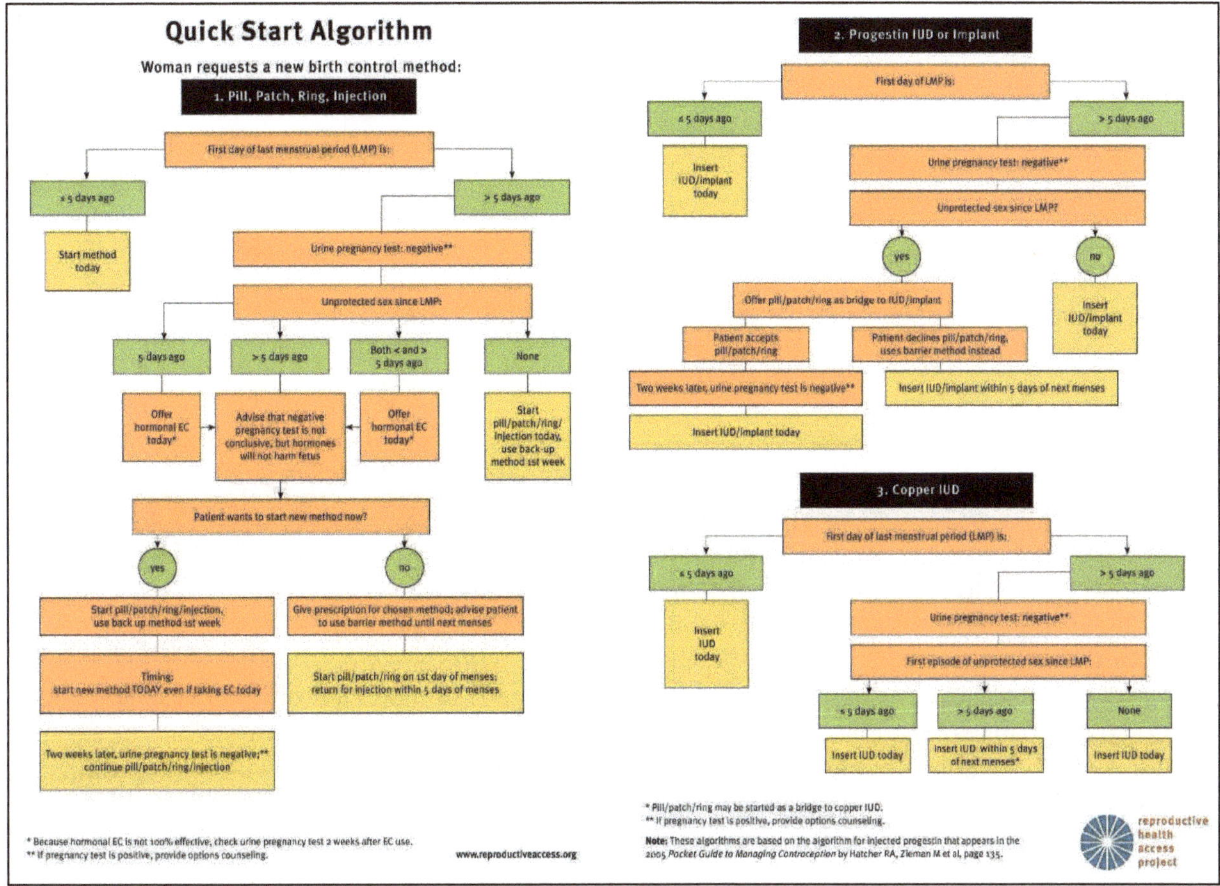

Figure 230 Management Algorithm for Contraception

8.8.4 Amenorrhea

Amenorrhea refers to the **absence of menstruation in women of reproductive age**. It is classified into two categories namely primary TRP and secondary TRP. Primary amenorrhoea refers to absence of menstruation in a **young lady by age 16 provided** that she has normal body stature and secondary sexual characteristics. **Secondary amenorrhea is defined as the failure of the menstruation at least for three cycles in a female who once had regular periods**. There are several reasons for amenorrhea and they include hormonal imbalance, stress, excessive exercise, malnutrition, PCOS, thyroid diseases, congenital anomalies of the reproductive tract. The causes of a weakened spine and lowered resilience include a low-calorie diet, obesity, weight fluctuations, and heavy exercise. The specific therapy directed at the management of the condition depends on the **actual causal factor and may include hormone treatment or therapy, change in lifestyle, or surgery.** There is a need to diagnose it during its early stages and treat it so as to avoid future serious complications related to health issues.

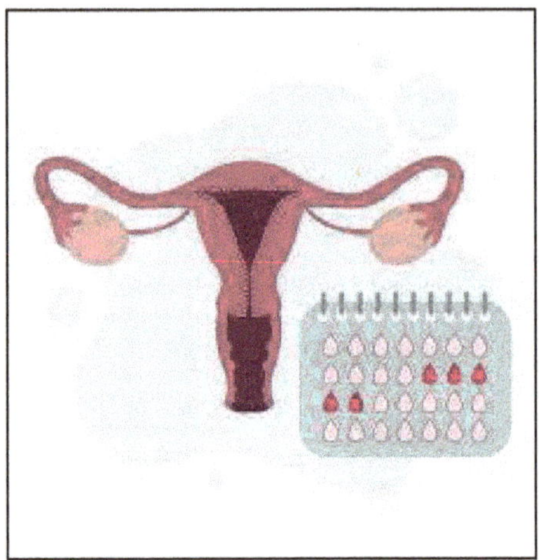

Figure 231 Amenorrhea

8.8.4.1 Classification of Amenorrhea

The algorithm below explains the diagnostic strategy of a female patient with primary amenorrhea which can be defined as the absence of menses. The **first examination** that has to be conducted includes a **historical and medical examination** to ascertain if the secondary sexual characteristics are developed or not. The first action is taken is to determine the **level of FSH and LH** so as to factor the **type of amenorrhea present**. Therefore, on the basis of the results, the patient can have hypogonadotropic hypogonadism when both FSH and LH levels are low and hypergonadotropic hypogonadism when **FSH and LH levels are high**. A karyotype analysis is also carried out in order to detect for instance, Turner syndrome or other chromosomal disorders. If there is no evidence, the next take is imaging examination such as ultrasound exam of the uterus and check for structural changes. The treatment options will, therefore, vary with the cause such **as hormonal treatment** if the problem is hormonal or surgery if there are abnormalities with the reproductive organs.

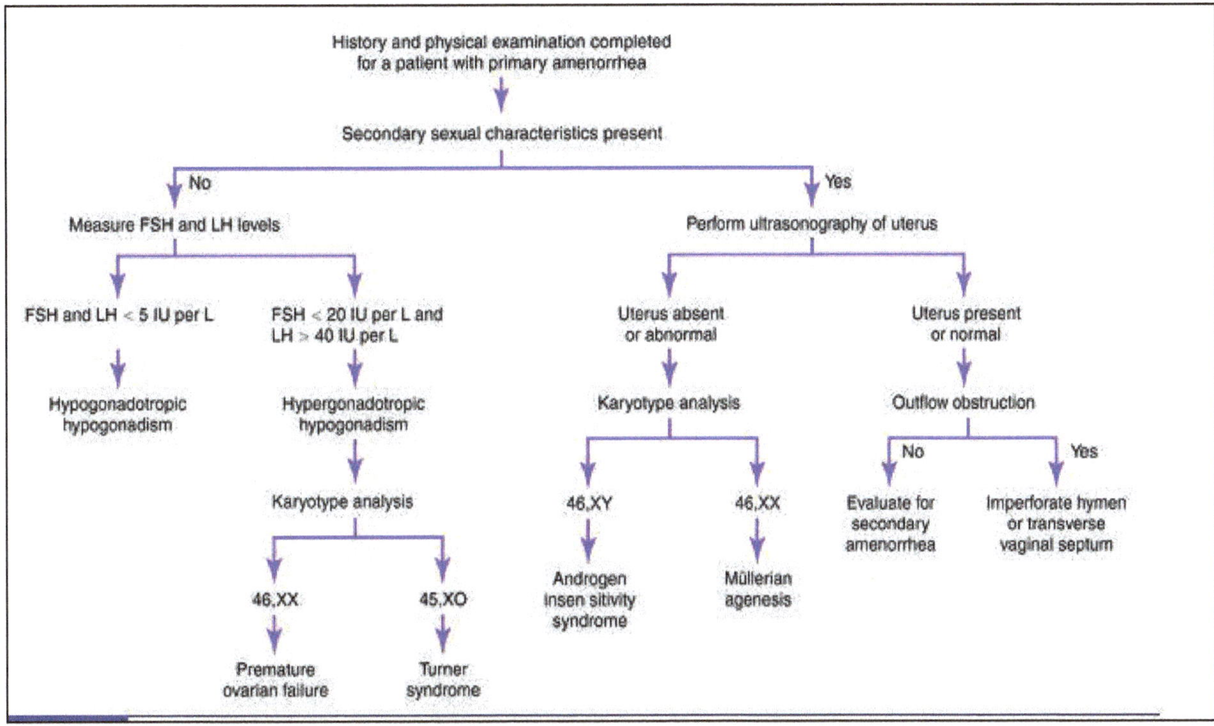

Figure 232 Evaluation of Primary Amenorrhea

8.8.4.2 Types of Amenorrhea

The image presented shows the categories found in cases of amenorrhea differentiating between physiological and pathological causes and effects. Amenorrhea can be physiological in that may stem from conditions that do not **require medical intervention such as before the onset of puberty (primary), during pregnancy, lactation, or after menopause (secondary).** These are some conditions that are normal changes that occur in our physiological systems and therefore are not illnesses. However, there can also be pathological amenorrhea, which is caused by certain health related complications. The disorder is subdivided into concealed, also called **cryptomenorrhea, and real, also known as true anomenorrhoea**. Secondary amenorrhea can be observed when menstruation is physically present but cannot be seen because it has been obstructed by a congenital or acquired disorder. **Secondary amenorrhea** means no menstruation is the result of pathological causes such as hormonal imbalance, stress etc and thus needs a medical evaluation.

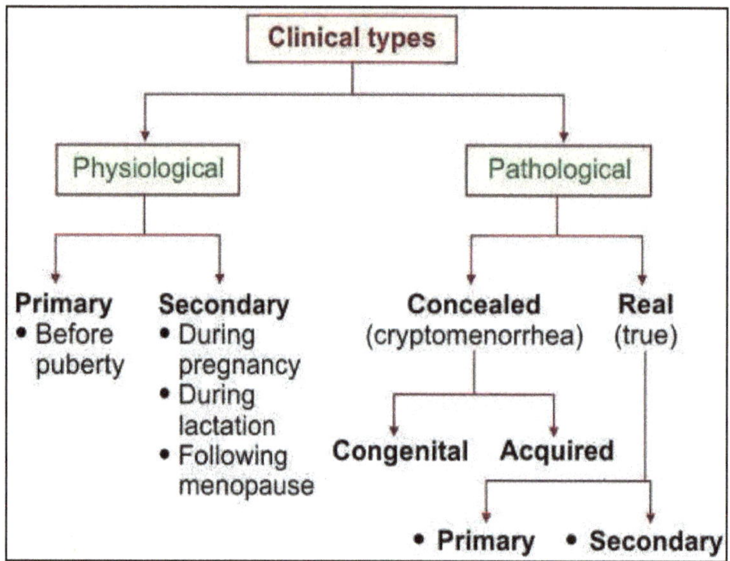

Figure 233 Clinical types of Amenorrhea

8.8.4.3 Antibiotics for Amenorrhea

The table provides details on several drugs used in the treatment of **amenorrhea**, a condition characterized by the absence of menstruation. Medications like **medroxyprogesterone**, **Provera**, and **Prometrium** are commonly used for managing amenorrhea. **Medroxyprogesterone** (rating: 7.2) and **Provera** (rating: 7.4) are prescription-only medications (Rx) and are often prescribed to induce menstruation in women with irregular periods. Both are not recommended for use during pregnancy and are not classified as controlled substances. Other drugs like **progesterone** (rating: 5.8) and **norethindrone** (rating: 6.7) are also used but are available as both **prescription and over-the-counter** (Rx/OTC) options, giving patients more flexibility in treatment. **Progesterone** has a lower rating compared to others and is considered **B** for pregnancy, indicating moderate risk. **Norethindrone** is also used for managing hormonal imbalances causing amenorrhea. Overall, these drugs are aimed at restoring regular menstrual cycles, with considerations for their safety during pregnancy and potential effects on alcohol use and controlled substance status.

Table 144 Drugs used to treat Amenorrhea

Drug name	Rating	Reviews	Activity	Rx/OTC	Preg	CSA	Alcohol
medroxyprogesterone	7.2	201 reviews		Rx	X	N	
Provera	7.4	117 reviews		Rx	X	N	
progesterone	5.8	6 reviews		Rx/OTC	B	N	
norethindrone	6.7	18 reviews		Rx	X	N	X
Prometrium	7.3	4 reviews		Rx/OTC	B	N	
Endometrin	Rate	Add review		Rx/OTC	B	N	
Crinone	Rate	Add review		Rx/OTC	B	N	
Gallifrey	Rate	Add review		Rx	X	N	X

8.8.4.4 SOAP Notes for Amenorrhea

Table 145 SOAP Notes for Amenorrhea

Component	Details
Subjective (S)	A 21-year-old female presents with the complaint of no menstrual periods for the past 6 months. She reports a history of irregular periods but has never had a regular cycle. The patient denies any pain, abnormal discharge, or other associated symptoms. She is not pregnant, and there is no history of recent weight changes, stress, or significant illness. She is sexually active and not using any contraception. No significant family history of reproductive disorders is reported.
Objective (O)	The patient appears healthy with no signs of distress. Physical examination is unremarkable, with normal vital signs. No signs of hirsutism, acne, or galactorrhea. Pelvic exam reveals no obvious abnormalities. FSH and LH levels were obtained, and an ultrasound of the uterus and ovaries has been scheduled to evaluate for any abnormalities.
Assessment (A)	The patient's absence of menstruation for 6 months, coupled with the lack of secondary sexual characteristics, is suggestive of primary amenorrhea. Differential diagnosis includes hypothalamic dysfunction, polycystic ovary syndrome (PCOS), and possible anatomical abnormalities. Further testing is required to confirm the underlying cause.
Plan (P)	**Pharmacological:** Consider hormonal therapy depending on the results of the ultrasound and blood tests (See algorithm below). **Non-**

	pharmacological: Advise stress reduction techniques and maintain a healthy diet. **Follow-up:** Return visit in 2 weeks to review test results and consider referral to a gynecologist or endocrinologist if necessary. **Education:** Educate the patient on the possible causes of amenorrhea and the importance of follow-up care to determine appropriate treatment options.

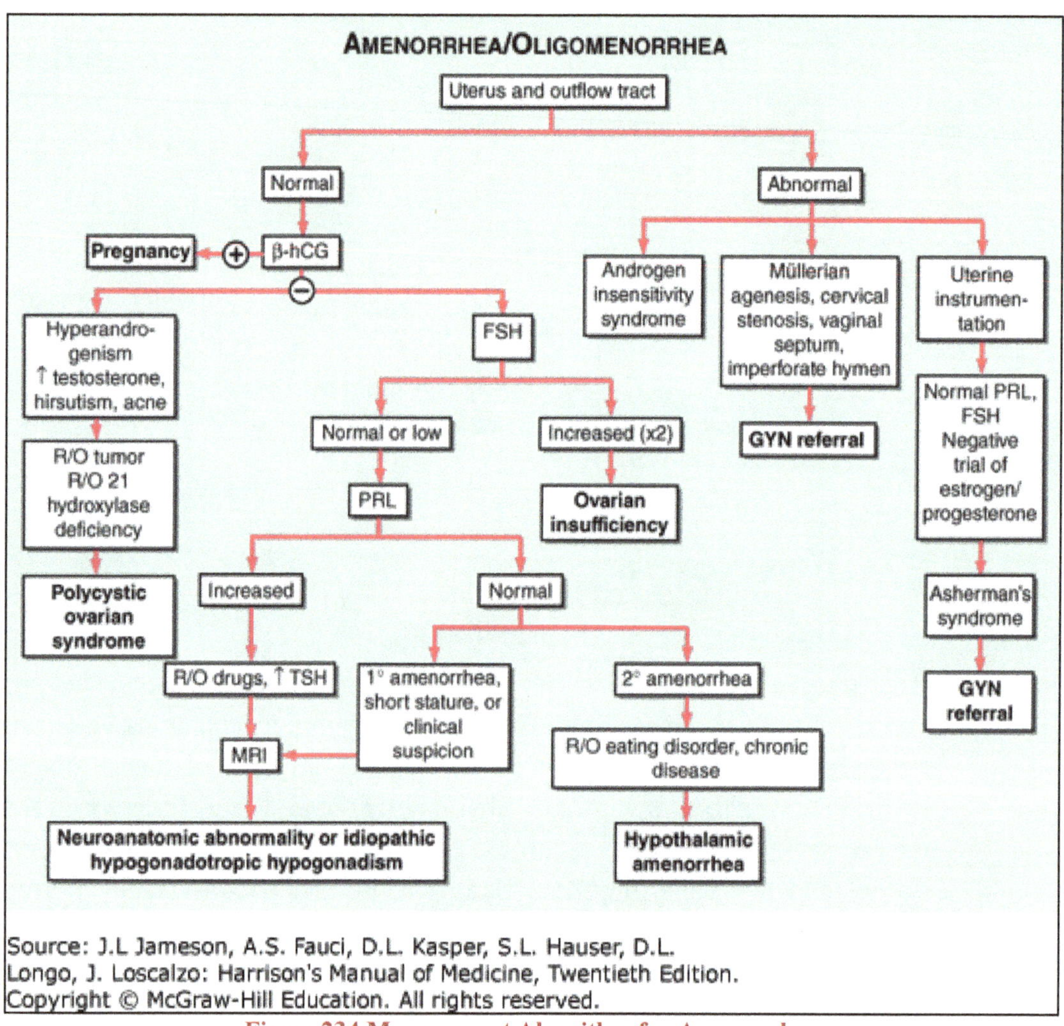

Source: J.L Jameson, A.S. Fauci, D.L. Kasper, S.L. Hauser, D.L. Longo, J. Loscalzo: Harrison's Manual of Medicine, Twentieth Edition.

Figure 234 Management Algorithm for Amenorrhea

8.8.5 All Breast Cancer Types and Benign Masses

Breast cancer encompasses a variety of types, each with distinct characteristics and behaviors. The common varieties of it is **invasive ductal carcinoma, invasive lobular carcinoma, and ductal carcinoma in situ.** IDC starts in the **milk ducts** in the breast tissue and is more likely to have the cancer cells spread to other parts of the breast tissue and other body organs while **ILC originates from the milk producing cells** in the lobules in the breast and can spread in a more random manner to the surrounding cells in the breast and other organs. DCIS is a cancer that has not spread outside the milk ducts and has not invaded other tissues of the body. There are other other rare **types of breast cancer for instance inflammatory breast cancer, medullary carcinoma, mucinous carcinoma, among others.** Benign breast mass, therefore, are those growths which resemble cancerous ones but are not fatal and cannot spread through the body. Other times, the conditions are benign which present themselves as **Fibroadenoma, cysts, and fibrocystic changes**. These masses are more often discovered when taking mammograms or ultrasounds. Thus, **benign tumors** are not normally removed through surgery, but they need to be watched for a change in size or characteristics. Both breast cancer and benign masses are diagnosed and managed with the help of imaging studies, fine **needle aspirations or biopsies and histopathological examination.** The distinction between malignant and benign neoplasms at an early stage has lots of prognostic significance in terms of treatment management. **Self-breast examination** can also be used as an education tool by empowering individuals to understand their own bodies and identify potential changes, leading to early detection of breast cancer

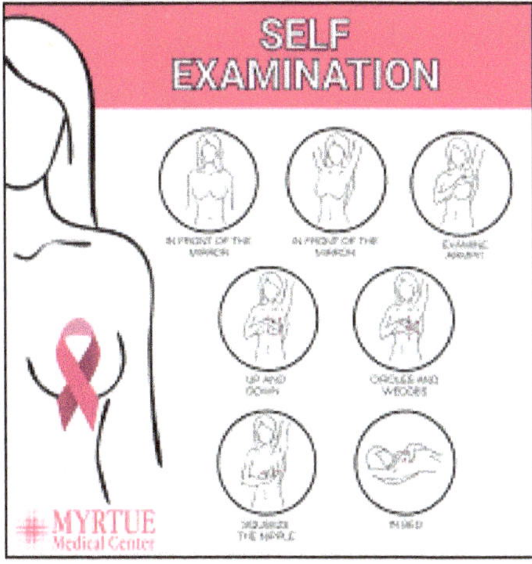

Figure 235 Self-Examination of Breast

8.8.5.1 Types of Breast Cancers

The diagram outlines the two primary categories of breast cancer: non-invasive (or in-situ) and invasive types. **Non-invasive breast cancer includes conditions such as Lobular Carcinoma In Situ (LCIS) and Ductal Carcinoma In Situ (DCIS).** LCIS is considered a benign condition that does not spread outside the lobules of the breast, although it increases the risk of developing invasive breast cancer in the future. On the other hand, DCIS, which begins in the ducts, is still confined to the ducts and has not spread to surrounding tissues but can eventually develop into invasive cancer if left untreated. Invasive breast cancer, which has spread beyond its original tissue, includes Invasive **Ductal Carcinoma (IDC) and Invasive Lobular Carcinoma (ILC).** IDC accounts for approximately 80% of all breast cancer cases and originates in the ductal tissue of the breast, spreading into the surrounding tissue. ILC, making up about 10% of cases, starts in the lobules and also spreads to surrounding tissues. Additionally, there are rare types of invasive breast cancer, including **inflammatory breast cancer and Paget's disease**, both of which are aggressive and present unique challenges in diagnosis and treatment.

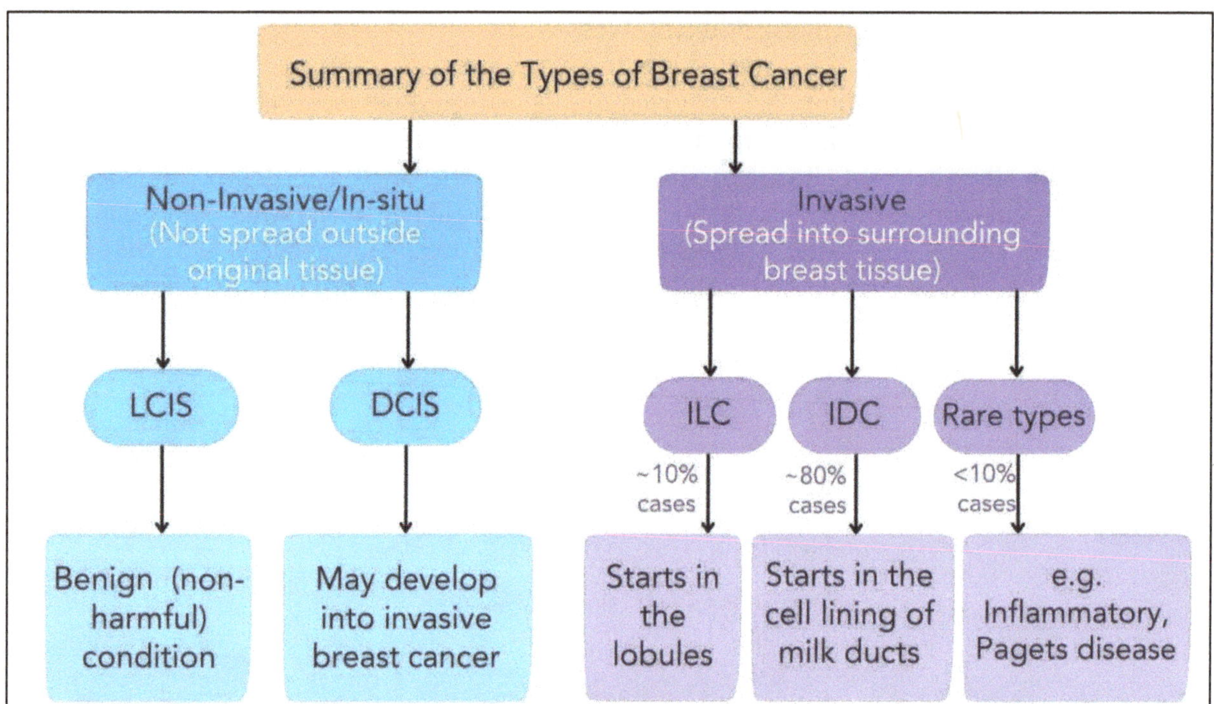

Figure 236 Types of Breast Cancers

8.8.5.2 Types of Benign Masses

The diagram shows that there are **several subclasses to breast masses** in terms of features, symptoms or implication to the patient's health. Some masses are harmless while others may indicate cases like the breast cancer, among others. **An abscess is a type of breast lump filled with pus,** which is a pus pocket located in the breast due to bacterial infection. This illness usually manifests itself by causing inflammation, redness, and tenderness, and, sometimes, the affected area needs to be drained and receive antibiotics. At the same time**, a tumor can be either good or bad depending on its nature or type. Fibroadenomas are usual benign tumor** in nature while invasive breast cancers are malignant tumors which have the ability to spread to other tissues round the tumor. They are round cavities found in the breast and most of them are not cancerous. They are unlikely to be painful, but can be uncomfortable or painful if they get to a larger size and can normally be managed through aspiration or just observation**. Fibroadenomas affect young women and are tumors containing glandular as well as fibrous tissue**. These are usually smooth, movable and non-tender and may be observed or sometimes shavings are done on them. Finally, cystic dysplasia of the breast is the pathological and morphological changes that may lead to the **formation of cysts and cicatrices**. These actions lead to such symptoms like breast pain and lumps, these are mostly caused by hormonal changes. Treatment could be analgesia and some modifications of one's habits and living pattern. These masses point to the need to perform routine breast examination and for proper testing to establish the nature of the masses and how they should be handled.

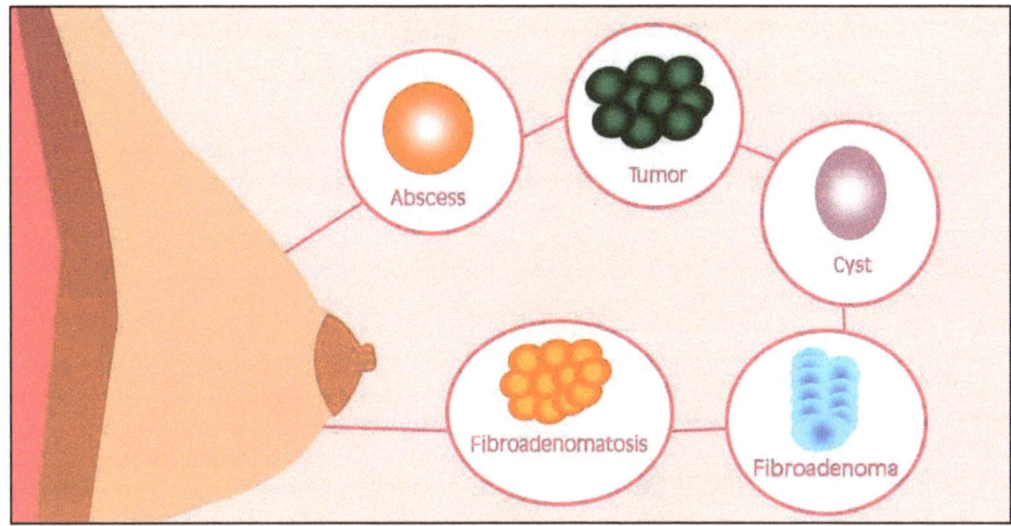

Figure 237 Benign Breast Masses/Diseases

8.8.5.3 SOAP Notes for Breast Cancer Types

Table 146 SOAP Notes for Breast Cancer

Component	Details
Subjective (S)	A 50-year-old female presents with a new, hard, non-mobile lump in the right breast noticed during routine self-examination. She reports mild discomfort around the lump but no significant pain. The patient has a family history of breast cancer (mother diagnosed at age 55).
Objective (O)	On physical examination, there is a firm, irregular, non-tender mass approximately 3 cm in diameter located in the upper inner quadrant of the right breast. Skin changes, such as dimpling or erythema, are noted over the mass. No palpable axillary lymph nodes are found.
Assessment (A)	The presentation is concerning for breast cancer, possibly an invasive ductal carcinoma (IDC). The mass characteristics, along with the family history, warrant further investigation through imaging (mammogram and ultrasound) and biopsy for histopathological examination.
Plan (P)	**Pharmacological:** If breast cancer is confirmed, initiate treatment protocols which may include chemotherapy, hormonal therapy, or targeted therapy based on the subtype (See algorithm below). **Non-pharmacological:** Refer to oncology for further management, including surgery (lumpectomy or mastectomy) and possible radiation therapy. **Follow-up:** Schedule follow-up for biopsy results and refer to oncologist for treatment plan. **Education:** Educate the patient on breast cancer, the importance of

	early detection, and possible treatment options. Discuss genetic counseling given the family history, along with patient self-breast exam

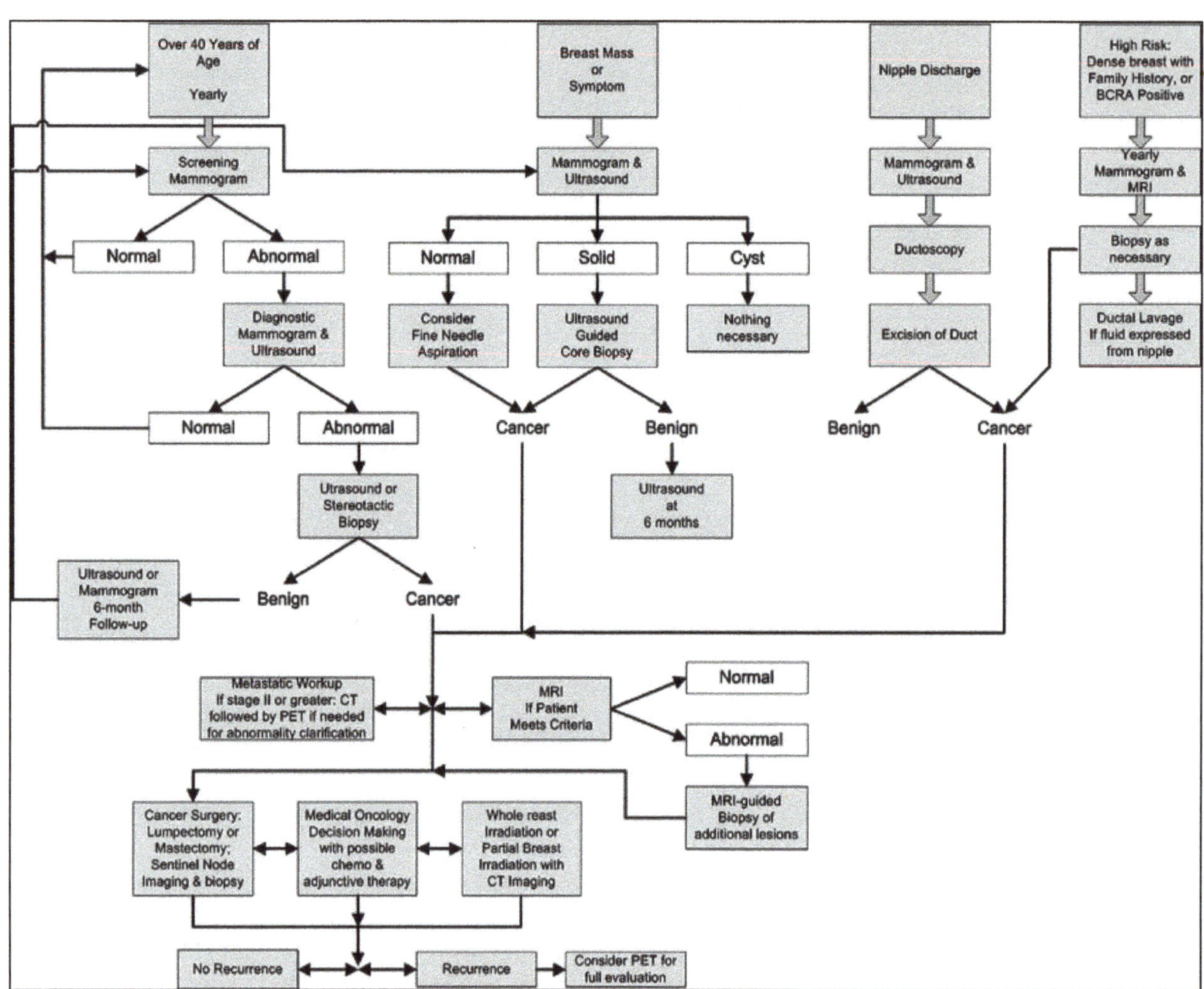

Figure 238 Management Algorithm for Breast Cancer

8.8.5.4 SOAP Notes for Benign Masses

Table 147 SOAP Notes for Benign Masses

Component	Details
Subjective (S)	A 30-year-old female presents with a non-painful, firm lump in the left breast noticed during self-examination a few weeks ago. The lump has remained the same size. She denies any changes in breast size, skin changes, or nipple discharge. There is no family history of breast cancer.
Objective (O)	Physical examination reveals a well-defined, mobile, firm mass approximately 2 cm in diameter located in the upper outer quadrant of the left breast. No signs of erythema, skin dimpling, or nipple discharge. The axillary lymph nodes are not enlarged.
Assessment (A)	The patient likely has a benign breast mass, possibly a fibroadenoma. This is a common non-cancerous growth in young women. Further imaging, such

	as mammography or ultrasound, and possibly biopsy, are recommended for confirmation.
Plan (P)	**Pharmacological:** No treatment needed unless symptomatic (e.g., pain management with acetaminophen or ibuprofen) (See algorithm below). **Non-pharmacological:** Monitor the mass for changes, and advise the patient to perform regular breast self-exams. **Follow-up:** Schedule a follow-up visit in 3-6 months to monitor the mass. If the mass increases in size or if any concerning symptoms develop, further imaging or biopsy should be considered. **Education:** Educate the patient on benign breast masses and the importance of early detection and regular breast exams.

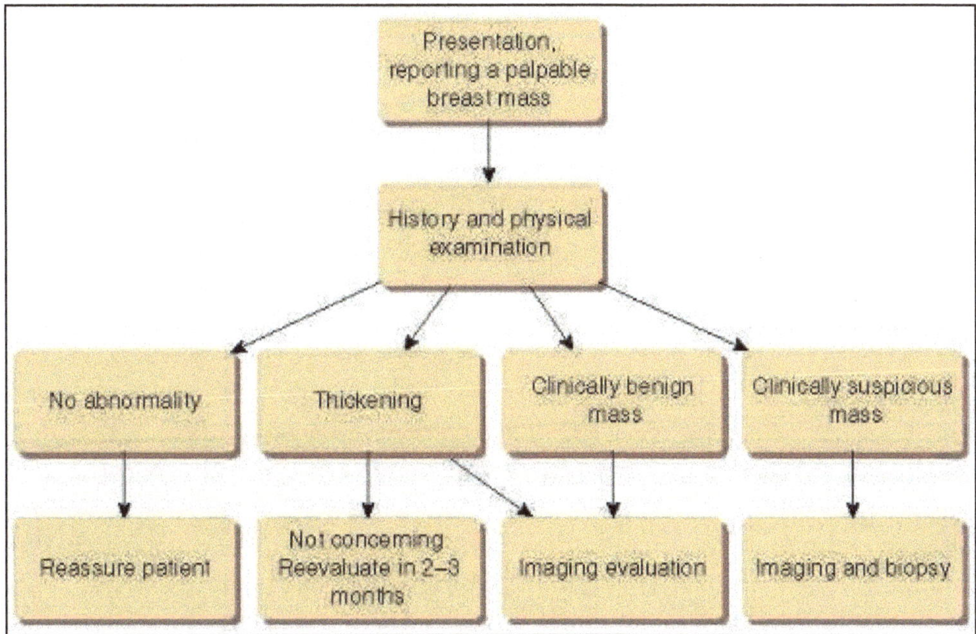

Figure 239 Management Algorithm for Benign Mass

8.8.6 Dysmenorrhea

Dysmenorrhea is commonly defined as painful menstruation that tends to occur in a woman during the menstrual cycle. In its definitions it can be divided into two forms: **Primary dysmenorrhea and secondary dysmenorrhea.** The most common type is the **primary dysmenorrhea** and this does not have any relation or connection with any disease in the pelvic region. It is most commonly starts within several years of sexual maturity and is commonly attributed to **increased production of prostaglandin which causes uterine contractions, pain and inflammation**. These cramps are usually felt in the lower abdomen yet may spread to the lower back or thighs sometimes. The secondary dysmenorrhea is characterized by diseases including endometriosis, fibroid or Pelvic inflammatory disease. This kind of **dysmenorrhea commonly develops at a later age** and is more long-standing, the pain rises in the extent to which it persists. The usual manifestations of Dysmenorrhea are pain in **the lower abdomen, vomiting, nausea, general body weakness and excessive passing of urine or stool.** The management of dysmenorrhea involves the use of NSAIDs with the aim of decreasing pain and inflammation, hormonal contraceptive pills that help in regulation of the menstrual cycle and in severe cases of secondary dysmenorrhea, surgery may be used.

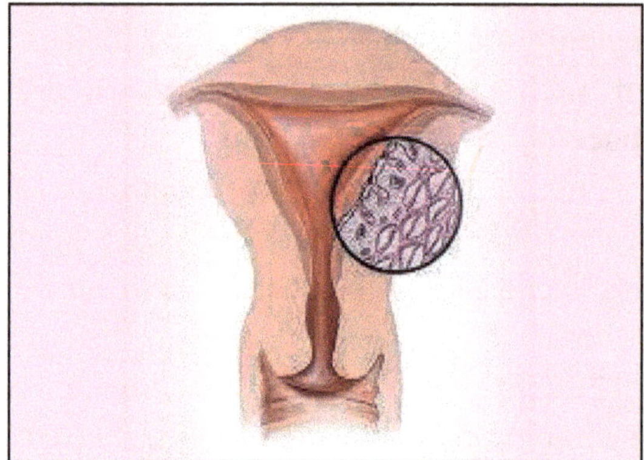

Figure 240 Dysmenorrhea

8.8.6.1 Assessment of Severity of Dysmenorrhea

The following cross tabulations display grading system of dysmenorrhea based on the degree and its disabling ability in performing daily and work activities. The grading reflects the official data identifying the relationship between the grades and pain measured on the **linear analog scale, using the numeric scale from 0 to 10 cm.**

- **Grade 0 represents no dysmenorrea, i**n other words, patient does not feel any pain and does not experience restriction by the pain in her normal functioning. Grade 1 pertains to the situation wherein the patient experiences pain during menstruation though this does not interfere with her daily activities or work. In this case there are few general signs, and **NSAIDs are seldom required, but when they are taken they are useful**.
- **The grade 2 is a moderate pain that limits the activities of the daily life** but is not very severe when it comes to the work life. It may be lacking in many ways the purely 'systemic' clinical signs and **symptoms are limited, and NSAIDs are inevitably required and often useful as analgesics.**
- **Moderate menstrual pain is depicted under grade 3** which means that the pain is disruptive to daily and working life. Symptomatic changes are extensive, and although pharmacological interventions might be required, they might not be sufficient to bring the patient back to work. It becomes advantageous in **determining how severe the dysmenorrhea is and the kind of treatment needed.**

Grade	Description of dysmenorrhea	Impact of dysmenorrhea on work life	Systemic symptoms	Use and efficacy of nonsteroidal anti-inflammatory analgesics
0	No dysmenorrhea	None	None	None needed
1	Pain is present during menses, but life activities not significantly impacted	Minimal to none	None	Rarely needed, and effective when taken
2	Moderate pain, daily activities are affected	Moderate	Few	Medications needed and often effective
3	Severe menstrual pain, major impact on life	Severe	Prevalent	Medications needed, but seldom effective enough to return patient to full function

Source: Adapted from Andersch B, Milson I. An epidemiologic study of young women with dysmenorrhea. Am J Obstet Gynecol 1982;144:655–660.

Figure 241 Assessment Severity Grading of Dysmenorrhea

8.8.6.2 SOAP Notes for Dysmenorrhea

Table 148 SOAP Notes for Dysmenorrhea

Component	Details
Subjective (S)	A 22-year-old female presents with complaints of moderate to severe crampy pelvic pain that occurs during her menstrual cycle. She reports that the pain begins on the first day of menstruation and lasts for 2-3 days. The pain is associated with nausea, headache, and lower back pain. The patient states that the pain is severe enough to affect her ability to carry out daily activities, including work and exercise. She denies any abnormal vaginal discharge or fever. Her menstrual cycle is regular, and she has no significant medical history or known gynecological conditions.
Objective (O)	The patient appears mildly distressed but is in no acute distress. Vital signs: BP 120/75 mmHg, HR 78 bpm, Temp 36.8°C (98.2°F). On abdominal examination, there is mild tenderness in the lower abdomen, especially on palpation of the lower quadrants. No signs of abnormal vaginal discharge or fever. Pelvic exam is normal with no signs of pathology.
Assessment (A)	The patient's symptoms of crampy pelvic pain during menstruation, with associated systemic symptoms such as nausea and headache, are consistent with primary dysmenorrhea (Grade 2). There is no evidence of secondary causes, such as endometriosis or fibroids, based on the patient's history and examination findings.
Plan (P)	**Pharmacological:** Start over-the-counter NSAIDs (ibuprofen 400 mg every 4-6 hours as needed for pain relief). Consider hormonal contraceptive options (oral contraceptive pills) for longer-term management if symptoms persist (See algorithm below). **Non-pharmacological:** Advise the patient to apply heat pads to the lower abdomen and to rest during menstruation. Recommend lifestyle changes such as regular exercise to improve overall menstrual health. **Follow-up:** Schedule a follow-up appointment in 3-4 months to assess symptom improvement and consider further management if pain persists. **Education:**

	Educate the patient about dysmenorrhea, its symptoms, and the effectiveness of NSAIDs and hormonal contraceptives. Discuss the importance of seeking medical advice if the pain worsens or if abnormal symptoms, such as irregular bleeding, occur.

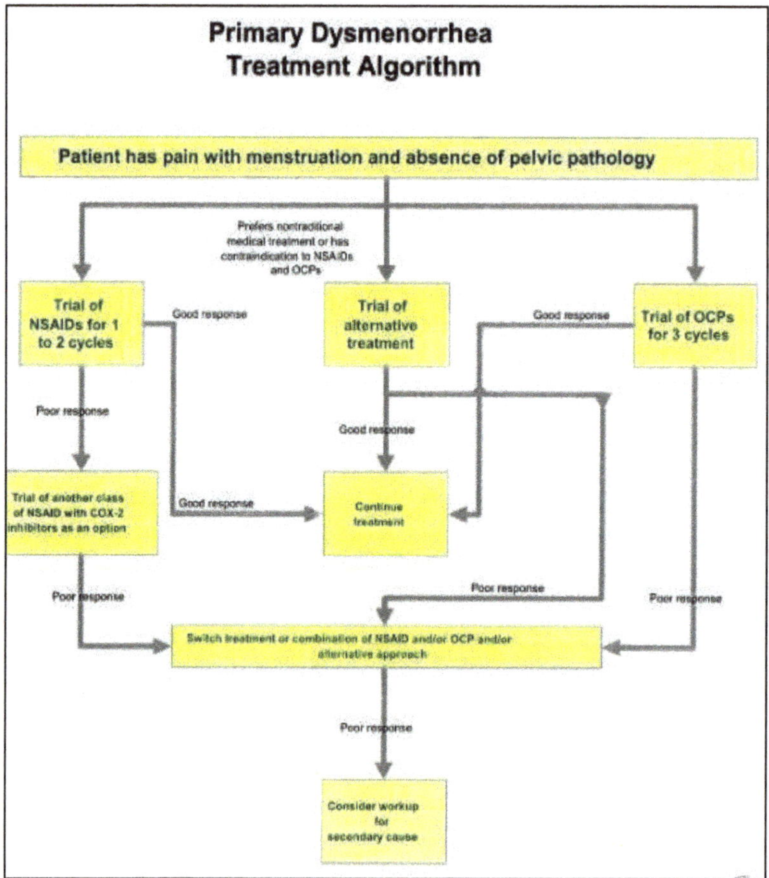

Figure 242 Management Algorithm for Primary Dysmenorrhea

8.8.7 Polycystic Ovary Syndrome

Polycystic Ovary Syndrome is known to be a common hormonal problem among women of reproductive age and is **characterized by ovary abnormalities.** This condition is described by the amenorrhoea which might be **irregular or absent, increased levels of androgens, and multiple benign ovarian cysts on the cysts.** Some of the manifestations of this condition in women are acne, increased **hair growth especially on the face (hirsutism), thinning of the hair, and fertility issues.** The occurrence of PCOS is not well understood, but it is considered to be hereditary and influenced by several factors such as insulin resistance and hormonal imbalance specifically androgen excess. The diagnosis is usually clinical, clinical signs, ultrasonography and blood tests of hormonal activity. **This is actually a chronic condition** without any cure but the emphasis is placed on relief of pervading symptoms. This means, contraceptives for periods and menstrual cramps, androgen blocker to fade body hairs, diet and exercise for **insulin resistance.**

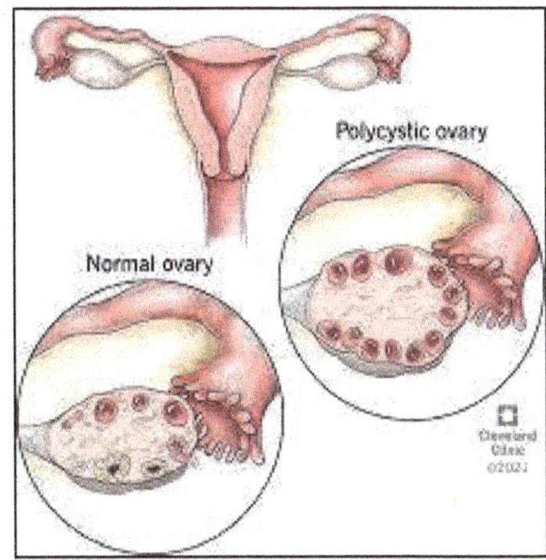

Figure 243 Normal VS. PCOs

8.8.7.1 Types of PCOs

There are different types of **Polycystic Ovary Syndrome (PCOS)** depending on the **signs and symptoms a person** has, and they include; It is from the above-mentioned categories that clinicians gain direction on the particular displays to be expected, as well as develop client-centered treatment plans. **Type A include irregularity in ovulation, high level of male hormone, and small cysts in the ovaries. Type 3 is characterized by high androgen level and irregular ovulation** but does not meet the criteria for PCOS, meaning it does not possess the polycystic ovary. **Type C has hyperandrogenism and polycystic ovaries** but the women do not have irregular menses and ovulating problems. Nevertheless, another type of **PCOS is called type D,** which is characterized by irregular ovulation, polycystic ovaries, but no hyperandrogenism. This type has different hormonal disorders and the characteristics of the ovary. Although, the exact cause of PCOS is not yet clear, these types are useful tools in its classification and deciding on the right course of action. **Because there exist various types,** the management adopted to deal with it involves aspects like hormonal therapy in cases of menstrual disorders and androgen signs. It also includes modification of lifestyle such as dietary changes and physical training as part of management since it enhances the status of patients.

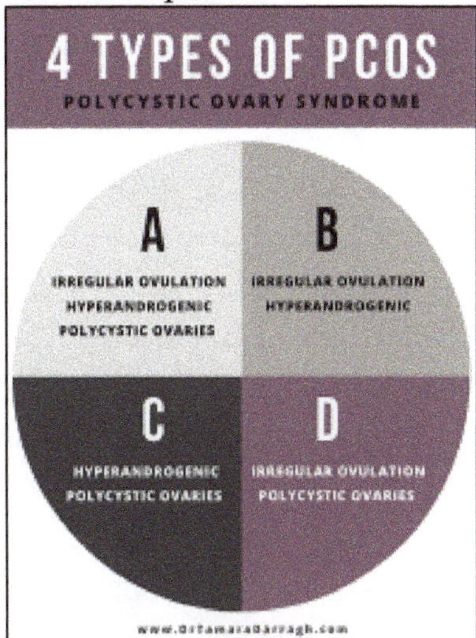

Figure 244 Types of PCOs

This flowchart shows the various subtypes of Polycystic Ovary Syndrome **depending on the features presented by the condition.** With regard to the first outcome, identifying whether the disorder actually exists in particular cases is the basic step for analysing it. To summarize, if it is not PCOS, **then the person cannot fall under any category I** have described. If PCOS diagnosis is yes, the next factor that has to be checked is insulin resistance. **When insulin resistance is present** in the individual, then it is referred to as insulin-resistant PCOS. For those with no insulin resistance, the **flow proceeds to elicit the individual's menstrual history** before use of contraceptive pills. When they are using the normal cycle before they started the use of the pill then they are said to be **having post-pill PCOS.** If the menstrual cycle irregularity was present before the usage of birth control, it is by means of signs of chronic inflammation or of elevated DHEAS, which are distinctive of inflammatory or adrenal PCOS, respectively. This classification system allows for the determination of the causes of the PCOS symptoms and treatment pattern according to the type.

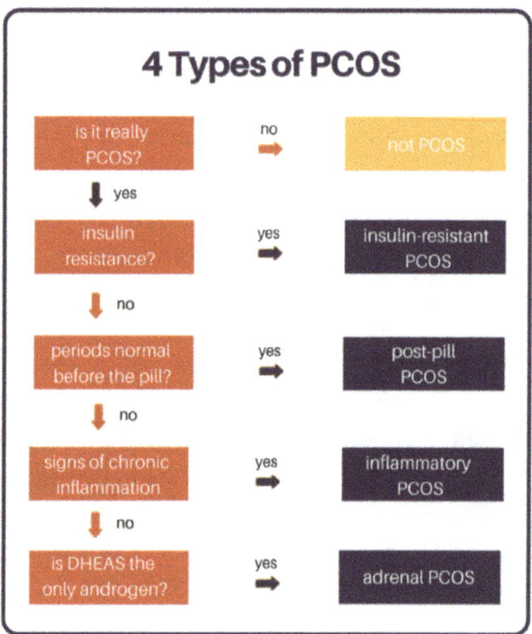

Figure 245 Types of PCOs

8.8.7.2 SOAP Notes for PCOs

Table 149 SOAP Notes for PCOs

Component	Details
Subjective (S)	A 26-year-old female presents with complaints of irregular menstrual cycles, increased facial hair, and difficulty losing weight. She mentions that her periods have been irregular for the past two years, with intervals ranging from 35 to 60 days. The patient also reports occasional acne flare-ups and thinning hair on her scalp. She is concerned about her fertility and has been trying to conceive for the past year without success. The patient denies any significant medical history other than these symptoms.
Objective (O)	On physical examination, the patient appears healthy but has mild hirsutism (excessive facial hair on chin and upper lip) and acne on her cheeks and jawline. Vital signs are normal, and there are no signs of abdominal distention or tenderness. Pelvic examination reveals no abnormalities, and ultrasound imaging shows multiple small cysts on both ovaries. Laboratory

	tests show elevated testosterone and insulin resistance, confirming the clinical suspicion of PCOS.
Assessment (A)	The patient's irregular menstrual cycles, hirsutism, acne, and ultrasound findings of multiple ovarian cysts, along with elevated testosterone levels and insulin resistance, are consistent with a diagnosis of Polycystic Ovary Syndrome (PCOS). She is also experiencing infertility, which is a common complication of the condition.
Plan (P)	**Pharmacological:** Initiate oral contraceptives to regulate menstrual cycles and reduce androgenic symptoms (acne, hirsutism). Metformin may be prescribed to address insulin resistance (See algorithm below). **Non-pharmacological:** Advise weight management through diet and exercise, as this can help improve insulin sensitivity and menstrual regularity. **Follow-up:** Schedule a follow-up in 3 months to evaluate treatment response and reassess fertility options. **Education:** Educate the patient on the long-term risks of PCOS, including diabetes, heart disease, and infertility, and emphasize the importance of maintaining a healthy weight and adhering to the prescribed treatment plan.

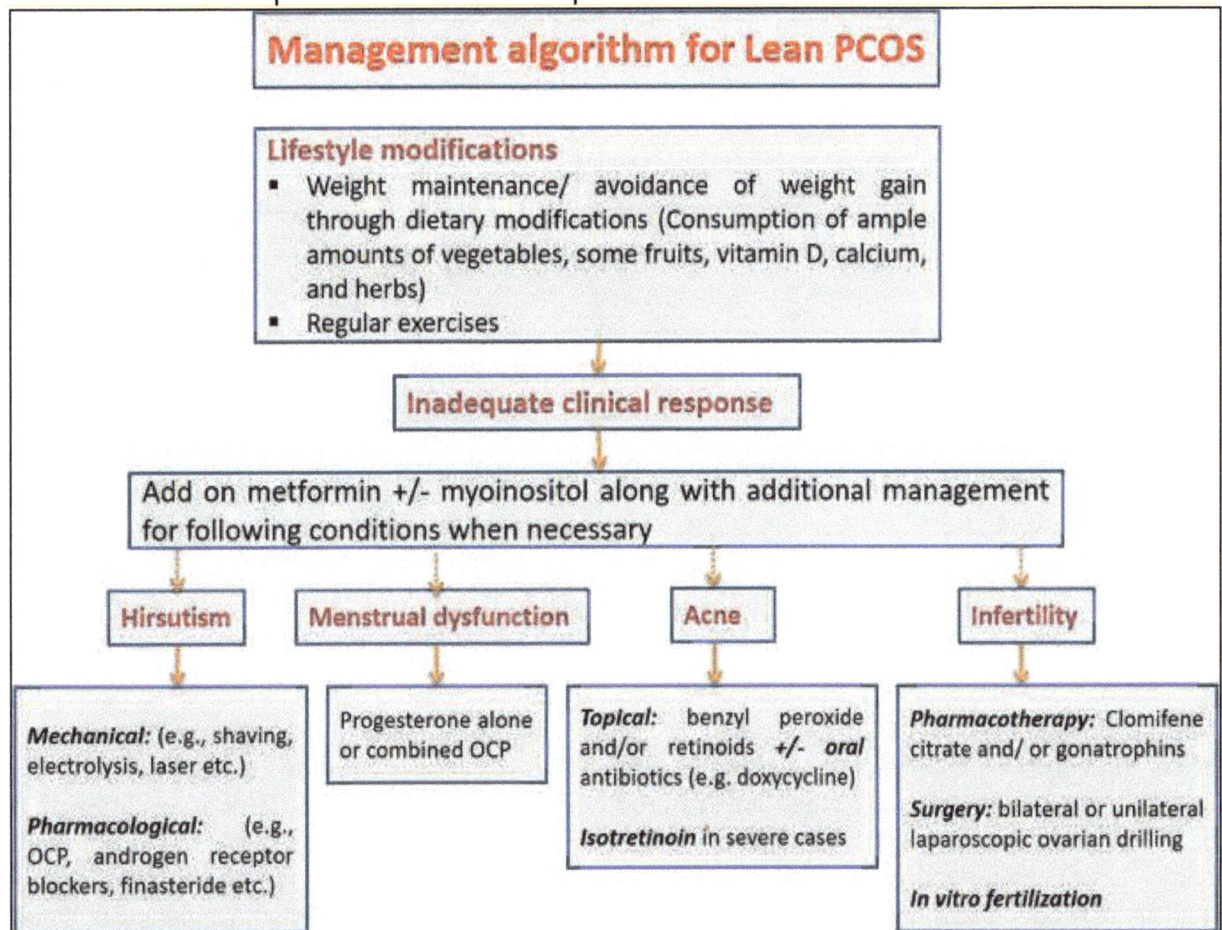
Management algorithm for Lean PCOS
Lifestyle modifications
▪ Weight maintenance/ avoidance of weight gain through dietary modifications (Consumption of ample amounts of vegetables, some fruits, vitamin D, calcium, and herbs)
▪ Regular exercises
Inadequate clinical response
Add on metformin +/- myoinositol along with additional management for following conditions when necessary
Hirsutism
Menstrual dysfunction
Acne
Infertility
Mechanical: (e.g., shaving, electrolysis, laser etc.)
Pharmacological: (e.g., OCP, androgen receptor blockers, finasteride etc.)
Progesterone alone or combined OCP
Topical: benzyl peroxide and/or retinoids +/- oral antibiotics (e.g. doxycycline)
Isotretinoin in severe cases
Pharmacotherapy: Clomifene citrate and/ or gonatrophins
Surgery: bilateral or unilateral laparoscopic ovarian drilling
In vitro fertilization

Figure 246 Management Algorithm for Lean PCOs

8.8.8 Vulvovaginal Infections

Vulvovaginitis refers to infections of the **female genitourinary system by bacteria, fungi or virus.** The major ones are ***Candida albicans*** which is behind yeast infections, ***Gardnerella vaginalis*** which results to bacterial vaginosis and ***Trichomonas vaginalis*** which gives rise to **trichomoniasis**. This condition has symptoms that include, **change of color, thin or thick vagina discharge, itching, burning sensation in the vaginal area and pain while urinating or during intercourse**. They can be 'precipitated' by some factors like hormonal factors; these include pregnancy and menopause, **the use of antibiotics, diabetes and poor hygiene**. This is normally done through published analyses of patient history, clinical assessment of the patient, and laboratory analysis using, among others, **wet mount microscopy, pH test and culture**. Depending on the type of infection, the treatment will be deployed. Yeast infection has antifungal solutions while bacterial has **antibiotics and trichomoniasis has antiprotozoal treatment**. Some things that can be done in order to avoid such infections are washing, dressing properly and proper management of diseases such as diabetes.

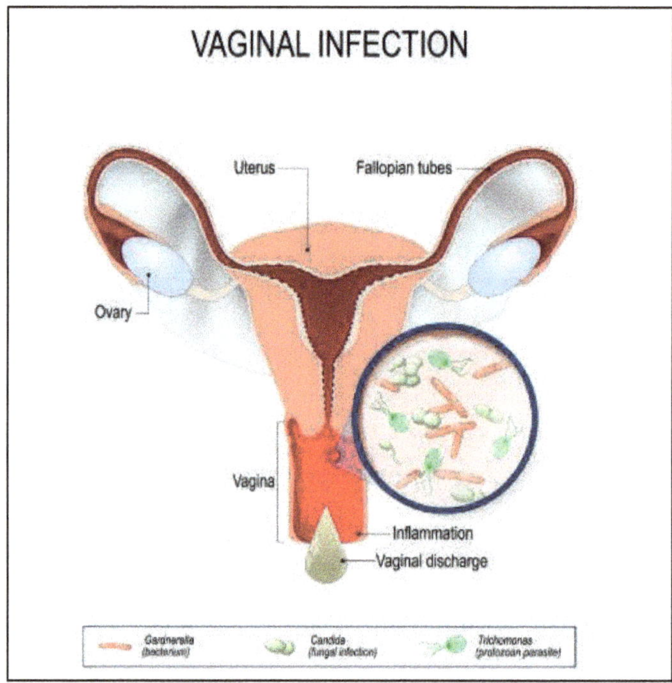

Figure 247 Vaginal Infection

8.8.8.1 Classification of Vaginal Infection

Bacterial vaginosis, yeast infections and trichomoniasis are some of the common diseases that affect the vulvovaginal system and although they are similarly located in the **same region of the female reproductive system**, they are differently caused and presented. It is a condition that occurs when there is a vaginal infection with the bacteria that are always present in the human body, it is characterized by the **smell of fish and a thin and white or grey discharge**. This is majorly associated **signs like itching, burning, and the raising of its Ph level**. On the other hand, the smelly discharge is due to the overgrowth of the yeast, Candida and has a thicker white or creamy consistency like cottage cheese. It causes itching, burning sensation that is rather intense but **the woman's vaginal pH is not affected regardless of these infections**. Trichomonas vaginitis is sexually transmitted disease that results due to Trichomonas vaginalis and symptoms include **foul-smelling, grey, frothy discharge**. It also raises the primary vaginal pH, most of the symptoms are similar to BV such as itching, and burning. It is done according to the symptoms and signs, investigations are done to know the exact reason, in order to treat the specific condition.

Table 150 Classification of Vaginal Infections

	Bacterial Vaginosis (BV)	Yeast Infection	Trichomoniasis
Cause	Overgrowth of bacteria naturally found in the vagina	Overgrowth of fungus in the vagina and/or vaginal opening	Sexually transmitted infection in vagina caused by parasite
Odor	Fishy or Unpleasant	None	Musty or Unpleasant
Discharge	Thin, milky white or grey	Thick, white, cottage, cheese-like	Frothy, yellowish or greenish
Itching, Burning, Irritation	Sometimes	Usually	Sometimes
Increased pH	Yes	No	Yes

8.8.8.2 Antibiotics for Vaginal Infections

Table 151 List of Antibiotics for Vaginal Infection

Infection Type	Antibiotic/Treatment	Form	Dosage	Precautions/Notes
Trichomoniasis	Metronidazole	Oral Tablet	Twice a day for 5-7 days	Avoid alcohol during treatment
		Oral Tablet (Large Dose)	Single Large Dose (Higher risk)	Avoid alcohol during treatment
		Single Dose Oral	Single Large Dose	Avoid alcohol during treatment
Bacterial Vaginosis	Antibiotic Tablets or Gels	Tablets/Gels/Creams	Varies, Usually for 5-7 days	Partners may also need treatment
	Antibiotic Tablets or Gels	Tablets/Gels/Creams	Varies, Usually for 5-7 days	Partners may also need treatment
	Antibiotic Gel (Long-term use)	Gel (Vaginal Use)	Daily for several months	Prolonged treatment may be necessary

Yeast Infection	Short-course Vaginal Therapy (Cream/Ointment)	Cream/Ointment/Suppositories	3-7 days	Over-the-counter options available
	Oral Medicine (Fluconazole)	Oral Tablet	Single Dose	May be used for recurrent infections
	Oral Medicine (Vivjoa, Brexafemme)	Oral Tablet	Single Dose (or 2-3 doses)	Used for recurrent infections
	Long-course Vaginal Therapy	Cream/Ointment	Daily for 2 weeks, then weekly for 6 months	Avoid in pregnancy

8.8.8.3 SOAP Notes for Vaginal Infections

Table 152 SOAP Notes for Vaginal Infection

Component	Details
Subjective (S)	A 30-year-old female presents with complaints of vaginal itching, burning, and unusual discharge for the past 4 days. She describes the discharge as thin, grayish-white, and with a fishy odor. She denies any pain during urination or intercourse. She has not had recent antibiotic use, and no history of sexually transmitted infections. She is concerned about the unusual odor and itching.
Objective (O)	The patient appears in no acute distress. On pelvic examination, there is a thin, milky white discharge with a fishy odor on speculum exam. The vaginal mucosa appears slightly erythematous. No lesions or signs of trauma are observed. The cervix is healthy with no discharge or tenderness.
Assessment (A)	The patient's symptoms, including the odor and discharge, are consistent with bacterial vaginosis (BV). Differential diagnoses include a yeast infection or trichomoniasis, but the fishy odor and discharge characteristics are more indicative of BV.
Plan (P)	**Pharmacological**: Initiate treatment with oral metronidazole (500 mg twice daily for 7 days) or vaginal metronidazole gel (See algorithm below). **Non-pharmacological**: Advise the patient to avoid douching or using scented hygiene products. **Follow-up**: Follow-up in one week if symptoms persist or worsen. **Education**: Educate the patient on the importance of completing the full course of antibiotics, avoiding irritants, and practicing safe sex to prevent recurrence of infections.

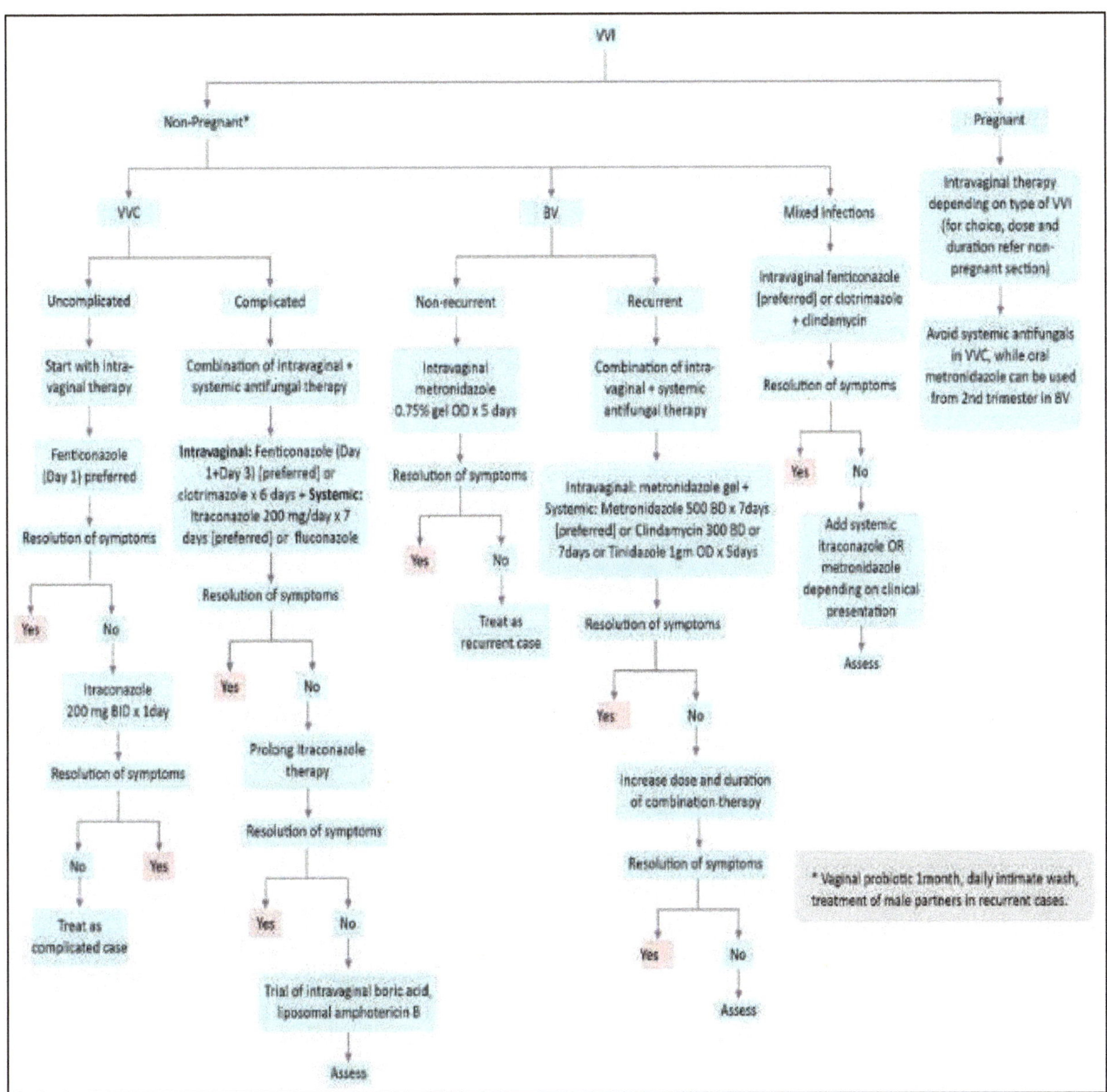

Figure 248 Algorithm for the Management of Vaginal Infections

8.8.9 Atrophic Vaginitis

Atrophic vaginitis is commonly known as **vaginal atrophy** which is characterized by the thinning of the vaginal walls, dryness and decrease elasticity of the vagina, primarily resulting from **decreased estrogen levels.** It happens often in postmenopausal women but occasionally it may happen in women with hysterectomy or even breastfeeding mothers. Lack of **estrogen results into a decrease in the secretion of natural wetness in the vagina hence; dryness, inflammation and pain during sexual activity.** Itching and burning sensation are some of the signs which women are likely to have and may include dyspareunia or pain while having intercourse and changes in the urinary system, whereby a woman may need to **urinate more than usual.** The condition may also make the vaginal walls more vulnerable to contracting such diseases as urinary tract diseases or candidiasis resulting from decreased secretion of **vaginal fluids and low acidity.** Atrophic vaginitis can be diagnosed through patient's history and clinical examination The clinical signs and symptoms of atrophic vaginitis therefore include. Vaginal irritants and inflammatory medications can be administered in the form of a vaginal moisturizer or lubricant, or estrogen in the form of **a cream, ring or vaginal tablet to rebuild the vaginal lining.** There are non hormonal therapies such as; use of **Vaginal Dehydroepiandrosterone (DHEA).** In some rare instances, continuous HRT is used, in as a systemic manner, and it involves adding estrogen and progestogen. Subsequent visits should be planned to track how the symptoms are and how the patient is reacting to treatment.

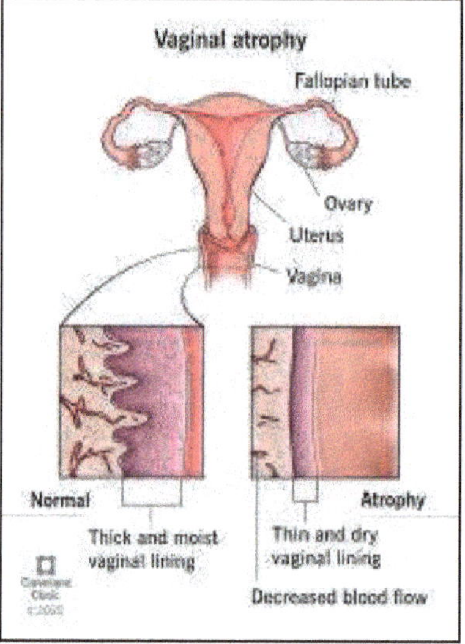

Figure 249 Vaginal Atrophy

8.8.9.1 Classification of Atrophic Vaginitis

Vaginitis is a condition that is as a result of the inflammation of the vaginal tissue and this event can be **occasioned by many causes and thereby bringing some level of discomfort**. It is also classified as infectious and non infectious. Infectious vaginitis can result from bacterial infection, fungal infection and parasitic infection including the **Candida (yeast) and Trichomoniasis** respectively. The infections present so many symptoms including abnormal discharge in the **female reproductive system, itching, and irritation. Non-Infective vaginitis on the other hand comprises conditions like atrophic vaginitis,** this is mostly related with low estrogen levels that lead to vaginal discharge and rawness especially in postmenopausal women. Some of the non-infectious diseases are a**llergic contact dermatitis, chemical induced dermatitis, and lichen planus,** which is precipitated by an immune response. Another form of non-infectious vaginitis includes desquamative vaginitis which requires peeling of vaginal tissue. Both conditions should be diagnosed and **treated according to the cause of vaginitis to control the symptoms** and lack of needed treatment.

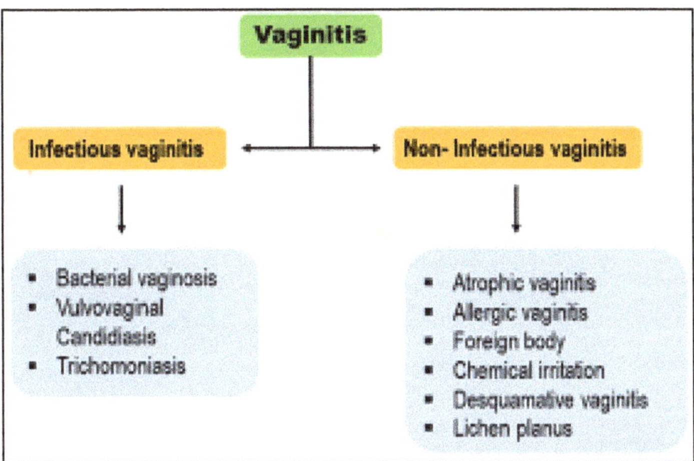

Figure 250 Classification of Vaginitis

8.8.9.2 SOAP Notes for Atrophic Vaginitis

Table 153 SOAP Notes for Atrophic Vaginitis

Component	Details
Subjective (S)	A 60-year-old postmenopausal female presents with a complaint of vaginal dryness, irritation, and discomfort during sexual intercourse. She reports an increase in vaginal itching and burning sensation, especially after urination. The patient denies any abnormal vaginal discharge, fever, or pelvic pain. She has a history of menopause 5 years ago and has not been on any hormone replacement therapy (HRT). She is concerned about these symptoms affecting her quality of life.
Objective (O)	The patient appears well-nourished and in no acute distress. On pelvic examination, there is noticeable vaginal dryness and a thin, pale vaginal mucosa. No active infection is observed. There is a decrease in vaginal elasticity, and the labia appear atrophic. No significant tenderness or masses are palpated.
Assessment (A)	The patient's symptoms and clinical findings are consistent with atrophic vaginitis, likely secondary to decreased estrogen levels post-menopause. This condition is often associated with vaginal dryness, irritation, and discomfort, particularly during sexual activity.
Plan (P)	**Pharmacological:** Recommend vaginal estrogen therapy, either in the form of a cream, tablet, or ring. Consider non-hormonal lubricants for symptomatic relief (See algorithm below). **Non-pharmacological:** Advise the use of water-based lubricants during sexual intercourse and discuss the benefits of vaginal moisturizers. **Follow-up:** Schedule a follow-up visit in 6-8 weeks to assess the patient's response to therapy. If symptoms persist or worsen, further evaluation may be needed to rule out other conditions. **Education:** Educate the patient on the nature of atrophic vaginitis, the benefits of estrogen therapy, and the importance of managing vaginal dryness to improve sexual health and comfort.

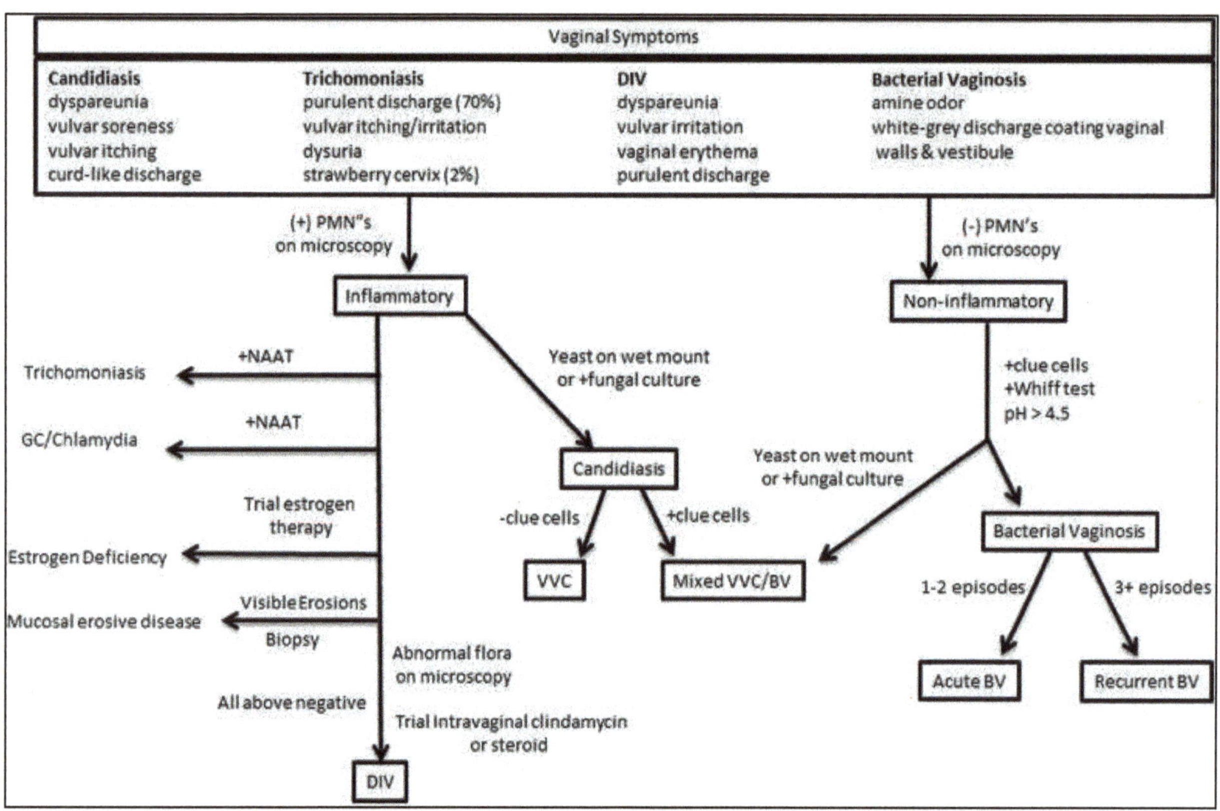

Figure 251 Algorithm for the Diagnosis and Management for Atrophic Vaginitis

8.8.10 Endometritis, Myometritis, and Fibroids

Table 154 Comprehensive Analysis of Endometritis, Myometritis, and Fibroids

Feature	Endometritis	Myometritis	Fibroids
Definition	Inflammation of the endometrium (uterine lining)	Inflammation of the myometrium (uterine muscle)	Non-cancerous growths in the myometrium
Causes	Bacterial infection (often post-childbirth, abortion, or IUD use); STIs	Bacterial infection (often post-childbirth, surgical procedures like C-sections)	Genetic and hormonal factors, influenced by estrogen
Risk Factors	Cesarean section, prolonged labor, multiple vaginal exams, IUD use	Cesarean section, hysterectomy, or D&C surgery	Obesity, family history, early menarche, African American descent

Symptoms	Fever, lower abdominal pain, abnormal vaginal discharge, heavy menstrual bleeding	Fever, uterine tenderness, abnormal discharge, abdominal pain, pain during intercourse	Heavy menstrual bleeding, pelvic pressure/pain, frequent urination, constipation
Diagnosis	Pelvic exam, ultrasound, blood cultures, pelvic MRI	Pelvic exam, ultrasound, blood cultures, MRI	Pelvic ultrasound, MRI, hysteroscopy/laparoscopy
Treatment	Antibiotics (oral or IV), sometimes surgical removal of retained tissue	Antibiotics (oral or IV), surgical removal if needed	Medications (hormonal), myomectomy, hysterectomy, uterine artery embolization
Complications	Sepsis, chronic pelvic pain, fertility issues (if untreated)	Sepsis, infertility, chronic pelvic pain, complications during pregnancy	Infertility, pregnancy complications, anemia (due to heavy bleeding)
Prevention	Prompt treatment of infections, proper post-birth care	Timely treatment of infections post-surgery or childbirth	There is no guaranteed prevention, but managing risk factors can help
Recurrence	May recur, especially if underlying causes are not addressed	May recur if underlying causes are not treated	Fibroids may recur even after treatment, especially if not surgically removed
Impact on Pregnancy	Can cause miscarriage, preterm labor, or infection during delivery	Can lead to preterm labor, miscarriage, or delivery complications	Can cause complications like miscarriage, preterm labor, and abnormal fetal positioning

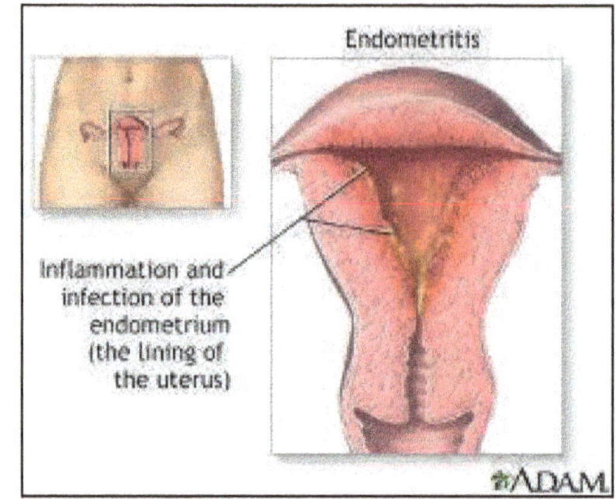

Figure 252 Endometritis

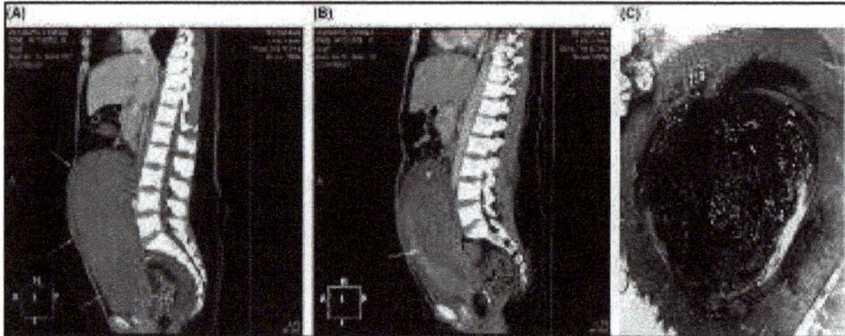

Figure 253 Myometritis

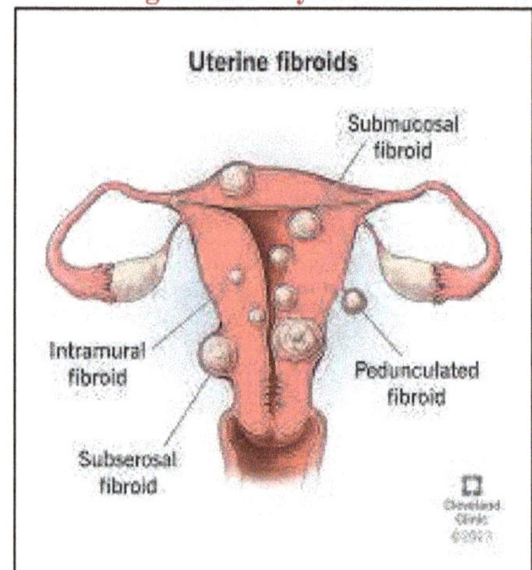

Figure 254 Fibroids

8.8.10.1 SOAP Notes for Endometritis

Table 155 SOAP Notes for Endometritis

Component	Details
Subjective (S)	A 32-year-old female presents with fever, lower abdominal pain, foul-smelling vaginal discharge, and fatigue following a miscarriage. Denies abnormal vaginal bleeding or urinary symptoms. Concerned about possible infection.
Objective (O)	Fever of 101°F. On pelvic examination, tenderness in the lower abdomen, malodorous discharge, and enlarged, tender uterus. No active bleeding. Cervical swab collected for culture.

Assessment (A)	Likely endometritis due to recent miscarriage and bacterial infection. Common postpartum complication associated with retained tissue or bacterial infections.
Plan (P)	**Pharmacological:** Initiate broad-spectrum IV antibiotics (e.g., clindamycin, gentamicin) pending culture results. Adjust based on sensitivity (See algorithm below). **Non-pharmacological:** Rest and hydration. Avoid sexual intercourse until resolution. **Follow-up:** Follow-up in 48-72 hours for symptom improvement. Ultrasound if needed. **Education:** Educate on completing antibiotic course, risks of untreated infection, and recurrence in future pregnancies.

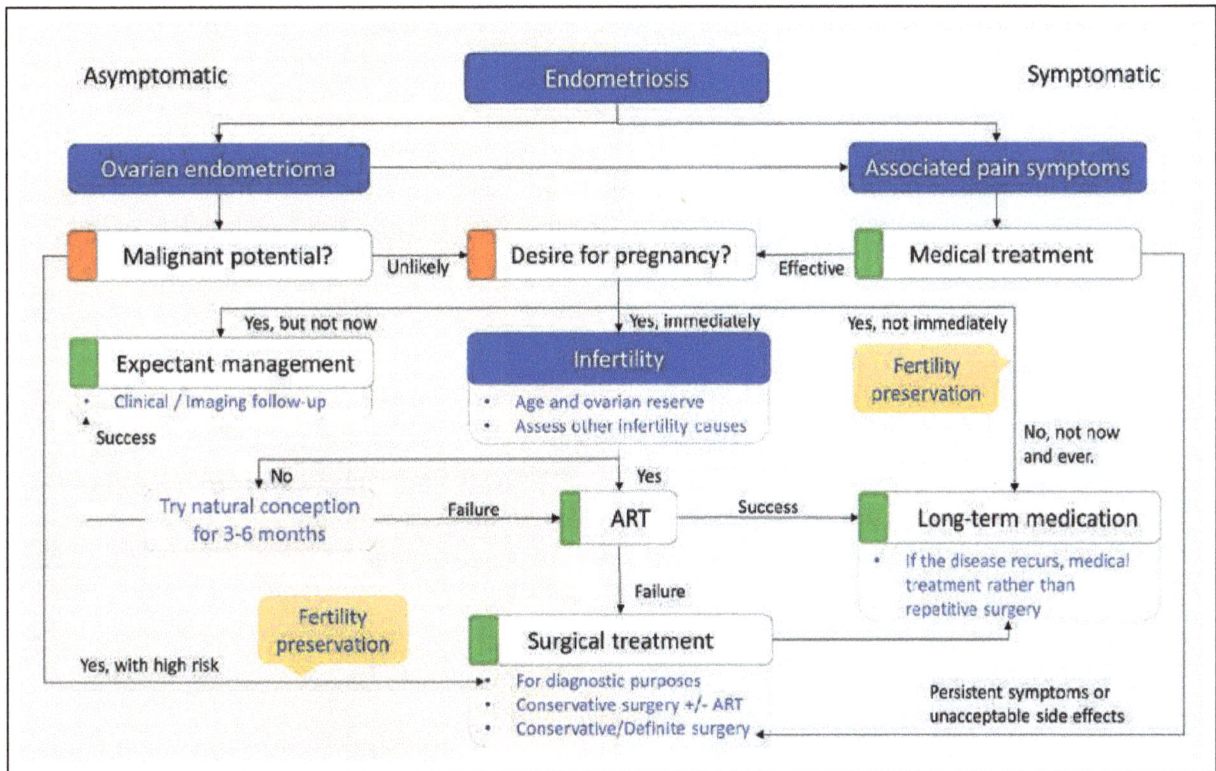

Figure 255 Treatment Algorithm for Endometritis

8.8.10.2 SOAP Notes for Myometritis

Table 156 SOAP Notes for Myometritis

Component	Details
Subjective (S)	A 28-year-old female presents with fever, pelvic pain, and uterine tenderness after cesarean section. No significant vaginal discharge or abnormal bleeding, but reports malaise.
Objective (O)	Mild fever of 100.5°F. Uterus tender to palpation with no abnormal discharge. Cesarean incision site clean. CBC shows elevated WBC.
Assessment (A)	Likely myometritis due to postpartum infection following cesarean delivery. Common after cesarean sections or prolonged labor.

Plan (P)	**Pharmacological:** IV antibiotics (e.g., ampicillin, gentamicin) for broad-spectrum coverage. Adjust based on cultures. **Non-pharmacological:** Hydration, rest, and monitoring of vital signs. **Follow-up:** Follow-up in 24-48 hours for response to antibiotics. Ultrasound if symptoms worsen. **Education:** Discuss antibiotic adherence, potential complications like sepsis, and the importance of follow-up care.

8.8.10.3 SOAP Notes for Fibroids

Table 157 SOAP Notes for Uterine Fibroids

Component	Details
Subjective (S)	A 45-year-old female presents with heavy menstrual bleeding, pelvic pressure, and frequent urination for the past 3 months. Menstrual periods have become longer and heavier. Denies significant pain or fever. Concerned about quality of life.
Objective (O)	Well-nourished, no acute distress. Palpable mass in lower abdomen, consistent with uterine enlargement. Normal cervix and no abnormal vaginal discharge. Pelvic ultrasound shows multiple fibroids.
Assessment (A)	Uterine fibroids (leiomyomas), benign tumors causing symptoms like heavy menstrual bleeding, pelvic pressure, and urinary frequency. Common in women of reproductive age.
Plan (P)	**Pharmacological:** Hormonal therapy (e.g., combined oral contraceptives, progestin IUD) to manage bleeding. Consider GnRH agonists if symptoms are severe (See algorithm below). **Non-pharmacological:** Regular monitoring with pelvic ultrasounds to track fibroid growth. **Follow-up:** Follow-up in 6-8 weeks to assess treatment response. Consider myomectomy or uterine artery embolization if necessary. **Education:** Discuss fibroid nature, treatment options, symptom management, and complications (e.g., infertility, miscarriage).

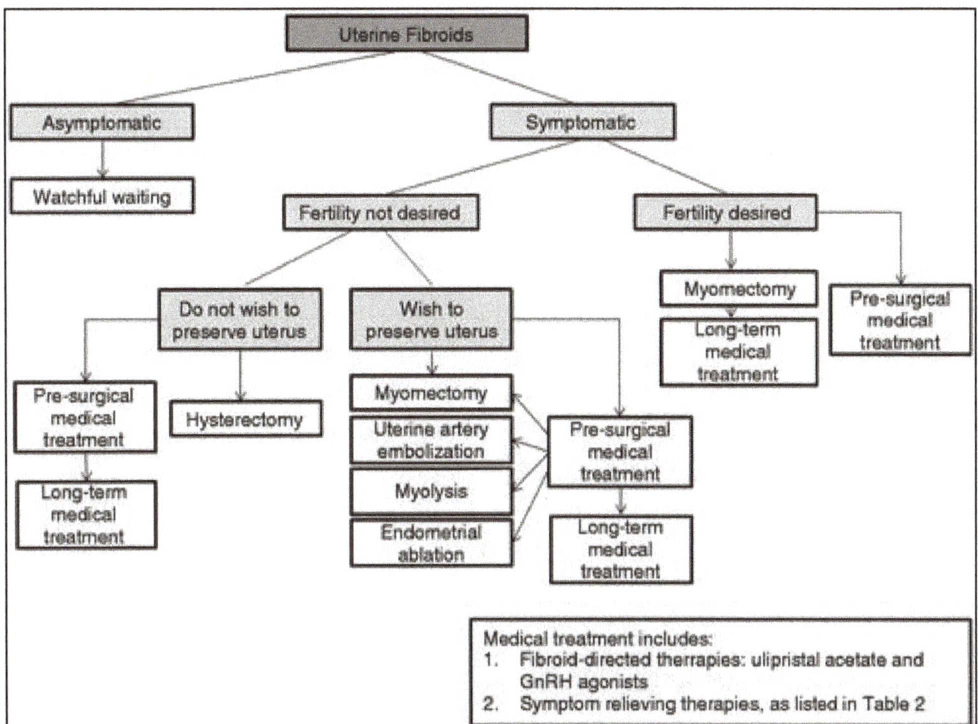

Figure 256 Algorithm for the Management of Uterine Fibroids

8.8.11 Ovarian Cancer

Table 158 SOAP Notes for Ovarian Cancer

Component	Details
Subjective (S)	A 52-year-old female presents with a 2-month history of bloating, feeling full quickly, and occasional pelvic pain. She reports fatigue and mild lower back pain. Her menstrual cycle has become irregular in the past year, and she has noticed a slight increase in abdominal girth. She has a family history of ovarian cancer (mother), but denies significant weight loss or changes in bowel habits.
Objective (O)	The patient appears mildly uncomfortable but in no acute distress. Vital signs are stable: BP 126/80 mmHg, HR 74 bpm, Temp 98.2°F. Pelvic examination reveals mild abdominal distention and tenderness in the lower abdomen. A pelvic ultrasound shows a complex ovarian mass. Serum CA-125 levels are elevated.
Assessment (A)	The patient's symptoms of bloating, fullness, and pelvic pain, combined with the ultrasound findings and elevated CA-125, are concerning for ovarian cancer. The family history further raises suspicion. A biopsy and CT scan will be needed to confirm diagnosis and assess staging.
Plan (P)	Pharmacological: Prepare for surgery (oophorectomy) if ovarian cancer is confirmed. Consider chemotherapy or radiation therapy post-surgery depending on the staging results. Non-pharmacological: Refer to an oncologist for further management. Follow-up: Schedule a follow-up appointment after diagnostic workup to discuss treatment options.

	Education: Educate the patient on the next steps for diagnosis and treatment, and provide information on managing symptoms and potential side effects of treatment.

8.8.12 Paget's disease of the breast

Table 159 SOAP Notes for Paget's Disease

Component	Details
Subjective (S)	A 60-year-old female presents with itching, redness, and flaking of the skin around the nipple of her left breast. She also reports occasional burning sensations and tenderness in the affected area. The patient has no history of breast cancer, but her mother had breast cancer. She is concerned about the changes in her breast skin.
Objective (O)	The patient appears well, though mildly distressed by the discomfort. Vital signs are stable: BP 130/85 mmHg, HR 72 bpm, Temp 98.4°F. On examination, there is erythema, scaling, and crusting of the nipple with slight nipple retraction. There is no palpable mass, but the area is tender to touch. Mammography and biopsy are scheduled for further evaluation.
Assessment (A)	The patient's symptoms, including skin changes around the nipple, are suggestive of Paget's disease of the breast, which is often associated with underlying breast carcinoma. Biopsy is needed for definitive diagnosis and to assess whether there is associated invasive breast cancer.
Plan (P)	Pharmacological: If a malignancy is confirmed, treatment options may include surgery (mastectomy), chemotherapy, or radiation therapy. Non-pharmacological: Referral to a breast specialist for biopsy and further management. Follow-up: Schedule follow-up post-biopsy to discuss results and treatment options. Education: Educate the patient on Paget's disease of the breast, the importance of biopsy for diagnosis, and potential treatments depending on biopsy results.

Golden MOH Points

1. **Testicular Torsion is a Surgical Emergency**: Immediate diagnosis and intervention are critical. Delay in detorsion of the testicle can lead to irreversible damage and loss of function. Classic symptoms include sudden, severe scrotal pain, swelling, and the absence of the cremasteric reflex.
2. **Primary Dysmenorrhea Management**: Nonsteroidal anti-inflammatory drugs (NSAIDs) are commonly used for pain management in primary dysmenorrhea. Hormonal contraceptives can be beneficial for those with recurring symptoms. Laparoscopic procedures should be considered for cases unresponsive to medical management.
3. **Polycystic Ovary Syndrome (PCOS) and Infertility**: PCOS is a leading cause of anovulatory infertility. Management includes weight management, insulin sensitizers like metformin, and ovulation induction agents such as clomiphene citrate.
4. **Atrophic Vaginitis Post-Menopause**: Atrophic vaginitis is caused by estrogen deficiency, leading to vaginal dryness, irritation, and dyspareunia (painful intercourse). Topical estrogen treatment is the first-line therapy, and vaginal moisturizers or lubricants are also commonly recommended.
5. **Bacterial Vaginosis and Treatment**: Bacterial vaginosis (BV) is caused by an imbalance in vaginal flora. It is often treated with antibiotics such as metronidazole or clindamycin. The main symptoms are a fishy odor and thin, grayish discharge.
6. **Cervical Cancer Screening and Pap Smear**: The Pap smear is a critical screening tool for detecting abnormal cervical cells, including those indicative of precancerous changes or cervical cancer. Regular screening can significantly reduce the incidence and mortality of cervical cancer.

MCQs with Answers and Rationale:

1. What is the most common cause of testicular torsion in adolescents?

a) Trauma
b) Excessive exercise
c) Spontaneous torsion
d) Infection

Answer: c) Spontaneous torsion **Rationale**: Testicular torsion often occurs without trauma or any specific trigger. It is caused by abnormal rotation of the spermatic cord, typically in adolescents and young men.

---

2. Which of the following is the first-line treatment for primary dysmenorrhea?

a) Hormonal contraceptives
b) Nonsteroidal anti-inflammatory drugs (NSAIDs)
c) Antidepressants
d) Surgery

Answer: b) Nonsteroidal anti-inflammatory drugs (NSAIDs) **Rationale**: NSAIDs are the most commonly recommended first-line treatment for managing primary dysmenorrhea, as they reduce inflammation and alleviate pain.

---

3. Which of the following is the most common form of breast cancer?

a) Ductal carcinoma in situ (DCIS)
b) Invasive ductal carcinoma (IDC)
c) Lobular carcinoma
d) Inflammatory breast cancer

Answer: b) Invasive ductal carcinoma (IDC) **Rationale**: IDC is the most common type of breast cancer, accounting for about 80% of all breast cancer cases. It starts in the milk ducts and spreads to surrounding tissue.

---

4. What is the most common type of vaginal infection associated with a fishy odor and thin, grayish discharge?
a) Yeast infection
b) Trichomoniasis
c) Bacterial vaginosis
d) Atrophic vaginitis
Answer: c) Bacterial vaginosis **Rationale**: BV is characterized by a fishy odor and thin, grayish discharge due to an overgrowth of bacteria. It is typically treated with antibiotics like metronidazole.

---

5. A 60-year-old postmenopausal woman presents with vaginal dryness and discomfort during sexual intercourse. What is the most likely diagnosis?
a) Atrophic vaginitis
b) Vaginal yeast infection
c) Bacterial vaginosis
d) Endometrial cancer
Answer: a) Atrophic vaginitis **Rationale**: Atrophic vaginitis is commonly seen in postmenopausal women due to decreased estrogen levels, leading to vaginal dryness, irritation, and discomfort.

---

6. A 25-year-old woman presents with irregular periods, excess facial hair, and weight gain. On ultrasound, she has polycystic ovaries. What is the most likely diagnosis?
a) Endometriosis
b) Polycystic ovary syndrome (PCOS)
c) Ovarian cancer
d) Hyperthyroidism
Answer: b) Polycystic ovary syndrome (PCOS) **Rationale**: PCOS is a common endocrine disorder associated with irregular periods, hyperandrogenism (e.g., facial hair), and polycystic ovaries on ultrasound.

---

7. What is the most appropriate first-line treatment for bacterial vaginosis (BV)?
a) Oral fluconazole
b) Oral metronidazole
c) Topical hydrocortisone
d) Intravaginal estrogen
Answer: b) Oral metronidazole **Rationale**: BV is treated with antibiotics, and metronidazole is the first-line option, either orally or intravaginally, to restore the balance of vaginal flora.

---

8. Which of the following is NOT a risk factor for ovarian cancer?
a) Family history of ovarian cancer
b) Early menarche
c) Nulliparity
d) Use of oral contraceptives

Answer: d) Use of oral contraceptives **Rationale**: Oral contraceptives are known to reduce the risk of ovarian cancer by inhibiting ovulation. The other options are risk factors for ovarian cancer.

---

9. What is the primary cause of secondary amenorrhea in women of reproductive age?
a) Polycystic ovary syndrome (PCOS)
b) Pregnancy
c) Ovarian failure
d) Thyroid dysfunction
Answer: b) Pregnancy **Rationale**: Pregnancy is the most common cause of secondary amenorrhea. Other causes include PCOS, ovarian failure, and thyroid disorders.

---

10. Which of the following is a characteristic feature of trichomoniasis?
a) Thick, white, cottage-like discharge
b) Frothy, yellowish, or greenish discharge
c) Itching and burning but no discharge
d) A strong, fishy odor without discharge
Answer: b) Frothy, yellowish, or greenish discharge **Rationale**: Trichomoniasis is a sexually transmitted infection caused by a parasite, leading to frothy, yellowish or greenish discharge and a strong odor.

These questions cover various topics including contraception, dysmenorrhea, PCOS, breast cancer, vulvovaginal infections, and atrophic vaginitis, providing a comprehensive review and understanding of these conditions.

9 Chapter 9: Integumentary System

9.1 Anatomy and Physiology of Integumentary System

The integumentary system operates as the **body's biggest organ system** while mainly consisting of skin and hair along with nails together with different glands. Its fundamental task exists in **providing body defense** through creating a **protective shield versus infectious agents** along with corrosive substances and external objects. This system functions as an essential organ by controlling body temperature yet helps **vitamin D synthesis** as well as **sensory signal detection**. The skin displays three distinct structural layers which progress from the top as epidermis to the bottom as hypodermis with dermis in the middle. Superficially situated above other skin layers **stands the epidermis which consists of stratified squamous epithelium and primarily contains keratinocytes**. The skin receives protection from water and develops its color through melanocytes which live within the layers. Beneath the epidermis **the dermis stands with its connective tissue** along with its blood vessels and its tissue units of hair and sweat glands. Nutrient exchange happens through the vascular network of the dermis while the dermis supports the epidermis structure. **The hypodermis contains mainly adipose tissue** that functions to protect the body as insulation and also functions as an energy reserve. The sebum fluids generated by skin sebaceous glands prevent drying and sweat glands support body temperature control through sweating. Touch sensation and pressure together with temperature sensation are processed by skin-based sensory receptors including **Meissner's corpuscles and Pacinian corpuscles**. The integumentary system supports both homeostasis preservation plus internal organ protection as well as sensory reception.

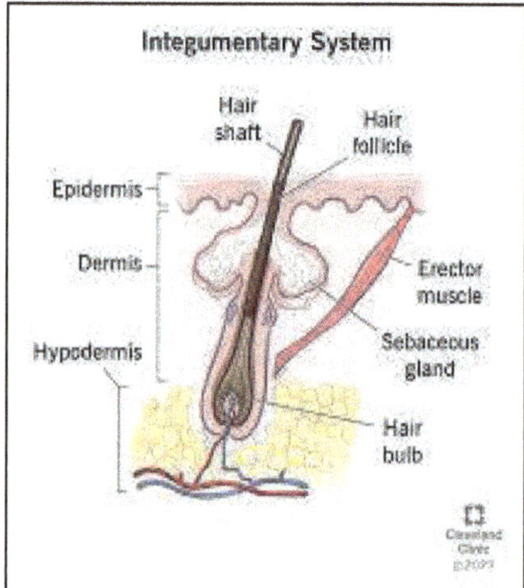

Figure 257 Integumentary System Overview

9.2 Common Conditions of Integumentary System

"PAH-SCI-IEF-LRV-HAT-CSC-FFC-EBM-SAR-MBSW" P: Psoriasis, A: Atopic Dermatitis, H: Hidradenitis Suppurativa, S: Cellulitis, C: Necrotizing Fasciitis, I: Impetigo, L: Lyme Disease, R: Rocky Mountain Spotted Fever, V: Varicella-Zoster Virus Infections, H: Herpetic Whitlow, A: Actinic Keratosis, T: Tineas (All 6 types), C: Contact Dermatitis, S: Superficial Candidiasis, C: Clenched Fist Injuries, FFC: Folliculitis, Furuncles, Carbuncles, E: Erysipelas, B: Bites (Human and Animals), M: Meningococcemia, S: Scabies, A: Acne Vulgaris, R: Rosacea, M: Molluscum Contagiosum, BS: Bioterrorism & Smallpox, and W: Wound Management & Primary Practice Procedures

Table 160 Common Conditions of Integumentary System

Condition	Description	Key Symptoms	Diagnostic Tools	Treatment Options
Psoriasis	A chronic autoimmune condition causing the rapid buildup of skin cells, leading to thick, scaly patches.	Red, inflamed patches of skin, often with silvery scales, common on elbows, knees, and scalp.	Clinical examination, biopsy if needed.	Topical corticosteroids, vitamin D analogs, phototherapy, systemic treatments like methotrexate or biologics.
Atopic Dermatitis	A chronic, inflammatory skin condition often associated with asthma and hay fever, causing itchy rashes.	Dry, itchy patches of skin, commonly on the face, elbows, and knees, often worse at night.	Clinical examination, skin biopsy if needed.	Topical corticosteroids, antihistamines for itching, emollients, immunosuppressive treatments for severe cases.
Hidradenitis Suppurativa	A chronic skin condition involving the formation of painful abscesses and tunnels under the skin.	Painful lumps under the skin, often in areas where skin rubs together, such as the armpits, groin, or buttocks.	Clinical examination, biopsy for severe cases.	Topical antibiotics, oral antibiotics, immunosuppressants, laser therapy, and surgical interventions for abscesses.
Cellulitis	An acute bacterial skin infection, often caused by *Streptococcus* or *Staphylococcus* bacteria, affecting the	Red, swollen, tender, and warm skin, often with fever and chills.	Clinical examination, blood cultures, ultrasound if abscess suspected.	Oral antibiotics (e.g., cephalexin), IV antibiotics for severe cases, supportive care.

	deeper layers of the skin.			
Necrotizing Fasciitis	A rapidly progressing, life-threatening soft tissue infection that can spread to muscles and organs.	Severe pain, swelling, fever, rapid progression of skin necrosis, and signs of shock.	Clinical examination, MRI or CT for deep involvement, blood cultures.	Immediate IV antibiotics (e.g., penicillin, clindamycin), surgical debridement, supportive care in ICU.
Impetigo	A highly contagious bacterial infection, typically caused by *Streptococcus* or *Staphylococcus* bacteria, affecting the outer layers of the skin.	Blistering sores that burst and form a yellowish crust, commonly around the mouth or nose.	Clinical examination, wound culture.	Topical antibiotics (e.g., mupirocin), oral antibiotics for severe or widespread cases.
Lyme Disease	A tick-borne infection caused by *Borrelia burgdorferi*, leading to multisystem involvement.	Erythema migrans (bull's-eye rash), fever, fatigue, and joint pain.	Clinical examination, ELISA test, Western blot for confirmation.	Oral antibiotics (e.g., doxycycline), IV antibiotics for severe cases, symptomatic treatment.
Rocky Mountain Spotted Fever	A tick-borne illness caused by *Rickettsia rickettsii*, presenting with fever, rash, and systemic involvement.	Fever, headache, petechial rash starting at wrists and ankles, history of tick exposure.	Clinical examination, serologic testing (PCR).	Doxycycline, supportive care, and fluid management.

Varicella-Zoster Virus Infections	Viral infection causing chickenpox in children and shingles in adults.	Itchy, vesicular rash with red spots and fluid-filled blisters, typically in clusters.	Clinical examination, PCR testing, direct fluorescent antibody.	Antiviral medications (e.g., acyclovir), symptomatic relief (e.g., calamine lotion, pain management).
Herpetic Whitlow	A painful infection of the finger caused by the herpes simplex virus.	Painful, swollen, and red area on the finger, often with blisters.	Clinical examination, PCR for HSV.	Antiviral medications (e.g., acyclovir), supportive care.
Actinic Keratosis	Pre-cancerous lesions caused by UV exposure.	Rough, scaly patches, often on sun-exposed skin.	Clinical examination, biopsy if needed.	Cryotherapy, topical treatments (5-FU, imiquimod), laser therapy.
Tineas (All 6 types)	Fungal infections affecting various parts of the body.	Red, itchy rashes in circular patterns, often with raised borders.	Clinical presentation, skin scraping for fungal cultures.	Topical antifungals (clotrimazole, terbinafine), oral antifungals for severe cases.
Contact Dermatitis	Inflammation due to allergens or irritants.	Red, itchy patches, sometimes blistering or crusting.	Patch testing for allergens, clinical examination.	Topical corticosteroids, antihistamines, avoiding irritants.
Superficial Candidiasis	Fungal infection often in moist areas, caused by *Candida* species.	Red, itchy rashes with white, curd-like patches in moist areas.	KOH prep for fungal elements, clinical examination.	Topical antifungals (clotrimazole, miconazole), oral antifungals for severe cases.
Clenched Fist Injuries	Injuries from punching, causing wounds	Painful, swollen, and sometimes infected	Physical examination, X-rays if fractures	Wound care, antibiotics, tetanus prophylaxis.

	and potential infections.	hand or finger injuries.	are suspected.	
Folliculitis, Furuncles, Carbuncles	Bacterial infections of hair follicles (folliculitis) or deeper (furuncles, carbuncles).	Red, painful bumps (folliculitis) or larger, pus-filled boils (furuncles, carbuncles).	Culture and sensitivity, clinical exam, drainage for abscess.	Topical antibiotics (mupirocin), oral antibiotics for abscesses, drainage.
Erysipelas	Acute skin infection caused by *Group A Streptococcus*, often with fever.	Red, raised patches of skin with fever and chills.	Clinical presentation, culture of skin lesion.	Oral antibiotics (penicillin), warm compresses.
Bites (Human and Animals)	Wounds caused by human or animal bites, can cause infection.	Painful, swollen, possibly infected bite wounds.	Physical examination, wound culture.	Wound cleaning, tetanus prophylaxis, oral antibiotics.
Meningococcemia	Bloodstream infection caused by *Neisseria meningitidis*, potentially leading to meningitis.	High fever, chills, rash (petechial), and shock.	Blood cultures, lumbar puncture for meningitis.	IV antibiotics (ceftriaxone, penicillin), supportive care.
Lyme Disease	A tick-borne infection caused by *Borrelia burgdorferi*, leading to multisystem involvement.	Erythema migrans (bull's-eye rash), fever, fatigue, and joint pain.	Clinical examination, ELISA test, Western blot for confirmation.	Oral antibiotics (e.g., doxycycline), IV antibiotics for severe cases.
Rocky Mountain Spotted Fever	Tick-borne illness caused by *Rickettsia*	Fever, headache, petechial	Clinical examination, serologic	Doxycycline, supportive care, and fluid management.

	rickettsii, presenting with fever, rash, and systemic involvement.	rash starting at wrists and ankles, history of tick exposure.	testing (PCR).	
Scabies	Parasitic infestation caused by *Sarcoptes scabiei*, leading to intense itching.	Intense itching, small red bumps or burrows on skin.	Skin scraping for mites, clinical examination.	Permethrin cream, oral ivermectin for severe cases.
Acne Vulgaris	Chronic skin condition characterized by pimples, cysts, pustules, and scars.	Pimples, cysts, pustules, and scarring on the face and body.	Clinical exam, hormonal analysis, and imaging if severe.	Topical retinoids (tretinoin), antibiotics, systemic treatments for severe cases.
Rosacea	Chronic inflammatory skin condition with redness, flushing, and visible blood vessels.	Redness, visible blood vessels, and pustules on the face.	Clinical examination, biopsy for definitive diagnosis.	Topical metronidazole, oral antibiotics for severe cases.
Molluscum Contagiosum	Viral infection that causes raised, waxy papules on the skin.	Small, raised, waxy papules, usually with a central dimple.	Skin scraping, PCR, culture if needed.	Cryotherapy, imiquimod for severe cases, watchful waiting.
Bioterrorism & Smallpox	Rare diseases, including smallpox, involving specific bioterrorism responses.	Rashes, fever, and possible history of exposure to bioterrorism agents.	Clinical evaluation, appropriate testing for specific agent.	Smallpox vaccination, antivirals, quarantine, bioterrorism response protocols.
Wound Management &	General wound care and primary	Wound healing, wound	Clinical examination, appropriate	Wound care, suturing, local

Primary Practice Procedures	procedures like suturing and anesthesia.	closure via sutures, local anesthesia.	imaging for complex cases.	anesthesia, antibiotic ointments.

9.3 Major Medical Conditions of Integumentary System

CHRONIC CONDITIONS

9.3.1 Psoriasis

The skin disorder which **demonstrates autoimmune nature and fast cell skin turnover** results in unpleasant **scaly skin layers called psoriasis**. During psoriasis the immune system produces incorrect skin cell targeting which accelerates both cell reproduction and inflammatory responses. Plaque psoriasis stands as the most prevalent form which produces red elevated areas that display silvery-white scales and usually appears on **elbows, knees, scalp and lower back**. **Guttate stands apart from the other types of psoriasis** including inverse and pustular and erythrodermic. Psoriasis develops due to unknown factors although healthcare professionals think the condition arises from both **genetic factors alongside outside elements such as infections and medications and stress.** The condition tends to occur in people who have relatives dealing with autoimmune diseases. The treatment aims to reduce inflammation and control skin cell reproduction for patients experiencing psoriasis despite the condition being incurable. The therapeutic plan for psoriasis treatment includes the application of **topical corticosteroids in combination with vitamin D analogs and phototherapy along with systemic therapies** as needed for severe conditions that include methotrexate and biologic medications. To effectively manage psoriasis patients should practice regular skincare care along with stress management techniques and minimize exposure to known triggers.

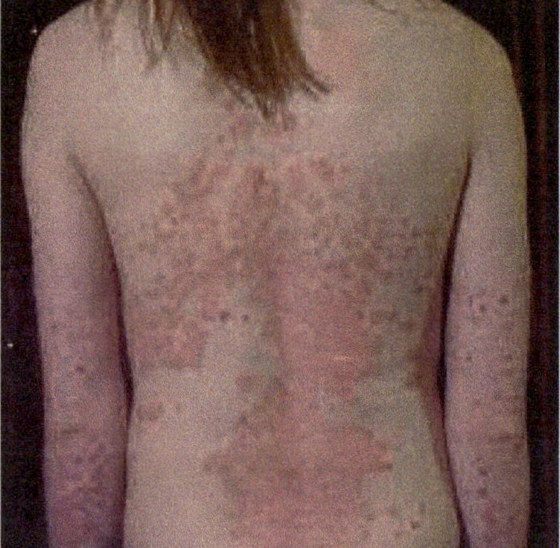

Figure 258 Psoriasis

9.3.1.1 Types of Psoriasis

The picture displays all psoriasis forms which represent **a persistent autoimmune skin condition**. **Plaque psoriasis** stands out as the most prevalent form since it causes elevated red skin surfaces with silvery scales which typically develop on knees elbows and backbone. The skin condition of **Guttate psoriasis** produces droplike shaped rash outbreaks which arise from infections such as strep throat and primarily affects the areas extending from the trunk to the limbs. The **white pustule appearance** with surrounding red skin surfaces marks pustular psoriasis and usually manifests on hands and feet. The condition of **scalp psoriasis** results in red patches accompanied by scalp skin flakiness which commonly triggers dandruff symptoms. **Nail psoriasis** causes damage to both fingernails and toenails by creating depressions and discolorations which sometimes detach fingers from the nail bed surfaces. **Psoriatic erythroderma** stands as a serious form of psoriasis because it results in severe widespread redness and intense skin shedding which poses possible lethal risks to patients. The different forms of psoriasis affect people differently through their varying severity and skin locations even though all share fast cell proliferation and skin swelling. The main goal of treatment is symptom control together with the prevention of future outbreaks.

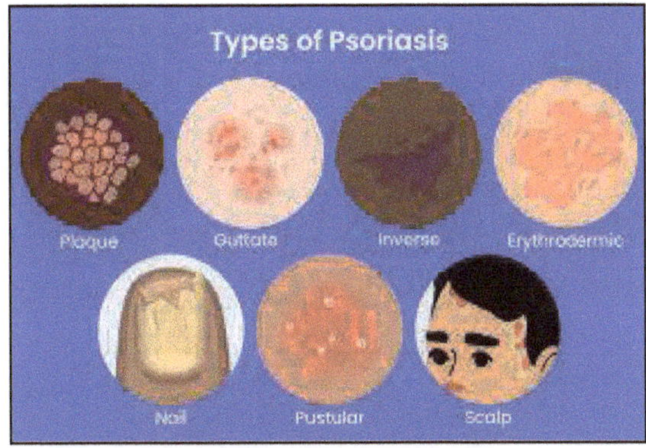

Figure 259 Types of Psoriasis

9.3.1.2 SOAP Notes for Psoriasis

Table 161 SOAP Notes for Psoriasis

Component	Details
Subjective (S)	A 32-year-old male presents with a complaint of red, scaly patches on his elbows, knees, and scalp. The patient reports that these lesions have been present for several months and have worsened in the last few weeks, with increased itching and irritation. He denies any significant pain or fever. The patient has a family history of psoriasis and mentions experiencing increased stress in the past month.
Objective (O)	The patient appears well-nourished and in no acute distress. On physical examination, well-defined, erythematous plaques with silvery scales are noted on the elbows, knees, and scalp. No signs of infection or bleeding are observed. Nail pitting is present, but there are no signs of pustules or extensive erythema. The skin lesions do not exhibit signs of secondary bacterial infection.
Assessment (A)	The patient's symptoms and clinical findings are consistent with plaque psoriasis, which is a chronic autoimmune disorder characterized by the rapid turnover of skin cells. Given the family history and stress as a potential trigger, this exacerbation is likely stress-related.
Plan (P)	**Pharmacological:** Recommend topical corticosteroids (e.g., betamethasone) for localized lesions. Consider topical vitamin D analogs (e.g., calcipotriene) to slow down cell turnover. For extensive lesions, phototherapy (UVB therapy) or systemic treatments (methotrexate or biologics) may be considered (See algorithm below). **Non-pharmacological:** Recommend regular moisturizing to reduce dryness and prevent flare-ups. Encourage

stress management techniques such as mindfulness or therapy. **Follow-up:** Schedule a follow-up visit in 4-6 weeks to assess response to treatment and adjust if necessary. **Education:** Educate the patient about the chronic nature of psoriasis, potential triggers (like stress), and the importance of adherence to treatment to manage flare-ups.

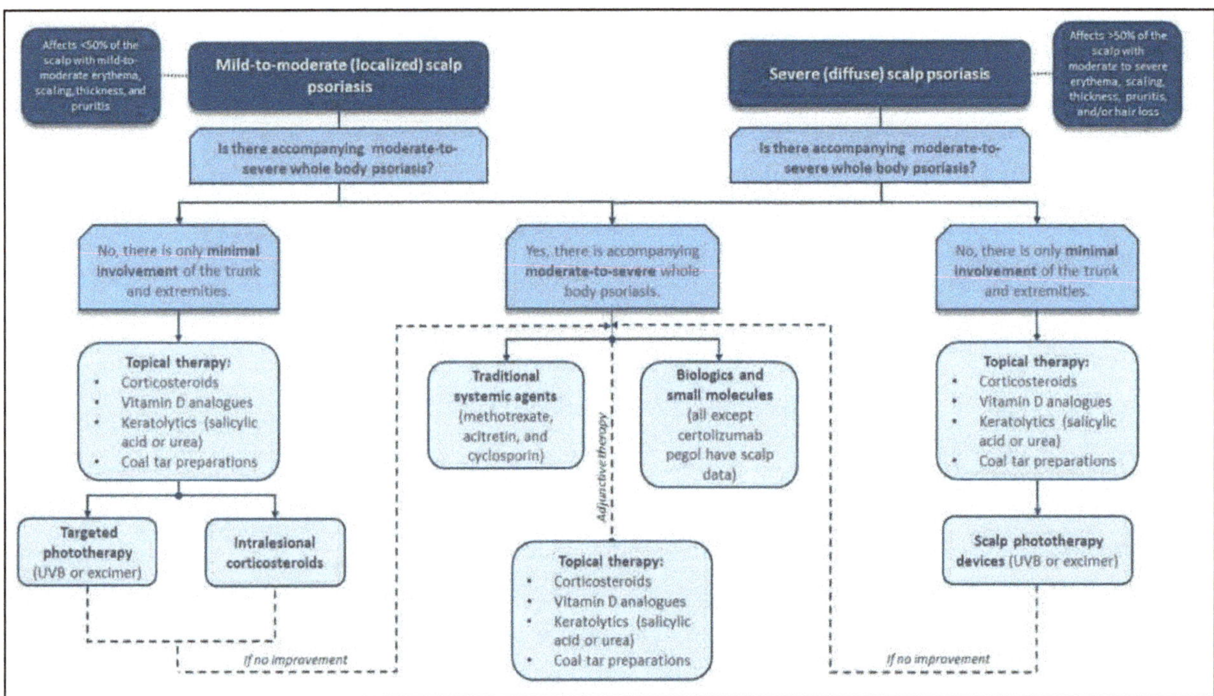

Figure 260 Treatment Algorithm for Scalp Psoriasis

9.3.2 Atopic Dermatitis

The skin condition **Atopic Dermatitis (AD) commonly referred to as eczema** exists as a persistent **inflammatory condition** that shows itself through d**ry red skin areas which experience intense itching.** The skin condition starts in early childhood and people with this condition commonly develop asthma and hay fever. Multiple factors produce the exact cause of atopic dermatitis which stems from genetic predisposition together with environmental influences and immune system function. P**eople with AD face increased risks of allergens and skin sensitizers** as well as infections because their barrier function remains impaired. The visible indicators of this condition consist of severe itchy sensations together with skin dryness and red skin with visible scaling which **commonly appear on the face alongside elbows and knees.** The condition of atopic dermatitis worsens when patients encounter allergy-producing substances and environmental irritants or experience stress from changes in climate. The care for atopic dermatitis consists of **minimizing flare-ups combined with skin barrier protection**. The standard medical strategy for AD requires topical corticosteroids along with calcineurin inhibitors together with emollients. Doctors will prescribe either oral antihistamines or immunosuppressive drugs which contain **cyclosporine to patients who have extreme symptoms**. The treatment includes skin hydration practice because patients need to prevent possible flare-ups and learn about trigger avoidance strategies.

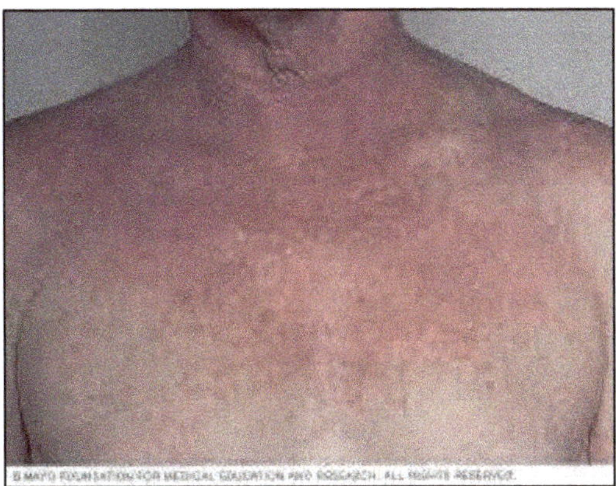

Figure 261 Atopic Dermatitis

9.3.2.1 Types of Atopic Dermatitis

The skin **presents with inflammation together with itching and irritability** because hereditary and environmental elements cause these conditions. Research indicates that **idiopathic eczema arises when doctors cannot identify the cause but experts link it to natural genetic inheritance or environmental elements**. Seborrheic eczema shows itself in skin regions with many sebaceous glands specifically the **scalp and facial areas and the chest** because overactive sebaceous glands lead to both redness and flaking of the skin. People with atopic eczema tend to also develop asthma or hay fever along with their condition and this condition primarily affects children. The condition creates **severe skin itch** along with dry skin which develops into cracked regions. The most frequent form of eczema in young children occurs on visible parts of their body **including their face and skin surfaces exposed to irritants**. The main areas affected by the condition known as **dyshidrotic eczema** are hands and feet where it produces blisters that lead to intense itching particularly when patients encounter stress or encounter allergens. Worker exposure to workplace irritants as well as allergens leads to **professional eczema but microbial eczema** develops from bacterial, fungal or viral infections that trigger both skin inflammation and infection. The types of **eczema have unique triggers** that need adjusted treatment approaches consisting of hydrating therapies and corticosteroid creams alongside the elimination of certain substances.

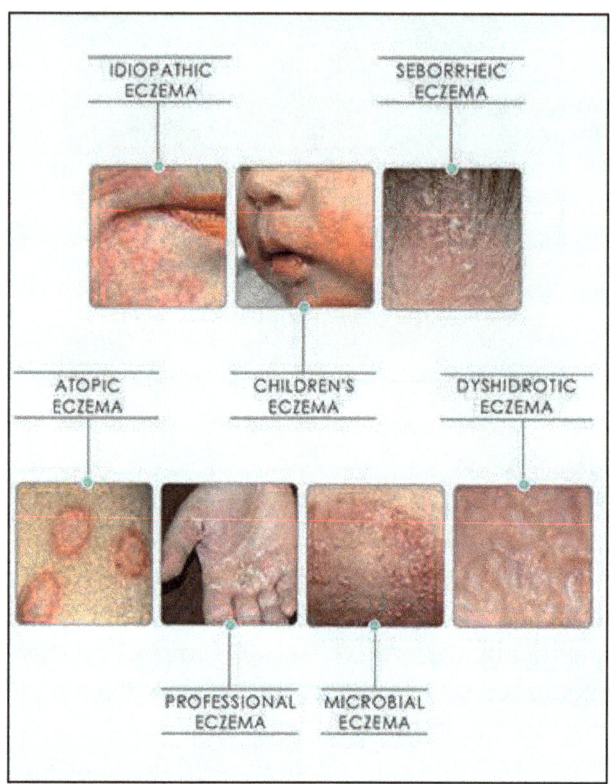

Figure 262 Types of Atopic Dermatitis

9.3.2.2 SOAP Notes of Atopic Dermatitis

Table 162 SOAP Notes for Atopic Dermatitis

Component	Details
Subjective (S)	A 5-year-old child presents with complaints of itchy, dry skin on the face, elbows, and behind the knees, which has worsened over the past few weeks. The mother reports that the child has a family history of asthma and hay fever. The child scratches frequently, especially at night, leading to red, inflamed patches of skin. No fever or discharge is noted. The mother mentions that the child has had similar episodes in the past.
Objective (O)	The child appears in no acute distress but has noticeable redness and scaling on the face, inner elbows, and knees. The lesions are well-demarcated with dry, cracked skin. No secondary infection or oozing is observed. The skin is rough, with some areas exhibiting fine, dry flakes. There is no sign of systemic involvement (e.g., fever or lymphadenopathy).
Assessment (A)	The patient's symptoms and clinical presentation are consistent with Atopic Dermatitis (Eczema), likely triggered by a combination of genetic factors (family history of atopy) and environmental factors (e.g., seasonal changes). The lesions are typical of childhood eczema, commonly seen on the face and flexural areas (elbows and knees).
Plan (P)	**Pharmacological:** Start with topical corticosteroids (e.g., hydrocortisone 1%) for inflammation control and emollients to hydrate and protect the skin. Consider calcineurin inhibitors (e.g., tacrolimus) for sensitive areas

like the face. If the eczema worsens or a secondary infection develops, consider oral antibiotics or stronger corticosteroids (See algorithm below). **Non-pharmacological:** Advise the mother on the importance of regular moisturizing and avoiding known irritants or allergens (e.g., soaps, certain fabrics). Recommend mild, non-scented skin care products and gentle, lukewarm baths. **Follow-up:** Schedule a follow-up appointment in 4-6 weeks to monitor progress and assess the need for changes in therapy. **Education:** Educate the mother about the chronic nature of atopic dermatitis, the importance of early intervention, and strategies to manage flare-ups, including avoiding triggers and using moisturizers regularly.

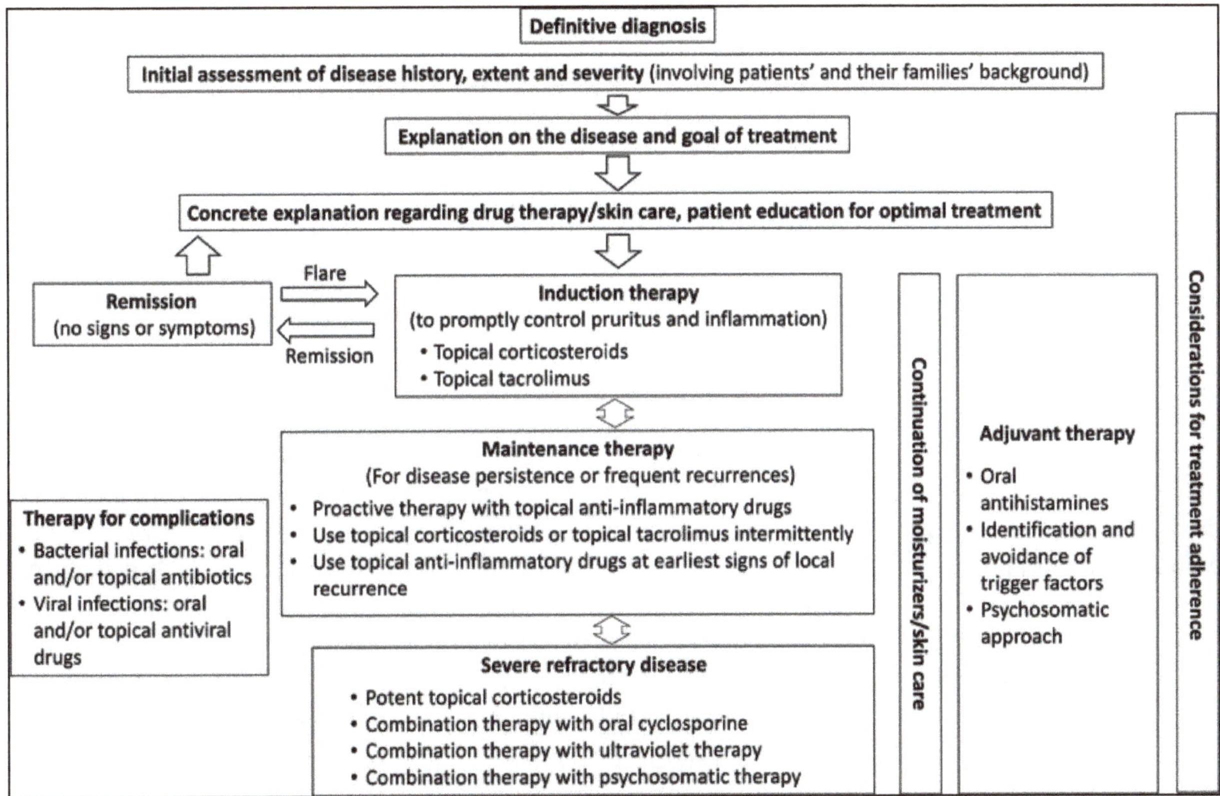

Figure 263 Algorithm for the Treatment and Management of Atopic Dermatitis

9.3.3 Hidradenitis Suppurative

As a **chronic inflammatory disorder Hidradenitis Suppurativa** creates painful abscesses with **under-surface tunnels beneath the skin** which develop specifically in contact zones between body areas like armpits and groin alongside buttocks and under the breast regions. When hair follicles and sweat glands become blocked during the condition the situation produces inflammation and infection. The skin of **individuals with HS develops permanent scarring** with the additional formation of sinus tracts or tunnels underneath the skin surface after multiple flare-ups occur. Current research suggests **HS develops from the interaction between heredity, immune system malfunction and external factors including physical rubbing and mental**

stress as well as sweating. Medical authorities recognize HS as a condition that often occurs alongside **obesity and metabolic syndrome plus Crohn's disease**. Medication strategies for Hidradenitis Suppurativa treatment involve applying antibiotics and taking medications both orally and topically in addition to using corticosteroids and immunosuppressants to control infections and inflammation. Medical procedures involving drain procedures and tissue removal become necessary when HS reaches severe stages. **Reducing flare-ups in HS** requires both proper weight management alongside personal hygiene tracking.

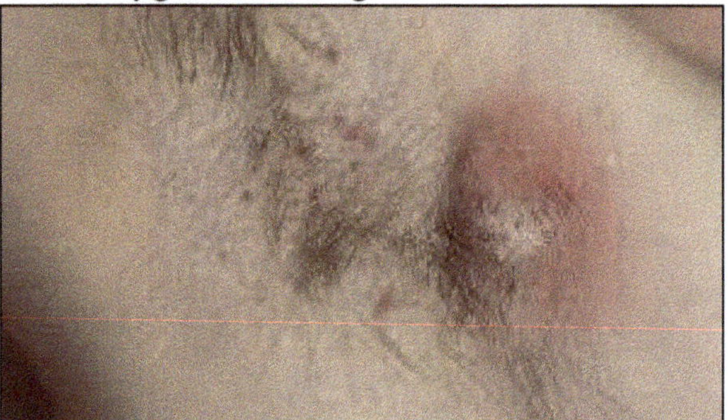

Figure 264 Hidradenitis Suppurative

9.3.3.1 Stages of Hidradenitis Suppurativa

A picture depicts the **progression of Hidradenitis Suppurativa (HS) from Stage 1 to Stage 2 and Stage 3** through its presentations of abscesses combined with skin tunnels. **The first stage of this skin condition shows one or multiple abscesses** which do not cause scarring alongside sinus tract development. Such abscesses stay limited to one area of the body and cause tenderness but lead to simpler health outcomes. **At Stage 2 of HS recurrence happens with abscesses** separated by normal skin tissue accompanied by scar tissue development. Stage 2 manifestation involves wider territorial spread that raises both flare-up frequency and the level of distress for patients. A **large extent contamination in Stage 3** causes many abscesses to appear over extensive regions which results in major scarring in combination with multiple sinus tracts underneath skin surfaces. The third stage proves damaging to tissue structures and causes permanent deformities of the affected area. **Each patient experiences different stages of the condition** along its evolutionary path while early medical treatment with antibiotics alongside anti-inflammatory drugs and operations assist with managing the condition and slowing disease advancement.

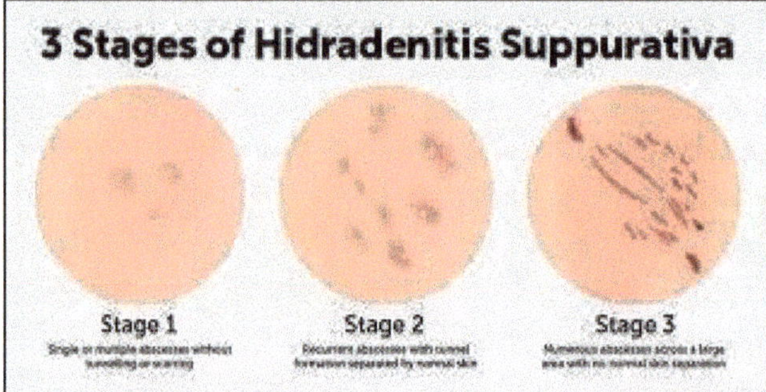

Figure 265 Stages of Hidradenitis Suppurative

9.3.4 SOAP Notes for Hidradenitis Suppurative

Table 163 SOAP Notes for Hidradenitis Suppurative

Component	Details
Subjective (S)	A 28-year-old female presents with recurrent painful lumps in her armpits, groin, and buttocks, which have been present for several months. The patient reports that the lumps have been progressively worsening, with more frequent flare-ups over the past few weeks. She also notes increased discomfort during physical activity and sweating. She has a family history of similar skin issues and is concerned about scarring. No fever or systemic symptoms are reported.
Objective (O)	On physical examination, there are multiple tender, erythematous lumps located in the axillary, groin, and perianal areas. Some lumps have drainage of pus, and there is mild scarring and hyperpigmentation noted in the affected areas. No significant systemic involvement (fever, lymphadenopathy). There is evidence of sinus tract formation in some areas, indicating a more advanced stage.
Assessment (A)	The patient's symptoms and physical findings are consistent with Hidradenitis Suppurativa, likely in Stage 2, with recurrent abscesses and the formation of scar tissue. The condition is characterized by the blockage of hair follicles and sweat glands, leading to inflammation, infection, and the formation of abscesses.
Plan (P)	**Pharmacological:** Initiate oral antibiotics (e.g., clindamycin) to treat active infection and reduce inflammation. Consider topical corticosteroids for localized flare-ups. For more severe cases, consider biologic agents (e.g., adalimumab) to reduce disease activity (See algorithm below). **Non-pharmacological:** Recommend warm compresses to reduce swelling, proper hygiene, and avoidance of friction in affected areas. Encourage the patient to wear loose-fitting clothing to reduce irritation. **Follow-up:** Schedule a follow-up visit in 4-6 weeks to assess response to treatment and manage any flare-ups. If symptoms worsen or persist, discuss further options such as surgical drainage or excision of abscesses. **Education:** Educate the patient on the chronic nature of HS, the importance of early intervention to prevent further damage, and strategies to manage flare-ups, including weight management, stress reduction, and lifestyle changes.

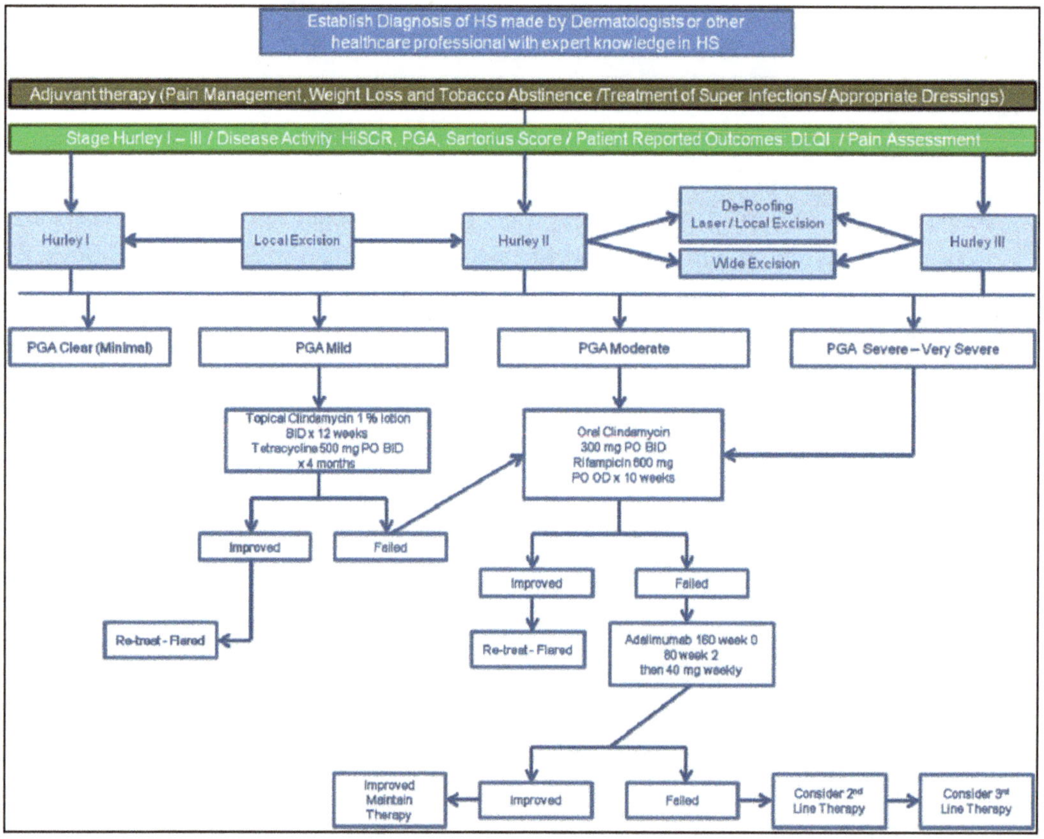

Establish Diagnosis of HS made by Dermatologists or other healthcare professional with expert knowledge in HS

Adjuvant therapy (Pain Management, Weight Loss and Tobacco Abstinence /Treatment of Super Infections/ Appropriate Dressings)

Stage Hurley I – III / Disease Activity: HiSCR, PGA, Sartorius Score / Patient Reported Outcomes: DLQI / Pain Assessment

Hurley I

Local Excision

Hurley II

De-Roofing Laser / Local Excision

Wide Excision

Hurley III

PGA Clear (Minimal)

PGA Mild

PGA Moderate

PGA Severe – Very Severe

Topical Clindamycin 1 % lotion BID x 12 weeks Tetracycline 500 mg PO BID x 4 months

Oral Clindamycin 300 mg PO BID Rifampicin 600 mg PO OD x 10 weeks

Improved

Failed

Re-treat - Flared

Improved

Failed

Re-treat - Flared

Adalimumab 160 week 0 80 week 2 then 40 mg weekly

Improved Maintain Therapy

Improved

Failed

Consider 2nd Line Therapy

Consider 3rd Line Therapy

Figure 266 Treatment and Management Algorithm for Hidradenitis Suppurative

9.3.5 Cellulitis

The bacterial **skin infection cellulitis** primarily targets skin layers extending from dermis down into subcutaneous tissues. The bacterial agents ***Streptococcus or Staphylococcus*** use skin cuts or insect bites to enter and lead to this condition. The infection leads to red skin which becomes swollen with tenderness while feeling hot to the touch although it quickly spreads to new areas if a patient does not receive treatment. **Cellulitis symptoms consist mainly of fever combined with body chills and local infection site discomfort that generates pain and tenderness**. Visible red streaks will extend from the infected spot while skin surface appears shiny. Medical authorities determine that handling an untreated skin infection leads to dangerous medical outcomes such as abscesses and sepsis while **lymphangitis emerges as a third potential complication**. Most cases require oral antibiotic medications but severe infections need intravenous antibiotics as treatment. The affected area should be raised above heart level while attention must be paid to any signs of infection worsening. In cases of repeat cellulitis that becomes severe additional medical care will be required.

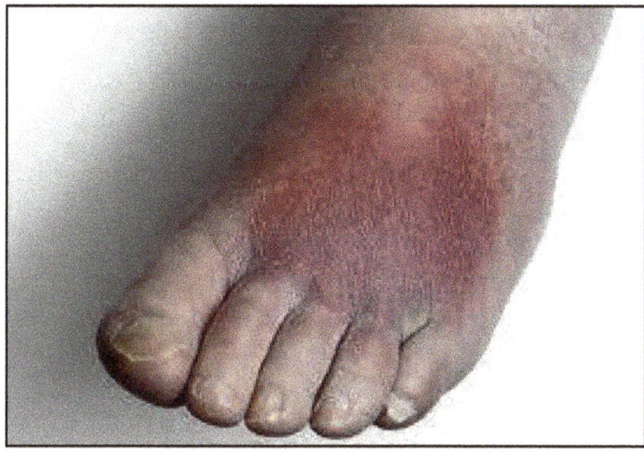

Figure 267 Cellulitis

9.3.5.1 Classification of Cellulitis

The image uses a **classification method for cellulitis assessment** which considers both patient health status and disease level severity. The classification includes **patients with systemic toxicity absence as well as patients who maintain good control of their long-term health conditions**. Most patients receive effective oral antibiotic treatment inside their homes while experiencing an uncomplicated infection. **Patients classified as Class Two** show minimal sickness signs or full health status unless they present with peripheral vascular disease or morbid obesity or chronic venous insufficiency conditions that would impact their healing process. Intensive medical treatment with closer monitoring will usually be needed for these patients. **Patients within Class Three exhibit multiple serious signs** such as acute confusion combined with tachycardia and breathlessness and hypotension because these symptoms point to a systemic infection response. People with these medical conditions either experience unstable health problems that hinder their response to medical treatment or face serious limb-threatening infections due to problematic blood circulation. **The most severe category of cases falls under Class Four** as patients show septicemia along with necrotizing fasciitis or deadly infections which demand quick medical care at high levels of intensity.

Table 164 Classification of Cellulitis

Class	Description
One	Patients have no signs of systemic toxicity, have no uncontrolled long-term conditions and can usually take oral antibiotics at home
Two	Patients are either unwell or well but have a condition such as peripheral vascular disease, chronic venous insufficiency or morbid obesity which affects recovery
Three	Patients may be unwell and have symptoms such as acute confusion, tachycardia, breathlessness, hypotension or may have unstable conditions that may interfere with a response to therapy or have a limb-threatening infection due to vascular compromise
Four	Patients have septicaemia (blood poisoning) or severe life-threatening infection such as necrotizing fasciitis

9.3.5.2 SOAP Notes for Cellulitis

Table 165 SOAP Notes for Cellulitis

Component	Details

Subjective (S)	A 58-year-old male presents with redness, swelling, and pain on his left lower leg. The patient reports that the symptoms began 2 days ago after a small scratch from gardening. He also mentions feeling feverish with chills and general fatigue. The patient has a history of Type 2 Diabetes Mellitus and peripheral vascular disease. He is concerned about the spreading redness.
Objective (O)	On physical examination, the left lower leg is erythematous, swollen, and tender to the touch. The skin is warm, and there is no visible break in the skin apart from a small scratch. The patient's temperature is 101°F. The area of redness appears to be expanding, and the borders are not well defined. There is mild lymphangitis visible with streaks of redness extending proximally. No signs of abscess formation or systemic signs of shock.
Assessment (A)	The patient's symptoms and findings are consistent with **Cellulitis**, likely exacerbated by the patient's underlying diabetes and peripheral vascular disease, which complicates recovery. The condition appears to be in Class Two, as the patient has a chronic condition that may affect recovery but does not have severe systemic toxicity.
Plan (P)	**Pharmacological:** Initiate oral antibiotics (e.g., cephalexin or clindamycin) to treat the infection. Consider a broader spectrum antibiotic if there is no improvement in 48-72 hours (See algorithm below). **Non-pharmacological:** Encourage the patient to elevate the leg to reduce swelling, apply warm compresses to the affected area, and maintain good hygiene. Monitor blood sugar levels due to the patient's diabetes. **Follow-up:** Schedule a follow-up in 3-5 days to monitor for improvement and ensure no systemic involvement. If symptoms worsen or new signs appear, consider IV antibiotics and hospitalization. **Education:** Educate the patient on recognizing signs of worsening infection, such as increased redness, warmth, or spreading of symptoms, and the importance of controlling blood sugar to improve healing.

9.3.6 Necrotizing Fasciitis

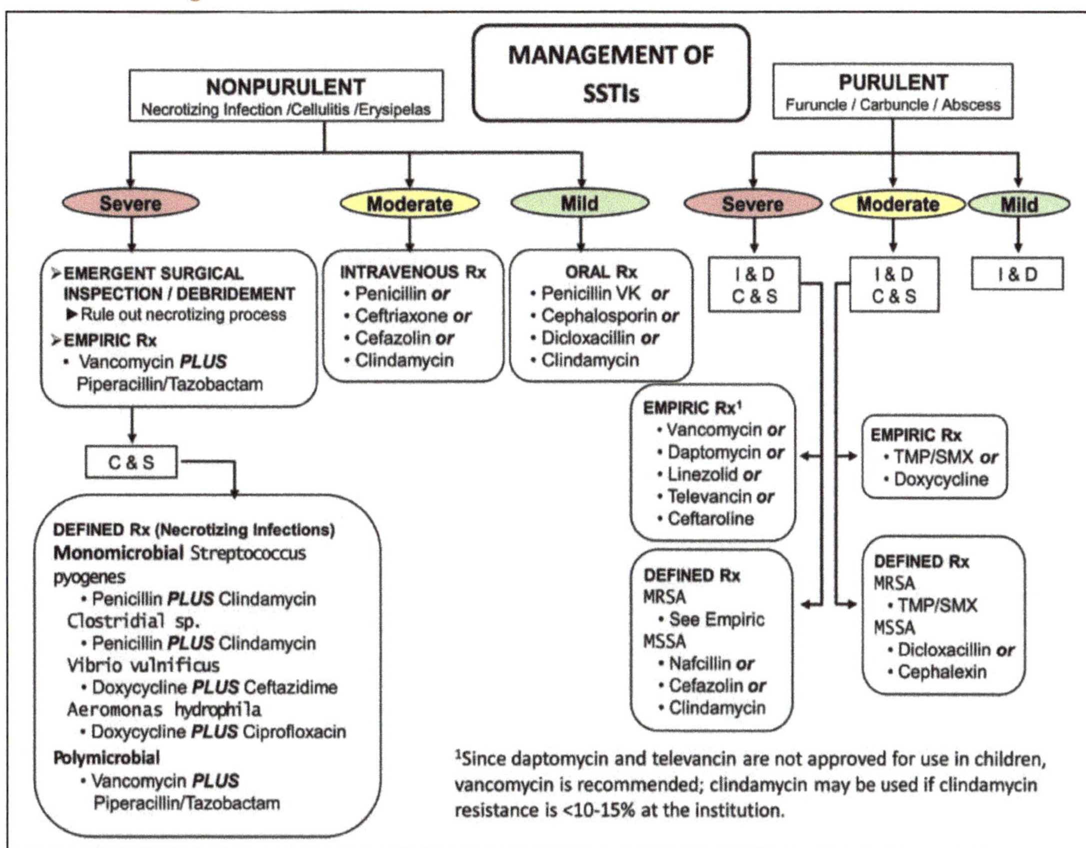

Figure 268 Treatment and Management Algorithm of Cellulitis

Necrotizing Fasciitis (NF) represents a very unusual and dangerous soft tissue infection which attacks the skin together with muscle and fat tissues in a quick destructive manner. NF develops wh**en both GAS and Clostridium bacteria accompany other unspecified species into the body through injuries or surgical procedures or damaged skin**. Fascial plane infection occurs swiftly because it crosses the connective tissue structure that envelops muscles and organs thus **earning it the nickname "flesh-eating bacteria."** Necrotizing fasciitis demonstrates its presence through extreme localized pain that exceeds what the skin shows together with sudden tissue enlargement and facial redness as well as **subcutaneous gas bubble formation**. During disease advancement tissue destruction infects the area before causing tissue to darken into **purplish or black hues while patients develop serious symptoms including body temperature increase and shock and organ failure.** The condition requires fast medical attention through complete surgical removal of dying tissue combined with powerful intravenous antibiotics administered in an **intensive care unit (ICU).** The essential condition for achieving better patient outcomes involves both early medical diagnosis combined with immediate intensive treatment interventions.

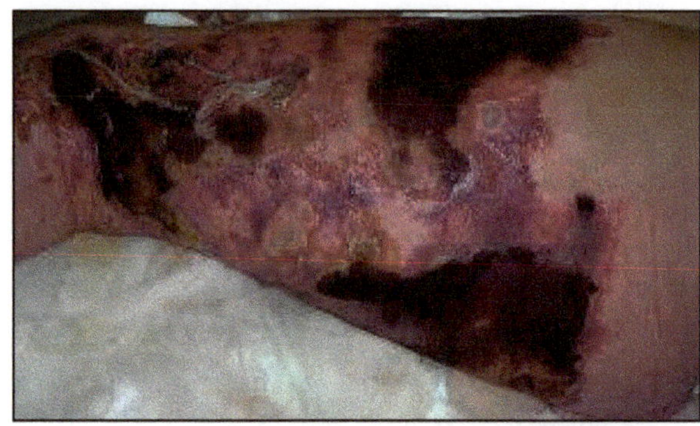

Figure 269 Necrotizing Fasciitis

9.3.6.1 Classification of Necrotizing Fasciitis

A comprehensive flowchart in the image offers in-depth details about **Necrotizing Fasciitis (NF) management together with its different types.** The treatment of this dangerous infection requires prompt aggressive tissue removal as its main management approach. **The first stage of treatment includes emergency resuscitation** measures along with antibiotic medications that treat the systemic infection. The identification of specific causative organisms depends on correct specimen analysis. Two main categories define Necrotizing Fasciitis according to this chart.

- **NF Type I occurs from mixed environments of aerobes and anaerobes** that produce conditions such as nonclostridial crepitant cellulitis, synergistic necrotizing cellulitis and progressive bacterial synergistic gangrene. The infection presents with multiple bacteria strains thus requires advanced microbiological investigation of both Gram-positive and Gram-negative bacteria species.
- **NF Type II arises from Gram-positive cocci bacteria composed mainly of *Streptococcus pyogenes, Staphylococcus aureus,* and Group A *streptococcal myonecrosis* agents**. The infection can also cause tissue destruction through aeromonas bacteria found in freshwater environments and through vibrio bacteria detected in saltwater environments.

Proper patient outcomes rely on early intervention which includes appropriate debridement followed by correct identification of infecting microorganisms and specialized antibiotic treatment.

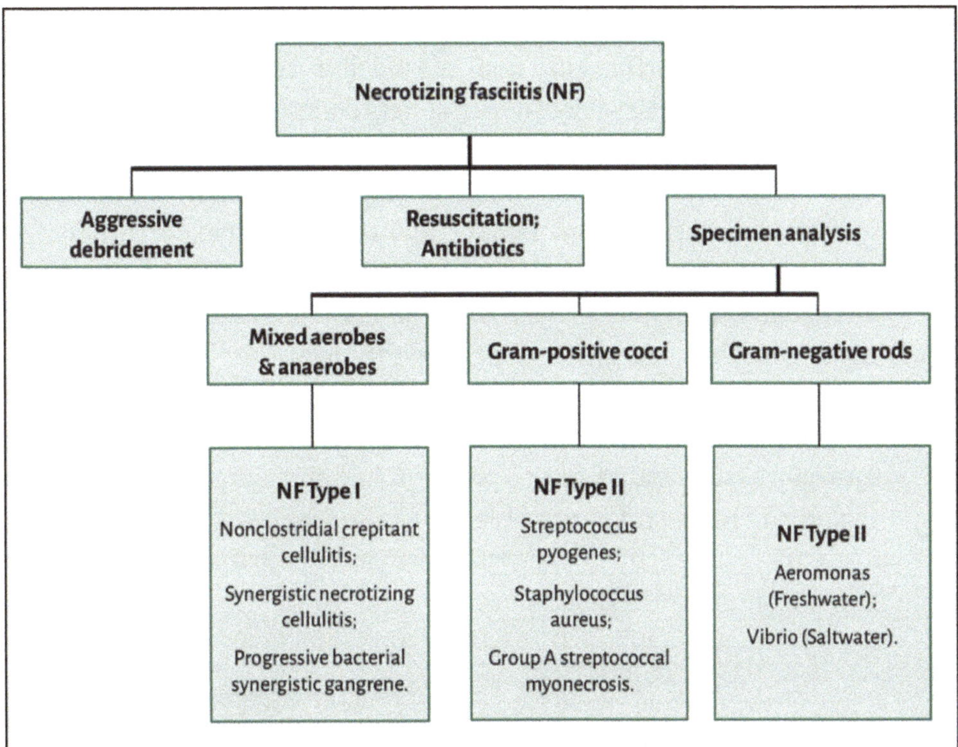

Figure 270 Classification of Necrotizing Fasciitis

9.3.6.2 SOAP Notes for Necrotizing Fasciitis

Table 166 SOAP Notes for Necrotizing Fasciitis

Component	Details
Subjective (S)	A 45-year-old male presents with severe, rapidly progressing pain in his lower abdomen following a recent abdominal surgery. The patient reports that the pain began as mild discomfort but has worsened over the last 24 hours. He describes the area as becoming increasingly swollen and red. The patient also has fever and chills, with a history of diabetes mellitus and hypertension. The patient expresses concern about the worsening pain and visible changes in the skin.
Objective (O)	The patient is febrile with a temperature of 102°F. On physical examination, the abdominal area is erythematous, swollen, and extremely tender to touch. There is crepitus in the affected area, indicating the presence of gas under the skin. The skin has progressed to a purplish discoloration, with signs of necrosis. There is no significant drainage, but the tissue appears increasingly compromised. Blood pressure is low, and the patient appears to be in mild shock.
Assessment (A)	The clinical presentation, including severe localized pain, erythema, crepitus, systemic symptoms, and tissue necrosis, is consistent with Necrotizing Fasciitis (NF). This is likely caused by Gram-positive cocci, including Streptococcus pyogenes or Staphylococcus aureus, considering the rapid progression of the infection. This condition is classified as NF Type II, which typically involves these organisms.

Plan (P)	**Pharmacological:** Start broad-spectrum IV antibiotics immediately (e.g., vancomycin, clindamycin, and piperacillin-tazobactam) to cover Gram-positive cocci, Gram-negative rods, and anaerobes. Once culture results are available, adjust antibiotics based on sensitivity. Surgical: Aggressive debridement of necrotic tissue is required to control the spread of the infection. **Resuscitation:** Begin aggressive fluid resuscitation and monitor vital signs closely, as the patient is showing signs of shock. **Follow-up:** Immediate transfer to the ICU for continued monitoring and supportive care. Further surgical debridement may be needed based on the progression of the infection. **Education:** Discuss the severity and urgency of the condition with the patient's family. Explain the importance of early and aggressive treatment to prevent further tissue loss and complications, including the need for possible future surgeries.

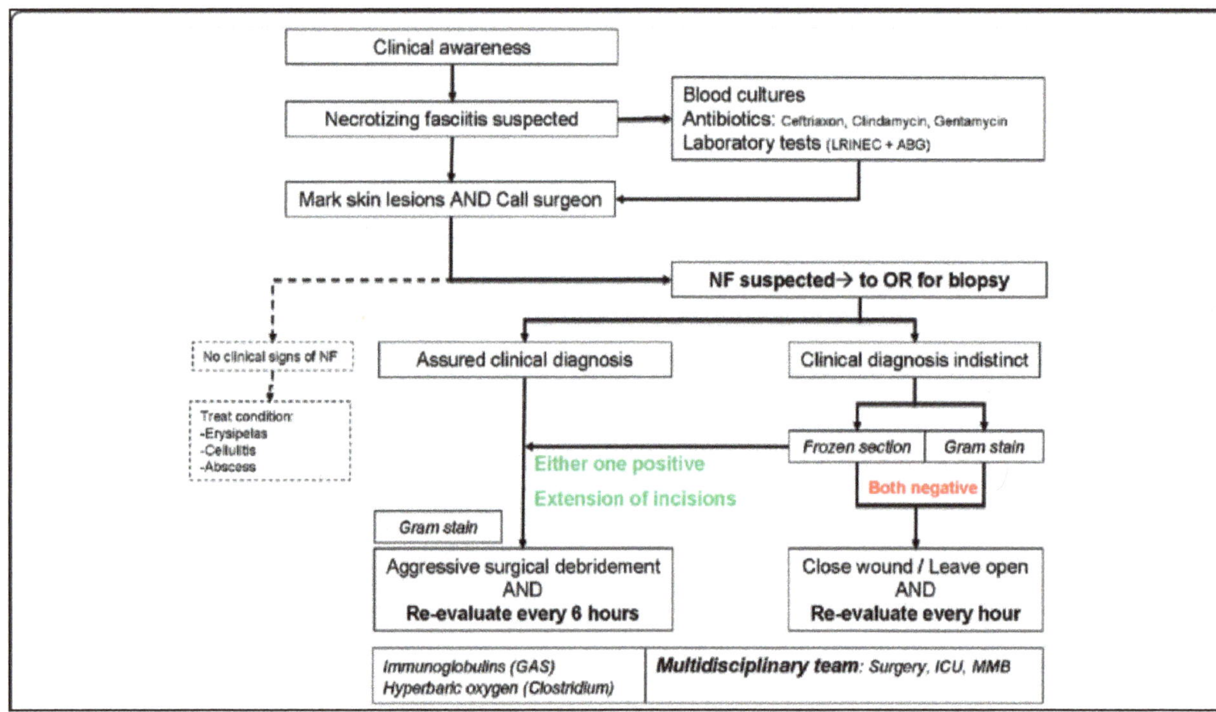

Figure 271 Management Algorithm for Necrotizing Fasciitis

9.3.7 Impetigo

Impetigo exists as a **highly contagious bacterial skin condition** which typically happens when Streptococcus pyogenes or ***Staphylococcus aureus*** bacteria infect the body tissue. The bacterial skin infection affects **children in particular** but it can develop in people throughout their lifetime. The illness usually starts as tiny red blisters that eventually break open and produce yellowish-**brown scabbed over surfaces that define its signature appearance**. The lesions appear mainly surrounding nasal areas and mouth regions along with potential occurrences on arms and legs. The bacterial illness **Impetigo spreads across populations because of physical interaction** with sick people together with contact with infected materials. Such infections arise from current skin health states including eczema together with insect bite irritation. **Ring-shaped skin lesions** combine with discomfort together with intense itching to form the symptoms of this condition. The most common therapeutic approach for **localized impetigo infections includes the application of mupirocin antibiotics on the skin surface.** Correct treatment of major and severe infections requires patients to take oral cephalexin antibiotics. **Regular hand washing with proper hygiene** together with resistance to scratching serve as essential strategies to stop impetigo from spreading between people. Uncured impetigo may end up causing both cellulitis and deleterious kidney effects.

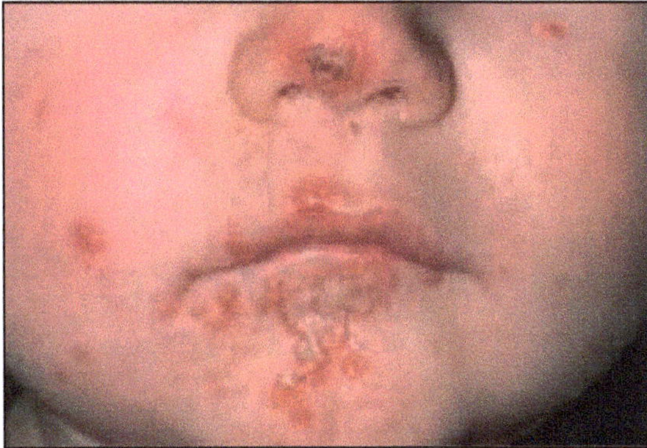

Figure 272 Impetigo

9.3.7.1 Types of Impetigo

The image presents various presentations of the contagious skin infection Impetigo that originates from bacteria including ***Streptococcus pyogenes*** or ***Staphylococcus aureus***. This most prevalent variant **of Impetigo starts as pin-sized red ulcers** that quickly turn into areas of yellow-brown crust one finds in the top section of the image. The **skin infection type commonly develops on the mouth region together with the nose area and any skin that receives direct sunlight.** The bullous form presents middle stage larger fluid-filled blisters which break open to produce similar crust but create bigger skin breakages. The unique **variant of impetigo exists at low frequencies and appears as a result of *Staphylococcus aureus* infections**. The ecthyma form found below the other sections deepens into the skin tissue to create ulcers which form scars. The bacteria responsible for both **impetigo variants cause Ecthyma** which damages skin tissue extensively since it occurs among neglected cases or unclean individuals. Different severities of impetigo need either topical or oral antibiotic treatment while maintaining proper hygiene practices for prevention of spread.

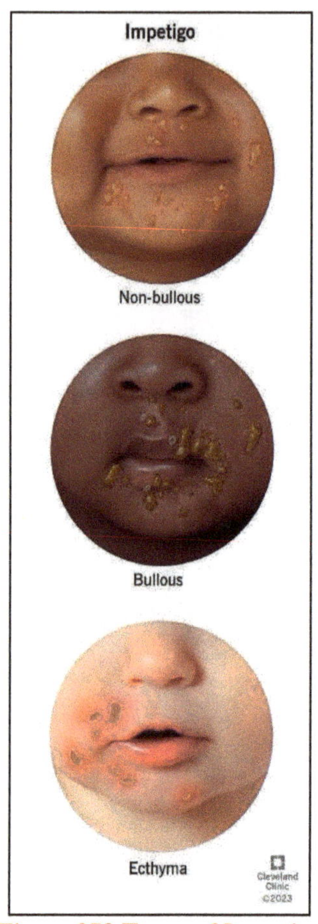

Figure 273 Types of Impetigo

9.3.7.2 SOAP Notes for Impetigo

Table 167 SOAP Notes for Impetigo

Component	Details
Subjective (S)	A 4-year-old child presents with a rash around the mouth and nose that has been present for the last 2-3 days. The mother reports that the rash started as small red spots, which then began to blister and ooze, forming a yellowish crust. The child is not experiencing pain but is frequently scratching the affected areas. There is no fever, but the mother is concerned about the infection spreading to other areas or family members. The child has no significant past medical history and is up to date on vaccinations.
Objective (O)	On physical examination, there are multiple erythematous, crusted lesions around the mouth, nose, and chin. The lesions are characteristic of non-bullous impetigo, with yellow-brown crusts covering broken blisters. There is no evidence of systemic infection or fever. No lymphadenopathy is noted. There are no signs of deeper infection or cellulitis.
Assessment (A)	The clinical presentation is consistent with Non-bullous Impetigo, a highly contagious superficial bacterial skin infection. The patient likely has an

	infection caused by *Streptococcus pyogenes* or *Staphylococcus aureus*, and the rash is localized around the face.
Plan (P)	**Pharmacological:** Prescribe topical mupirocin ointment to be applied to the affected areas twice daily for 7-10 days. If the infection is widespread or does not improve, consider prescribing oral antibiotics (e.g., cephalexin) (See algorithm below). **Non-pharmacological:** Instruct the mother to keep the affected areas clean and avoid touching the lesions to prevent the spread of infection. Encourage the child to wash their hands regularly. **Follow-up:** Schedule a follow-up appointment in 5-7 days to assess the response to treatment. If symptoms persist or worsen, oral antibiotics may be necessary. **Education:** Educate the mother on the contagious nature of impetigo, the importance of completing the full course of antibiotics, and measures to prevent the spread of the infection to others, including not sharing towels or other personal items.

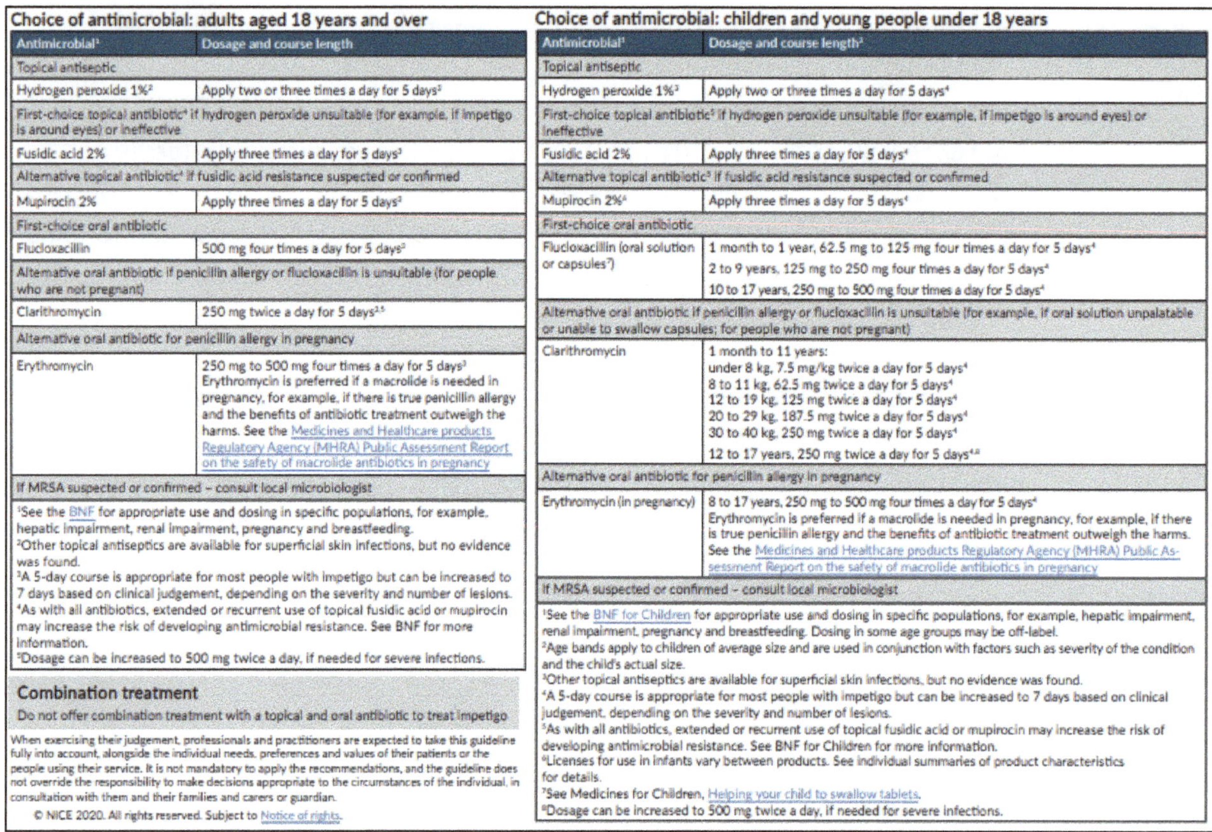

Choice of antimicrobial: adults aged 18 years and over

Antimicrobial[1]	Dosage and course length
Topical antiseptic	
Hydrogen peroxide 1%[2]	Apply two or three times a day for 5 days[3]
First-choice topical antibiotic[4] if hydrogen peroxide unsuitable (for example, if impetigo is around eyes) or ineffective	
Fusidic acid 2%	Apply three times a day for 5 days[3]
Alternative topical antibiotic[4] if fusidic acid resistance suspected or confirmed	
Mupirocin 2%	Apply three times a day for 5 days[3]
First-choice oral antibiotic	
Flucloxacillin	500 mg four times a day for 5 days[3]
Alternative oral antibiotic if penicillin allergy or flucloxacillin is unsuitable (for people who are not pregnant)	
Clarithromycin	250 mg twice a day for 5 days[3,5]
Alternative oral antibiotic for penicillin allergy in pregnancy	
Erythromycin	250 mg to 500 mg four times a day for 5 days[3] Erythromycin is preferred if a macrolide is needed in pregnancy, for example, if there is true penicillin allergy and the benefits of antibiotic treatment outweigh the harms. See the Medicines and Healthcare products Regulatory Agency (MHRA) Public Assessment Report on the safety of macrolide antibiotics in pregnancy
If MRSA suspected or confirmed – consult local microbiologist	

[1]See the BNF for appropriate use and dosing in specific populations, for example, hepatic impairment, renal impairment, pregnancy and breastfeeding.
[2]Other topical antiseptics are available for superficial skin infections, but no evidence was found.
[3]A 5-day course is appropriate for most people with impetigo but can be increased to 7 days based on clinical judgement, depending on the severity and number of lesions.
[4]As with all antibiotics, extended or recurrent use of topical fusidic acid or mupirocin may increase the risk of developing antimicrobial resistance. See BNF for more information.
[5]Dosage can be increased to 500 mg twice a day, if needed for severe infections.

Combination treatment

Do not offer combination treatment with a topical and oral antibiotic to treat impetigo

When exercising their judgement, professionals and practitioners are expected to take this guideline fully into account, alongside the individual needs, preferences and values of their patients or the people using their service. It is not mandatory to apply the recommendations, and the guideline does not override the responsibility to make decisions appropriate to the circumstances of the individual, in consultation with them and their families and carers or guardian.

Choice of antimicrobial: children and young people under 18 years

Antimicrobial[1]	Dosage and course length[2]
Topical antiseptic	
Hydrogen peroxide 1%[3]	Apply two or three times a day for 5 days[4]
First-choice topical antibiotic[5] if hydrogen peroxide unsuitable (for example, if impetigo is around eyes) or ineffective	
Fusidic acid 2%	Apply three times a day for 5 days[4]
Alternative topical antibiotic[5] if fusidic acid resistance suspected or confirmed	
Mupirocin 2%[6]	Apply three times a day for 5 days[4]
First-choice oral antibiotic	
Flucloxacillin (oral solution or capsules[7])	1 month to 1 year, 62.5 mg to 125 mg four times a day for 5 days[4] 2 to 9 years, 125 mg to 250 mg four times a day for 5 days[4] 10 to 17 years, 250 mg to 500 mg four times a day for 5 days[4]
Alternative oral antibiotic if penicillin allergy or flucloxacillin is unsuitable (for example, if oral solution unpalatable or unable to swallow capsules; for people who are not pregnant)	
Clarithromycin	1 month to 11 years: under 8 kg, 7.5 mg/kg twice a day for 5 days[4] 8 to 11 kg, 62.5 mg twice a day for 5 days[4] 12 to 19 kg, 125 mg twice a day for 5 days[4] 20 to 29 kg, 187.5 mg twice a day for 5 days[4] 30 to 40 kg, 250 mg twice a day for 5 days[4] 12 to 17 years, 250 mg twice a day for 5 days[4,8]
Alternative oral antibiotic for penicillin allergy in pregnancy	
Erythromycin (in pregnancy)	8 to 17 years, 250 mg to 500 mg four times a day for 5 days[4] Erythromycin is preferred if a macrolide is needed in pregnancy, for example, if there is true penicillin allergy and the benefits of antibiotic treatment outweigh the harms. See the Medicines and Healthcare products Regulatory Agency (MHRA) Public Assessment Report on the safety of macrolide antibiotics in pregnancy
If MRSA suspected or confirmed – consult local microbiologist	

[1]See the BNF for Children for appropriate use and dosing in specific populations, for example, hepatic impairment, renal impairment, pregnancy and breastfeeding. Dosing in some age groups may be off-label.
[2]Age bands apply to children of average size and are used in conjunction with factors such as severity of the condition and the child's actual size.
[3]Other topical antiseptics are available for superficial skin infections, but no evidence was found.
[4]A 5-day course is appropriate for most people with impetigo but can be increased to 7 days based on clinical judgement, depending on the severity and number of lesions.
[5]As with all antibiotics, extended or recurrent use of topical fusidic acid or mupirocin may increase the risk of developing antimicrobial resistance. See BNF for Children for more information.
[6]Licenses for use in infants vary between products. See individual summaries of product characteristics for details.
[7]See Medicines for Children, Helping your child to swallow tablets.
[8]Dosage can be increased to 500 mg twice a day, if needed for severe infections.

Figure 275 Antimicrobial Prescribing for Impetigo

9.3.8 Lyme Disease

Lyme disease is a tick-borne illness caused by the bacterium *Borrelia burgdorferi*, transmitted to humans through the bite of an infected black-legged tick, also known as the deer tick. The main areas where Lyme disease exists include northern parts of North America and Europe and Asian regions and these territories have high concentrations of deer ticks. A bull's-eye rash called **erythema migrans usually develops at the tick bite location three to thirty days following the infection transmission.** After the tick bite the rash forms as a red circular spot at the entry point which spreads outward presenting a clear area inside such as a bull's-eye. Early Lyme disease manifestation includes both fever together with chills coupled with fatigue and headache and muscle aches. The lack of **proper treatment for Lyme disease** enables the condition to advance through various stages where it affects the nervous system **(leading to symptoms such as facial palsy or meningitis)** and damages the heart by causing heart block or irregular heartbeat and leads to arthritis in the joints. Medical professionals administer oral doxycycline or amoxicillin antibiotics to patients with Lyme disease during the initial stages of infection while intravenous antibiotics become necessary for severe cases. Treatment success **depends on early detection of Lyme disease** to prevent advanced health issues. People should minimize their risk exposure by implementing protective measures when in tick-prone environments and through proper use of repellents and protective clothing as well as tick inspections after outdoor activities.

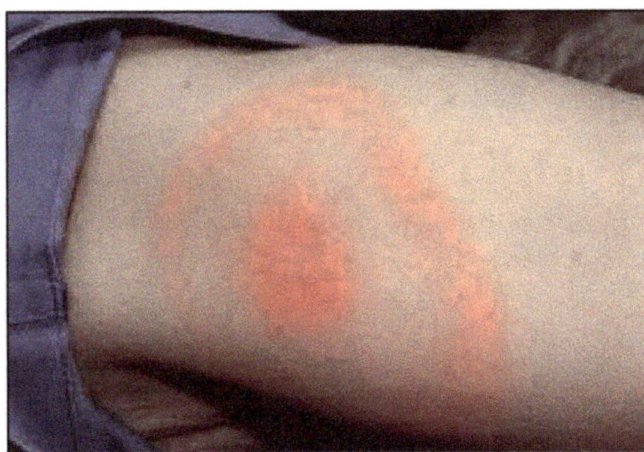

Figure 276 Lyme Disease

9.3.8.1 Stages of Lyme Disease

Lyme disease has three stages according to the image and this tick-borne sickness results from scarce Borrelia burgdorferi pathogen infections. **During Lyme disease's first stage** the most notable symptom clients exhibit is erythema migrans which develops into an oval-shaped flat and bordered red patch that becomes white when blanched. The eruption shows up **between three and thirty days following a tick bite.** The typical symptom picture of Lyme disease includes muscle pain together with fatigue and fever as well as headache and hepatitis and pharyngitis complaints. The infection moves into the acute disseminated infection stage three to five weeks after erythema migrans rash develops and appears if untreated. **The next stage presents several circular skin spots with ring-like patterns andbroken circular center design**. Neurological manifestations appear as meningoencephalitis accompanied by cranial neuropathy through Bell's palsy and radiculopathy as well as cardiac manifestations that lead to AV block development. Patients presenting with the late stage of Lyme disease develop chronic fatigue together with chronic encephalopathy and memory impairment and show symptoms of hypersomnolence along with psychiatric disturbances. **A major sign of late-stage Lyme disease involves arthritis that particularly affects the knee joints** and could negatively develop into ongoing chronic arthritis which would persist unless patients receive treatment. The successful resolution of Lyme disease demands prompt medical diagnosis combined with appropriate treatment to stop its advancement into more advanced stages.

Table 168 Stages of Lyme Disease

3 Stages of Lyme Disease		
Early Lyme Disease	Erythema migrans	• Most characteristic clinical manifestation • Well demarcated, flat-bordered, blanching erythematous oval patch • Hematogenous spread leads to secondary lesions
	Constitutional symptoms	• Fatigue, myalgia, fever
	Meningeal irritation	• Headache
	Gastrointestinal symptoms	• Hepatitis • Pharyngitis
Acute Disseminated Infection	Cutaneous	• Multiple annular/target-shaped lesions (Early)
	Neurologic manifestations	• Meningoencephalitis • Cranial neuropathy (Bell palsy) (Bilateral in 33%) • Radiculopathy
	Cardiac manifestations	• Occurs 3-5 weeks from erythema migrans • AV block
Late Lyme Disease	Neurologic manifestations	• Fatigue • Chronic encephalopathy • Memory impairment • Hypersomnolence • Psychiatric disturbances
	Arthritis	• Most often affects the knee, can be oligoarticular • Can lead to chronic Lyme arthritis (recurring arthritis)

9.3.8.2 SOAP Notes for Lyme Disease

Table 169 SOAP Notes for Lyme Disease

Component	Details
Subjective (S)	A 35-year-old male presents with a bull's-eye rash on his left leg that appeared 5 days ago after returning from a hiking trip in a known tick-endemic area. The patient reports feeling fatigued, with muscle aches and mild fever over the past few days. He also mentions a headache and a sore throat. The patient is concerned that the rash and symptoms may be linked to Lyme disease, as he has heard about tick-borne illnesses. He denies any significant medical history but does mention that he has had no prior tick bites.
Objective (O)	The patient has a well-demarcated erythematous oval patch on the left thigh, with a central area of clearing and a red ring surrounding it, consistent with erythema migrans. The rash is not raised or indurated. The patient has a temperature of 100°F. No other rashes are noted, but the lymph nodes are mildly enlarged. The patient is alert but exhibits mild fatigue and myalgia. No neurological deficits or cardiac irregularities are noted.
Assessment (A)	The patient's symptoms and the characteristic erythema migrans are consistent with early-stage Lyme disease. The patient's exposure to tick-endemic areas and the presence of systemic symptoms such as fatigue and headache further support this diagnosis. The absence of neurological or severe cardiac involvement at this stage suggests it is an early infection.
Plan (P)	**Pharmacological:** Start **oral doxycycline** (100 mg twice daily) for 14 days, as the patient presents with early-stage Lyme disease (See table below). **Non-pharmacological:** Recommend rest and hydration. Advise the patient

to monitor for any new or worsening symptoms, especially neurological or cardiac signs. **Follow-up:** Schedule a follow-up in 2 weeks to assess progress and check for potential complications. If symptoms worsen or new signs develop (e.g., facial paralysis, heart irregularities), consider referral to a specialist. **Education:** Educate the patient on the importance of completing the full course of antibiotics. Discuss the potential complications of untreated Lyme disease, including chronic arthritis and neurological involvement. Emphasize the need to take precautions in tick-prone areas, such as using insect repellent and checking for ticks regularly.

Table 170 Treatment options for Early Lyme Disease

Table 2. Treatment Options for Early Lyme Disease

Sign	Characteristic	Drug	Dosage (adult)	Length of Therapy (days)
EM	Without neurologic manifestations, advanced AV heart block	Doxycycline	100 mg po twice/day	14 (range 10-21)
		Amoxicillin	500 mg po three times/day	14 (range 14-21)
		Cefuroxime axetil	500 mg po twice/day	14 (range 14-21)
		Azithromycin	500 mg po once/day	7-10
		Clarithromycin	Nonpregnant: 500 mg po twice/day	14-21
		Erythromycin	500 mg po four times/day	14-21
	Undistinguishable from community-acquired cellulitis	Cefuroxime axetil	500 mg po twice/day	14-21
		Amoxicillin/ clavulanic acid	500 mg three times/day	14-21
Lyme meningitis, other manifestations of early neurologic Lyme disease	Acute neurologic disease manifested by meningitis, radiculopathy	1st: ceftriaxone	2 g IV once/day	14 (range 10-28)
		Alternative: cefotaxime	2 g IV q8h	10-28
		Alternative: penicillin G	Normal renal function: 18-24 million U/day q4h	10-28
		Doxycycline	Intolerant to beta-lactam antibiotics: 200-400 mg/day po in 2 divided doses	10-28
Lyme carditis, AV heart block, myopericarditis	Outpatient basis	Same as EM, without advanced AV heart block, plus ICD placement		

AV: atrioventricular; EM: erythema migrans; ICD: intercardiac defibrillator.
Source: Reference 3.

9.3.9 Burns

The **tissues and skin experience injuries** from thermal exposure along with chemical contact or electrical shock and radiation and abrasion events. **All burn wound severity falls under three different categories: first-degree and second-degree and third-degree.** The skin layer called epidermis represents the only tissue damaged in first-degree burns although it leads to redness together with pain and slight swelling. **Burns which reach up to the dermis along with the epidermis produce blisters while bringing extreme pain coupled with swelling.** Third-degree burns penetrate all layers of the skin while damaging deeper tissues and produce either charred or white skin which does not experience pain because nerve damage happened. **Fluid loss along with infection and scarring remains damaging enough to require patients to receive immediate medical attention when suffering from burns**. Medical care should be pursued immediately after using cool (not cold) water to cool the burn area and applying a clean nonstick dressing on the burned skin. The **treatment requires topical antibiotics and pain relief together** with possible skin grafts or intravenous fluids when the condition becomes serious. Long-term care for burn patients includes rehabilitation along with scar prevention as part of the treatment protocol.

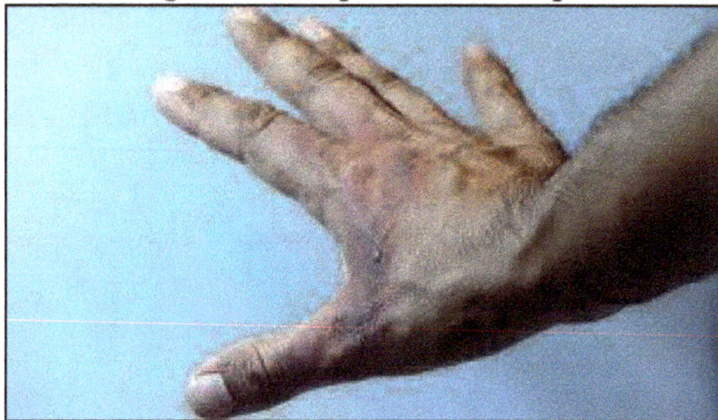

Figure 277 Burns

9.3.9.1 Classification of Burns

The image demonstrates **four burn severity levels** determined by how deeply injuries penetrate into the skin layers and underlying tissues. First-degree burns impact only the **top layer of skin (epidermis)** yet they result in skin redness together with pain and swelling. Such burn injuries remain commonly light and recover in less than one week while preserving normal skin appearance. The skin damage from **second-degree burns (partial or intermediate thickness)** reaches the dermis which causes intense pain along with blister formation and tissue swelling. The healing process extends longer because such burns tend to result in scarring. **Third-degree burns totally obliterate the skin tissue** extending from the epidermis through the dermis and beyond to penetrate deeper body structures including fat tissues and muscles and bones. The burned tissues appear either white or charred or leathery while no feeling of pain exists in the area because nerve damage has occurred. **Fourth-degree burns wipe out all layers of skin and impact muscles and underlying tissue structures** that result in permanent damage which requires treatment through skin grafts or amputation procedures. Intensive medical intervention along with rapid medical treatment becomes crucial for patients with such burns to minimize risks of failure or loss of fluids and tissue infections.

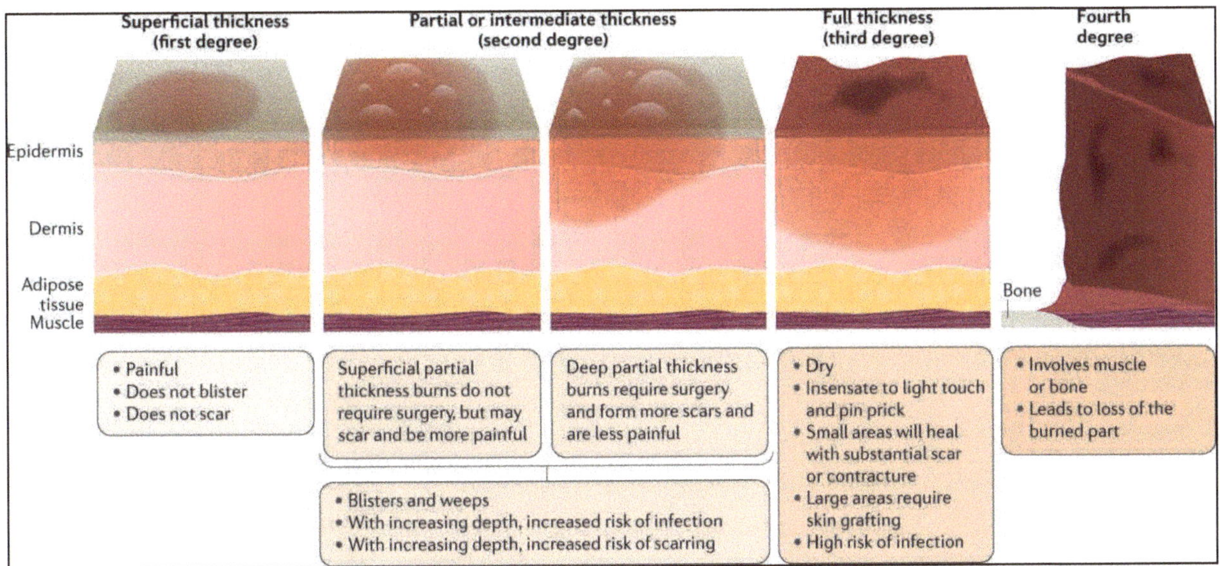

Figure 278 Classification of Burns

9.3.9.2 Degree of Burns

The picture displays the **basic burn classifications according to their injury level.** The least severe form of burn **injuries affects only the epidermis as depicted on the left side of the image**. First-degree burns produce an effect of surface tissue redness with pain and light swelling that heals up in less than a week without leaving behind any enduring damage or atrophic marks. The middle part of the image reveals second-degree burns that destroy the two skin layers of epidermis and dermis. **The affected skin develops painful blisters together with intense swelling because of such burns.** In addition to healing that spans a few weeks, the severity of the burn will determine whether scars form or stay away. The most serious burns appear on the right side because they penetrate deep into the **skin beyond epidermis and dermis to affect tissue layers** including fat and muscles as well as bone deposits. Because nerve destruction occurs the burned area becomes white with leather-like texture while **exhibiting no sensation to pain**. Healing processes usually demand medical attention through skin grafts yet this treatment leads to high scars formation risks and enduring tissue destruction.

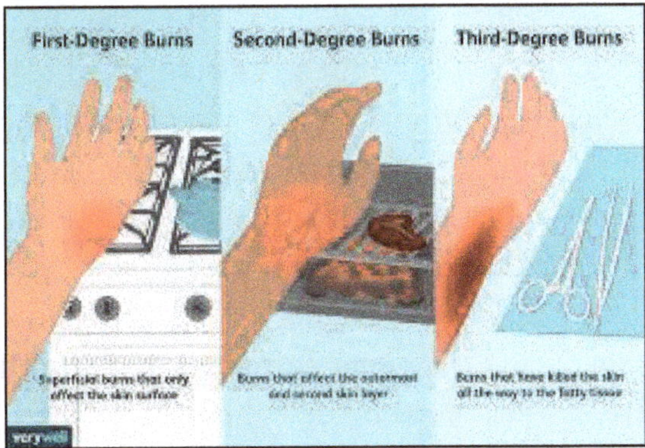

Figure 279 Degree of Burns

9.3.9.3 SOAP Notes for Burns

Table 171 SOAP Notes for Burns

Component	Details
Subjective (S)	A 30-year-old male presents with a burn injury on his left forearm. He reports that he accidentally touched a hot stove, causing the burn. The

	injury occurred about 2 hours ago. The patient describes feeling immediate pain and notices redness and blistering on the affected area. He is concerned about possible scarring and is unsure of the severity of the burn. He has no significant medical history.
Objective (O)	On physical examination, the affected area on the left forearm shows the following: First-degree burn (superficial): Redness and mild swelling over a small area. Second-degree burn (partial thickness): Several small blisters are present with clear fluid, along with erythema and moderate swelling. Third-degree burn (full thickness): A small portion of the forearm displays white, leathery skin with no pain sensation, indicating deeper tissue involvement.
Assessment (A)	The patient has a mixed degree burn injury: A first-degree burn on the upper part of the forearm with superficial redness. A second-degree burn with blistering on the mid-section of the forearm. A third-degree burn on a small portion of the lower forearm, with full-thickness injury extending to deeper tissues. The extent of third-degree burns suggests significant damage that may require specialized care.
Plan (P)	**Pharmacological:** For the first-degree burn: Use cool compresses and topical aloe vera gel to soothe the skin. Over-the-counter pain relievers (e.g., ibuprofen) can be taken for mild pain. For the second-degree burn: Apply a topical antibiotic ointment (e.g., mupirocin) and cover with a sterile dressing. If the blisters break, apply hydrocortisone cream for inflammation. For the third-degree burn: Immediate wound care with sterile dressings and IV fluids to prevent shock. Referral to a burn specialist for potential skin grafts and further management (See algorithm below). **Non-pharmacological:** Keep the affected areas clean and covered with sterile gauze to avoid infection. Avoid popping blisters to reduce the risk of infection. **Follow-up:** Schedule a follow-up appointment in 3-5 days to evaluate healing and assess any need for further wound care. For third-degree burns, hospital admission for specialized care is required. **Education:** Educate the patient on burn care, signs of infection (redness, pus, increased pain), and the importance of avoiding direct sunlight on the affected skin during the healing process. Inform the patient about scarring risks and the potential need for rehabilitation if skin grafts are required.

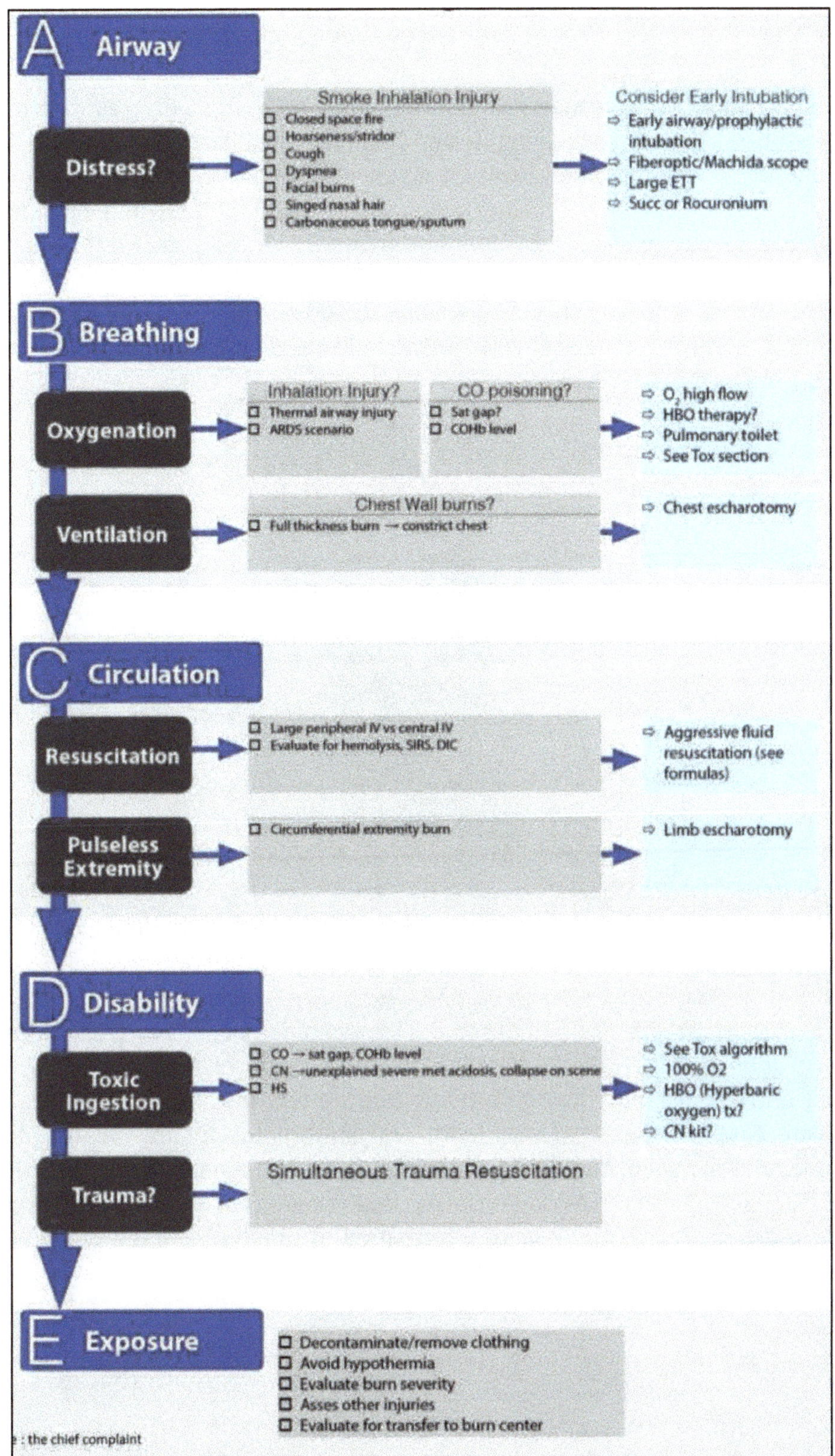

Figure 280 Algorithm for Burn

OTHER CONDITIONS

9.3.10 Actinic Keratosis

Actinic keratosis (AK) is a precancerous skin lesions which clinically manifest themselves as scaly, hyperkeratotic skin lesion occurring in sun-damaged skin. They may be pink, red, or brown and more commonly seen on the sun exposed areas such as the **face, ears, neck, scalp, chest, backs of hands, forearms, or lips.** They are not malignant at first and may transform into squamous cell carcinoma in case they are not treated. AK is generally dealt primarily by cryotherapy where the **skins growth is frozen using liquid nitrogen**. Systems of medication that can be used to treat areas requiring specific focusing include 5-fluorouracil also known as 5-FU as well as imiquimod to kill the abnormal cells. In chronic cases, laser therapy or the use of electro surgery may be used as the last resort.

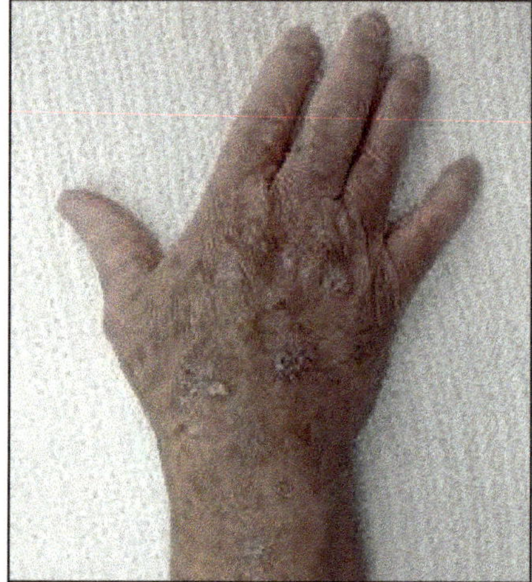

Figure 281 9.3.6 Actinic Keratosis

9.3.11 Tineas (All 6 types)

Tinea are skin infections due to dermatophytes and the involved anatomic areas are different. All the tinea infections appear as **circular, itchy rashes with erythematous margins and have different naming based on the area affected, namely**: ***tinea corporis, tinea cruris, tinea pedis, tinea capitis, tinea unguium and tinea barbae.*** Tinea capitis is characterized by hair loss while *tinea unguium* results to thickening of the nails. The treatment of this skin condition is usually through topical antifungals specifically **clotrimazole or terbinafine for mild conditions**. For chronic or severe cases, systemic therapy with oral antifungals for the treatment of. systemic infection is done, and the agents used include terbinafine or itraconazole. Other measures which can also help check reoccurrence include ensuring that the areas of skin are always dry and avoid using powders or creams which might lead to formation of fungus.

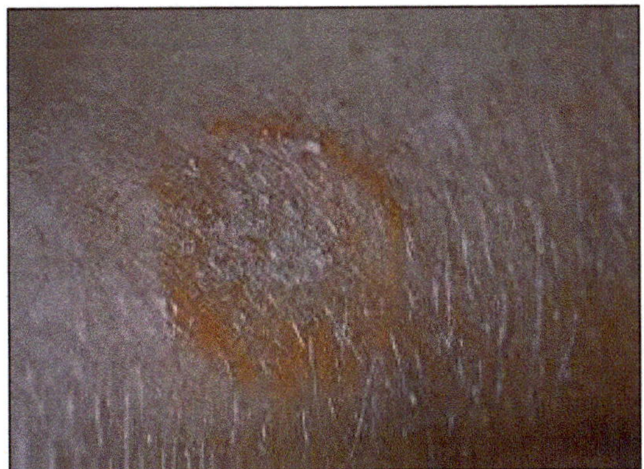

Figure 282 Tinea Corporis

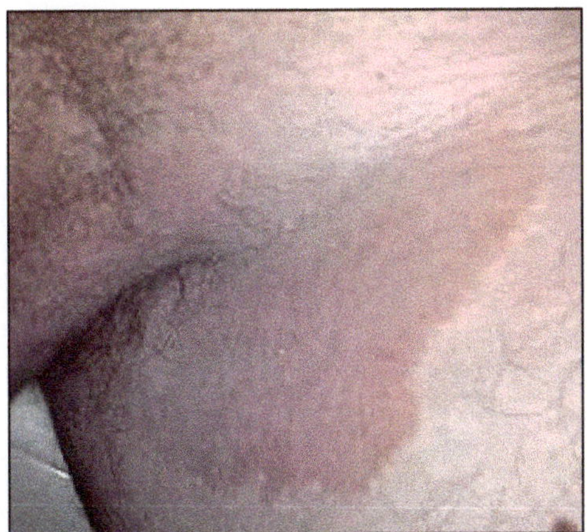

Figure 283 Tinea Cruris

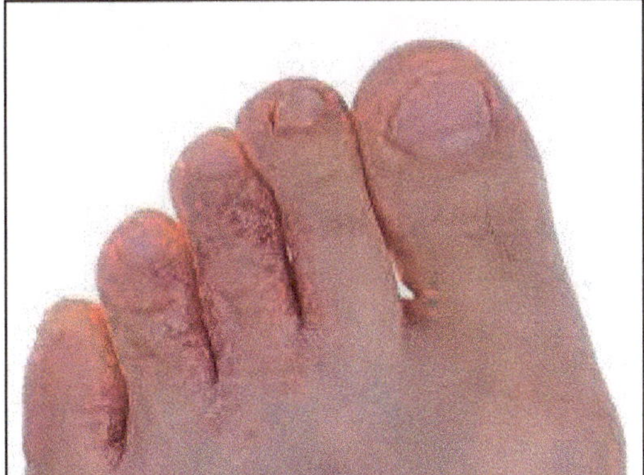

Figure 284 Tinea Pedis

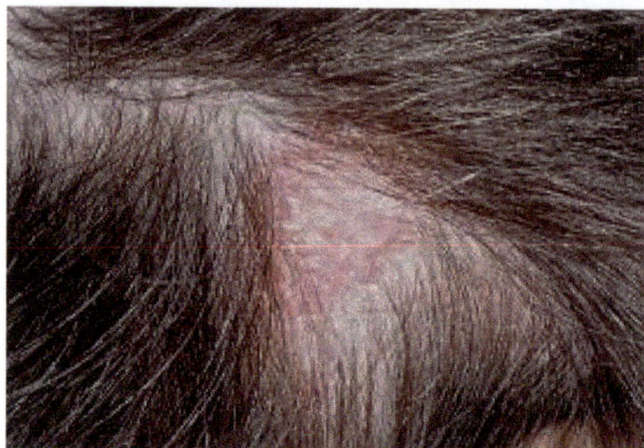

Figure 285 Tinea Capitis

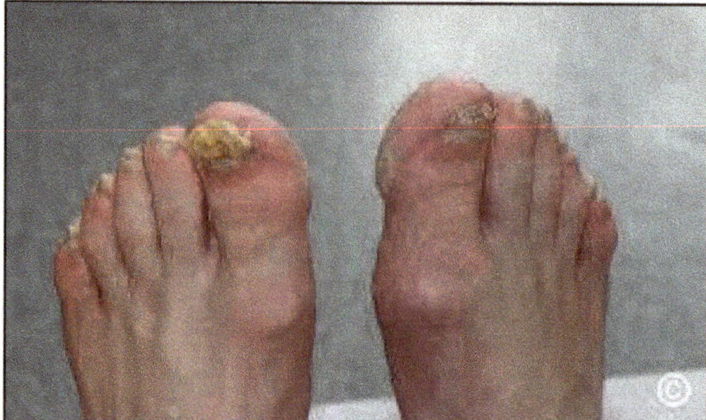

Figure 286 Tinea Unguium

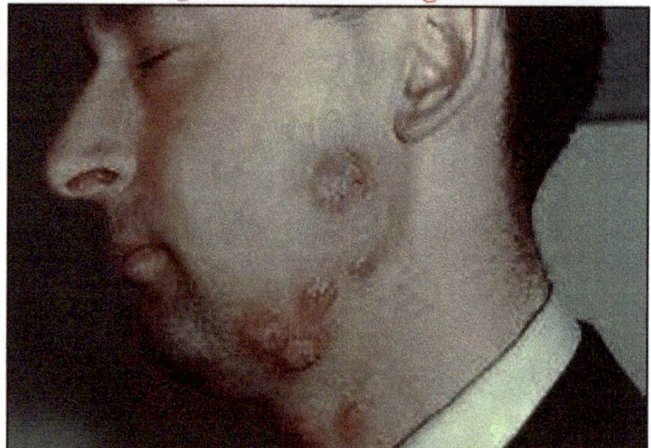

Figure 287 Tinea Barbae

9.3.12 Contact Dermatitis

Contact dermatitis refers to an inflammation of the skin that results from exposure to agents that can be allergic or irritants. Clinically, eczema appears as patches which may be erythematous, scaly, weeping, oozing or crusted, and may reach as far as the regional lymphadenitis. Allergic contact dermatitis results from such **plants as poison ivy, fragrances, or nickels while on the part of irritant contact dermatitis** it results from substances such as harsh chemicals or wetness. management of this disease includes excluding the irritant from the patient's environment and applying topical corticosteroids. More serious cases may call for oral steroid such as prednisolone. Therefore, the use of antihistamines may decrease itching and the use of emollients may help to rebuild the skin barrier. In chronic **type, patch testing might reveal which of the chemicals** should be avoided.

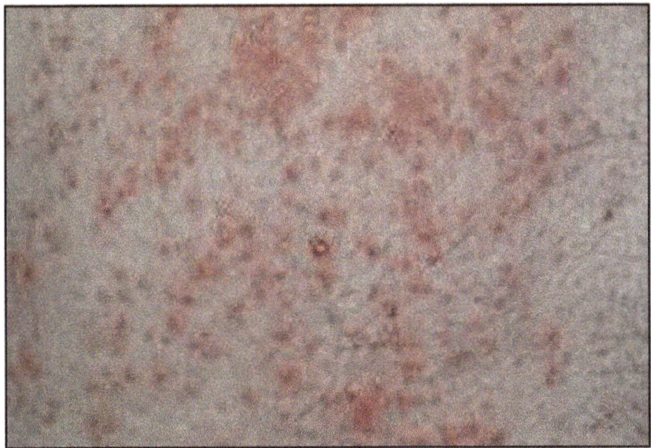

Figure 288 Contact Dermatitis

9.3.13 Superficial Candidiasis

Superficial candidiasis is among the **fungal infections** that affect the skin by **Candida species** especially at areas that are either warm or exposed to moisture such as the oral cavity, skin folds and the genital area. It is reddened, itchy rashes that may also have creamy, curd-like deposit on the lining of the **mouth or the private area (oral thrush or vaginal yeast infections).** Numerous in those with **AIDS or other immunologic diseases** and in patients with a history of an antibacterial treatment. Creams such as clotrimazole or miconazole are used to treat mild infection on the skin surface. Other systemic antifungals such Itraconazole may be prescribed for invasive or recurrent conditions including oral thrush. **Maintaining dryness** and cleaning the areas or using antifungal powders are some of the possibilities that can help avoid the return of the issue.

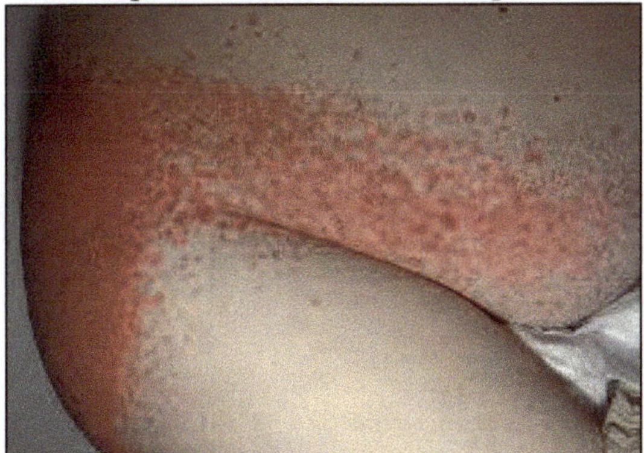

Figure 289 Superficial Candidiasis

9.3.14 Clenched Fist Injuries

Clenched fist injuries refer to injuries caused when an individual puts his or she fist in an object, eliciting skin, soft tissue or bone injury. These injuries may cause puncture injuries or fractures of bones and there is a tendency of having **bacteria penetrate through to the deeper tissues and cause an infection.** There is no time to waste when it comes to wound care, and this requires cleaning and administration of antibiotics as a form of prevention against infection. Fractures may require an **X-ray to help evaluate for the presence of fracture(s).** Infection has to be treated with oral or intravenous antibiotics; in case of deep wound or involvement of the bone, the wound requires surgical intervention.

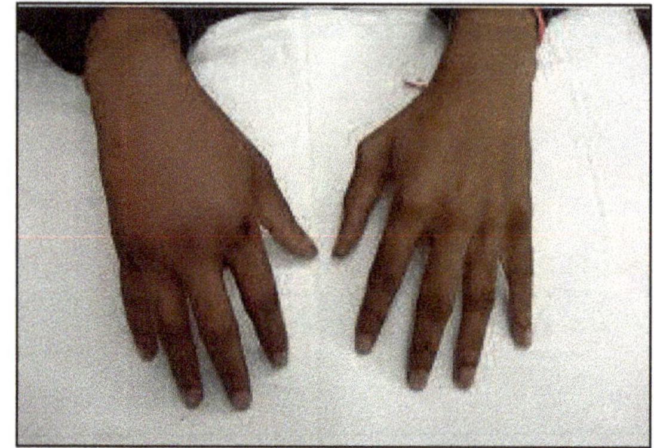

Figure 290 Clenched Fist Injuries

9.3.15 Folliculitis, Furuncles, Carbuncles

Folliculitis is the inflammation of hair follicles and manifests as small pimple-like or red pimples. A furuncle is an intense, a painful infection of **hair follicles filled with pus, while carbuncle is small and connected furuncle.** These are usually associated with ***Staphylococcus aureus*** bacterium. Applying warm compresses to the region is helpful due to its ability for reducing inflammation and encouraging the process of drainage. For mild ones, **mupirocin is prescribed for topically used agents and drugs**. In more serious or cases or a recurrent nature may call for oral antibiotics such as dicloxacillin or perhaps the drained of abscess. Antiseptic soaps can be useful to avoid a new infection in the infected areas of the body.

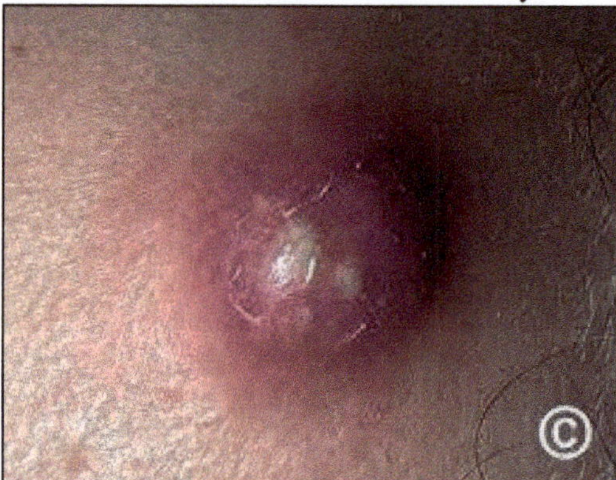

Figure 291 Folliculitis, Furuncles, Carbuncles

9.3.16 Erysipelas

Erysipelas is a mild, acute type of **cellulitis caused by Group A Streptococcus** whereby the affected skin becomes bright red, smooth, and well-defined and is usually accompanied by fever and chills. The skin at the affected areas stands and appears **glossy can be located at any part of the body but sometimes it is found on the face and legs.** For mild cases, the patient's doctor may prescribe oral antibiotics such as penicillin or amoxicillin for moderate cases, intravenous antibiotics may be required. Managing the affected limb by keeping it off the ground and regular washing is also good in this regard.

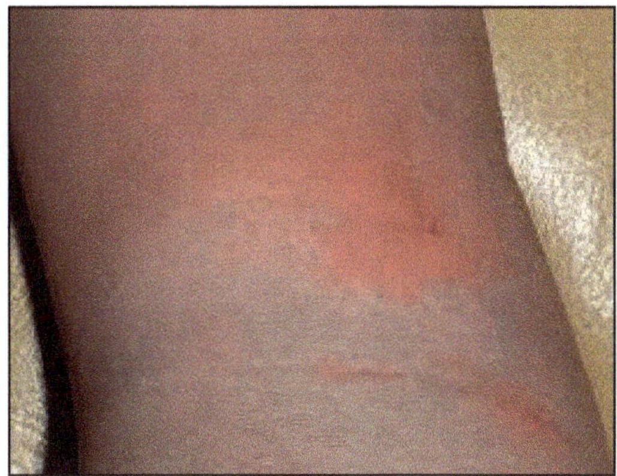

Figure 292 Erysipelas

9.3.17 Bites (Human and Animals)

In human and animal bites, there are usually puncture wounds that make a **pathway for bacteria to enter the tissues hence, infection.** Dog and cat bites are prone to deeper infections because of the type of teeth they have, while human bite usually occurs in hands. Washing the wound with soap and water should not be avoided. **Tetanus prophylaxis** may be needed. Antibiotics including **amoxicillin-clavulanate** are administered to prevent and in some circumstances, the skin layer is not sutured so as not to hold bacteria. Some animal bites may need rabies vaccination.

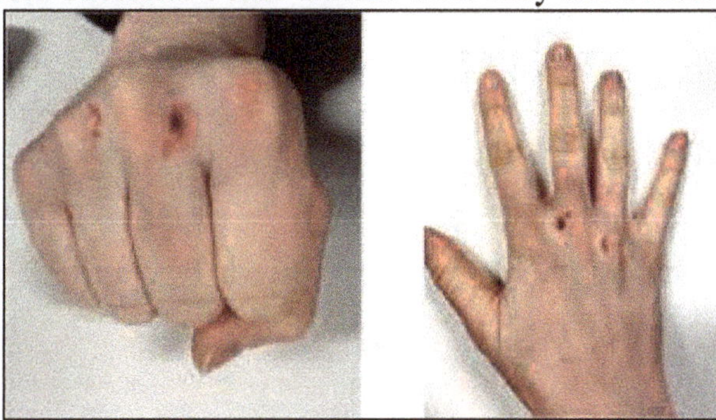

Figure 293 Bites

9.3.18 Meningococcemia

Meningococcemia is an intra-vascular infection due to ***Neisseria meningitidis*** with fever, rigor, **rash pin point spots, and symptoms of shock**. it may advance to meningitis soon that is associated with considerable morbidity. Initial management involves intravenous antibiotics such as ceftriaxone or penicillin because of the nature of meningococcemia. Anti-inflammatory agents may be used to add some corticosteroids to the patient's regimen. A similar monitoring is required in an **ICU setting** because of the danger of septic shock.

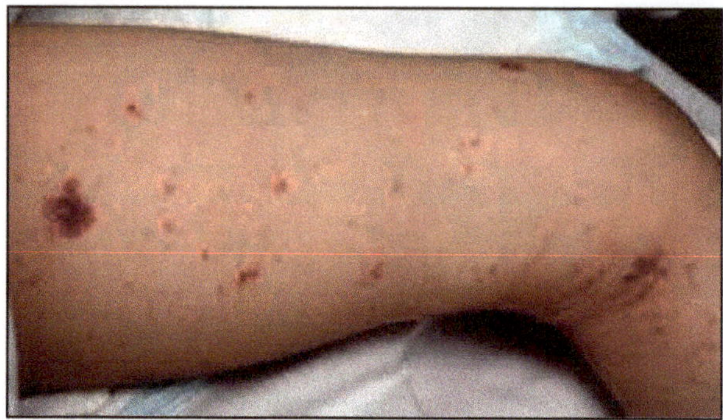

Figure 294 Meningococcemia

9.3.19 Rocky Mountain Spotted Fever

Tick-borne, it is caused by ***Rickettsia rickettsii*** and its symptoms are as follows: **fever, rash that begins from the wrist and ankle, and history of exposure to tick.** Further development of rash can be petechial ones, and the disease is potentially lethal in the absence of proper treatment. Specific **antimicrobial treatment is Doxycycline** which has been observed to be effective even in children and should be started as early as possible. Interventions for the severe cases involve giving fluids and assessing for any involvement of organs.

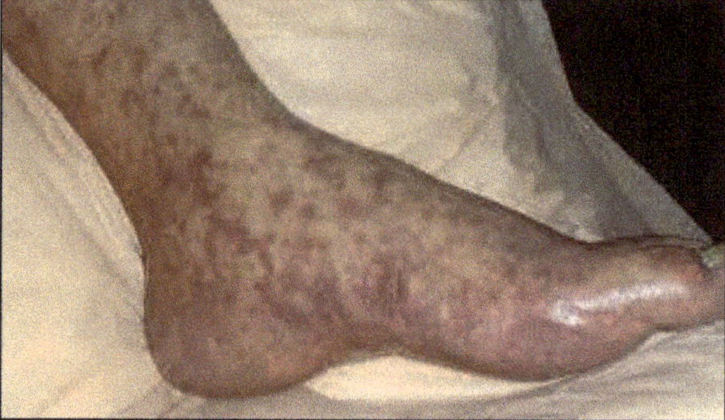

Figure 295 Rocky Mountain Spotted Fever

9.3.20 Varicella-Zoster Virus Infections

Varicella also called chickenpox presents with an itchy rash that develops from macules becoming papules and then vesicles and later crusts are formed and predominate in the truncal area. Varicella zoster commonly manifests as a unilateral painful and vesicular rash dermatomal in distribution. In order to decrease the **severity of the symptoms and cut the duration of the session elaborated below medications are used**; The drugs such as antihistamines help in treating the itching while Acetaminophen treats fever. For shingles, in some cases, there is post-herpetic neuralgia and will need further pain treatment.

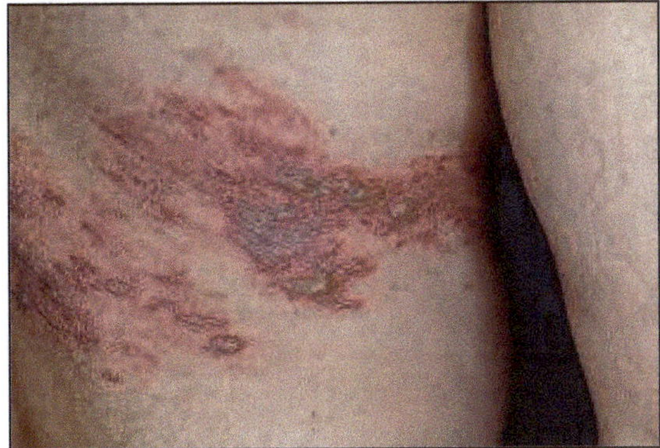

Figure 296 Varicella-Zoster Virus Infections

9.3.21 Herpetic Whitlow

Herpetic whitlow is an acutely infected finger condition that results from **Herpes simplex virus (HSV) characterized** by **swelling, erythema, and vesicular formation**. This is observed in both the health care providers or people with oral herpes. Acyclovir therapy may be effective in cutting down on symptoms as well as the amount of the virus spread among patients. Some of the supportive care may include**: treatment of pain, and antisepsis** to be made to the wound so as to avoid secondary infection.

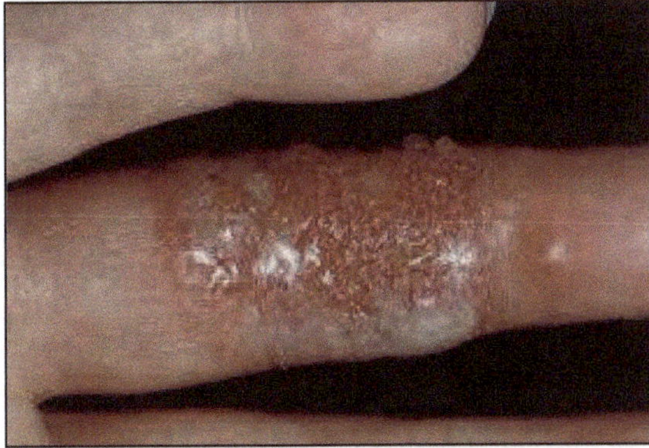

Figure 297 Herpetic Whitlow

9.3.22 Paronychia

Paronychia is an inflammation involving the nail fold usually due to bacterial or fungal infection, presenting **features being redness, swelling and pain near the nail**. It may be acute or chronic. The mild cases of this skin condition do not require invasive treatment; you can try warm compress and topical antibiotics. If the **abscess is formed, this requires incision and emptying**, and then the medication with antibiotics for bacterial infections is needed.

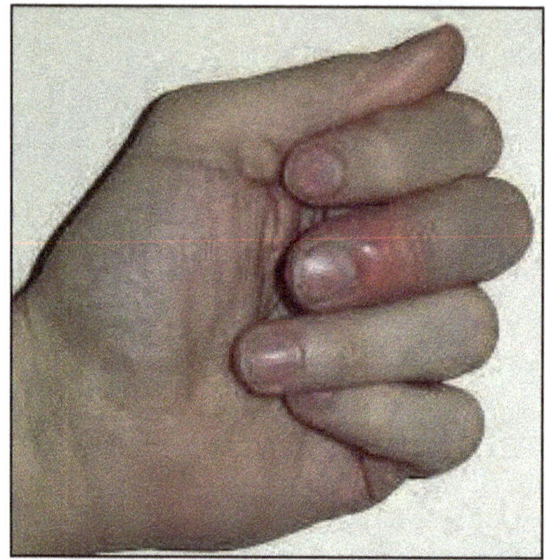

Figure 298 Paronychia

9.3.23 Scabies

Scabies can be defined as a parasitic skin disease that is caused by the ***Sarcoptes scabiei*** mite; it manifests itself as a **severe itching and a pimple like eruption usually in the folds of the skin**. It is transmitted through direct contact with the affected individual. **Permethryn cream** is the first and foremost remedy that should be employed in treating this condition. Other measures that were mentioned are oral ivermectin for those with severe cases. On the same note, itching may take several weeks to resolve after treatment has been administered.

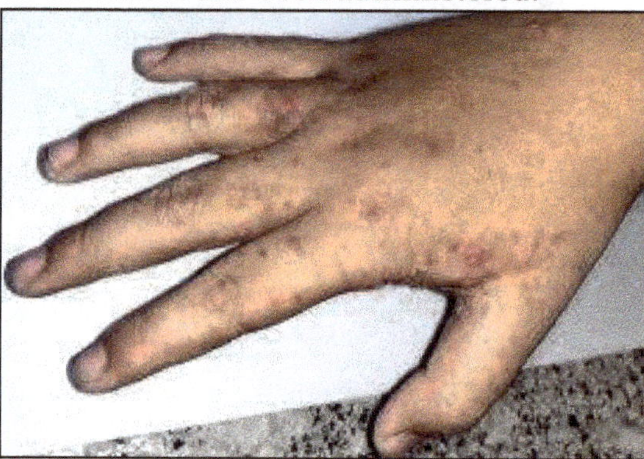

Figure 299 Scabies

9.3.24 Acne Vulgaris

Acne vulgaris is a persistent dermatological condition that manifest itself by formations as **comedones, papules, pustules and cysts** occurring mainly in the **face, back and shoulder areas**. It also has an influence with some psychological disorders and is most commonly associated with the hormone changes that accompany puberty. Moderate to severe skin conditions are treated with **topical retinoids (tretinoinin), benzoyl peroxide and oral antibiotics such as doxycycline**. In several circumstances, therefore, oral isotretinoin can be administered for persistent and severe cystic acne.

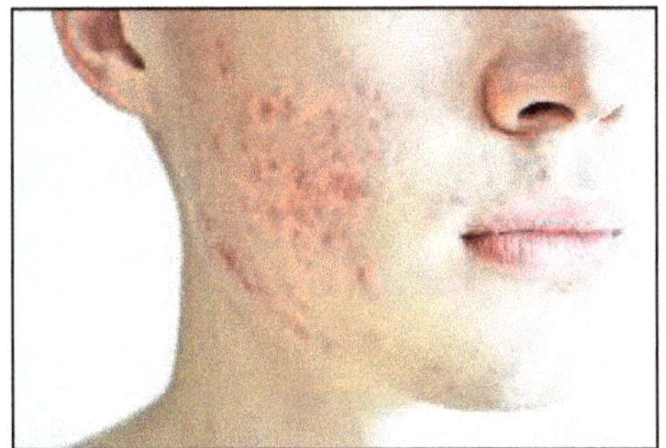

Figure 300 Acne Vulgaris

9.3.25 Rosacea

Rosacea is a chronic skin disease characterized by persistent **erythema and edema with telangiectasia, occasional papules and pustules formation.** It affects particularly the freedom-skinned individuals and it is usually caused by various factors such as. Irritants such as cigarettes, alcohol, certain foods must be reduced by **an acute alcohol consumption, spicy foods, and cigarette smoking.** In extreme cases, there are other related treatments through mouth drugs such as **tetra cyclin**. Some cases have pointed out that the visible light source of the laser therapeutic device may have an advantage in targeting blood vessels.

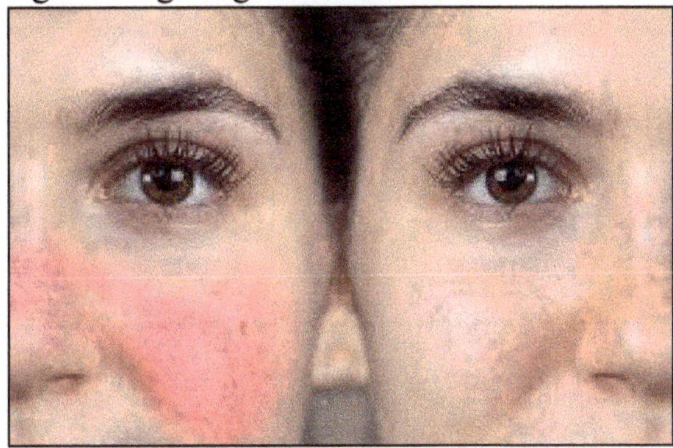

Figure 301 Rosacea

9.3.26 Molluscum Contagiosum

Molluscum contagiosum is a viral skin disease; **manifesting as small (2-7mm), firm, round or oval lesion with central umbilication.** It is an infection by the molluscum virus and is known to have a propensity to clear the skin on its own. **Cryotherapy or curettage** can be suggested for the prolonged type of the disease. These topical agents also assist in the removal of lesions through an application of imiquimod or cantharidin.

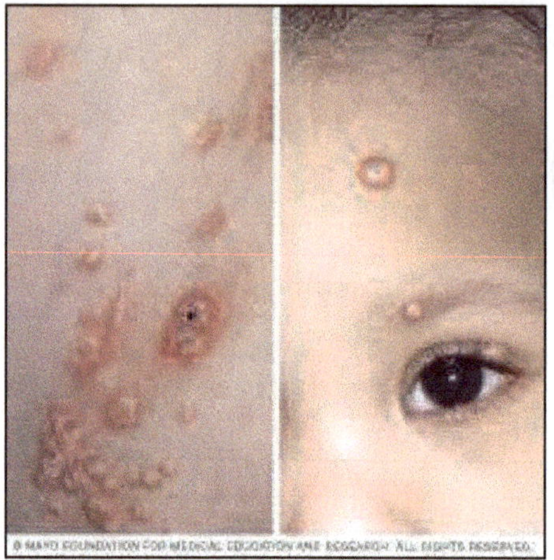

Figure 302 Molluscum Contagiosum

9.3.27 Bioterrorism & Smallpox

There are differences between the smallpox virus and variola virus starting with the fact that smallpox is a serious disease that is **accompanied by fever, general discomfort, and a rashed pustular eruption.** Some of the agents of bioterrorism are diseases that can be used to terrorize the people. Smallpox does not have a specific cure and is treated with antiviral medicines while vaccination is used to prevent the diseases. **Bioterrorism management is unique** since identification is needed quickly for the specific agent and certain antibiotics or antivirals must be used.

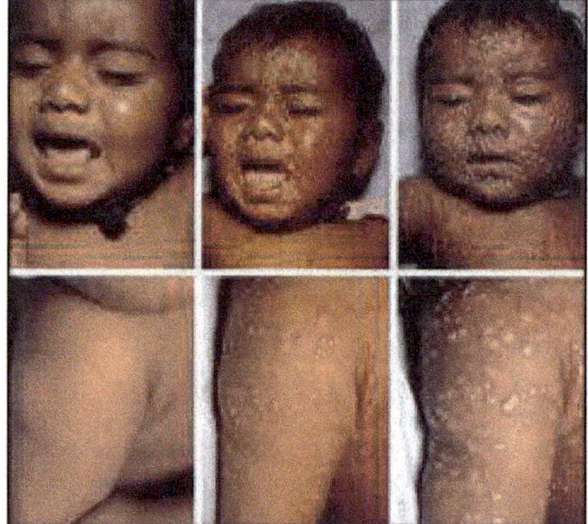

Figure 303 Bioterrorism and Small Box

9.3.28 Wound Management & Primary Practice Procedures

Wound care is illumination, by washing, removing of dead tissue and applying various dressings to different types of injuries for **example cuts, scrapes, and puncture wounds.** These are the simple procedures that are performed in this field, these include suturing in order to suture the **wounds and local anesthesia to numb the area** before the performance of any operation. Wound care involves washing with antiseptic solutions, application of **antibiotics and use of dressing**. Stitching is required for major or wide injuries so that proper healing of the skin can be achieved to prevent infections.

9.4 Moh Golden Points and Summary Question Answers

9.4.1 Moh Golden Points

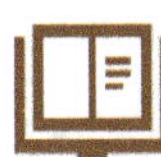
Necrotizing Fasciitis (NF) is a life-threatening infection that requires aggressive surgical debridement, IV antibiotics, and intensive fluid resuscitation to prevent systemic shock and further tissue damage.

Lyme disease is caused by *Borrelia burgdorferi*, transmitted by tick bites, with the hallmark erythema migrans (bull's-eye rash) in early stages, and oral antibiotics like doxycycline are used to treat it effectively.

Cellulitis presents with red, swollen, and painful skin, commonly caused by *Streptococcus* or *Staphylococcus*. Early treatment with oral antibiotics can prevent complications like abscess formation or sepsis.

Impetigo is a highly contagious bacterial skin infection characterized by red sores that turn into yellowish crusts. Treatment typically involves topical mupirocin or oral antibiotics for more widespread cases.

Burn injuries are classified into first-degree, second-degree, and third-degree burns based on skin depth. Immediate cooling, wound care, and fluid resuscitation are critical for management.

Hidradenitis Suppurativa (HS) is a chronic inflammatory condition leading to abscesses in areas with hair follicles and sweat glands. Treatment involves antibiotics, immunosuppressants, and sometimes surgical drainage.

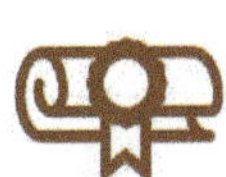
Psoriasis is an autoimmune condition that causes rapid skin cell turnover, presenting with silvery plaques. Topical treatments such as corticosteroids and vitamin D analogs are commonly used.

9.4.2 Summary Questions & Answers

1. What is the most characteristic clinical manifestation of Lyme disease? a) Fever and chills b) Erythema migrans c) Diarrhea d) Bullous lesions
2. Which type of burn affects all layers of the skin and may require skin grafting? a) Fist-degree burn b) Second-degree burn c) Third-degree burn d) Fourth- degree burn
3. What is the first-line treatment for non-bullous impetigo? a) Oral antibiotics b) Topical mupirocin c) Topical antifungals d) Systemic corticosteroids
4. Which of the following is a common complication of untreated cellulitis? a) Sepsis b) Tinnitus c) Arthritis d) Hemorrhage
5. What is the primary method for diagnosing Necrotizing Fasciitis (NF)? a) MRI b) Skin biopsy c) Blood cultures d) X-rays
6. Which of the following is a key symptom of Hidradenitis Suppurativa (HS)? a) Chronic swelling of the legs b) Painful lumps under the skin in areas with hair follicles and sweat glands c) Multiple red, scaly patches d) Itchy, dry skin patches
7. What type of microorganism typically causes second-degree burns to become infected? a) Bacteria b) Virus c) Fungus d) Parasites
8. What is the main cause of Lyme disease? a) Tick bites from Borrelia burgdorferi b) Airborne virus exposure c) Ingestion of contaminated water d) Mosquito bites
9. Which of the following treatments is essential for third-degree burns? a) Applications of Aloe Vera gel b) IV antibiotics c) Skin grafting d) Oral hydration

10. Which type of immunosuppressant is commonly used to treat Hidradenitis Suppurativa (HS)?

a) Methotrexate
b) Prednisone
c) Adalimumab
d) Tacrolimus

9.4.3 Rationales

1. **Answer: b) Erythema migrans**

Rationale: **Erythema migrans**, a bull's-eye rash, is the hallmark of Lyme disease in the early stages and appears at the site of a tick bite.

2. **Answer: c) Third-degree burn**

Rationale: **Third-degree burns** extend through the epidermis, dermis, and into deeper tissues, often requiring **skin grafting** for healing.

3. **Answer: b) Topical mupirocin**

Rationale: **Topical mupirocin** is the treatment of choice for localized **non-bullous impetigo**.

4. **Answer a) Sepsis**

Rationale: **Cellulitis** can progress to **sepsis** if left untreated, due to the spread of infection into the bloodstream.

5. **Answer: a) MRI**

Rationale **MRI** is the most effective diagnostic tool for identifying the spread and depth of **Necrotizing Fasciitis**.

6. **Answer: b) Painful lumps under the skin in areas with hair follicles and sweat glands**

Rationale: **Hidradenitis Suppurativa (HS)** involves painful abscesses or lumps typically in the armpits, groin, or under the breasts.

7. **Answer: a) Bacteria**

Rationale: **Bacterial infections**, particularly from **Staphylococcus aureus** or **Streptococcus pyogenes**, can infect **second-degree burns**, leading to complications like cellulitis.

8. **Answer a) Tick bites from Borrelia burgdorferi**

Rationale: **Lyme disease** is caused by ***Borrelia burgdorferi***, which is transmitted through the bite of an infected **deer tick**.

9. **Answer: c) Skin grafting**

Rationale: **Third-degree burns** often require **skin grafting** to promote healing and restore skin function due to deep tissue damage.

10. **Answer: c) Adalimumab**

Rationale: **Adalimumab** is a **biologic agent** commonly used for the treatment of **Hidradenitis Suppurativa** to reduce inflammation and prevent flare-ups.

10 Chapter 10: Hematologic System

10.1 Anatomy and Physiology of Hematologic System

Blood and its components move through the body because the hematologic system produces blood while **regulating its distribution and managing its components**. The system consists of bone marrow coupled with blood vessels together with spleen and lymph nodes and blood. The main function of the **hematologic system supports homeostasis** through the transport of gases, nutrients, hormones, waste products and protection against infection as well as temperature regulation. **Blood cells are produced within the spongy bones** especially in the pelvis and ribs and the sternum where bone marrow resides. Hematopoiesis stands for the method through which three specific blood cells develop including **erythrocytes (red blood cells), leukocytes (white blood cells) and thrombocytes (platelets).** Erythrocytes carry oxygen with their hemoglobin molecule yet they perform transport duties whereas leukocytes protect the body through immunity functions and thrombocytes assist blood clot formation. Blood vessels function as parts of the cardiovascular system to tr**ansport blood throughout the body through an oxygenated blood flow in arteries leading to tissue delivery followed by a deoxygenated blood return through venous circulation.** Old red blood cells pass through the spleen for filtration and the organ also produces antibodies simultaneously. **The lymph nodes execute lymph filtration and maintain residence for immune cells.** The liver functions in hematologic operations through its ability to generate proteins for blood clotting along with its job as a toxin filter.

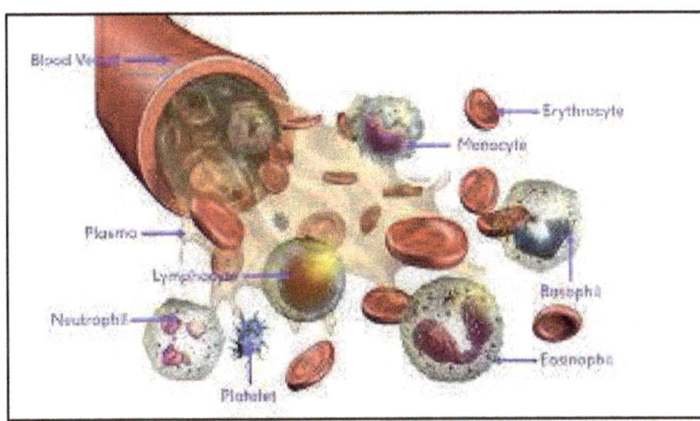

Figure 304 Anatomy of Hematologic System

The picture visualizes blood development from stem cells through their journey to peripheral bloodstream. The first stage of hematopoiesis happens within bone marrow where **hematopoietic stem cells (HSCs)** exist so they can split into different blood cell types. The stem cell pool transforms progenitor cells into **multiple blood cell types after producing them**. The progenitor cells access the bone marrow pool for proliferation and maturation as they expand in numbers. Through its production line in bone marrow the tissue generates substantial numbers of **granulocytes and erythrocytes as well as thrombocytes** for protecting immunity and facilitating blood clotting and delivering oxygen. The pool retains cells before these elements are eventually distributed through circulation. The fully matured cells travel to p**eripheral blood to execute their necessary roles.** Neutrophils together with eosinophils and basophils function as granulocytes in immune defense while thrombocytes contribute to blood clotting to minimize bleeding and **erythrocytes carry oxygen throughout the entire body**. The chart displays how blood maintains equilibrium between cell storage in addition to their capacity for functional activity to sustain continuous cell availability for body systems.

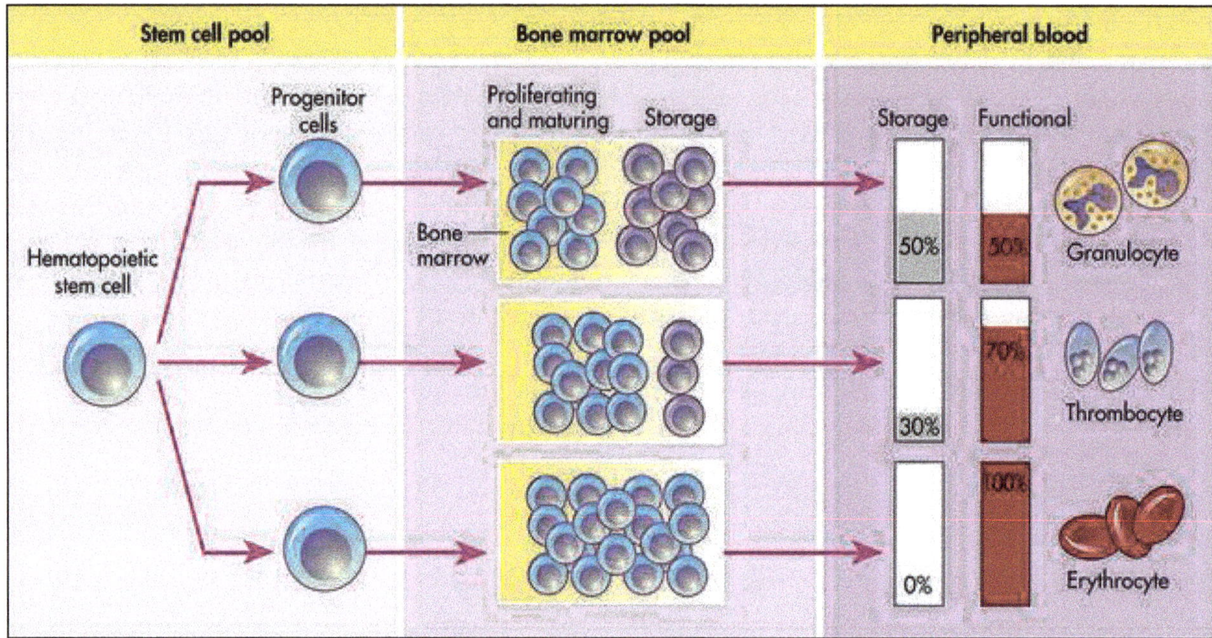

Figure 305 Hematopoiesis from the stem cell pool

The graphic displays the precise division of whole blood elements that make up 8% of total body mass. The blood composition includes two fundamental elements where plasma represents 55% by volume and **formed elements occupy 45% by volume**. Plasma has a **high water content (91%) together with three significant proteins: albumins (57%) and globulins (38%) and fibrinogen (4%). Plasma contains water (91%) together with proteins albumins (57%), globulins (38%), and fibrinogen (4%) as well as various solutes** including ions and nutrients along with waste products and gases and regulatory substances. The **formed elements occupy 45% of blood volume and contain erythrocytes (red blood cells) together with leukocytes (white blood cells) and platelets.** All formed elements mainly consist of erythrocytes since they represent over 99% of these components while playing a primary role in oxygen transport. The formed elements' leukocyte group includes neutrophils as well as **lymphocytes and monocytes and eosinophils and basophils and all combined make up minimal than 1% of total blood elements** but they play essential roles in defense mechanisms. Clotting essentials come primarily from platelets alongside the remaining less than 1% of formed elements. The leukocytes together with platelets exist in the buffy coat which stands between plasma and red blood cells. The blood composition demonstrates vital elements responsible for executing important bodily functions such as oxygen delivery and immune defense processes and coagulation mechanisms.

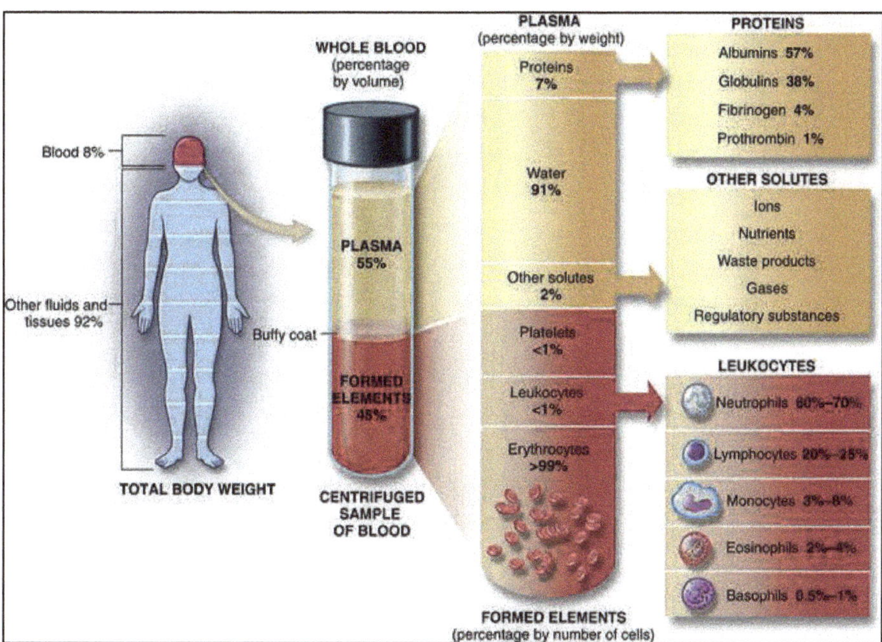

Figure 306 Composition of Whole Blood

The image shows detailed information about the **blood cell production process called hematopoiesis** that begins with stem cells and generates multiple mature blood cell varieties. Within the initial development process the **totipotent stem cell initiates first before pluripotent stem** cells appear followed by **multipotent stem cells** which possess the capacity to develop precise cell types. The **hematopoietic stem cell** proves crucial from all multipotent stem cells because it produces every type of blood cell. The hematopoiesis mechanism differentiates into two principal progenitor lines that **produce lymphoid and myeloid progenitors**. The myeloid progenitor cells produce different blood cells including basophils and eosinophils with **monocytes and granulocytes and megakaryocytes which create platelets.** The **lymphoid progenitor cells create B cells together with T cells and natural killer (NK) cells.** The differentiation and proliferation of specific progenitor cells function under regulation from the cytokines and growth factors which comprise **IL-3, IL-5, GM-CSF, and SCF.** The bone marrow functions as a site for immune cell differentiation and the spleen together with lymph nodes finalize the maturation of **T and B cells** as well as other immune cells. The diagram showcases how stem cells use an intricate route to produce numerous specialized blood cells and immune cells which both support body system operations and assist in fighting infections.

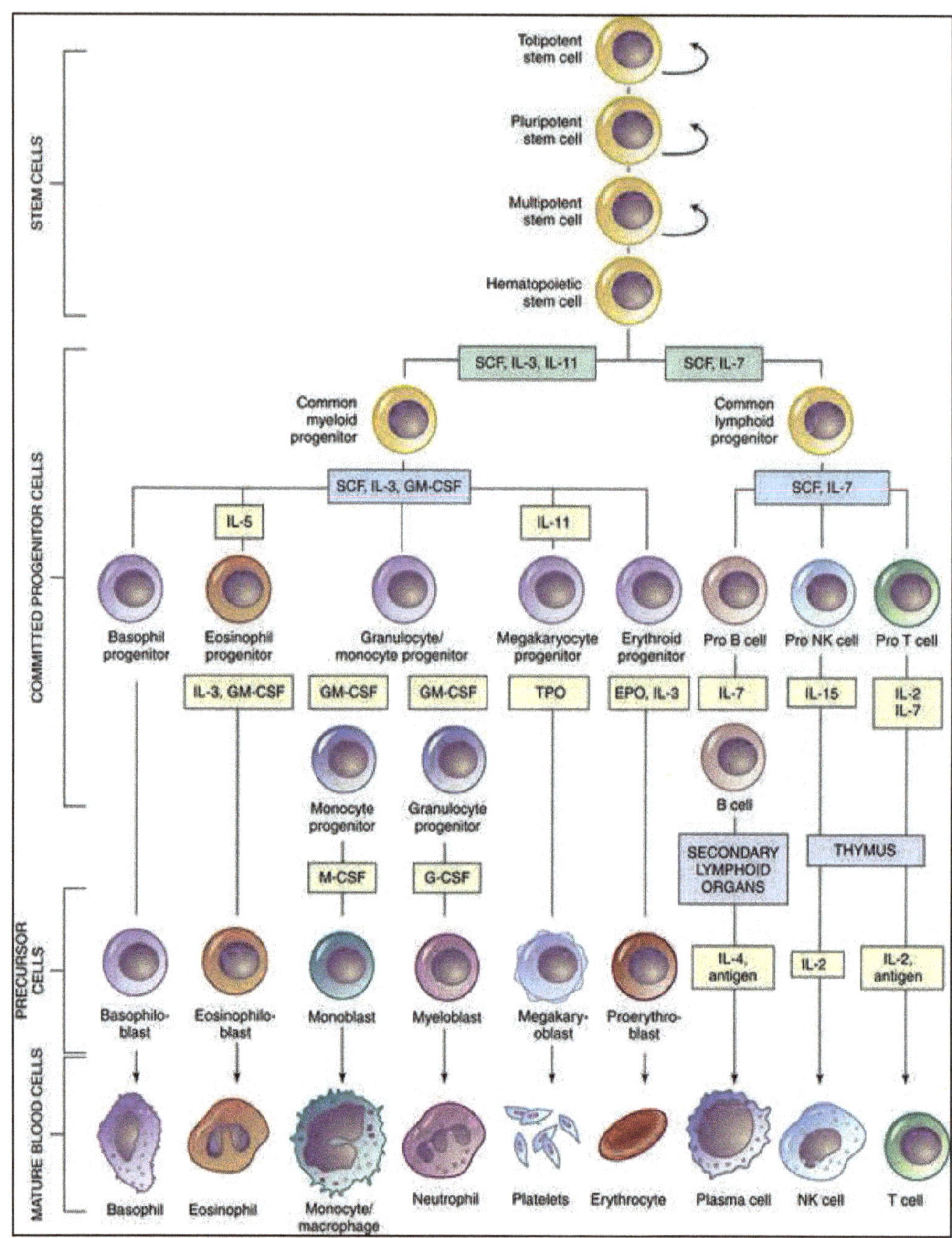

Figure 307 Differentiation of Hematopoietic Cells

10.2 Common Conditions of Hematologic System

Table 172 Common Conditions of Hematologic System

Condition	Description	Key Symptoms	Diagnostic Tools	Treatment Options
Anemia	A condition characterized by a deficiency of red blood	Fatigue, pallor, shortness of breath, dizziness,	Complete blood count (CBC), reticulocyte count, iron	Iron supplements, vitamin B12 or folic acid supplementation,

	cells or hemoglobin, leading to inadequate oxygen delivery to tissues.	weakness, cold extremitie s.	studies, bone marrow biopsy.	blood transfusions, erythropoiesis-stimulating agents.
Hemophilia A	A genetic disorder caused by a deficiency in **Factor VIII**, leading to impaired blood clotting.	Excessive bleeding or bruising, spontaneou s joint or muscle bleeds.	Coagulation studies (PT, aPTT), Factor VIII activity assay, genetic testing.	Factor VIII infusions, desmopressin (mild cases), gene therapy.
Hemophilia B	A genetic disorder caused by a deficiency in **Factor IX**, leading to impaired blood clotting.	Excessive bleeding or bruising, spontaneou s joint or muscle bleeds, similar to Hemophilia A but with different factor deficiency.	Coagulation studies (PT, aPTT), Factor IX activity assay, genetic testing.	Factor IX infusions, desmopressin (mild cases), gene therapy.
Thrombocytopen ia	A condition where there is a reduced number of platelets, leading to difficulty in blood clotting.	Easy bruising, prolonged bleeding, petechiae, heavy menstrual periods.	Platelet count (CBC), bone marrow biopsy, bleeding time, clotting tests.	Platelet transfusion, corticosteroids, immunoglobulin therapy, treatment of underlying cause.

Multiple Myeloma	A cancer of the plasma cells, which are a type of white blood cell, causing abnormal production of antibodies.	Bone pain, fatigue, weight loss, frequent infections, weakness, abnormal bleeding.	CBC, serum protein electrophoresis, bone marrow biopsy, imaging (X-rays, MRI).	Chemotherapy, stem cell transplant, immunomodulatory drugs, proteasome inhibitors.
Hodgkin's Lymphoma Disease	A type of cancer that originates in the lymphatic system, characterized by the presence of **Reed-Sternberg cells.**	Painless swelling of lymph nodes, fever, night sweats, weight loss, fatigue.	Excisional biopsy of lymph node, CT/PET scans, blood tests, Reed-Sternberg cell identification.	Chemotherapy, radiation therapy, stem cell transplant, targeted therapy.
Non-Hodgkin Lymphoma Disease	A group of cancers that originate in the lymphatic system, not involving **Reed-Sternberg cells.**	Painless swelling of lymph nodes, fever, night sweats, weight loss, fatigue, similar to Hodgkin's lymphoma.	Excisional biopsy of lymph node, CT/PET scans, blood tests, no Reed-Sternberg cells.	Chemotherapy, radiation therapy, stem cell transplant, targeted therapy.
Neutropenia	A condition characterized by low	Frequent infections, fever,	CBC, absolute neutrophil count (ANC),	Granulocyte colony-stimulating

	neutrophil count, increasing susceptibility to infections.	chills, mouth ulcers, weakness, fatigue.	bone marrow biopsy.	factor (G-CSF), antibiotics, bone marrow stimulants.
Acute Hemorrhage	A condition in which there is significant blood loss, leading to reduced blood volume and oxygen delivery.	Dizziness, weakness, pale skin, cold extremities, rapid heart rate, low blood pressure.	CBC, assessment of hemoglobin and hematocrit, assessment of blood loss, vital signs monitoring.	Blood transfusions, IV fluids, surgical interventions to stop bleeding, blood volume replacement.

10.3 Major Medical Conditions of Hematologic System

10.3.1 Anemia

Anemic patients experience a **deficit of healthy red blood cells** along with insufficient hemoglobin which results in inadequate oxygen delivery to body tissues. Hemoglobin represents the iron-containing protein present in red blood cells which performs the vital body-wide oxygen transport function. **The insufficient amount of red blood cells or their associated hemoglobin** results in impaired organ and tissue oxygen delivery which produces symptoms that include tiredness and weakness along with **paleness of skin, light headedness and breathlessness**. Anemia develops when the body lacks sufficient iron, vitamin B12, folate nutrients, suffers from kidney disease, cancer, experiences blood loss from injuries, surgeries, or experiences menstruation while also including **genetic sickle cell anemia as a cause of anemia.** Anemia diagnosis requires both a CBC test and specialty testing for proper assessment of its root cause and severity level. The treatment plan depends on the specific cause of anemia and includes choosing **dietary alterations or medication together with nutritional supplements.**

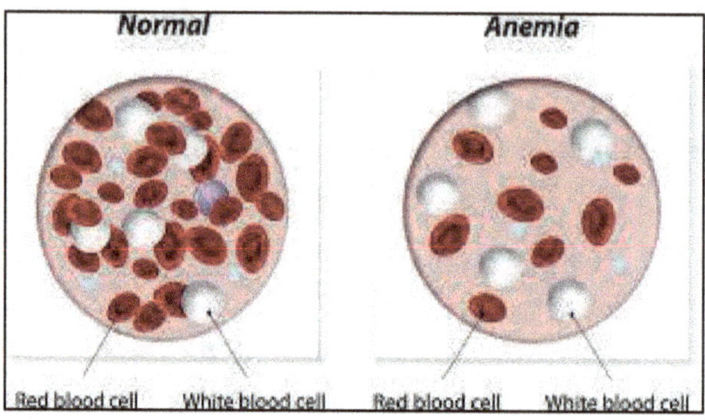

Figure 308 Normal Vs. Anemia

10.3.1.1 Types of Anemia

Different types of anemia exist with their own unique root causes and biological patterns. There exist three main categories of anemia:

- **Iron Deficiency Anemia** stands as the dominant form of anemia which develops due to reduced body iron levels resulting in poorly made hemoglobin. Antiethiogenic factors including inadequate dietary intake and severe menstruation yet also inadequate iron absorption account for its development. Microcytic small red blood cells together with hypochromic pale red blood cells appear through blood testing.
- **The deficiency of Vitamin B12 or Folate** leads to the development of this type of anemia since both nutrients play essential roles in red blood cell production. Insufficient levels of vitamin B12 lead to the development of macrocytic red blood cells which are also megaloblastic in nature. Three major factors responsible for this type of anemia include dietary deficiencies along with malabsorption or particular medications.
- **This anemia develops from chronic inflammation and infections and chronic kidney** diseases since they prevent normal iron storage usage by the body. Normal-sized red blood cells together with their normal red hue make up the profile of this type of anemia even though iron levels tend to decrease and ferritin levels increase.
- **Red blood cell destruction exceeds production rates during situations of Hemolytic Anemia**. Hemolytic anemia develops due to autoimmune disorders together with infections and inherited medical conditions including sickle cell anemia and thalassemia. The blood test results indicate higher reticulocyte levels as well as increased bilirubin and broken red blood cells found in blood smears.
- **Aplastic Anemia stands as a severe and infrequent disorder** which stops bone marrow from generating sufficient levels of all blood components including red cells and white cells and platelets. The disease appears due to autoimmune disorders along with specific drugs and exposure to radiation. All types of blood cells demonstrate extremely reduced counts in blood tests along with red blood cells.
- **Sickle Cell Anemia** appears as a genetic disorder which shapes red blood cells into sickle forms while increasing their vulnerability to breaking. The disease produces a long-lasting state of anemia with recurring painful conditions. Medical diagnosis of sickle cell anemia requires both sickle-shaped red blood cells in lab tests and hemoglobin electrophoresis results.
- **The genetic disorder of Thalassemia produces abnormal substances named hemoglobins** in the blood. The condition causes small red blood cells together with diminished hemoglobin levels. The anemia severity in patients depends on whether they have alpha or beta thalassemia.

- **Fanconi Anemia functions as an uncommon inherited disease** which results in bone marrow failure together with physical structural problems. The disorder results in pancytopenia symptoms together with its childhood onset.

Different anemias require diagnosis through clinical evaluation and blood tests such as complete blood count with iron studies and vitamin examinations in addition to genetic tests occasionally. Healthcare plans depend on the fault behind anemia to include dietary supplements alongside medications or blood transfusions and perhaps bone marrow transplants.

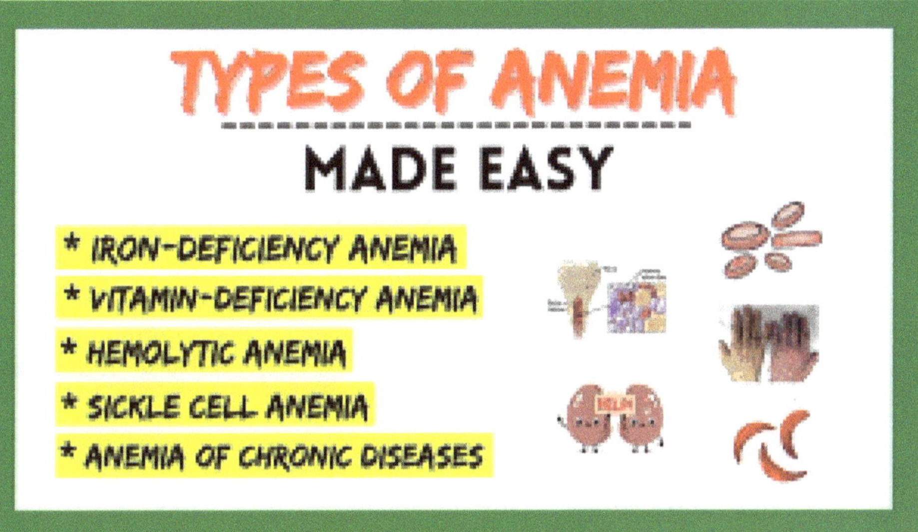

Figure 309 Types of Anemia

10.3.1.2 Classification of Anemia

This illustration displays how various anemia types like **microcytic versus normocytic versus macrocytic are classified through red blood cell size measurements.** The analysis of red blood cells shows microcytic **anemia when MCV measures below 80 fL and** causes small cell structures which tend to appear due to iron deficiency anemia or thalassemia. The anemia type normocytic presents normal red blood cell size measured between 80 and 100 fL while it typically reveals **anemia of chronic disease, acute blood loss or renal disease**. The presence of macrocytic anemia occurs with enlarged red blood cells (MCV greater than 100 fL) caused by vitamin B12 or folate deficiencies in megaloblastic anemia alongside alcoholism and liver disease and myelodysplasia. Healthcare providers can diagnose anemia better and provide appropriate treatments through **evaluation of MCV levels.**

Mean corpuscular volume (MCV) is a measure of the average size of red blood cells and used to classify different types of anemia (measured in femtoliter)

Microcytic Anemia	Normocytic Anema	Macrocytic Anema
MCV less than 80 fl	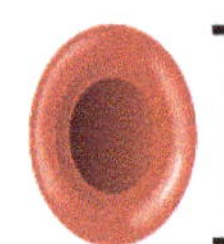 MCV 80-100 fl	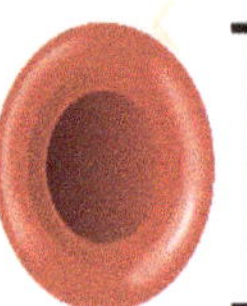 MCV greater than 100 fl
Small Red Blood Cell	**Normal Red Blood Cell**	**Large Red Blood Cell**
• Iron-deficiency anemia • Thalassemia	• Anemia of chronic disease • Aplastic anemia • Hemolytic anemia	• Vitamin B12 deficiency anemia • Folate deficiency anemia

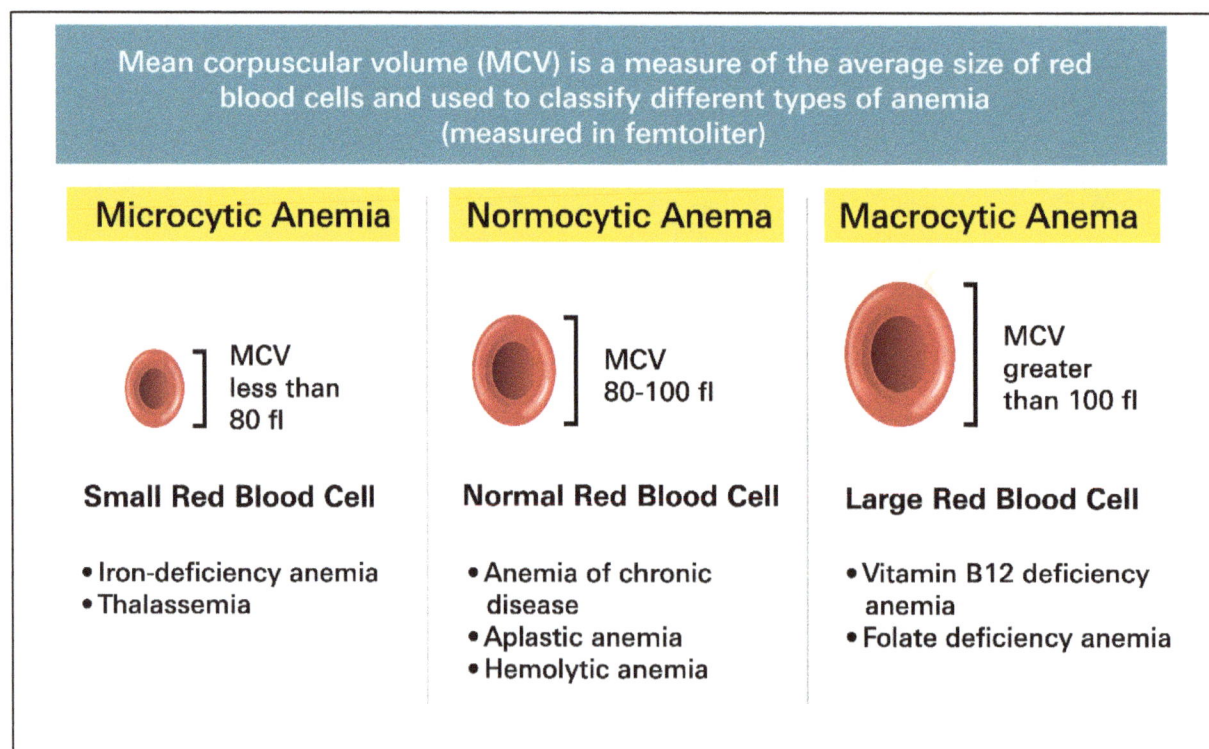

Figure 310 Anemia Classification Based on MCV Values

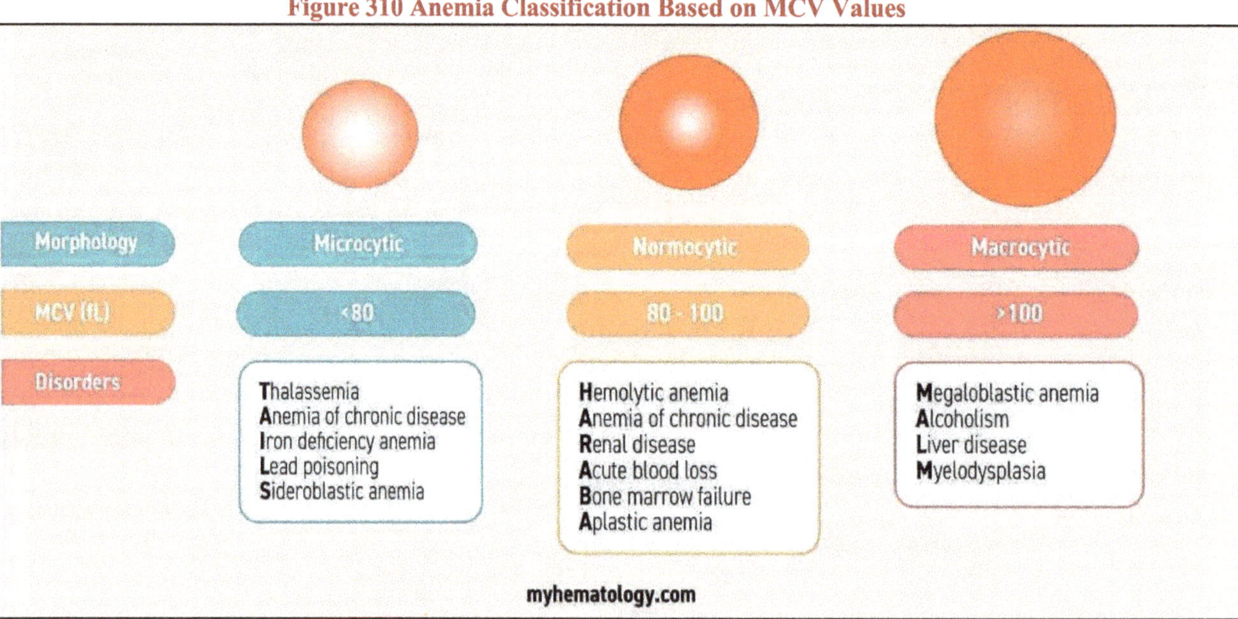

Figure 311 Morphological Classification of Anemia

10.3.1.3 How to Read Comprehensive Blood Work to Determine the Type of Anemia

1. Hemoglobin (Hb) and Hematocrit (Hct) Levels

Hemoglobin assessment together with hematocrit represents the diagnostic tools for identifying anemia cases. Medical testing directly measures the amount of oxygen-transporting protein hemoglobin which exists in red blood cells. **The percentage of red blood cells in blood volume is shown through the measurement of hematocrit level.** The blood levels of both hemoglobin and hematocrit will be low in anemia cases. A reduction in oxygen-carrying ability shows up through low hemoglobin counts while simultaneously decreased red blood cells become visible through low hematocrit results. **The diagnostic values help recognize anemia** along with its intensity however more testing will identify which type of anemia exists.

2. Mean Corpuscular Volume (MCV)

The Mean Corpuscular Volume (MCV) measures the average size of red blood cells. MCV measurements enable medical staff to differentiate between three different forms of anemia according to their cell dimension size. Tests reveal microcytic anemia through MCV measurements less than **80 fL which indicates small blood cells commonly occur** because of iron deficiency or thalassemia. Red blood cells with normal dimensions exist in normocytic anemia causing an **MCV between 80 and 100 fL** and develop most commonly from chronic disease and acute blood loss events. The development of macrocytic anemia with an MCV greater than 100 fL can be attributed to vitamin B12 and folate deficiencies that cause megaloblastic anemia.

3. Reticulocyte Count

Reticulocytes represent immature red blood cells which the bone marrow activates during their **transport to bloodstream**. The bone marrow produces reticulocytes according to the amount of anemia present. When blood cells suffer destruction during hemolysis or when blood loss occurs the **bone marrow generates extra red blood cells** that raise the reticulocyte count. Active bone marrow functioning is indicated through high reticulocyte levels which is characteristic of hemolytic anemia or acute blood loss conditions. The bone marrow suffers from dysfunction when the reticulocyte count remains low since patients either have aplastic anemia or anemia of chronic disease.

4. Red Cell Distribution Width (RDW)

RDW provides measurements about the dissimilarities in red blood cell size distribution. Patient blood cells present size variations when their RDW results are high hence pointing to iron **deficiency anemia or various mixed anemia types that involve multiple blood cell disorders**. The red cell distribution width of anemia of chronic disease remains normal and it reflects the typically uniform red blood cells. The early detection of iron deficiency anemia can be facilitated through **Red Cell Distribution** Width since this test reveals abnormalities before other measurements do which helps medical providers determine appropriate diagnostic tests and treatment approaches.

5. Iron Studies

Tests measuring **bodily iron levels** along with iron distribution help physicians determine both iron deficiency anemia and anemia of chronic disease. A complete set of iron studies includes **measurements of serum iron together with ferritin and total iron-binding capacity and transferrin saturation.** A patient with iron deficiency anemia will exhibit low serum iron levels in combination with reduced ferritin levels **as well as elevated TIBC** which indicates the body lacks sufficient iron stores. The body's inflammation response in anemia of chronic disease might lead to normal or elevated ferritin levels and simultaneously low serum iron and normal or low TIBC values.

6. B12 and Folate Levels

Vitamin B12 together with folate are essential for red blood cell formation because their deficiencies trigger macrocytic anemia which enlarges normal red blood cell dimensions. Blood analysis of **B12 and folate levels assists in detecting megaloblastic anemia** which causes cells to produce large and underdeveloped red blood cells. An improper DNA synthesis from **low vitamin B12 or folate causes disruptions during normal red blood cell production**. Early diagnosis of these conditions is crucial for preventing permanent nerve damage because vitamin supplements either through injections or as oral medications can typically treat anemic conditions effectively.

7. Peripheral Blood Smear

Peripheral blood microscopic evaluation serves as an important diagnostic method to study red blood cell form including **size and color and detection of physical anomalies**. The peripheral blood smear examination reveals smaller red blood cells together with pale-staining cells which point to **insufficient hemoglobin content in iron deficiency anemia**. Anemia of the spherocyte type produces unevenly shaped and destroyed red blood cells detectable through blood smear analysis. **Megaloblastic anemia** appears through the adult blood analysis as megaloblasts which represent abnormally enlarged red blood cells. Through the analysis of the smear healthcare providers acquire important information which helps distinguish different anemia types and reveals their base causes.

8. CBC Indices

The Complete Blood Count (CBC) indices are essential for diagnosing and classifying anemia, a condition characterized by a deficiency of red blood cells or hemoglobin. Key CBC indices include: **Hemoglobin (Hb):** A protein in red blood cells that carries oxygen. Low levels indicate anemia. **Hematocrit (Hct):** The percentage of blood volume composed of red blood cells. A low hematocrit is suggestive of anemia. **Mean Corpuscular Volume (MCV):** Measures the average size of red blood cells. A low MCV (<80 fL) suggests microcytic anemia (e.g., iron deficiency anemia), while a high MCV (>100 fL) suggests macrocytic anemia (e.g., vitamin B12 or folate deficiency). **Mean Corpuscular Hemoglobin (MCH):** Represents the average amount of hemoglobin in a red blood cell. Low MCH indicates hypochromic anemia. **Red Cell Distribution Width (RDW):** Measures the variation in red blood cell size. An elevated RDW indicates anisocytosis, commonly seen in iron-deficiency anemia.

9. Additional Tests

Hemoglobin electrophoresis and bone marrow biopsy tests provide diagnosis for particular kinds of anemia when additional testing becomes required. Hemoglobin electrophoresis serves for sickle cell anemia and thalassemia diagnosis because it detects abnormal hemoglobin types that include **HbS in sickle cell disease**. Doctors perform a bone marrow biopsy when they need to check blood cell production ability because aplastic anemia and myelodysplastic syndromes are suspected. The **testing of haptoglobin levels** combined with bilirubin levels can reveal signs of hemolysis in hemolytic anemia as well as diagnose the underlying causes of anemia.

10.3.1.4 SOAP Notes for Pancytopenia

Table 173 SOAP Notes for Pancytopenia

Component	Details
Subjective (S)	A 32-year-old female presents with fatigue, weakness, and frequent infections over the past two months. She reports easy bruising and occasional nosebleeds. She denies any recent illnesses or trauma. No significant past medical history is noted.
Objective (O)	On physical examination, the patient appears pale and has mild bruising on her arms and legs. No lymphadenopathy or hepatosplenomegaly is noted. Blood work shows a hemoglobin of 8.5 g/dL, white blood cell count of 2,000/μL, and platelet count of 50,000/μL. The peripheral blood smear reveals hypocellular bone marrow and pancytopenia.

Assessment (A)	The patient's symptoms of fatigue, weakness, frequent infections, easy bruising, and the laboratory findings of low hemoglobin, leukocytes, and platelets are consistent with pancytopenia. Further evaluation is needed to determine the underlying cause, such as bone marrow disorders, aplastic anemia, or leukemia.
Plan (P)	**Pharmacological**: Initiate treatment for underlying cause once identified (e.g., hematopoietic growth factors, immunosuppressive therapy for aplastic anemia) (See algorithm below). **Non-pharmacological**: Monitor blood counts frequently and provide supportive care (e.g., blood transfusions, infection prevention). **Follow-up**: Refer to a hematologist for further investigation, including bone marrow biopsy, and review blood work regularly. **Education**: Educate the patient on the need for close monitoring and the potential for serious complications such as infections or bleeding.

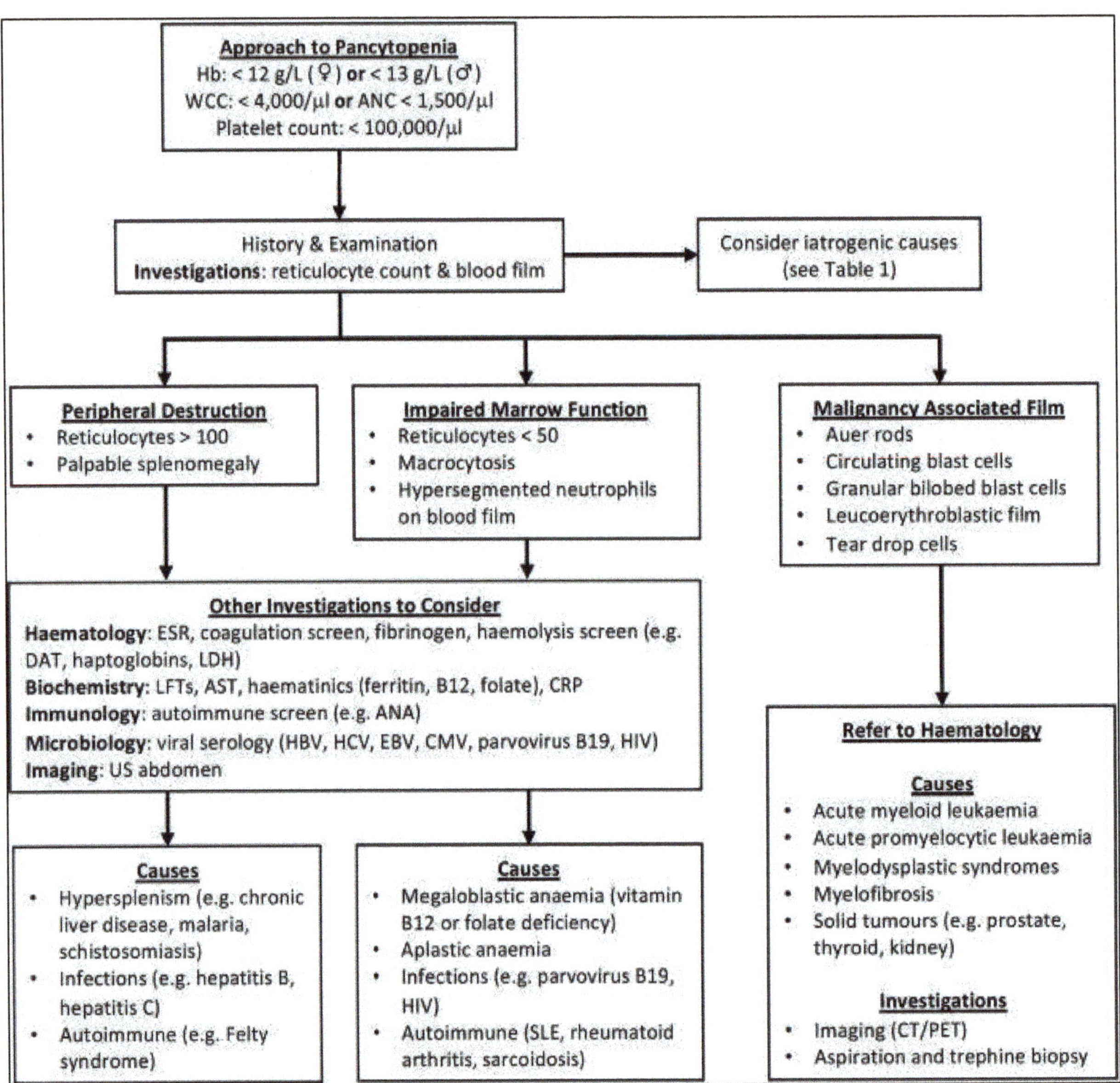

Approach to Pancytopenia
Hb: < 12 g/L (♀) or < 13 g/L (♂)
WCC: < 4,000/μl or ANC < 1,500/μl
Platelet count: < 100,000/μl
History & Examination
Investigations: reticulocyte count & blood film
Consider iatrogenic causes (see Table 1)
Peripheral Destruction
• Reticulocytes > 100
• Palpable splenomegaly
Impaired Marrow Function
• Reticulocytes < 50
• Macrocytosis
• Hypersegmented neutrophils on blood film
Malignancy Associated Film
• Auer rods
• Circulating blast cells
• Granular bilobed blast cells
• Leucoerythroblastic film
• Tear drop cells
Other Investigations to Consider
Haematology: ESR, coagulation screen, fibrinogen, haemolysis screen (e.g. DAT, haptoglobins, LDH)
Biochemistry: LFTs, AST, haematinics (ferritin, B12, folate), CRP
Immunology: autoimmune screen (e.g. ANA)
Microbiology: viral serology (HBV, HCV, EBV, CMV, parvovirus B19, HIV)
Imaging: US abdomen
Refer to Haematology
Causes
• Acute myeloid leukaemia
• Acute promyelocytic leukaemia
• Myelodysplastic syndromes
• Myelofibrosis
• Solid tumours (e.g. prostate, thyroid, kidney)
Investigations
• Imaging (CT/PET)
• Aspiration and trephine biopsy
Causes
• Hypersplenism (e.g. chronic liver disease, malaria, schistosomiasis)
• Infections (e.g. hepatitis B, hepatitis C)
• Autoimmune (e.g. Felty syndrome)
Causes
• Megaloblastic anaemia (vitamin B12 or folate deficiency)
• Aplastic anaemia
• Infections (e.g. parvovirus B19, HIV)
• Autoimmune (SLE, rheumatoid arthritis, sarcoidosis)

10.3.1.5 SOAP Notes for Anemia

Table 174 SOAP Notes for Anemia

Component	Details
Subjective (S)	A 45-year-old female presents with complaints of fatigue, weakness, and shortness of breath, which have been progressively worsening over the past month. The patient reports feeling dizzy when standing up and has noticed paleness of her skin. She has a history of heavy menstrual periods but denies any recent trauma or gastrointestinal bleeding. She mentions that she often feels cold, particularly in her extremities. The patient has no significant past medical history other than menstrual irregularities.
Objective (O)	On physical examination, the patient appears fatigued but in no acute distress. The skin appears pale, and her conjunctivae are also pale. Her pulse is 88 bpm, and blood pressure is 110/70 mmHg. There is no

	lymphadenopathy, and the lungs are clear on auscultation. Cardiovascular exam is normal, though a slight tachycardia is noted when standing. The abdomen is soft with no hepatosplenomegaly.
Assessment (A)	The patient's symptoms, including fatigue, pallor, and shortness of breath, are consistent with **anemia**. Given her history of heavy menstrual periods and the absence of other causes of blood loss, **iron deficiency anemia** is the most likely diagnosis. However, further tests are needed to confirm this, including a complete blood count (CBC) and iron studies.
Plan (P)	**Pharmacological:** Begin oral iron supplements (ferrous sulfate 325 mg) daily to address the suspected iron deficiency anemia (See algorithm). **Non-pharmacological:** Advise the patient to consume more iron-rich foods such as lean meats, leafy greens, and fortified cereals. **Follow-up:** Schedule a follow-up appointment in 2-3 weeks to assess the response to iron supplementation and to review the results of the CBC and iron studies. If symptoms persist or worsen, further evaluation for other causes of anemia will be necessary. **Education:** Educate the patient on the importance of taking iron supplements as prescribed and adhering to dietary recommendations. Discuss possible side effects of iron supplements, such as constipation, and encourage hydration and fiber intake to alleviate this.

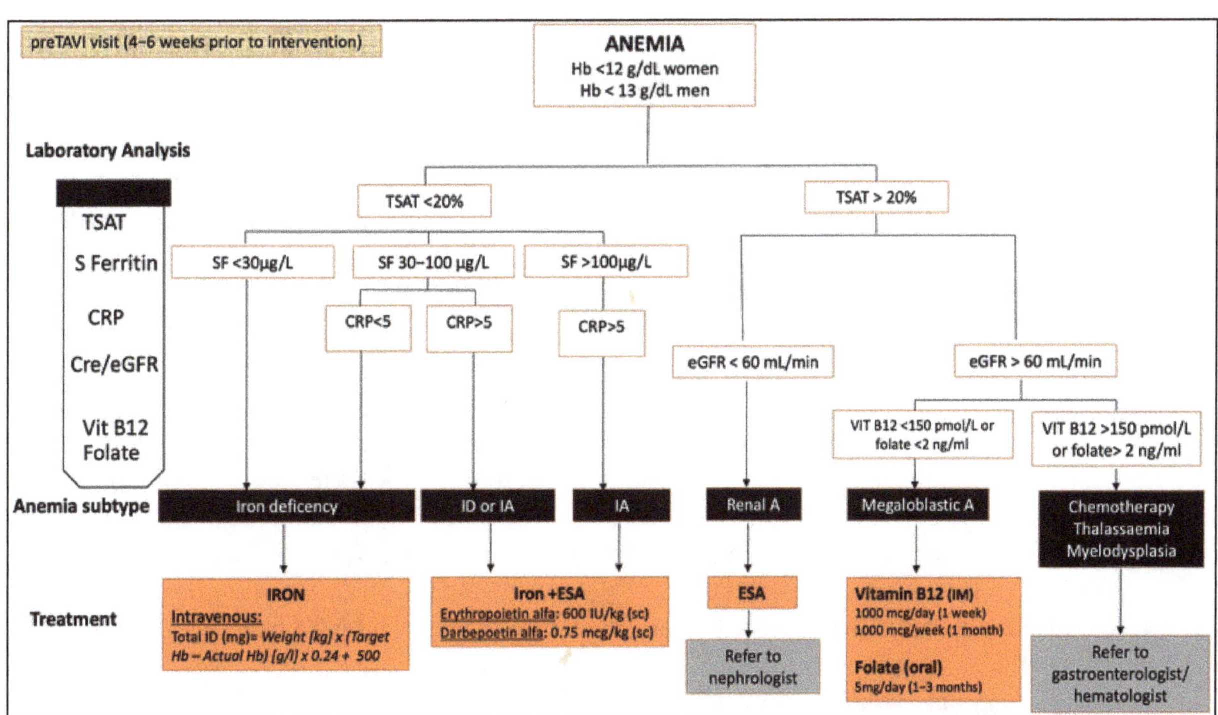

Figure 312 Management Algorithm for Anemia

10.3.2 Hemophilia A and B

The genetic diseases Hemophilia A and B cause excessively prolonged bleeding through **Factor VIII and Factor IX deficiencies** which disrupts the blood clotting process. The most frequent form of hemophilia **A manifests as Factor VIII protein deficiency which is essential to create**

blood clots. Majority **of X-linked recessive inheritance** causes this disorder to affect specifically males rather than females. The condition produces symptoms such as unexpected bleeding that occurs in joints and muscles and sustained bleeding after injuries or medical procedures. The condition of **Hemophilia B which goes by the name Christmas disease** results from decreased levels of Factor IX. **Hemophilia A and B present with comparable clinical symptoms** which include bruising easily and automatic joint bleeding as well as bleeding that lasts excessively. Hemophilia B exists as an X-linked recessive inherited condition which primarily causes problems in male individuals. The diagnosis of both diseases occurs through tests that evaluate clotting factor activity in blood samples. The medical management of Hemophilia A or Hemophilia B requires replacement therapy with **Factor VIII when treating Hemophilia A patients and Factor IX when treating patients with Hemophilia B** so they can prevent or control bleeding situations. Novel medical research into gene therapy shows potential for future medical treatments.

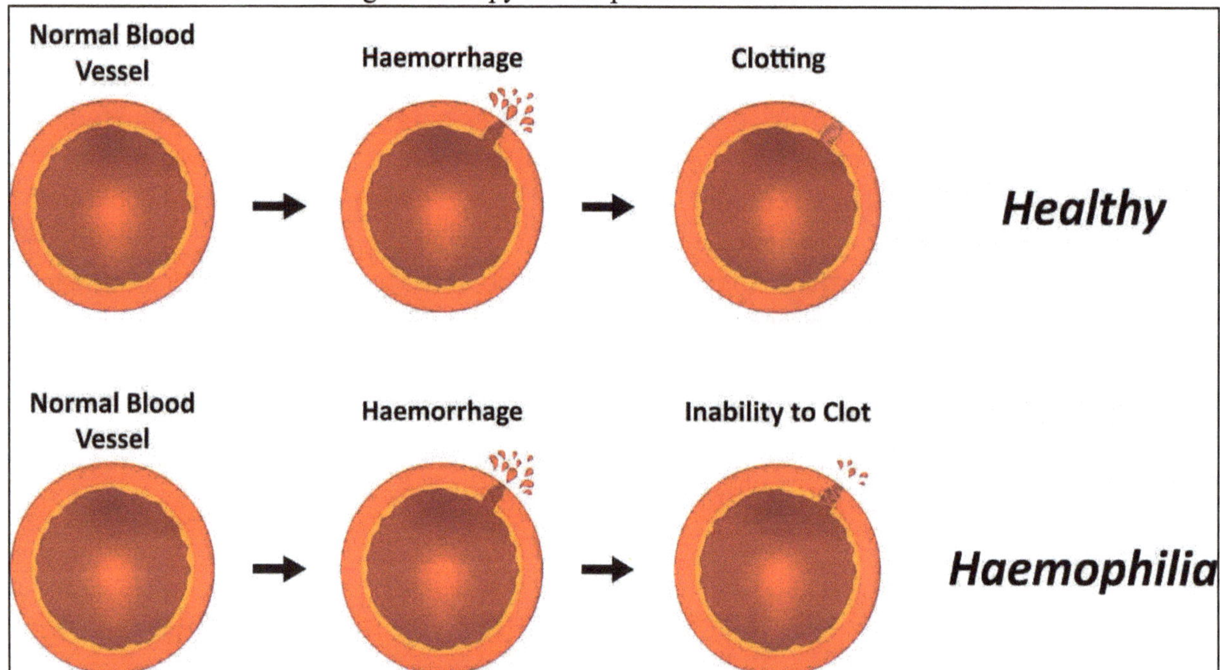

Figure 313 Hemophilia

The picture presents an introduction to inherited bleeding conditions Hemophilia A and B that result from insufficient clotting **factors VIII and IX. Type A Hemophilia represents 80-85% of all hemophilia** types because patients with this condition have insufficient Factor VIII levels needed to achieve normal blood clotting capability. Hemophilia B which physicians commonly refer to as **Christmas disease exists as 15-20%** of all cases because patients lack Factor IX. Most cases of these diseases manifest in male patients because inheritance is X-linked recessive. Females predominantly serve as carriers of these genetic disorders. Both Hemophilia A and B lead to different disease causes; Hemophilia A occurs because Factor VIII levels become reduced **while Factor IX levels decline in Hemophilia B.** The two groups of hemophilic conditions produce similar tragic symptoms which include unexpected bleeding along with bleeding in muscles and joints and extended bleeding times following injuries or surgical procedures. The treatment for both conditions requires factor replacement therapy to provide the missing clotting factor.

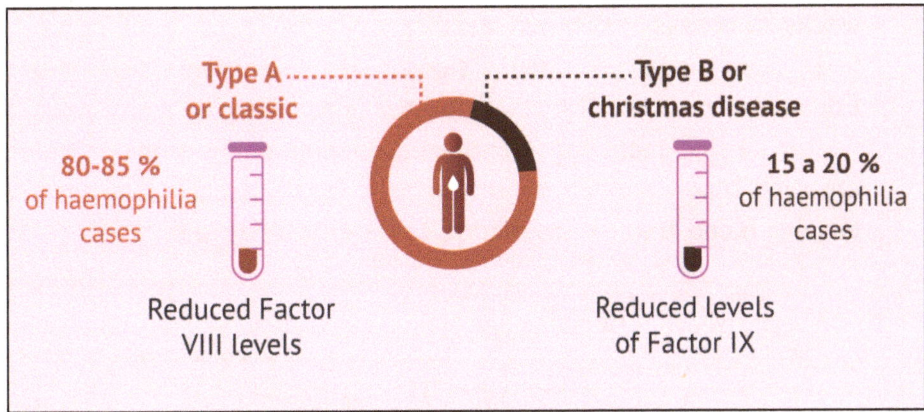

Figure 314 Hemophilia A and B

10.3.2.1 SOAP Notes for Hemophilia

Table 175 SOAP Notes for Hemophilia

Component	Details
Subjective (S)	A 10-year-old male presents with a history of recurrent spontaneous joint bleeds, especially in the knees and elbows. The patient reports frequent bruising even with minor trauma and prolonged bleeding after dental procedures. He also has a family history of hemophilia, with his father diagnosed with Hemophilia B and his maternal uncle diagnosed with Hemophilia A. The patient denies any recent trauma but has been experiencing increased pain and swelling in his left knee after playing sports.
Objective (O)	On physical examination, the patient appears well-nourished but is visibly in mild distress due to pain in his left knee. There is noticeable swelling and tenderness in the knee joint, with reduced range of motion. The patient's skin shows multiple bruises on the legs and arms. The left knee joint appears inflamed with no open wounds. There is no significant lymphadenopathy or hepatosplenomegaly.
Assessment (A)	The patient's symptoms and family history are consistent with a diagnosis of Hemophilia, likely Hemophilia A or Hemophilia B. Given the recurrent joint bleeds and family history, factor level testing is essential to confirm the diagnosis. The patient likely has Hemophilia A (Factor VIII deficiency) or Hemophilia B (Factor IX deficiency), both of which are X-linked recessive conditions.
Plan (P)	**Pharmacological:** Start Factor VIII replacement therapy for suspected Hemophilia A or Factor IX replacement therapy for Hemophilia B. The patient should receive prophylactic factor infusions to prevent further joint bleeds and manage acute bleeding episodes (See algorithm below). **Non-pharmacological:** Advise the patient and family on safe physical activity levels, limiting activities that could result in injury or bleeding. Recommend regular follow-up with a hematologist for ongoing management and monitoring of factor levels. **Follow-up:** Schedule a follow-up visit in 2

	weeks to assess treatment efficacy, review factor replacement regimens, and monitor for any signs of bleeding or side effects. **Education:** Educate the family on the importance of maintaining a supply of factor replacement at home, recognizing early signs of bleeding, and ensuring timely medical intervention when necessary. Discuss the need for ongoing blood tests to monitor clotting factor levels.

Figure 315 SOAP Notes for Hemophilia

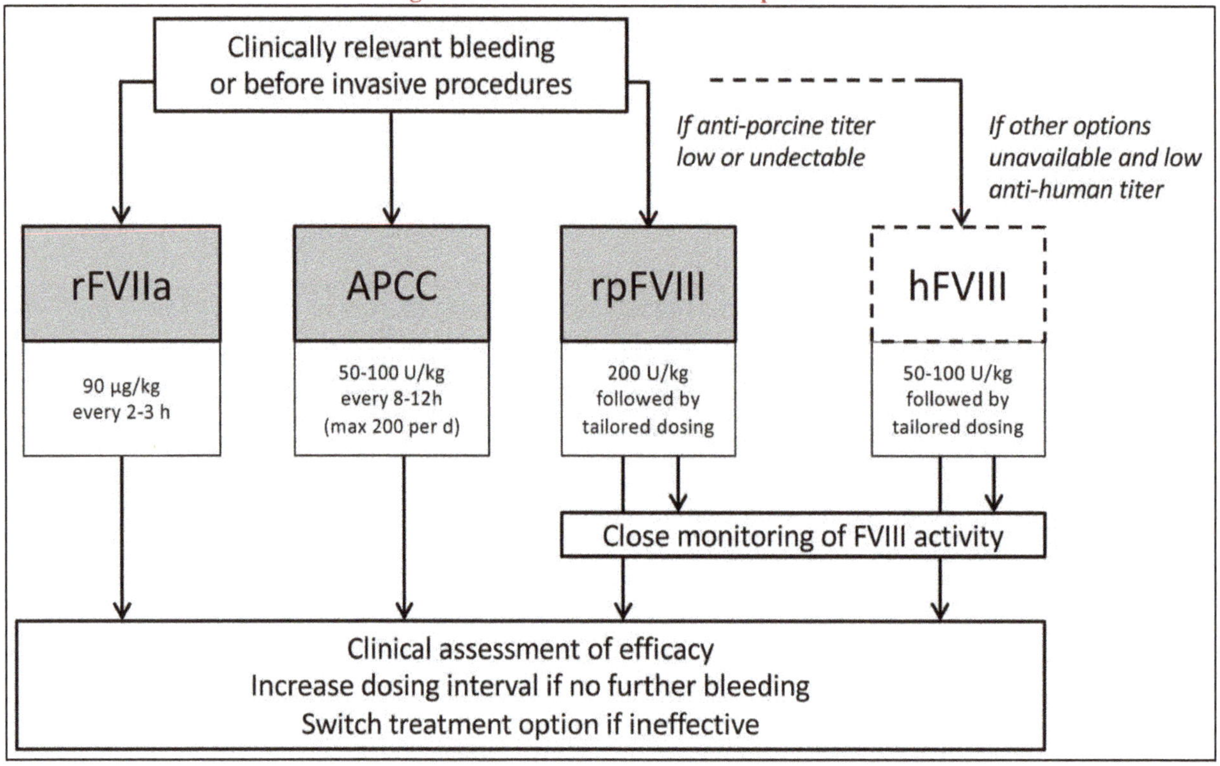

Clinically relevant bleeding
or before invasive procedures
If anti-porcine titer low or undectable
If other options unavailable and low anti-human titer
rFVIIa
90 μg/kg
every 2-3 h
APCC
50-100 U/kg
every 8-12h
(max 200 per d)
rpFVIII
200 U/kg
followed by
tailored dosing
hFVIII
50-100 U/kg
followed by
tailored dosing
Close monitoring of FVIII activity
Clinical assessment of efficacy
Increase dosing interval if no further bleeding
Switch treatment option if ineffective

Figure 316 Management Algorithm for Hemophilia

10.3.3 Thrombocytopenia

When the blood contains insufficient platelets the medical condition known as thrombocytopenia develops **leading to poor blood clotting ability and increased risk of bleeding.** The formation of blood clots for stopping bleeding depends heavily on platelets since they act as the key components in clot formation. Several conditions including **bone marrow disorders (aplastic anemia) and platelet destruction from autoimmune diseases (ITP or infections) and spleen platelet trapping will cause thrombocytopenia.** The main characteristics of thrombocytopenia come as easy bruising alongside delayed bleeding after small cuts along with nosebleeds and gums bleeding as well as **small red or purple skin spots known as petechiae**. Medical personnel use complete blood count results to diagnose this condition by identifying low platelet levels. Medical intervention for thrombocytopenia begins with identification of the fundamental cause and includes treatment with steroids for **autoimmune disorders or hospital-based platelet transfusions** and the utilization of therapy appropriate for the underlying illness. Patients need continuous evaluation alongside supportive treatment for managing this condition properly.

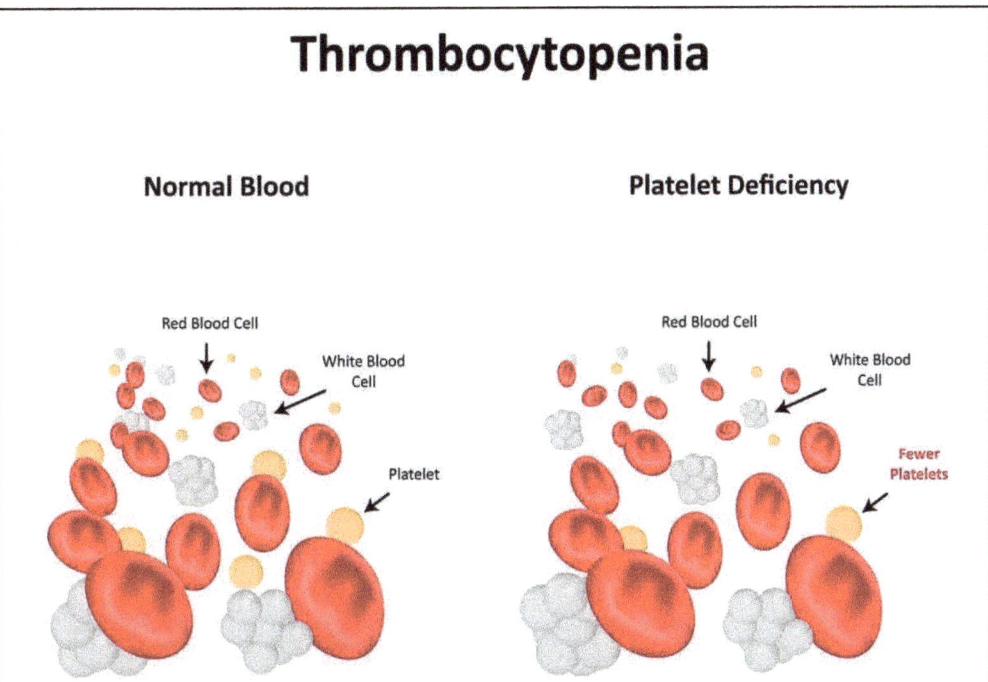

Figure 317 Thrombocytopenia

10.3.3.1 Classification of Thrombocytopenia

The provided image presents a thorough explanation **of thrombocytosis with thrombocytopenia** which represent disorders characterized by irregular platelet numbers in blood. Thrombocytosis occurs when platelet counts become excessive and it exists as primary or secondary varieties. The occurrence of primary thrombocytosis primarily affects adult patients because this condition develops alongside **excessive hematopoiesis and a JAK2 gene somatic mutation** that typically appears in medical conditions including **polycythemia vera and essential thrombocythemia and idiopathic myelofibrosis**. The **pediatric population experiences secondary thrombocytosis** more frequently since this condition develops as a result of chronic inflammation alongside infections and iron deficiency and tissue-damage symptoms in Kawasaki disease. A decrease in platelet count represents thrombocytopenia while this condition occurs because of either elevated platelet damage or reduced platelet generation. Of all thrombocytopenia cases, **the isolated type known as primary occurs in 80% of patients whereas secondary thrombocytopenia appears with other health conditions in the remaining 20% of cases.** Secondary thrombocytopenia develops from autoimmune diseases and infections as well as particular medications which affect platelet creation along with platelet survival lasting periods. The required treatment approach for both conditions depends on identifying their root cause

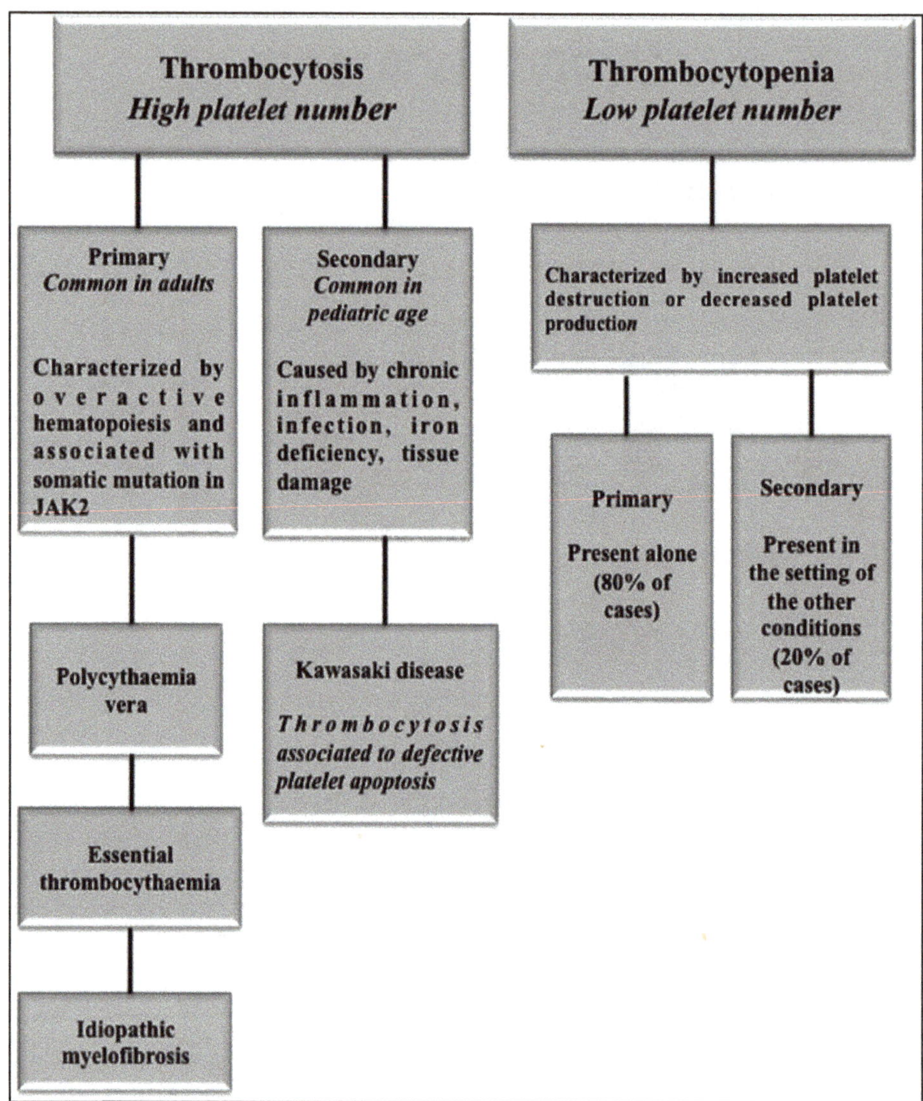

Figure 318 Classification of Thrombocytopenia

10.3.3.2 SOAP Notes for Kawasaki disease

Table 176 SOAP Notes for Kawasaki disease

Component	Details
Subjective (S)	A 4-year-old male presents with a 5-day history of high fever (39°C), irritability, red, swollen rash on palms and soles, red eyes (conjunctivitis), swollen tongue (strawberry tongue), and cracked lips. No significant past medical history. Family history includes upper respiratory infections.
Objective (O)	Fever (38.5°C), erythema of conjunctivae without discharge, strawberry tongue, cracked lips, maculopapular rash on the trunk, palms, and soles, bilateral cervical lymphadenopathy. The child is irritable but alert. No other significant findings.
Assessment (A)	The clinical presentation of fever, conjunctivitis, strawberry tongue, rash, and lymphadenopathy is highly suggestive of **Kawasaki disease**, a vasculitic

	condition that affects medium-sized arteries and can lead to coronary artery aneurysms.
Plan (P)	**Pharmacological**: Initiate intravenous immunoglobulin (IVIG) and aspirin therapy. **Non-pharmacological**: Provide supportive care (fever management and hydration). Monitor vital signs, particularly heart rate. Perform an initial echocardiogram. **Follow-up**: Refer to pediatric cardiology for ongoing assessment. Follow-up echocardiogram in 1-2 weeks. **Education**: Educate the parents on Kawasaki disease, its potential complications (such as coronary artery aneurysms), and the need for regular follow-up for heart monitoring.

10.3.3.3 SOAP Notes for Thrombocytopenia

Table 177 SOAP Notes for Thrombocytopenia

Component	Details
Subjective (S)	A 32-year-old male presents with easy bruising, prolonged bleeding after minor cuts, and frequent nosebleeds over the past week. He also reports feeling fatigued and notices small red or purple spots (petechiae) on his legs. The patient has no history of recent trauma or heavy bleeding, but he recently started taking a new medication for a respiratory infection. He denies any fever or weight loss but is concerned about the bruising. No significant past medical history or family history of bleeding disorders.
Objective (O)	On physical examination, the patient appears well-nourished but shows signs of bruising on the forearms and legs. Petechiae are visible on both legs, and there is mild conjunctival pallor. No active bleeding is observed. The spleen and liver are not palpable. Vital signs are stable with blood pressure 118/76 mmHg, heart rate 80 bpm, and temperature 98.6°F.
Assessment (A)	The patient's symptoms, including easy bruising, petechiae, and prolonged bleeding, are consistent with thrombocytopenia. Given the recent medication use, the thrombocytopenia may be drug-induced, though further testing is needed to confirm the cause. The patient's platelet count is likely to be low based on the clinical presentation. Other possible causes of thrombocytopenia, such as immune thrombocytopenic purpura (ITP), will need to be considered.
Plan (P)	**Pharmacological:** Order a complete blood count (CBC) with platelet count to confirm thrombocytopenia. If confirmed, consider discontinuing the new medication if it is determined to be the cause. If the platelet count is significantly low, platelet transfusion may be necessary (See algorithm below). **Non-pharmacological:** Advise the patient to avoid activities that may cause injury or bleeding (e.g., contact sports or heavy lifting). Educate the patient about recognizing signs of active bleeding and when to seek emergency care. **Follow-up:** Schedule a follow-up appointment in 1 week to reassess platelet counts and monitor for signs of bleeding. If platelet

counts do not improve or worsen, further investigations, including **bone marrow biopsy**, may be needed. **Education:** Discuss the potential causes of thrombocytopenia, including drug-induced thrombocytopenia and autoimmune conditions. Inform the patient about the importance of reporting any new symptoms such as severe bleeding or signs of infection.

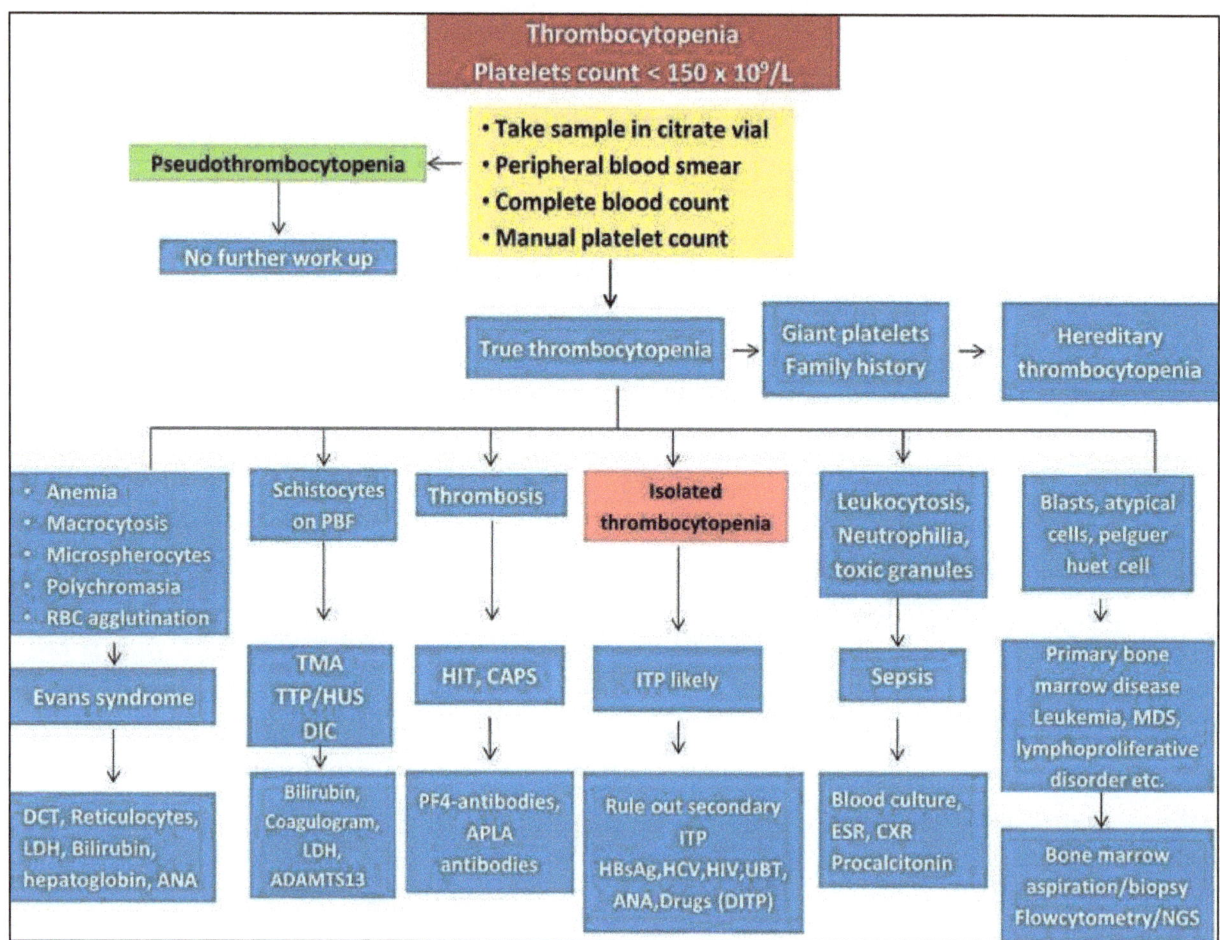

Figure 319 Algorithm for the Management of Thrombocytopenia

10.3.4 Multiple Myeloma

Multiple Myeloma manifests when cancer develops in the plasma cells that exist inside the bone marrow. The white blood cell type plasma cells functions to produce antibodies as immune defenders against infections. **Cancerous transformations of these cells** along with their uncontrolled proliferation in multiple myeloma result in the production of abnormal antibodies which we **refer to as M-proteins or monoclonal proteins**. The continued development of cancerous plasma cells in the bone marrow leads them to replace healthy blood cells thus creating anemia and causing infections and bleeding problems. The abnormal proteins build up in kidney tissue which causes this organ to malfunction. The development of bone lesions in **multiple myeloma patients causes back and rib bone pain** that is common among these patients. The symptoms of multiple myeloma also present with fatigue along with unexpected weight loss while patients develop frequent infections that lead to elevated blood calcium levels named hypercalcemia. The weakened state of bones leads to pathologic fractures. Doctors use M-protein blood tests alongside bone marrow biopsy results to detect plasma cells and X-ray/MRI studies **combined with serum protein electrophoresis to confirm monoclonal proteins** in multiple myeloma diagnosis. Stem cell transplant combined with chemotherapy medications and proteasome inhibitors and immunomodulatory drugs make up the available treatment options for multiple myeloma. Monoclonal antibodies together with CAR T-cell therapy represent newer therapeutic approaches that hold potential for handling the disease. The multiple myeloma disease leads to a variable survival outlook since it exists as a persistent illness yet doctors have trouble predicting how patients will fare. Patients need both prompt identification of multiple myeloma and consistent medical treatment to enhance both life quality and survival duration.

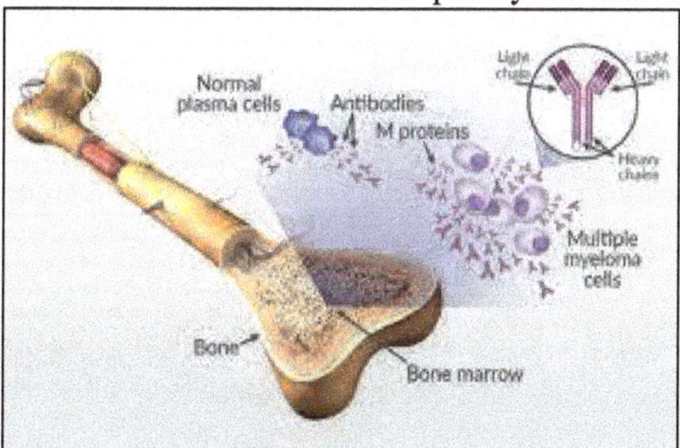

Figure 320 Multiple Myeloma

10.3.4.1 Types of Multiple Myeloma

The diagram presents a summary of multiple myeloma types since this illness affects plasma cells found in bone marrow. Multiple myeloma has two main precursor conditions beginning with **MGUS (Monoclonal Gammopathy of Undetermined Significance)** which shows plasma cell increases apart from disease symptoms. Multiple Myeloma rarely develops from MGUS even though this condition carries potential to become myeloma. The second category includes **SMM (Smoldering Multiple Myeloma)** as a progressive stage that leads to multiple myeloma. The condition includes greater numbers of faulty plasma cells than MGUS yet patients avoid symptoms and no evidence shows organ damage. SMM stays in an observation period called "watch and wait" since it leads to multiple myeloma development in some cases. The last condition shown in the image represents **MM (Multiple Myeloma)** as a form of blood cancer that affects plasma cells located in the bone marrow. The disease exists when abnormal plasma cells overgrow in the body resulting in bone pain alongside renal dysfunction and anemia as well as hypercalcemia. A diagnosis of **multiple myeloma only emerges from progression through either MGUS or SMM conditions** which indicates the development of malignant cancer that demands medical intervention and continued monitoring.

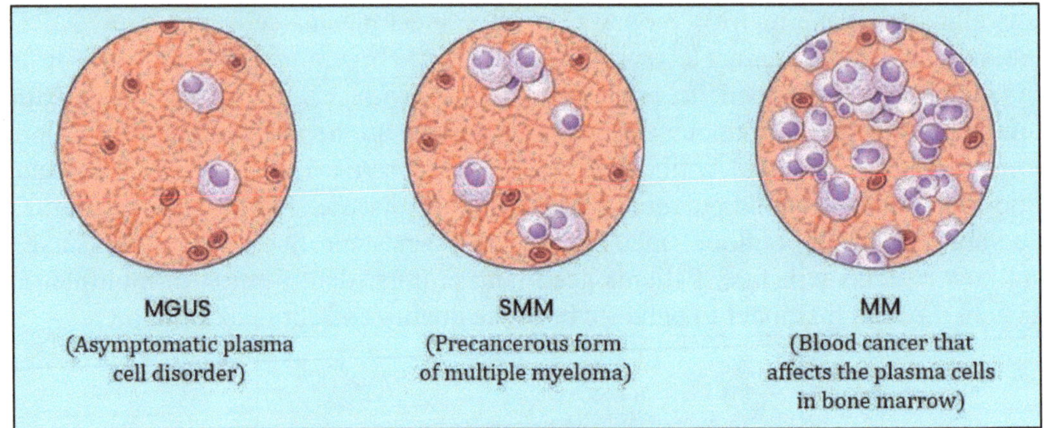

Figure 321 Types of Multiple Myeloma

10.3.4.2 SOAP Notes for Multiple Myeloma

Table 178 SOAP Notes for Multiple Myeloma

Component	Details
Subjective (S)	A 62-year-old male presents with a history of persistent back pain, fatigue, and weakness that has gradually worsened over the past two months. The patient also reports unintentional weight loss and recurrent infections. He has noticed bruising easily and has had frequent nosebleeds. He has a family history of cancer, but no known history of multiple myeloma. He mentions feeling more fatigued than usual, and his mobility is limited due to pain. He has not undergone recent trauma or injury.
Objective (O)	On physical examination, the patient appears frail and fatigued. There is noticeable tenderness in the lower back and ribs. No palpable lymphadenopathy or hepatosplenomegaly is observed. The skin is pale, and petechiae are seen on the arms. Blood pressure is 120/75 mmHg, heart rate is 88 bpm, and temperature is normal at 98.4°F. Neurological exam is unremarkable.
Assessment (A)	The patient's clinical presentation, including bone pain, fatigue, easy bruising, and recurrent infections, is suggestive of multiple myeloma. Given the combination of symptoms and risk factors, further investigation is warranted to confirm the diagnosis. Blood tests and imaging studies will be ordered to assess for monoclonal proteins (M-proteins), bone lesions, and impaired kidney function, all of which are indicative of multiple myeloma.
Plan (P)	**Pharmacological:** Order a complete blood count (CBC), serum protein electrophoresis to detect M-proteins, and bone marrow biopsy to assess for abnormal plasma cells. Renal function tests and imaging studies (X-ray, CT, or MRI) will be done to check for bone lesions (See algorithm below). **Non-pharmacological:** Advise the patient to limit weight-bearing activity to avoid fractures and falls. **Follow-up:** Schedule a follow-up visit in 1 week to review lab results and imaging findings. If confirmed, initiate chemotherapy, stem cell transplant, or immunomodulatory drugs depending on disease stage.

Education: Educate the patient about the potential for bone damage, renal impairment, and the importance of adhering to treatment protocols. Discuss possible side effects of treatment, including fatigue and infections, and the need for regular follow-ups for monitoring disease progression.

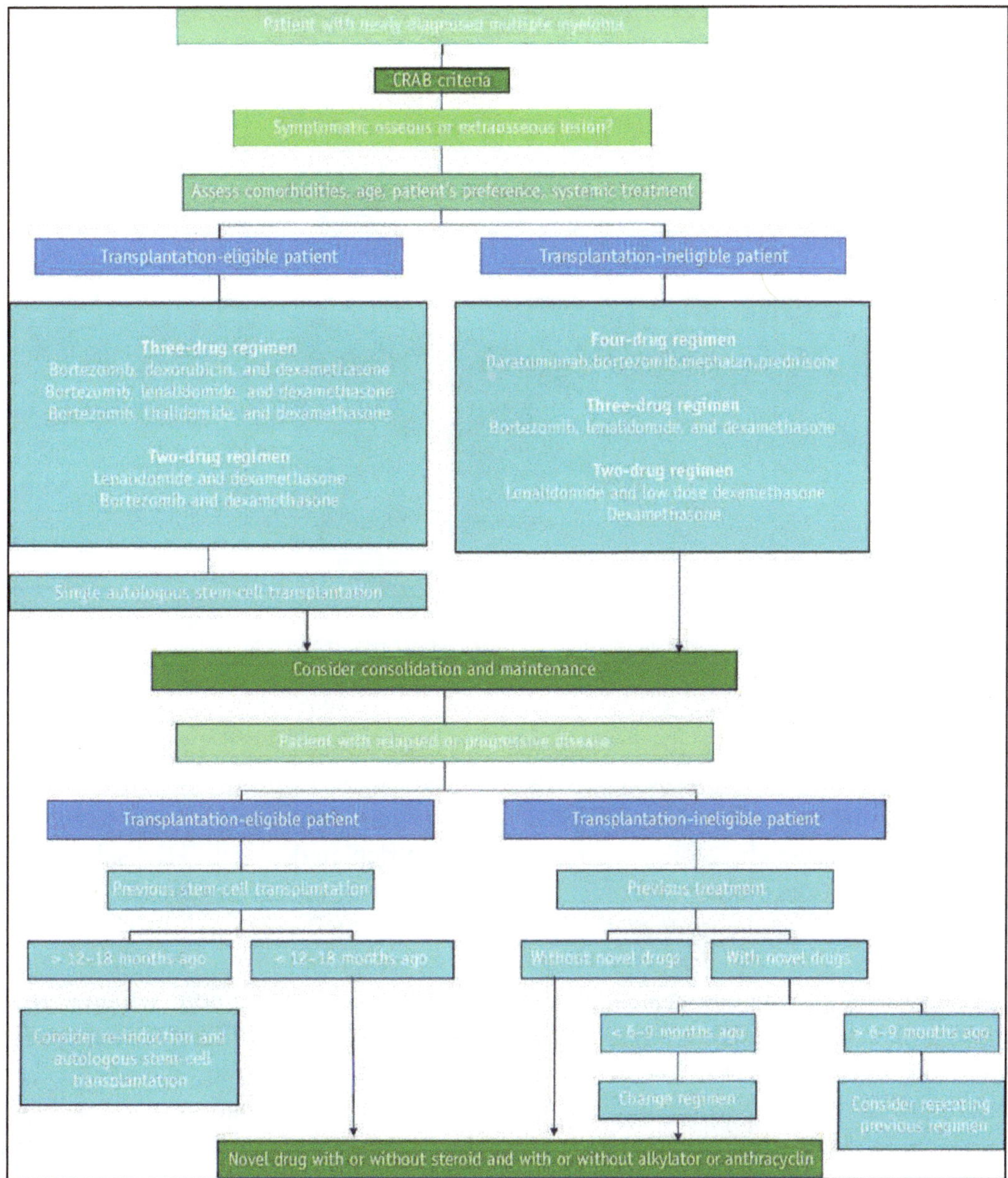

Figure 322 Treatment Algorithm for Myeloma

10.3.5 Hodgkin's Lymphoma Disease

The cancer of **Hodgkin's Lymphoma develops in the lymphatic system** which functions as a crucial component of the body's immune system. Reed-Sternberg cells serve as diagnostic markers of the disease because they appear inside tissue samples during this type of lymphoma. The major symptoms of Ho**dgkin's Lymphoma include painless lymph node swelling in neck or armpit**

or groin regions combined with fever, night sweats, unusual weight loss, general tiredness and itchy skin (also known as B symptoms). HL causes remain unclear because scientists believe that both genetics and **Epstein-Barr virus (EBV)** infection play a role in its development. Doctors confirm Hodgkin lymphoma diagnosis by testing the lymph nodes through biopsy techniques while they stage the **cancer using CT scans combined with PET** scans and bone marrow biopsy. Patients receive chemotherapy and radiation therapy for their treatment which leads to high recovery rates when diagnosis occurs early. The therapy of choice for treatment-resistant situations requires stem cell transplantation. The projection for survival is better for patients under 40 years old.

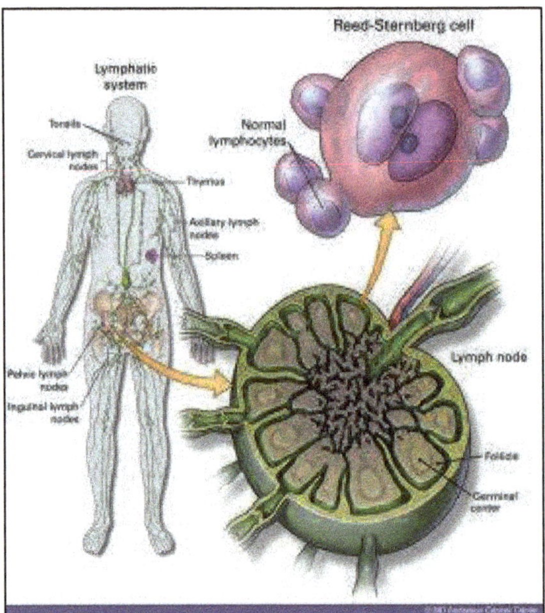

Figure 323 Hodgkin Lymphoma

10.3.5.1 Types of Hodgkin Lymphoma

The image presents both **Classical Hodgkin's Lymphoma and Nodular Lymphocyte-Predominant Hodgkin's Lymphoma (NLPHL)** as the primary forms of **Hodgkin's Lymphoma (HL).** The most usual subtype of Classical HL exists in four subtypes: Nodular sclerosis, Mixed cellularity, Lymphocyte-rich, along with Lymphocyte-depleted. Each HL subtype presents different patterns of **Reed-Sternberg cells in the lymph nodes** which help differentiate them. Nodular sclerosis stands as the most prevalent subtype because it contains fibrotic tissue patterns within lymph nodes. The rare disease Nodular lymphocyte-predominant **Hodgkin's lymphoma (NLPHL)** presents popcorn cells as a distinct variant of Reed-Sternberg cells which helps doctors differentiate it from other Hodgkin's lymphoma types. Therefore NLPHL shows a more favorable prognosis than classical types. **NLPHL mainly appears in younger patients** since its development proceeds slowly compared to classical HL. The identification of HL subtype helps medical staff understand which treatments will work best and what patients can expect regarding their chances of recovery.

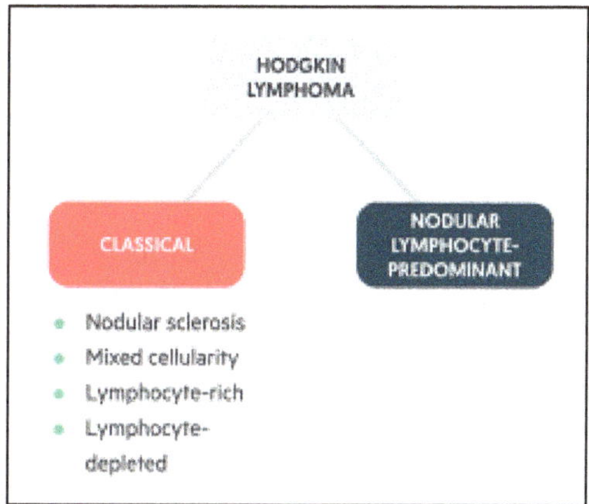

Figure 324 Types of Hodgkin Lymphoma

10.3.5.2 SOAP Notes for Hodgkin Lymphoma

Table 179 SOAP Notes for Hodgkin's Lymphoma

Component	Details
Subjective (S)	A 28-year-old male presents with a painless swelling in his neck, which he noticed about three weeks ago. He also reports feeling fatigued and having night sweats. He has lost approximately 10 pounds in the past month without trying. He denies any recent infections, trauma, or significant medical history, although his paternal uncle was diagnosed with lymphoma. The patient has no significant past medical history other than seasonal allergies. He is concerned about the swelling and symptoms.
Objective (O)	On physical examination, the patient appears well-nourished but slightly fatigued. There is a noticeable, non-tender lymphadenopathy in the left cervical region. The spleen and liver are not palpated. The skin is warm and dry, with no visible rashes. Vital signs are stable with blood pressure 120/78 mmHg, heart rate 85 bpm, and temperature 99.2°F. There is no jaundice or pallor observed. No signs of other systemic involvement are noted.
Assessment (A)	The patient's symptoms, including painless lymphadenopathy, night sweats, weight loss, and fatigue, are suggestive of Hodgkin's Lymphoma. The pattern of symptoms, especially in the absence of infection or other known causes, raises concern for lymphoma. Given his age and family history, further evaluation is warranted to confirm the diagnosis and subtype, which could be classical HL or Nodular Lymphocyte-Predominant HL.
Plan (P)	**Pharmacological:** Order a biopsy of the enlarged lymph node to confirm the diagnosis and identify Reed-Sternberg cells. Additionally, CT scan and PET scan will be performed to assess for

other areas of involvement (See algorithm below). **Non-pharmacological:** Advise the patient on symptom management, including rest and hydration, and educate him on the potential side effects of treatment if confirmed. **Follow-up:** Schedule a follow-up visit in 1 week to discuss the biopsy results and treatment plan based on staging. If diagnosed with HL, discuss possible treatments such as chemotherapy, radiation, or stem cell transplant. **Education:** Explain the nature of Hodgkin's lymphoma, the importance of early treatment, and potential outcomes. Emphasize the need for regular monitoring and supportive care during treatment.

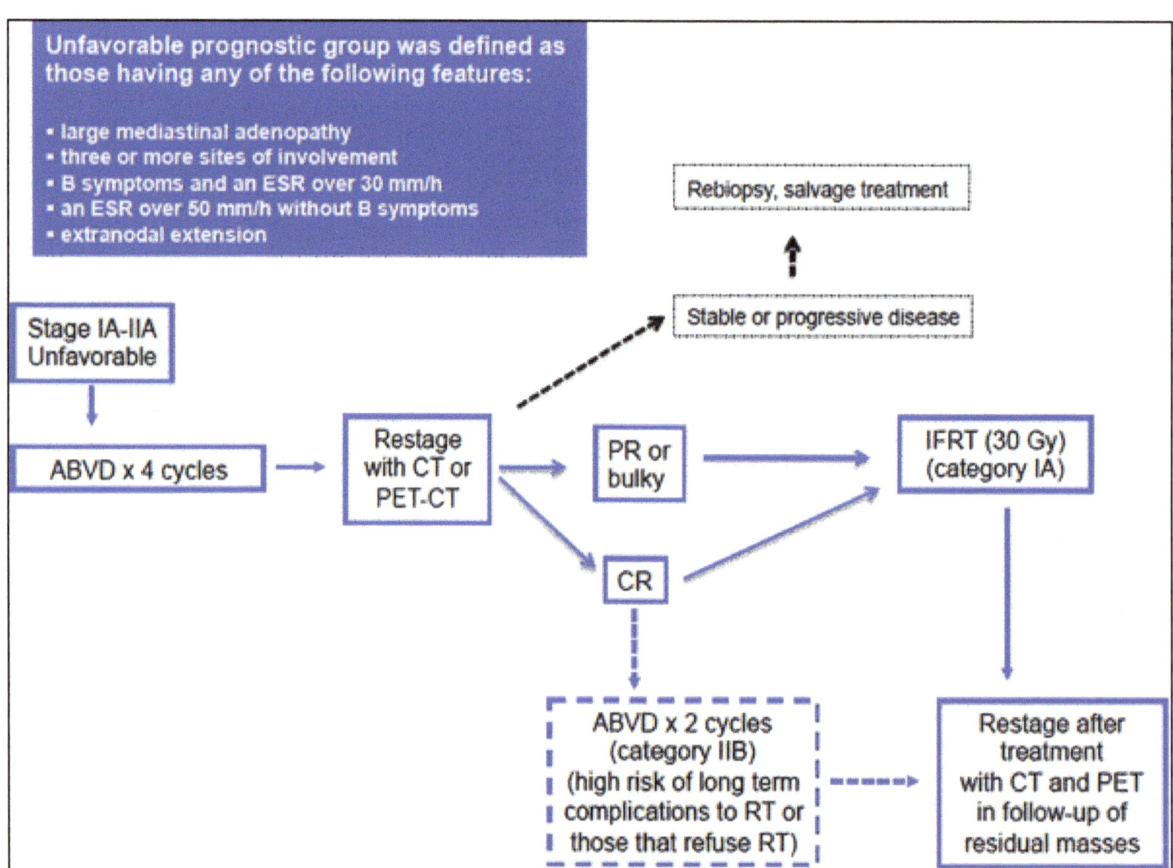

Figure 325 Management Algorithm Guidelines for Hodgkin Lymphoma

10.3.6 Non-Hodgkin Lymphoma Disease

Non-Hodgkin Lymphoma (NHL) develops as a wide range of blood cancers that begin in the body's immune system lymphatic tissues. **During NHL only the specific Reed-Sternberg** cells are absent as a disease characteristic. Any region of the lymphatic system beginning from lymph nodes through spleen to bone marrow can develop NHL before the cancer spreads to other body parts. **Adults face a higher risk for developing NHL** and the disease occurrence steadily grows as people become older. The medical signs of NHL consist of enlarged but non-painful lymph nodes along with fevers, night sweats, unexpected weight reduction and weariness and stomach pain when the spleen or intestines show involvement. The different NHL subtypes group into two main categories consisting of indolent disease that grows slowly and aggressive disease that develops rapidly. **Doctors validate an NHL diagnosis by conducting a biopsy** combined with visual examinations and blood tests. The disease treatment depends on specific NHL features and disease stages using combinations of chemotherapy and radiation therapy and immunotherapy and stem cell transplants. **The survivability depends on the type of NHL** as indolent cases tend to have lengthier patient outcomes.

10.3.6.1 Types of Non Hodgkin Lymphoma Disease

The visual

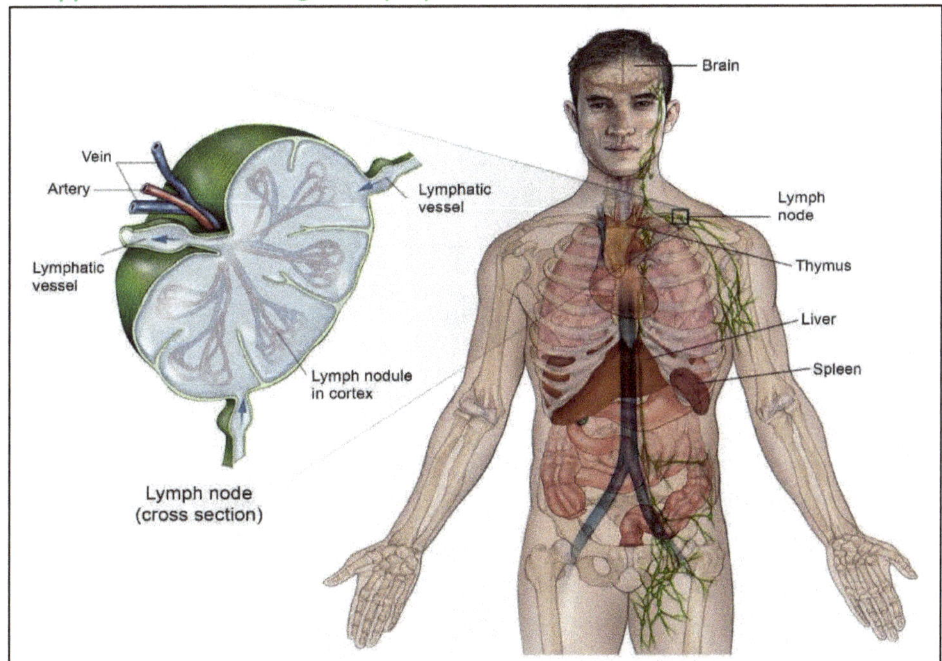

Figure 326 Non-Hodgkin Lymphoma Disease

representation highlights how **Hodgkin's Lymphoma (HL) and Non-Hodgkin's Lymphoma (NHL)** differ specifically through the absence of Reed-Sternberg cells in NHL cells. One main difference between Hodgkin's lymphoma and non-Hodgkin's lymphoma occurs because Hodgkin's lymphoma contains **Reed-Sternberg cells yet NHL lacks these cells**. The origin of NHL starts with lymphocytes whose primary function belongs to white blood cells of the immune system. Both B-cells and T-cells belong to the lymphocyte family and their malignant transformation results in tumors throughout different areas of the lymphatic system. The disease subtype of NHL depends on whether it infects B-cells or T-cells since each cell type leads to distinct developmental profiles. **A heterogeneous group of lymphomas named NHL presents** different clinical paths and doctors confirm its diagnosis by identifying malignant lymphocytes in examined tissue samples. The particular lymphoma subtype together with its stage determines the necessary treatment protocols and patient outcomes.

Figure 327 Differentiation of Non Hodgkin Lymphoma

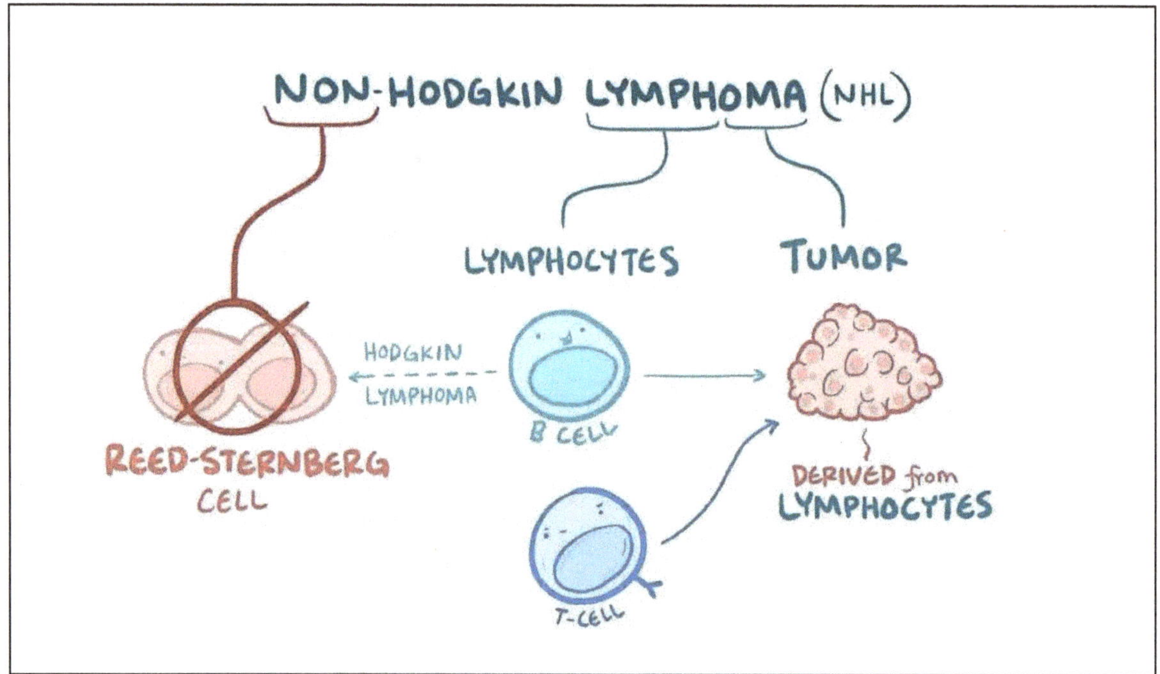

10.3.6.2 SOAP Notes for Non Hodgkin Lymphoma Disease

Table 180 SOAP Notes for Non Hodgkin Lymphoma

Component	Details
Subjective (S)	A 58-year-old male presents with painless swelling of lymph nodes in the neck and abdomen, which he has noticed over the past month. He also reports recent fatigue, unexplained weight loss of 10 pounds in the last 3 weeks, and intermittent night sweats. The patient has a history of hypertension but is otherwise healthy. He denies fever, pain, or any recent infections. No known family history of cancer.
Objective (O)	On physical examination, the patient appears fatigued but in no acute distress. There is noticeable, non-tender lymphadenopathy in the cervical and inguinal regions. The abdomen is soft, with no organomegaly, but there is slight tenderness in the left lower quadrant. Vital signs: BP 130/85 mmHg, HR 76 bpm, temperature 98.7°F. No hepatosplenomegaly or other significant findings.
Assessment (A)	The patient's clinical presentation, including painless lymphadenopathy, weight loss, night sweats, and fatigue, is suggestive of Non-Hodgkin's Lymphoma (NHL). Given the lymph node involvement and systemic

	symptoms, further investigation is required to confirm the diagnosis and subtype. Possible causes include B-cell or T-cell lymphoma, with the most likely diagnosis being an aggressive form of NHL based on symptom presentation.
Plan (P)	**Pharmacological:** Order a biopsy of the affected lymph node to confirm the presence of malignant lymphocytes and determine the subtype of NHL. Also, order CT scan and PET scan to assess the extent of the disease (See algorithm below). **Non-pharmacological:** Advise the patient to monitor for any new or worsening symptoms and seek immediate care for any signs of bleeding or infection. **Follow-up:** Schedule a follow-up visit in 1 week to discuss biopsy results and staging. If confirmed as NHL, initiate treatment with chemotherapy or radiation based on staging and lymphoma subtype. <br

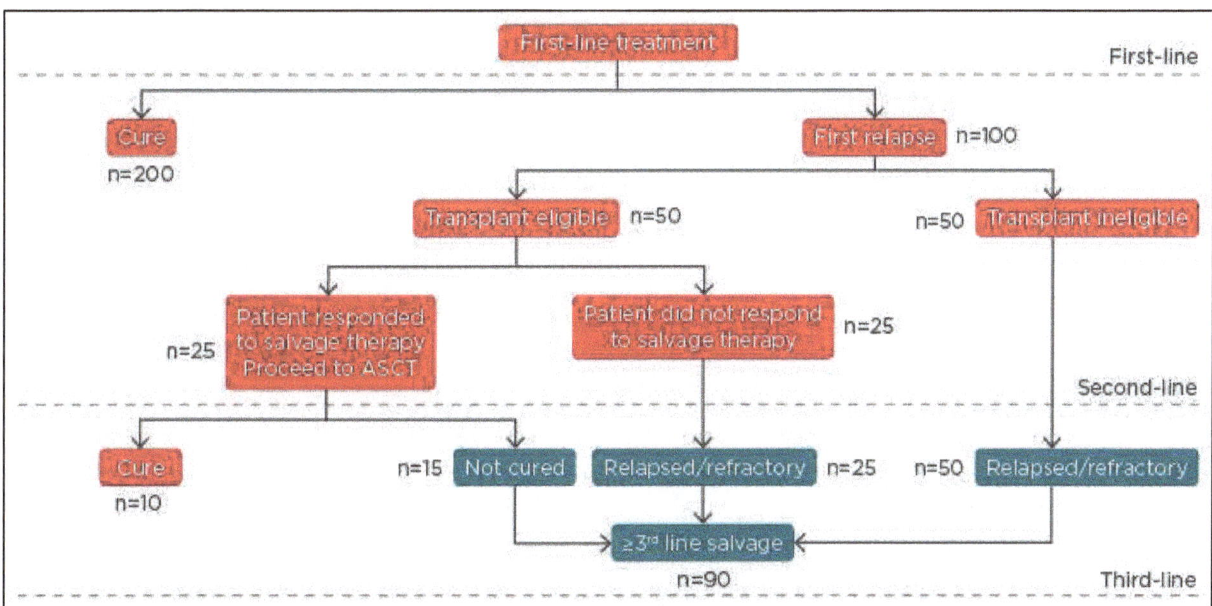

Figure 328 Algorithm for the Management of Non Hodgkin Lymphoma

10.3.7 Neutropenia

Neutropenia manifests as a medical condition where the body has insufficient neutrophils which serve as white blood cells vital for combating bacterial along with fungal infections. An insufficient number of immune system neutrophils increases vulnerability to infections in the body. The human body can develop neutropenia from several components such as bone marrow disorders, autoimmune diseases, chemotherapy, radiation therapy, viral infections or medications. Doctors group the severity of neutropenia into three levels which depend on the absolute neutrophil count results: mild with **1,000-1,500 cells/µL, moderate with 500-1,000 cells/µL and severe with less than 500 cells/µL.** People with this condition often experience fevers together with chills and infections that develop in the mouth as well as throat and skin areas. A diagnosis of neutropenia becomes certain after running a **complete blood count (CBC) test with differential results**. The treatment approach for neutropenia depends on both the origin and intensity of the condition and may consist of antibiotics together with growth factor usage or extraction of responsible medications. Patients with severe neutropenia should seek hospital treatment because it enables prevention of fatal bloodstream infections.

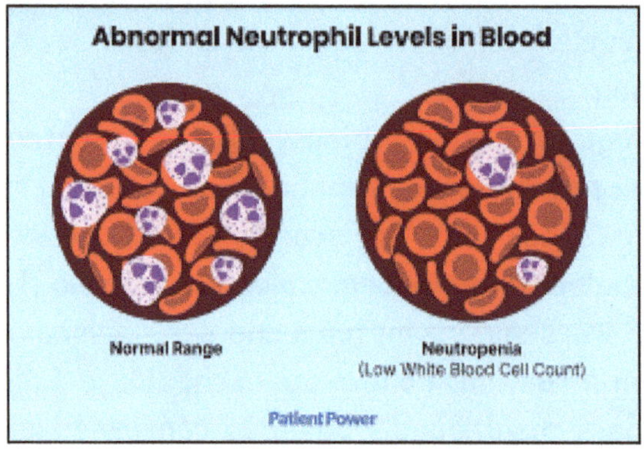

Figure 329 Neutropenia

10.3.7.1 SOAP Notes for Neutropenia

Table 181 SOAP Notes for Neutropenia

Component	Details
Subjective (S)	A 45-year-old female with a history of **breast cancer**, currently undergoing chemotherapy, presents with a fever of 101°F and reports feeling fatigued. She mentions that she has had a sore throat and mouth ulcers for the past few days but no cough or shortness of breath. The patient denies any recent infections or noticeable bruising. She has been on chemotherapy for the past month and is concerned about the increased risk of infection.
Objective (O)	On physical examination, the patient appears fatigued but is alert and oriented. Temperature is 101°F. There is visible redness and sores on the inner cheeks and gums. No lymphadenopathy is noted. Her abdomen is soft with no tenderness or organomegaly. Lung examination is clear. The rest of the exam is unremarkable.
Assessment (A)	The patient's fever, mouth ulcers, and history of chemotherapy are concerning for neutropenia. Given her recent chemotherapy, it is likely that her neutrophil count is low, putting her at risk for infection. A complete blood count (CBC) with differential will be ordered to confirm neutropenia and assess its severity.
Plan (P)	**Pharmacological:** Order a CBC with differential to assess the neutrophil count. If neutropenia is confirmed, initiate broad-spectrum antibiotics to prevent any infections. Consider growth factors like G-CSF (Granulocyte Colony-Stimulating Factor) to stimulate neutrophil production if neutropenia is severe (See algorithm below). **Non-pharmacological:** Advise the patient to practice strict hygiene and avoid crowded places to reduce infection risk. **Follow-up:** Contact the patient within 24-48 hours to assess if the fever subsides and if blood counts improve. If symptoms worsen or the neutrophil count remains low, further interventions or hospitalization may be needed. **Education:** Educate the patient about neutropenia,

	infection prevention, and the importance of seeking medical help immediately if fever or signs of infection worsen.

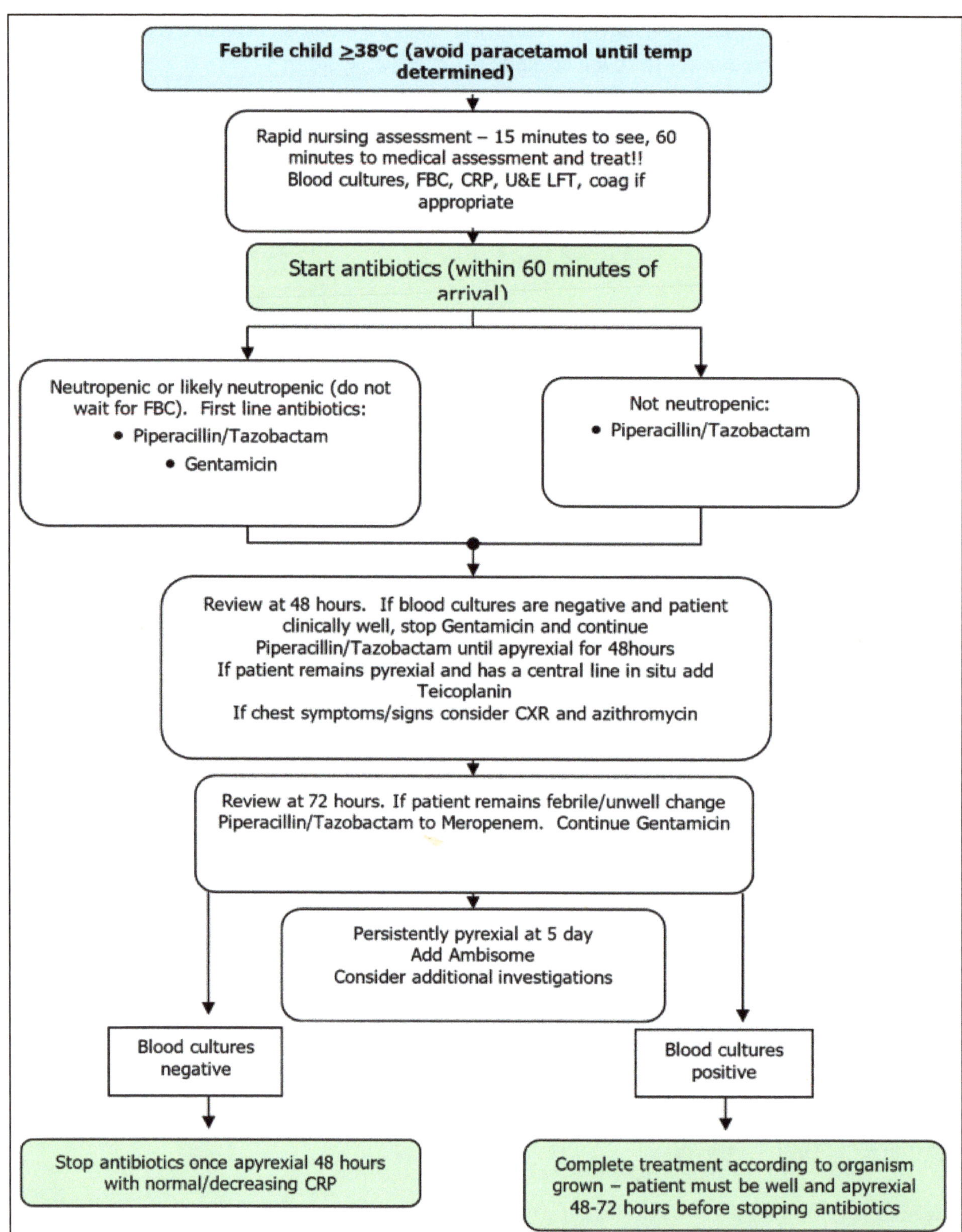

Febrile child ≥38°C (avoid paracetamol until temp determined)
Rapid nursing assessment – 15 minutes to see, 60 minutes to medical assessment and treat!!
Blood cultures, FBC, CRP, U&E LFT, coag if appropriate
Start antibiotics (within 60 minutes of arrival)
Neutropenic or likely neutropenic (do not wait for FBC). First line antibiotics:
• Piperacillin/Tazobactam
• Gentamicin
Not neutropenic:
• Piperacillin/Tazobactam
Review at 48 hours. If blood cultures are negative and patient clinically well, stop Gentamicin and continue Piperacillin/Tazobactam until apyrexial for 48hours
If patient remains pyrexial and has a central line in situ add Teicoplanin
If chest symptoms/signs consider CXR and azithromycin
Review at 72 hours. If patient remains febrile/unwell change Piperacillin/Tazobactam to Meropenem. Continue Gentamicin
Persistently pyrexial at 5 day
Add Ambisome
Consider additional investigations
Blood cultures negative
Blood cultures positive
Stop antibiotics once apyrexial 48 hours with normal/decreasing CRP
Complete treatment according to organism grown – patient must be well and apyrexial 48-72 hours before stopping antibiotics

Figure 330 Management Algorithm for Neutropenia

10.3.8 Acute Hemorrhage

Acute hemorrhage results from immediate and fast blood loss through the circulation system when trauma, surgical procedures or ruptured blood vessel occurs. Acute hemorrhage severity depends on both the extent of blood volume loss as well as the speed of blood loss from the body. **The symptoms of hypotension with tachycardia along with pallor and weakness accompanied by dizziness and confusion and cool clammy skin indicate acute hemorrhage**. Patients who experience severe blood loss will go into shock which might result in organ failure and probably death unless medical care is provided immediately. Blood pressure and perfusion stay stable through initial vasoconstriction and heart rate acceleration however these compensatory functions become inadequate with extended hemorrhage. Auditing the degree of blood loss depends on **clinical signs and laboratory tests which include measuring hemoglobin and hematocrit levels** for patient assessment. Acute bleeding requires instant treatment through fluid resuscitation together with blood transfusions and possible surgical procedures to stop the bleeding. Emergent procedures become vital for both preventing dangerous medical emergencies and improving patient results.

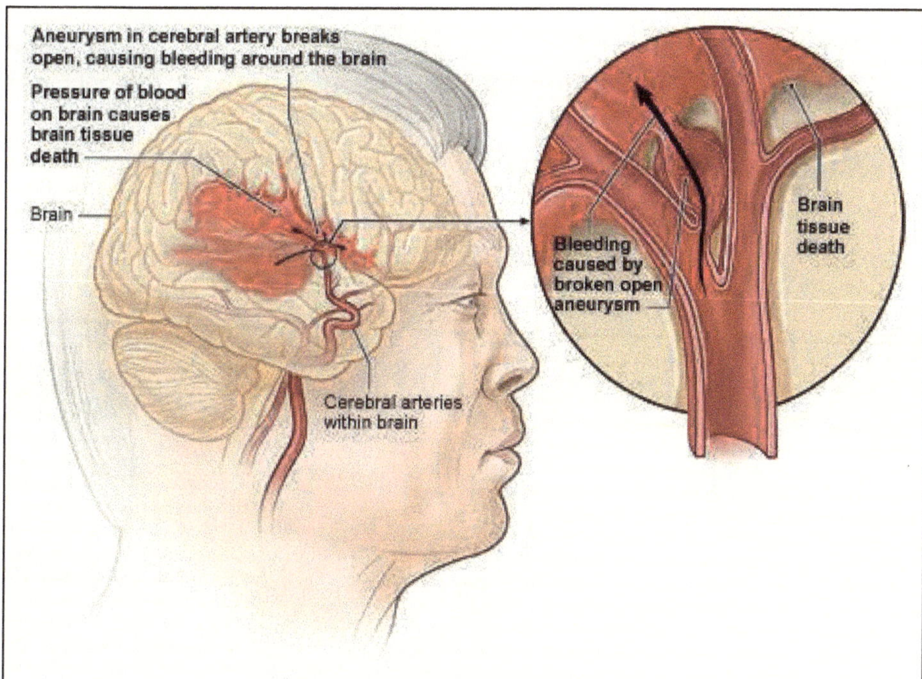

Figure 331 Acute Hemorrhage

10.3.8.1 SOAP Notes for Acute Hemorrhage

Table 182 SOAP Notes for Acute Hemorrhage

Component	Details
Subjective (S)	A 34-year-old male presents with significant **blood loss** after a motor vehicle accident. He reports feeling lightheaded, dizzy, and weak since the accident. He noticed **severe bleeding** from a laceration on his left thigh and was unable to stop it despite applying pressure. The patient is anxious and feels faint. He denies any past medical history of bleeding disorders.
Objective (O)	On examination, the patient is **pale** and **diaphoretic**, with **tachycardia** (heart rate of 120 bpm) and **hypotension** (blood pressure 90/60 mmHg). The left thigh has a large laceration with active bleeding. The wound is

	deep, and **pressure dressing** is in place. The patient's skin is cold, and **capillary refill** is delayed in the extremities. There is **mild confusion** but no loss of consciousness.
Assessment (A)	The patient is presenting with **acute hemorrhage** secondary to trauma (motor vehicle accident) and **active bleeding** from the left thigh laceration. The patient's **tachycardia** and **hypotension** indicate significant blood loss, potentially approaching **hypovolemic shock**. Immediate management is required to control the bleeding, stabilize vital signs, and prevent further complications.
Plan (P)	**Pharmacological:** Administer **IV fluids** (normal saline or lactated Ringer's) immediately for volume resuscitation. Prepare for **blood transfusion** based on hemoglobin and hematocrit levels. **Non-pharmacological:** Apply **pressure dressing** to control bleeding. Ensure continuous monitoring of **vital signs** (heart rate, blood pressure, respiratory rate) and **oxygen saturation**. **Follow-up:** Transfer the patient to the **operating room** for surgical exploration and wound closure if bleeding cannot be controlled. Reevaluate blood counts, and assess for any signs of internal bleeding. **Education:** Educate the patient on the importance of early treatment and monitoring during the recovery phase, emphasizing the need for follow-up visits to check for complications such as infection or delayed bleeding.

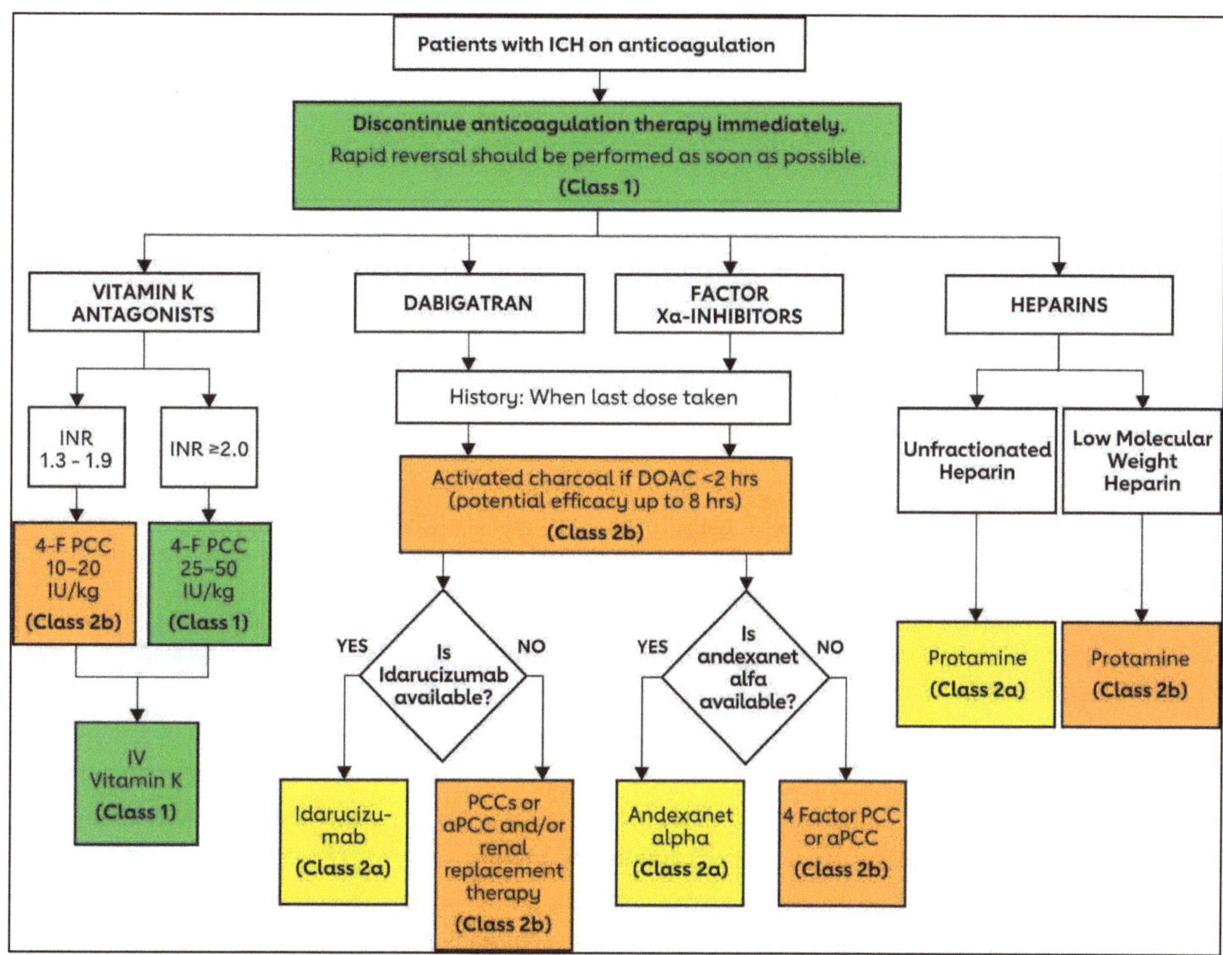

Figure 332 Algorithm for the Management of Acute Hemorrhage (Intracranial)

10.4 Moh Golden Points and Summary Question Answers

10.4.1 Moh Golden Points

Anemia is characterized by a decrease in the number of red blood cells or hemoglobin, which impairs oxygen delivery. It can be classified as microcytic, normocytic, or macrocytic, based on red blood cell size (MCV).

The most common type of anemia, caused by inadequate iron to produce hemoglobin. Diagnosed with a low serum ferritin, serum iron, and high total iron-binding capacity (TIBC).

Vitamin B12 and Folate Deficiency Anemia cause macrocytic anemia with elevated MCV and a low reticulocyte count. The diagnosis is confirmed through serum B12 or folate levels.

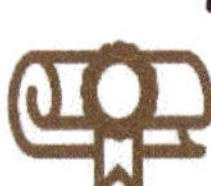

Hemophilia A is a deficiency of Factor VIII, while Hemophilia B is a deficiency of Factor IX. Both conditions lead to impaired blood clotting and require factor replacement therapy to manage bleeding episodes.

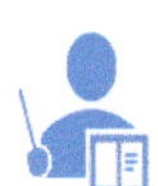

Characterized by a low platelet count, leading to easy bruising, bleeding, and petechiae. It can result from bone marrow failure, platelet destruction, or sequestration in the spleen.

Leukemia is a cancer of the bone marrow and blood, leading to excessive production of abnormal white blood cells. It is classified into acute and chronic forms, with acute leukemia requiring urgent treatment due to rapid progression.

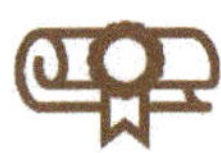

A cancer of plasma cells in the bone marrow, causing bone pain, anemia, and renal impairment. Treatment involves chemotherapy, stem cell transplants, and newer immunomodulatory drugs.

10.4.2 Summary Questions & Answers

1. Which of the following is the most common cause of microcytic anemia?
a) Vitamin B12 deficiency
b) Iron deficiency
c) Chronic disease
d) Folate deficiency

2. What is the primary deficiency in Hemophilia A?
a) Factor II
b) Factor VIII
c) Factor IX
d) Factor X

3. Which blood test is most commonly used to diagnose Vitamin B12 deficiency anemia?
a) Serum iron
b) Serum B12 levels
c) Ferritin levels
d) Red blood cell count

4. A low platelet count in a patient with petechiae and easy bruising is characteristic of which condition?
a) Hemophilia
b) Thrombocytopenia
c) Leukemia
d) Sickle Cell Anemia

5. The presence of Reed-Sternberg cells in a lymph node biopsy is diagnostic of which condition?
a) Non-Hodgkin’s Lymphoma
b) Acute leukemia
c) Hodgkin’s Lymphoma
d) Multiple Myeloma

6. In Multiple Myeloma, which of the following is commonly elevated?
a) Hemoglobin
b) M-protein (Monoclonal protein)
c) Platelet count
d) Reticulocyte count

7. The most common cause of macrocytic anemia is:
a) Iron deficiency
b) Vitamin B12 or Folate deficiency
c) Hemolysis
d) Chronic disease

8. What is the hallmark finding in the peripheral blood smear of a patient with sickle cell anemia?
a) Schistocytes
b) Sickle-shaped red blood cells
c) Hypochromic red blood cells
d) Spherocytes

9. Which of the following is a characteristic feature of Non-Hodgkin's Lymphoma?
a) Presence of Reed-Sternberg cells

b) Lymphadenopathy without Reed-Sternberg cells
c) Bone pain as a primary symptom
d) Marked splenomegaly in early stages

10. The main treatment for acute leukemia is:
a) Blood transfusions
b) Chemotherapy
c) Stem cell transplant
d) Bone marrow biopsy

10.4.3 Rationales

1. Answer: b) Iron deficiency

Rationale: **Iron deficiency anemia** is the most common cause of **microcytic anemia**, where the red blood cells are smaller than normal, and the hemoglobin content is reduced due to insufficient iron.

---

2. Answer: b) Factor VIII

Rationale: **Hemophilia A** is caused by a deficiency in **Factor VIII**, a clotting factor necessary for proper blood clotting. Hemophilia B, in contrast, is caused by a deficiency in **Factor IX**.

---

3. Answer: b) Serum B12 levels

Rationale: **Serum B12 levels** are used to diagnose **Vitamin B12 deficiency anemia**, which causes **macrocytic** anemia. Low B12 levels are indicative of the deficiency causing the abnormality in red blood cell production.

---

4. Answer b) Thrombocytopenia

Rationale: **Thrombocytopenia** refers to a low platelet count and is characterized by symptoms such as **petechiae**, easy bruising, and bleeding due to insufficient platelets for clot formation.

---

5. Answer: c) Hodgkin's Lymphoma

Rationale: **Reed-Sternberg cells** are a hallmark of **Hodgkin's Lymphoma**, a type of cancer that originates in the lymphatic system. Their presence in a lymph node biopsy helps differentiate it from **Non-Hodgkin's Lymphoma**.

---

6. Answer: b) M-protein (Monoclonal protein)

Rationale: **Multiple Myeloma** is characterized by the overproduction of abnormal **M-protein** by malignant plasma cells. This protein can be detected in the blood or urine, which is a key diagnostic marker for the disease.

---

7. Answer: b) Vitamin B12 or Folate deficiency

Rationale: **Vitamin B12** or **folate deficiency** leads to **macrocytic anemia**, where red blood cells are larger than normal, often due to impaired DNA synthesis, resulting in the production of abnormally large red blood cells.

---

8. Answer b) Sickle-shaped red blood cells

Rationale: **Sickle cell anemia** is characterized by the presence of **sickle-shaped red blood cells** on a **peripheral blood smear**, caused by **abnormal hemoglobin (HbS)**, which results in the deformation of red blood cells under low oxygen conditions.

---

9. Answer: b) Lymphadenopathy without Reed- Sternberg cells

Rationale: **Non-Hodgkin's Lymphoma** is characterized by lymphadenopathy, often involving **B-cells** or **T-cells**, but unlike **Hodgkin's lymphoma**, it does not contain **Reed-Sternberg cells**. The lymphoma can be indolent or aggressive.

---

10. Answer: b) Chemotherapy

Rationale: **Chemotherapy** is the primary treatment for **acute leukemia** as it is designed to quickly target and kill the rapidly proliferating cancerous white blood cells. For certain cases, **stem cell transplant** may be considered as part of long-term treatment

11 Chapter 11: Endocrine System

11.1 Anatomy and Physiology of Endocrine System

The endocrine system maintains body functions through hormone secretion to operate various physical operations. Through the bloodstream these hormones function as chemical signals that **guide physiological operations in target organs and tissues.** The endocrine system contains several primary glands which comprise the hypothalamus together with its pituitary gland and thyroid gland and parathyroid glands followed by the adrenal glands and the pancreas and the gonads (testes and ovaries) and the pineal gland. As **brain-based control center the hypothalamus unites** the functions of the nervous system with those of the endocrine system. The hypothalamus uses hormones to control pituitary gland hormone releases that lead to the regulation of other endocrine glands. The **thyroid gland** which exists in the neck produces thyroid hormones that govern metabolic processes along with energy expenditure. The stress response ability of the body relies on adrenal glands which rest atop the kidneys to generate cortisol and adrenaline hormone production. The pancreas sits behind the **stomach to regulate blood sugar through its production of insulin and glucagon.** The gonads generate three hormones including estrogen and progesterone and testosterone to control both reproductive activities and secondary sexual characteristics.

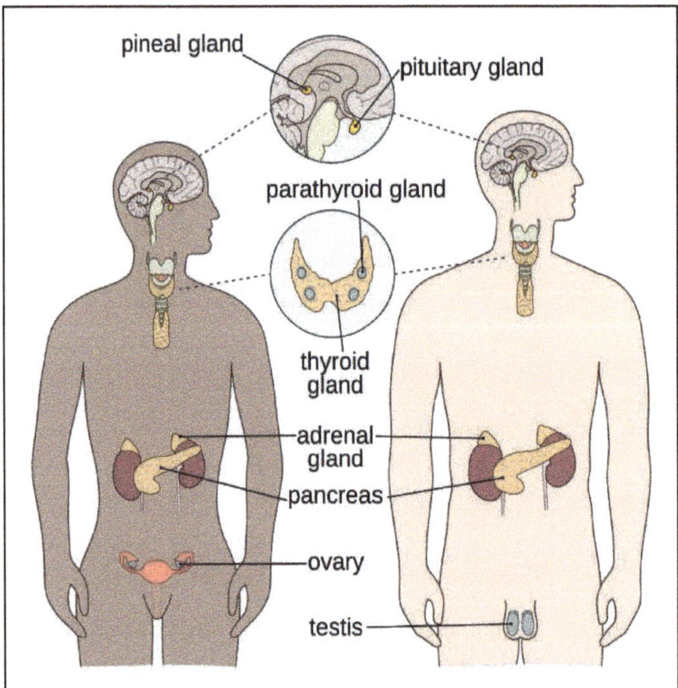

Figure 333 Anatomy and Physiology of Endocrine System

11.2 Role of the Hypothalamus and Pituitary Gland in Hormone Regulation

The **endocrine system regulation depends on the hypothalamus and pituitary gland** which function as the main body centers to control hormone release. The **hypothalamus positions inside the brain** maintains surveillance on different body processes while producing hormones to control pituitary gland functioning. T**he endocrine system uses this structure to communicate signals between the nervous system and endocrine system** to process information related to stress and temperature and hunger. Within the body's leading organ resides the anterior and posterior regions which together form the pituitary gland. Several vital body processes receive regulatory control by

anterior pituitary hormones which manage growth hormone production for growth together with thyroid-stimulating hormone regulation of metabolism and gonadotropins for reproductive functions comprising FSH and LH. **The posterior pituitary** serves as a hormone reservoir for hypothalamic oxytocin and antidiuretic hormone (ADH) that determine birth processes and water regulation and lactation. Through their interconnected system both hypothalamus and pituitary regulate hormonal releases that control bodily functions for homeostasis upkeep and to support growth along with reproduction and stress management.

11.3 Anatomy of Hypothalamus and Pituitary Gland

The image presents a thorough depiction of the hypothalamus along with the pituitary gland which indicates their **essential parts as well as their close connection.** At the top portion of the diagram the **hypothalamus stands near both brainstem and optic chiasm.** This part of the brain manages various bodily functions through hormone control which leads it to communicate directions to the pituitary gland. Two primary divisions make up the pituitary gland through its anterior and posterior sections. The anterior pituitary includes **three defined sections which are paras tuberalis together with pars intermedia and pars distalis.** As parts of the pituitary gland they activate the release of growth hormone and thyroid-stimulating hormone and gonadotropins type hormones. **Oxytocin and antidiuretic hormone** escape from the posterior pituitary area under the infundibulum through the direct action of the hypothalamus. The close anatomical link between hypothalamus and pituitary **gland through the infundibulum becomes** visible in the image while demonstrating their essential role in hormone regulation and homeostasis control.

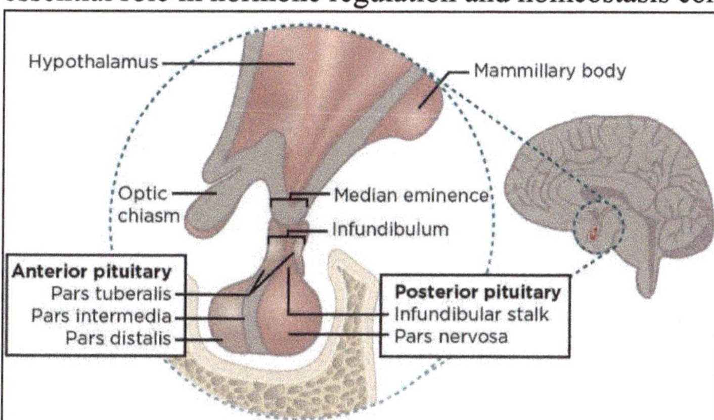

Figure 334 Anatomy of Hypothalamus and Pituitary Gland

11.4 Hormonal Regulation by the Hypothalamus and Pituitary Gland

The image shows the intricate hormonal communication between hypothalamus and pituitary gland which controls both anterior and posterior pituitary operations. The diagram's upper segment **demonstrates hormones that emerge from the posterior pituitary**. The hypothalamus generates **antidiuretic hormone (ADH)** which resides in the posterior pituitary until it sends this hormone into bloodstream circulation. The primary targets of ADH hormone include the **kidneys, sweat glands and circulatory system** which promote water reabsorption to regulate body water balance. As a second hormone from the **posterior pituitary Oxytocin (OT)** is made in the hypothalamus before its storage occurs in the posterior pituitary. The hormone exists to stimulate contractions of the uterus throughout childbirth in female reproductive processes.

The anterior pituitary hormones follow guidance from hypothalamus-released hormones according to the lower section in the graphic. **GnRH hormone from the hypothalamus stimulates the anterior pituitary to release both LH and FSH hormones** that control reproductive system functions by regulating gametes and sex hormone production. The brain hormone **Thyrotropin-**

releasing hormone (TRH) causes production of thyroid-stimulating hormone (TSH) to activate thyroid gland hormone output which maintains metabolic balance. The hormone prolactin-releasing hormone stimulates mammary glands through prolactin inhibitory hormone to produce prolactin that activates milk production. **Growth hormone releasing hormone (GHRH) triggers growth hormone (GH)** production through inhibiting growth hormone inhibiting hormone (GHIH) while the GH stimulates liver and bone as well as muscle growth and metabolic function. The brain hormone **Corticotropin-releasing hormone (CRH) activates the release of adrenocorticotropic hormone (ACTH)** that stimulates glucocorticoid production from adrenal glands to regulate stress responses and metabolism. The image represents the specific feedback operations which the hypothalamus and pituitary perform to achieve homeostasis together with essential body control functions.

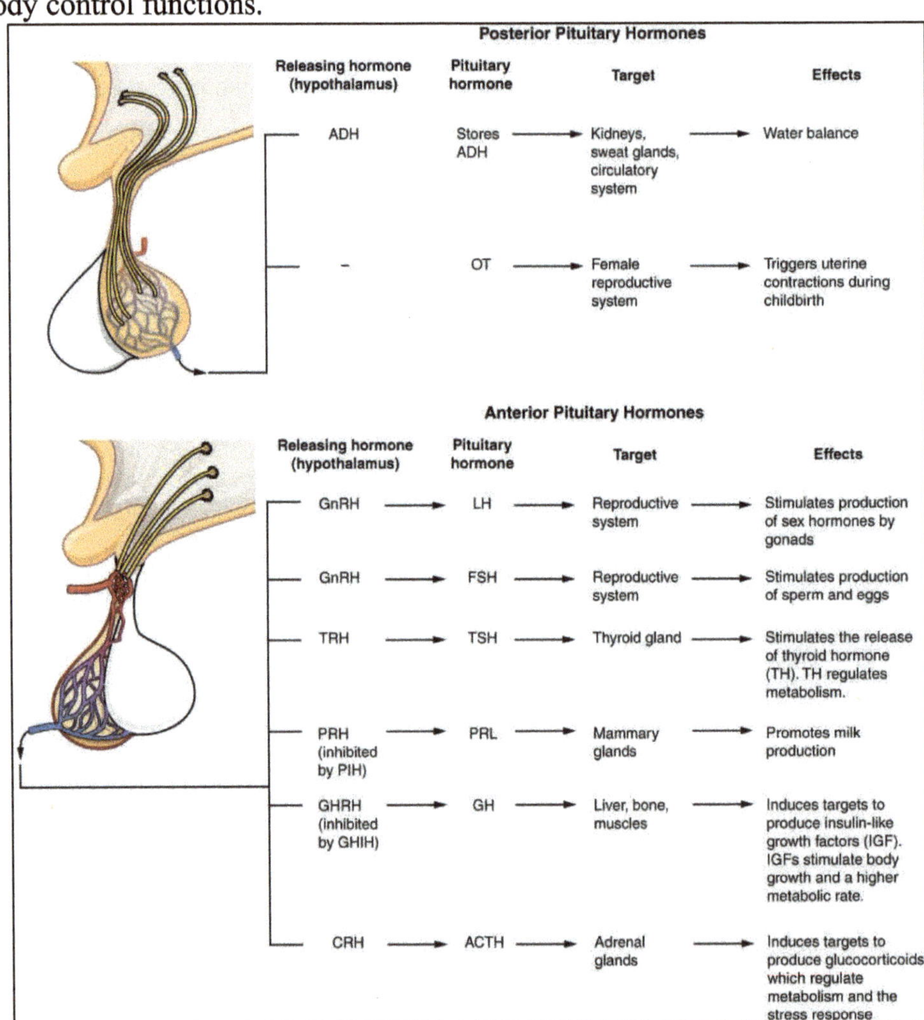

Figure 335 Classification of Pituitary Gland Hormones

11.5 Regulation of Hormone Secretion and Feedback Mechanisms

The illustration displays the complex ne**rvous system-to-hypothalamus-to-anterior pituitary-to-target glands network** which explains the effects of physical and emotional pressure on hormone regulation. The hypothalamus receives input from both the central nervous system and **immune system which starts a sequence of hormonal reactions**. The hypothalamus receives direct stimulation from physical and emotional stress elements which modifies hormone production patterns. From the hypothalamus originates a signal to activate the anterior pituitary which produces different hormones like thyrotropin and corticotropin. Following the release from the **hypothalamus the pituitary hormones travel to target glands such as thyroid gland, adrenal cortex, testes along with ovaries and liver to activate hormonal releases which include thyroid hormones (triiodothyronine and thyroxine) steroid hormones and the hormones estrogens and androgens.** Through feedback loops hormone secretion can be regulated by high hormone concentrations at the local level thus maintaining homeostasis according to the diagram. Bloodstream hormones generally connect with carrier proteins that control hormone concentrations to limit their amount of variation. Androgen levels decrease the amount of carrier proteins in blood but estrogen levels increase their presence. The system shows that hormones release through pulsating patterns which a pineal gland regulate using melatonin. The unique pulsatile hormone release **mechanism plays an essential role** in preserving uniform physiological processes across the entire body. The diagram showcases how numerous systems work together with different glands to establish a balanced reaction toward body-specific and environmental triggers.

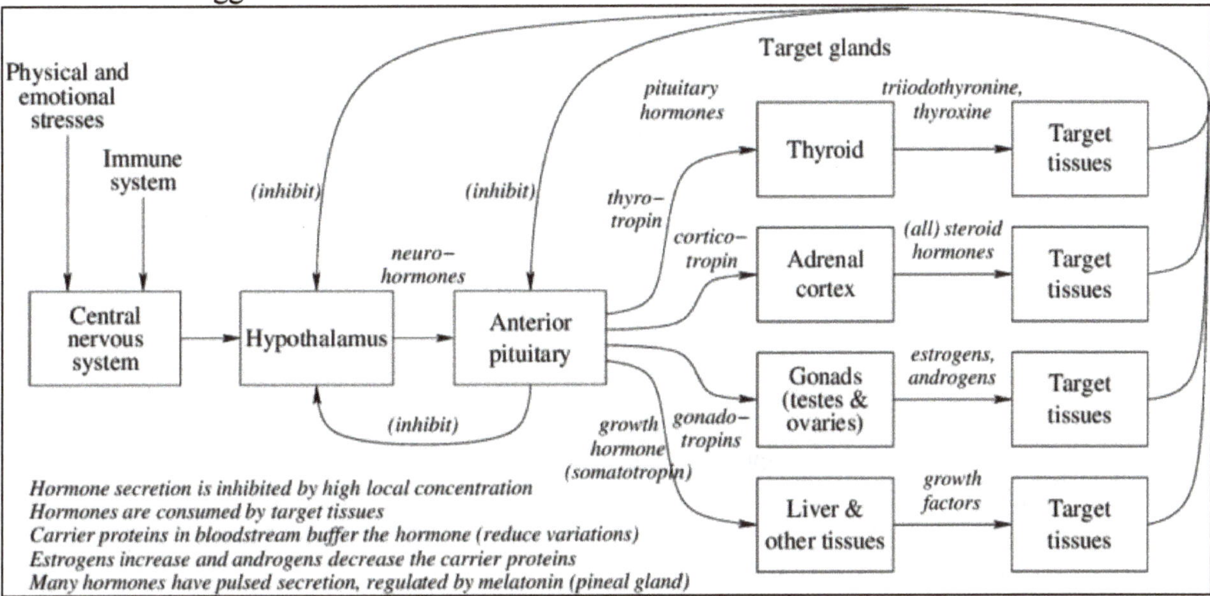

Figure 336 The hypothalamus-pituitary-target organ axis (in human endocrine system)

11.6 Hypothalamic and Pituitary Hormone Regulation and Related Disorders

The hormonal pathways perform vital functions by controlling growth reactions and managing metabolism while overseeing reproductive abilities and processing stress mechanisms. Pituitary tumors frequently lead to dysregulation which produces a wide spectrum of health conditions demonstrating the fundamental importance of controlling hormone levels for wellness.

11.6.1 CRH to ACTH Flowchart

The hypothalamus controls the CRH release that stimulates the anterior pituitary to secrete the hormone ACTH. When stimulated by ACTH the adrenal glands produce cortisol. The steroid hormone cortisol plays an essential role in sustaining homeostasis while regulating immune-system functions alongside its stress management capabilities. Cortisol reaches high amounts in the body to maintain blood sugar control and reduce inflammation and stabilize metabolism. Genetically incorrect growth of **ACTH-cell adenoma causes Cushing's disease** that leads to elevated cortisol levels thus **generating central obesity and striae and hyperglycemia and osteoporosis and hirsutism**.

11.6.2 TRH to TSH Flowchart

The hypothalamus produces **Thyrotropin-releasing hormone (TRH)** to trigger the anterior pituitary's production of **Thyroid-stimulating hormone (TSH).** The thyroid gland produces thyroid hormones **T3/T4 in response to stimulation by TSH** which controls metabolism together with thermogenesis and protein synthesis. The abnormally functioning TSH-cell adenoma produces thyroidular abnormalities that result in **thyroid goiter and hyperthyroxinemia conditions which disturb metabolic operations**.

11.6.3 GHRH to GH Flowchart

The **anterior pituitary produces Growth hormone (GH)** through the stimulation of **Growth hormone-releasing hormone (GHRH) released by the hypothalamus.** The primary target of Growth hormone (GH) lies within the liver to produce Insulin-like Growth Factor 1 (IGF-1). The growth factor IGF-1 triggers developmental processes that expand tissues throughout the body including both bone length growth and organ maturation. The overproduction of growth hormone from GH-cell adenoma cases in patients with Acromegaly causes symptoms which include **acral enlargement together with soft tissue swelling and cardiac hypertrophy and hypertension and hyperglycemia and sleep apnea.**

11.6.4 GnRH to LH and FSH Flowchart

The Gonadotropin-releasing hormone (GnRH) emitted by the hypothalamus activates Luteinizing hormone (LH) and Follicle-stimulating hormone (FSH) release from the anterior pituitary. LH and FSH control reproductive processes by determining gonadal function to produce estradiol and progesterone and testosterone which manage sexual hormone production. A disruption in this hormonal flow which occurs in **PRL-cell adenoma (prolactinoma) leads to infertility together with amenorrhea and hypogonadism resulting in reproductive and fertility complications.**

11.6.5 Dopamine Regulation of Prolactin

The hypothalamus releases dopamine to block prolactin release from the anterior pituitary. The main function of prolactin includes stimulating milk production in mammary glands. Reproductive complications develop from PRL-cell adenoma's prolactin overproduction because it causes both **galactorrhea and infertility and hypogonadism.**

11.6.6 Non-Functional Adenomas

Non-functional adenomas represented in the diagram are hormone-deficient pituitary tumors that create important effects in the body canal. The central effects from these tumors include **hypogonadism or hypergonadism although many silent tumors do not cause symptoms linked to hormone overproduction**.

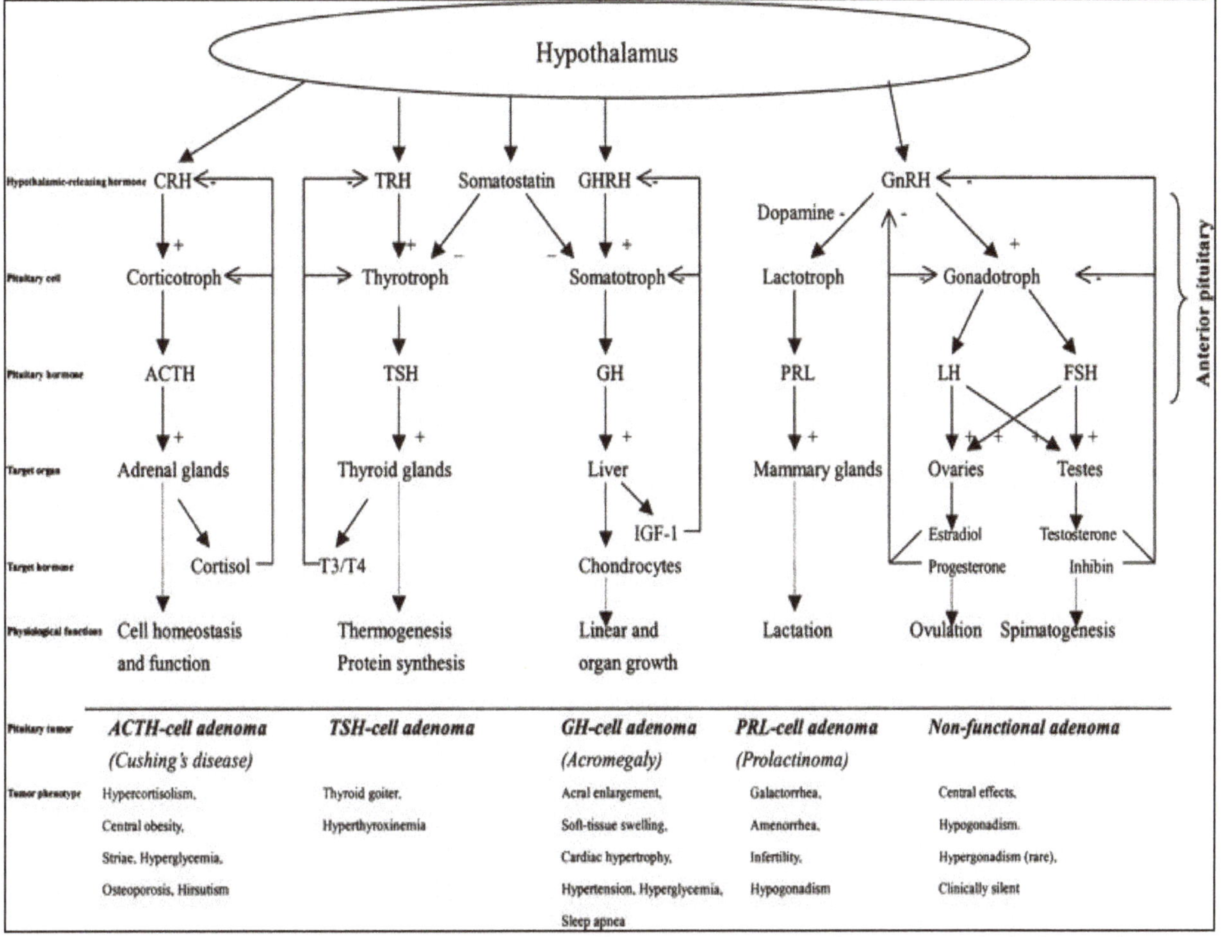

Figure 337 Scheme of the hypothalamic-anterior pituitary-target organ axis systems and pituitary adenoma pathogenesis

11.6.7 Insulin Classification

Table 183 Comprehensive Analysis of Insulin Hormone

Class	Mechanism of Action	Examples	Side Effects
Sulfonylureas	Stimulate the pancreas to release more insulin by binding to the sulfonylurea receptor on beta cells.	Glibenclamide, Glipizide	Hypoglycemia, weight gain, GI disturbances, allergic reactions.
Biguanides	Reduce hepatic glucose production and improve insulin sensitivity in muscle and fat cells.	Metformin	GI disturbances (e.g., diarrhea, nausea), lactic acidosis (rare), vitamin B12 deficiency.
Alpha-Glucosidase Inhibitors	Inhibit enzymes in the intestine that break down carbohydrates, slowing glucose absorption.	Acarbose, Miglitol	Flatulence, diarrhea, abdominal discomfort.

Amylin Mimetics	Mimic amylin to regulate postprandial glucose by slowing gastric emptying and promoting satiety.	Pramlintide	Nausea, vomiting, hypoglycemia (when used with insulin).
Incretin Mimetics	Mimic the action of incretin hormones (GLP-1) to increase insulin release in response to meals and reduce glucagon secretion.	Exenatide, Liraglutide	GI upset (e.g., nausea, diarrhea), risk of pancreatitis.
DPP-4 Inhibitors	Inhibit DPP-4 enzyme, which breaks down incretin hormones, thus enhancing insulin secretion and reducing glucagon levels.	Sitagliptin, Saxagliptin	Upper respiratory tract infections, headache, GI disturbances.
SGLT-2 Inhibitors	Inhibit sodium-glucose co-transporter 2 in the kidneys, reducing glucose reabsorption and increasing urinary glucose excretion.	Empagliflozin, Canagliflozin	Genital infections, urinary tract infections, dehydration, hypotension.

11.6.7.1 Types of Insulin

The chart provides an overview of the different types of insulin based on their duration and intensity of action. It classifies insulin into four categories: **Rapid Acting, Short Acting, Intermediate Acting, and Long Acting. Rapid Acting** insulin starts working within minutes and peaks within 1-2 hours, making it ideal for managing post-meal blood sugar spikes. Short Acting insulin, with a slightly delayed peak, also targets post-meal blood sugar but has a longer duration compared to **Rapid Acting insulin.** Intermediate Acting insulin has an even slower onset and provides a more gradual release of insulin, making it suitable for basal control over a longer period. Finally, Long Acting insulin is designed to work for up to **24 hours**, offering continuous basal insulin coverage. This chart helps to visualize how each type of insulin works over time, assisting healthcare professionals and patients in selecting the appropriate insulin for effective diabetes management.

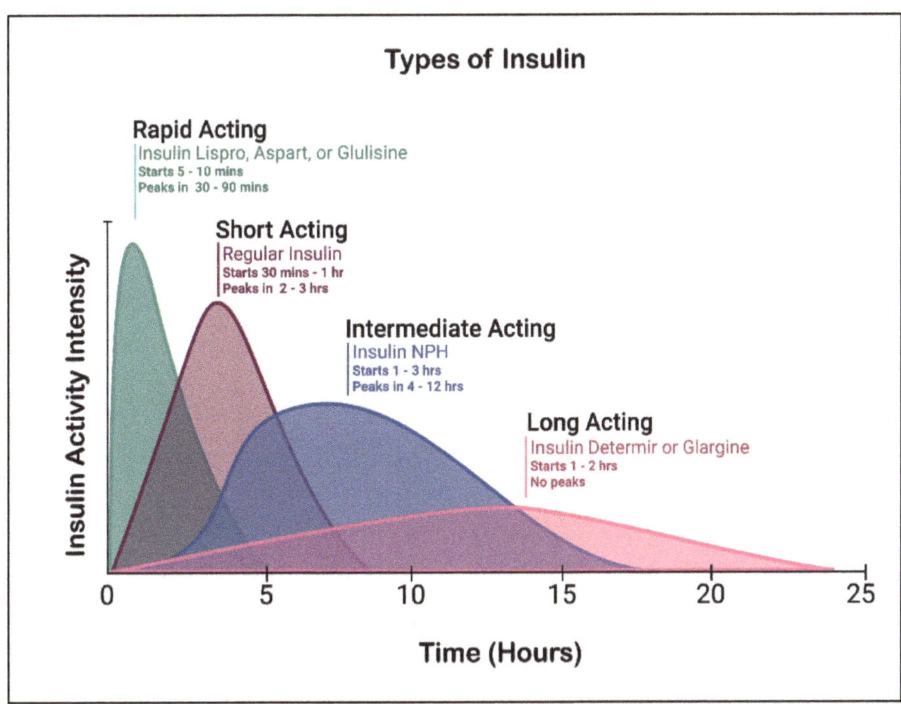

Figure 338 Types of Insulin

11.7 Common Conditions of Endocrine System

Helen's Hungry, Don't Take All Cuddly Snacks." Helen's = Hypothyroidism Hungry = Hyperthyroidism Don't = Diabetes Mellitus Take = Thyroid Cancer All = Addison Disease Cuddly Snacks = Cushing Disease

Table 184 Common Conditions of Endocrine System

Condition	Description	Key Symptoms	Diagnostic Tools	Treatment Options
Hypothyroidism	A condition in which the thyroid gland doesn't produce enough thyroid hormones.	Fatigue, weight gain, cold intolerance, constipation, depression.	Thyroid function tests (TSH, T3, T4), ultrasound, thyroid biopsy.	Levothyroxine replacement therapy, lifestyle changes.
Hyperthyroidism	A condition where the thyroid gland produces too much thyroid hormone.	Weight loss, rapid heartbeat, excessive sweating, tremors, anxiety.	Thyroid function tests (TSH, T3, T4), radioactive iodine uptake test, thyroid scan.	Anti-thyroid medications (methimazole), radioactive iodine therapy, surgery.
Diabetes Mellitus	A condition where the	Increased thirst,	Blood glucose test, HbA1c,	Insulin therapy (Type 1), oral

	body either can't produce enough insulin or can't effectively use the insulin it produces.	frequent urination, unexplained weight loss, fatigue.	oral glucose tolerance test.	medications (Type 2), lifestyle management.
Thyroid Cancer	Cancer of the thyroid gland, typically involving abnormal cell growth.	Lump in the neck, difficulty swallowing, hoarseness, neck pain.	Physical exam, thyroid ultrasound, biopsy, blood tests (calcitonin).	Surgery (thyroidectomy), radioactive iodine therapy, chemotherapy.
Addison Disease	A disorder of the adrenal glands where they produce insufficient cortisol.	Fatigue, weight loss, low blood pressure, salt cravings, skin darkening.	ACTH stimulation test, blood tests (cortisol levels), ACTH levels.	Corticosteroid replacement (hydrocortisone), mineralocorticoids.
Cushing Disease	A condition where the adrenal glands produce excessive cortisol, often due to tumors.	Obesity, high blood pressure, muscle weakness, purple striae, mood changes.	Dexamethasone suppression test, cortisol levels, ACTH levels, imaging (CT/MRI).	Surgical removal of tumors, corticosteroid therapy, medications to control cortisol production.

11.8 Major Medical Conditions of Endocrine System

11.8.1 Hypothyroidism

The medical condition hypothyroidism develops when the thyroid gland produces insufficient levels of **thyroid hormones including thyroxine (T4) and triiodothyronine (T3)**. The body needs these hormones to control metabolic rates as well as assist growth and developmental processes. Such low hormonal levels in the body cause metabolic processes to normalize which results in fatigue and weight gain alongside sensitivity to cold temperatures and constipation and feelings of depression. **Dry skin along with hair thinning and muscle weakness** are additional indications in hypothyroidism manifesting in patients. Hypothyroidism mainly occurs because of **Hashimoto's thyroiditis** which represents an immune system disorder that attacks the thyroid gland. Iodine deficiency together with specific medications and surgical or radiation-induced thyroid gland damage make up other causes of this condition. Medical tests of **thyroid-stimulating hormone (TSH)** and thyroid hormones provide doctors with the evidence needed to confirm hypothyroidism in patients. Patients who receive **hypothyroidism treatment** utilize synthetic thyroid hormone medications including levothyroxine to recover thyroid functionality and lessen their symptoms.

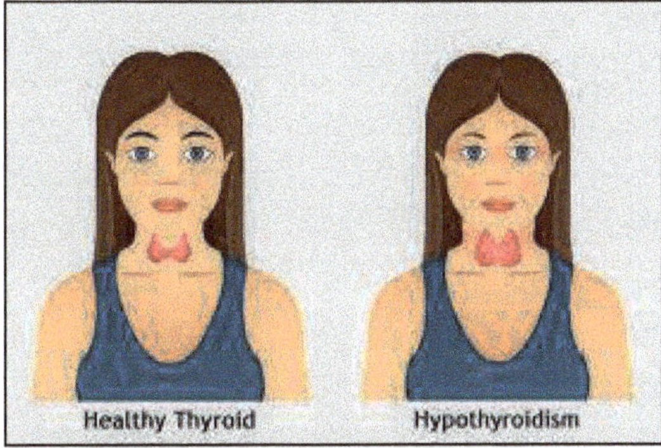

Figure 339 Hypothyroidism

11.8.1.1 Types of Hypothyroidism

The illustration demonstrates primary secondary and tertiary hypothyroidism through their position within the thyroid hormone production pathway. Patients with primary hypothyroidism exhibit a glandular origin that causes insufficient production of thyroid hormones (T4 and T3). When the thyroid fails to **produce enough T4 and T3 hormones**the body releases more TSH to stimulate further hormone production as a compensatory response. The pituitary gland malfunction leads to insufficient TSH release which blocks thyroid stimulation and causes the levels of **T4 and T3** to decrease in secondary hypothyroidism. A problem in the hypothalamus leads to inadequate **thyrotropin-releasing hormone (TRH)** release that diminishes **pituitary TSH production and ultimately results in a deficiency of T4 and T3.** Every classification demonstrates where a failure occurs within the thyroid hormone regulatory system.

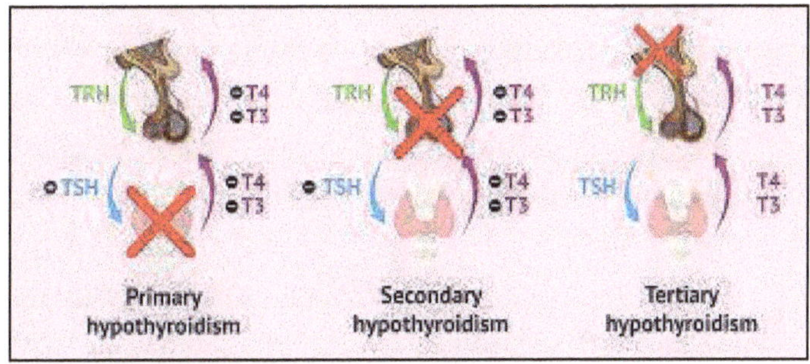

Figure 340 Different Types of Hypothyroidism

[illegible] otes for Hypothyroidism

Table 185 SOAP Notes for Hypothyroidism

Component	Details
Subjective (S)	A 45-year-old female presents with complaints of fatigue, weight gain, and cold intolerance, which have been progressively worsening over the past 2 months. The patient reports feeling constipated and has noticed dry skin and thinning hair. She also mentions experiencing joint pain and muscle weakness. She has no significant past medical history, except for menstrual irregularities, and denies any recent trauma or gastrointestinal symptoms.
Objective (O)	On physical examination, the patient appears fatigued but in no acute distress. Her skin is dry, and her hair is thinning. The pulse is 72 bpm, and blood pressure is 115/75 mmHg. There is no lymphadenopathy, and the lungs are clear on auscultation. Cardiovascular exam is normal, though a slight bradycardia is noted. The abdomen is soft with no hepatosplenomegaly. Reflexes are diminished.
Assessment (A)	The patient's symptoms, including fatigue, weight gain, cold intolerance, constipation, dry skin, and thinning hair, are consistent with hypothyroidism. Given her clinical presentation, further tests are needed to confirm the diagnosis, including thyroid function tests (TSH, T3, T4). If confirmed, primary hypothyroidism due to autoimmune thyroiditis (Hashimoto's thyroiditis) is the most likely etiology.
Plan (P)	**Pharmacological**: Begin levothyroxine (starting dose based on weight and TSH level) to address the suspected hypothyroidism (See algorithm below). **Non-pharmacological**: Advise the patient to maintain a balanced diet, exercise regularly, and manage stress to support thyroid function. **Follow-up**: Schedule a follow-up appointment in 6-8 weeks to reassess TSH levels and evaluate the patient's clinical response to levothyroxine. If symptoms persist, further diagnostic workup may be required. **Education**: Educate the patient on the importance of daily medication adherence, taking levothyroxine on an empty stomach, and avoiding iron or calcium supplements within 4 hours of taking the thyroid medication. Discuss the potential side effects of levothyroxine, such as palpitations or weight loss, and instruct the patient to report any unusual symptoms promptly.

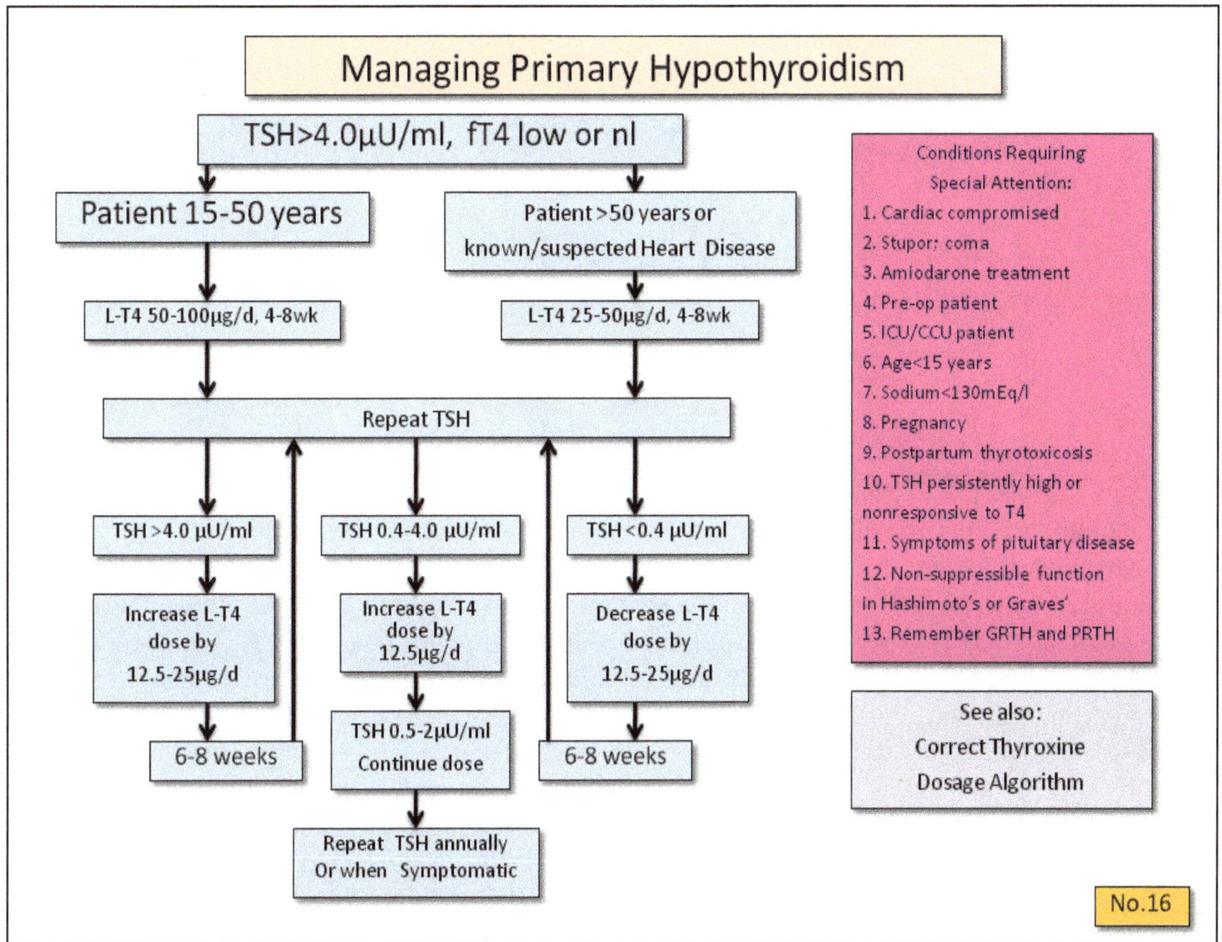

Figure 341 Algorithm for the Management of Hypothyroidism

11.8.2 Hyperthyroidism

The thyroid gland generates excessively high levels of thyroid hormones T4 and T3 during a condition named hyperthyroidism. Body functions increase rapidly because of excessive thyroid hormones which serve to manage body metabolism. Symptoms of hyperthyroidism include unusual weight changes, cardiovascular acceleration and heavy perspiration and shaking movements along with nervousness combined with intolerance to heat. People with hyperthyroidism typically represent themselves through symptoms such as anxiety, fatigue, muscle weakness and bowel movements which occur too often. **Grave's disease represents the main reason behind hyperthyroidism** because it functions as an autoimmune condition that makes the thyroid tissue target itself causing excessive thyroid hormone development. Excessive hormone production occurs in patients with toxic multinodular goiter as well as patients who have toxic adenoma because of a thyroid tumor's benign nature. Secondary hyperthyroidism develops through pituitary gland **TSH overproduction that comes from a pituitary adenoma** thus enacting increased thyroid hormone production. People typically validate a diagnosis by testing blood to check T4 or T3 levels that rise above normal and TSH levels that remain normal or decrease below average. Treatment methods consist of utilizing anti-thyroid medications or performing radioactive iodine therapy or performing surgery based on the specific source of hyperthyroidism. **The treatment of hyperthyroidism requires immediate attention to prevent severe complications including heart disease and osteoporosis alongside thyroid storm** which is an unsafe escalation of symptoms.

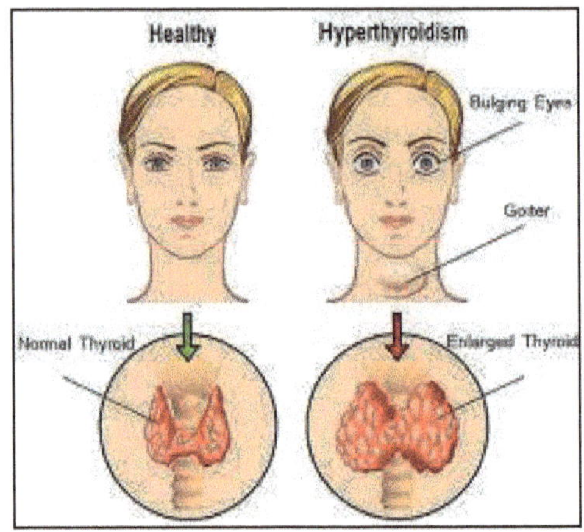

Figure 342 Hyperthyroidism

11.8.2.1 Classification of Hyperthyroidism

The diagram presents fundamental understanding of hyperthyroidism through its primary and secondary classifications followed by an explanation of respective causes alongside diagnostic indications. **Patients with primary hyperthyroidism develop high T4 levels and low TSH levels because their thyroid gland produces too much thyroid hormone T4. Grave's disease** together with toxic multinodular goiter and toxic adenomas represent the main conditions that result in primary hyperthyroidism. The presence of diagnostic markers TSHR-Ab or Anti-TPO Ab serves as evidence to confirm that **Grave's disease causes hyperthyroidism**. Secondary hyperthyroidism happens when TSH goes up resulting in overactive thyroid hormone production at the thyroid gland. A pituitary tumor known as TSH-secreting pituitary adenoma leads to the unwanted secretion of excessive TSH. When pituitary dysfunction arises as the cause of **secondary hyperthyroidism T4 levels increase and TSH stays either normal or elevated**. The diagram establishes key hyperthyroidism origins and diagnostic steps needed to distinguish between main and secondary forms.

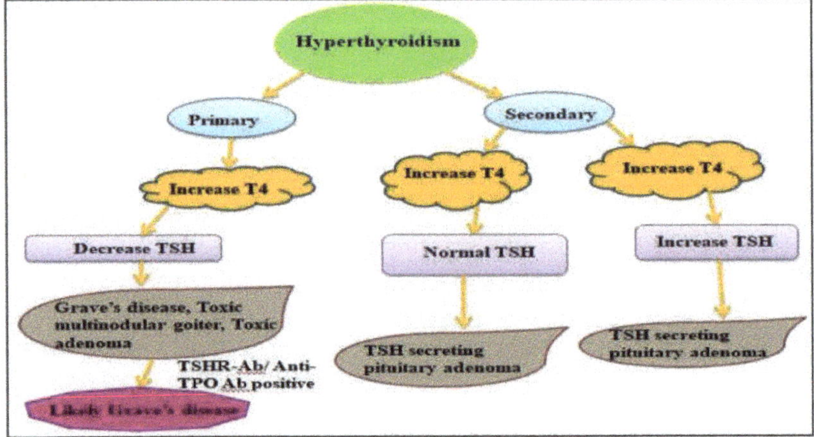

Figure 343 Classification of Hyperthyroidism

11.8.2.2 SOAP Notes for Hyperthyroidism

Table 186 SOAP Notes for Hyperthyroidism

Component	Details
Subjective (S)	A 38-year-old female presents with complaints of weight loss, rapid heartbeat, and increased sweating, which have been progressively worsening over the past 2 months. The patient reports feeling anxious and

	restless, with difficulty sleeping at night. She also notes increased appetite but still has unexplained weight loss. She denies any recent trauma or gastrointestinal issues. Her past medical history is unremarkable.
Objective (O)	On physical examination, the patient appears anxious and restless. Her pulse is 120 bpm, and blood pressure is 130/80 mmHg. Her skin is warm and moist, and there is mild tremor in her hands. The thyroid gland is enlarged with a smooth texture. Cardiovascular exam reveals tachycardia, but no murmurs. The abdomen is soft with no hepatosplenomegaly, and the neurological exam is otherwise normal.
Assessment (A)	The patient's symptoms, including weight loss, tachycardia, increased sweating, anxiety, and tremors, are consistent with hyperthyroidism. Given the clinical presentation, Grave's disease is the most likely diagnosis, though other causes such as toxic multinodular goiter or toxic adenoma should be considered. Further tests, including thyroid function tests (T3, T4, TSH) and thyroid antibodies (TSHR-Ab, Anti-TPO Ab), are needed for confirmation.
Plan (P)	**Pharmacological**: Begin anti-thyroid medications (methimazole or propylthiouracil) to reduce thyroid hormone production (See algorithm below). **Non-pharmacological**: Advise the patient to avoid stimulants (such as caffeine) and manage stress. **Follow-up**: Schedule a follow-up appointment in 4-6 weeks to assess treatment response and monitor thyroid function. If symptoms persist or worsen, consider radioactive iodine therapy or refer for surgical evaluation. **Education**: Educate the patient on the importance of medication adherence, potential side effects of anti-thyroid medications (such as rash or liver toxicity), and the need for regular monitoring of thyroid function.

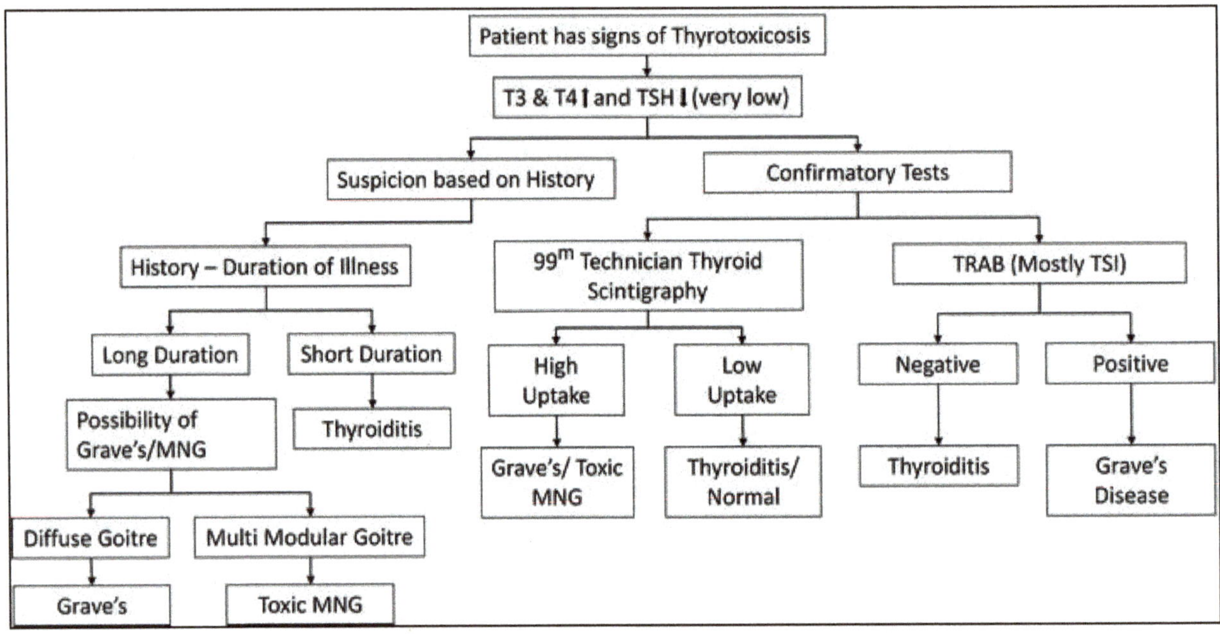

Figure 344 Management Algorithm for Hyperthyroidism

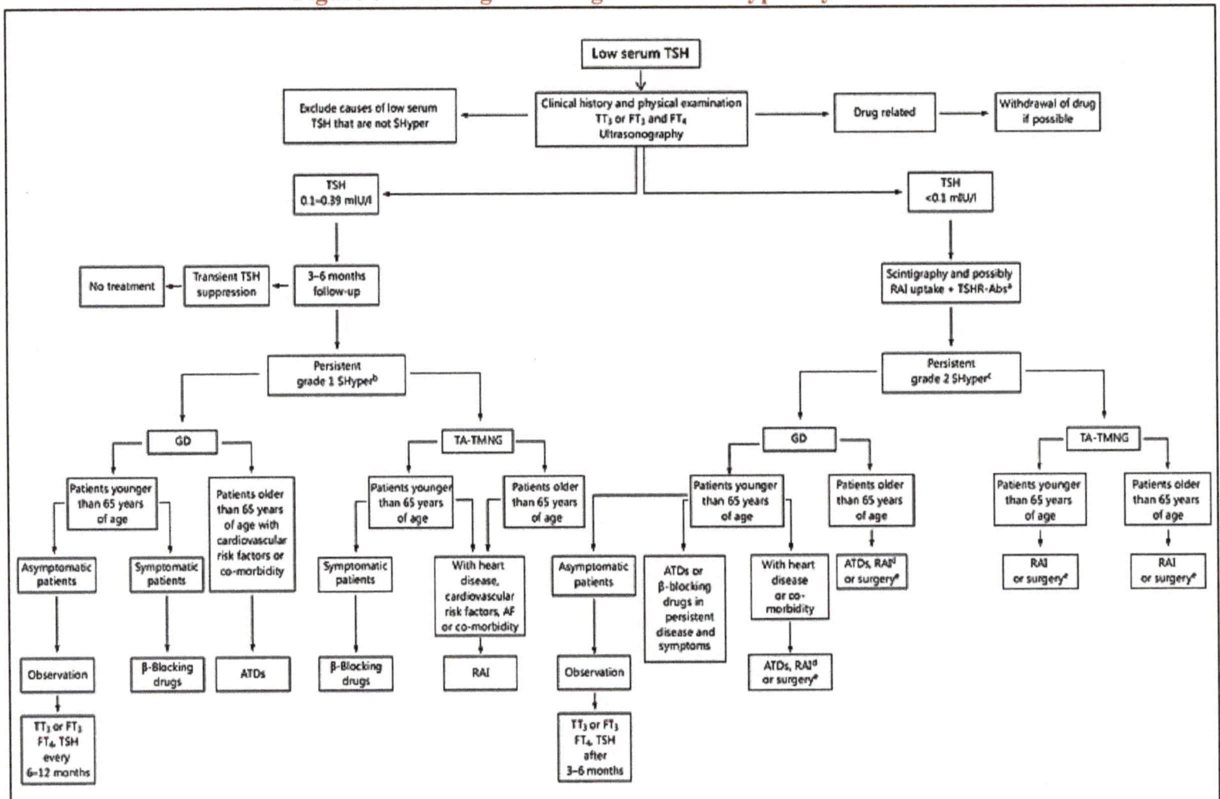

Figure 345 Algorithm for The Management of Subclinical Hyperthyroidism

11.8.3 Diabetes Mellitus

Diabetes mellitus presents as a chronic metabolic condition which manifests when blood glucose reaches elevated levels because the body either lacks sufficient insulin or fails to properly use insulin. The two major types of diabetes include **Type 1 along with Type 2.** The immune system assaults and destroys pancreatic beta cells that produce insulin resulting in Type 1 diabetes which causes little or no insulin production. People with this type develop diabetes either during their childhood years or through their adolescent period. **Type 2 diabetes exists as the most prevalent form of diabetes** because one of two conditions develops: insulin resistance or complete pancreatic insulin deficiency before the body reaches its requirements. Medical indications of diabetes include intense thirst and repeated urination together with unexplained body weight reduction and feeling drained and impaired vision clarity. People with uncontrolled diabetes develop dangerous medical complications which include **heart disease as well as kidney failure, nerve damage and blindness**. Diagnosis is usually made through **blood tests, such as fasting blood glucose, HbA1c, or an oral glucose tolerance test.** Treatment depends on the type of diabetes. Patients with Type 1 diabetes need lifelong insulin therapy yet those with Type 2 diabetes typically control the condition with lifestyle adjustments augmented by oral medications together with possible insulin supplements. The core aspects of diabetes care entail patients to monitor blood glucose levels frequently and **keep diets balanced and exercise regularly** and watch their weight. Medical interventions using insulin injections help treat critical diabetes cases alongside maintaining stable blood glucose levels that reduce health problems.

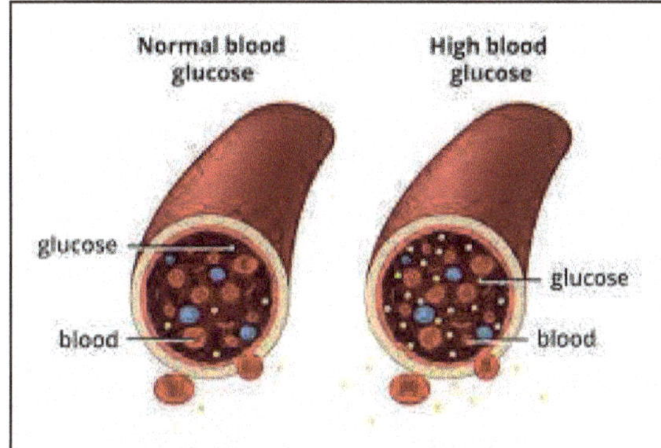

Figure 346 Diabetes Mellitus

11.8.3.1 Pancreas and Diabetes Mellitus

The pancreas exists as a flat gland that sits behind the stomach where its endocrine components regulate blood sugar levels. Inside its structure are the islets of Langerhans that contain beta cells which serve to produce insulin together with alpha cells which create glucagon and delta cells which generate somatostatin. **Hormones from these three cell types work synchronously** to balance blood glucose concentration thus controlling energy metabolism in the body. High blood sugar levels known as hyperglycemia constitute the central features of metabolic disorders which develop because of insulin secretion and action deficiencies. The two categories of diabetes mellitus consist of **Type 1 diabetes that develops from beta cell destruction** through autoimmune processes and **Type 2 diabetes that results from insulin resistance**. Women who develop diabetes during pregnancy go through similar health conditions as Type 2 diabetes patients do. Hyperglycemia that persists over time results in serious medical problems which affect the kidney organs and cause eye damage and nerve damage and tissue loss which requires amputations. **Diagnosis of diabetes relies on high blood glucose values that require reading of fasting plasma glucose ≥ 126 mg/dL coupled with random glucose ≥ 200 mg/dL and HbA1c ≥ 6.5%.** Mid-level diabetic conditions called pre-diabetes can be identified through impaired fasting glucose or glucose tolerance tests. The worldwide health crisis of diabetes receives its highest contributions from India and China.

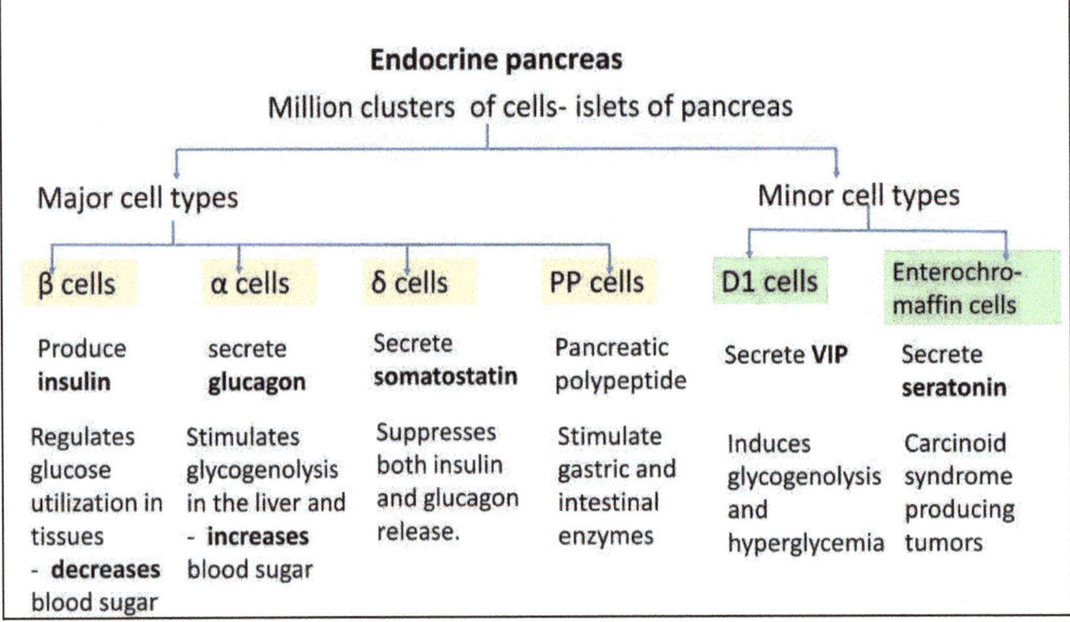

11.8.3.2 Types of Diabetes Mellitus

The images provide an overview of the classification and subtypes of diabetes mellitus. The second figure presents a broad classification of diabetes, including **Type 1 and Type 2 diabetes**, as well as other less common causes such as genetic defects in beta-cell function, genetic defects in **insulin action, exocrine pancreatic defects, endocrinopathies, infections, certain medications, genetic syndromes, and gestational diabetes mellitus.** This highlights the complex and multifactorial nature of diabetes, where various causes contribute to the development of the disease. The second image provides a more detailed breakdown of diabetes mellitus, particularly focusing on Type 1 and Type 2 diabetes. Type 1 diabetes is characterized by absolute **insulin deficiency and destruction of beta cells,** which can further be divided into two subtypes: Type 1A (immune-mediated) and Type 1B (idiopathic). In contrast, Type 2 diabetes is marked by relative insulin deficiency and insulin resistance, which leads to difficulties in glucose regulation. Additionally, gestational diabetes mellitus, a condition that occurs **during pregnancy**, is also classified under this broader category of diabetes. Together, these figures illustrate the diverse nature of diabetes and its classification based on causes, pathophysiology, and progression.

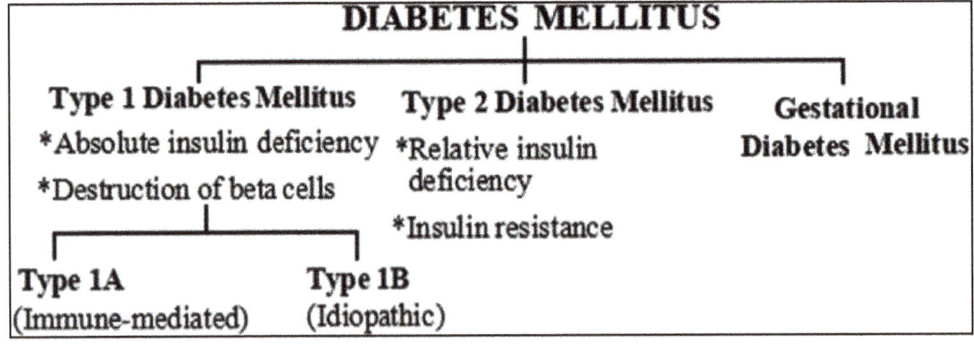

Figure 347 Types of Diabetes Mellitus

CLASSIFICATION OF DIABETES
• Type 1 Diabetes
• Type 2 Diabetes
• Genetic defects of β cell function
• Genetic defects in insulin action
• Exocrine pancreatic defects
• Endocrinopathies
• Infections
• Drugs
• Genetic syndromes associated with Diabetes
• Gestational Diabetes mellitus

Figure 348 Classification of Diabetes

11.8.3.3 Model for the Management of Diabetes

The image establishes an extensive framework for weight management by combining measurement of **body mass index (BMI) with progressive stages of obesity complications and individualized treatment solutions.** The assessment of BMI serves as the initial step in the model to create different groups for individuals based on their BMI values that span from ≤25 to >35. Moving on from BMI assessment comes the process of evaluating complication stages which divide into three stages. The stage assessment **includes unaffected individuals in Stage 1 while Stage 2 applies to patients with prediabetes or hypertension and Stage 3 addresses severe complications.** Follow-up actions for intervention exist for all stages of assessment. Users in Stage 1 receive instructions to maintain their weight or reach it through nutritious eating combined with daily exercise. Levels of complication severity determine appropriate interventions because Stage 2 and Stage 3 patients need intentional caloric deprivation together with structured diets and weight-loss medications which could lead to surgical referral. This system demonstrates that patients need individualized therapeutic approaches to deal with obesity and its connected health issues.

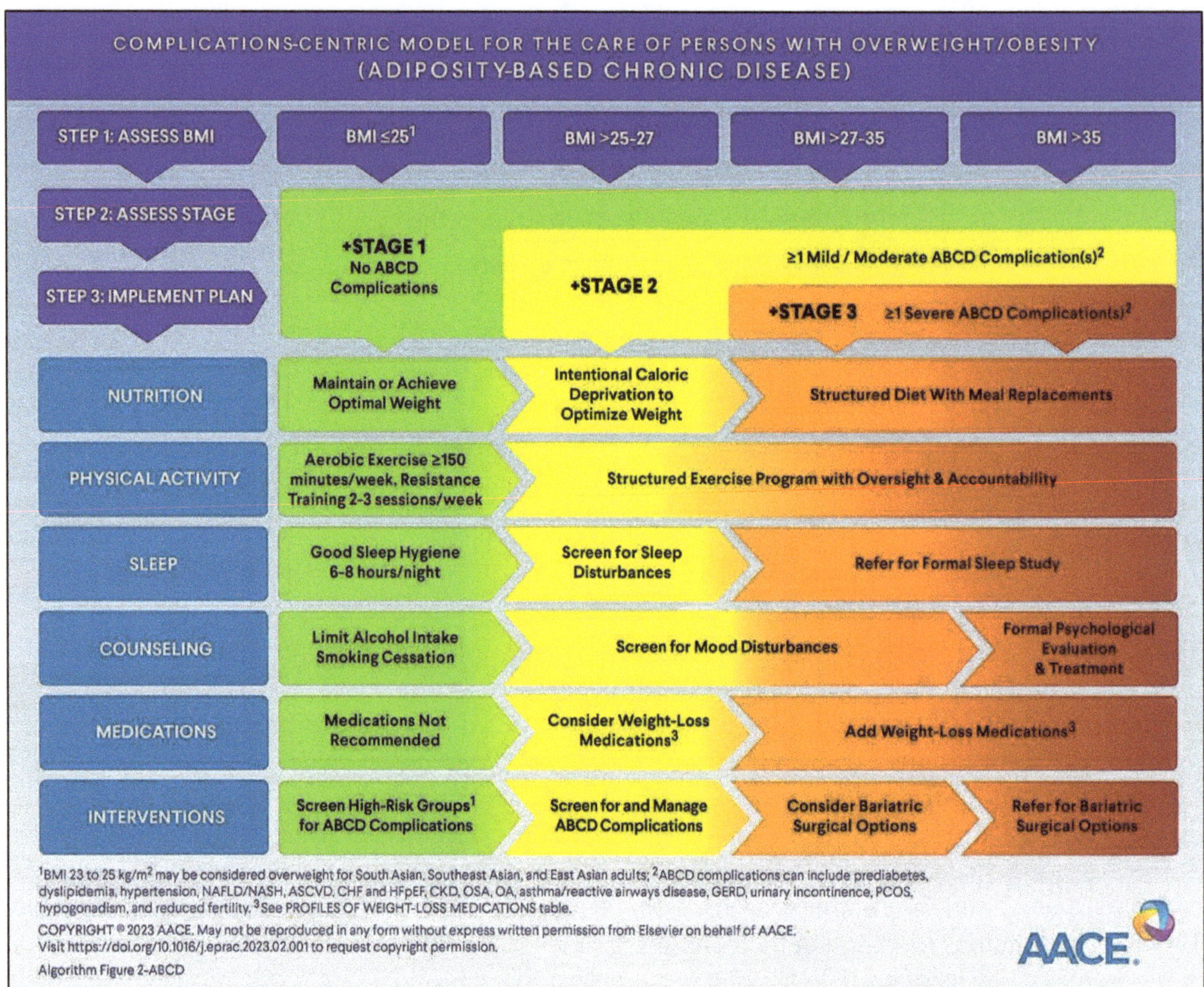

Figure 349 Comprehensive model for managing individuals with overweight or obesity

11.8.3.4 Diabetes Mellitus Medications: Classes, Mechanisms, and Side Effects

Table 187 DM Model of Medication

Class of DM Medication	How It Works	Side Effects
Insulin	- Aspart (fast acting) - Lispro (Humalog) - Glulisine - Humulin R (only for IV use) - Humulin N (Intermediate acting) - Lantus (long acting)	Hypoglycemia, weight gain
Sulfonylureas (e.g., Amaryl)	Increases insulin release from pancreas	Headache, dizziness, weight gain
Glinides	Increases insulin release from the pancreas	Hypoglycemia, weight gain
Biguanides (e.g., Metformin)	Decreases hepatic glucose production, increases insulin sensitivity	GI issues (nausea, diarrhea), lactic acidosis

Thiazolidinediones (TZDs)	Increases insulin sensitivity	Weight gain, edema, increased risk of heart failure
Alpha-glucosidase Inhibitors (e.g., Acarbose)	Inhibits carbohydrate breakdown in the gut	GI issues (flatulence, diarrhea)
Amylin Mimics (e.g., Pramlintide)	Slows gastric emptying, reduces appetite	Nausea, hypoglycemia
Incretin Mimics (e.g., GLP-1 Agonists like Exenatide)	Stimulates insulin release, slows gastric emptying, reduces appetite	Nausea, vomiting, weight loss
Dipeptidyl Peptidase-4 Inhibitors (DPP-4 Inhibitors) (e.g., Januvia)	Increases incretin levels, which stimulate insulin release	Headache, upper respiratory infections
SGLT-2 Inhibitors (e.g., Canagliflozin)	Increases glucose excretion via the kidneys	Increased urination, dehydration, urinary tract infections

11.8.3.5 SOAP Notes for Diabetes Mellitus

Table 188 SOAP Notes for Diabetes

Component	Details
Subjective (S)	A 50-year-old male presents with complaints of increased thirst, frequent urination, unexplained weight loss, and fatigue over the past few months. He reports feeling more tired than usual and has noticed a delay in wound healing. He also mentions blurred vision occasionally. The patient has a family history of diabetes and has been eating a high-carbohydrate diet. He denies any recent trauma or infections.
Objective (O)	On physical examination, the patient appears slightly fatigued but in no acute distress. His skin is dry, and there are mild signs of dehydration. The pulse is 88 bpm, and blood pressure is 135/85 mmHg. No lymphadenopathy is noted, and the lungs are clear on auscultation. His abdomen is soft with no hepatosplenomegaly. Neurological examination reveals no abnormal findings, although a slight reduction in sensation in the feet is observed.
Assessment (A)	The patient's symptoms, including polyuria, polydipsia, weight loss, fatigue, and blurred vision, are highly suggestive of diabetes mellitus. Given his family history and lifestyle factors, Type 2 diabetes is the most likely diagnosis. Diagnostic tests, including fasting blood glucose, HbA1c, and an oral glucose tolerance test, are recommended for confirmation.
Plan (P)	**Pharmacological**: Initiate metformin 500 mg daily to help manage blood glucose levels. **Non-pharmacological**: Advise the patient on lifestyle changes, including dietary modifications (low glycemic index foods), regular exercise, and weight management. **Follow-up**: Schedule a follow-up

	appointment in 2 weeks to assess glucose control and evaluate any potential side effects from medication. **Education**: Educate the patient about diabetes management, including monitoring blood glucose levels, the importance of medication adherence, recognizing symptoms of hypoglycemia, and maintaining a healthy diet and exercise routine. Encourage the patient to attend a diabetes education program for further guidance.

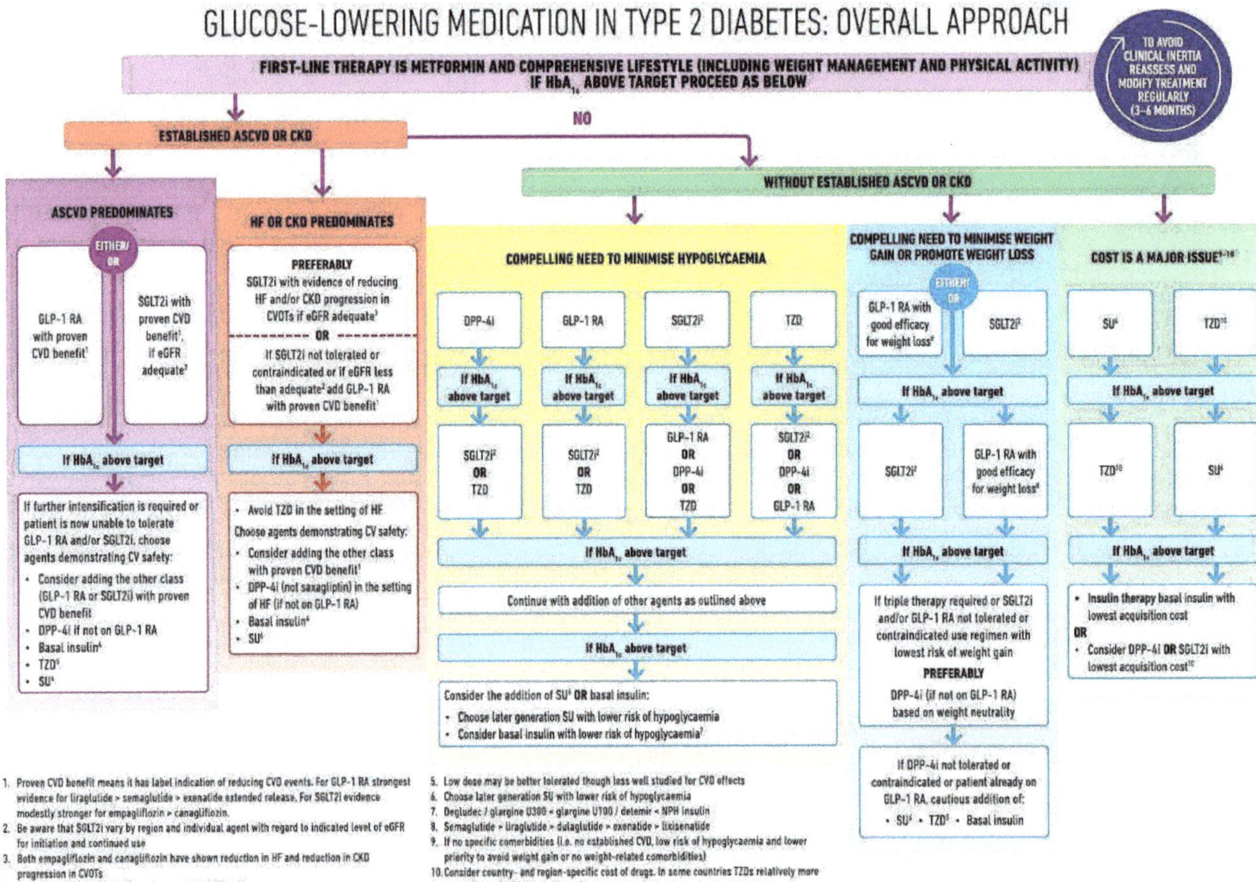

Figure 350 Overall Approach for the Management of Diabetes

11.8.4 Thyroid Cancer

Thyroid cancer emerges within the thyroid gland which exists in the neck region to produce the hormones required for regulating metabolism and growth. Thyroid tissue contains follicular cells that generate **thyroid hormones together with parafollicular cells that release calcitonin**. The follicular cells normally produce thyroid cancer because genetic mutations combine with exposure to radiation and environmental elements. **The condition normally occurs in adult women within the 30 to 50-year age range**. The main thyroid cancer types include papillary thyroid cancer that occurs frequently and carries beneficial results while follicular thyroid cancer exists as a less common variety which medical teams can effectively treat. The two less common types of thyroid cancer include **medullary thyroid cancer that develops from parafollicular cells and anaplastic thyroid cancer** which is an extremely aggressive with severe outcomes.

The typical indicators of having thyroid cancer consist of a lump without discomfort in the **neck region along with problems in swallowing, breathing issues, hoarseness and occasionally pain that affects the neck or throat.** Most thyroid cancer cases identify without producing any symptoms thus getting discovered during regular medical tests performed to evaluate other health problems. A physical examination combined with blood hormone testing together with **ultrasound imaging and biopsy through FNA determines thyroid cancer diagnosis.** Medical professionals sometimes utilize genetic testing to detect mutations which are specific to specific thyroid cancer types. The treatment plan for thyroid cancer requires consideration of patient health status combined with disease stage and diagnostic type. A thyroidectomy stands as the principal treatment for most thyroid cancer cases **because it removes the thyroid gland from the body**. The medical procedure of giving radioactive iodine therapy follows surgery to destroy cancerous cells which remain in the body. When dealing with anaplastic thyroid cancers physicians need to **combine chemotherapy with radiation therapy**. Thyroid cancer shows favorable outcomes when considering its following stages especially for patients with papillary and follicular types because they experience high survival rates. **Continuous monitoring must be maintained because recurrence might occur.**

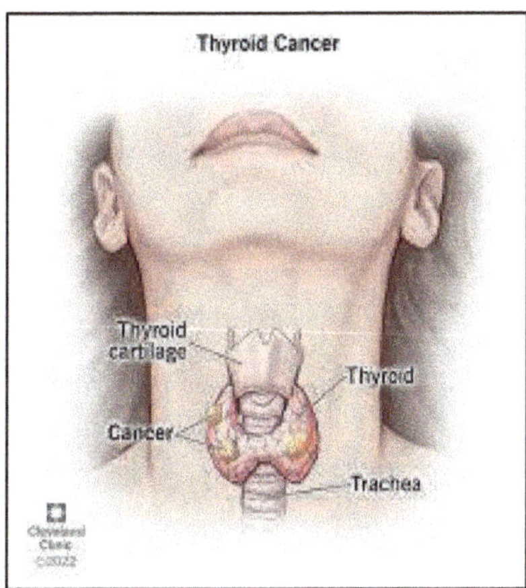

Figure 351 Thyroid Cancer

11.8.4.1 Types of Thyroid Cancer

The diagram presents a summary of thyroid cancer subtypes which depend on the cellular origin within thyroid gland tissue. Main thyroid gland tissue contains both follicular epithelial cells and **parafollicular (C) cells.** The hormone-producing follicular epithelial cells determine the origin of **differentiated thyroid cancer (DTC)** because they give rise to this cancer type. DTC encompasses two main types: **papillary thyroid cancer (PTC)** that makes up 70%-80% of cases together with **follicular thyroid cancer (FTC)** which forms 10%-15% of cases. Most thyroid cancer cases develop from well-differentiated cells leading to favorable treatment outcomes. Other thyroid cancers make up a tiny portion of total cases because they appear less frequently. The majority of thyroid cancer cases arise from parafollicular C cells leading to a condition known as **medullary thyroid cancer (MTC)** while this cancer represents only 5%-10% of all thyroid cancers. Undifferentiated thyroid cancer has two rare but aggressive forms in the diagram including **anaplastic thyroid cancer (ATC)** that exists as less than 2% of all cases.

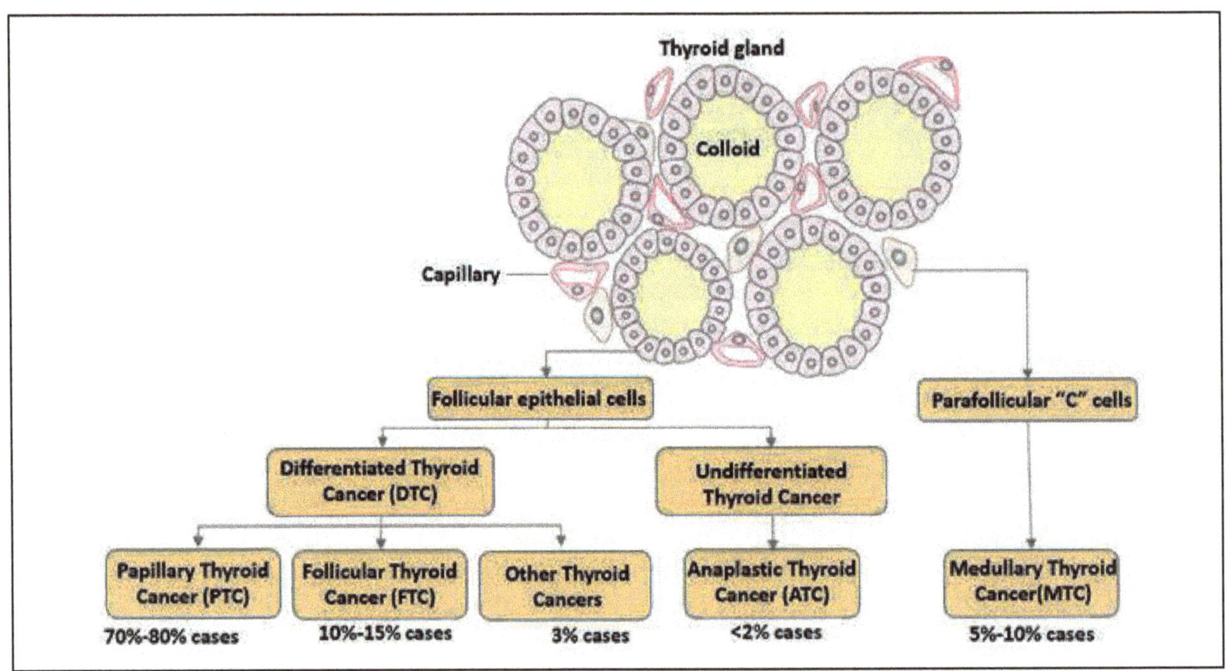

Figure 352 Types of Thyroid Cancer

11.8.4.2 SOAP Notes for Thyroid Cancer

Table 189 SOAP Notes for Thyroid Cancer

Component	Details
Subjective (S)	A 50-year-old female presents with a painless lump in the neck, which she noticed a few weeks ago. She also reports recent difficulty swallowing and occasional hoarseness. The patient denies pain, trauma, or recent infections. She has no significant medical history but mentions a family history of thyroid problems. She is concerned about the lump and is seeking further evaluation.
Objective (O)	On physical examination, a firm, non-tender nodule is palpated on the right side of the neck. No signs of lymphadenopathy are noted. The patient's vital signs are stable, with a blood pressure of 120/78 mmHg and a pulse rate of 80 bpm. The thyroid gland is enlarged, and a slight hoarseness is noted upon speaking. No signs of respiratory distress or stridor are present.
Assessment (A)	The patient's symptoms, including a painless neck lump and hoarseness, are concerning for possible thyroid cancer. Based on the physical exam, a thyroid nodule is present, which warrants further investigation with imaging (ultrasound) and a fine-needle aspiration biopsy (FNA) for a definitive diagnosis. The differential diagnosis includes papillary thyroid cancer (PTC), follicular thyroid cancer (FTC), or medullary thyroid cancer (MTC), with PTC being the most likely.
Plan (P)	**Pharmacological**: No medications are indicated at this time (See algorithm below). **Non-pharmacological**: Recommend ultrasound imaging of the thyroid to assess the nodule size, characteristics, and any lymph node involvement. **Follow-up**: Schedule a follow-up appointment to discuss the

results of the ultrasound and FNA biopsy. **Education**: Educate the patient on the importance of biopsy for diagnosing thyroid cancer and explain the next steps in treatment, which may include surgery (thyroidectomy) depending on the biopsy results. Discuss the potential side effects of surgery and the likelihood of good prognosis if the cancer is detected early.

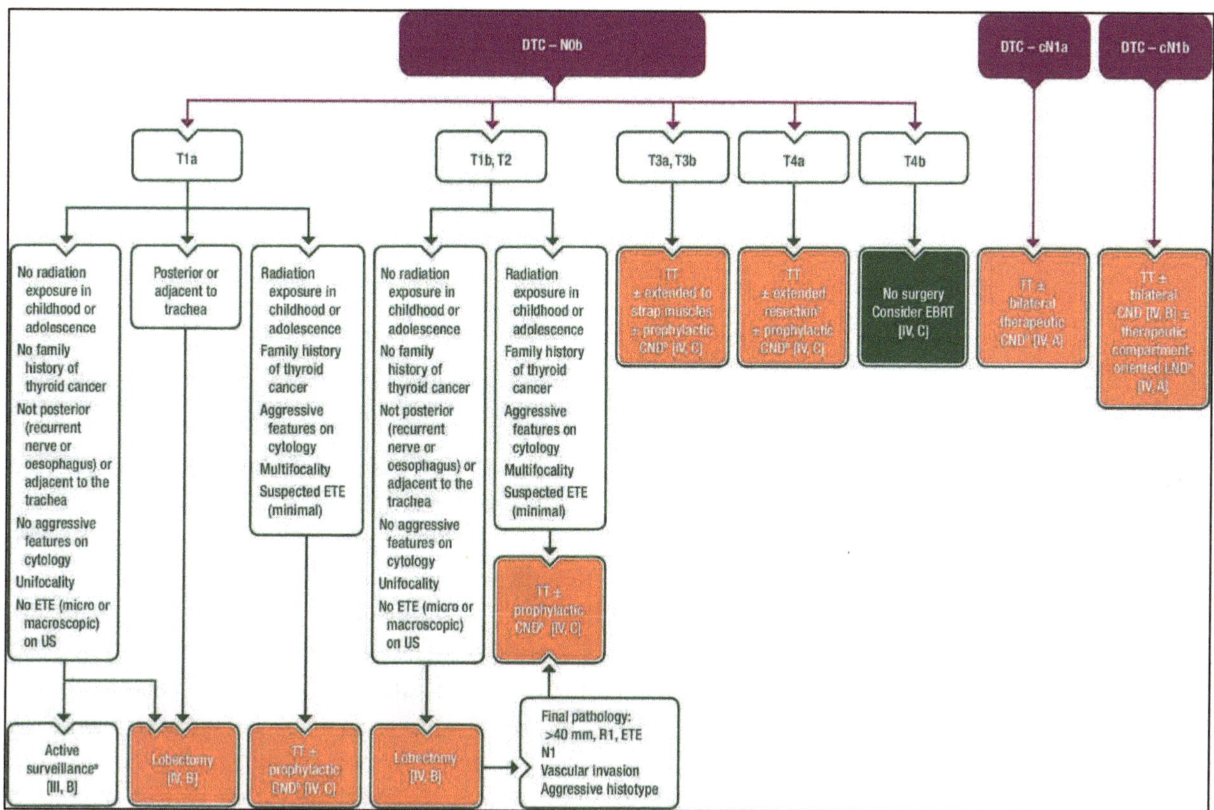

Figure 353 Algorithm for the Management of Differentiated Thyroid Cancer

11.8.5 Addison Disease

The medical condition Addison's disease also known as primary adrenal insufficiency represents a **rare disorder characterized by low cortisol and aldosterone production** in the adrenal glands. The two adrenal glands situated above the kidneys create necessary hormones which **modulate metabolic processes and immune** function and stress response. Addison's disease happens when the adrenal cortex sustains damage from an **autoimmune response** which makes the body attack its own adrenal glands. Other possible causes for this condition are infections along with tuberculosis or when cancer spreads to the area. Patients with Addison's disease develop their **symptoms slowly and experience** persistent tiredness alongside body weakness and weight reduction and blood pressure decrease and light-headedness after standing up and increased salt appetite together with skin pigmentation changes. The human body develops these symptoms when cortisol and aldosterone remain in insufficient levels. Medical tests show low cortisol activity together with high **ACTH activity to establish diagnosis and sometimes reveal low aldosterone levels.** Patients with this diagnosis receive two types of hormone replacement therapy through oral corticosteroids which duplicate cortisol structure as well as the need for mineralocorticoids that serve as aldosterone substitutes. Addison's disease becomes life-threatening when it leads to adrenal crisis which needs prompt IV fluids and corticosteroids for emergency treatment.

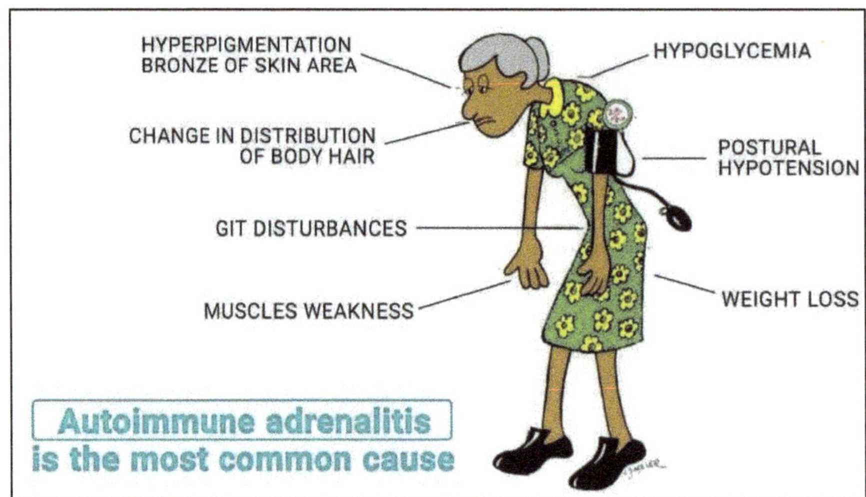

Figure 354 Addison's Disease

11.8.5.1 Addison's Disease Classification

This schematic illustration demonstrates the primary reasons that cause Addison's disease through autoimmune disorders and infections alongside other potential factors. **The Western world mainly records autoimmune adrenalitis as the primary reason behind Addison's disease**. The immune system of the body attacks the adrenal glands without reason in this form leading to diminished cortisol and aldosterone production. The most prevalent infectious mechanism which causes adrenal gland damage is **tuberculosis (TB)** under the specific condition of infective adrenalitis. Apart from TB the disease can stem from HIV infections as well as fungal and syphilis infections. **Hemorrhage from meningitis and malignant cancer** spread to adrenal tissue are among the other listed causes under this category. Insufficient hormone production resulting from adrenal gland damage caused by the various causes of this **disease produces symptoms and complications similar to Addison's disease.**

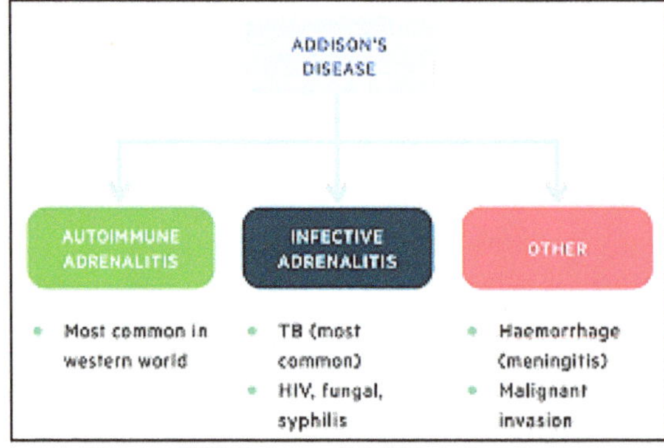

Figure 355 Types of Addison's Disease

11.8.5.2 SOAP Notes for Addison's Disease

Table 190 SOAP Notes for Addison's Disease

Component	Details
Subjective (S)	A 45-year-old female presents with complaints of chronic fatigue, weight loss, muscle weakness, and dizziness, which have been progressively

	worsening over the past 2 months. She mentions experiencing salt cravings and has noticed darkening of her skin, particularly around her joints. The patient reports that she often feels lightheaded, especially when standing up. She denies any recent infections, trauma, or significant medical history except for occasional joint pain.
Objective (O)	On physical examination, the patient appears fatigued but is in no acute distress. Her skin appears hyperpigmented, especially on her elbows, knuckles, and the folds of her skin. Blood pressure is 90/60 mmHg, with a slight postural drop. Pulse is 85 bpm. No signs of lymphadenopathy or organomegaly are noted. Reflexes are normal, but the patient reports mild muscle weakness. The abdominal exam reveals no tenderness or masses.
Assessment (A)	The patient's symptoms, including fatigue, weight loss, salt cravings, and hyperpigmentation, are suggestive of Addison's disease. The most likely etiology is autoimmune adrenalitis, as it is the most common cause in the Western world. Infectious causes such as tuberculosis, HIV, or fungal infections could also be considered, though the patient has no relevant exposure history. Further tests, including ACTH stimulation tests, serum cortisol levels, and adrenal antibody testing, are necessary for confirmation.
Plan (P)	**Pharmacological**: Begin hydrocortisone replacement therapy (15-25 mg/day), and consider fludrocortisone for mineralocorticoid replacement if necessary (See algorithm below). **Non-pharmacological**: Advise the patient to increase sodium intake to compensate for aldosterone deficiency. **Follow-up**: Schedule follow-up in 2 weeks to assess the patient's response to treatment and monitor for side effects. **Education**: Educate the patient about Addison's disease, the importance of medication adherence, and how to manage an adrenal crisis. Discuss how to recognize symptoms of acute adrenal insufficiency and the need for emergency care. Consider testing for infectious causes, such as tuberculosis, depending on the results of initial tests.

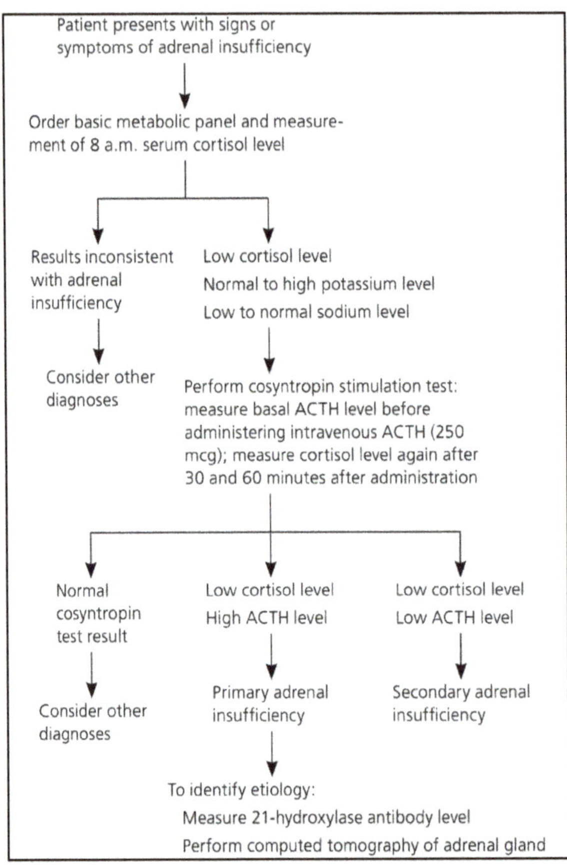

Figure 356 Treatment Management Algorithm for Addison's Disease

11.8.6 Cushing Disease

Cushing's syndrome arises due to ongoing high cortisol levels in body systems which emerge from continuing corticosteroid drugs or tumors that make **cortisol or adrenocorticotropic hormone (ACTH).** The hormone cortisol originates from adrenal glands and serves as a regulatory agent for metabolism and immune responses as well as stress reaction control. A high amount of cortisol production causes different health complications to appear. **Cushing's syndrome creates two distinctive symptoms because patients gain weight rapidly above their chests and stomach areas but maintain lean extremities.** This pattern results in moon face along with buffalo hump. The combination of high blood pressure with muscle weakness and easy bleeding and skin thinning and purple stretch marks form among the symptoms of this condition. The hormone imbalance causes menstrual irregularities and leads to excessive hair growth in women. **Osteoporosis and diabetes** along with **infection susceptibility as potential complications of severe Cushing's syndrome.** A healthcare professional diagnoses Cushing syndrome through blood tests and urine tests that measure cortisol and imaging scans that **identify tumor locations**. The main approach to treatment depends on the cause that requires the reduction of steroids and the removal of tumors by surgical procedures or medications which block cortisol release in the body.

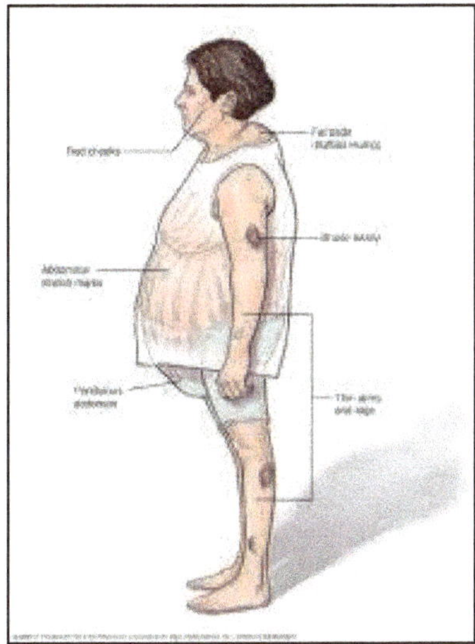

Figure 357 Cushing Syndrome

11.8.6.1 Types of Cushing Syndrome

Cushing's syndrome exists in two major forms that are ACTH-dependent and ACTH-independent as indicated in this diagram. Cushing's syndrome with ACTH dependence develops when **adrenocorticotropic hormone (ACTH)** secretion increases leading to excessive cortisol production by the adrenal glands. A pituitary adenoma represents the main reason for ACTH-dependent Cushing's syndrome and medical experts call it Cushing's disease because benign **pituitary gland tumors release elevated levels of ACTH.** Bronchial carcinomas along with other tumors can produce ACTH independently from the pituitary gland thus becoming known as ectopic ACTH-producing tumors. The occurrence of Cushing's syndrome without ACTH participation represents the condition known as **ACTH-independent Cushing's syndrome**. Long-term therapeutic administration of corticosteroids results in overproduction of cortisol leading to this condition. The production of cortisol becomes uncontrolled when an adrenal tumor like **an adrenal adenoma or carcinoma** exists within the body. People with Cushing's syndrome experience similar clinical signs from cortisol excess although their specific origins and treatment plans differ between each subgroups.

11.8.6.2 SOAP Notes for Cushing Syndrome

Table 191 SOAP Notes for Cushing Syndrome

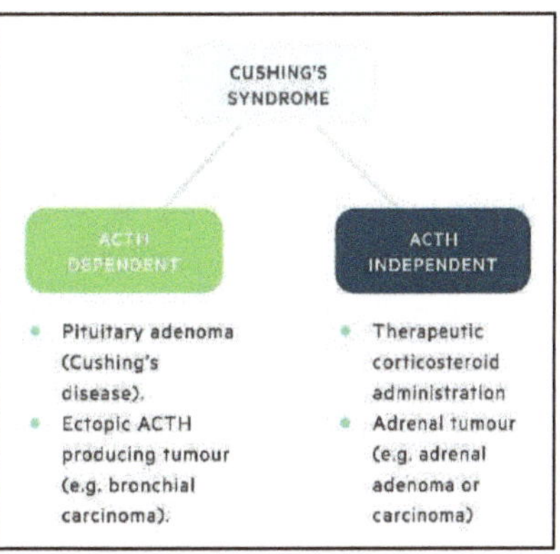

Figure 358 Types of Cushing Syndrome

Component	Details

Subjective (S)	A 45-year-old male presents with complaints of recent weight gain, particularly in the abdomen and face, and reports a "moon face" appearance. He mentions experiencing fatigue, increased thirst, frequent urination, and difficulty sleeping. He also notes that his skin has become more fragile, with easy bruising and the development of purple stretch marks on his abdomen. He has a history of long-term corticosteroid use for asthma.
Objective (O)	On physical examination, the patient appears overweight with noticeable central obesity and a rounded face (moon face). Skin shows multiple purple striae and easy bruising. Blood pressure is 145/90 mmHg, and pulse is 95 bpm. The abdomen is soft, with no signs of hepatomegaly. The neurological exam is unremarkable, but there is mild muscle weakness noted in the lower extremities. Reflexes are normal.
Assessment (A)	The patient's symptoms, including weight gain, "moon face," abdominal striae, skin thinning, and easy bruising, are indicative of Cushing's syndrome. Given his history of prolonged corticosteroid use, this is likely ACTH-independent Cushing's syndrome due to therapeutic corticosteroid administration. However, further testing is needed to confirm this, including 24-hour urinary free cortisol, late-night salivary cortisol, and imaging studies to rule out any adrenal tumors.
Plan (P)	**Pharmacological**: Recommend tapering corticosteroid use under medical supervision, if applicable, and consider adjusting asthma management (See algorithm below). **Non-pharmacological**: Advise weight management, a balanced diet, and regular exercise to help manage symptoms. **Follow-up**: Schedule follow-up in 2-3 weeks to assess the patient's response to medication changes and to discuss results of diagnostic tests (e.g., cortisol levels and adrenal imaging). **Education**: Educate the patient about the effects of prolonged corticosteroid use and the importance of monitoring symptoms. Discuss possible alternative treatments for asthma to reduce cortisol exposure.

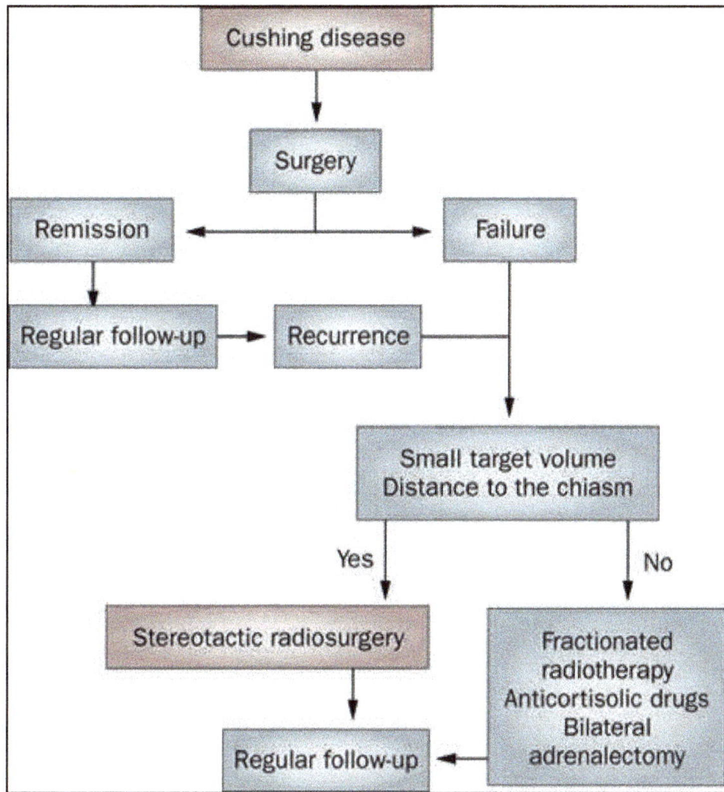

Figure 359 Algorithm for the Management of Cushing Syndrome

11.9 Moh Golden Points and Summary Question Answers

11.9.1 Moh Golden Points

Thyroid cancer diagnosis and types: Papillary thyroid cancer (PTC) is the most common type, while medullary thyroid cancer (MTC) arises from parafollicular cells. Fine-needle aspiration (FNA) and ultrasound are essential for diagnosis.

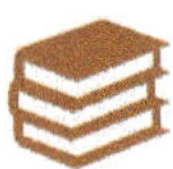

Addison's disease management: Addison's disease results from adrenal insufficiency and is most commonly caused by autoimmune adrenalitis. Corticosteroid replacement is the primary treatment.

Cushing's syndrome: Can be classified into ACTH-dependent and ACTH-independent categories. ACTH-dependent includes pituitary adenomas (Cushing's disease), while ACTH-independent can result from exogenous corticosteroid use or adrenal tumors.

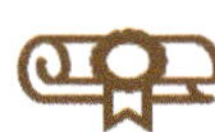

Diabetes Mellitus: Type 1 diabetes is an autoimmune condition leading to beta cell destruction, whereas Type 2 diabetes is primarily due to insulin resistance and is commonly associated with obesity and lifestyle factors.

Hypothyroidism: Characterized by fatigue, weight gain, and cold intolerance, hypothyroidism is often caused by autoimmune thyroiditis (Hashimoto's). Levothyroxine is the mainstay treatment.

Hyperthyroidism: Often caused by Grave's disease or toxic goiter, hyperthyroidism leads to weight loss, palpitations, and tremors. Treatment includes anti-thyroid medications, radioactive iodine therapy, or surgery.

Pancreatic endocrine function: The pancreas regulates blood glucose through insulin (from beta cells) and glucagon (from alpha cells). Dysregulation leads to diabetes mellitus.

11.9.2 Summary Questions & Answers

1 Which of the following is the most common cause of hyperthyroidism?
a) Hashimoto's thyroiditis
b) Graves' disease
c) Toxic multinodular goiter
d) Thyroid carcinoma

2. Which hormone is primarily deficient in Addison's disease?
a) Thyroxine
b) Insulin
c) Cortisol
d) Aldosterone

3. The most common type of thyroid cancer is:
a) Anaplastic thyroid cancer
b) Medullary thyroid cancer
c) Papillary thyroid cancer
d) Follicular thyroid cancer

4. What is the mainstay treatment for hypothyroidism?
a) Methimazole
b) Radioactive iodine
c) Levothyroxine
d) Prednisone

5. Which condition is associated with moon face and central obesity?
a) Addison's disease
b) Hyperthyroidism
c) Cushing's syndrome
d) Diabetes mellitus

6. Which of the following is a common cause of secondary hypothyroidism?
a) Pituitary adenoma
b) Hashimoto's thyroiditis
c) Thyroidectomy
d) Iodine deficiency

7 In Type 2 diabetes, what is the primary pathophysiological defect?
a) Insulin resistance
b) Insulin deficiency
c) Beta cell destruction
d) Excess glucagon secretion

8. Which of the following is a characteristic of Addison's disease?
a) Hyperpigmentation
b) Weight gain
c) Tachycardia
d) Hypertension

9. The diagnostic test for Cushing's syndrome includes which of the following?
a) ACTH stimulation test
b) Serum cortisol levels
c) Thyroid function test
d) HbA1c

10. Which type of thyroid cancer originates from parafollicular cells?
a) Follicular thyroid cancer
b) Medullary thyroid cancer
c) Papillary thyroid cancer
d) Anaplastic thyroid cancer

11.9.3 Rationales

1.Answer: b) Graves' disease
Rationale: Graves' disease is the most common cause of hyperthyroidism, characterized by autoimmune stimulation of the thyroid gland.

2. **Answer: c) Cortisol**
Rationale: Addison's disease is characterized by adrenal insufficiency, resulting in a deficiency of cortisol, and sometimes aldosterone.

3. **Answer: c) Papillary thyroid cancer**
Rationale: Papillary thyroid cancer (PTC) is the most common form, accounting for 70%-80% of thyroid cancers.

4. **Answer c) Levothyroxine**
Rationale: Levothyroxine is the synthetic form of thyroid hormone used to replace deficient thyroid hormones in hypothyroidism.

5. **Answer: c) Cushing's syndrome**
Rationale: Cushing's syndrome, due to excess cortisol, leads to distinctive features such as moon face and central obesity.

6. **Answer: a) Pituitary adenoma**
Rationale: Secondary hypothyroidism is typically caused by pituitary dysfunction, such as a pituitary adenoma, leading to reduced TSH production.

7. **Answer a) Insulin resistance**
Rationale: Type 2 diabetes is primarily due to insulin resistance, with the pancreas initially producing sufficient insulin but the body failing to respond properly.

8. Answer: **a) Hyperpigmentation**
Rationale: Hyperpigmentation, particularly in skin folds, is a hallmark feature of Addison's disease due to increased ACTH levels.

9. Answer: b) Serum cortisol levels
Rationale: Elevated cortisol levels, especially after testing, help diagnose Cushing's syndrome, and the dexamethasone suppression test may be used to confirm the diagnosis.

10. Answer: **b) Medullary thyroid cancer**
Rationale: Medullary thyroid cancer originates from the parafollicular cells of the thyroid, which secrete calcitonin.

12 Chapter 12: Head, Eyes, Ears, Nose, and Throat (HEENT)

12.1 Anatomy and Physiology of HEENT System

The HEENT system refers to the head, eyes, ears, nose, and throat, which are interconnected structures that play crucial roles in various bodily functions such as sensory perception, breathing, communication, and immune defense.

Head: The head houses the brain, which is the central control system for the body. The skull, made up of several bones, protects the brain, eyes, and ears. Additionally, the face contains the muscles responsible for facial expressions and masticatory function (chewing).

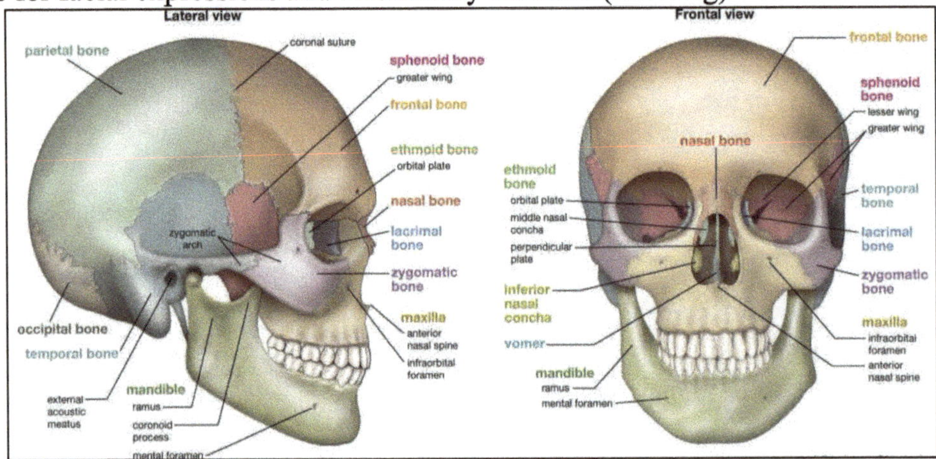

Figure 360 Anatomy of Head

Eyes: The eyes are the organs responsible for vision. They consist of structures like the cornea, lens, retina, and optic nerve, all of which work together to capture light and convert it into visual signals that are sent to the brain for interpretation. The eyelids and lacrimal glands also provide protection and moisture to the eyes.

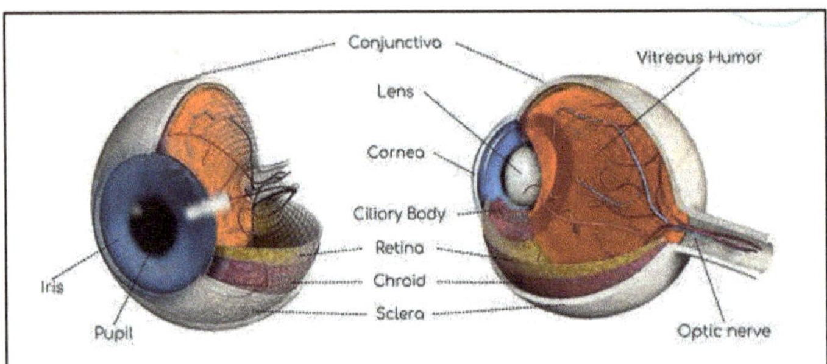

Figure 361 Anatomy of an Eye

Ears: The ears are responsible for hearing and balance. The outer ear collects sound waves, which are then transmitted through the middle ear to the inner ear, where sound is converted into nerve impulses for the brain. The inner ear also contains the vestibular system, which helps with maintaining balance and spatial orientation.

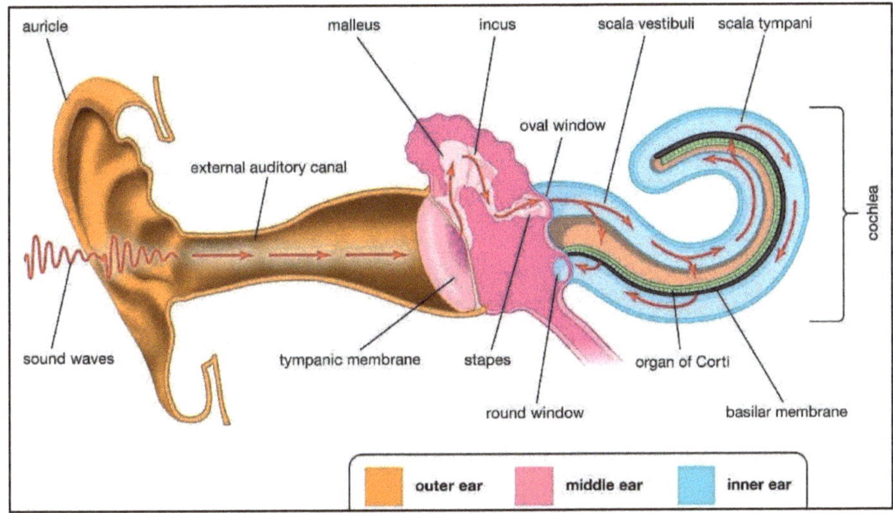

Figure 362 Anatomy and Physiology of Ear

Nose: The nose serves as the primary organ for breathing and smelling. It filters, warms, and humidifies the air before it enters the lungs. The nasal cavity also houses the olfactory receptors, which are responsible for the sense of smell.

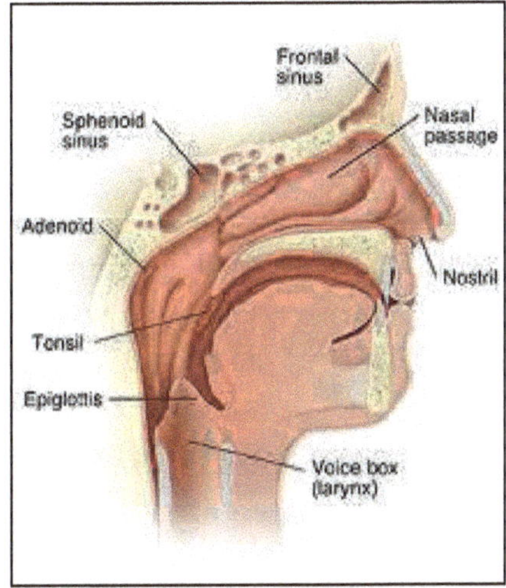

Figure 363 Anatomy of Nose

Throat: The throat, or pharynx, is a passageway for air, food, and liquids. It connects the nose and mouth to the larynx and esophagus. The throat is also involved in speech production, thanks to the larynx, which houses the vocal cords. The tonsils in the throat play a role in immune defense by trapping pathogens.

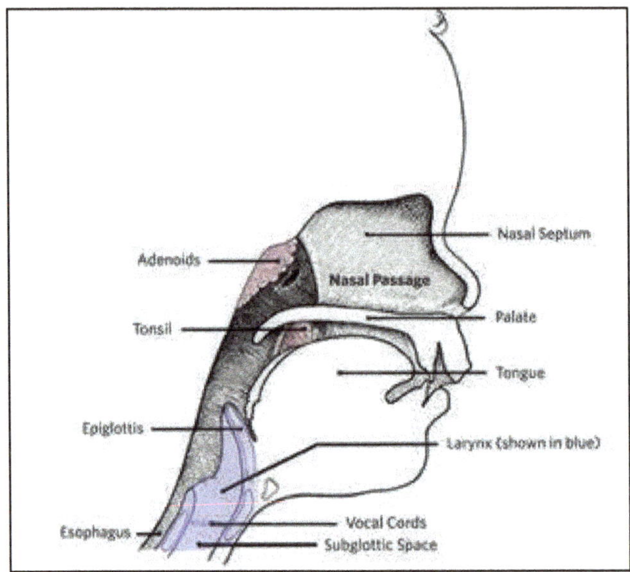

Figure 364 Anatomy and Physiology of Throat

12.2 Evaluation Tests

12.2.1 Vision Test

Evaluation of eye health functions alongside visual impairment detection requires vision tests to be performed. Visual acuity measurement through **Snellen chart testing** requires patients to read letters or symbols at a set distance for assessing their vision quality. Regular vision results in a **recorded value of 20/20.** The recognition of different colors between red and green appears in color vision tests through the **Ishihara exam** since it detects **cases of color blindness**. **The Amsler grid tests** helps monitor central vision as a tool for **macular degeneration detection**. The refraction test serves as a standard procedure to establish appropriate corrective lens prescriptions through evaluations of light focusing abilities of the eyes. **Tonometry** uses documented techniques to detect glaucoma and measure the level of intraocular pressure. The identification of early eye diseases depends on consistent vision tests for preserving healthy eyesight.

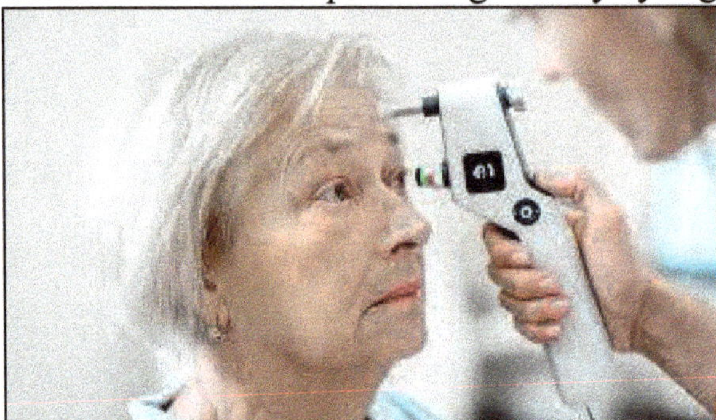

Figure 365 Tonometry Test

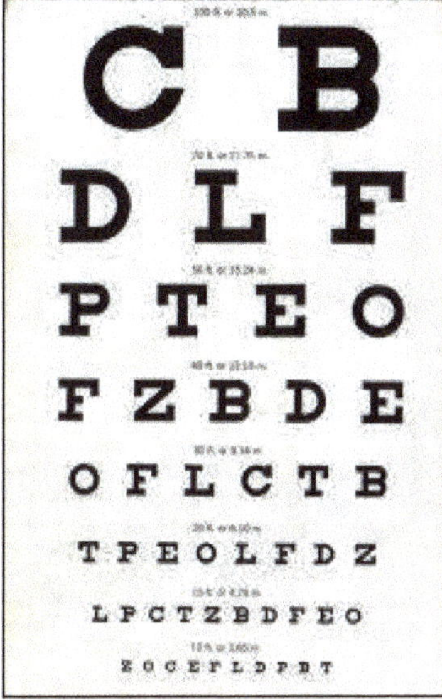

Figure 366 Snellen Chart Test

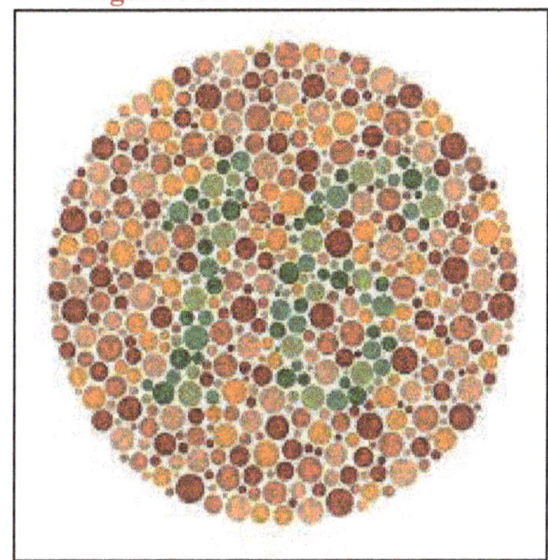

Figure 367 Ishihara Test

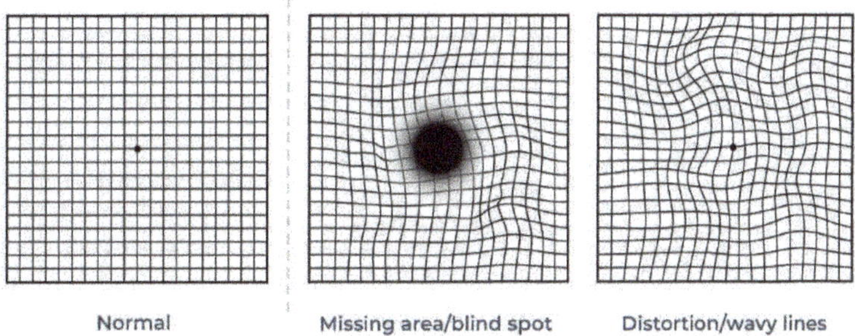

Figure 368 Amsler grid tests

12.2.2 Hearing Tests

Auditory system function testing through hearing examinations determines hearing loss detection. The pure-tone audiometry test employs headphones to play sounds of multiple frequencies and volumes to determine which sounds a person detects at the lowest level. The ability to perceive speech at different magnitudes is measured through speech audiometry to determine speech understanding abilities. The hearing specialist uses Rinne tests and Weber tests with tuning forks to determine whether hearing loss is conductive or sensorineural in nature. Testing with

Otoacoustic emissions (OAE) allows healthcare professionals to measure sounds emitted by the cochlea while the ear responds to different stimuli to identify inner ear functionality. Healthcare professionals use Auditory Brainstem Response tests to evaluate hearing pathways and auditory nerve operating condition through newborn screenings and tests with patients unable to do standard hearing evaluations. It is essential to conduct prompt hearing tests to detect hearing problems as these assessments help stop developmental delays from occurring.

12.3 Common Conditions for Head in HEENT System

"HHSTB" **H** for Head Injury **H** for Headache **S** for Stroke **T** for Brain Tumors **B** for Traumatic Brain Injuries (TBI)

Table 192 Common Head Conditions

Condition	Description	Key Symptoms	Diagnostic Tools	Treatment Options
Head Injury	Head injury refers to any trauma to the skull or brain, which can range from mild concussions to severe brain damage.	Loss of consciousness, confusion, dizziness, headaches, nausea, vomiting, memory issues, and possibly seizures.	CT scan, MRI, neurological examination, and physical assessment to determine the extent of the injury.	Rest, pain relievers, anti-seizure medications, and, in severe cases, surgery or rehabilitation.
Headache	Headaches are common, involving pain in the head, and can be caused by various factors, from stress to underlying neurological conditions.	Pain, pressure, or throbbing in the head, sensitivity to light or sound, nausea, and sometimes visual disturbances.	Clinical evaluation, patient history, neurological exam, MRI/CT for chronic or severe cases.	Pain relievers, anti-inflammatory medications, stress management, and in some cases, migraine-specific treatments like triptans.
Stroke	A stroke occurs when blood flow to the brain is interrupted, either by a blockage (ischemic) or rupture (hemorrhagic), causing brain damage.	Sudden numbness or weakness, difficulty speaking, confusion, loss of coordination, severe headache, and vision changes.	CT scan or MRI, physical and neurological examination, blood tests, and angiography in some cases.	Thrombolytics for ischemic stroke, surgery for hemorrhagic stroke, rehabilitation, and long-term medication for recovery.

Brain Tumors	Brain tumors are abnormal growths in the brain that can be benign or malignant, affecting brain function and structures.	Headache, seizures, nausea, vomiting, memory loss, changes in personality, and weakness or paralysis.	MRI, CT scan, biopsy for confirmation, neurological examination to assess function and location.	Surgery to remove or biopsy the tumor, radiation therapy, chemotherapy, and possibly corticosteroids to reduce swelling.
Traumatic Brain Injuries (TBIs)	Traumatic brain injuries (TBI) are injuries to the brain caused by external physical forces, often resulting from accidents, falls, or violence.	Confusion, dizziness, headache, nausea, vomiting, memory loss, difficulty concentrating, and changes in mood or behavior.	CT scan, MRI, neurological assessment, Glasgow Coma Scale (GCS) for evaluating severity.	Rest, physical therapy, cognitive therapy, medications to manage symptoms, and in severe cases, surgery or rehabilitation.

12.4 Major Medical Conditions for HEENT System of Head

12.4.1 Head Injury

Brain injuries present as both mild concussions together with severe forms of brain trauma. Head injuries **classified as mild will produce symptoms which include dizziness** along with headache and confusion but do not result in unconsciousness. People suffering severe brain traumas **experience both memory loss plus nausea together with vomiting and neurologic impairment** in addition to short-term unconsciousness. Rest usually heals most concussion instances although repeated concussions can trigger enduring problems. Emergency medical response becomes necessary when serious **head trauma gives rise to skull fractures and brain bleeding**. CT scan or MRI provides doctors with necessary imaging to determine how extensive the injury has become. Medical interventions for soft tissue knee injuries vary based on severity levels and could involve rest only up to **surgical procedures for serious conditions.**

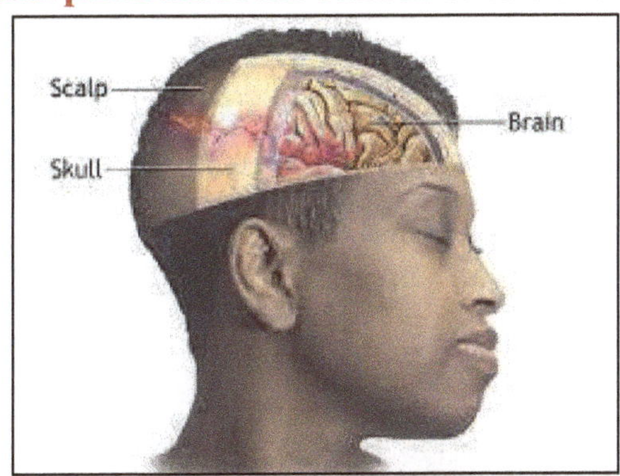

Figure 369 Head Injury

12.4.1.1 SOAP Notes for Head Injury

Table 193 SOAP Notes for Head Injury

Component	Details

Subjective (S)	A 30-year-old male presents with a history of a recent fall resulting in a blow to the head. He reports dizziness, mild headache, and difficulty concentrating. He denies any loss of consciousness but has noticed some memory lapses. No vomiting or seizures reported. He has no prior history of head trauma.
Objective (O)	On physical examination, the patient is alert and oriented but appears mildly confused. Vital signs are stable: BP 120/80 mmHg, pulse 76 bpm. The head has a small contusion, and there is tenderness on palpation of the scalp. No signs of intracranial hemorrhage or skull fractures. Neurological exam is normal with no signs of focal deficits.
Assessment (A)	The patient's symptoms, including headache, dizziness, and mild confusion after trauma, are consistent with a mild head injury or concussion. Given the lack of more serious symptoms (e.g., loss of consciousness or focal neurological signs), this is likely a mild traumatic brain injury. A CT scan may be needed if symptoms worsen.
Plan (P)	**Pharmacological**: Over-the-counter pain relievers (acetaminophen) for headache. **Non-pharmacological**: Rest and observation for 24 hours to monitor for worsening symptoms. **Follow-up**: Follow-up in 1-2 days to reassess neurological status and repeat imaging if symptoms persist or worsen. **Education**: Advise the patient to avoid activities that could lead to another head injury, such as contact sports, for at least 2 weeks.

12.4.2 Headache

Most people endure headaches as part of their everyday life which exists between primary and secondary types. Primary headaches including tension-type headaches and migraines and cluster headaches emerge without medical **medical causes and typically present in distinct periods**. The migraine headache features profound pain combined with vomiting and extreme sensitivity to light whereas cluster headaches appear as intense pain that focuses on a single eye. The underlying factors of brain tumors, strokes and sinus infections lead to secondary headaches. Doctors use detailed **history-taking, physical examination along with imaging tests** if required to diagnose patients. Different treatment plans exist for different headache types and levels of severity that go from OTC medications to specialized medical therapies for persistent conditions (Discussed in detail in chapter 6).

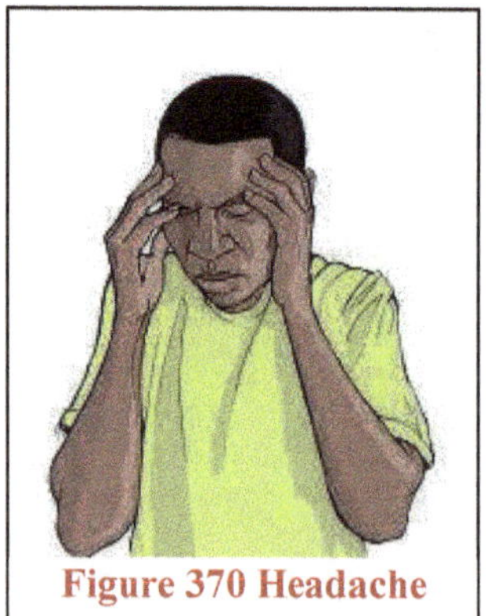

Figure 370 Headache

12.4.2.1 SOAP Notes for Headache

Table 194 SOAP Notes for Headache

Component	Details
Subjective (S)	A 40-year-old female presents with a 3-day history of a severe, throbbing headache located around the temples. She reports nausea, sensitivity to light, and occasional vomiting. The pain worsens with physical activity and is associated with a history of migraines. No visual disturbances noted.
Objective (O)	On physical examination, the patient is visibly uncomfortable due to headache. Vital signs are BP 130/85 mmHg, pulse 82 bpm. No fever or neck stiffness is present. Neurological examination is normal with no focal deficits.
Assessment (A)	The patient's symptoms, including severe, throbbing headache with nausea and vomiting, are consistent with a migraine. The history of similar symptoms and absence of other neurological findings suggest that this is a primary headache disorder.
Plan (P)	**Pharmacological**: Prescribe triptans (sumatriptan) for acute migraine relief and consider prophylactic medication if attacks are frequent. **Non-pharmacological**: Encourage regular sleep, hydration, and avoiding known migraine triggers. **Follow-up**: Follow-up in 1 week if symptoms persist or worsen. **Education**: Educate the patient on lifestyle changes, including stress management, and the proper use of migraine medication to avoid overuse headaches.

12.4.3 Stroke

The interruption of blood flow to the brain triggers a stroke through two mechanisms including **blockages (ischemic stroke) and vessel ruptures (hemorrhagic stroke).** Over half of strokes restache under the ischemic category with blood clots that block arteries as their main cause. A **hemorrhagic stroke emerges when blood vessels** inside the brain suddenly break open thereby causing bleeding to occur. The onset of stroke produces three groups of symptoms which include **numbness or weakness, speaking difficulties, confusion, coordination problems and intense headaches.** Doctors normally verify stroke diagnosis through clinical imaging exams which show the specific region and form of a stroke. The medical approach for stroke involves using thrombolytics as well as surgery along with recovery programs to prevent potential sequelae (Discussed in detail in Chapter 6).

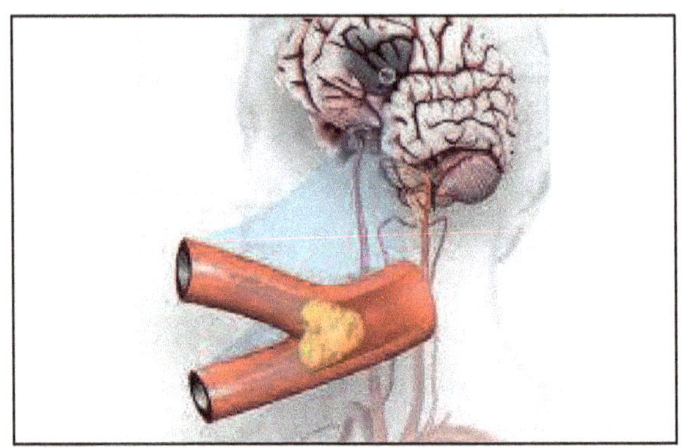

Figure 371 Stroke

12.4.3.1 SOAP Notes for Stroke

Table 195 SOAP Notes for Stroke

Component	Details
Subjective (S)	A 68-year-old male presents with sudden-onset right-sided weakness, slurred speech, and difficulty walking. He also reports numbness in the right arm and leg. He denies any previous history of stroke or transient ischemic attack (TIA).
Objective (O)	On physical examination, the patient has right-sided hemiparesis, dysarthria, and facial drooping on the right side. BP is 160/90 mmHg, pulse 90 bpm. The patient is alert but confused. Neurological exam shows impaired right-sided motor function and decreased sensation in the right arm and leg.
Assessment (A)	The patient's sudden-onset right-sided weakness, slurred speech, and facial drooping are consistent with an acute ischemic stroke, likely affecting the left hemisphere of the brain. Immediate CT scan is needed to determine the presence of hemorrhage or ischemia and initiate appropriate treatment.
Plan (P)	**Pharmacological**: Administer thrombolytics (rtPA) if ischemic stroke is confirmed and within the therapeutic window. **Non-pharmacological**: Begin monitoring in a stroke unit for further interventions. **Follow-up**: Immediate follow-up for rehabilitation once the acute phase is managed. **Education**: Educate the patient and family on stroke symptoms, prevention strategies, and the importance of rehabilitation for recovery.

12.4.4 Brain Tumors

Brain tumors develop as abnormal masses throughout the brain tissue while these lesions can exist as benign tumors and malignant varieties. **Brain cell tumors develop naturally** within the brain tissue yet other body areas can spread tumors to the brain (metastatic tumors). People with brain tumors may show **different symptoms based on tumor dimensions and anatomical placement** together with tumor classification yet they often present with headache symptoms along with queasiness and seizure activity and changes in vision and mental function deterioration. Medical practitioners usually diagnose brain tumors using **MRI and CT scans** along with supplementary biopsies to properly classify the tumor type. Treatment options depend on tumor characteristics which can include surgery with necessary radiation therapy and chemotherapy prescriptions. The **timely discovery of tumors** proves essential for enhancing medical results particularly with malignant cancerous growths (Discussed in detail in chapter 6).

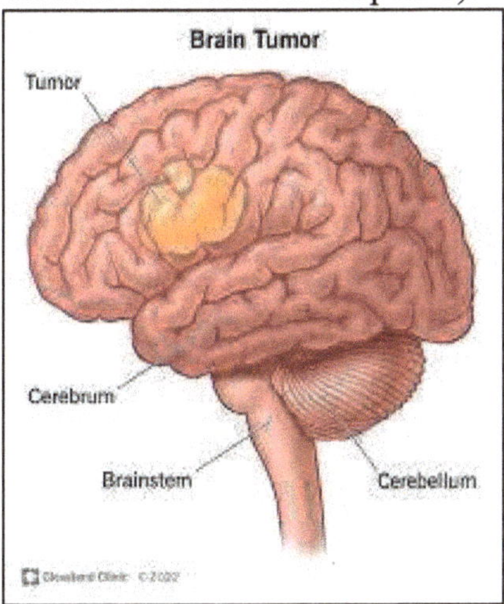

Figure 372 Brain Tumor

12.4.4.1 SOAP Notes for Brain Tumors

Table 196 SOAP Notes for Brain Tumors

Component	Details
Subjective (S)	A 55-year-old female presents with progressive headaches, nausea, and difficulty with balance. She reports intermittent vision disturbances and memory problems over the past month. She denies any history of head trauma or neurological disease.
Objective (O)	On physical examination, the patient appears fatigued with mild ataxia and difficulty maintaining balance. BP is 125/80 mmHg, pulse 78 bpm. Neurological exam reveals mild dysphasia and a positive Romberg sign. Fundoscopic examination shows papilledema.
Assessment (A)	The patient's symptoms, including progressive headaches, vision changes, and balance issues, suggest the possibility of a brain tumor, likely affecting the cerebellum or occipital lobes. MRI of the brain is recommended for confirmation.
Plan (P)	**Pharmacological**: Prescribe corticosteroids to reduce cerebral edema and alleviate symptoms. **Non-pharmacological**: Arrange for urgent MRI of the brain to confirm the diagnosis and locate the tumor. **Follow-up**: Follow-up in 1-2 days after imaging results. **Education**: Educate the patient on the possible diagnosis, treatment options, and the importance of timely intervention.

12.4.5 Traumatic Brain Injuries (TBIs)

A Traumatic Brain Injury (TBI) develops because an outside force applied to the head causes disruptions in typical brain operation. Patients can sustain any combination of concussion injuries which range from simple cerebral trauma to permanent brain destruction. Patients who experience traumatic brain injuries might display confusion in addition to dizziness and headache while also

experiencing nausea and vomiting and showing signs of memory impairment and problems with attention and exhibiting mood or behavioral changes. Serious traumatic brain injuries will cause patients to lose consciousness or produce major impairments to their neurological functions. Medical professionals **diagnose TBI by combining CT scans or MRI** results with brain function evaluations which they conduct using neurological assessments. The treatment options for sports-related TBIs consist of monitoring basic cases with rest or require surgical intervention combined with intensive **rehabilitation for major injuries.** Adequate medical care stands essential for avoiding both mental and physical disabilities which emerge within long periods following brain trauma (Discussed in detail in chapter 6).

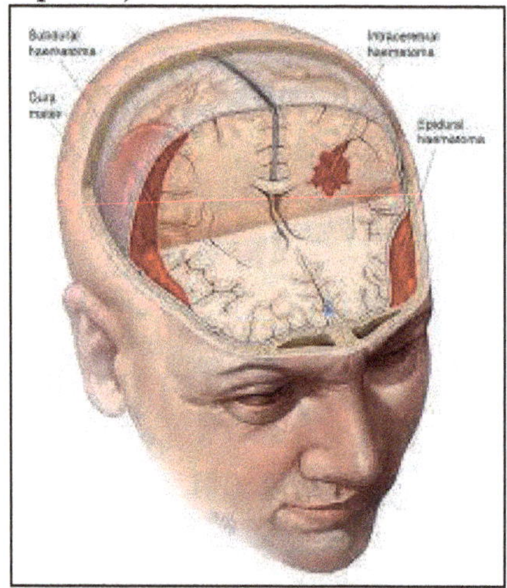

Figure 373 Traumatic Brain Injury

12.4.5.1 SOAP Notes for TBIs

Table 197 SOAP Notes for TBI

Component	Details
Subjective (S)	A 22-year-old male presents after a motor vehicle accident with a headache, dizziness, and difficulty concentrating. He denies loss of consciousness but reports feeling confused and lightheaded. No vomiting or seizures reported.
Objective (O)	On physical examination, the patient appears mildly confused and disoriented but is alert and oriented to person, place, and time. Vital signs are BP 120/75 mmHg, pulse 88 bpm. Neurological exam reveals mild difficulty with short-term memory recall, but cranial nerves are intact. No focal motor deficits.
Assessment (A)	The patient's symptoms following a motor vehicle accident suggest a mild traumatic brain injury or concussion. The absence of loss of consciousness and focal neurological deficits makes the likelihood of severe brain injury low, but a CT scan is recommended to rule out bleeding or fractures.
Plan (P)	**Pharmacological**: Over-the-counter analgesics (acetaminophen) for headache. **Non-pharmacological**: Recommend rest and observation for 24-48 hours. **Follow-up**: Follow-up in 2-3 days to reassess neurological status and repeat imaging if symptoms worsen. **Education**: Advise the patient to

	avoid physical exertion and return to normal activities slowly, as symptoms may fluctuate.

12.5 Common Conditions for Eyes in HEENT System

"CHC-AA-MO-RO-AGE-SS-BEEP-PE-DHDC" C = Corneal Ulcers, H = Herpes Keratitis, C = Contact-Lens Related Keratitis, A-A = Acute Angle-Closure Glaucoma and Acute Angle-Open Glaucoma, M = Multiple Sclerosis (Optic Neuritis), O = Orbital Cellulitis, R = Retinal Detachment, A-G = Age-related Macular Degeneration, S = Sjogren's Syndrome, B = Blepharitis, E = Entropion, E = Ectropion, P = Pinguecula, P = Pterygium, D = Disc Cupping, H = Hypersensitivity Retinopathy, D = Diabetic Retinopathy, and C = Cataracts

Table 198 Common Conditions for Eyes in HEENT System

Condition	Description	Key Symptoms	Diagnostic Tools	Treatment Options
Corneal Ulcers	Open sores on the cornea caused by infection, trauma, or dry eyes.	Pain, redness, blurred vision, sensitivity to light, and watery eyes.	Slit-lamp examination, fluorescein staining, corneal cultures.	Antibiotics, corticosteroid eye drops, pain management, and sometimes surgery.
Herpes Keratitis	An eye infection caused by herpes simplex virus affecting the cornea.	Eye pain, redness, blurred vision, tearing, and light sensitivity.	Slit-lamp examination, fluorescein staining, PCR for herpes simplex virus.	Antiviral medication (acyclovir), corticosteroid eye drops, and pain management.
Contact-Lens Related Keratitis	Infection of the cornea caused by improper contact lens use.	Redness, pain, and blurred vision, often with a history of poor contact lens hygiene.	Slit-lamp examination, corneal cultures, patient history of contact lens use.	Antibiotic eye drops, contact lens hygiene education, and possibly discontinuing lens use.
Acute Angle-Closure Glaucoma	Condition where the drainage angle of the eye becomes blocked, leading to	Severe eye pain, headache, nausea, vomiting, and rapid loss of vision.	Tonometry for measuring intraocular pressure, gonioscopy, dilated eye exam.	Immediate ophthalmic emergency treatment, including medications to reduce intraocular

	increased intraocular pressure.			pressure and possibly surgery.
Acute Angle-Open Glaucoma	Gradual increase in eye pressure, often without symptoms until significant damage occurs.	Gradual vision loss, peripheral vision loss, and elevated intraocular pressure.	Tonometry for measuring intraocular pressure, visual field tests, optic nerve imaging.	Medications to reduce intraocular pressure, laser therapy, or surgery.
Multiple Sclerosis (Optic Neuritis)	Inflammation of the optic nerve, leading to vision loss or discomfort.	Vision loss or dimming, eye pain, and reduced color vision.	OCT (Optical Coherence Tomography), visual acuity tests, MRI of the brain.	Corticosteroids, optic nerve protection therapy, and rehabilitation for vision loss.
Orbital Cellulitis	Severe infection of the tissues surrounding the eye, often following a sinus infection.	Pain, swelling, redness around the eyes, fever, and sometimes vision changes.	CT scan or MRI of the orbit, blood cultures, and ophthalmologic exam.	Antibiotic therapy (oral or IV), corticosteroid treatment, and surgery if needed.
Retinal Detachment	Occurs when the retina separates from the underlying layer, causing potential permanent vision loss.	Sudden vision loss, flashes of light, and floaters in the vision.	Fundoscopy, B-scan ultrasound, OCT.	Laser surgery, cryotherapy, or surgery to repair the retinal detachment.
Age-related Macular Degeneration	A degenerative condition affecting the central part of the retina	Blurred or distorted central vision, difficulty recognizing	Amsler grid, fundoscopy, optical coherence tomography (OCT).	Anti-VEGF injections, laser therapy, and lifestyle changes to slow disease progression.

	(macula), leading to central vision loss.	faces or reading.		
Sjogren's Syndrome	An autoimmune disorder that affects moisture-producing glands, including the eyes, leading to dry eyes.	Dry eyes, burning sensation, eye irritation, and difficulty wearing contact lenses.	Schirmer test, tear break-up time, patient history of autoimmune disorders.	Artificial tears, immunosuppressive therapy, and treatment of underlying autoimmune conditions.
Blepharitis	Inflammation of the eyelids, often involving the eyelashes and causing redness and irritation.	Red, swollen eyelids with crusting, itching, and burning sensations.	Eyelid examination, slit-lamp evaluation, and bacterial cultures if necessary.	Lid hygiene, warm compresses, antibiotic ointment, and corticosteroid drops.
Entropion	A condition where the eyelid turns inward, causing the eyelashes to rub against the cornea.	Inward-turning eyelids causing irritation, redness, and tearing.	Physical examination, slit-lamp examination, eyelid eversion test.	Surgical correction, artificial tears, and lubrication therapy.
Ectropion	Occurs when the eyelid turns outward, leading to exposure of the inner eyelid and eye irritation.	Eyelids turning outward, leading to irritation, dryness, and redness.	Physical examination, slit-lamp examination, and evaluation of the eyelid position.	Surgical correction of the eyelid position, lubrication therapy.
Pinguecula	A benign growth on the conjunctiva	Yellowish, slightly raised	Slit-lamp examination, fluorescein	No treatment needed for mild cases, but surgery

	of the eye, often due to UV light exposure.	growth on the conjunctiva, usually near the cornea.	staining, and visual acuity testing.	if it interferes with vision.
Pterygium	A growth of tissue from the conjunctiva onto the cornea, often due to prolonged sun exposure.	Red, fleshy growth on the conjunctiva, often extending onto the cornea.	Slit-lamp examination, fluorescein staining, and visual acuity tests.	Surgical removal if necessary, and corticosteroid treatment if inflamed.
Disc Cupping	Refers to the appearance of the optic disc in glaucoma, where the cup of the optic nerve becomes enlarged.	Enlarged optic disc, deeper cup, and increased cup-to-disc ratio, often associated with glaucoma.	Ophthalmoscopy, OCT, fundus photography.	Glaucoma treatment (medications, laser therapy, surgery), optic nerve monitoring.
Hypersensitivity Retinopathy	Damage to the retina caused by immune system reactions, often due to systemic conditions.	Blurred vision, flashing lights, and visual disturbances due to retinal immune response.	Fluorescein angiography, fundoscopy, and optical coherence tomography (OCT).	Anti-inflammatory treatment, retinal laser therapy, or steroids.
Diabetic Retinopathy	Damage to the blood vessels in the retina due to diabetes, leading to vision problems.	Blurry vision, difficulty seeing at night, and seeing halos around lights.	Slit-lamp examination, visual acuity test, fundoscopy, and cataract grading.	Surgical removal or cataract surgery for vision correction.

Cataracts	Clouding of the lens of the eye, causing blurry vision and difficulty seeing in low light.	Cloudy or blurry vision, glare, and difficulty with night vision.	Slit-lamp examination, visual acuity test, fundoscopy, and cataract grading.	Surgical removal or cataract surgery for vision correction.

12.6 Major Medical Conditions of Eyes in HEENT System

12.6.1 Corneal Ulcers

Corneal ulcers are open sores on the cornea caused by infection, trauma, or dry eyes. They lead to **pain, redness, blurred vision, and sensitivity to light** and can be serious if untreated, leading to permanent vision loss.

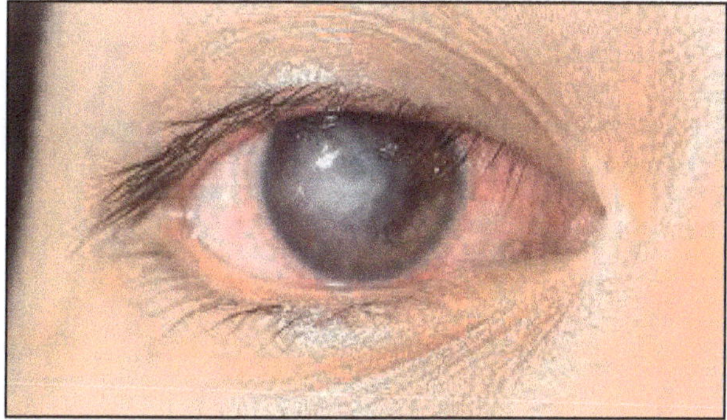

Figure 374 Corneal Ulcer

12.6.1.1 SOAP Notes for Corneal Ulcers

Table 199 SOAP Notes for Corneal Ulcer

Component	Details
Subjective (S)	A 25-year-old female presents with eye pain, redness, and blurred vision after wearing contact lenses for an extended period without cleaning them. She reports sensitivity to light and excessive tearing.
Objective (O)	On physical examination, the patient has a red, inflamed eye with a visible ulcer on the cornea. Visual acuity is reduced. Slit-lamp examination reveals a circular ulcer in the central cornea with fluorescein staining.
Assessment (A)	The patient's symptoms, including eye pain, blurred vision, and sensitivity to light, are consistent with a corneal ulcer. The condition is likely caused by bacterial infection due to improper contact lens hygiene.
Plan (P)	**Pharmacological**: Prescribe antibiotics (ciprofloxacin eye drops) to treat the bacterial infection. **Non-pharmacological**: Advise the patient to discontinue contact lens use until the ulcer resolves. **Follow-up**: Reassess in 2-3 days to monitor healing and evaluate for complications. **Education**: Educate the patient on proper contact lens hygiene and the importance of avoiding lens wear during treatment.

12.6.2 Herpes Keratitis

Herpes keratitis is an infection of the cornea caused by the herpes simplex virus, resulting in eye **pain, redness, and blurred vision**. It can lead to scarring of the cornea and permanent vision loss if not treated with antiviral medications. **Contact-lens related keratitis** is an infection of the cornea caused by improper contact lens use, such as wearing them too long or failing to clean them properly. **Symptoms include pain, redness, and blurred vision**, and it requires immediate treatment to prevent permanent damage.

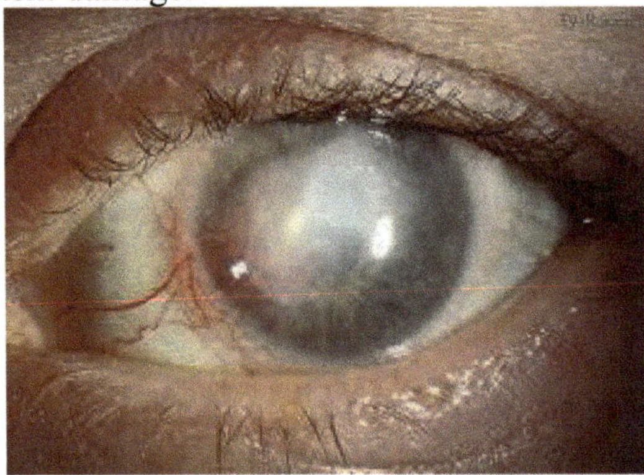

Figure 375 Herpes Keratitis

12.6.2.1 SOAP Notes for Herpes Keratitis

Table 200 SOAP Notes for Herpes Keratitis

Component	Details
Subjective (S)	A 30-year-old male presents with pain in the left eye, blurred vision, and sensitivity to light. He reports a history of cold sores and now has eye pain and redness in the same eye.
Objective (O)	On physical examination, the left eye is red, and the patient exhibits pain upon palpation. Slit-lamp examination shows dendritic ulcers on the cornea, consistent with herpes simplex virus infection.
Assessment (A)	The patient's symptoms, including eye pain, blurred vision, and a history of cold sores, are consistent with herpes keratitis. The dendritic ulcer observed on slit-lamp examination confirms the diagnosis.
Plan (P)	**Pharmacological**: Prescribe antiviral eye drops (acyclovir) and oral antivirals. **Non-pharmacological**: Advise the patient to avoid touching or rubbing the eye to prevent viral spread. **Follow-up**: Follow-up in 1-2 weeks to assess resolution and check for complications such as corneal scarring. **Education**: Educate the patient on managing herpes simplex virus outbreaks and the importance of early treatment to prevent vision loss.

12.6.3 Acute Angle- Closer Glaucoma

Acute angle-closure glaucoma occurs when the drainage angle of the eye becomes blocked, leading to a **sudden rise in intraocular pressure**. Symptoms include severe eye pain, headache, nausea, vomiting, and a rapid loss of vision, **requiring immediate treatment to prevent blindness**.

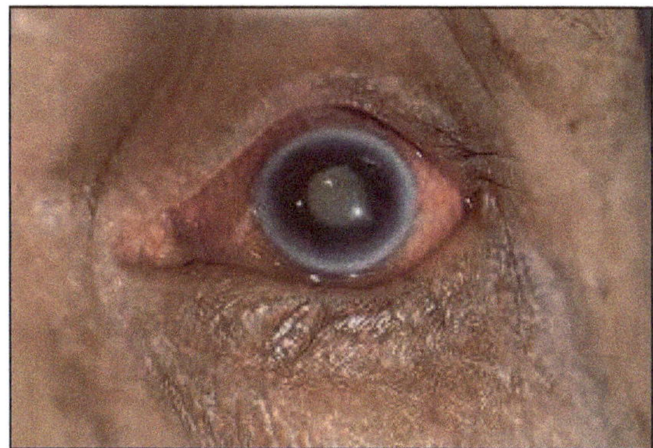

Figure 376 Acute Angle - Closer Glaucoma

12.6.3.1 SOAP Notes for Acute Angle Closer Glaucoma

Table 201 SOAP Notes for Acute Angle Closer Glaucoma

Component	Details
Subjective (S)	A 60-year-old male presents with sudden onset of severe eye pain, headache, nausea, and vomiting. He reports blurred vision and seeing halos around lights.
Objective (O)	On physical examination, the patient has a markedly red eye and a dilated, non-reactive pupil. Tonometry reveals elevated intraocular pressure of 40 mmHg. Gonioscopy shows closed angles.
Assessment (A)	The patient's symptoms, including sudden eye pain, headache, nausea, vomiting, and elevated intraocular pressure, are consistent with acute angle-closure glaucoma.
Plan (P)	**Pharmacological**: Administer medications to lower intraocular pressure (e.g., acetazolamide, beta-blockers, prostaglandin analogs). **Non-pharmacological**: Arrange for laser iridotomy to relieve the blockage and prevent further attacks. **Follow-up**: Immediate follow-up after treatment to reassess eye pressure and consider prophylactic treatment for the other eye. **Education**: Educate the patient on the importance of prompt treatment to prevent permanent vision loss.

12.6.4 Acute Angle-Open Glaucoma

Acute angle-open glaucoma is a condition where eye pressure increases gradually over time, often without **noticeable symptoms until significant damage occurs**. It can lead to peripheral vision loss and, if untreated, complete blindness, with treatments aimed at reducing intraocular pressure

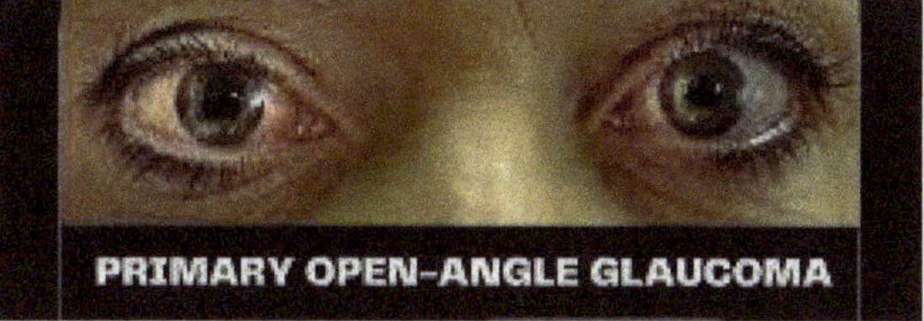

Figure 377 Acute Angle Open Glaucoma

12.6.4.1 SOAP Notes for Acute Angle Open Glaucoma

Table 202 SOAP Notes for Acute Angle Open Glaucoma

Component	Details

Subjective (S)	A 65-year-old female presents with a gradual loss of peripheral vision over the past few months. She denies any pain or acute discomfort but reports difficulty seeing in low light.
Objective (O)	On physical examination, the patient shows signs of optic nerve cupping. Tonometry reveals elevated intraocular pressure of 28 mmHg. Visual field testing shows a loss of peripheral vision.
Assessment (A)	The patient's gradual vision loss and elevated intraocular pressure are consistent with acute angle-open glaucoma, a form of chronic glaucoma that leads to optic nerve damage.
Plan (P)	**Pharmacological**: Prescribe topical eye drops to reduce intraocular pressure (e.g., latanoprost, timolol). **Non-pharmacological**: Regular monitoring of intraocular pressure and visual fields. **Follow-up**: Reassess in 1 month to monitor intraocular pressure and visual fields. **Education**: Educate the patient on adherence to medication to prevent further optic nerve damage and the importance of regular eye exams.

12.6.5 Multiple Sclerosis (Optic Neuritis)

Optic neuritis, often associated with multiple sclerosis, involves inflammation of the optic nerve, **leading to vision loss or discomfort.** It typically presents as pain with eye movement, dimming vision, and sometimes color vision loss.

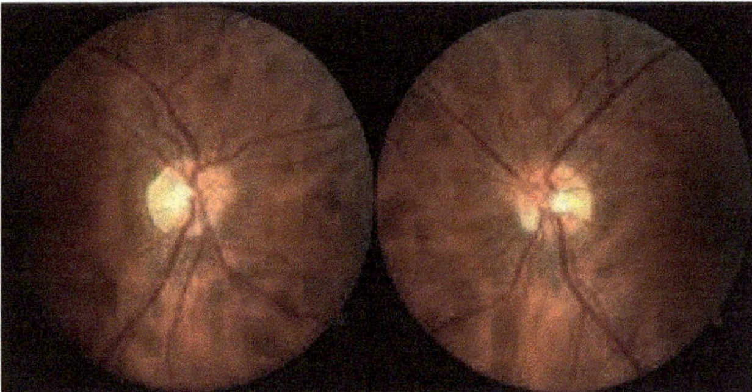

Figure 378 Optic Neuritis

12.6.5.1 SOAP Notes for Optic Neuritis

Table 203 SOAP Notes for Optic Neuritis

Component	Details
Subjective (S)	A 32-year-old female presents with blurred vision in her right eye and pain upon eye movement. She reports having episodes of numbness and weakness in her limbs over the past few months, with a history of similar symptoms.
Objective (O)	On physical examination, the patient has a visual acuity of 20/40 in the right eye and mild pain on eye movement. Fundoscopy reveals a swollen optic disc, and a visual field test shows a central scotoma.
Assessment (A)	The patient's symptoms, including eye pain with movement and vision loss, are consistent with optic neuritis, which is often associated with multiple sclerosis.

Plan (P)	**Pharmacological**: Start high-dose corticosteroids (methylprednisolone) to reduce inflammation. **Non-pharmacological**: Recommend rest and follow-up care. **Follow-up**: Reassess vision and neurological status in 1 week. **Education**: Educate the patient on MS and the potential for future relapses, emphasizing the importance of early treatment and monitoring.

12.6.6 Orbital Cellulitis

Orbital cellulitis is a serious infection of the tissues surrounding the **eye, often resulting from a sinus infection or trauma**. It presents with **pain, swelling, redness around the eyes, fever, and possibly vision changes**, and requires immediate medical attention.

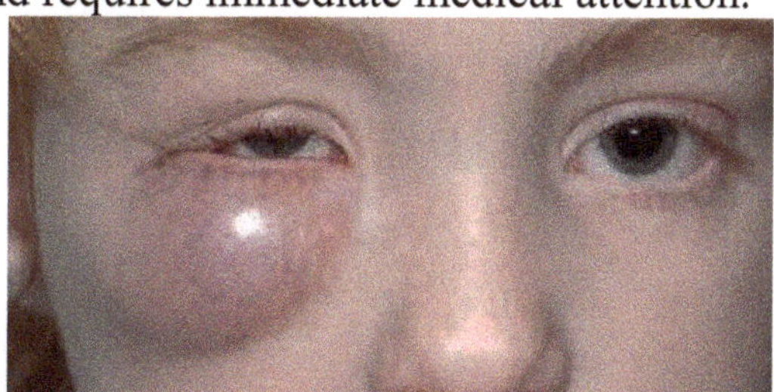

Figure 379 Orbital Cellulitis

12.6.6.1 SOAP Notes for Orbital Cellulitis

Table 204 SOAP Notes for Orbital Cellulitis

Component	Details
Subjective (S)	A 40-year-old male presents with severe pain, redness, and swelling around the left eye. He has a recent history of a sinus infection and reports fever and difficulty moving the eye.
Objective (O)	On physical examination, the patient has erythema, swelling, and tenderness around the left eye with restricted ocular movements. There is also mild proptosis. CT imaging of the orbit confirms soft tissue inflammation around the eye.
Assessment (A)	The patient's symptoms, including fever, pain, and swelling around the eye, suggest orbital cellulitis, likely due to a sinus infection.
Plan (P)	**Pharmacological**: Initiate broad-spectrum IV antibiotics (vancomycin, ceftriaxone). **Non-pharmacological**: Hospitalization for IV antibiotics and close monitoring. **Follow-up**: Reassess in 48-72 hours to evaluate response to treatment and consider surgical drainage if no improvement. **Education**: Educate the patient on the importance of completing the full course of antibiotics to prevent complications.

12.6.7 Retinal Detachment

Retinal detachment occurs when the retina separates from the underlying layer, which can lead to **permanent vision loss if not treated promptly.** Symptoms include sudden vision loss, flashes of light, and floaters in the vision.

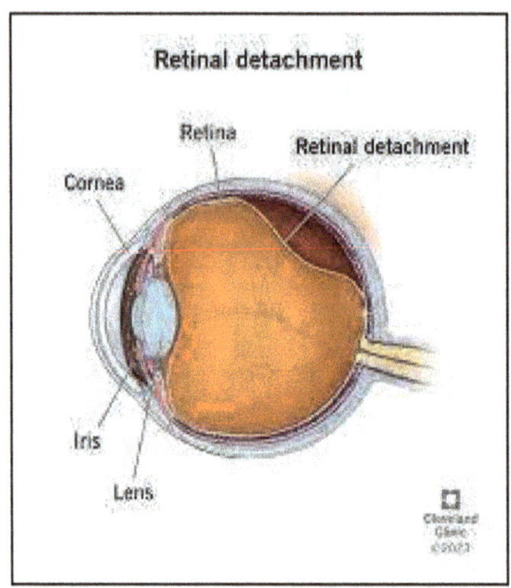

Figure 380 Retinal Detachment

12.6.7.1 SOAP Notes for Retinal Detachment

Table 205 SOAP Notes for Retinal Detachment

Component	Details
Subjective (S)	A 50-year-old female presents with sudden onset of vision loss in her right eye, along with flashes of light and floaters. She denies any trauma but has a history of myopia.
Objective (O)	On physical examination, the right eye has decreased visual acuity, and fundoscopy reveals a retinal tear and detachment. The macula appears displaced, confirming retinal detachment.
Assessment (A)	The patient's sudden vision loss with flashes of light and floaters is consistent with retinal detachment, likely related to her myopia.
Plan (P)	**Pharmacological**: No specific pharmacological treatment, but analgesics for pain. **Non-pharmacological**: Urgent referral to an ophthalmologist for laser therapy or surgery (cryotherapy or pneumatic retinopexy). **Follow-up**: Immediate follow-up for surgical management. **Education**: Explain the need for urgent surgical intervention to prevent permanent vision loss.

12.6.8 Age-related to Macular Degeneration

Age-related macular degeneration is a degenerative condition affecting the macula, the **central part of the retina, leading to central vision loss**. Symptoms include blurred or distorted vision and difficulty recognizing faces or reading, particularly in older adults.

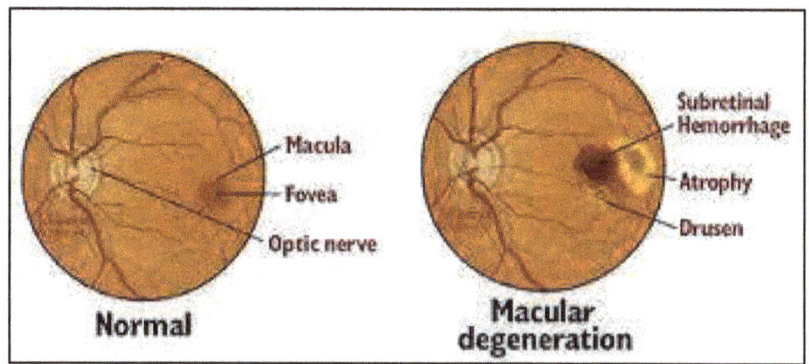

Figure 381 Macular Degeneration

12.6.8.1 SOAP Notes for Macular Degeneration

Table 206 SOAP Notes for Macular Degeneration

Component	Details
Subjective (S)	A 68-year-old male presents with blurred central vision, making it difficult to read or recognize faces. He reports noticing that straight lines appear wavy in his vision.
Objective (O)	On physical examination, visual acuity is reduced, and fundoscopy reveals drusen (yellow deposits) and pigment changes in the macula. OCT shows thinning of the retina.
Assessment (A)	The patient's symptoms, including blurred central vision and visual distortions, are consistent with age-related macular degeneration (AMD). The presence of drusen on fundoscopy and retinal thinning further confirms the diagnosis.
Plan (P)	**Pharmacological**: Anti-VEGF injections (e.g., ranibizumab, aflibercept) for wet AMD to slow progression and manage fluid buildup. **Non-pharmacological**: Recommend lifestyle changes such as a diet rich in antioxidants (e.g., dark leafy greens) and vitamins. **Follow-up**: Follow-up every 4-6 weeks to monitor for disease progression and manage any complications, with potential repeat anti-VEGF injections. **Education**: Educate the patient on managing AMD with the importance of regular eye exams, healthy diet, and the potential benefits of anti-VEGF treatment to prevent severe vision loss.

12.6.9 Sjogren's Syndrome

Sjogren's syndrome is an autoimmune disorder that affects moisture-producing glands, including those in the **eyes, leading to dryness, irritation, and a burning sensation**. It can significantly impact quality of life and is often associated with other autoimmune conditions.

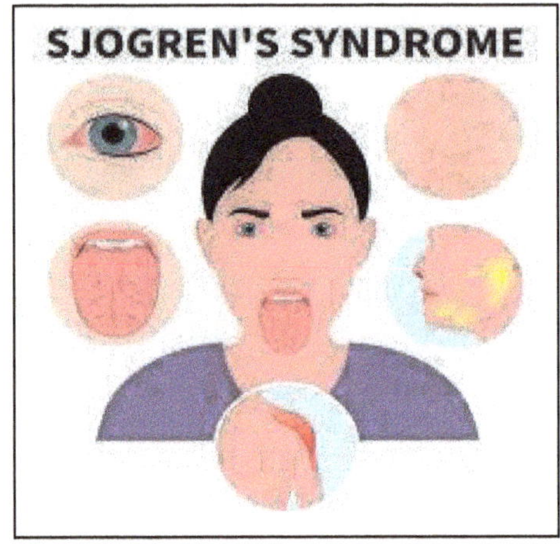

Figure 382 Sjogren's Syndrome

12.6.9.1 SOAP Notes for Sjogren's Syndrome

Table 207 SOAP Notes for Sjogren's Syndrome

Component	Details
Subjective (S)	A 55-year-old female presents with complaints of dry eyes and mouth, along with difficulty swallowing and a persistent dry cough. She has a history of fatigue and joint pain.
Objective (O)	On physical examination, the patient has dry, red eyes and a dry oral mucosa. Schirmer's test confirms decreased tear production. There is no palpable lymphadenopathy, but she has mild joint tenderness.
Assessment (A)	The patient's symptoms of dry eyes, mouth, and systemic fatigue, along with positive Schirmer's test, suggest Sjogren's syndrome, an autoimmune disorder.
Plan (P)	**Pharmacological**: Prescribe artificial tears and saliva substitutes for symptomatic relief. **Non-pharmacological**: Recommend increased hydration, use of humidifiers, and avoidance of dry environments. **Follow-up**: Regular follow-up for symptom management and to monitor for complications like dental decay. **Education**: Educate the patient on the chronic nature of Sjogren's syndrome, its autoimmune nature, and the importance of eye and oral hygiene to prevent further complications.

12.6.10 Blepharitis

Blepharitis is an inflammation of the eyelids, often **involving the eyelashes and causing redness, swelling, and irritation.** It is typically chronic and can cause discomfort, itching, and crusting along the eyelid margins.

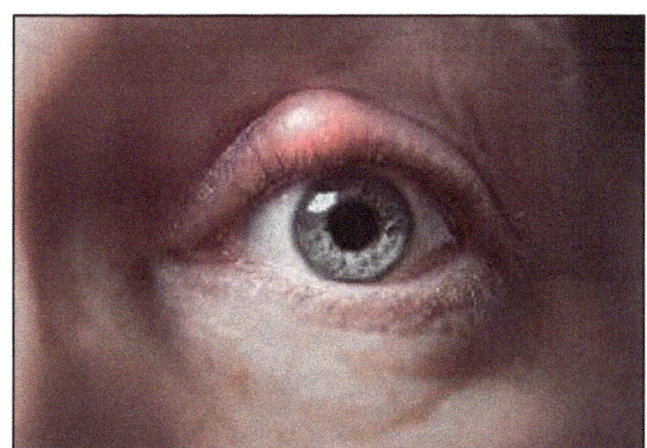

Figure 383 Blepharitis

12.6.10.1 SOAP Notes for Blepharitis

Table 208 SOAP Notes for Blepharitis

Component	Details
Subjective (S)	A 40-year-old female presents with redness, swelling, and itching in both eyelids. She reports crusting along her eyelashes, especially upon waking, and a burning sensation in her eyes throughout the day.
Objective (O)	On physical examination, the patient's eyelids are erythematous with crusting and flakes along the lash line. The conjunctiva appears mildly injected, but there is no sign of corneal involvement.
Assessment (A)	The patient's symptoms of eyelid inflammation, crusting, and irritation are consistent with blepharitis, an inflammation of the eyelid margins often caused by bacterial infection or seborrheic dermatitis.
Plan (P)	**Pharmacological**: Prescribe antibiotic ointment (e.g., erythromycin or bacitracin) for eyelid application and corticosteroid eye drops if inflammation is severe. **Non-pharmacological**: Advise daily eyelid hygiene with warm compresses and gentle cleaning of the eyelid margins. **Follow-up**: Follow-up in 2-3 weeks to monitor symptom resolution and adjust treatment if necessary. **Education**: Educate the patient on proper eyelid hygiene, the chronic nature of blepharitis, and the importance of ongoing management to prevent flare-ups.

12.6.11 Entropion

Entropion is a condition where the eyelid turns inward, causing the eyelashes to rub against the cornea. This **leads to irritation, redness, tearing, and can cause damage** to the cornea if left untreated.

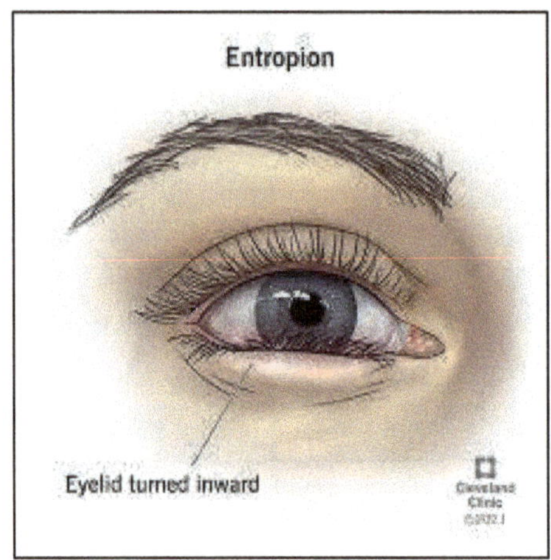

Figure 384 Entropion

12.6.11.1 SOAP Notes for Entropion

Table 209 SOAP Notes for Entropion

Component	Details
Subjective (S)	A 70-year-old male presents with complaints of eye irritation, redness, and excessive tearing in his left eye. He reports that his lower eyelid has been turning inward, causing his eyelashes to rub against his cornea.
Objective (O)	On physical examination, the left lower eyelid is turned inward, and the eyelashes are in direct contact with the cornea. The patient shows signs of conjunctival irritation and mild corneal abrasion.
Assessment (A)	The patient's symptoms and the inward-turning eyelid are consistent with entropion, which is causing mechanical irritation of the cornea.
Plan (P)	**Pharmacological**: Artificial tears and lubricating ointments to relieve eye irritation. **Non-pharmacological**: Recommend warm compresses and eyelid protection. Surgical correction is recommended if symptoms persist or worsen. **Follow-up**: Follow-up in 1-2 weeks to monitor eyelid position and corneal health. **Education**: Educate the patient on the risks of corneal damage and the potential need for surgery if the condition does not improve.

12.6.12 Ectropion

Ectropion occurs when the **eyelid turns outward, leading to exposure of the inner eyelid and eye irritation.** It results in dryness, discomfort, and excessive tearing and may require surgery to correct.

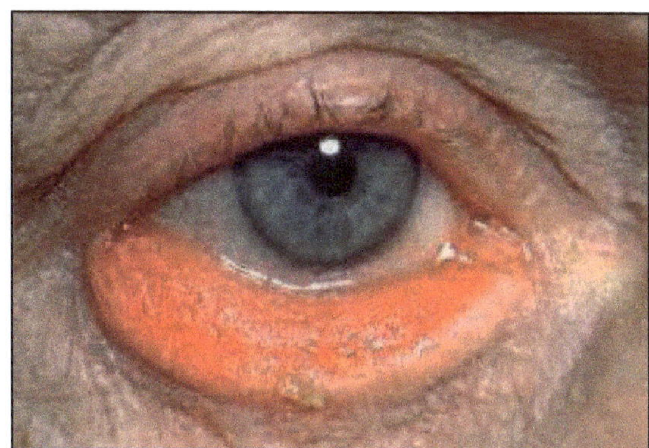

Figure 385 Ectropion

12.6.12.1 SOAP Notes for Ectropion

Table 210 SOAP Notes for Ectropion

Component	Details
Subjective (S)	A 65-year-old female presents with complaints of dry eyes, irritation, and excessive tearing in her right eye. She reports that her lower eyelid has been turning outward, causing her inner eyelid to be exposed.
Objective (O)	On physical examination, the patient's right lower eyelid is turned outward, exposing the conjunctiva. There is mild conjunctival redness and dryness, but no active infection or corneal damage.
Assessment (A)	The patient's symptoms, along with the outward-turning eyelid, are consistent with ectropion, which is causing exposure and irritation of the inner eyelid and eye.
Plan (P)	**Pharmacological**: Prescribe artificial tears to relieve dryness and irritation. **Non-pharmacological**: Recommend lubricating ointments for night-time use and eyelid protection. Surgical correction may be needed if symptoms persist or worsen. **Follow-up**: Follow-up in 1-2 weeks to evaluate the response to treatment. **Education**: Educate the patient on the potential for corneal damage if untreated and the importance of surgical intervention if conservative measures do not provide relief.

12.6.13 Pinguecula

Pinguecula is a benign growth on the **conjunctiva, often due to UV light exposure, aging, or irritation.** It presents as a yellowish, raised area on the white part of the eye, usually near the cornea, but rarely causes vision problems.

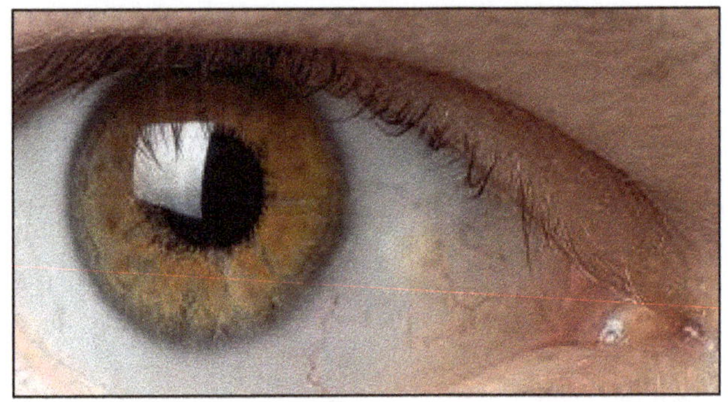

Figure 386 Pinguecula

12.6.13.1 SOAP Notes for Pinguecula

Table 211 SOAP Notes for Pinguecula

Component	Details
Subjective (S)	A 55-year-old male presents with a yellowish growth on the white part of his eye, near the cornea. He reports no significant pain or irritation but has noticed the growth becoming more noticeable over time, especially in bright sunlight.
Objective (O)	On physical examination, the patient has a yellowish, raised growth on the conjunctiva, usually near the nasal side of the cornea. The cornea itself appears unaffected, and visual acuity is normal.
Assessment (A)	The patient's symptoms and the appearance of a yellow, raised growth on the conjunctiva are consistent with pinguecula, a benign lesion commonly caused by UV light exposure or aging.
Plan (P)	**Pharmacological**: Prescribe artificial tears for dryness if necessary. **Non-pharmacological**: Advise wearing UV-protective sunglasses and minimizing sun exposure. **Follow-up**: Follow-up in 6-12 months to monitor for any changes in size or symptoms. **Education**: Educate the patient on the benign nature of pinguecula and the importance of protecting the eyes from further UV damage to prevent progression to more serious conditions like pterygium.

12.6.14 Pterygium

Pterygium is a fleshy growth of tissue from the **conjunctiva onto the cornea, often due to prolonged sun exposure or environmental irritants**. It can cause redness, irritation, and, in severe cases, affect vision if it grows large enough to cover the cornea.

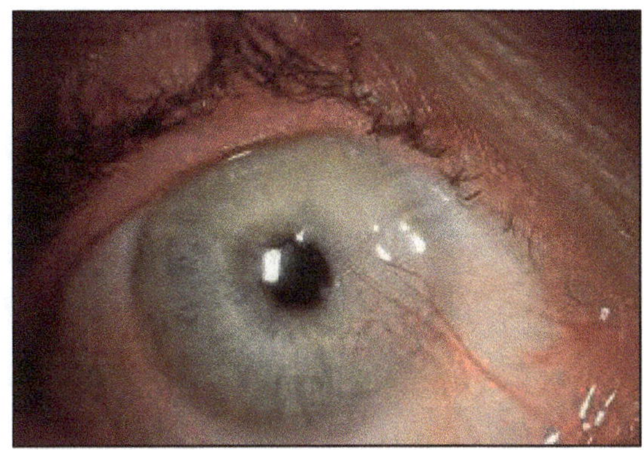

Figure 387 Pterygium

12.6.14.1 SOAP Notes for Pterygium

Table 212 SOAP Notes for Pterygium

Component	Details
Subjective (S)	A 50-year-old male presents with a fleshy growth on the white part of his eye, near the cornea. He reports occasional irritation and redness, especially after prolonged sun exposure.
Objective (O)	On physical examination, the patient has a fleshy, triangular growth on the conjunctiva extending onto the cornea. The cornea shows mild irritation, but the patient has normal visual acuity.
Assessment (A)	The patient's symptoms, along with the presence of a triangular growth extending from the conjunctiva onto the cornea, are consistent with pterygium. This condition is often associated with UV exposure or environmental factors.
Plan (P)	**Pharmacological**: Prescribe artificial tears to relieve irritation and corticosteroid eye drops for inflammation if needed. **Non-pharmacological**: Advise wearing UV-protective sunglasses and limiting sun exposure to prevent progression. **Follow-up**: Follow-up in 6-12 months to monitor for growth progression and potential vision interference. **Education**: Educate the patient on the need for UV protection and the potential for surgical removal if vision is affected by the growth.

12.6.15 Disc Cupping

Disc cupping refers to the enlargement of the optic nerve head's cup, commonly seen in glaucoma. It is **associated with vision loss due to optic nerve damage and is monitored using ophthalmoscopy** and OCT to track progression.

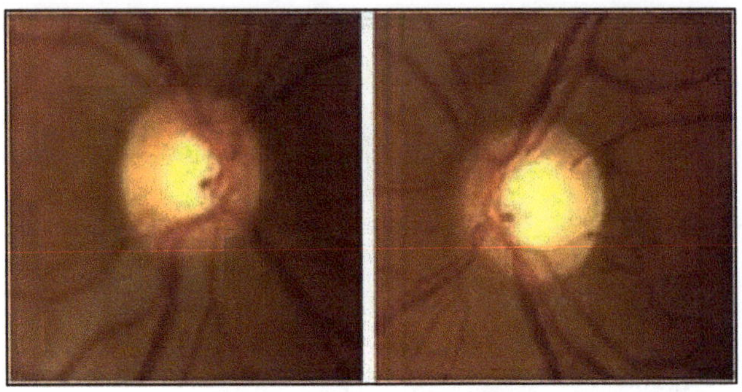

Figure 388 Disc Cupping

12.6.15.1 SOAP Notes for Disc Cupping

Table 213 SOAP Notes for Disc Cupping

Component	Details
Subjective (S)	A 60-year-old male presents with a gradual loss of peripheral vision over the past few months. He has a family history of glaucoma and reports difficulty seeing in low-light conditions.
Objective (O)	On fundoscopy, the patient shows an enlarged optic disc with a deeper cup, indicating disc cupping. Tonometry reveals elevated intraocular pressure (IOP) of 28 mmHg. Visual field testing shows loss of peripheral vision.
Assessment (A)	The patient's symptoms, along with disc cupping and elevated intraocular pressure, are consistent with glaucoma. Disc cupping is a hallmark sign of optic nerve damage due to glaucoma.
Plan (P)	**Pharmacological**: Prescribe medications to reduce intraocular pressure (e.g., latanoprost, timolol). **Non-pharmacological**: Recommend regular eye exams to monitor progression of glaucoma and prevent further optic nerve damage. **Follow-up**: Follow-up in 4-6 weeks to reassess intraocular pressure and monitor visual fields. **Education**: Educate the patient on the importance of medication adherence and regular eye exams to prevent further damage to the optic nerve and preserve vision.

12.6.16 Hypersensitivity Retinopathy

Hypersensitivity retinopathy is a form of retinal damage caused by immune system reactions, often **triggered by systemic conditions like autoimmune disorders**. It results in blurred vision, flashing lights, and visual disturbances that require management of the underlying condition.

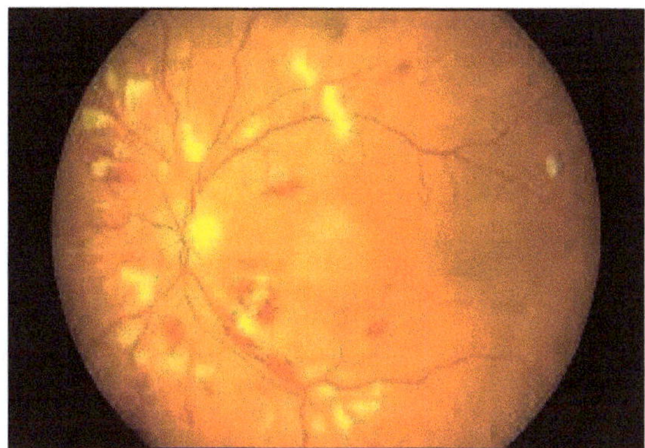

Figure 389 Hypersensitivity Retinopathy

12.6.16.1 SOAP Notes for Hypersensitivity Retinopathy

Table 214 SOAP Notes for Hypersensitivity Retinopathy

Component	Details
Subjective (S)	A 45-year-old female with a history of autoimmune disease presents with blurred vision, flashing lights, and difficulty focusing. She reports recent changes in her health and new medications.
Objective (O)	On fundoscopy, there are signs of retinal damage with hemorrhages and exudates, suggesting hypersensitivity retinopathy. Optical coherence tomography (OCT) shows retinal swelling.
Assessment (A)	The patient's symptoms and retinal findings are consistent with hypersensitivity retinopathy, likely due to her autoimmune condition.
Plan (P)	**Pharmacological**: Prescribe anti-inflammatory medications (e.g., corticosteroids) to address retinal inflammation. **Non-pharmacological**: Manage the underlying autoimmune condition to prevent further retinal damage. **Follow-up**: Follow-up in 1-2 weeks to monitor retinal condition and assess the response to treatment. **Education**: Educate the patient on managing their autoimmune condition and the potential effects on eye health.

12.6.17 Diabetic Retinopathy

Diabetic retinopathy is a complication of diabetes where **damage to the retinal blood vessels causes vision problems**. It can lead to blurry vision, difficulty seeing at night, and, in severe cases, blindness if left untreated.

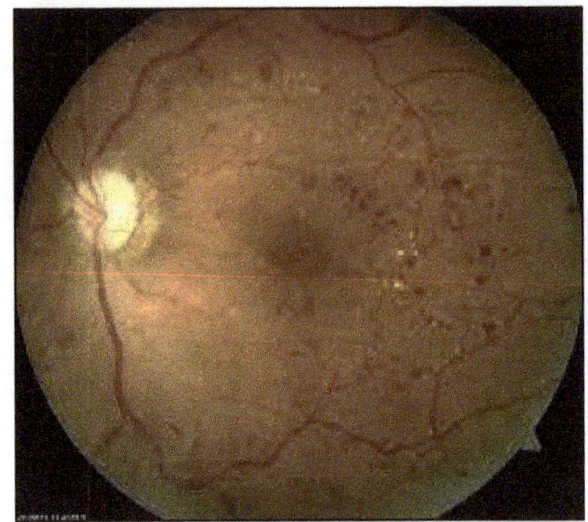

Figure 390 Diabetic Retinopathy

12.6.17.1 SOAP Notes for Diabetic Retinopathy

Table 215 SOAP Notes for Diabetic Retinopathy

Component	Details
Subjective (S)	A 55-year-old male with a history of poorly controlled diabetes presents with blurred vision and difficulty seeing at night. He reports noticing these issues progressively over the past few months, with an increase in floaters.
Objective (O)	On physical examination, visual acuity is reduced, and fundoscopy reveals microaneurysms, retinal hemorrhages, and exudates in the retinal vessels, consistent with diabetic retinopathy. There is no evidence of macular edema.
Assessment (A)	The patient's symptoms, along with retinal findings of microaneurysms and hemorrhages, are consistent with diabetic retinopathy, a complication of chronic diabetes affecting retinal blood vessels.
Plan (P)	**Pharmacological**: If applicable, recommend anti-VEGF (vascular endothelial growth factor) injections or laser treatment for macular edema or proliferative diabetic retinopathy. **Non-pharmacological**: Tight control of blood glucose levels and blood pressure to prevent progression. **Follow-up**: Regular follow-up every 3-6 months to monitor the progression of retinopathy and manage any associated complications. **Education**: Educate the patient on the importance of strict blood glucose management and regular eye exams to prevent vision loss from diabetic retinopathy.

12.6.18 Cataracts

Cataracts occur when the lens of **the eye becomes cloudy, leading to blurry vision and difficulty seeing in low light.** It is a common age-related condition and is treated effectively with surgery to remove the clouded lens and replace it with an artificial one.

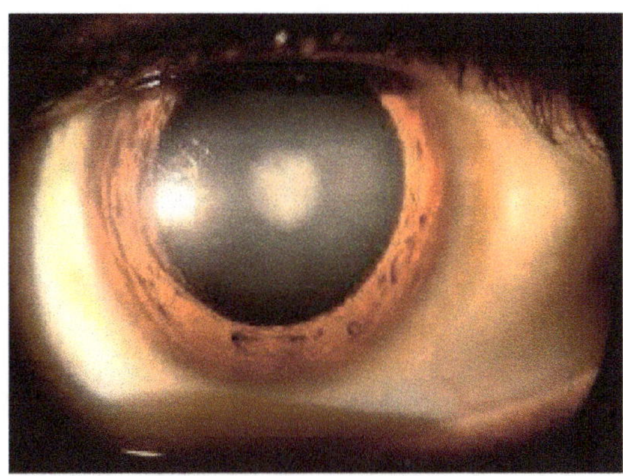

Figure 391 Cataract

12.6.18.1 SOAP Notes for Cataract

Table 216 SOAP Notes for Cataract

Component	Details
Subjective (S)	A 70-year-old female presents with blurry vision, difficulty seeing at night, and sensitivity to glare, especially when driving. She reports noticing these symptoms progressively over the past year.
Objective (O)	On physical examination, visual acuity is reduced, and the lens appears cloudy upon slit-lamp examination. There are no signs of acute eye infections or inflammation, and the retina appears healthy.
Assessment (A)	The patient's symptoms, including blurry vision, difficulty with night vision, and glare, are consistent with cataracts, a common age-related condition causing clouding of the eye's natural lens.
Plan (P)	**Pharmacological**: No specific pharmacological treatment is needed for cataracts. **Non-pharmacological**: Advise the use of magnifying glasses or stronger lighting to aid vision temporarily. **Surgical intervention**: Discuss cataract surgery for lens removal and replacement with an intraocular lens (IOL) once the cataract begins to significantly impact daily activities. **Follow-up**: Schedule follow-up in 6 months to monitor progression and discuss surgical options if necessary. **Education**: Educate the patient on cataract progression, surgical treatment options, and the expected benefits of cataract surgery in restoring vision.

12.7 Common Conditions of Ears and Sinuses

"A CAB A OOV" **A** = Auricular Hematoma, **C** = Acoustic Neuroma, **C** = Cholesteatoma, **B** = Battle Sign, **A** = Acute Otitis Media, **A** = Acute Bacterial Rhinosinusitis, **O** = Otitis Media with Effusion, **O** = Otitis Externa, **V** = Vertigo (Maneuvers)

Table 217 Common Conditions of Ears and Sinuses

Condition	Description	Key Symptoms	Diagnostic Tools	Treatment Options
Auricular Hematoma	Auricular hematoma is a collection of	Pain, swelling, and redness	Physical examination, possible	Drainage of blood and compression

	blood between the ear's cartilage and skin, usually caused by trauma.	of the ear, possible deformity if untreated.	drainage or aspiration of fluid, and ultrasound.	bandage, sometimes surgical intervention.
Acoustic Neuroma	Acoustic neuroma is a benign tumor on the vestibulocochlear nerve, affecting balance and hearing.	Hearing loss, tinnitus (ringing in the ear), and dizziness.	MRI of the brain and auditory canal to detect tumor presence.	Surgical removal of the tumor, sometimes followed by radiation or hearing aids.
Cholesteatoma	Cholesteatoma is an abnormal skin growth in the middle ear, often due to recurrent ear infections.	Hearing loss, ear drainage, dizziness, and possible facial nerve weakness.	Physical examination, CT or MRI for detailed imaging of the ear.	Surgical removal of the cholesteatoma, possible hearing aids for hearing loss.
Battle Sign	Battle sign refers to bruising behind the ear, often associated with a skull fracture.	Bruising behind the ear, indicating potential skull fracture.	Physical examination, with emphasis on bruising and neurological assessment.	No specific treatment, but immediate investigation for skull fracture and potential imaging.
Acute Otitis Media	Acute otitis media is an infection of the middle ear, usually caused by bacteria or viruses.	Ear pain, fever, difficulty hearing, and sometimes fluid discharge	Otoscope for examining the ear, tympanometry, and cultures for bacteria.	Antibiotics for bacterial infections, pain relief with over-the-counter medications.

		from the ear.		
Acute Bacterial Rhinosinusitis	Acute bacterial rhinosinusitis occurs when the sinuses become infected with bacteria after a viral infection.	Facial pain, nasal congestion, thick nasal discharge, and fever.	Sinus X-rays, CT scans, or nasal endoscopy for sinus examination.	Antibiotics (if bacterial), nasal saline irrigation, and decongestants.
Otitis Media with Effusion	Otitis media with effusion is fluid buildup in the middle ear without infection signs.	Hearing difficulties , particularly in children, and a sensation of fullness in the ear.	Otoscopic examination and hearing tests.	Observation and monitoring, with possible myringotomy if fluid persists.
Otitis Externa	Otitis externa, also known as swimmer's ear, is an infection of the outer ear canal.	Itching, pain, swelling of the ear canal, and possible discharge.	Otoscope for canal examination, swab for culture if necessary.	Antibiotic ear drops for bacterial infection, pain management.
Vertigo (Maneuvers)	Vertigo is a spinning sensation, often caused by inner ear disturbances like BPPV, treated with specific maneuvers.	Dizziness or a spinning sensation, especially when changing head positions.	Dix-Hallpike test or other positional tests to diagnose BPP	

12.8 Major Medical Conditions of Ears and Sinuses in HEENT System

12.8.1 Auricular Hematoma

Auricular hematoma is a collection of blood between the ear's cartilage and skin, usually caused by trauma, such as blunt force or a blow to the ear. If untreated, it can lead to fibrosis and deformity of the ear, often referred to as **"cauliflower ear."**

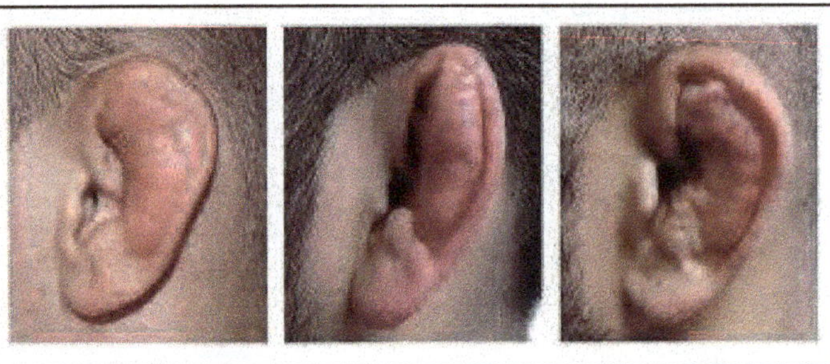

Figure 392 Auricular Hematoma

12.8.1.1 SOAP Notes for Auricular Hematoma

Table 218 SOAP Notes for Auricular Hematoma

Component	Details
Subjective (S)	A 28-year-old male presents with swelling and pain in his right ear following a traumatic injury during a contact sport. He reports that the swelling has been present for several hours and that the pain has increased gradually.
Objective (O)	On physical examination, the right ear is swollen, red, and tender. The swelling is confined to the external ear, and there is no active bleeding or discharge. The ear's appearance suggests an auricular hematoma.
Assessment (A)	The patient's symptoms, including ear swelling and tenderness after trauma, are consistent with an auricular hematoma.
Plan (P)	**Pharmacological**: Pain management with NSAIDs (e.g., ibuprofen). **Non-pharmacological**: Drainage of the hematoma to prevent fibrosis and deformity. Apply compression dressing post-drainage. **Follow-up**: Recheck in 1-2 days to ensure proper drainage and prevent recurrence. **Education**: Educate the patient on the importance of early intervention to avoid permanent ear deformity ("cauliflower ear").

12.8.2 Acoustic Neuroma

Acoustic neuroma is a benign tumor that develops on the vestibulocochlear nerve, affecting balance and hearing. Symptoms may include **hearing loss, tinnitus (ringing in the ear), and dizziness, and it is typically diagnosed through MRI.**

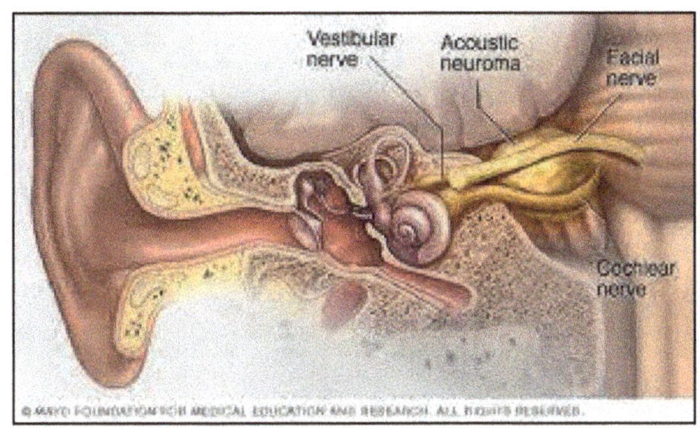

Figure 393 Acoustic Neuroma

12.8.2.1 SOAP Notes for Acoustic Neuroma

Table 219 SOAP Notes for Acoustic Neuroma

Component	Details
Subjective (S)	A 55-year-old female presents with progressive hearing loss in her right ear, along with tinnitus and occasional dizziness. She has noticed the symptoms worsening over the last six months.
Objective (O)	On physical examination, the patient has normal external ear findings. Audiometry confirms sensorineural hearing loss in the right ear. Neurological exam is normal, but vestibular testing reveals slight imbalance.
Assessment (A)	The patient's symptoms, including unilateral hearing loss, tinnitus, and vestibular dysfunction, are suggestive of acoustic neuroma (vestibular schwannoma).
Plan (P)	**Pharmacological**: No specific pharmacological treatment for the tumor itself. **Non-pharmacological**: MRI of the brain and internal auditory canal to confirm the diagnosis. **Surgical intervention**: Consider surgical resection of the tumor, depending on size and location. **Follow-up**: Schedule follow-up in 1-2 weeks after MRI results for a surgical consultation. **Education**: Educate the patient on the benign nature of acoustic neuromas but stress the need for surgical removal to prevent further hearing loss and complications.

12.8.3 Cholesteatoma

Cholesteatoma is an abnormal skin growth in the middle ear, often caused by repeated ear infections. It can lead to hearing loss, dizziness, and potential damage to the bones of the middle ear if left untreated.

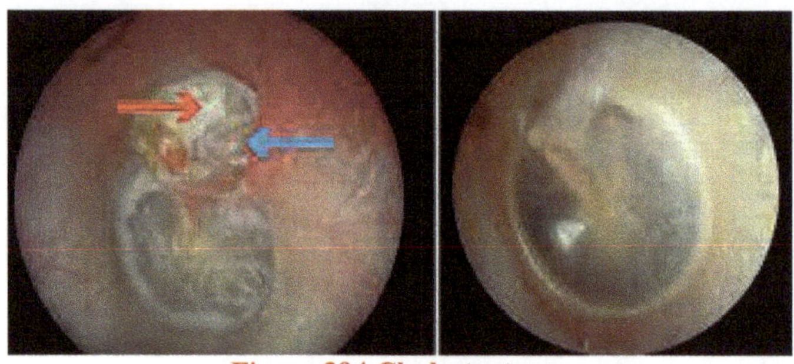

Figure 394 Cholesteatoma

12.8.3.1 SOAP Notes for Cholesteatoma

Table 220 SOAP Notes for Cholesteatoma

Component	Details
Subjective (S)	A 45-year-old male presents with a history of recurrent ear infections and a sensation of fullness in his right ear. He reports occasional drainage from the ear and decreased hearing over the past year.
Objective (O)	On physical examination, the right ear is mildly tender, with a noticeable discharge. Otoscopy reveals a white, pearly mass in the middle ear, likely indicative of a cholesteatoma. Tympanometry shows conductive hearing loss.
Assessment (A)	The patient's symptoms and findings, including recurrent ear infections, discharge, and a middle ear mass, are consistent with cholesteatoma.
Plan (P)	**Pharmacological**: Prescribe antibiotics if infection is present in the ear. **Non-pharmacological**: Refer the patient for a CT scan to assess the extent of the cholesteatoma and evaluate for damage to the ossicles. **Surgical intervention**: Surgical removal of the cholesteatoma, which may involve tympanoplasty or mastoidectomy. **Follow-up**: Follow-up in 1-2 weeks after surgery to ensure complete removal and monitor for recurrence. **Education**: Educate the patient on the potential for hearing loss and complications if the cholesteatoma is left untreated.

12.8.4 Battle sign

Battle sign refers to bruising behind the ear, often **associated with a skull fracture**. It can be a sign of traumatic injury to the skull and requires immediate medical attention to rule out intracranial injuries.

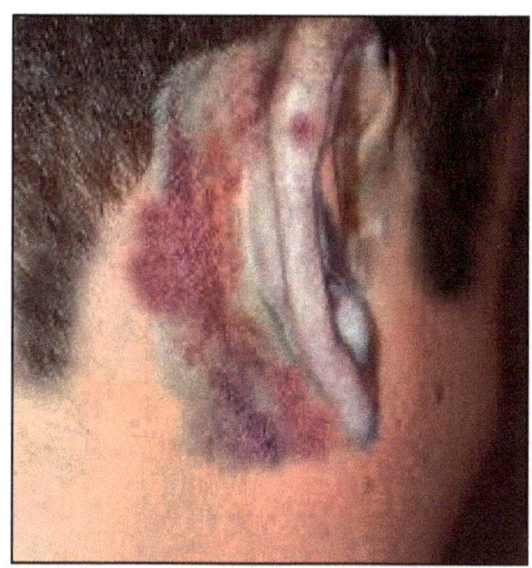

Figure 395 Battle Sign

12.8.4.1 SOAP Notes for Battle Sign

Table 221 SOAP Notes for Battle Sign

Component	Details
Subjective (S)	A 35-year-old male presents with bruising behind his left ear following a head injury from a fall. He reports a history of trauma but denies loss of consciousness or any obvious external head wounds.
Objective (O)	On physical examination, the patient has bruising behind the left ear (Battle sign), which is tender to palpation. No visible skull fractures or lacerations are observed, and neurological examination is normal.
Assessment (A)	The presence of Battle sign suggests a possible basilar skull fracture, often associated with significant trauma.
Plan (P)	**Pharmacological**: Pain management with analgesics (e.g., acetaminophen or ibuprofen). **Non-pharmacological**: Order a CT scan of the head to rule out any skull fractures or intracranial injuries. **Follow-up**: Immediate follow-up after imaging results to address potential fractures or complications. **Education**: Educate the patient on the importance of monitoring for signs of intracranial injury (e.g., worsening headache, vomiting, or confusion).

12.8.5 Acute Otitis Media

Acute otitis media is an infection of the m**iddle ear, typically caused by bacteria or viruses, leading to pain, fever, and sometimes hearing loss.** It is more common in children and may resolve with antibiotics or pain management, depending on severity.

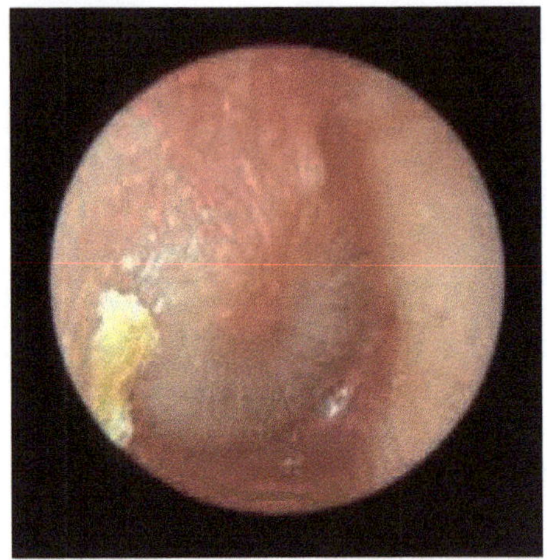

Figure 396 Acute Otitis Media

12.8.5.1 SOAP Notes for Otitis Media

Table 222 SOAP Notes for Otitis Media

Component	Details
Subjective (S)	A 4-year-old child presents with complaints of ear pain, fever, and irritability for the past two days. The child has a history of recurrent ear infections.
Objective (O)	On physical examination, the child appears ill and is crying when the ear is touched. Otoscopic examination reveals a red, bulging tympanic membrane with effusion.
Assessment (A)	The patient's symptoms, including fever, ear pain, and tympanic membrane findings, are consistent with acute otitis media, likely bacterial in origin.
Plan (P)	**Pharmacological**: Prescribe amoxicillin or alternative antibiotics if allergic (See algorithm below). **Non-pharmacological**: Pain management with acetaminophen or ibuprofen. **Follow-up**: Reassess in 2-3 days to evaluate response to treatment and ensure resolution. **Education**: Educate the parents on the importance of completing the full course of antibiotics to prevent complications and recurrent infections.

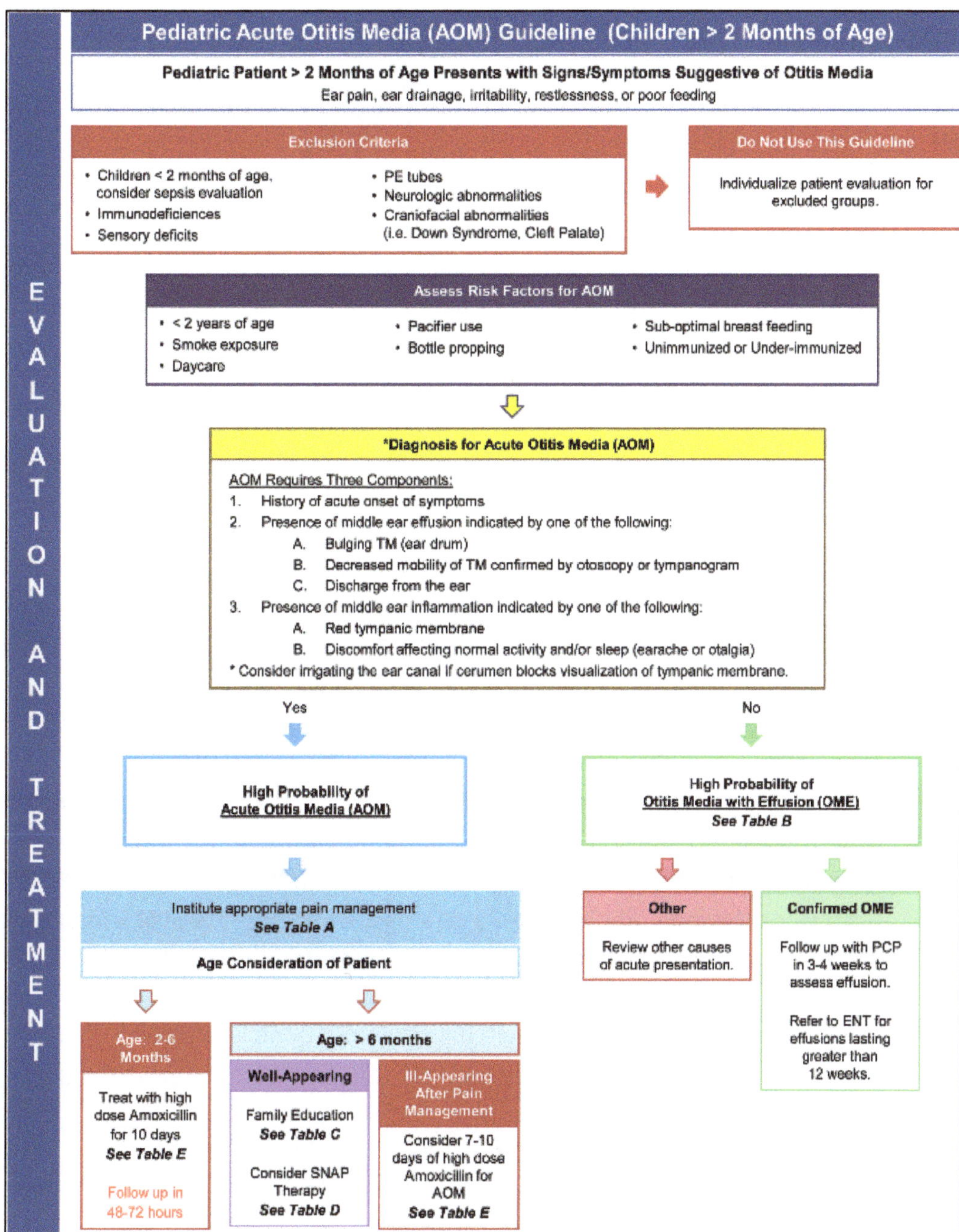

Figure 397 Algrithm for the Management of Pediatric Acute Otitis Media

12.8.6 Acute Bacterial Rhinosinusitis

Acute bacterial rhinosinusitis occurs when the sinuses become infected with bacteria, often following a viral upper respiratory infection. Symptoms **include facial pain, nasal congestion, and a thick nasal discharge, and antibiotics** may be required if bacterial infection is confirmed.

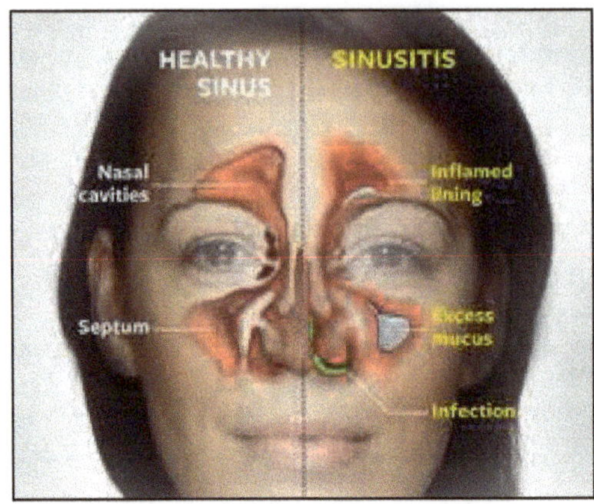

Figure 398 Acute Bacterial Rhinosinusitis

12.8.6.1 SOAP Notes for Acute Rhinosinusitis

Table 223 SOAP Notes for Acute Rhinosinusitis

Component	Details
Subjective (S)	A 30-year-old male presents with facial pain, nasal congestion, and a thick yellow nasal discharge that has persisted for the last 10 days. He reports worsening symptoms after an initial cold.
Objective (O)	On physical examination, there is tenderness over the maxillary sinuses, and the patient has thick nasal discharge. Nasal endoscopy shows purulent secretion from the middle meatus.
Assessment (A)	The patient's symptoms and examination findings suggest acute bacterial rhinosinusitis, likely following a viral upper respiratory infection.
Plan (P)	**Pharmacological**: Prescribe antibiotics (e.g., amoxicillin-clavulanate). **Non-pharmacological**: Recommend nasal saline irrigation and decongestants. **Follow-up**: Reassess in 7-10 days if symptoms do not improve. **Education**: Educate the patient on managing symptoms and the importance of completing the antibiotic course to prevent complications.

12.8.7 Otitis media with effusion

Otitis media with effusion is a condition where fluid accumulates in the middle ear without signs of infection. It can cause hearing difficulties, particularly in children, and often resolves on its own, though persistent cases may require medical intervention.

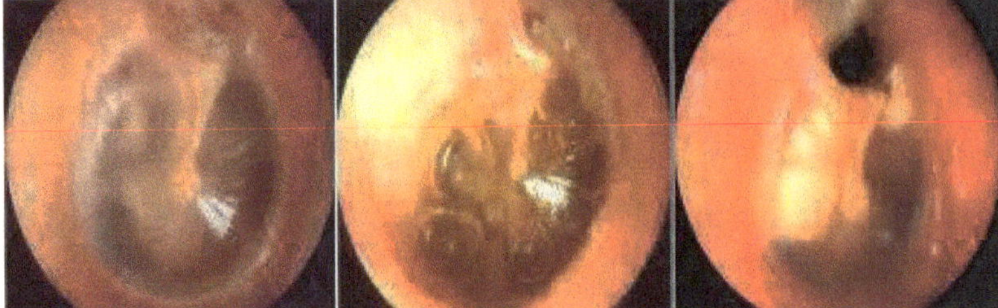

Figure 399 Otitis Media with Effusion

12.8.7.1 SOAP Notes for Otitis Media with Effusion

Table 224 SOAP Notes for Otitis Media with Effusion

Component	Details

Subjective (S)	A 3-year-old child presents with a history of recurrent ear infections and a sensation of fullness in the right ear. Parents report no fever or acute pain but note difficulty in hearing.
Objective (O)	On physical examination, the child is alert but has mild irritability. Otoscopic examination reveals a dull tympanic membrane with a visible fluid level behind the membrane.
Assessment (A)	The patient's symptoms and otoscopic findings are consistent with otitis media with effusion, characterized by fluid in the middle ear without signs of acute infection.
Plan (P)	**Pharmacological**: No antibiotics are needed unless an infection is suspected. **Non-pharmacological**: Observe the condition for 4-6 weeks, and provide pain relief if necessary. **Follow-up**: Reassess in 1-2 months to check for resolution or persistent effusion. **Education**: Educate parents on the usual self-limiting course of this condition and the importance of follow-up to prevent hearing loss.

12.8.8 Otitis Externa

Otitis externa, commonly known as swimmer's ear, is an infection or inflammation of the outer ear canal caused by bacteria or fungi. Symptoms include itching, pain, and discharge from the ear, often aggravated by water exposure.

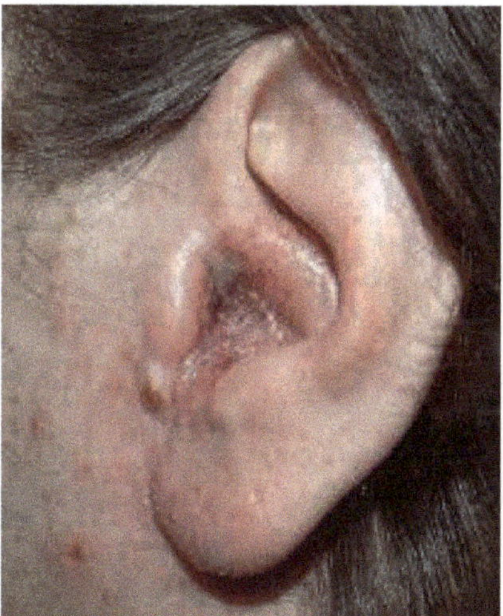

Figure 400 Otitis Externa

12.8.8.1 SOAP Notes for Otitis Externa

Table 225 SOAP Notes for Otitis Externa

Component	Details
Subjective (S)	A 25-year-old female presents with itching, pain, and swelling in her right ear after swimming in a pool. She reports a feeling of fullness and occasional discharge.
Objective (O)	On physical examination, the outer ear canal is swollen, red, and tender to touch, with yellowish discharge. No tympanic membrane abnormalities are noted.

Assessment (A)	The patient's symptoms and findings are consistent with otitis externa, often caused by bacterial infection, commonly following water exposure.
Plan (P)	**Pharmacological**: Prescribe antibiotic ear drops (e.g., ciprofloxacin). **Non-pharmacological**: Recommend avoiding water exposure and gentle cleaning of the ear canal. **Follow-up**: Follow-up in 1 week if symptoms persist or worsen. **Education**: Educate the patient on proper ear hygiene and the importance of keeping ears dry to prevent recurrence.

12.8.9 Vertigo (Maneuvers)

Vertigo is a sensation of spinning or dizziness, commonly caused by inner ear disturbances like **benign paroxysmal positional vertigo (BPPV)**. Specific maneuvers, such as the Epley maneuver, are used to reposition debris in the ear and relieve symptoms.

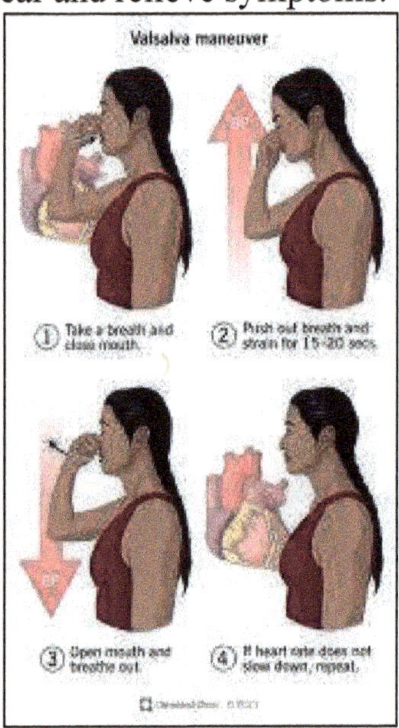

Figure 401 Maneuvers

12.8.9.1 SOAP Notes for Maneuvers

Table 226 SOAP Notes for Maneuvers

Component	Details
Subjective (S)	A 60-year-old female presents with a sensation of spinning and dizziness when changing head positions, which started suddenly after getting out of bed this morning.
Objective (O)	On physical examination, the patient has no signs of neurological deficit. The Dix-Hallpike test reproduces the vertigo and nystagmus, confirming benign paroxysmal positional vertigo (BPPV).
Assessment (A)	The patient's symptoms and the positive Dix-Hallpike test are consistent with BPPV, a common cause of vertigo.
Plan (P)	**Pharmacological**: No specific medications are required for BPPV, but antihistamines or benzodiazepines may be used for symptomatic relief if needed (See algorithm below). **Non-pharmacological**: Perform the Epley maneuver to reposition the displaced otoconia in the inner ear. **Follow-up**:

	Follow-up in 1-2 weeks to monitor progress and repeat maneuvers if necessary. **Education**: Educate the patient on the benign nature of BPPV and the effectiveness of maneuvers in managing symptoms.

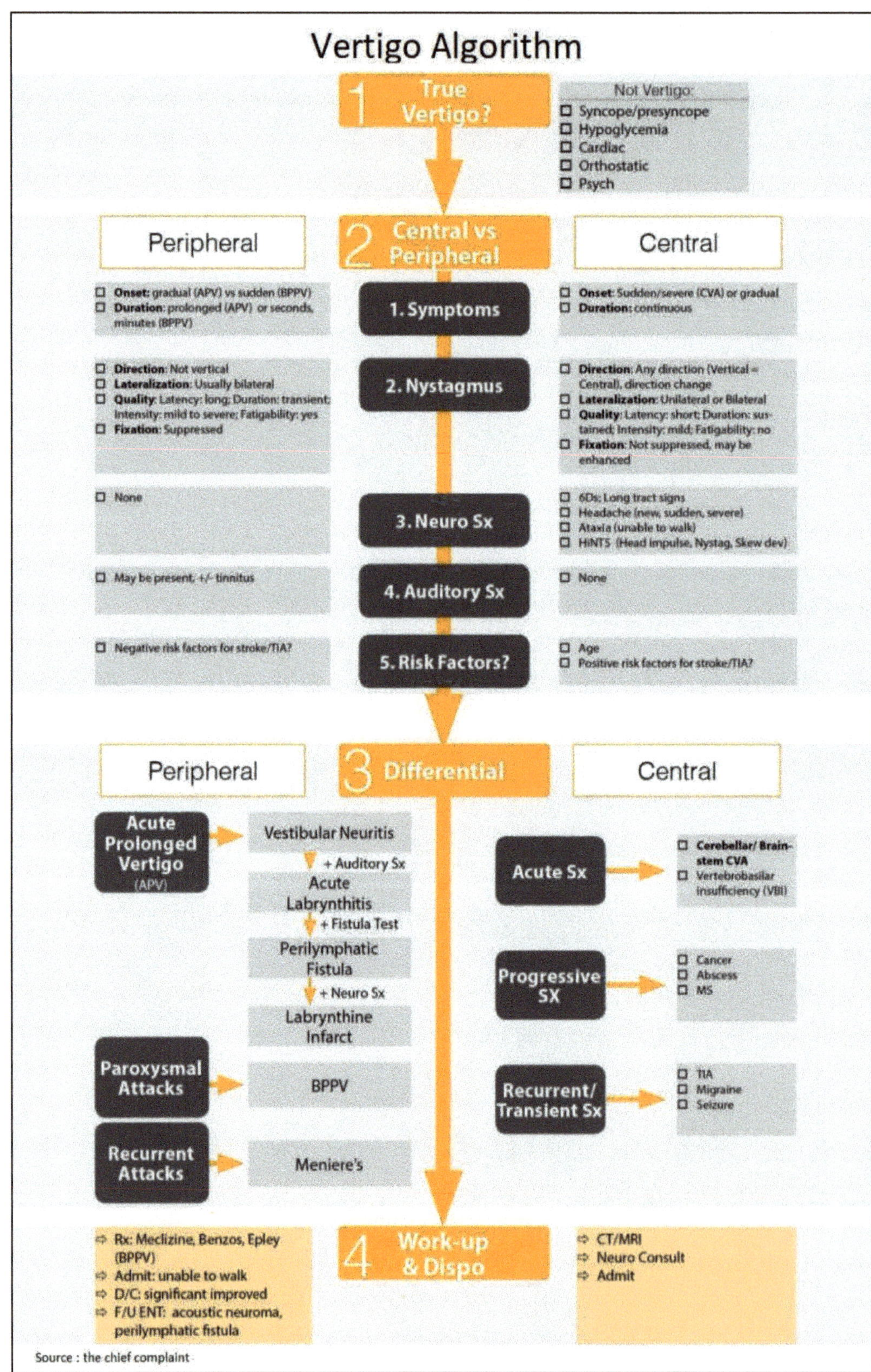

Figure 402 Algorithm for the Management of Vertigo

12.9 Common Conditions of Nose in HEENT System

"Astonishing Experts See People." A = Allergic Rhinitis, E = Epistaxis, S = Septal Perforation, and **P = Nasal Polyps**

Table 227 Common Conditions of Nose in HEENT System

Condition	Description	Key Symptoms	Diagnostic Tools	Treatment Options
Allergic Rhinitis	Allergic rhinitis is an inflammation of the nasal passages caused by allergens such as pollen, dust, or pet dander.	Sneezing, nasal congestion, runny nose, and itching, particularly during allergy seasons.	Physical examination, skin prick tests, or serum IgE testing for specific allergens.	Prescribe antihistamines (e.g., loratadine) and intranasal corticosteroids (e.g., fluticasone). Recommend allergen avoidance.
Epistaxis	Epistaxis, or nosebleeds, occur when blood vessels in the nasal passages break, leading to bleeding from one or both nostrils.	Sudden nosebleed, often from one nostril. May be triggered by dry air, trauma, or underlying medical conditions.	Physical examination, possibly nasal endoscopy if bleeding is recurrent or severe.	Apply nasal decongestant (e.g., oxymetazoline), petroleum jelly, and recommend using a humidifier.
Septal Perforation	A septal perforation is a hole or defect in the nasal septum, which separates the nostrils.	Nasal obstruction, crusting, and occasional bleeding from the nose.	Anterior rhinoscopy to identify the septal defect, and sometimes CT scans to evaluate the extent.	Recommend nasal saline sprays, advise discontinuing nasal decongestant sprays. Follow-up in 1 month for evaluation.
Nasal Polyps	Nasal polyps are benign growths in the nasal passages or sinuses that can cause chronic congestion and frequent infections.	Chronic nasal congestion, loss of smell, and frequent sinus infections. Difficulty breathing through the nose.	Endoscopic examination revealing soft, pale polyps in nasal passages. Sometimes, CT scans to assess sinus involvement.	Intranasal corticosteroids (e.g., fluticasone), antihistamines for symptom control. Consider surgery if symptoms persist.

12.10 Major Medical Conditions of Nose

12.10.1 Allergic Rhinitis

Allergic rhinitis is an inflammation **of the nasal passages caused by allergens such as pollen, dust, or pet dander.** Symptoms include sneezing, nasal congestion, runny nose, and itching, particularly during allergy seasons.

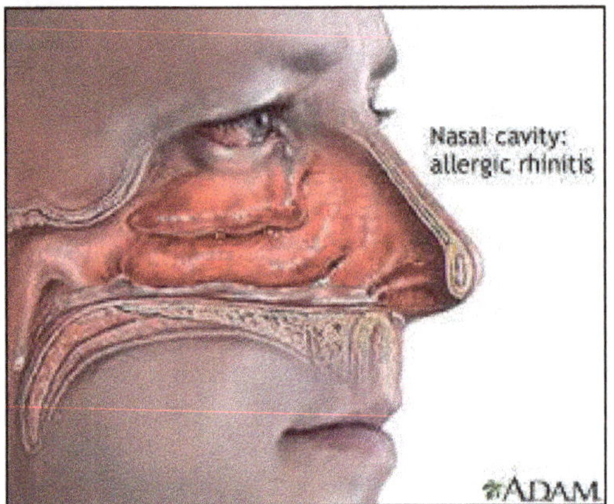

Figure 403 Allergic Rhinitis

12.10.1.1 SOAP Notes for Allergic Rhinitis

Table 228 SOAP Notes for Allergic Rhinitis

Component	Details
Subjective (S)	A 30-year-old male presents with sneezing, nasal congestion, and a runny nose for the past two weeks. He reports that symptoms are worse during the day and outdoors, especially when exposed to pollen.
Objective (O)	On physical examination, the patient has pale, swollen nasal mucosa, clear nasal discharge, and watery eyes. There is no fever, and the throat is clear.
Assessment (A)	The patient's symptoms, including sneezing, nasal congestion, and clear rhinorrhea, are consistent with allergic rhinitis, likely triggered by pollen.
Plan (P)	**Pharmacological**: Prescribe antihistamines (e.g., loratadine) and intranasal corticosteroids (e.g., fluticasone). **Non-pharmacological**: Recommend avoiding allergens, using a saline nasal rinse, and keeping windows closed during high pollen seasons. **Follow-up**: Reassess in 2-4 weeks to evaluate symptom control. **Education**: Educate the patient on allergen avoidance strategies and proper use of medications.

12.10.2 Epistaxis

Epistaxis, or nosebleeds, occur when blood vessels in the **nasal passages break, leading to bleeding from one or both nostrils.** Common causes include dry air, trauma, or underlying medical conditions, and treatment typically involves controlling the bleeding and addressing the underlying cause.

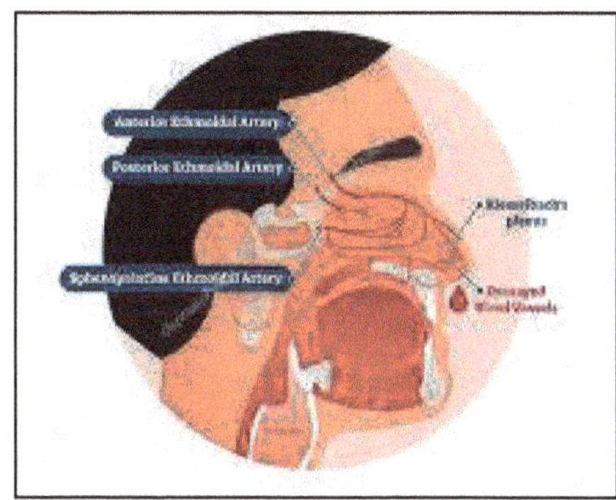

Figure 404 Epistaxis

12.10.2.1 SOAP Notes for Epistaxis

Table 229 SOAP Notes for Epistaxis

Component	Details
Subjective (S)	A 45-year-old female presents with sudden onset of nosebleed from the left nostril that started while she was at work. She denies any trauma or recent upper respiratory infections.
Objective (O)	On physical examination, the patient is not in distress. Active bleeding is noted from the anterior nasal septum. There is no evidence of facial trauma, and the nasal mucosa is dry.
Assessment (A)	The patient's symptoms of spontaneous nosebleeding, combined with dry nasal mucosa, are consistent with epistaxis, likely due to dry air.
Plan (P)	**Pharmacological**: Apply nasal decongestant (oxymetazoline) and recommend petroleum jelly to the nasal passages. **Non-pharmacological**: Use a humidifier at home, and avoid vigorous nose blowing. **Follow-up**: Follow-up in 1 week if bleeding recurs or does not resolve. **Education**: Educate the patient on nasal care to prevent dryness and recurrence of nosebleeds.

12.10.3 Septal Perforation

A septal perforation is a hole or defect in the nasal septum, which separates the nostrils. It can result **from trauma, chronic use of nasal sprays, or certain infections,** leading to symptoms like nasal obstruction, crusting, and bleeding.

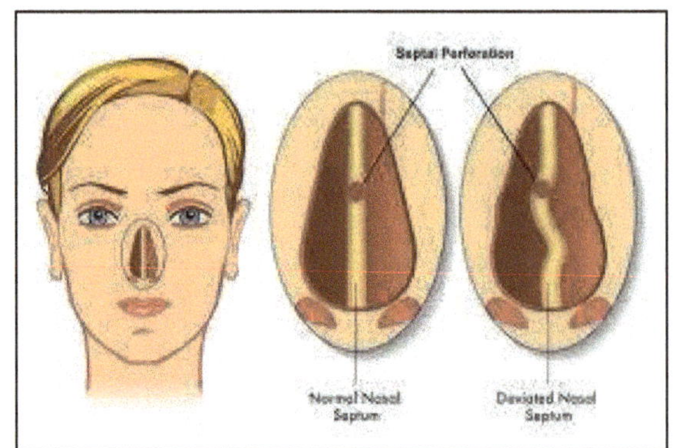

Figure 405 Septal Perforation

12.10.3.1 SOAP Notes for Septal Perforation

Table 230 SOAP Notes for Septal Perforation

Component	Details
Subjective (S)	A 50-year-old male presents with nasal obstruction, crusting, and occasional bleeding from the nose. He reports a history of frequent nasal spray use for sinus congestion.
Objective (O)	On physical examination, a visible hole is noted in the nasal septum on anterior rhinoscopy. There is moderate nasal crusting and minimal bleeding.
Assessment (A)	The patient's history of chronic nasal spray use, combined with symptoms of nasal obstruction, crusting, and a visible septal defect, is consistent with septal perforation.
Plan (P)	**Pharmacological**: Recommend nasal saline sprays to help with dryness and crusting. **Non-pharmacological**: Advise discontinuing the use of nasal decongestant sprays. **Follow-up**: Follow-up in 1 month to monitor for further symptoms and evaluate the need for surgical intervention if the perforation worsens. **Education**: Educate the patient on the risks of prolonged nasal spray use and the potential for permanent damage.

12.10.4 Nasal Polyps

Nasal polyps are benign, non-cancerous growths in the nasal passages or sinuses that can cause **chronic congestion, loss of smell, and frequent sinus infections**. They are commonly associated with conditions like asthma, sinusitis, or allergic rhinitis.

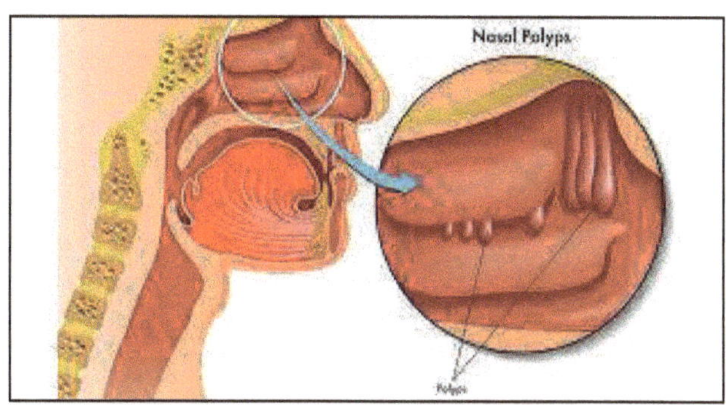

Figure 406 Nasal Polyps

12.10.4.1 SOAP Notes for Nasal Polyps

Table 231 SOAP Notes for Nasal Polyps

Component	Details
Subjective (S)	A 40-year-old female presents with chronic nasal congestion, loss of smell, and frequent sinus infections over the past year. She reports difficulty breathing through her nose, especially at night.
Objective (O)	On physical examination, the patient has clear nasal discharge and swollen nasal mucosa. Endoscopy reveals multiple soft, pale polyps in the nasal passages, particularly around the middle turbinate.
Assessment (A)	The patient's symptoms of chronic congestion, loss of smell, and nasal polyps on examination are consistent with nasal polyposis, likely related to underlying allergic rhinitis or chronic sinusitis.
Plan (P)	**Pharmacological**: Prescribe intranasal corticosteroids (e.g., fluticasone) and antihistamines for symptom control. **Non-pharmacological**: Recommend nasal saline rinses and avoiding known allergens. **Follow-up**: Reassess in 4-6 weeks to monitor for symptom improvement. **Surgical intervention**: Consider referral to an ENT specialist for potential surgical removal if symptoms persist or worsen. **Education**: Educate the patient on long-term management strategies, including medication adherence and avoiding triggers.

12.11 Common Conditions of Mouth and Neck in HEENT System

12.12 Major Medical Conditions of Mouth and Neck

12.12.1 Avulsed Tooth

An avulsed tooth refers to a tooth that has been completely displaced from its socket, usually due to trauma. Immediate action, such as **replanting the tooth or storing it in milk,** is critical to save the tooth.

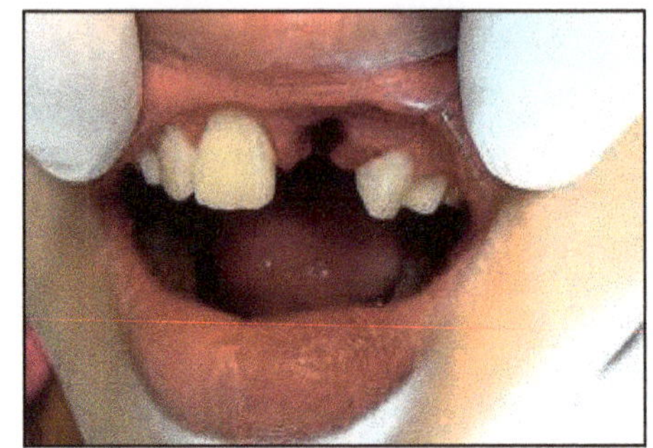

Figure 407 Avulsed Tooth

12.12.1.1 SOAP Notes for Avulsed Tooth

Table 232 SOAP Notes for Avulsed Tooth

Component	Details
Subjective (S)	A 6-year-old child presents with a dislodged front tooth following an accidental fall while playing. The tooth was completely displaced from its socket.
Objective (O)	On examination, there is visible trauma to the upper dental arch with no bleeding from the socket. The tooth is missing, but no signs of other facial trauma are noted.
Assessment (A)	The patient's condition is consistent with an avulsed tooth, a dental emergency requiring immediate intervention to maximize the chance of successful replantation.
Plan (P)	**Pharmacological**: No specific medications unless infection is suspected. **Non-pharmacological**: Immediately replant the tooth if possible, or store it in milk or saline for transport to a dentist. **Follow-up**: Referral to a dentist or emergency care for replantation or a dental implant if replantation is not possible. **Education**: Educate the parents on the importance of quick action and storing the tooth correctly for possible replantation.

12.12.2 Peritonsillar Abscess

A peritonsillar abscess is a pus-filled pocket that forms near the tonsils, often as a complication of a tonsillitis infection. **Symptoms include severe throat pain, fever, difficulty swallowing, and a muffled voice, and treatment typically** involves drainage and antibiotics.

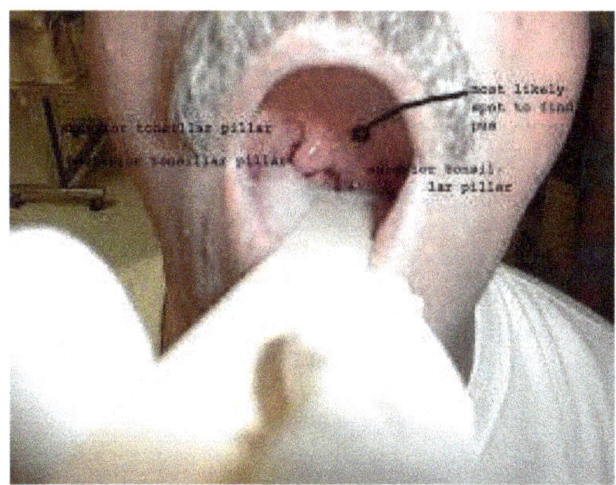

Figure 408 Peritonsillar Abscess

12.12.2.1 SOAP Notes for Peritonsillar Abscess

Table 233 SOAP Notes for Peritonsillar Abscess

Component	Details
Subjective (S)	A 25-year-old female presents with severe sore throat, difficulty swallowing, and fever for the past 3 days. She describes a muffled voice and unilateral neck pain.
Objective (O)	On physical examination, the patient has fever (101°F), severe pain on the right side of the throat, and a visible bulging tonsil. There is swelling and redness of the uvula, with deviation to the left.
Assessment (A)	The patient's presentation, including fever, unilateral tonsillar swelling, and muffled voice, is consistent with a peritonsillar abscess.
Plan (P)	**Pharmacological**: Start intravenous antibiotics (e.g., ampicillin-sulbactam) to cover both aerobic and anaerobic bacteria. **Non-pharmacological**: Perform incision and drainage (I&D) of the abscess, if necessary. **Follow-up**: Reassess in 24-48 hours to monitor for improvement or complications. **Education**: Educate the patient on completing the full course of antibiotics and the need for follow-up care.

12.12.3 Diphtheria

Diphtheria is a contagious bacterial infection affecting the mucous membranes of the **nose and throat, causing a thick grayish membrane to form**. It is a life-threatening condition that requires immediate antibiotic treatment and, in some cases, antitoxin administration.

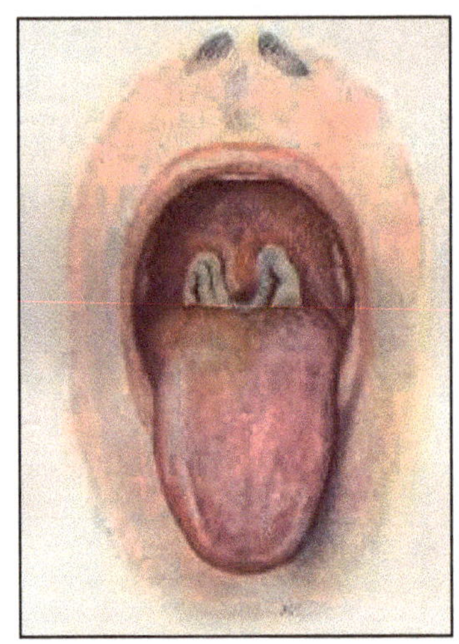

Figure 409 Diphtheria

12.12.3.1 SOAP Notes for Diphtheria

Table 234 SOAP Notes for Diphtheria

Component	Details
Subjective (S)	A 4-year-old child presents with fever, sore throat, and difficulty swallowing for the past two days. The child's mother reports noticing a grayish membrane in the throat.
Objective (O)	On physical examination, the child has a high fever (102°F) and a grayish-white membrane over the tonsils and pharynx, characteristic of diphtheria. There is tender cervical lymphadenopathy.
Assessment (A)	The patient's symptoms, including fever, sore throat, and the presence of a grayish membrane, suggest diphtheria, a serious bacterial infection caused by *Corynebacterium diphtheriae*.
Plan (P)	**Pharmacological**: Administer diphtheria antitoxin and appropriate antibiotics (penicillin or erythromycin). **Non-pharmacological**: Hospitalization for isolation and monitoring of airway obstruction. **Follow-up**: Immediate referral to an infectious disease specialist for further management. **Education**: Educate the parents on the severity of the disease and the importance of vaccination to prevent future cases.

12.12.4 Virchow's Node

Virchow's node is a swollen lymph node located in the left supraclavicular area, which can be a **sign of metastatic cancer, particularly from abdominal or thoracic malignancies**. It is often an indicator of advanced disease and warrants further diagnostic investigation.

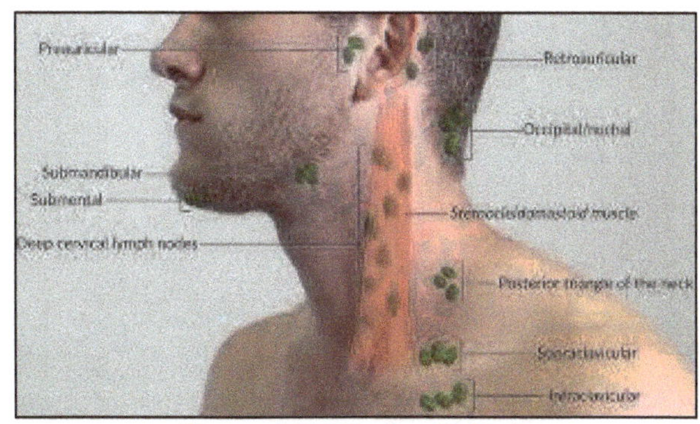

Figure 410 Virchow's Node

12.12.4.1 SOAP Notes for Virchow's Node

Table 235 SOAP Notes for Virchow's Node

Component	Details
Subjective (S)	A 60-year-old male presents with a painless swelling in the left side of the neck that has been gradually increasing in size over the past month.
Objective (O)	On physical examination, a hard, non-tender lymph node is palpated in the left supraclavicular region. No other enlarged lymph nodes are noted.
Assessment (A)	The patient's symptoms, including the presence of a single, non-tender lymph node in the left supraclavicular region (Virchow's node), are concerning for metastatic cancer, often from the abdomen or thorax.
Plan (P)	**Pharmacological**: No specific medications unless infection is suspected. **Non-pharmacological**: Refer the patient for imaging (CT or ultrasound) and possible biopsy to investigate the cause of the lymphadenopathy. **Follow-up**: Follow-up after diagnostic tests for cancer staging and treatment planning. **Education**: Educate the patient on the need for further evaluation, including possible cancer diagnosis and treatment.

12.12.5 Koplik's Spot

Koplik's spots are small, white spots with a red halo that appear on the inside of the cheeks and are a hallmark sign of measles. They usually **appear 2-3 days** before the rash and are diagnostic for the viral infection.

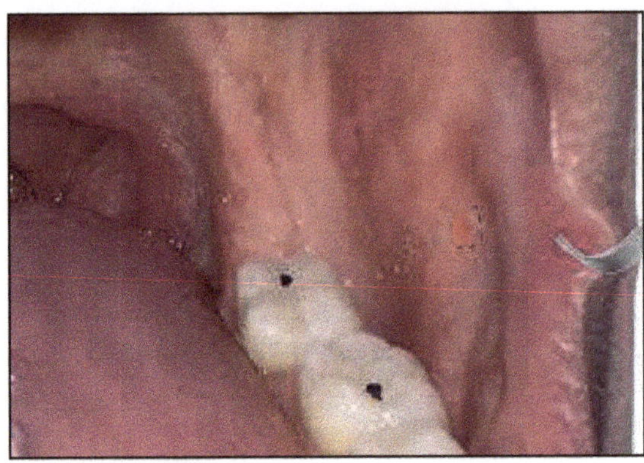

Figure 411 Koplik's Spot

12.12.5.1 SOAP Notes for Koplik's Spot

Table 236 SOAP Notes for Koplik's Spot

Component	Details
Subjective (S)	A 2-year-old child presents with a 3-day history of fever, cough, and runny nose. The child's mother reports noticing small white spots on the inside of the cheeks.
Objective (O)	On physical examination, the child has a characteristic rash of measles on the face and trunk. Koplik's spots are visible on the buccal mucosa, just opposite the molars.
Assessment (A)	The patient's symptoms, including fever, cough, and the presence of Koplik's spots, are diagnostic for measles, a highly contagious viral infection caused by the measles virus.
Plan (P)	**Pharmacological**: Symptomatic treatment with acetaminophen for fever and hydration. **Non-pharmacological**: Isolate the patient to prevent spread of the virus. **Follow-up**: Reassess in a few days to monitor for complications like secondary infections. **Education**: Educate the parents on the importance of vaccination and the expected course of the illness.

12.12.6 Hairy Leukoplakia

Hairy leukoplakia is a white, corrugated lesion typically found on the sides of the tongue, often seen in **individuals with HIV/AIDS**. It is caused by Epstein-Barr virus (EBV) and is not cancerous but can be a sign of immunosuppression.

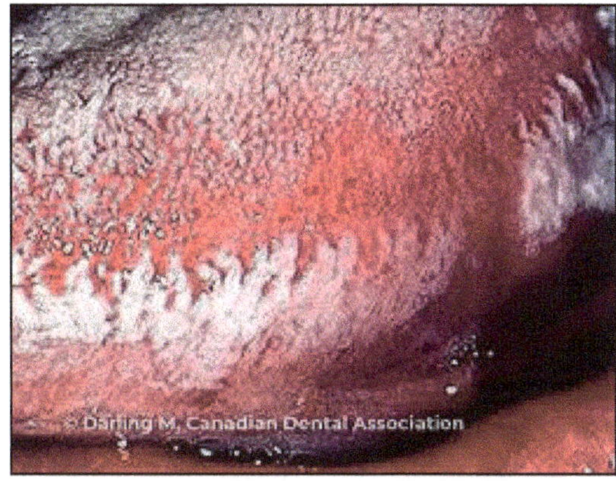

Figure 412 Hairy Leukoplakia

12.12.7 Cheilosis

Cheilosis, or angular cheilitis, is a condition characterized by painful cracks or sores at the corners of the mouth. It can be caused by fungal or bacterial infections, nutritional deficiencies (e.g., vitamin B2 or iron), or ill-fitting dentures.

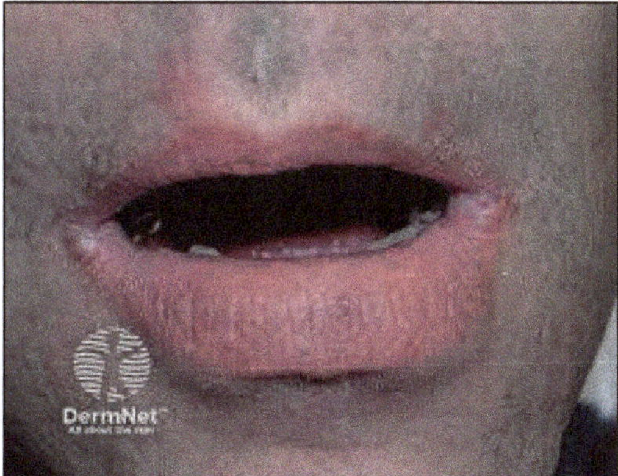

Figure 413 Cheilosis

12.13 Common Conditions of Throat in HEENT System

"Aunt Pat Does Very Kind Hobbies Carefully.", A = Avulsed Tooth, P = Peritonsillar Abscess, D = Diphtheria, V = Virchow's Node, K = Koplik's Spot, H = Hairy Leukoplakia, and C = Cheilosis

Table 237 Common Conditions of Throat in HEENT System

Condition	Description	Key Symptoms	Diagnostic Tools	Treatment Options
Avulsed Tooth	An avulsed tooth refers to a tooth that has been completely displaced from its socket, usually due to trauma.	Displaced tooth, trauma, possible swelling and bleeding in the oral cavity.	Physical exam, replantation or storage of tooth, ultrasound for further evaluation.	Replantation or storage of tooth in milk or saline, referral to dentist for replantation or dental implant.
Peritonsillar Abscess	A peritonsillar abscess is a	Severe sore throat, difficulty swallowing,	Physical examination,	IV antibiotics (e.g., ampicillin-

	pus-filled pocket near the tonsils, often due to tonsillitis.	fever, muffled voice, and unilateral neck pain.	possible drainage or culture of pus from abscess.	sulbactam), incision and drainage (I&D) of the abscess if needed.
Diphtheria	Diphtheria is a bacterial infection affecting the nose and throat, causing a grayish membrane.	Fever, sore throat, difficulty swallowing, grayish membrane in the throat, and tender lymph nodes.	Physical exam, throat culture, and sometimes blood tests for bacterial identification.	Administer diphtheria antitoxin, antibiotics (penicillin or erythromycin), isolation and airway management.
Virchow's Node	Virchow's node is a swollen lymph node in the left supraclavicular area, often a sign of metastatic cancer.	Painless, non-tender swelling in the left supraclavicular area, often associated with advanced disease.	Physical exam, imaging (CT or ultrasound), biopsy for confirmation.	Imaging for staging, referral to oncology, and possible biopsy or surgical intervention.
Koplik's Spot	Koplik's spots are small white spots with a red halo, characteristic of measles.	Fever, cough, runny nose, and small white spots on the inside of the cheeks (Koplik's spots).	Physical exam, often seen with measles rash, diagnostic for measles.	Symptomatic treatment with acetaminophen for fever, hydration, and isolation.
Hairy Leukoplakia	Hairy leukoplakia is a white, corrugated lesion on the tongue, commonly seen in HIV/AIDS patients and caused by EBV.	White, corrugated lesions on the sides of the tongue, commonly seen in immunocompromised individuals.	Physical exam, oral examination, and diagnosis confirmed in HIV/AIDS patients.	Symptomatic treatment for oral lesions, antivirals if EBV is suspected, managing HIV/AIDS.
Cheilosis	Cheilosis, or angular cheilitis, is	Painful cracks or sores at the corners of the mouth, often	Physical exam, diagnosis confirmed	Topical antifungal or antibacterial

	characterized by painful cracks at the corners of the mouth.	caused by fungal or bacterial infections.	with visual inspection.	treatment, maintaining oral hygiene, managing nutritional deficiencies.

12.14 Major Medical Conditions of Throat in HEENT System

12.14.1 Strep Throat

Strep throat is a **bacterial infection of the throat caused by *Group A Streptococcus***, leading to sore throat, fever, and difficulty swallowing. It is treated with antibiotics to prevent complications such as rheumatic fever.

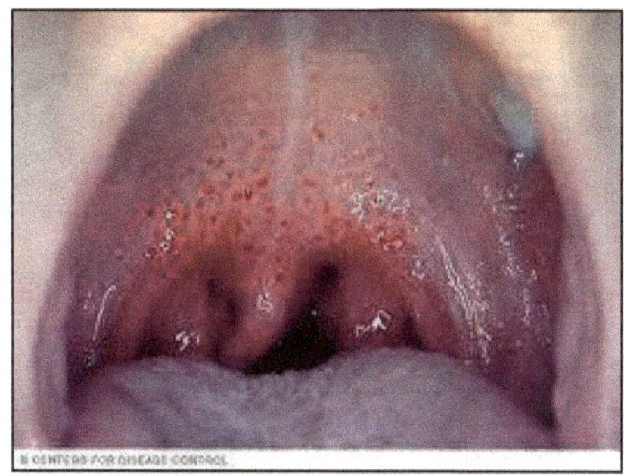

Figure 414 Strep Throat

12.14.1.1 SOAP Notes for Strep Throat

Table 238 SOAP Notes for Strep Throat

Component	Details
Subjective (S)	A 10-year-old child presents with a 2-day history of sore throat, fever, and difficulty swallowing. The child's mother reports a history of exposure to a sibling with similar symptoms.
Objective (O)	On physical examination, the child has erythematous tonsils with white exudates, a fever of 102°F, and tender anterior cervical lymphadenopathy.
Assessment (A)	The patient's symptoms, including fever, sore throat with exudates, and lymphadenopathy, are consistent with strep throat caused by Group A Streptococcus.
Plan (P)	**Pharmacological**: Prescribe antibiotics (e.g., amoxicillin or penicillin) to treat the bacterial infection and prevent complications (See algorithm below). **Non-pharmacological**: Recommend analgesics (e.g., acetaminophen or ibuprofen) for pain relief. **Follow-up**: Follow-up in 48 hours to monitor for response to treatment. **Education**: Educate the parent on the importance of completing the full course of antibiotics to prevent complications like rheumatic fever.

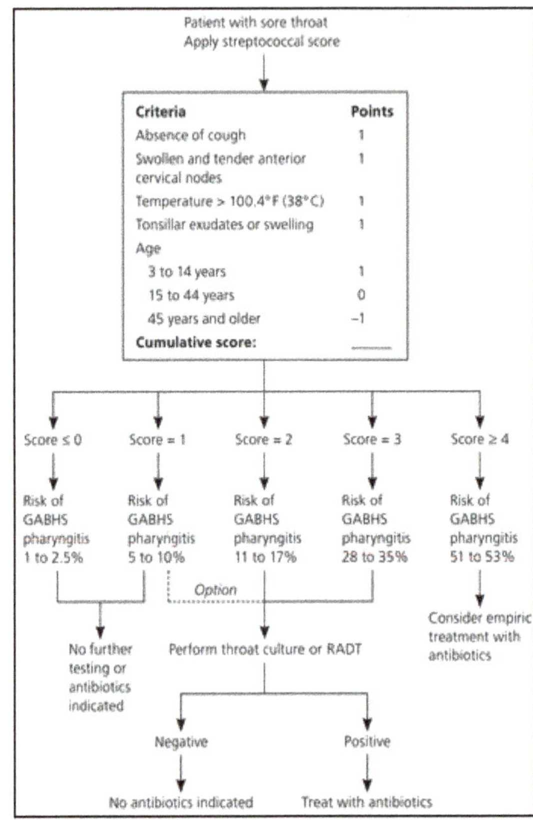

Figure 415 Management Algorithm for Strep Throat

12.14.2 Tonsilitis

Tonsillitis is the inflammation of the tonsils, often caused by viral or bacterial infections, resulting in a sore throat, **difficulty swallowing, and fever**. In severe cases, it may require antibiotics or surgery (tonsillectomy) if recurrent or chronic.

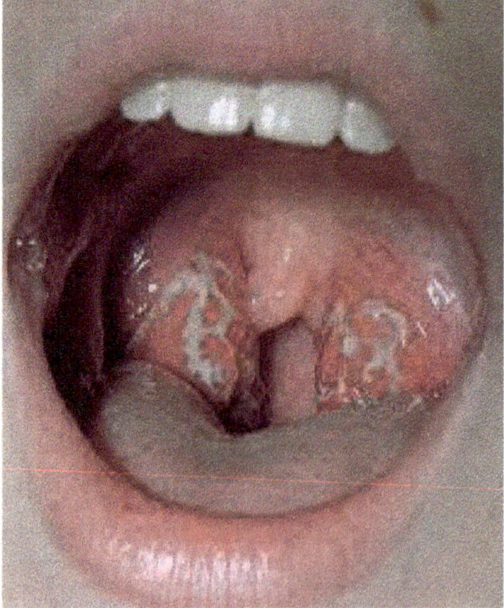
Figure 416 Tonsilitis

12.14.2.1 SOAP Notes for Tonsilitis

Table 239 SOAP Notes for Tonsilitis

Component	Details

Subjective (S)	A 22-year-old female presents with a sore throat, fever, and difficulty swallowing for the past 3 days. She reports a history of recurrent sore throats.
Objective (O)	On physical examination, the tonsils are erythematous and swollen, with yellowish exudate on both sides. The patient has a fever of 101°F and mild cervical lymphadenopathy.
Assessment (A)	The patient's symptoms and the findings of erythematous, exudative tonsils are consistent with acute tonsillitis, which may be viral or bacterial in origin.
Plan (P)	**Pharmacological**: If bacterial, prescribe antibiotics (e.g., penicillin or amoxicillin). If viral, recommend symptomatic treatment with pain relievers and fluids (See algorithm below). **Non-pharmacological**: Advise warm saline gargles and throat lozenges. **Follow-up**: Follow-up in 1-2 weeks if symptoms persist or worsen, and consider tonsillectomy for recurrent cases. **Education**: Educate the patient on the potential need for surgery if tonsillitis becomes chronic or recurrent.

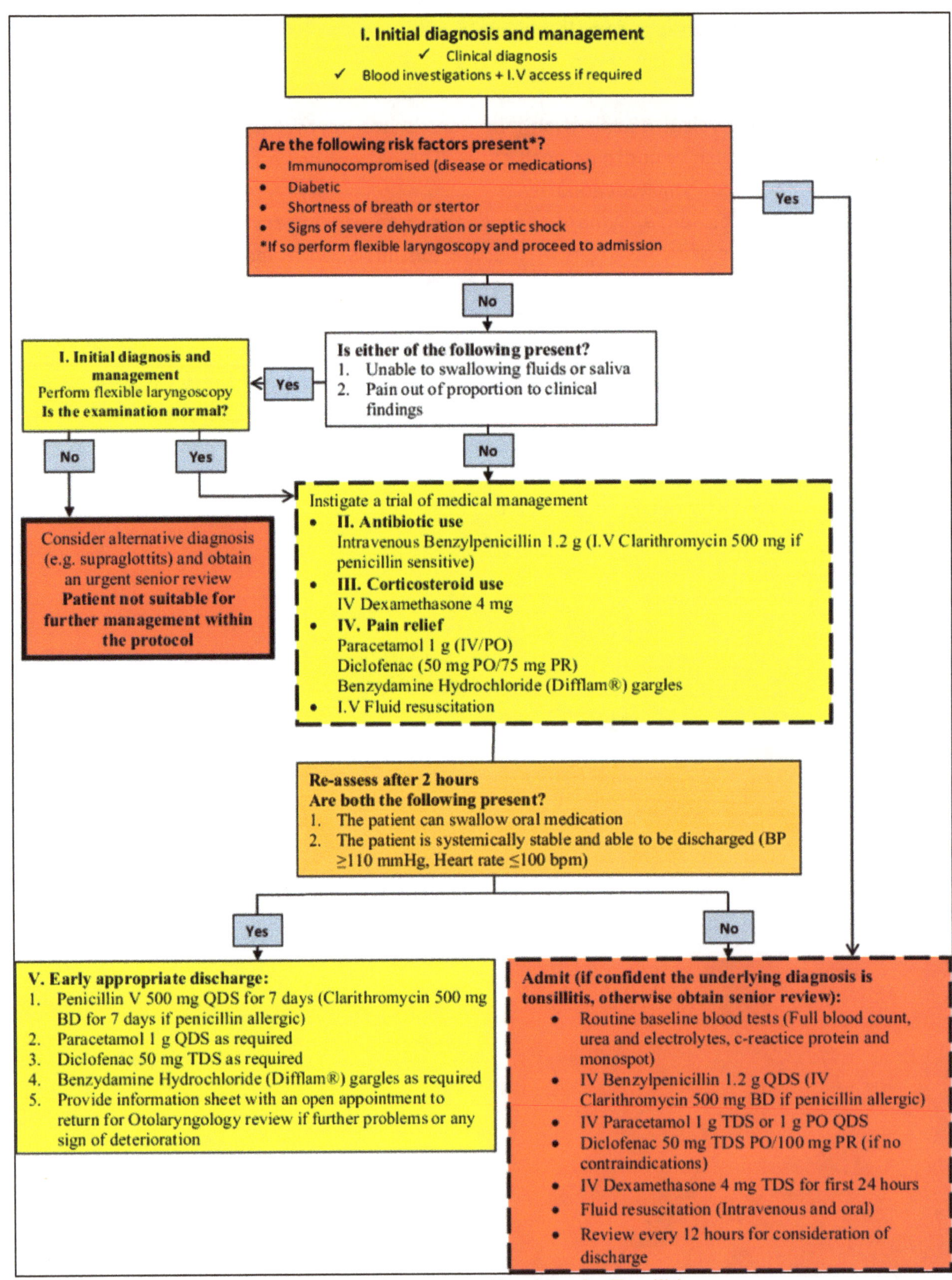

I. Initial diagnosis and management
✓ Clinical diagnosis
✓ Blood investigations + I.V access if required
Are the following risk factors present*?
• Immunocompromised (disease or medications)
• Diabetic
• Shortness of breath or stertor
• Signs of severe dehydration or septic shock
*If so perform flexible laryngoscopy and proceed to admission
Yes
No
Is either of the following present?
1. Unable to swallowing fluids or saliva
2. Pain out of proportion to clinical findings
Yes
I. Initial diagnosis and management
Perform flexible laryngoscopy
Is the examination normal?
No
Yes
No
Consider alternative diagnosis (e.g. supraglottits) and obtain an urgent senior review
Patient not suitable for further management within the protocol
Instigate a trial of medical management
• II. Antibiotic use
Intravenous Benzylpenicillin 1.2 g (I.V Clarithromycin 500 mg if penicillin sensitive)
• III. Corticosteroid use
IV Dexamethasone 4 mg
• IV. Pain relief
Paracetamol 1 g (IV/PO)
Diclofenac (50 mg PO/75 mg PR)
Benzydamine Hydrochloride (Difflam®) gargles
• I.V Fluid resuscitation
Re-assess after 2 hours
Are both the following present?
1. The patient can swallow oral medication
2. The patient is systemically stable and able to be discharged (BP ≥110 mmHg, Heart rate ≤100 bpm)
Yes
No
V. Early appropriate discharge:
1. Penicillin V 500 mg QDS for 7 days (Clarithromycin 500 mg BD for 7 days if penicillin allergic)
2. Paracetamol 1 g QDS as required
3. Diclofenac 50 mg TDS as required
4. Benzydamine Hydrochloride (Difflam®) gargles as required
5. Provide information sheet with an open appointment to return for Otolaryngology review if further problems or any sign of deterioration
Admit (if confident the underlying diagnosis is tonsillitis, otherwise obtain senior review):
• Routine baseline blood tests (Full blood count, urea and electrolytes, c-reactice protein and monospot)
• IV Benzylpenicillin 1.2 g QDS (IV Clarithromycin 500 mg BD if penicillin allergic)
• IV Paracetamol 1 g TDS or 1 g PO QDS
• Diclofenac 50 mg TDS PO/100 mg PR (if no contraindications)
• IV Dexamethasone 4 mg TDS for first 24 hours
• Fluid resuscitation (Intravenous and oral)
• Review every 12 hours for consideration of discharge

Figure 417 Management Algorithm for Tonsilitis

12.14.3 Mononucleosis

Mononucleosis, commonly called **"mono,"** is a viral infection caused by the Epstein-Barr virus (EBV), leading to fever, sore throat, swollen lymph nodes, and fatigue. It is usually self-limiting, and treatment is focused on symptom management, including rest and hydration.

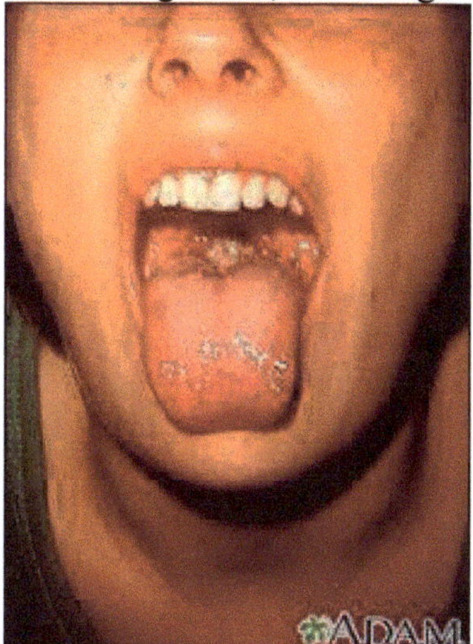

Figure 418 Mononucleosis

12.14.3.1 SOAP Notes for Mononucleosis

Table 240 SOAP Notes for Mononucleosis

Component	Details
Subjective (S)	A 19-year-old male presents with a 1-week history of sore throat, fatigue, and swollen lymph nodes. He also reports mild fever and decreased appetite.
Objective (O)	On physical examination, the patient has enlarged, tender posterior cervical lymph nodes, an inflamed throat with white exudates, and mild splenomegaly.
Assessment (A)	The patient's symptoms, including fever, sore throat, lymphadenopathy, and splenomegaly, are consistent with mononucleosis caused by Epstein-Barr virus (EBV).
Plan (P)	**Pharmacological**: Symptomatic treatment with analgesics (e.g., acetaminophen or ibuprofen) and hydration (See algorithm below). **Non-pharmacological**: Recommend adequate rest, hydration, and avoiding contact sports to prevent splenic rupture. **Follow-up**: Follow-up in 2-4 weeks if symptoms persist or worsen. **Education**: Educate the patient on the self-limiting nature of the infection and the importance of rest and hydration to support recovery.

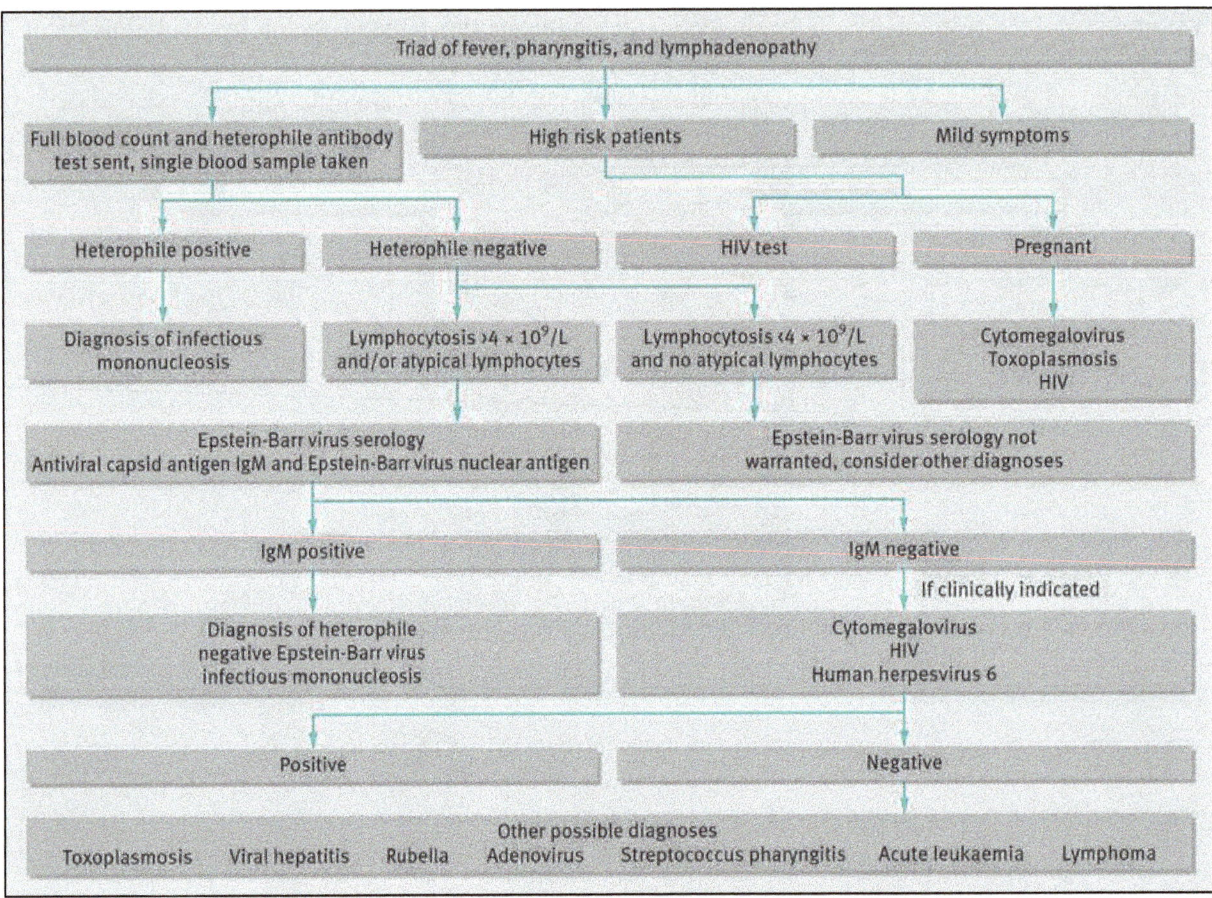

Figure 419 Algorithm for the Management of Mononucleosis

12.15 Moh Golden Points and Summary Question Answers

12.15.1 Moh Golden Points

HEENT Assessment: A thorough HEENT (Head, Eyes, Ears, Nose, Throat) examination is essential in evaluating a broad spectrum of conditions, ranging from infections to malignancies.

Eye Complaints: Any sudden vision changes, especially in older individuals, may indicate serious conditions like retinal detachment, acute angle-closure glaucoma, or diabetic retinopathy.

Hearing Loss: Sudden hearing loss, especially if associated with ear pain or drainage, can be indicative of conditions such as otitis media, otitis externa, or even an acoustic neuroma.

Nasal Obstruction: Persistent nasal congestion, particularly if accompanied by facial pain, can point to chronic sinusitis, nasal polyps, or even malignancy.

Sore Throat with Fever: A sore throat accompanied by fever should prompt a consideration of strep throat, tonsillitis, or infectious mononucleosis.

Lymphadenopathy: Swelling of the lymph nodes in the neck can be a sign of infection, malignancy, or systemic disease.

A new neck mass should be evaluated for malignancy, especially in patients with a history of smoking or alcohol use.

12.15.2 Summary Questions & Answers

1. Which of the following is the most common cause of acute otitis media (AOM) in children?
a) Streptococcus pneumoniae
b) Haemophilus influenzae
c) Respiratory syncytial virus (RSV)
d) Epstein-Barr virus (EBV)

2. A patient presents with unilateral sudden vision loss, a history of flashes of light, and a sensation of a curtain falling over their eye. What is the most likely diagnosis?
a) Retinal detachment
b) Acute angle-closure glaucoma
c) Optic neuritis
d) Macular degeneration

3. Which of the following is the most common cause of a sore throat in children?
a) Epstein-Barr virus (EBV)
b) Group A Streptococcus
c) Rhinovirus
d) Adenovirus

4. A 55-year-old patient with a history of smoking presents with hoarseness, a persistent cough, and unexplained weight loss. On examination, a hard, non-tender mass is noted on the neck. What is the most likely diagnosis?
a) Thyroid carcinoma
b) Acute laryngitis
c) Squamous cell carcinoma of the larynx
d) Lymphoma

5. Which of the following findings is characteristic of acute bacterial rhinosinusitis?
a) Clear nasal discharge and cough
b) Facial pain or pressure and purulent nasal discharge
c) Red, dry lips and sore throat
d) Rhinorrhea with clear fluid drainage

6. Which of the following is the hallmark sign of measles?
a) Koplik's spots
b) Pityriasis rosea
c) Scarlet fever rash
d) Petechial rash

7. A patient with nasal polyps is most likely to have which of the following conditions?
a) Asthma
b) Diabetes mellitus
c) Hypertension
d) Hyperthyroidism

8. A 60-year-old male presents with a swollen lymph node in the left supraclavicular region. What is the most concerning potential cause?
a) Acute bacterial infection
b) Metastatic cancer
c) Tuberculosis
d) Benign lymphadenopathy

9. Which of the following is the most common cause of viral pharyngitis?
a) Epstein-Barr virus (EBV)
b) Influenza virus
c) Adenovirus
d) Rhinovirus

10. A 30-year-old male presents with a painful, swollen, and tender external ear canal after swimming. He reports a sensation of fullness in the ear. What is the likely diagnosis?
a) Acute otitis media
b) Otitis externa
c) Acoustic neuroma
d) Otitis media with effusion

12.15.3 Rationales

1. **Answer: a) Streptococcus pneumoniae**

Rationale: Streptococcus pneumoniae is the most common bacterial pathogen causing acute otitis media in children. Other bacteria, like *Haemophilus influenzae*, also contribute but are less common.

---

2. **Answer: a) Retinal detachment**

Rationale: Retinal detachment is characterized by sudden vision loss, flashes of light, and the sensation of a curtain or veil coming down over the field of vision, which is a classic presentation.

---

3. **Answer: b) Group A Streptococcus**

Rationale: Group A Streptococcus is the most common bacterial cause of sore throat in children, leading to strep throat. It can be identified with rapid antigen testing or throat cultures.

---

4. **Answer: c) Squamous cell carcinoma of the larynx**

Rationale: In a patient with a history of smoking, hoarseness, persistent cough, and a neck mass, squamous cell carcinoma of the larynx is a strong consideration. Early detection is critical for effective management.

---

5. **Answer: b) Facial pain or pressure and purulent nasal discharge**

Rationale: Acute bacterial rhinosinusitis is typically characterized by facial pain or pressure, purulent nasal discharge, and nasal congestion, especially after a viral upper respiratory infection.

---

6. **Answer: a) Koplik's spots**

Rationale: Koplik's spots are small white spots with a red halo on the inside of the cheeks and are a hallmark sign of measles, often seen before the characteristic rash.

---

7. **Answer: a) Asthma**

Rationale: Nasal polyps are commonly associated with asthma, chronic sinusitis, and allergic rhinitis. The presence of nasal polyps often worsens asthma control.

---

8. **Answer: b) Metastatic cancer**

Rationale: A swollen left supraclavicular node (Virchow's node) is highly suggestive of metastatic cancer, especially from abdominal or thoracic malignancies.

---

9. **Answer: c) Adenovirus**

Rationale: Adenovirus is a common cause of viral pharyngitis, particularly in children, and is often associated with other symptoms like conjunctivitis and respiratory involvement.

---

10. **Answer: b) Otitis externa**

Rationale: Otitis externa, also known as swimmer's ear, is an infection of the external auditory canal, commonly caused by bacteria or fungi, often following water exposure.

13 Chapter 13: Psychiatric/Behavioral Health

13.1 Anatomy and Physiology of Psychiatric/Behavioral Health

Psychiatric and behavioral health involve the structural and functional aspects of the human body, specifically the brain, nerves and the chemistry of the body that influences the mental and emotional state of the patient. Mental disorders are generally founded in the origin of the mind as it controls passion, ideas, and behavior. **The limbic system, composed of the brain areas involved in the regulation of rage, fear, and lust, is also involved in PORN addiction, as well as those structures related to decision-making the prefrontal cortex.** These include; Serotonin , Dopamine, norepinephrine and norepinephrine which are vital in the mental health of people as they act as messengers in the brain cells. These can lead to conditions such as depression, anxiety or schizophrenia when their level is not in harmony. For example, less serotonin is usually found in a person with a depression illness while more dopamine is usually related to a case of schizophrenia. The ANS is also involved since it governs involuntary phasic responses, such as heart rate and stress responsiveness that are more pronounced in **PTSD and anxiety disorders, among others.** Also, hormones of the endocrine system that affect mood and stress responses have a bearing on psychiatric status. This is important for the reason that the development of medications for the treatment of psychiatric **disorders involve identifying the neurotransmitting** system while arriving at therapeutic ways of intervention includes involving changes of brain function and actions.

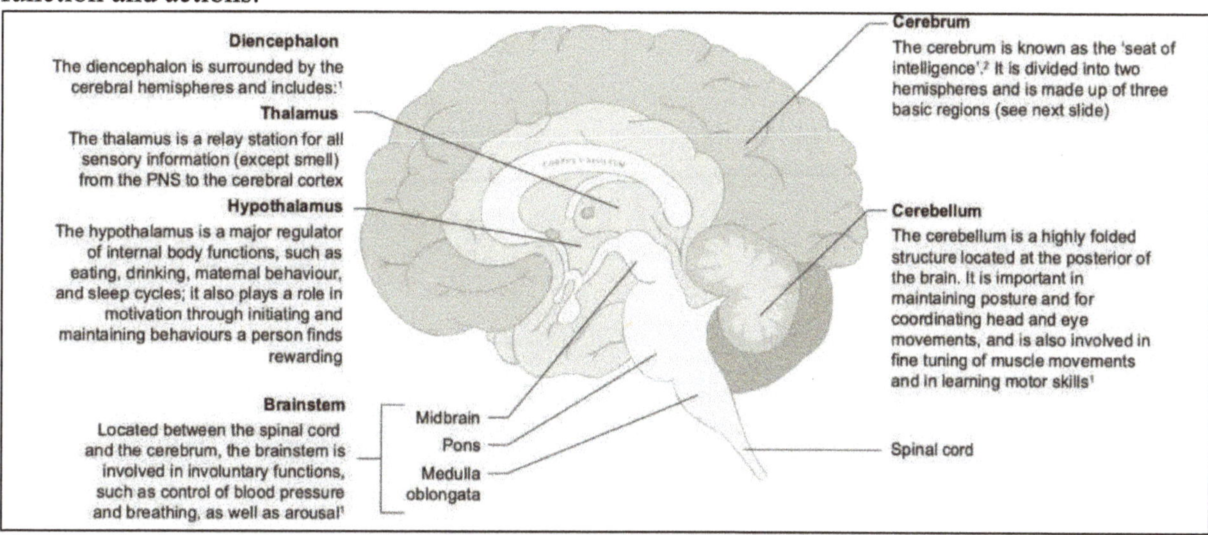

Diencephalon
The diencephalon is surrounded by the cerebral hemispheres and includes:[1]
Thalamus
The thalamus is a relay station for all sensory information (except smell) from the PNS to the cerebral cortex
Hypothalamus
The hypothalamus is a major regulator of internal body functions, such as eating, drinking, maternal behaviour, and sleep cycles; it also plays a role in motivation through initiating and maintaining behaviours a person finds rewarding
Brainstem
Located between the spinal cord and the cerebrum, the brainstem is involved in involuntary functions, such as control of blood pressure and breathing, as well as arousal[1]
Midbrain
Pons
Medulla oblongata
Cerebrum
The cerebrum is known as the 'seat of intelligence'.[2] It is divided into two hemispheres and is made up of three basic regions (see next slide)
Cerebellum
The cerebellum is a highly folded structure located at the posterior of the brain. It is important in maintaining posture and for coordinating head and eye movements, and is also involved in fine tuning of muscle movements and in learning motor skills[1]
Spinal cord

Figure 420 Anatomical Regions of the Brain

13.2 Common Conditions of Psychiatric/Behavioral Health

"People And Dogs Always Dig In Beds, And Sometimes Ant Snakes Migrate." **P**TSD, **A**nxiety, **D**epression, **A**lcoholism, **D**elirium, **S**moking Cessation, **I**nsomnia, **B**ipolar Disorder, **S**chizophrenia, **A**norexia Nervosa, **M**unchausen Syndrome, **A**ll Types of Abuses, **S**erotonin Toxicity, and **M**alignant Neuroleptic Syndrome

Table 241 Common Conditions of Psychiatric/ Behavioral Health

Condition	Description	Key Symptoms	Diagnostic Tools	Treatment Options
PTSD (Posttraumatic	A mental health	Flashbacks, nightmares,	Clinical interviews, PTSD	Cognitive Behavioral

Stress Disorder)	disorder triggered by experiencing or witnessing traumatic events.	hypervigilance, emotional numbness, avoidance.	checklist, Beck Depression Inventory.	Therapy (CBT), Eye Movement Desensitization and Reprocessing (EMDR), medications (SSRIs like sertraline).
Anxiety	A condition involving excessive worry or fear that disrupts daily life.	Restlessness, rapid heartbeat, excessive worrying, difficulty concentrating, panic attacks.	Generalized Anxiety Disorder scale (GAD-7), psychological evaluation.	Cognitive Behavioral Therapy (CBT), medications (benzodiazepines, SSRIs), relaxation techniques.
Depression	A mood disorder that causes persistent feelings of sadness and loss of interest.	Persistent sadness, lack of interest in activities, fatigue, difficulty concentrating, thoughts of death or suicide.	Beck Depression Inventory, PHQ-9, clinical interview.	Antidepressants (SSRIs, SNRIs), psychotherapy (CBT, IPT), lifestyle changes (exercise, sleep improvements).
Alcoholism	A chronic disease characterized by an inability to control alcohol consumption.	Craving alcohol, inability to cut down, neglect of responsibilities, withdrawal symptoms, blackouts.	CAGE Questionnaire, AUDIT (Alcohol Use Disorder Identification Test).	Detoxification, Cognitive Behavioral Therapy (CBT), 12-step programs (AA), medications (disulfiram, naltrexone).
Delirium	A rapid change in brain function that results in confusion, disorientation, and impaired attention.	Confusion, reduced awareness of surroundings, hallucinations, agitation, poor memory.	Clinical assessment, Confusion Assessment Method (CAM).	Treat underlying causes (infection, dehydration), sedatives if necessary, manage symptoms, address

				environmental factors.
Insomnia	Difficulty falling or staying asleep, or waking up too early and not being able to go back to sleep.	Difficulty falling asleep, waking up frequently during the night, waking up too early, daytime fatigue, irritability.	Sleep history, sleep diary, polysomnography, actigraphy.	Cognitive Behavioral Therapy for Insomnia (CBT-I), sleep hygiene practices, medications (zolpidem, melatonin).
Bipolar Disorder	A mood disorder involving extreme mood swings that include emotional highs (mania or hypomania) and lows (depression).	Extreme mood swings, periods of elevated mood (mania), irritability, risky behavior during manic episodes, depressive symptoms.	Clinical interview, mood charting, DSM-5 diagnostic criteria.	Mood stabilizers (lithium), antipsychotics, antidepressants, psychotherapy.
Schizophrenia	A chronic and severe mental disorder that affects how a person thinks, feels, and behaves.	Hallucinations, delusions, disorganized thinking, negative symptoms (apathy, lack of emotion, withdrawal).	Clinical interviews, DSM-5 criteria, neuroimaging, psychological testing.	Antipsychotic medications, CBT, supportive therapy, rehabilitation.
Anorexia Nervosa	An eating disorder characterized by an extreme fear of gaining weight and a distorted body image.	Severe restriction of food intake, excessive exercise, fear of gaining weight, distorted body image.	Physical examination, psychological assessment, DSM-5 criteria.	Nutritional rehabilitation, psychotherapy (CBT), family therapy, medications (SSRIs, antipsychotics).

Munchausen Syndrome	A condition in which a person repeatedly acts as if they have a physical or mental illness when they are not really sick.	Falsification of symptoms, frequent hospital visits, seeking attention or sympathy.	Medical history, psychological assessment, lab tests to rule out actual illness.	Psychiatric intervention, psychotherapy (CBT), managing underlying psychological issues.
All Types of Abuses	Physical, emotional, psychological, or sexual harm inflicted on an individual.	Visible injuries, withdrawal, fear of certain individuals, anxiety, depression, low self-esteem.	Clinical interviews, physical examination, forensic evidence, psychological assessment.	Counseling, crisis intervention, legal intervention, support groups, family therapy, safety planning.
Serotonin Toxicity	A potentially life-threatening condition caused by excessive serotonin levels in the brain, often from medication.	Agitation, confusion, rapid heart rate, high blood pressure, muscle rigidity, tremors, hyperreflexia.	Clinical presentation, blood tests (serotonin levels), urine tests for drugs.	

13.3 Major Medications Given in Psychiatric/Behavioral Conditions

Table 242 Categorization of Psychiatric Medications

Category	Drugs	Indications
NEW Antipsychotics	1. Risperidone (Risperdal), 2. Paliperidone (Invega), 3. Ziprasidone (Geodon), 4. Olanzapine (Zyprexa), 5. Quetiapine (Seroquel), 6. Clozapine (Clozaril), 7. Aripiprazole (Abilify)	Schizophrenia, Bipolar Disorder
Benzodiazepines	1. Alprazolam (Xanax), 2. Clonazepam (Klonopin), 3. Lorazepam (Ativan), 4. Clonazepam (Xanax), 5. Chlordiazepoxide (Librium)	Bipolar Disorder, Generalized Anxiety Disorder, Acute Alcohol Withdrawal, Panic, Schizophrenia

SSRI	1. Fluoxetine (Prozac), 2. Paroxetine (Paxil, Paxil CR), 3. Citalopram (Celexa), 4. Escitalopram (Lexapro), 5. Sertraline (Zoloft), 6. Fluvoxamine (Luvox)	Depression, Panic, Bipolar Disorder, OCD, Generalized Anxiety Disorder
SNRI	1. Venlafaxine (Effexor), 2. Desvenlafaxine (Pristiq)	Depression, Panic, OCD, Generalized Anxiety Disorder
Mood Stabilizers	1. Lithium carbonate (Eskalith, Lithobid), 2. Valproic acid (Depakote), 3. Carbamazepine (Tegretol), 4. Oxcarbazepine (Trileptal), 5. Lamotrigine (Lamictal), 6. Topiramate (Topamax)	Bipolar Disorder
Atypical Antidepressants	1. Nefazodone (Serzone), 2. Trazodone (Desyrel), 3. Bupropion (Wellbutrin), 4. Mirtazapine (Remeron)	Depression
Cyclic Antidepressants	1. Amitriptyline (Elavil), 2. Nortriptyline (Pamelor), 3. Desipramine (Norpramin)	Depression, Panic, OCD, Generalized Anxiety Disorder
MAOIs	1. Phenelzine (Nardil), 2. Tranylcypromine (Parnate), 3. Isocarboxazid (Marplan), 4. Selegiline (Eldepryl)	Depression, Panic, OCD, Generalized Anxiety Disorder
Anticonvulsants	1. Depakote (Valproic Acid), 2. Tegretol (Carbamazepine), 3. Lamictal (Lamotrigine)	Schizophrenia
Opioid Antagonists	1. Naloxone (Narcan), 2. Naltrexone (Revia, Depade)	Opiate Withdrawal Treatment

13.4 Major Medical Conditions of Psychiatric/Behavioral Health

13.4.1 Depression

Depression is a mental ailment wherein one experiences sad mood for most of the time, has loss of interest or pleasure in the majority of daily activities. The person's emotions, thought process, and even his physical conditions are influenced by it. Depression has several possible causes attributable to genetics, abnormal levels of serotonin and dopamine, stress, major life changes, and circumstances like abuse. These consist of tiredness, changes in appetite and sleep, seeming to have a hard time focusing, and thoughts about dying or suicide. There are some types of depression such as major depressive disorder, persistent depressive disorder which was earlier known as dysthymia and bipolar disorder especially when pessimism is preceded by a period of mania. Depression may be treated either with the help of an antidepressant and/or an antipsychotic drug in combination with counseling. Mood stabilizers, especially selective serotonin reuptake inhibitors (SSRIs) are commonly administered to ensure control of emotions. Another one is cognitive-behavioral therapy or CBT which is also effective in helping people alter their thinking patterns. It is very important to give a child a proper attention at the right time to aid him/her to gain better results.

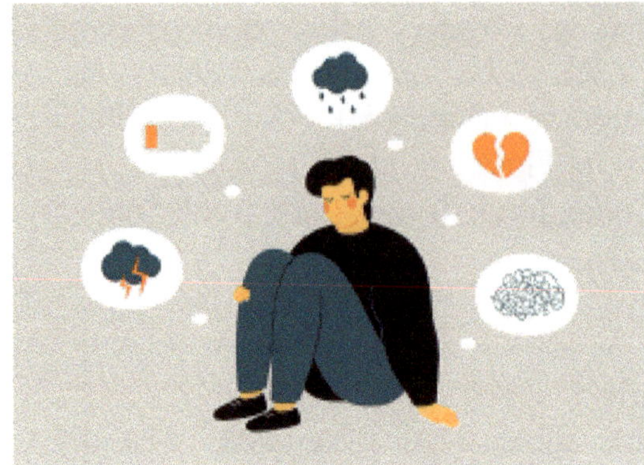

Figure 421 Depressive Symptoms

13.4.1.1 Symptoms of Depression

The picture depicts various signs and symptoms of depression, indicating that it causes sever emotions and physical psychological health issues. One of them is the depressed mood, which is characterized by low, or even severely low, mood, and the person seems to be depressed and may feel empty most of the time. There also is eye decreased interest in or pleasure from previously enjoyable activities which results in apathy and low motivation. It also causes change in appetite and weight in that a person will either tend to overeat or loss his appetite. Other factors that tend to worsen the situation include poor sleep patterns, whether in terms of insomnia, or oversleeping. Tiredness and weakness are taking hold, and even task that used to be creative have become herculean. Many individuals with depression also experience feelings of worthlessness or guilt, often over things beyond their control. Some of the symptoms may include agitation or slowed movements due to the physical side of depression and impaired concentration, which makes it difficult to focus on cognitive tasks. Sometimes the patient may begin fantasising about death in other forms, and this may call for urgent attention since it may lead to suicide thoughts. Such manifestations, if sustained, may significantly impair one's performance and should not be ignored by seeking appropriate help.

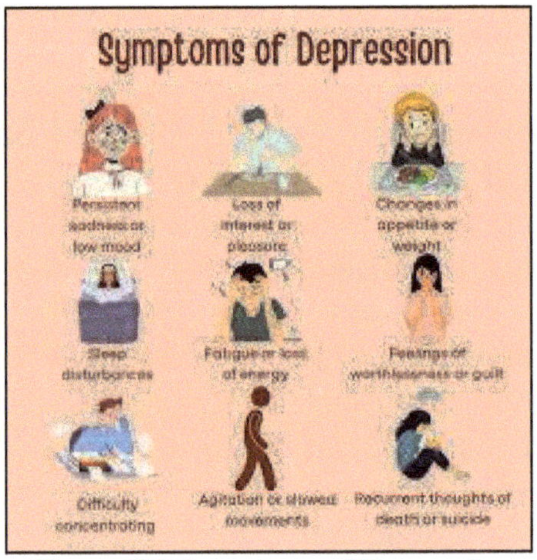

Symptoms of Depression

Persistent sadness or low mood
Loss of interest or pleasure
Changes in appetite or weight
Sleep disturbances
Fatigue or loss of energy
Feelings of worthlessness or guilt
Difficulty concentrating
Agitation or slowed movements
Recurrent thoughts of death or suicide

Figure 422 Symptoms of Depression

13.4.1.2 Types of Depression

In the image below, different types of depression are depicted. These are MDD, PDD, bipolar disorder, SAD, post-partum depression, psychotic depression and premenstrual dysphoric disorder respectively. In this case there are a number of types of depression and each of them has the peculiarities of its nature and potential outcomes. Major Depressive Disorder (MDD) can be described as having low mood and/or loss of interest that provides with some level of disability or incapacitation. Dysthymia, or Persistent Depressive Disorder (PDD) is a long term form of depression that etiologies for not less than two years, though symptoms are not as severe. Bipolar Disorder is characterized by mania and depression type of mood swings. Other types include the seasonal affective disorder where the symptoms are related to particular seasons; especially with the onset of the winter season with short daylight. Postpartum depression is a condition in which a woman suffers from severe sadness and helps exhaustion after giving birth. Psychotic Depression includes multiple features of depression such as missed appointment, loss of interests, and psychotic features such as hallucinations or paranoid thoughts. Last is Pre menstrual dysphoric disorder (PMDD), it is the severe form of PMS which results in depression symptoms in the days before menstration. ,Every one of them needs an individual approach and may include therapy, medication, or their use in equal shares.

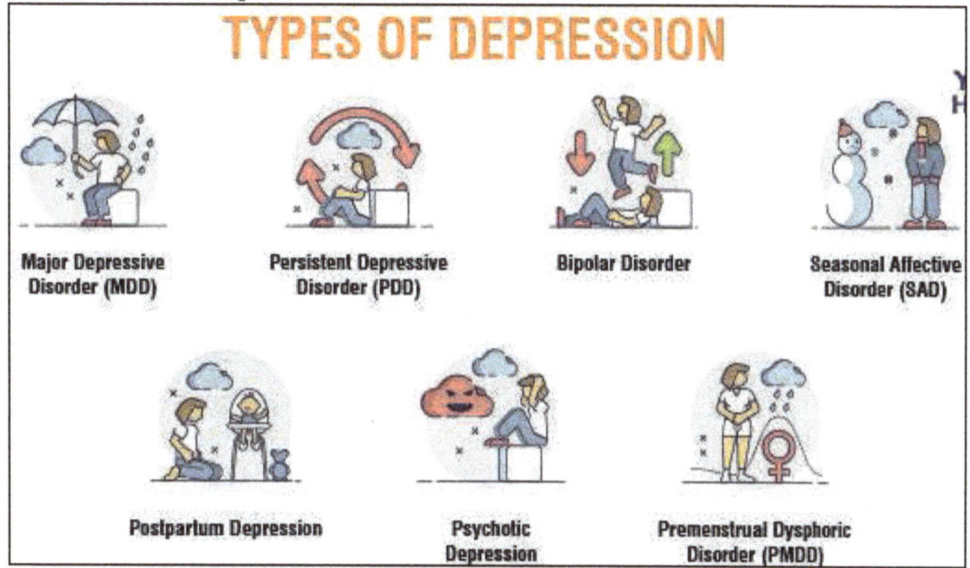

Figure 423 Types of Depression

13.4.1.3 SOAP Notes for Depression

Table 243 SOAP Notes for Depression

Component	Details
Subjective (S)	A 30-year-old male presents with complaints of persistent sadness, lack of interest in activities, and difficulty concentrating, which have been present for the past six weeks. The patient reports feeling fatigued most days and has noticed a significant decrease in appetite and weight. He mentions difficulty sleeping and feeling restless at night. The patient denies any history of trauma but expresses feelings of hopelessness. He has no significant past medical history.
Objective (O)	On physical examination, the patient appears downcast and has a flat affect. His pulse is 78 bpm, and blood pressure is 118/76 mmHg. No physical abnormalities were noted during the exam. The patient is alert but appears fatigued. There is no evidence of psychosis or suicidal behavior at the time of the exam. No other physical abnormalities are observed.
Assessment (A)	The patient's symptoms, including persistent sadness, loss of interest, fatigue, changes in appetite, and sleep disturbances, are consistent with

	major depressive disorder (MDD). The lack of other contributing factors suggests this as the primary diagnosis. Further evaluation, including a detailed mood assessment and possible screening tools such as the PHQ-9, will be necessary to confirm the diagnosis.
Plan (P)	**Pharmacological:** Initiate selective serotonin reuptake inhibitor (SSRI), such as sertraline 50 mg daily, to address the depressive symptoms (See algorithm below). **Non-pharmacological:** Recommend cognitive-behavioral therapy (CBT) to help address negative thought patterns. **Follow-up:** Schedule a follow-up appointment in 2-3 weeks to assess the response to treatment and discuss any side effects. **Education:** Educate the patient on the nature of depression and the importance of adhering to prescribed treatments. Discuss potential side effects of SSRIs, such as gastrointestinal upset or sexual dysfunction, and encourage open communication regarding side effects.

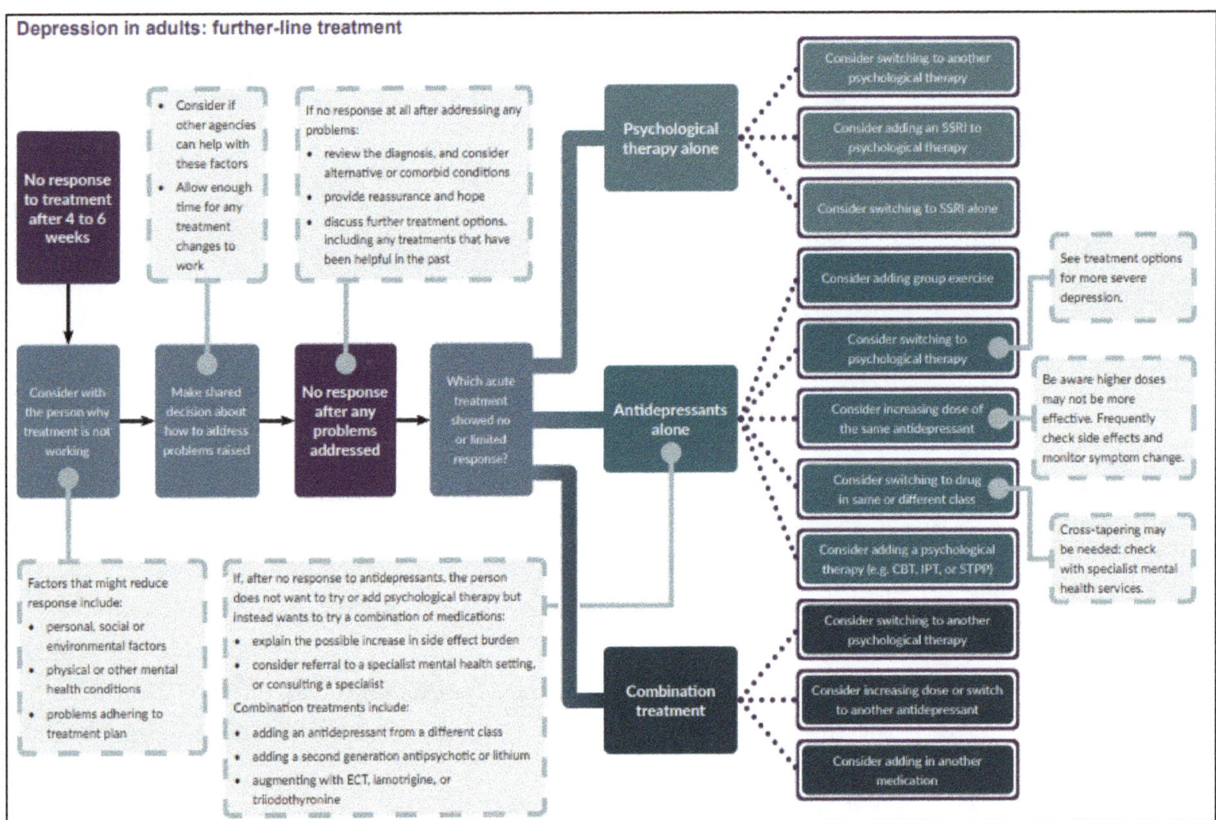

Figure 424 Algorithm for the Treatment and Management of Depression in Adults

13.4.2 Anxiety

Anxiety functions as a prevalent mental health disorder which causes beyond typical worry or fear or nervousness to become persistent and overwhelming. Anxiety manifests through a range of intensities that affect people from light anxiousness to overwhelming distress levels which hinder everyday activities. **Various genetic elements and environmental conditions together with psychological influences create the multiple causes of anxiety experienced by individuals**. Neurotransmitter imbalances between serotonin and dopamine inside the brain serve as biological risk factors for developing anxiety disorders. Several anxiety disorders exist along with **Generalized Anxiety Disorder (GAD), Social Anxiety Disorder and Panic Disorder** as well as Specific Phobias. Each disorder contains particular features which all include substantial worry and fear. People with GAD experience persistent worrying about different aspects of life yet panic disorder causes repeated unexpected panic episodes. People who suffer from social anxiety disorder experience extreme panic when around others because they fear being evaluated negatively yet those with specific phobias exhibit an unreasonable terror toward a specific thing or circumstance. **People with anxiety experience restlessness together with rapid heart rate, sweating, difficulty concentrating, muscle tension and sleep disturbances**. Anxiety at its most severe point creates panic attacks that cause people to feel heart pain and dizziness with a fearful sensation of doom approaching. A standardized approach to treating anxiety combines both **cognitive-behavioral therapy (CBT) to transform negative mental patterns and short-term use of select serotonin reuptake inhibitors (SSRIs) or benzodiazepines as medications**. People dealing with anxiety find relief through lifestyle adjustments which include both relaxation methods and regular exercise with mindfulness practice. Early access to right treatments accompanied by steady treatment practices lead to better quality of life and reduced likelihood of future complications.

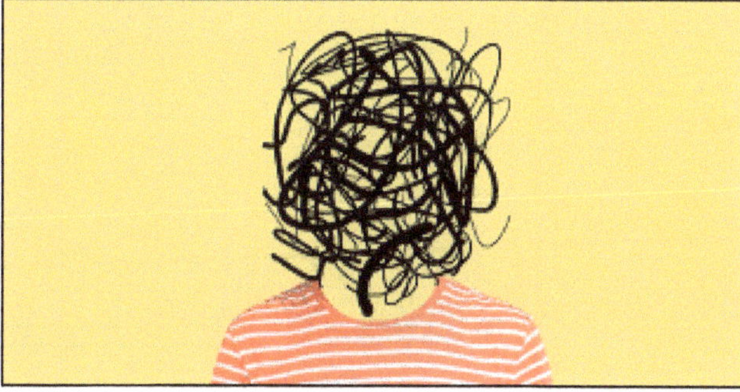

Figure 425 Anxiety

13.4.2.1 Types of Anxiety

- The psychological condition of **Separation Anxiety Disorder (SAD)** develops natural fear of detachment from essential individuals in childhood and might persist into adulthood. Someone with this disorder develops distressing reactions when they leave home or when they separate from their loved ones which interferes with their daily activities.
- **Generalized Anxiety Disorder (GAD)** forces people to experience prolonged intense worries regarding personal health together with work-related and social concerns. People with this type of anxiety experience persistent distress which becomes hard to manage because it creates physical symptoms including fatigue as well as muscle tension.
- **Panic Disorder** presents through multiple unexpected panic attacks that result in intense fear or discomfort surges. These sudden frightening episodes are recurrent and unexpected for those diagnosed with Panic Disorder. Physical manifestations of these panic attacks include an accelerated heartbeat combined with shortness of breath and dizziness to the extent that affected persons fear another attack.
- Selected patients with **Social Anxiety Disorder (SAD)** develop excessive social dread because they fear negative assessments and judgments from others during social situations.

People suffering from this condition generally lose their capability to maintain typical social contact within the community and to develop meaningful connections with others.

- **Specific Phobia** consists of an excessive and non-realistic fear of particular objects or situations including heights or animal encounters or flight. The intensifying anxiety makes people stay away from things that cause their reactions thus blocking both day-to-day activities and limiting their overall quality of life.
- Patients who have **Obsessive-Compulsive Disorder** display unwanted thought intrusions known as obsessions alongside compulsive need for repetitive actions or mental processes for anxiety reduction. The compulsive behaviors use up substantial time which results in functional limitations for the patient.
- The traumatic experience exposure that triggers **Post-Traumatic Stress Disorder (PTSD)** results in the development of flashbacks and nightmares and intense anxiety symptoms. Post-traumatic stress disorder generates two distinct symptoms in its patients including trauma-triggered avoidance behaviors alongside increased alertness signs like insomnia and restlessness.

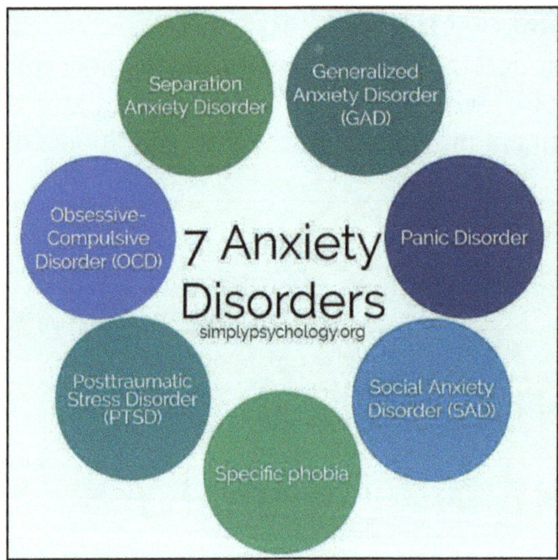

Figure 426 Anxiety Disorders

13.4.2.2 SOAP Notes for Anxiety

Table 244 SOAP Notes for Anxiety

Component	Details
Subjective (S)	A 28-year-old female presents with complaints of excessive worry and fear that have been present for the past two months. The patient reports feeling tense and on edge most days, with difficulty controlling her anxiety. She also mentions experiencing restlessness, difficulty concentrating, and muscle tension. Sleep is impaired, as she struggles to fall asleep due to racing thoughts. The patient denies any history of trauma or significant life stressors. She feels increasingly overwhelmed by her responsibilities at work.
Objective (O)	On physical examination, the patient appears anxious, with a slightly elevated heart rate of 88 bpm. Her blood pressure is 120/78 mmHg, and she appears fidgety during the exam. No physical abnormalities are noted,

	and she is alert and oriented. There is no evidence of psychosis or suicidal behavior. The patient denies any recent weight changes.
Assessment (A)	The patient's symptoms of excessive worry, restlessness, difficulty concentrating, and sleep disturbances are consistent with generalized anxiety disorder (GAD). The absence of other significant medical or psychiatric conditions supports this diagnosis. Further evaluation with standardized screening tools such as the GAD-7 would help confirm the diagnosis.
Plan (P)	**Pharmacological:** Initiate selective serotonin reuptake inhibitor (SSRI), such as escitalopram 10 mg daily, to manage anxiety symptoms (See algorithms below). **Non-pharmacological:** Recommend cognitive-behavioral therapy (CBT) to help address the patient's anxiety and coping mechanisms. **Follow-up:** Schedule a follow-up appointment in 2-3 weeks to assess the response to treatment and monitor for side effects. **Education:** Educate the patient about GAD, the role of SSRIs in managing anxiety, and the importance of therapy. Discuss potential side effects of SSRIs, including gastrointestinal issues and sexual dysfunction, and encourage ongoing communication regarding any concerns.

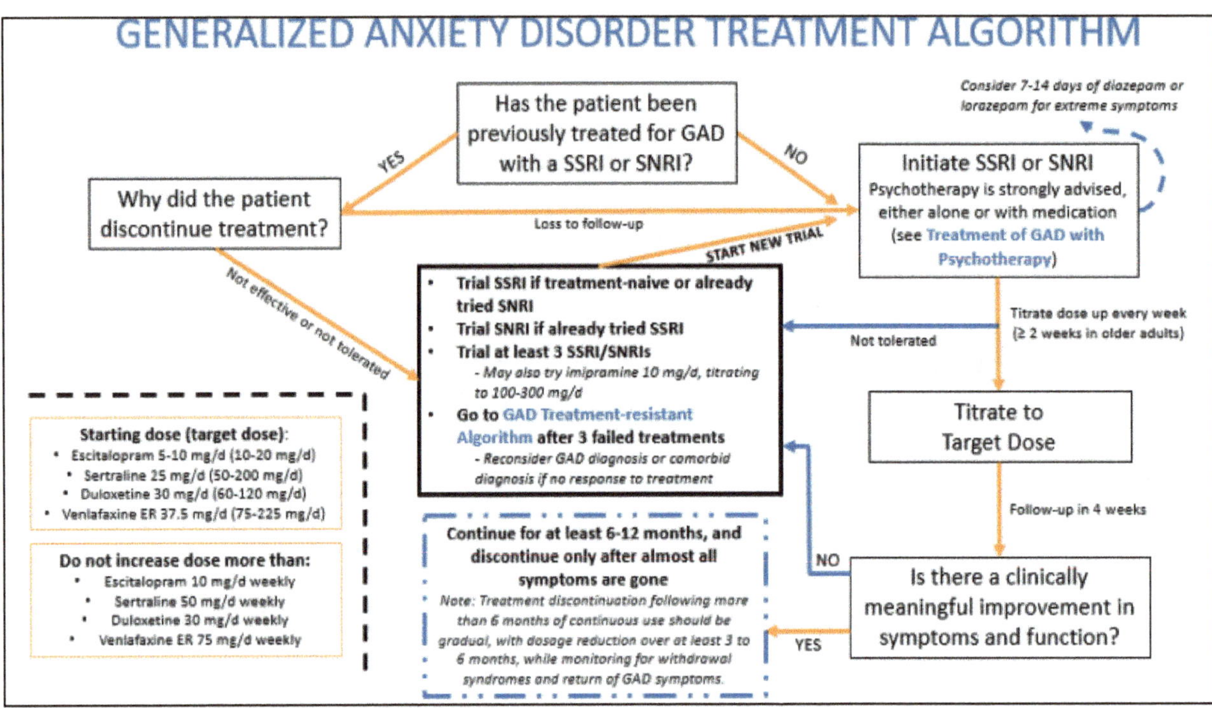

Figure 428 GAD Treatment Algorithm

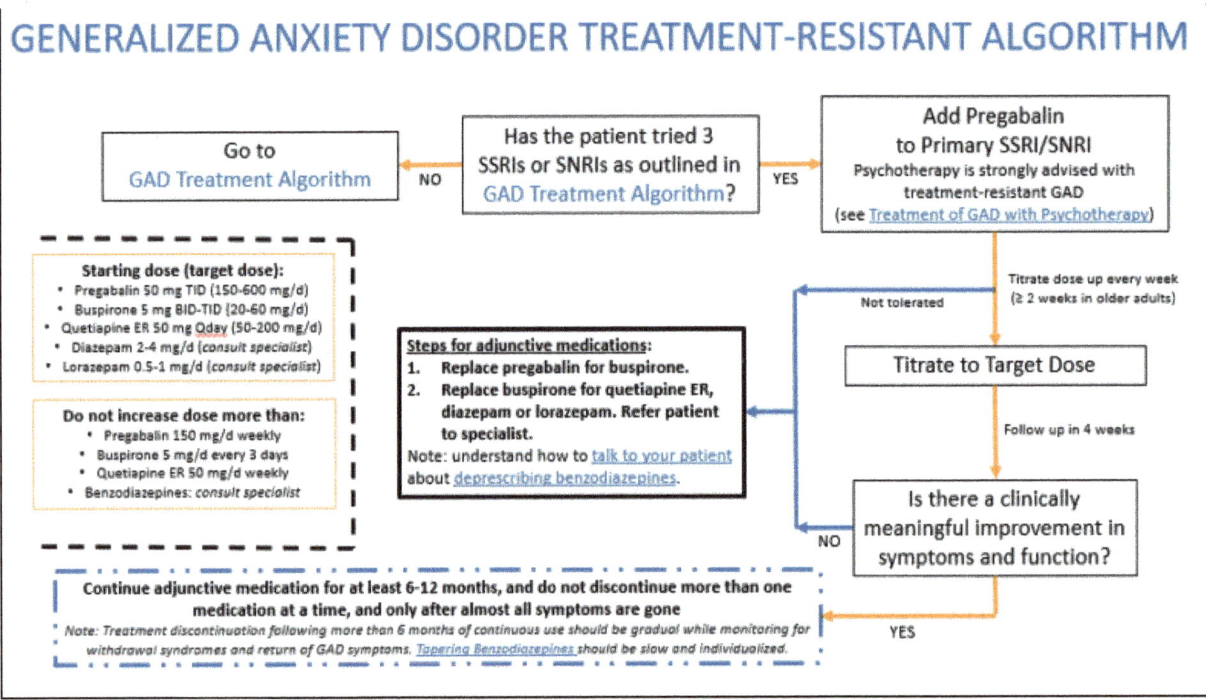

Figure 427 GAD Treatment-Resistant Algorithm

13.4.3 Alcohol Use Disorder/Alcoholism

Alcoholism is a chronic disease that is described by the compulsive and uncontrollable consumption of alcohol despite adverse effects to self and the society. It usually entails a urgent **desire to drink alcohol, the physical dependence among with alcohol, and coming up with withdrawal signs whenever alcohol consumption is cut or decreased**. Thus, the condition can result in serious psychological and physical complications, for example, kidney failure, heart diseases, and even depression or anxiety. Alcoholism is the problem that can be explained by the factors like genetic vulnerability, environmental aspects, and the presence of stress or trauma. Therapy used includes behavioural therapy, counselling, and use of drugs to curb the urges as well as avoid back sliding. Al**coholism is a chronic disease in which social, psychological, and physical factors** play a role and means that, in the treatment of the disorder, constant care is needed, and a strategic treatment plan should be adopted with highlighting the need for support at an early stage.

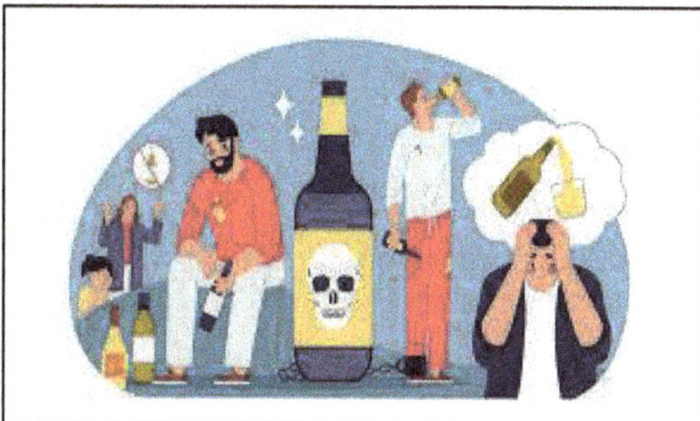

Figure 429 Alcoholism

13.4.3.1 Alcohol Use Disorder Spectrum

The image depicts the distribution of **Alcohol Use Disorder (AUD),** and estimates of different intensity levels which include mild, moderate, and severe. From the above chart, AUD is a disease that affects people, who are unable to moderate their intake of alcohol in a manner that is not hazardous to their personal/family, social, or occupational, and health. The spectrum starts with mild AUD, **which is a less severe form**, may involve from time to time overindulgence, or where the negative effects on the body are not very severe. Moderate and severe stage further develop where there are more **frequent and potentially hazardous use of alcohol,** and severe impact of the otherwise normal activities of life and region dependence. The image reinforces the fact that **AUD is not an absolute state and that it depends on the degree of loss of control**, which results from its consumption. The concept describing this condition and the relation of its severity to various treatment options depends on the stage of AUD is very important.

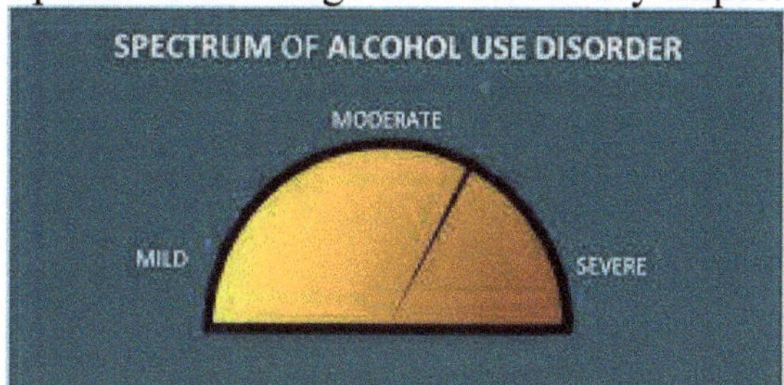

Figure 430 Alcoholism Spectrum

13.4.3.2 SOAP Notes for Alcoholism

Table 245 SOAP Notes for Alcoholism

Component	Details
Subjective (S)	A 34-year-old male presents with complaints of drinking alcohol regularly, about 5-6 times per week, with increasing consumption over the past 6 months. He reports difficulty limiting his alcohol intake, and has noticed that it is affecting his work performance and social relationships. The patient mentions feeling irritable when he is unable to drink, and

	occasionally experiences tremors and sweating after stopping drinking for a few hours. He has not been able to cut down despite multiple attempts. The patient denies any history of trauma or other significant medical conditions.
Objective (O)	On physical examination, the patient appears mildly disheveled but is alert and oriented. His vital signs include a pulse of 84 bpm and blood pressure of 122/80 mmHg. No physical abnormalities were noted, though the patient's speech is slightly slurred. There is no evidence of psychosis, and the patient is cooperative during the examination. No recent weight changes or visible withdrawal symptoms are noted at this time.
Assessment (A)	The patient's frequent alcohol use, inability to limit intake, and withdrawal symptoms such as tremors and irritability are consistent with moderate alcohol use disorder (AUD). These symptoms have led to impairments in both occupational and social functioning. Further evaluation with screening tools such as the AUDIT (Alcohol Use Disorders Identification Test) would be helpful to confirm the diagnosis and assess the severity.
Plan (P)	**Pharmacological**: Initiate a medication regimen, such as disulfiram or acamprosate, to assist with alcohol cessation (See algorithm below). **Non-pharmacological**: Recommend counseling, particularly cognitive-behavioral therapy (CBT), to address the patient's drinking patterns and triggers. **Follow-up**: Schedule a follow-up appointment in 2 weeks to assess the effectiveness of the medication and evaluate the patient's progress in treatment. **Education**: Educate the patient on the effects of alcohol on health and the importance of adhering to the prescribed treatment. Discuss potential side effects of medications and encourage support groups such as Alcoholics Anonymous (AA) for additional emotional support.

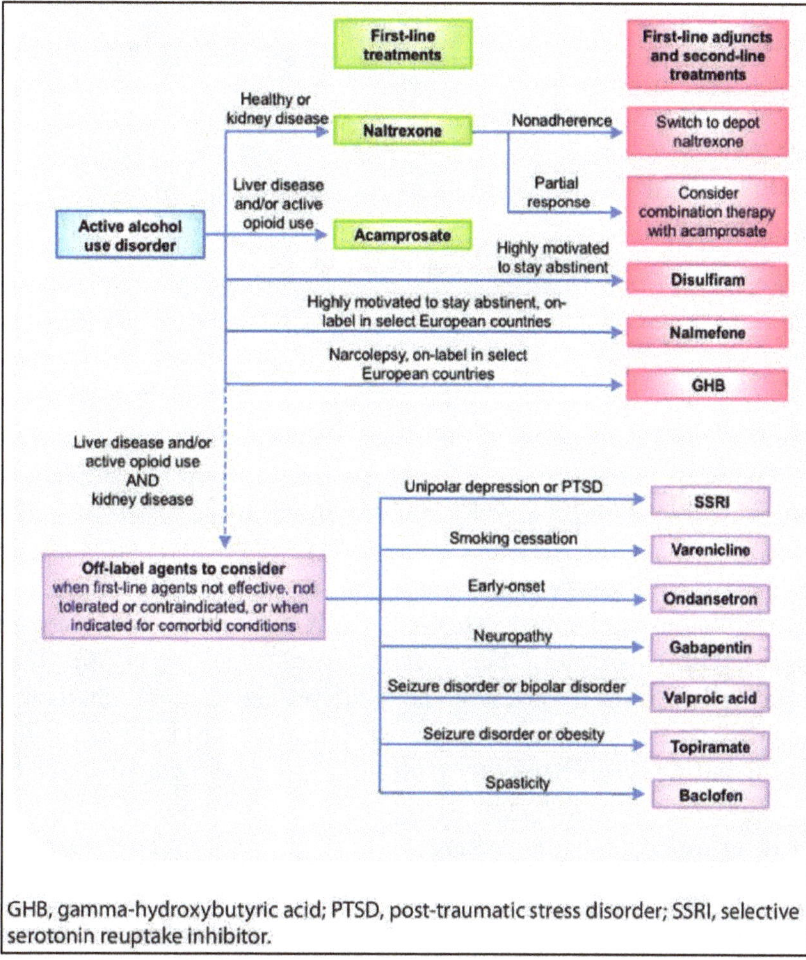

GHB, gamma-hydroxybutyric acid; PTSD, post-traumatic stress disorder; SSRI, selective serotonin reuptake inhibitor.

Figure 431 Algorithm for the Management of Alcoholism

13.4.4 Delirium

Delirium is a rapid onset and fluctuating process, in which the patient cannot focus, sustain attention, or think coherently. It is often acute and may originate from a multiplicity of engendering factors including **infections, metabolic disturbances, drugs, or alcohol.** The phenomenon of delirium is widespread among the hospitalised patients, especially the elderly and can be caused by surgery, illness or a shift in the environment. Some of the symptoms include confusion or lethargy, otherwise alternatives, disturbances in consciousness, illusionary experiences, and even aggression. **While dementia is a progressive and long-lasting disease, delirium is different** as it can be more or less severe sometime of the day and usually at night. Because of this, it is crucial to treat the root cause promptly, and manifest the symptoms in case of delirium because, if left untreated, it may eventually be fatal. **The management requires identifying a cause, stabilizing the environment and give supportive care that will enhance the healing process** of the damaged portion of the brain responsible for thinking. Specifically, early detection and treatment are important as they help lessen the chances of developing severe cases of dementia.

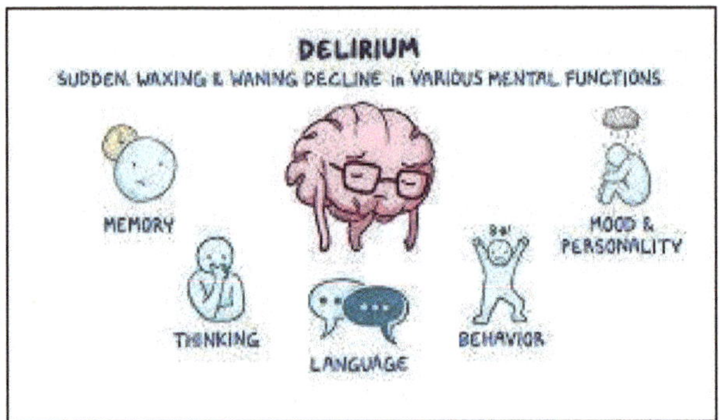

Figure 432 Delirium

13.4.4.1 Types of Delirium

The image depicts the three categories of delirium which include hypoactive, hyperactive and mixed categories. The most common type of subtypes of delirium is hypoactive delirium which manifests by slowness, reduced motor activity, and psychomotor retardation, and normally present with **anhedonia and apathy and hypoperformance. Hypersomnolent delirium,** which is less common than the hypoactive type, has agitation involving restless movement, decreased activity, and may have an irritable or angry effect. This is because hyperactive delirium patients are likely to **exhibit increased levels of emotions, as well as impulse-like behavior.** The mixed delirium in this case is a combination of the hypoactive and the hyperactive types, characterized by episodes in which the patient may be either drowsy or agitated. The affects of individuals in **mixed delirium** most of the time switches between being unemotional, and risky or aggressive behavior, thereby manifesting a more diverse expression. Knowledge of these subtypes is essential in managing the condition since it determines decision-making on the type of treatment to give the patient and nursing care, thus enabling individualized care.

Table 246 Types of Delirium

Hypoactive Delirium	Hyperactive Delirium	Mixed Delirium
• More common • Presentation: Slowed down, lethargic • Affect: Flat, withdrawn, lack of attention	• Less common • Presentation: Psychomotor agitation, restlessness • Affect: Disinhibition, aggressiveness	• Features consistent with both hypoactive and hyperactive delirium • Presentation: Variable with periods of lethargy and aggitation • Affect: Flat and alternating with impulsivity, and aggressive behavior

13.4.4.2 Difference Between 3Ds

The image differentiates between three conditions: Depression, Dementia, and Delirium, focusing on their symptoms, diagnostic criteria, treatments, and time courses. Depression is characterised **by persistent low mood, apathy, and fatigue, lasting at least two weeks, and is treated with antidepressants**. Dementia involves irreversible cognitive decline affecting daily activities, diagnosed through tests like **MoCA and treated with cholinesterase inhibitors**. Delirium, marked by acute confusion and inattention, lasts days to weeks and is often linked to substance imbalances, requiring antipsychotics. Diagnostic tools include **screening scales and imaging,**

while treatments involve a mix of pharmacological and non-pharmacological interventions tailored to each condition's unique features.

Table 247 Differential Summary of 3Ds

Differentiating Among the 3 Ds			
	Depression	**Dementia**	**Delirium**
Symptoms	• Apathy • Anhedonia • Depressed mood • Poor energy • Somatic concerns, fatigue, malaise	• Irreversible cognitive changes that interfere with ADLs	• Acute waxing and waning sensorium • Inattention
Time Course	• At least two weeks	• Months to years	• Days to weeks
Screening	• Geriatric Depression Scale	• MoCA • MMSE • SLUMS	• CAM
Recommended Labs	• CBC • Comprehensive metabolic panel (CMP) • Folate • RPR • TSH • Vit B_{12}	• CBC • CMP • Folate • RPR • TSH • Vit B_{12} • Vit D	• Blood alcohol level • CBC • CMP • Folate • TSH • Urinalysis • Urine drug screen • Vitamin B_{12}
Neuroimaging	• Brain MRI if concern for vascular depression	• Brain MRI	• CT head if focal neurological symptoms
Common Pharmacologic Treatment	• Antidepressants	• Cholinesterase inhibitors • Melatonin or ramelteon • Memantine	• Antipsychotics for agitation • Melatonin or ramelteon
Nonpharmacologic Treatment	• Cognitive behavioral therapy • ECT • Interpersonal therapy • Problem solving therapy • TMS	• Caregiver support • Problem-solving therapy • Psychosocial interventions	• Frequent reorientation • Maintaining sleep-wake cycle

13.4.4.3 SOAP Notes for Delirium

Table 248 SOAP Notes for Delirium

Component	Details
Subjective (S)	A 78-year-old male is brought in by his family, who report sudden changes in his behavior over the past 48 hours. The patient is noted to be more lethargic, difficult to wake, and unresponsive to basic commands. He has been disoriented at times, and family members express concerns over his fluctuating alertness. He also appears more withdrawn and less interested in engaging with them. The family denies any recent trauma or significant changes in his medication regimen.
Objective (O)	On physical examination, the patient is alert but displays a flat affect and exhibits slowed movements. His vital signs are stable with a pulse of 75

	bpm and blood pressure of 118/74 mmHg. The patient is unresponsive to some verbal stimuli and exhibits a lack of attention. No obvious signs of physical trauma are observed, and there are no apparent signs of hallucinations or agitation.
Assessment (A)	The patient's presentation is most consistent with hypoactive delirium, as evidenced by lethargy, flat affect, and withdrawn behavior. This may be related to an underlying medical condition, such as an infection or electrolyte imbalance, which will require further investigation. Additional screening tools such as the Confusion Assessment Method (CAM) should be used to further confirm the diagnosis and assess severity.
Plan (P)	**Pharmacological**: Consider discontinuing any potentially sedating medications and reassess the patient's pharmacological regimen (See algorithm below). **Non-pharmacological**: Provide supportive care, including hydration, pain management, and environmental modifications to reduce confusion. **Follow-up**: Order laboratory tests to evaluate for potential causes such as infections or metabolic disturbances. A follow-up reassessment of the patient's mental status is scheduled within 24-48 hours. **Education**: Educate family members about the nature of delirium, its common causes, and the importance of close monitoring. Discuss the need for a thorough investigation into the underlying cause to help address the delirium effectively.

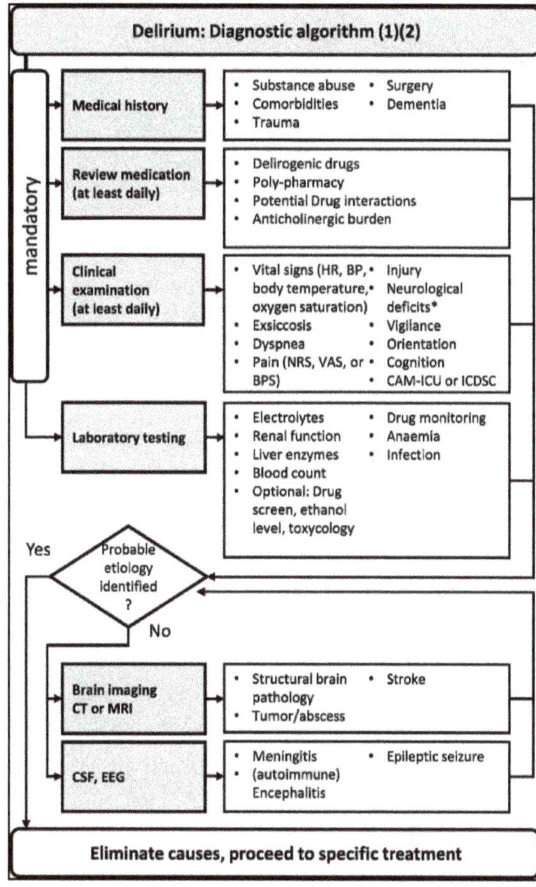

Figure 433 Management Algorithm for Delirium

Smoking Cessation

13.4.5 Insomnia

As a sleeping disorder, insomnia refers to the inability to fall asleep, to stay asleep, or waking up **too early and the inability to get back to sleep again.** It can be acute that lasts for several days or few weeks or chronic which is in existence for three nights per week for at least three months. There are many reasons behind insomnia such as stress, anxiety, and depression, bad habits, diseases, and some medicines. **Insomnia poses a considerable impact on the physical wellbeing** of an individual and well-being, which results to daytime tiredness, crankiness, blurred focus and productivity. It can also lead to the development of other aspects of mental disease, including mood disorders. Insomnia has the treatment by **cognitive-behavioral therapy for insomnia or CBT-I** intended to assist persons in changing their thoughts that affect sleep and waking hours routines. Sometimes sleep induction may be required to be carried out using some substances, and these may include sleeping pills although they are viewed as being for short term use only.

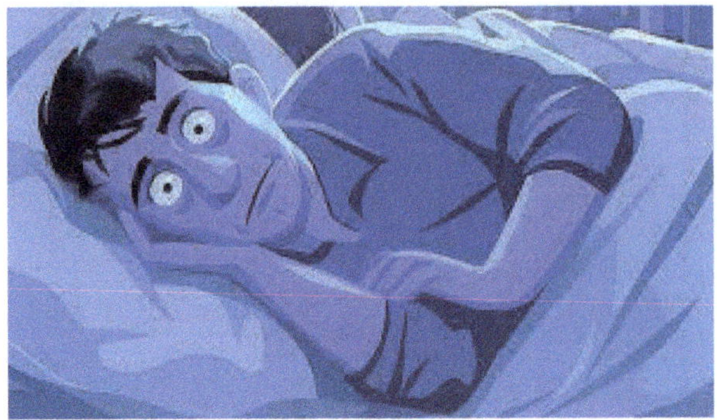

Figure 434 Insomnia

13.4.5.1 Types of Insomnia

The four categories of insomnia are depicted in the image below to show how this sleep problem can present itself. **The first type includes people who take time to go to sleep**; such a person may spend a lot of time in bed with little sleep until he or she fades off. **The second type is for those, who wakes up at night and cannot fall asleep again** and therefore, constantly has interrupted and interrupted night's sleep. **The third type captures persons who get up very early in the morning to only find that they cannot sleep again** which makes them have little or no sleep. **Thus, the fourth type is people who wake up in the morning still tired**, meaning that their night rest was interrupted, despite the fact that they got enough sleep. These forms of insomnia cause substantial disturbances in an individual's health and well-being and the efficacy of the two types of treatment depend on the nature of the sleep disturbance.

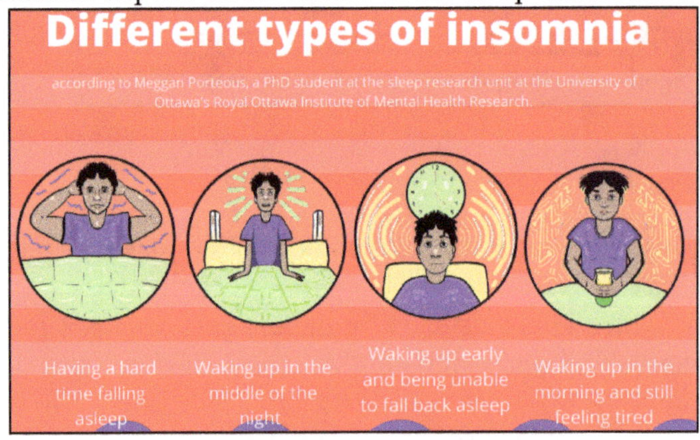
Different types of insomnia
according to Meggan Porteous, a PhD student at the sleep research unit at the University of Ottawa's Royal Ottawa Institute of Mental Health Research.
Having a hard time falling asleep
Waking up in the middle of the night
Waking up early and being unable to fall back asleep
Waking up in the morning and still feeling tired

Figure 435 Types of Insomnia

13.4.5.2 SOAP Notes for Insomnia

Table 249 SOAP Notes for Insomnia

Component	Details
Subjective (S)	A 40-year-old female presents with complaints of difficulty falling asleep for the past three weeks. She reports lying awake in bed for at least 30-60 minutes before she can fall asleep. In addition, she often wakes up in the middle of the night and struggles to return to sleep. The patient also notes that she wakes up early in the morning, typically around 4:00 AM, and is unable to fall back asleep. Despite spending a sufficient amount of time in bed, she feels fatigued and unrested upon waking. The patient denies any significant life stressors or medical conditions that may contribute to her symptoms.

Objective (O)	On physical examination, the patient appears well-groomed but is noticeably tired. Vital signs are within normal limits: pulse 76 bpm, blood pressure 118/76 mmHg. No signs of physical illness are noted. The patient is alert and oriented with no evidence of cognitive dysfunction or psychosis. No recent weight changes or health complaints are reported.
Assessment (A)	The patient's symptoms, including difficulty falling asleep, waking up in the middle of the night, early morning awakening, and feeling unrefreshed, are consistent with insomnia. The patient's presentation seems to involve multiple types of insomnia, including sleep-onset insomnia, middle-of-the-night awakening, and early morning awakening. No underlying medical conditions have been identified, suggesting that the insomnia is likely primary. A more thorough evaluation of sleep habits and potential psychological stressors is warranted.
Plan (P)	**Pharmacological**: Consider short-term use of a low-dose benzodiazepine (e.g., lorazepam 0.5 mg) or a non-benzodiazepine hypnotic (e.g., zolpidem 5 mg) for sleep assistance. **Non-pharmacological**: Recommend cognitive-behavioral therapy for insomnia (CBT-I) to address sleep hygiene, thoughts, and behaviors that may be contributing to the sleep disturbance. **Follow-up**: Schedule a follow-up appointment in 2-4 weeks to assess the patient's response to the treatment plan, as well as to monitor for any potential side effects. **Education**: Educate the patient on proper sleep hygiene practices, such as maintaining a regular sleep schedule, avoiding caffeine late in the day, and minimizing screen time before bed. Discuss the importance of treating underlying psychological factors if necessary.

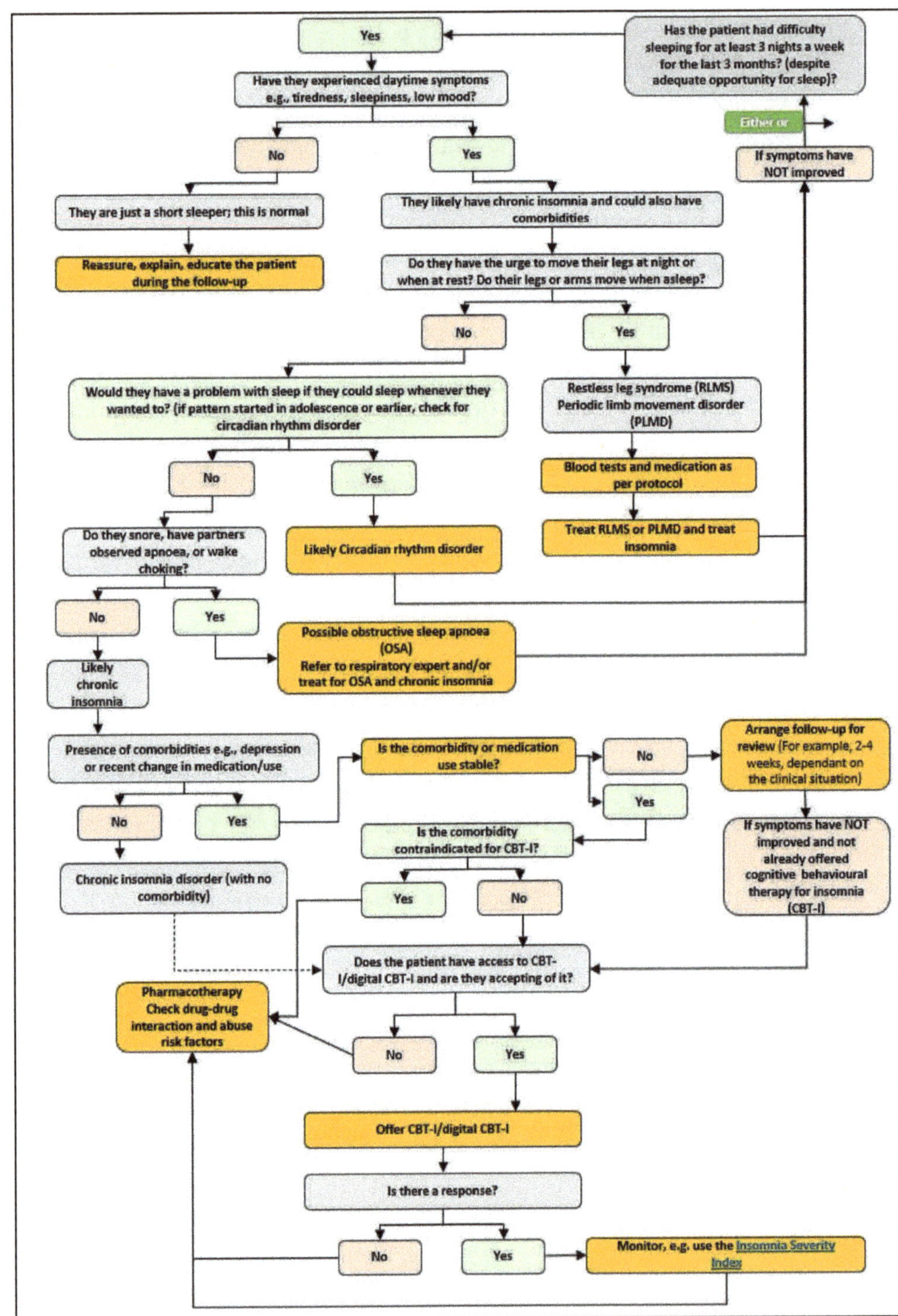

Figure 436 Algorithm for chronic insomnia disorder decision flow

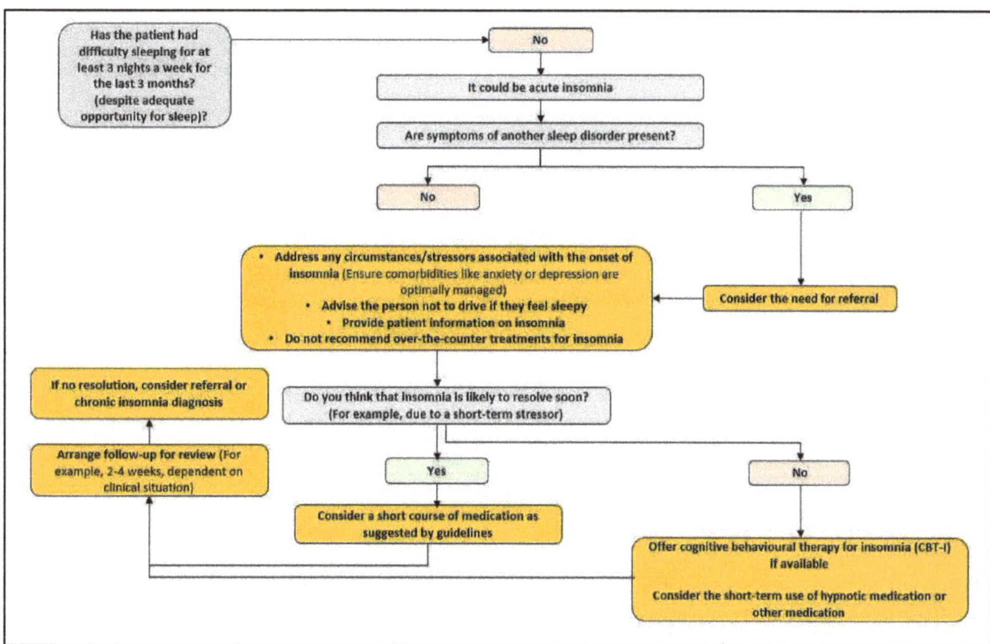

Figure 437 Algorithm for acute insomnia disorder decision flow

13.4.6 Bipolar Disorder

Bipolar disorder also known as manic-depressive illness is a disease which results to rapid **swinging of emotion from one extreme to another; mania and depression**. Such adjustments may render a person incapable of performing certain tasks in his/her day-to-day activities, jobs and interpersonal interactions. The different bipolar disorders are **Bipolar I, Bipolar II and Cyclothymic Disorder,** and they are all characterized by the **presence of mood swings**. It is characterized as having at least one manic episode, which can last for at least seven days or requires hospitalization, and may have a depressive episode. Bipolar II entails both hypomania, which is a less severe type of mania and depression but without the full-blown mania. Cyclothymic Disorder is characterised by hypomanic symptoms and depressed mood persisting for a period of two years, although the **full-blown manic or depressive episode is not experienced**. The researchers noted that the cause of bipolar disorder has not been fully explained; however, it is assumed that it has a genetic, environmental and neurobiological basis. The symptoms of mania are **over energy, impulsiveness, irritation, decrease in need of sleep, when depressive episodes include hopelessness, fatigue and decrease in interest in activities**. Within most treatment plans, mood stabilizers, antipsychotics, and psychotherapy are the key components to address mood swings and to avoid a relapse. It is essential to detect the disease at an early stage since if left untreated, bipolar disorder will affect one or both aspects of the individual's life – personal and professional. If properly managed, many persons with bipolar disorder are able to have normal existence and continued employment.

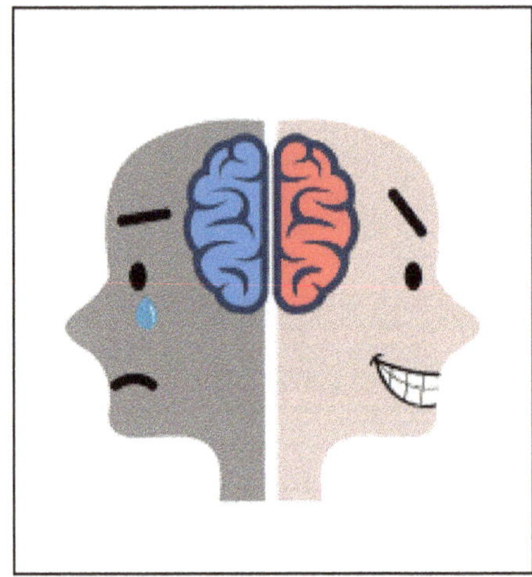

Figure 438 Bipolar Disorder

13.4.6.1 Types of Bipolar Disorder

This picture illustrates **Bipolar 1 vs Bipolar 2** to have a clear distinction of the kind of symptoms and how they are presented before the court**. Bipolar 1 is a diagnosis that includes at least one episode of manic or mixed episode of at least one week's duration,** which usually calls for hospitalization, and it can involve depressive episodes. The manic episodes which are characteristic of Bipolar 1 can cause moderate to severe disability and are expressed by the features such as increased energy, talkative, impulsive, and aggressive behavior, reduced need for sleep. On the other hand, **Bipolar 2 Disorder includes hypomania which is somewhat less serious than mania but last for shorter time- several days**. Bipolar 2 is distinguished from Bipolar 1 by the fact that there must be at least one instance of depressive episode; the hypomanic episodes are less severe compared to Bipolar 1. Like Bipolar 1, Bipolar 2 also presents similar symptoms of depressions comprising hopelessness, irritability, fatigue, etc. Bipolar 2 can sometimes be more difficult to diagnose **compared to bipolar 1 because the symptoms of hypomania** are much less conspicuous, which is why it is necessary to focus on the depressive episodes so as to determine Bipolar 2. Knowing these differences is beneficial in order to treat a patient properly given that the levels of mania and depression differ.

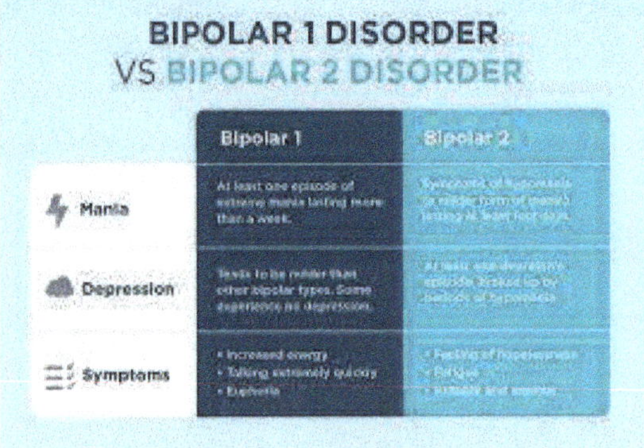

Figure 439 Types of Bipolar Disorder

13.4.6.2 SOAP Notes for Bipolar Disorder

Table 250 SOAP Notes for Bipolar Disorder

Component	Details
Subjective (S)	A 32-year-old female presents with a history of mood swings over the past several months. She reports episodes of increased energy, impulsivity, and

	irritability, often lasting for a few days at a time. During these periods, she has trouble sleeping, feels overly confident, and tends to make reckless decisions, such as spending large amounts of money. She also experiences prolonged periods of low mood, feelings of hopelessness, and fatigue, which interfere with her daily functioning. She denies any significant trauma or stressors but has a family history of mental health issues.
Objective (O)	On physical examination, the patient appears slightly agitated but is otherwise in no acute distress. Vital signs are stable: pulse 80 bpm, blood pressure 118/76 mmHg. The patient is alert and oriented, but exhibits a slightly elevated speech rate during the interview. No signs of physical illness are observed. There are no apparent cognitive impairments or psychosis during the examination.
Assessment (A)	The patient's presentation of mood fluctuations, including periods of excessive energy, impulsivity, and decreased need for sleep, coupled with depressive episodes characterized by fatigue, hopelessness, and irritability, is consistent with Bipolar 2 Disorder. The hypomanic episodes, though noticeable, are not as extreme as full manic episodes seen in Bipolar 1, which helps differentiate it from that disorder. Given the recurrent nature of these episodes, Bipolar 2 is the most likely diagnosis. A more thorough evaluation using mood tracking and standardized diagnostic tools such as the Mood Disorder Questionnaire (MDQ) is recommended.
Plan (P)	**Pharmacological**: Initiate a mood stabilizer, such as lithium or lamotrigine, to manage mood fluctuations and prevent relapse (See algorithm below). **Non-pharmacological**: Recommend cognitive-behavioral therapy (CBT) to help manage depressive symptoms and address behaviors associated with hypomania. **Follow-up**: Schedule a follow-up appointment in 2-3 weeks to monitor the patient's response to treatment and assess for any side effects. **Education**: Educate the patient about the nature of Bipolar 2 Disorder, the importance of medication adherence, and the potential benefits of therapy in managing mood swings. Discuss lifestyle modifications and the need for regular sleep patterns to help prevent mood instability.

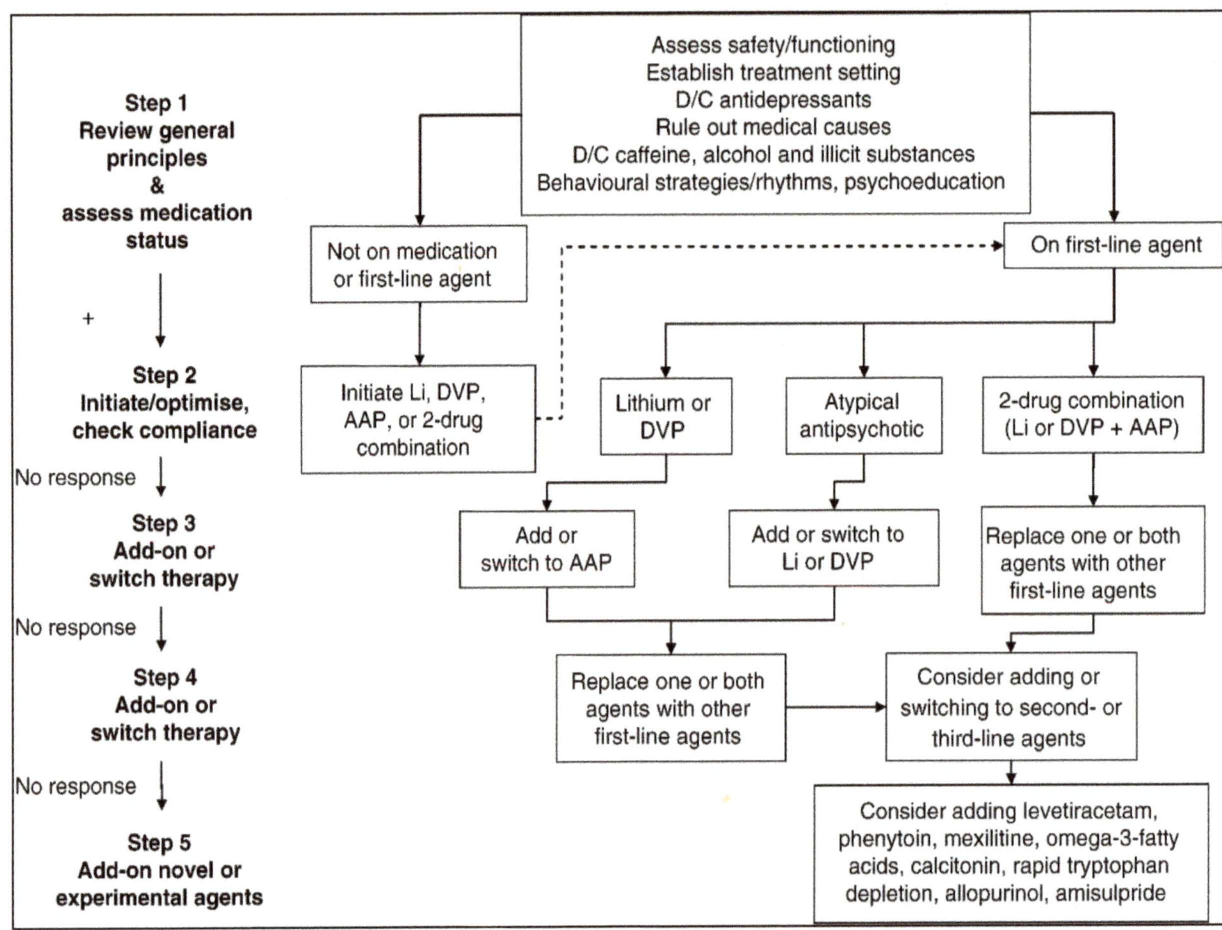

Figure 440 Management Algorithm for Bipolar Disorder

13.4.7 Schizophrenia

Schizophrenia is a severe mental illness diagnosed with psychotic features due to its symptoms that include altered perception of reality, behavior and emotional responses. It often has episodes of psychosis that are may be characterised by episodes were the person gets out of touch with reality. Major symptoms of schizophrenia include **paranoid beliefs (false beliefs), hallucinations (hearing or seeing things that are not real),** disorderly thinking and talking and having reduced mental abilities. These symptoms are particularly evident when the person is in the late **adolescence or early adulthood and manifests in gradual progression**. To this date, the reasons that lead to occurrence of schizophrenia are not known clearly, but it is believed that it has genetic, environmental and neurochemical influences. Dopamine and other neurotransmitters are also believed to be imbalanced because of the disorder. Schizophrenia poses a threat to an individual's functionality in the **society due to various complications that affect his/her ability to maintain social relationships, get a job, and perform activities, paranoid, disorganized, and catatonic, or by tangibles symptoms** that are most noticeable and prominent in the affected individual. The typical treatment includes the use of antipsychotic medication to control them and psychotherapy to help the patient with the strategies of **handling the symptoms and regaining social interactions**. This is due to the fact that if a person is started on a medication early, there is low chance that this will worsen the symptoms and the outcome will be better overall. In addition, other treatment interventions relating to the patient's support networks include family therapy and social reintegration to manage the condition and support the recovery process. Though schizophrenia is permanent, many patients can lead normal fulfilling lives if only proper treatment is provided to them and supported by appropriate psychosocial interventions.

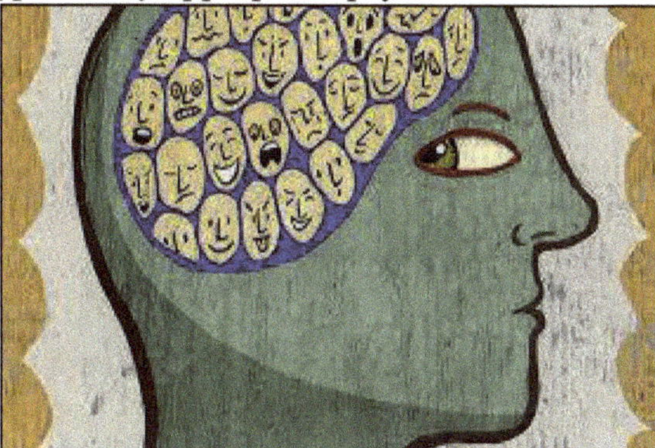

Figure 441 Schizophrenia

13.4.7.1 Classification of Schizophrenia

The figure is an illustration of the ICD-10 for schizophrenia, schizophreniform and paranoid disorders. **F20 to F29** range of the classification, outlines different types of schizophrenia; which is a complicated mental disorder described to be incapacitating. Schizophrenia is introduced under F20; the subdivisions include **paranoid schizophrenia F20.0** that involves the state with delusions of persecution or grandeur as well as hebephrenic schizophrenia F20.1, which is characterized by disorganized speech and behavior. **Catatonic schizophrenia (F20.2)** is also can be distinguished by highly expressed motor changes – a subject can be catatonic or hyperkinetic. There is also **unspecified schizophrenia or paranoid (F20.3)** which does not fall under other types of schizophrenia and others; **schizophrenic depressive (F20.4)** which occurs later after a person has developed a schizophrenic episode. This social disease definition is grouped under F20.5 and is deemed as schizophrenia in remission where the patient's symptoms are manageable but mild. F20.6 is simple schizophrenia that is characterized by the mild and chronic symptoms which are harder to identify. The classification is rounded off by **schizotypal disorder (F21),** which is a type of personality disorder that has much in common with schizophrenia but, usually, is less severe. These clerkship help the diagnosis and the subsequent treatment as it will help in identifying the right treatment for a particular patient depending on the symptoms exhibited.

Table 251 Classification of Schizophrenia

ICD – 10 CLASSIFICATION

F 20 – 29	Schizophrenia, Schizotypal & Delusional Disorders
F20	Schizophrenia
F20.0	Paranoid Schizophrenia
F20.1	Hebephrenic Schizophrenia
F20.2	Catatonic Schizophrenia
F20.3	Undifferentiated
F20.4	Post – Schizophrenic Depression
F20.5	Residual Schizophrenia
F20.6	Simple Schizophrenia
F21	Schizotypal Disorder

ICD – 10

13.4.7.2 SOAP Notes for Schizophrenia

Table 252 SOAP Notes for Schizophrenia

Component	Details
Subjective (S)	A 25-year-old male presents with a 6-month history of auditory hallucinations and delusions of persecution. The patient reports hearing voices telling him that people are plotting against him and that his thoughts are being controlled. He states that he often feels watched and believes that strangers are talking about him. The patient denies any significant history of trauma or substance abuse. He has become increasingly socially withdrawn, avoiding interactions with family and friends. He has difficulty maintaining employment due to his symptoms and often struggles to complete daily tasks.
Objective (O)	On physical examination, the patient appears disheveled and exhibits a flat affect. His speech is slow and fragmented, often losing coherence during conversation. No signs of acute physical illness are present, but his cognitive function appears impaired. The patient is alert and oriented to person, place, and time but shows difficulty maintaining attention during the interview. No overt motor disturbances are observed.
Assessment (A)	The patient's symptoms, including auditory hallucinations, delusions of persecution, and impaired cognitive function, are consistent with paranoid schizophrenia (ICD-10 F20.0). His social withdrawal, inability to maintain employment, and disorganized speech further support this diagnosis. The patient does not exhibit symptoms of other disorders, such as mood disorders or substance-induced psychosis. Given the severity of the symptoms and the impact on daily functioning, immediate intervention is necessary to manage the condition.
Plan (P)	**Pharmacological**: Initiate antipsychotic treatment with risperidone 2 mg daily to help manage the patient's delusions and hallucinations (See algorithm below). **Non-pharmacological**: Recommend cognitive-behavioral therapy (CBT) to address the patient's delusions and improve coping strategies. **Follow-up**: Schedule a follow-up appointment in 2 weeks to assess the effectiveness of the medication and monitor for side effects. **Education**: Educate the patient and his family about the nature of schizophrenia, the importance of medication adherence, and the potential side effects of antipsychotics. Discuss the role of therapy in improving social functioning and managing symptoms.

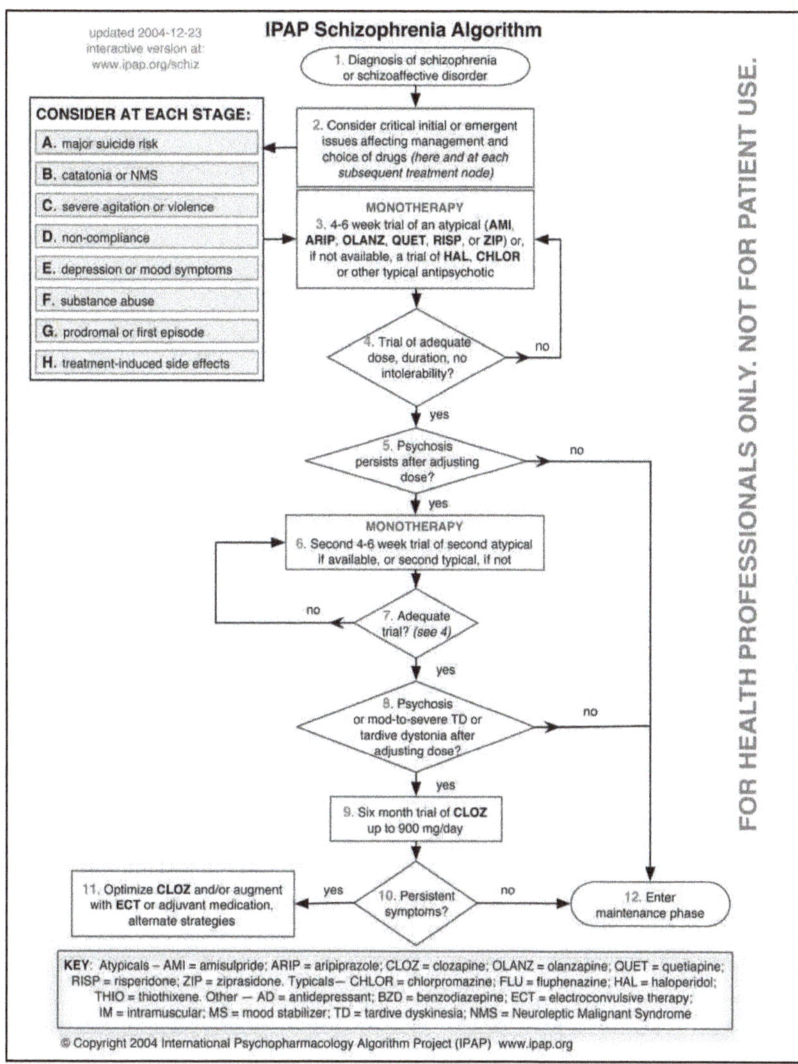
updated 2004-12-23
interactive version at:
www.ipap.org/schiz
IPAP Schizophrenia Algorithm
1. Diagnosis of schizophrenia or schizoaffective disorder
CONSIDER AT EACH STAGE:
A. major suicide risk
B. catatonia or NMS
C. severe agitation or violence
D. non-compliance
E. depression or mood symptoms
F. substance abuse
G. prodromal or first episode
H. treatment-induced side effects
2. Consider critical initial or emergent issues affecting management and choice of drugs (here and at each subsequent treatment node)
MONOTHERAPY
3. 4-6 week trial of an atypical (AMI, ARIP, OLANZ, QUET, RISP, or ZIP) or, if not available, a trial of HAL, CHLOR or other typical antipsychotic
4. Trial of adequate dose, duration, no intolerability?
no
yes
5. Psychosis persists after adjusting dose?
no
yes
MONOTHERAPY
6. Second 4-6 week trial of second atypical if available, or second typical, if not
no
7. Adequate trial? (see 4)
yes
8. Psychosis or mod-to-severe TD or tardive dystonia after adjusting dose?
no
yes
9. Six month trial of CLOZ up to 900 mg/day
11. Optimize CLOZ and/or augment with ECT or adjuvant medication, alternate strategies
yes
10. Persistent symptoms?
no
12. Enter maintenance phase
KEY: Atypicals – AMI = amisulpride; ARIP = aripiprazole; CLOZ = clozapine; OLANZ = olanzapine; QUET = quetiapine; RISP = risperidone; ZIP = ziprasidone. Typicals– CHLOR = chlorpromazine; FLU = fluphenazine; HAL = haloperidol; THIO = thiothixene. Other – AD = antidepressant; BZD = benzodiazepine; ECT = electroconvulsive therapy; IM = intramuscular; MS = mood stabilizer; TD = tardive dyskinesia; NMS = Neuroleptic Malignant Syndrome
© Copyright 2004 International Psychopharmacology Algorithm Project (IPAP) www.ipap.org
FOR HEALTH PROFESSIONALS ONLY. NOT FOR PATIENT USE.

Figure 442 Algorithm for the Management of Schizophrenia

13.4.8 Anorexia Nervosa

Anorexia nervosa is an eating disorder that entails compulsive **fear of being overweight or fat and may result into some eating habits and severe emaciation**. Patients suffering from anorexia nervosa are characterized by insistence on remaining thin, excessive food preoccupation and purging thus starving themselves. This disorder can appear at the period of adolescence or during young adult age and it tends to affect females, still, it can affect both sexes and any age. This is not **merely a disease of the physical body** but is coupled with severe mental and emotional disorder which includes one constantly feeling that one does not fit into the society or the world, being insecure, and having the urge to control or discipline one's body. If left unchecked, anorexia nervosa can **result in permanent harm to the body for instance, malnutrition, electrolyte imbalance, a broken immune system, organ failure, and in severe cases, death.** The sufferers of anorexia are also prone to other disorders like depressive, anxiety and obsessive-compulsive disorders. The observed anorexia nervosa treatment usually entails treatment by a qualified healthcare professional with a focus on medical complications and nutrition along with psychiatric evaluations with the counselor. **CBT is one of the dominant therapeutic interventions** assisting women in changing negative patterns of thoughts and perceiving eating and body image in a more realistic manner. Family therapy can also be recommended for support and intervention in relation to **family factors related to the disorder**. This is because anorexia nervosa is complex to treat and its treatment might last for an unnecessarily long duration before the patient is stable enough not to relapse.

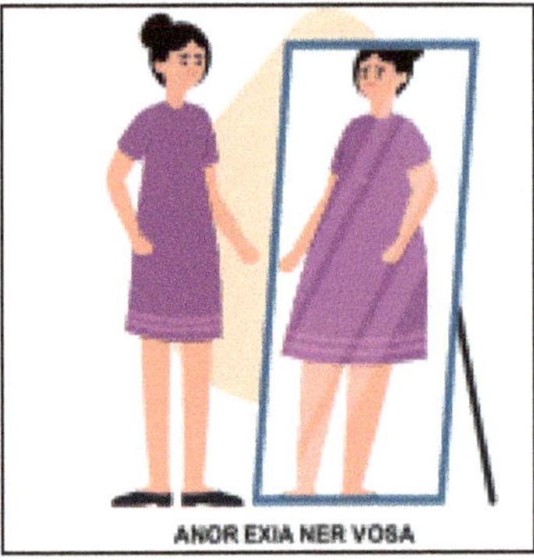

Figure 443 Anorexia Nervosa

13.4.8.1 SOAP Notes for Anorexia Nervosa

Table 253 SOAP Notes for Anorexia Nervosa

Component	Details
Subjective (S)	A 19-year-old female presents with concerns about significant weight loss over the past six months, accompanied by extreme preoccupation with food and body image. She reports restricting her caloric intake to fewer than 800 calories per day, despite having a healthy appetite. The patient expresses a constant fear of gaining weight and is dissatisfied with her body shape, particularly her stomach. She denies any binge eating behaviors or purging but has frequent thoughts about dieting. The patient also reports feeling fatigued, cold intolerance, and occasional dizziness. She has withdrawn socially and avoids family meals. She denies any history of trauma or substance use.
Objective (O)	On physical examination, the patient appears underweight, with a BMI of 16.5. Vital signs include a pulse of 56 bpm, blood pressure of 100/60 mmHg, and temperature of 97.6°F. No signs of acute illness are noted. The patient's skin appears dry, and her hair is thinning. There are no signs of edema, and her neurological exam is normal, but she appears fatigued. Psychological assessment reveals a distorted body image, with the patient expressing dissatisfaction with her appearance despite clear signs of underweight.
Assessment (A)	The patient's presentation, including extreme weight loss, dietary restriction, preoccupation with body image, and fear of gaining weight, is consistent with anorexia nervosa (ICD-10 F50.0). Her physical examination findings, including low BMI and signs of malnutrition, further support this diagnosis. The patient also exhibits significant psychological distress related to her appearance and food intake. The severity of her condition

	warrants immediate intervention to address both her physical and mental health needs.
Plan (P)	**Pharmacological**: Consider initiating a selective serotonin reuptake inhibitor (SSRI), such as fluoxetine, to address underlying anxiety and depressive symptoms that often accompany anorexia nervosa (See algorithm below). **Non-pharmacological**: Recommend cognitive-behavioral therapy (CBT) to address distorted body image and unhealthy eating patterns. **Nutritional intervention**: Refer the patient to a nutritionist for a personalized refeeding plan and nutritional counseling to safely regain weight. **Follow-up**: Schedule a follow-up appointment in 1-2 weeks to monitor weight restoration, physical health, and response to therapy. **Education**: Educate the patient and her family about anorexia nervosa, its risks, and the importance of adhering to treatment plans. Emphasize the need for gradual weight restoration and the role of therapy in addressing the psychological aspects of the disorder.

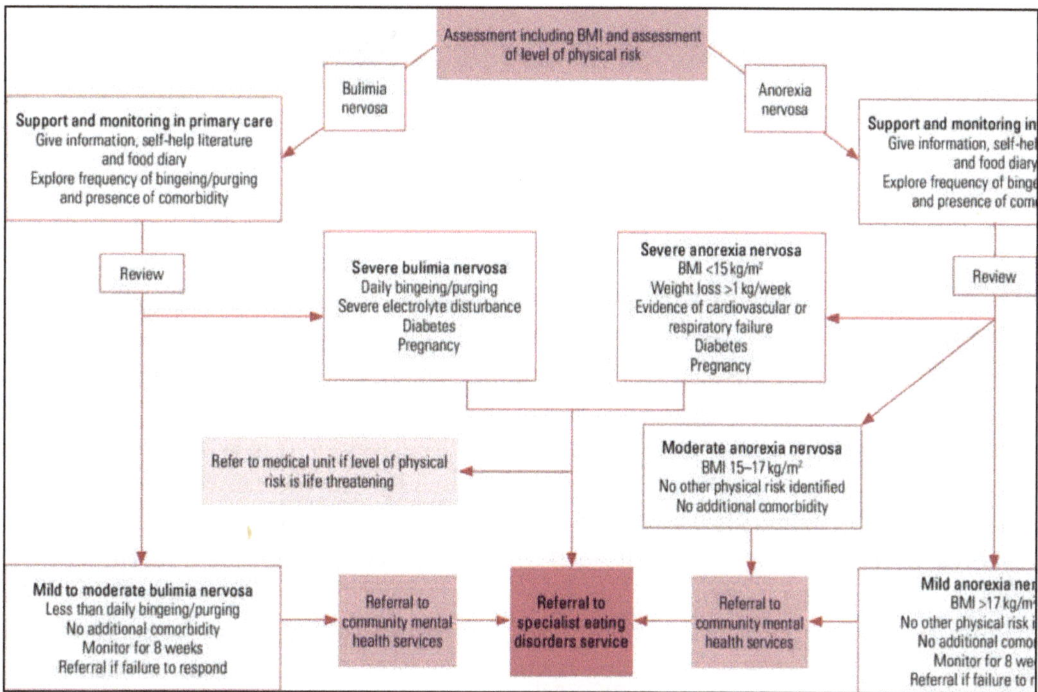

Figure 444 Management Algorithm for Anorexia Nervosa

13.4.9 Posttraumatic Stress Disorder (PTSD)

PTSD is a mental illness which affects individuals who live through a traumatic event or witness it, the trauma may include war, natural disasters, rape or other instances of physical violence. It has some of the features that have a duration of greater than one month and impairs an individual's functioning. The **signs related to PTSD** thus include the following: re-experiencing of the trauma through the cause, **flashbacks, and nightmares, increased alertness (anxiety, insomnia, agitation), avoidance of things that remind the victim of the trauma, and negative alteration in mood and cognitions (depression, guilt, and emotional numbing).** PTSD can occur at the time of the traumatic event or at some time later in the future after the traumatic event has occurred.

Specific characteristics of real-world trauma that put an individual at risk for developing PTSD include recurrent stressful life experiences, little social support, and other psychiatric disorders. Environmental factors, too: Other possible biological factors are changes on the chemical or anatomical level in the brain, for instance. It is frequently accompanied by depression, anxiety and addiction too, which makes diagnosis and management of the disorder difficult. The recommended treatment for PTSD is psychotherapy that **include cognitive-behavioral therapy (CBT), trauma focused CBT being common and widely recommended.** Another therapy used for traumatic event survivors is known as the **Eye Movement Desensitization and Reprocessing (EMDR).** Some of the drugs used in PTSD consist of selective serotonin reuptake inhibitors and these are administered since they assist in managing depression and anxieties resulting from the condition. If left untreated, PTSD results in severe and persistent handicaps in people's lives and increases likelihood of diagnoses of other major disorders. Through counseling, the use of drugs, and the support systems that are offered by close friends and family, one can be happy living with PTSD.

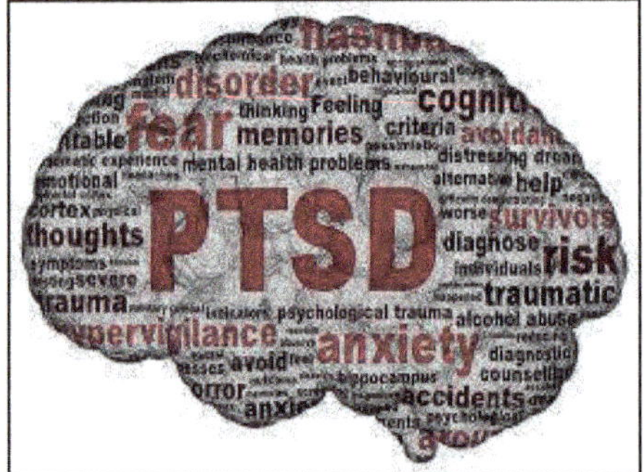

Figure 445 Post Traumatic Stress Disorder

13.4.9.1 Types of PTSD

The picture illustrates six forms of PTSD, which describes different degrees and manifestations of trauma. The first one is normal stress reaction which refers to the general reaction individuals make to stress; Although one might feel distressed for some time he/she does not develop any illness that is a cry for professional help as it is with the other types of stress. The second is **"Acute stress disorder",** which are symptoms occurring right after a traumatic event that may last from three days to a month. If these symptoms last for more than four weeks, it may develop into PTSD. As for the **" uncomplicated PTSD",** it refers to situations where the patient has no other issues beyond the PTSD symptoms they have developed due to the traumatic event. **"Dissociative PTSD"** therefore refer to symptoms of dissociation, or the feelings that the individual is detached from reality or that he/she has an inability to recall details of the trauma. **"Complex PTSD",** in turn, is a more severe form of PTSD that includes less recoverable and thus deeper emotional and psychological injuries resulting from long-term or repeated trauma, most often consisting of childhood abuse. Finally, there is **"Comorbid PTSD",** it is simply PTSD plus another mental illness like depression, or anxiety or any other illness and this makes diagnosis and treatment even difficult. It is crucial to apply a discreteness method when it comes to each type of PTSD to treat both trauma and patient's symptoms.

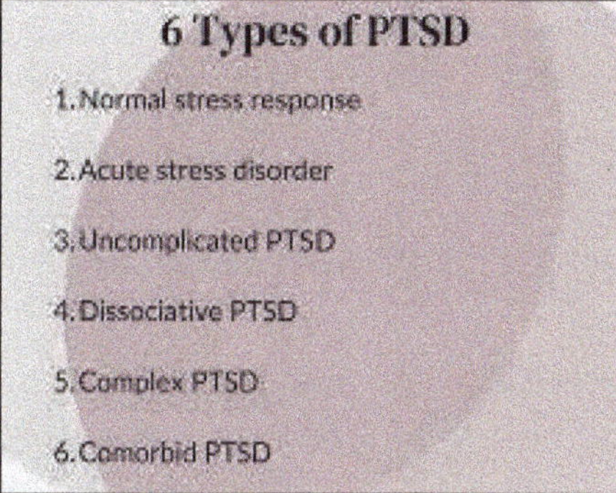

Figure 446 Types of PTSD

13.4.9.2 SOAP Notes for PTSD

Table 254 SOAP Notes for PTSD

Component	Details
Subjective (S)	A 30-year-old female presents with symptoms of anxiety, flashbacks, and sleep disturbances following a traumatic event one year ago. She reports feeling "on edge" most of the time and has frequent nightmares related to the trauma. The patient has difficulty concentrating and avoids places or people that remind her of the event. She feels detached from her surroundings and has trouble forming close relationships, feeling emotionally numb. She denies any history of substance abuse or major medical conditions. The patient is unsure whether her symptoms are a normal response to stress or if they are indicative of something more serious.
Objective (O)	On physical examination, the patient appears anxious but is well-groomed and oriented. Her vital signs are stable, with a pulse of 80 bpm and blood pressure of 120/80 mmHg. No signs of physical distress are noted, but the patient is visibly distressed when discussing the traumatic event. There are no signs of psychosis or acute physical illness. The patient is able to engage in the conversation but exhibits emotional numbing and difficulty with focus during the interview.
Assessment (A)	The patient's symptoms, including intrusive thoughts, nightmares, avoidance behavior, and emotional numbing, are consistent with PTSD. Based on the prolonged nature of her symptoms (lasting for one year) and the presence of dissociative features (emotional numbness, detachment), this presentation suggests Complex PTSD. The patient's difficulties in social relationships and emotional regulation further align with this diagnosis. A detailed trauma history and further psychological assessment, including the use of PTSD-specific screening tools (e.g., PCL-5), will be helpful for confirmation.
Plan (P)	**Pharmacological**: Initiate selective serotonin reuptake inhibitors (SSRIs), such as sertraline 50 mg daily, to help manage symptoms of anxiety and depression associated with PTSD (See algorithm below). **Non-**

pharmacological: Recommend trauma-focused cognitive-behavioral therapy (CBT) to address intrusive memories, emotional numbing, and avoidance behaviors. Additionally, consider Eye Movement Desensitization and Reprocessing (EMDR) therapy to help process the traumatic memories. **Follow-up**: Schedule a follow-up appointment in 2-3 weeks to evaluate the effectiveness of medication and therapy. **Education**: Educate the patient about PTSD, including the impact of trauma on mental health and the importance of adhering to treatment. Discuss self-care strategies and the role of therapy in managing emotional regulation. Encourage the patient to reach out for additional support as needed.

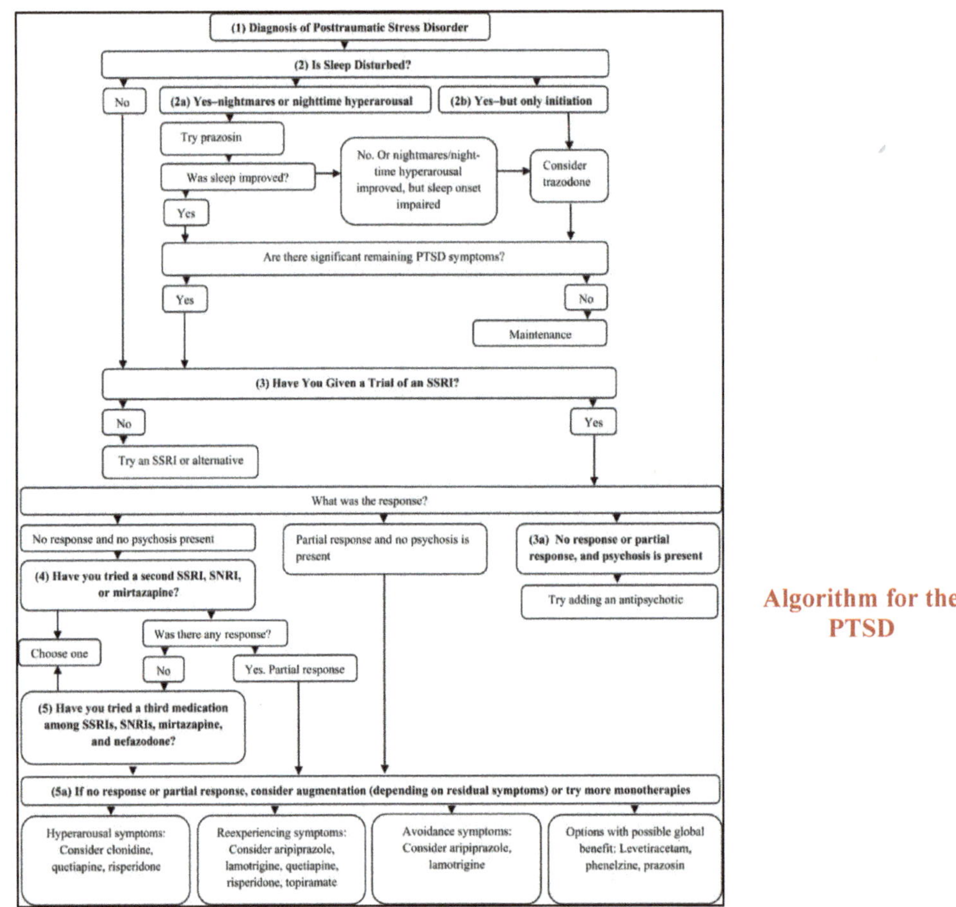

Figure 447 Management of Algorithm for the PTSD

13.4.10 Munchausen Syndrome

Munchausen Syndrome or Factitious Disorder Imposed on Self, is the mental disorder, which is characterized with feigning or exaggeration of the sickness in order to take on the role of a sick person in a bid to gain sympathy and attention from others. While in malingering, the symptoms are feigned so as to be awarded certain benefits such as monetary gain, Munchausen Syndrome **results from an inner psychological compulsion to be sick**. This condition can also present in different forms whereby the person will pretend that they have other physical symptoms or consciously develop or exaggerate injuries or diseases, or tamper with medical diagnostics tests. It refers to a situation where the individual with no **actual medical condition** is subjected to some procedures or treatments that are deemed unnecessary in the process. The real cause of the

Munchausen Syndrome is still unknown, but it was said to be related or associated with a history of abuse or trauma, psychological and psychosocial issues. The patient might have low self-esteem and excess drive for approval associated with self-demands of seeking medical attention. The impact of the disorder is that a patient may end up suffering from adverse health complications due to unnecessary treatment and interventions caused by fables. As for **Munchausen Syndrome,** this condition requires treatment through psychotherapy since it is believed that mental disorders are the cause of such **unnatural behavior.** CBT might assist in changing the patients' behaviour by helping them identify the causes behind their actions and find out more appropriate ways to deal with stressors. In other cases the patient may need a **prescription of drugs to treat other illnesses that may be affecting the mental health such as depression or anxiety.** The best time for treatment is as early as possible as this syndrome is chronic, and the behavior of the affected person may be dangerous if not controlled. Neglecting to develop a supportive therapeutic relationship with the patient is inopportune when treating **Munchausen Syndrome** patients due to the medical condition's possibility that the patient will reject the diagnosis.

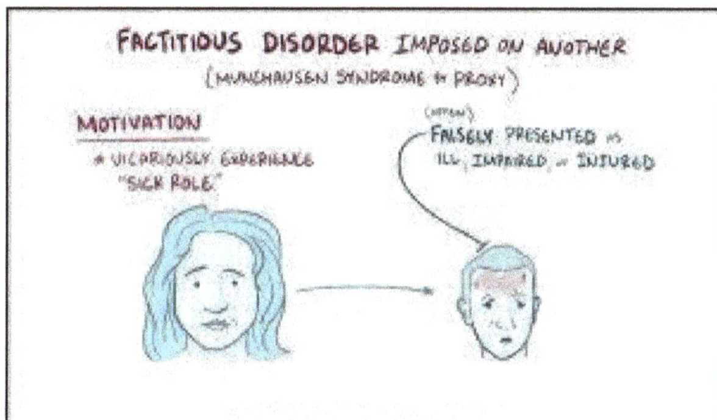

Figure 448 Munchausen Syndrome

13.4.10.1 SOAP Notes for Factitious Disorder

Table 255 SOAP Notes for Factitious Disorder

Component	Details
Subjective (S)	A 35-year-old female presents with a history of frequent hospital visits for various unexplained symptoms over the past two years. She reports ongoing complaints of severe abdominal pain, nausea, and dizziness, but diagnostic tests consistently return normal results. The patient admits to seeking multiple medical opinions but denies intentionally exaggerating her symptoms. She expresses frustration with her inability to get a definitive diagnosis and often requests invasive procedures, despite reassurances from healthcare providers. She reports a history of frequent hospitalizations for similar issues over the years but has not been diagnosed with any chronic conditions.
Objective (O)	On physical examination, the patient appears healthy and well-nourished, without signs of any acute illness. Vital signs are normal: pulse 72 bpm, blood pressure 118/76 mmHg. There are no physical signs of illness or distress during the examination. The patient does not exhibit any noticeable signs of malingering, but her behavior is concerning in light of the numerous normal diagnostic results and her repeated seeking of

	medical interventions. No signs of psychosis or cognitive impairment are observed.
Assessment (A)	The patient's repeated visits to medical facilities with symptoms that cannot be explained by medical tests or examinations, along with her insistence on unnecessary procedures, are indicative of Munchausen Syndrome (Factitious Disorder Imposed on Self). This behavior suggests an underlying psychological need for attention or sympathy, and there is a significant risk of harm due to unnecessary medical interventions. Psychological factors, such as a need for validation or attention, are likely contributing to her symptoms.
Plan (P)	**Pharmacological**: Consider referral to a psychiatrist to assess for underlying psychiatric conditions such as depression or anxiety that may be contributing to the behavior. Medication may be indicated if co-occurring disorders are diagnosed (See algorithm below). **Non-pharmacological**: Recommend psychotherapy, particularly cognitive-behavioral therapy (CBT), to explore the underlying emotional triggers for her behavior and work toward healthier coping strategies. **Follow-up**: Schedule a follow-up appointment in 2-4 weeks to assess progress and ensure that treatment plans are in place. **Education**: Educate the patient about the nature of Munchausen Syndrome, its psychological roots, and the potential harm caused by unnecessary medical treatments. Emphasize the importance of seeking appropriate psychological care to address the need for attention and validation in healthier ways.

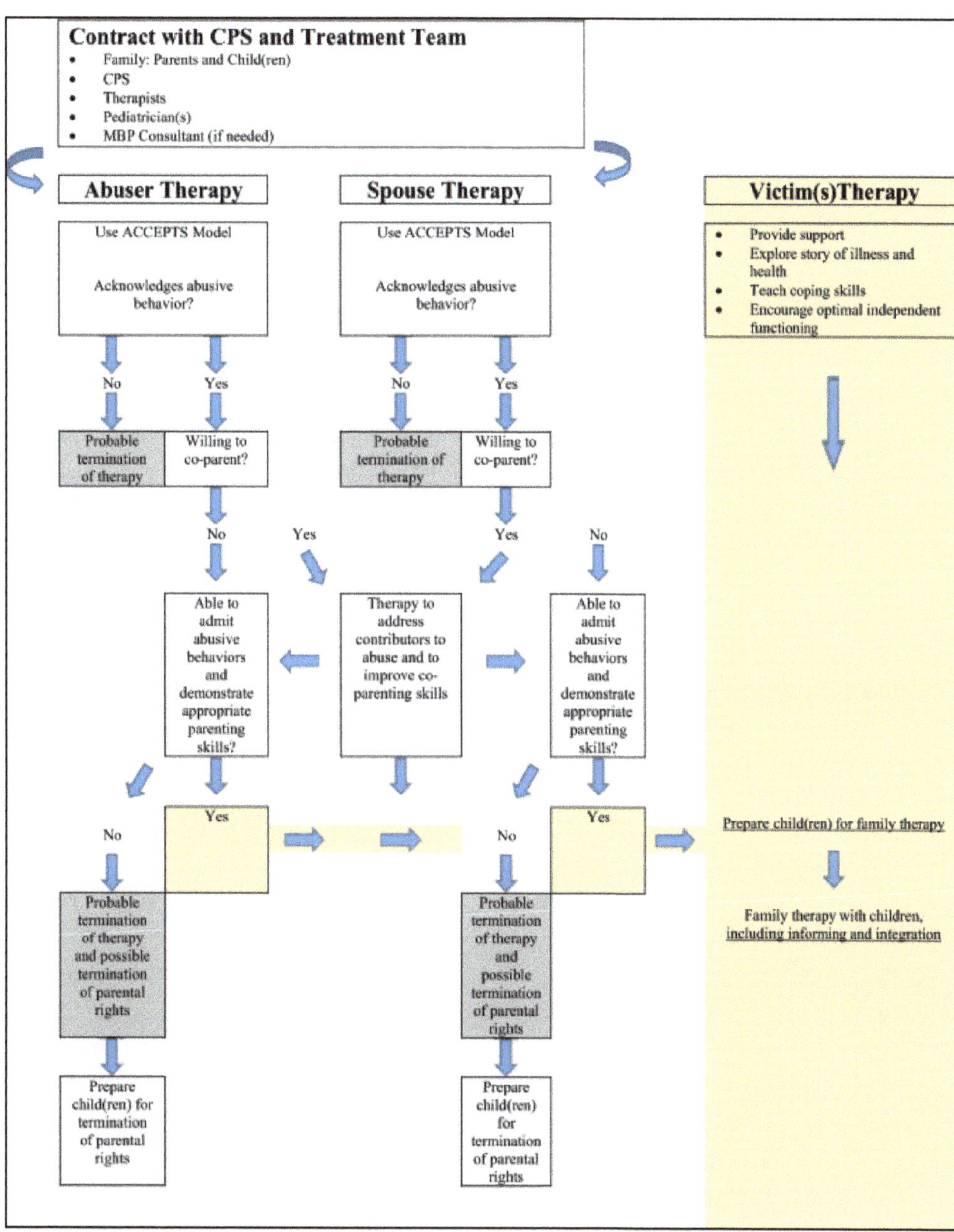

Figure 449 Algorithm for the Management of Factitious Disorder

13.4.11 Abuses

13.4.11.1 Types of Abuses

1. **Physical Abuse**

Physical abuse is when an agent injures another person, this could be in a form of striking, beating, physical punishment, and the use of unlawful or unreasonable physical restraints on another person. **Many a times physical abuse does not have physical signs or blows that will make other people easily notice it.** Explained from the medical perspective, one can also define physical abuse as when the person for whom care is being provided, or with whom the family member stays, does not receive the prescribed medications, or is deprived of the necessary medications by the carer.

2. **Sexual Abuse**

Sexual abuse is any act of putting **some sexual interest on you either through word or touch by someone who should not do that.** This is rape; if anyone has sex with you when you do not wish to engage in such an act. Still, it becomes rape if this person is your partner. Sexual abuse can also be sexually touching another person against their will or forcing the other person to touch one's genitals.

3. **Financial Abuse**

It is a common tactic in exercising power in the relationship to control finances of a vulnerable person. **Some of the financial abuse may be in the form of stealing money or property of a vulnerable person, financial deceit and refusal of a vulnerable person** to be entrusted with his or her money.

4. **Domestic Abuse**

Therefore, domestic abuse is a abuse that originates from a person living in the same home as the recipient of the abuse. **By definition, domestic abuse means that one person** in that particular domestic setting is abusing another person through psychological, physical, sexual, financial, or emotional abuse on a vulnerable person.

5. **Discrimination**

Discriminatory abuse is a situation whereby a certain person is treated unfairly because of a certain characteristic that he or she possesses. **Discriminatory abuse refers communicating to the sufferer insulting language, harassment or ill-treatment** as a result of these characteristics.

6. **Neglect and acts of omission**

Neglect is a type of abuse that involves many inaction's. Which can include neglect which is failing to meet ones **medical or physical needs, dehydration, failure to administer necessary medications, failure to maintain heat or even avoiding or leaving a person** alone.

7. **Self-neglect**

This is the stage when an individual is willing to do anything even to compromise his/her heath, personal cleanliness, and wellbeing. The level of self-neglect portrayed by the individual poses a serious risk to the health and safety of the afflicted persons. It could also be voluntary which is where a person deliberately decides to ignore **self-neglect such as refusal to seek assistance and services for health and social care.** Nonetheless, self-neglect is also sometimes referred to as unintentional, for instance, if an individual suffers from depression which increases their likelihood of self-neglect. An individual with a learning disability can have difficulties in paying attention and this may lead to forgetfulness and for example fail to take care of his or her appearance or the house, for instance forget to tidy up, have the chair and floor full of papers and dirt. **Self-neglect can result into some behaviors in the people that they cannot let go of certain items such as hoarding** . In physical sense, keeping clutter can be dangerous for the individual and has also serious repercussions on his mental health.

8. **Modern slavery**

There is evidence to suggest that the terms modern slavery is used to refer to slavery and human trafficking. People may be used to perform different kinds of work or house chores which are usually done by force and unpaid.

9. **Psychological Abuse**

Emotional abuse as a type of category d refers to a situation whereby an accused person deliberately frightens, torments, verbally humiliates or makes threats to another person. They can deny a particular person services, education or social contacts, or on the contrary, deny his acquaintanceship with friends. **Learning disability is also another factor that makes a person vulnerable to forced labor modern slavery.** They could be isolated in their communities for it has been identified that one in every ten citizens has a disability. They may be not have any eligibility to receive support services. Or it may be highly ignored if it does not fall under the-tag category of a 'big issue'.

10. Organisational or Institutional Abuse

Organisational and institutional abuse is where one is receiving care and he or she is being treated poorly in a certain care setting such as a care home. **It also may include a person receiving care in his or her own home**. It is an act that could be singular or multiple occurrences within a certain period and is outlined by lack of proper attention and care.

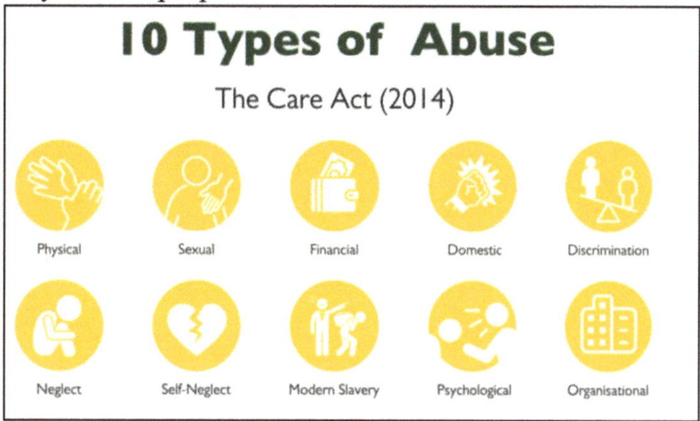

Figure 450 Types of Abuse

13.4.11.2 SOAP Notes for Abuse

Table 256 SOAP Notes for Abuse

Component	Details
Subjective (S)	A 45-year-old female presents with a history of frequent hospital visits for injuries, including bruises, cuts, and fractures, which she attributes to "clumsiness." She reports feeling increasingly anxious and fearful at home, especially around her spouse. The patient confides in the healthcare provider that her partner has been verbally abusive, belittling her and calling her names in front of their children. She denies any direct threats of violence but feels emotionally trapped and isolated. The patient reports feeling unsafe in her own home, with limited access to money or decision-making power.
Objective (O)	On physical examination, the patient has multiple unexplained bruises and healing cuts on her arms, consistent with a history of physical trauma. Her vital signs are stable: pulse 76 bpm, blood pressure 120/80 mmHg. The patient appears anxious, with tense posture and avoids eye contact. Her speech is coherent, but she appears emotionally distressed when discussing her home life. There are no obvious signs of acute physical trauma, but the patient exhibits signs of emotional distress.
Assessment (A)	The patient's presentation, including unexplained injuries, emotional distress, and reports of verbal abuse, suggests a case of domestic abuse (physical and emotional). The patient shows signs of both physical and psychological abuse, with possible ongoing harm in the home environment.

	The emotional distress and fear experienced by the patient indicate the need for further intervention to ensure her safety and well-being.
Plan (P)	**Pharmacological**: Consider referral to a psychiatrist or mental health professional for evaluation and support regarding the patient's emotional distress. Medication, such as an SSRI, may be considered for managing anxiety or depressive symptoms (See algorithm below). **Non-pharmacological**: Refer the patient to a domestic violence support service for counseling and assistance with safety planning. Provide resources on local shelters and legal services. **Follow-up**: Schedule a follow-up appointment in 1-2 weeks to monitor the patient's emotional well-being and safety, and assess the effectiveness of the support services. **Education**: Educate the patient about the dynamics of domestic abuse, including signs of emotional and physical abuse, and discuss available resources to protect her. Provide information about safety planning and legal options, including restraining orders.

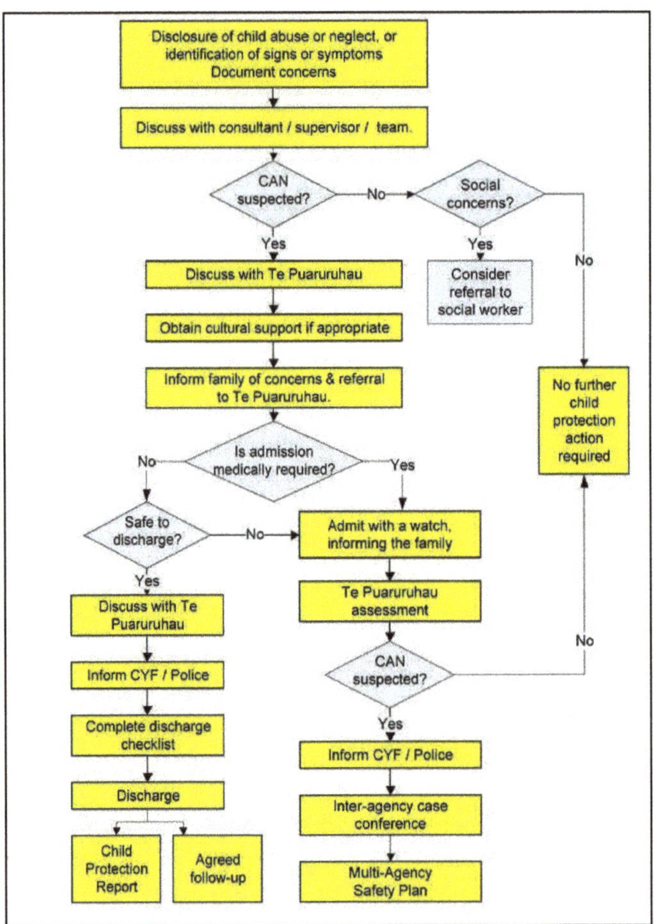

Figure 451 Algorithm for the Management of Suspected Child Abuse or Neglect

13.4.12 Serotonin Toxicity

Serotonin toxicity is also **referred to as serotonin syndrome** and is a severe complication that occurs as a result of excessive levels of serotonin, a neurotransmitter, in the body. It is most commonly associated with Intoxication most often as a result of drugs that stimulate serotonin receptors or enhance the level of serotonin in bloodstream either alone or in combination with other substances. This may result from the cause by the use of antidepressants such as SSRIs, and **SNRIs, MAOIs and the use of multiple drugs** which enhance serotonin at the same time and other recreational drugs like **MDMA**. Serotonin toxicity puts a person through a range of syndromes that affect the brain and the body in general. Common cognitive features manifested therefore include agitation, confusion, hallucination and/or delirium. **Autonomic dysfunctions may entail tachycardia, hyperthermia, fluctuating blood pressure levels, profuse sweating and shivering.** Somatic signs include stiffness, stiffness of the muscles caused by spasticity, muscle twitches, and contracted movements of muscles in response to stimulation. It can further develop to complications such as status epilepticus, metabolic acidosis system and organ failure thereby making it a medical emergency condition.

Management of serotonin toxicity mainly focuses on **removing the offending agent and supportive measures that include fluid therapy and reduction of fever in case of hyperthermia**. In more severe cases, certain drugs like serotonin antagonists such as cyproheptadine are given to block serotonergic receptors in the body. Common IV medication used in this case is **Benzodiazepines to reduce the level of agitation and muscle stiffness.** The patient should also be observed for any complication that may arise and this will require his/her stay to be in the intensive care unit. To avoid serotonin toxicity, special attention should be paid when setting the **beginning dose rates and/or adding the medications that affecting serotonin levels**. It is therefore necessary for healthcare practitioners to understand and anticipate polypharmacy and the signs of serotonin toxicity to be able to act accordingly. An early diagnosis and sequence of action regarding acute, uncomplicated mis-judgments may lead to severe consequences.

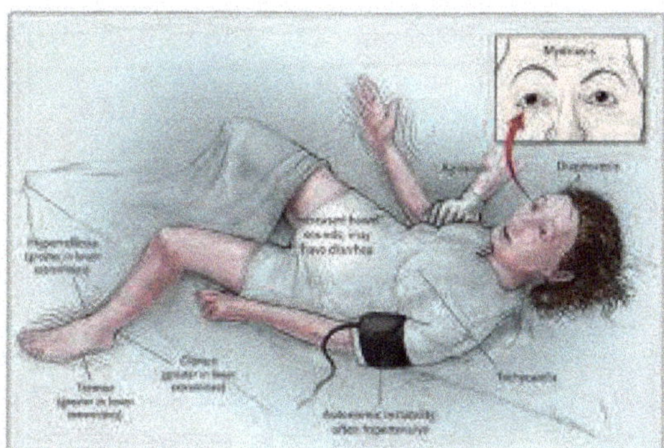

Figure 452 Serotonin Toxicity

13.4.12.1 Hunter Criteria for Serotonin Syndrome

The Hunter Criteria is an established method that helps in diagnosing serotonin syndrome, which is said to be potentially fatal due to elevated levels of serotonin in the brain. This flowchart of **serotonin syndrome decision making is used to establish if a patient falls** under the said syndrome. It starts with the first question on whether the patient is on any medicine that would raise serotonin levels; Serotonergic agents. Requirement for diagnosing the syndrome is an absence or **presence of clonus, spontaneous or inducible**. If clonus is present, other manifestations like agitation, diaphoresis or hyperreflexia endorse the diagnosis. This chart also brought into focus hyperthermia which is above 38 degrees Celsius and muscle stiffness. If a patient **exhibits these signs, then they fit into the serotonin syndrome and need treatment**

immediately. It identifies serotonin toxicity and guides the clinicians on the correct treatment that needs to be taken.

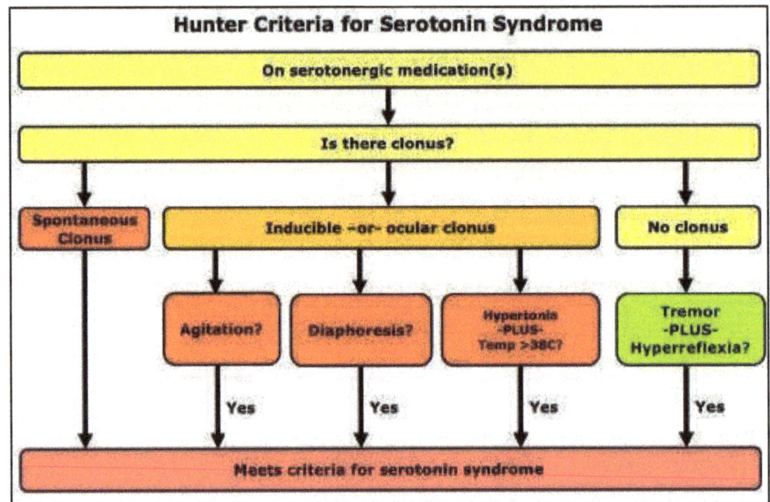

Figure 453 Hunter Criteria for Serotonin Syndrome

13.4.12.2 SOAP Notes for Serotonin Syndrome

Table 257 SOAP Notes for Serotonin Syndrome

Component	Details
Subjective (S)	A 28-year-old male presents to the emergency department after experiencing confusion, agitation, and muscle rigidity following the recent increase in his SSRI dosage. He reports feeling excessively hot, sweating profusely, and has noticed tremors in his hands. The patient also describes feeling restless and unable to sit still. His symptoms began within 12 hours of the dose adjustment and have progressively worsened. The patient denies any recent trauma, fever, or new medications, apart from the recent SSRI dosage change.
Objective (O)	On physical examination, the patient appears agitated and diaphoretic, with a temperature of 39°C (102.2°F). Muscle rigidity is noted in the upper and lower extremities, along with hyperreflexia and visible tremors. Spontaneous clonus is observed in the lower limbs, and inducible clonus is present upon slight manipulation. The patient's vital signs include a pulse of 110 bpm, blood pressure of 145/90 mmHg, and respirations of 22 per minute.
Assessment (A)	The patient's symptoms of agitation, hyperthermia, muscle rigidity, tremor, hyperreflexia, and clonus, along with his recent SSRI dosage adjustment, meet the Hunter Criteria for serotonin syndrome. Given the rapid onset of symptoms following the medication change and the presence of physical signs consistent with serotonin toxicity, this diagnosis is highly likely.
Plan (P)	**Pharmacological**: Discontinue the SSRI immediately and any other serotonergic medications. Administer intravenous fluids to address dehydration and support systemic function. Consider administering

cyproheptadine, a serotonin antagonist, to mitigate symptoms (See algorithm below). **Non-pharmacological**: Monitor the patient in a controlled setting, such as the ICU, for continuous monitoring of vital signs, temperature, and response to treatment. **Follow-up**: Reassess in 2-4 hours for improvement of symptoms. If the patient does not improve or symptoms worsen, further interventions may be required. **Education**: Educate the patient on the potential risks of serotonergic medications and the importance of reporting unusual symptoms following medication changes.

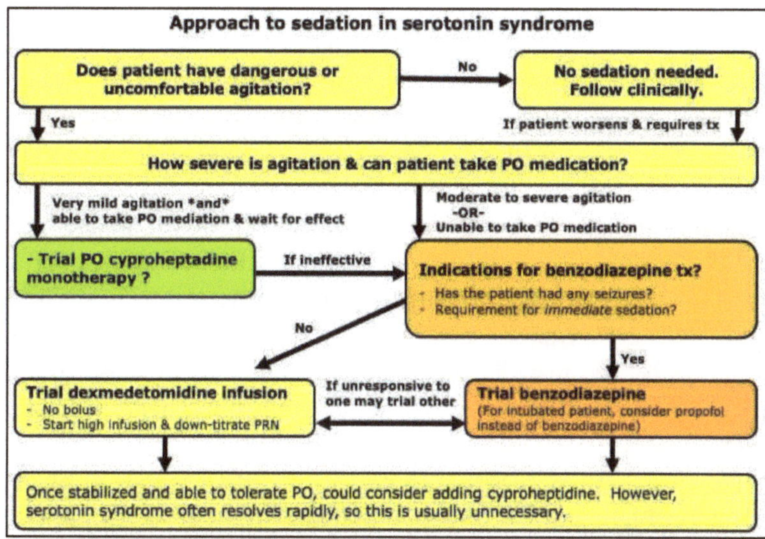

Figure 454 Management Algorithm for Serotonin Syndrome

13.4.13 Malignant Neuroleptic Syndrome

Neuroleptic Malignant Syndrome (NMS) is a possibly fatal side effect of antipsychotic drugs particularly those that belong to the first generation, although second generation can also cause the condition. **Typical signs of NMS include fever, muscle stiffness, instability in the patient's autonomic functioning (shifting blood pressure, racing heart rate, greatly increased sweating), confusion and altered mental state, and increased serum creatine kinase, pointing to muscle tissue and cellular damage.** The precise pathophysiology of NMS remains unclear; however, it is a supposed to be caused due to blockade of dopamine receptors, mainly in the CNS. The incidence of NMS is most frequent early in treatment or after a change in the dosage of antipsychotic drugs, and the symptoms may manifest within days to weeks after the initiation of treatment. It is an uncommon condition that, however, has implications of high morbidity and mortality in the event of neglected early treatment. **NMS is also believed to be caused by the blockage of dopamine receptors in the basal ganglia** resulting to abnormal thermoregulation, rigidity and change of mental status. The autonomic dysfunction, which occurs in NMS, may have some severe consequences, including organ failure, rhabdomyolysis with kidney failure, and cardiovascular imbalance. **Pharmacological treatment of NMS** includes stopping the use of the antipsychotic drug that has been consumed by the patient. Management focuses on supportive care, including rehydration with intravenous fluids to correct dehydration, measures to lower temperatures in **hyperthermic individuals, and administration of drugs like dantrolene,**

bromocriptine, or amantadine for dopamine blockade. In serious cases the patient should be admitted to the intensive care unit where the results will be closely monitored and aggressive interventions will be applied. Prompt identification of the problem and its early management is imperative to increase the patient's condition quality. Otherwise, the outlook is good; however, failure to seek early appropriate management results in complications and potentially fatal outcomes. **NMS requires constant observation of patients who are on antipsychotic drugs particularly those with other risks factors including old age** and other health complications. If NMS is suspected, the offending agent should be stopped and other interventions that are necessary to treat this condition should be given.

13.4.13.1 Difference Between Malignant Neuroleptic Syndrome and Serotonin Syndrome

This figure presents and analyzes Serotonin Syndrome Simple Comparison with the Neuroleptic Malignant Syndrome, **two severe conditions with similar manifestation but different onset and management. Serotonin Syndrome usually occurs within several hours** after ingestion of serotonergic drug and manifest with hyperreflexia, clonus particularly of lower limbs, agitation and autonomic instability**. The treatment of serotonin syndrome** is primarily supportive care and the drug of choice given for treatment is cyproheptadine, a serotonin antagonist. On the other hand, **NMS is a more slow and progressive syndrome** that can take between several days after the use of antipsychotic medications. Dopaminergic psychic identifies itself as NMS and it is characterized by **muscle rigidity, bradyreflexia, autonomic instability, and altered mental state**. The management of NMS usually requires the use of dantrolene and bromocriptine as an antidote to the dopamine antagonism. Hypothermia and hyperthermia both need rigorous supportive care; significant **intravenous fluids, and sedation using benzodiazepines, external cooling required for hyperthermia.** Therefore, it is important to understand differences between these syndromes in order to diagnose the problem at an early stage and start relevant treatment.

13.4.13.2 SOAP Notes for NMS

Table 258 SOAP Notes for NMS

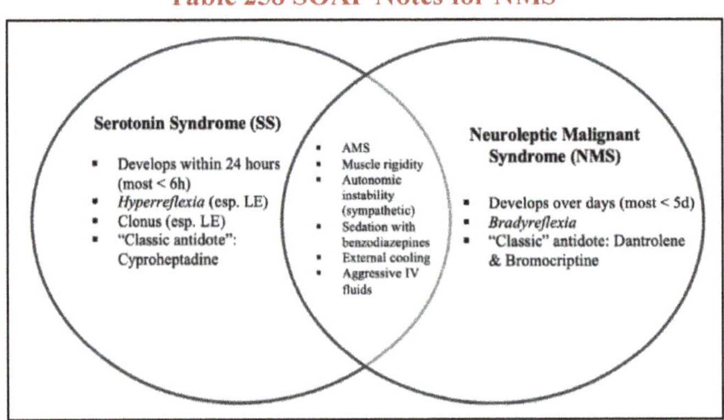

Figure 455 Overlapping Features of NMS and SS

Component	Details
Subjective (S)	A 40-year-old male presents to the emergency department with confusion, agitation, and muscle rigidity after starting a new antidepressant medication (SSRI) five days ago. The patient reports feeling increasingly restless and overheated, with profuse sweating, and states that his muscles have been stiff, especially in his arms and legs. He also describes

	feeling anxious and having difficulty staying still. The symptoms have progressively worsened over the last 24 hours. He denies any history of trauma or recent infections but has been on SSRIs for depression in the past.
Objective (O)	On physical examination, the patient appears agitated, diaphoretic, and has a fever of 39.5°C (103.1°F). He exhibits muscle rigidity, particularly in his lower limbs, and hyperreflexia. Clonus is inducible in both the lower and upper extremities. His pulse is 110 bpm, and blood pressure is 145/90 mmHg. There is no evidence of tremors, and the patient's speech is coherent but pressured. He is oriented but clearly distressed.
Assessment (A)	The patient's rapid onset of symptoms, including agitation, hyperthermia, muscle rigidity, and hyperreflexia following the initiation of an SSRI, is consistent with Serotonin Syndrome (SS). The presence of clonus and the progression of symptoms within 24 hours further support this diagnosis. Differential diagnosis includes Neuroleptic Malignant Syndrome (NMS), but the timeline and response to serotonergic medication favor serotonin syndrome.
Plan (P)	**Pharmacological**: Discontinue the SSRI immediately. Administer cyproheptadine 12 mg orally or intravenously as a serotonin antagonist. Start benzodiazepines (lorazepam 2 mg IV) to manage agitation and muscle rigidity (See algorithm below). **Non-pharmacological**: Begin supportive care with aggressive intravenous hydration, cooling measures to address hyperthermia, and monitoring of vital signs. **Follow-up**: Reassess the patient in 2-3 hours for improvement or worsening of symptoms. If no improvement, consider ICU admission for further monitoring. **Education**: Educate the patient about serotonin syndrome and its association with medications. Discuss the importance of promptly reporting any unusual side effects when starting new medications.

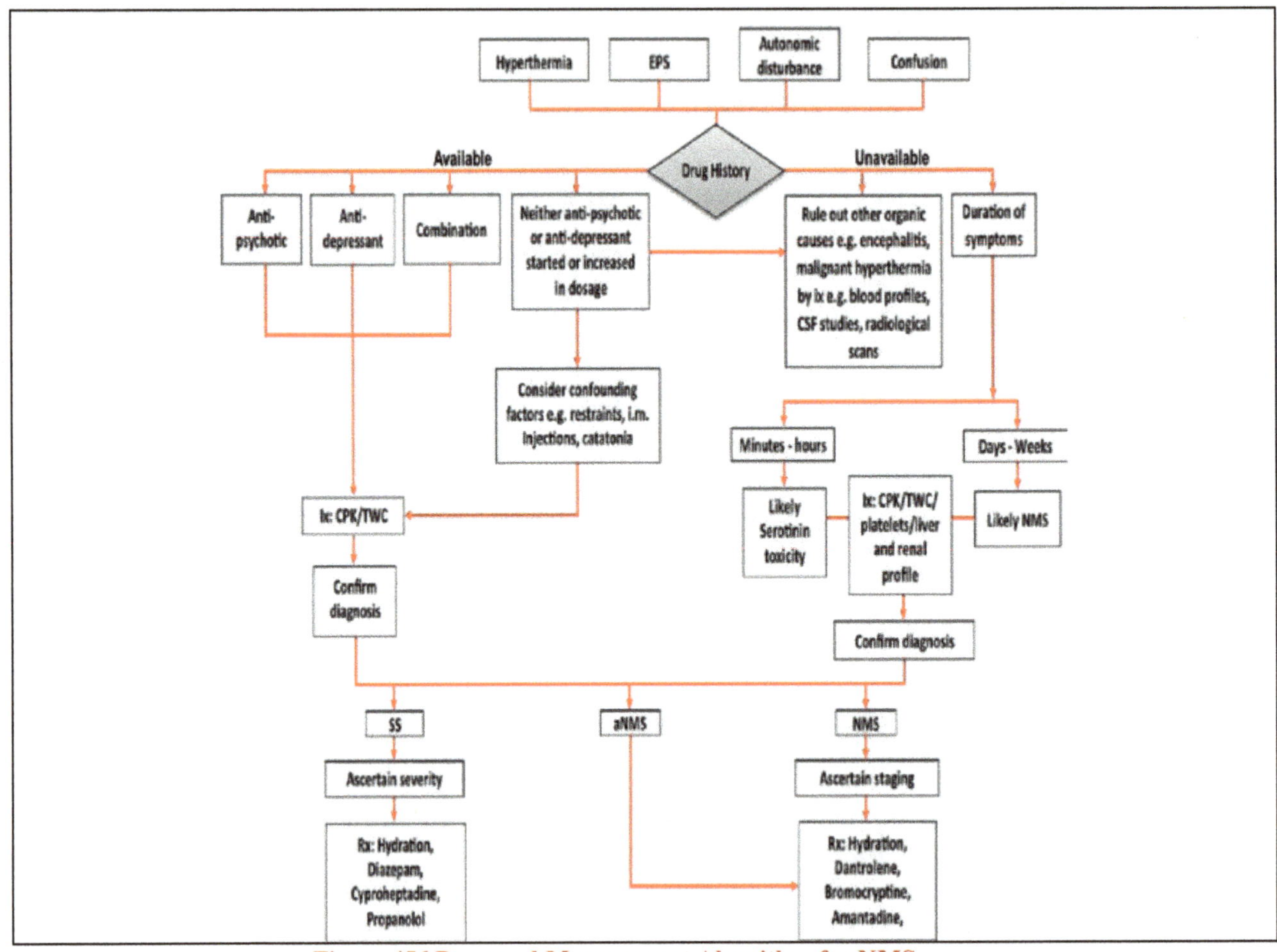

Figure 456 Proposed Management Algorithm for NMS

13.4.14 Epilepsy

Epilepsy is a neurological disorder characterized by recurrent, unprovoked seizures caused by abnormal electrical activity in the brain. Seizures can vary in severity and type, ranging from brief **lapses in consciousness (absence seizures) to intense convulsions (tonic-clonic seizures).** The condition may result from genetic factors, brain injury, or other underlying health issues. Symptoms include loss of consciousness, muscle jerking, or unusual sensations. Epilepsy is typically **managed with antiepileptic drugs (AEDs), lifestyle adjustments, and in some cases, surgery.** Treatment aims to control seizures and improve quality of life. Early diagnosis and proper management are essential for effective care.

13.4.14.1 Types of Epilepsy

Epilepsy Type	Signs and Symptoms	Treatment
Focal Seizures	- Can affect one side of the brain.	**Medications:**
(Partial Seizures)	- Symptoms depend on the area of the brain affected.	- **Carbamazepine**
	- Motor symptoms (e.g., jerking or stiffening of a limb).	- **Lamotrigine**
	- Sensory symptoms (e.g., tingling or visual changes).	- **Levetiracetam**

	- Aura (e.g., strange sensations before the seizure).	- **Topiramate**
	- Can evolve into generalized seizures (secondary generalized).	**Surgery**: Considered if seizures are drug-resistant and affect a specific area of the brain.
Generalized Seizures	- Affects both sides of the brain.	**Medications**:
	- Loss of consciousness.	- **Valproate (Valproic acid)**
Tonic-Clonic Seizures	- Stiffening (tonic phase) followed by rhythmic jerking (clonic phase).	- **Levetiracetam**
	- Biting of the tongue or cheek.	- **Lamotrigine**
	- Loss of bladder control.	- **Carbamazepine**
	- Postictal confusion or fatigue.	**Surgery**: Considered for refractory cases.
Absence Seizures (Petit Mal)	- Brief lapses in consciousness (usually only for seconds).	**Medications**:
	- Staring episodes.	- **Ethosuximide**
	- No postictal confusion.	- **Valproate**
Myoclonic Seizures	- Sudden, brief jerking of muscles, often occurring in clusters.	**Medications**:
	- May occur upon waking up.	- **Valproate**
	- No loss of consciousness.	- **Levetiracetam**
Atonic Seizures	- Sudden loss of muscle tone, causing the person to collapse or fall.	**Medications**:
	- Typically occur in children.	- **Valproate**
	- May cause head drops or falls.	- **Lamotrigine**
Status Epilepticus	- Continuous or rapidly recurring seizures without full recovery of consciousness in between.	**Treatment**:
	- Medical emergency requiring immediate intervention.	- **Benzodiazepines** (e.g., lorazepam, diazepam) for acute seizure management.
	- May lead to brain damage if untreated.	- **Phenytoin**, **Valproate**, or **Levetiracetam** for long-term seizure control.

13.4.14.2 SOAP Notes for Epilepsy

Table 259 SOAP Notes for Epilepsy

Component	Details

Subjective (S)	A 29-year-old male presents with a 2-year history of generalized tonic-clonic seizures. He reports having about two to three seizures per month, typically occurring at night during sleep. The patient describes experiencing a warning sensation (aura) before seizures, which includes a strange metallic taste and visual disturbances. He reports feeling fatigued and confused after seizures, with no memory of the event. The patient is currently on levetiracetam 500 mg twice daily, but he feels the seizures are not well-controlled. He denies any recent head trauma or changes in medication.
Objective (O)	The patient appears alert and oriented during the exam. Vital signs: BP 120/78 mmHg, HR 72 bpm, Temp 36.9°C (98.4°F). Neurological exam reveals no focal deficits. The patient demonstrates normal muscle strength, reflexes, and coordination. There is no evidence of recent trauma. The patient's medication adherence is consistent. An EEG shows generalized spike-and-wave activity, suggesting ongoing seizure activity.
Assessment (A)	The patient's history of generalized tonic-clonic seizures, along with the aura and EEG findings, is consistent with epilepsy. Despite being on levetiracetam, his seizures remain inadequately controlled, indicating the need for medication adjustment.
Plan (P)	**Pharmacological**: Increase levetiracetam dose to 1000 mg twice daily. Consider adding a second antiepileptic drug (AED) such as lamotrigine if seizures remain uncontrolled (See algorithm below). **Non-pharmacological**: Educate the patient on seizure safety precautions, including avoiding driving until seizures are better controlled. Encourage a regular sleep schedule and stress management techniques to minimize triggers. **Follow-up**: Schedule follow-up in 4 weeks to assess the efficacy of the medication adjustment. If seizures persist, consider further changes in medication or explore surgical options for drug-resistant epilepsy. **Education**: Educate the patient on the importance of medication adherence and recognizing warning signs of seizures.

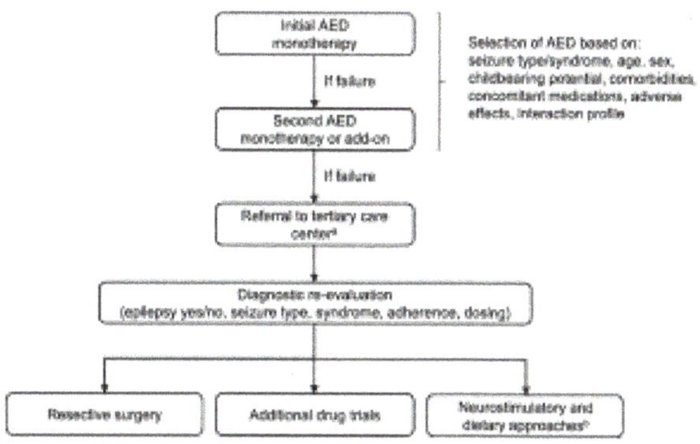

Figure 457 Algorithm for the Management of Epilepsy

13.4.15 Comprehensive Convulsion

Convulsions, also known as seizures, are sudden, involuntary movements or abnormal electrical activity in the brain that can result in a range of symptoms. They can be generalized, involving both sides of the brain, or focal, affecting one part of the brain. **Generalized seizures often lead to loss of consciousness and can involve rhythmic muscle jerking (tonic-clonic seizures), while focal seizures may cause localized twitching, sensory changes, or brief lapses in consciousness.** Convulsions can be triggered by a variety of factors, including epilepsy, head trauma, high fever (especially in children), infections, or metabolic imbalances. Symptoms vary depending on the type of seizure, but common signs include muscle rigidity, jerking, loss of consciousness, confusion, and fatigue post-seizure. **Treatment typically involves antiepileptic medications, lifestyle modifications, and in some cases, surgery for drug-resistant seizures**. Early diagnosis and appropriate treatment are crucial to managing the condition and reducing the frequency of episodes.

Table 260 SOAP Notes for Comprehensive Convulsions

Component	Details
Subjective (S)	A 42-year-old female presents with a 6-month history of generalized convulsions. She reports having 1-2 episodes per month, lasting approximately 2-3 minutes, where she loses consciousness and experiences whole-body muscle jerking. The patient describes postictal confusion and fatigue following the seizures. She also mentions occasional "aura" episodes, including a strange feeling of nausea and visual disturbances, just before a seizure. The patient is currently on carbamazepine, but her seizures remain poorly controlled. She has no significant history of head trauma or neurological disorders.
Objective (O)	The patient appears in no acute distress but is fatigued following a recent seizure episode. Vital signs: BP 125/80 mmHg, HR 70 bpm, Temp 36.7°C (98.1°F). Neurological exam shows no focal deficits between seizures. The patient has normal strength, reflexes, and coordination. Postictal findings show mild confusion, which resolves in about 30 minutes. The EEG shows generalized spike-and-wave activity indicative of convulsive seizures. No signs of injury from recent seizures were observed.
Assessment (A)	The patient's history of generalized convulsions, loss of consciousness, and the EEG findings suggest generalized tonic-clonic seizures. Despite being

	on carbamazepine, the seizures remain poorly controlled, indicating a need for medication adjustments.
Plan (P)	**Pharmacological**: Increase carbamazepine dosage and consider adding a second antiepileptic drug (AED), such as levetiracetam, for better control (See algorithm below). **Non-pharmacological**: Advise the patient to follow seizure safety measures, including avoiding driving and operating heavy machinery. Recommend regular sleep patterns and stress management. **Follow-up**: Schedule a follow-up appointment in 4 weeks to assess the effectiveness of medication adjustments. If seizures persist or worsen, consider a referral for further investigations, such as MRI, or evaluate the possibility of surgical options for drug-resistant epilepsy. **Education**: Educate the patient on the importance of adhering to prescribed medications, recognizing seizure triggers, and seeking medical help immediately if seizures increase in frequency or severity.

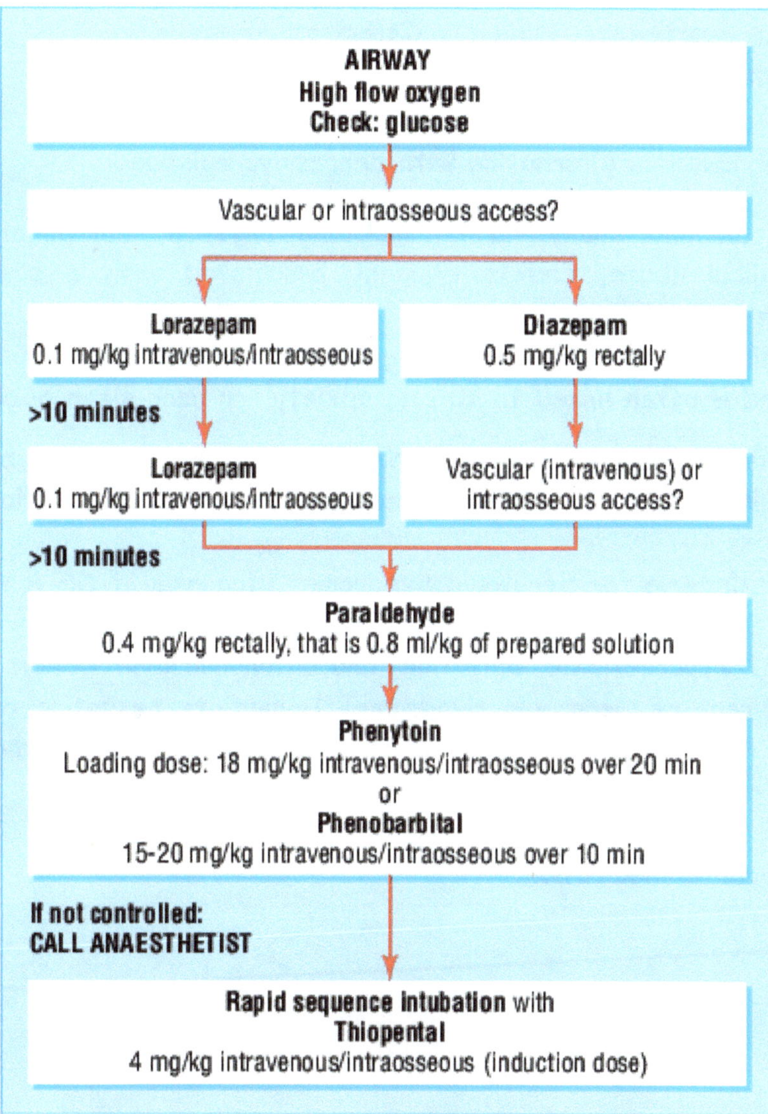

Figure 458 Algorithm for the Management of Seizures

13.5 Moh Golden Points and Summary Question Answers

13.5.1 Moh Golden Points

Bipolar disorder is characterized by extreme mood swings, with manic or hypomanic episodes alternating with depressive episodes.

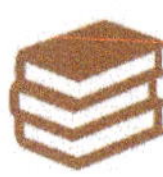

Abuse can take many forms, including physical, emotional, sexual, and psychological abuse, and is typically associated with a significant power imbalance

Insomnia involves difficulty falling asleep, staying asleep, or waking up too early and is often linked to stress, anxiety, or poor sleep hygiene.

Anorexia nervosa is a serious eating disorder characterized by intense fear of gaining weight and restrictive eating, leading to malnutrition and extreme weight loss.

Hunter Criteria for Serotonin Syndrome: Diagnosis of SS is made using the Hunter Criteria, which includes the presence of clonus (spontaneous or inducible), hyperreflexia, agitation, and autonomic dysfunction.

Management of Serotonin Syndrome: Immediate cessation of serotonergic medications, supportive care (hydration, cooling), and administration of cyproheptadine are crucial in managing serotonin syndrome.

Management of NMS: For NMS, the first step is to discontinue the antipsychotic medication.

13.5.2 Summary Questions & Answers

1. Which of the following is the classic antidote for Serotonin Syndrome (SS)?
A) Dantrolene
B) Bromocriptine
C) Cyproheptadine
D) Flumazenil

2. Which of the following symptoms is most commonly associated with Neuroleptic Malignant Syndrome (NMS)?
A) Hyperreflexia
B) Bradyreflexia
C) Inducible clonus
D) Tremors

3. What is the primary difference in the onset of Serotonin Syndrome and Neuroleptic Malignant Syndrome?
A) SS develops within days, NMS develops within hours.
B) SS develops within hours, NMS develops within days.
C) SS and NMS both develop within days.
D) SS develops in weeks, NMS develops in hours.

4. A 22-year-old female with a BMI of 16.5 and a history of extreme dieting, excessive exercise, and an intense fear of gaining weight is most likely suffering from:
A) Bipolar disorder
B) Schizophrenia
C) Anorexia nervosa
D) Delirium

5. What is the primary treatment for Neuroleptic Malignant Syndrome?
A) Cyproheptadine
B) Bromocriptine and dantrolene
C) Benzodiazepines
D) Supportive care with IV fluids only

6. Which of the following medications is most likely to cause Neuroleptic Malignant Syndrome?
A) SSRI
B) Antipsychotics
C) MAOI
D) Anticonvulsants

7. Which condition is most commonly associated with the use of first-generation antipsychotics?
A) Serotonin syndrome
B) Neuroleptic Malignant Syndrome (NMS)
C) Anorexia nervosa
D) Bipolar disorder

8. Which of the following is the first step in the treatment of Serotonin Syndrome?
A) Administer bromocriptine
B) Discontinue serotonergic drugs
C) Start cooling measures

D) Administer dantrolene

9. Which symptom is most characteristic of Neuroleptic Malignant Syndrome?

A) Hyperthermia with extreme agitation
B) Muscle rigidity with bradyreflexia
C) Hyperreflexia with spontaneous clonus
D) Diaphoresis with hyperactivity

10. Which of the following is a hallmark feature of Bipolar I Disorder?

A) Hypomanic episodes without major depressive episodes
B) Full manic episodes with or without depressive episodes
C) Predominantly depressive episodes
D) Occasional periods of elevated mood without mania

13.5.3 Rationales

1. **Answer: C) Cyproheptadine**

Rationale: Cyproheptadine is the classic antidote for serotonin syndrome as it is a serotonin antagonist.

---

2. **Answer: B) Bradyreflexia**

Rationale: NMS is characterized by bradyreflexia (slower reflexes), whereas serotonin syndrome presents with hyperreflexia.

---

3. **Answer: B) SS develops within hours, NMS develops within days.**

Rationale: Serotonin Syndrome typically develops within 6 hours, while NMS develops gradually over several days.

---

4. **C) Anorexia nervosa**

Rationale: **Anorexia nervosa** involves restrictive eating, intense fear of weight gain, and an altered body image, leading to significant weight loss and malnutrition.

---

5. **Answer: B) Bromocriptine and dantrolene**

Rationale: Bromocriptine (dopamine agonist) and dantrolene (muscle relaxant) are used to treat NMS.

---

6. **Answer: B) Antipsychotics**

Rationale: Antipsychotic medications, particularly first-generation antipsychotics, are the most common cause of NMS.

---

7. **Answer: B) Neuroleptic Malignant Syndrome (NMS)**

Rationale: NMS is a rare but serious side effect of **antipsychotic medications**, especially first-generation antipsychotics, characterized by hyperthermia, muscle rigidity, and autonomic instability.

---

8. **Answer: B) Discontinue serotonergic drugs**

Rationale: The first step in managing serotonin syndrome is to stop the use of serotonergic medications to prevent further serotonin accumulation.

---

9. **Answer: B) Muscle rigidity with bradyreflexia**

Rationale: NMS is characterized by muscle rigidity and bradyreflexia, unlike serotonin syndrome, which presents with hyperreflexia and clonus.

---

10. **Answer: B) Full manic episodes with or without depressive episodes**

Rationale: Bipolar I Disorder is characterized by manic episodes that can last at least a week and may or may not be accompanied by depressive episodes.

14 Chapter 14: Therapeutics for FNPs

14.1 Differential Diagnosis and Critical Thinking

14.1.1 How to approach clinical decision-making

Clinical decision-making is one of the most important processes that are carried out in the healthcare sector with implying significant consequences for the general quality of the treatment and patients' result. It entails the use of feelings, past performances, facts, and available data through professional standards to arrive at decisions that can promote safe treatment delivery. **For its part, clinical decision-making spans from immediate prior judgment when decision-making occurs with routine or probable event to slow deliberate reasoning when circumstances are not very certain.** The reality is that decision making also differs in terms of the level of complexity, depending on the situations within an organization and outside, some of which must be undertaken and implemented within a short span of time while there are some that may call for more consideration, consultations and analysis.

A critical procedure, which an effective practitioner has to undergo in order to provide quality care to the patient, involves the identification of a suitable pattern of care from past experiences, critical thinking skills to question the perceived facts and able to interpret the needs of the patient. **Evidence based practice is crucial to the decision making process since the guidelines give directions and the findings to be followed in clinical practice.** Finally, **effective North Carolina** healthcare communication involves the interdependence conception as it integrates teamwork in the evaluation of information, with healthcare experts deciding outcomes together with other healthcare experts. The implementation of the goal is to diversify care in the treatment process.

Besides the above mentioned clinical competences, several aspects contributes to clinical decision making. **These may range from the health care facility and the resources at its disposal, the patient's desires and the prescriber information base.** Also important is knowledge of one's shortcomings and asking for help when needed, as the healthcare practitioners require knowing when they need help or information. The process is interactive and iterative, and may involve definition of a problem, data collection, decision making, consultation with other stakeholders and reconsideration of a decision in the light of new information gained.

Among the concepts which have greatly influenced the clinical decisions, the shift towards shared decisions has been deemed significant. **Earlier, decision-making process was carried by the healthcare professionals for the beneficiaries, but the current practice is based on patient's involvement.** This, therefore, means that through explaining the illness and prognosis in language that the patient can understand, the patient has the opportunity to make an informed decision of the kind of treatment s/he would wish to take. This kind of cooperation results in patients' confidence, increased satisfaction, and eventually – positive health outcomes.

14.1.2 Using evidence-based practice in diagnosis

EBP is applied in the diagnostic process where decisions made regarding the care of patients are **based on research findings, knowledge, and values of the individuals.** EBP is a process, which entails using the best practice evidence from research studies which are up-to-date and peer-reviewed by other professionals to make decisions pertaining to service delivery. Regarding the diagnostic aspect, **EBP helps clinician use the right methods, tools and criteria for diagnosis and also the most current mechanisms for diagnosis, hence; improving on diagnosis and patients' general health condition.**

In employing the evidence-based practice in diagnosing, the healthcare practitioners first evaluate the latest information that has been produced as a result of research, including systematic reviews, guidelines, and other such research papers. **These resources contain the information that describes the efficiency and efficacy of a number of diagnostic procedures and allows choosing that diagnostics method which is most appropriate in a specific situation.** For instance, when practitioners are doing diagnosis of the diseases such as diabetes or hypertension, they will base their diagnosis on diagnostic indicators which are well founded from clinical trials and the longitudinal history, which provides a high level of certainty of diagnostic precision.

In addition, EBP entails taking into account of the patient care factors such as the history of the patient, symptoms and their preferences on the diagnosis. **Clinician also needs to involve personal experience to explain test results and compare it with the patient's characteristics.** This approach avoids the possibility of either concluding that the patient is healthy or sick based only on the test results, thus making the diagnosis as close as possible to the reality and patient's circumstances.

14.1.3 Observing red flags and referral to other healthcare specialists

Red flags are precise warning signs that may suggest that a patient has a significant pathology. They should not be ignored since they signal the possibility of severe disease or pathology in the patient, which could cause some adverse effects. **The identification of red-flag symptoms needs information gathering which probably involves coming up with open ended questions about the patient's medical history.** They can be vague, as in weak or weighted feeling or loss of weight and appetite, or more apparent, as in hemoptysis which could suggest diseases like cancer, infection, cardiovascular diseases and so on.

Patients first approach pharmacists, hence making it easy for them to note the symptoms they exhibit. **They should be aware of the diseases, presentation, and differential of benign symptoms from serious ones.** Through recognising the nominative signs during consultations pharmacists can be in a position to prevent occurrences by immediately intervening since they have a major impact on the safety of a patients.

Thus, should the patient exhibit such red-flag symptoms, the pharmacist is duty-bound to send the patient to a relevant healthcare provider for further assessment. **For less severe cases, the doctor may refer the patient to a general practitioner GP**. In cases where the situation calls for an emergency, for example the patient presents with chest pain or is exhibiting signs of a stroke, the pharmacist has to refer the case to an emergency department or call an emergency service. The situation background assessment recommendation tool or SBAR is sometimes used to make certain that any medical informations is effectively relayout with the referring professional.

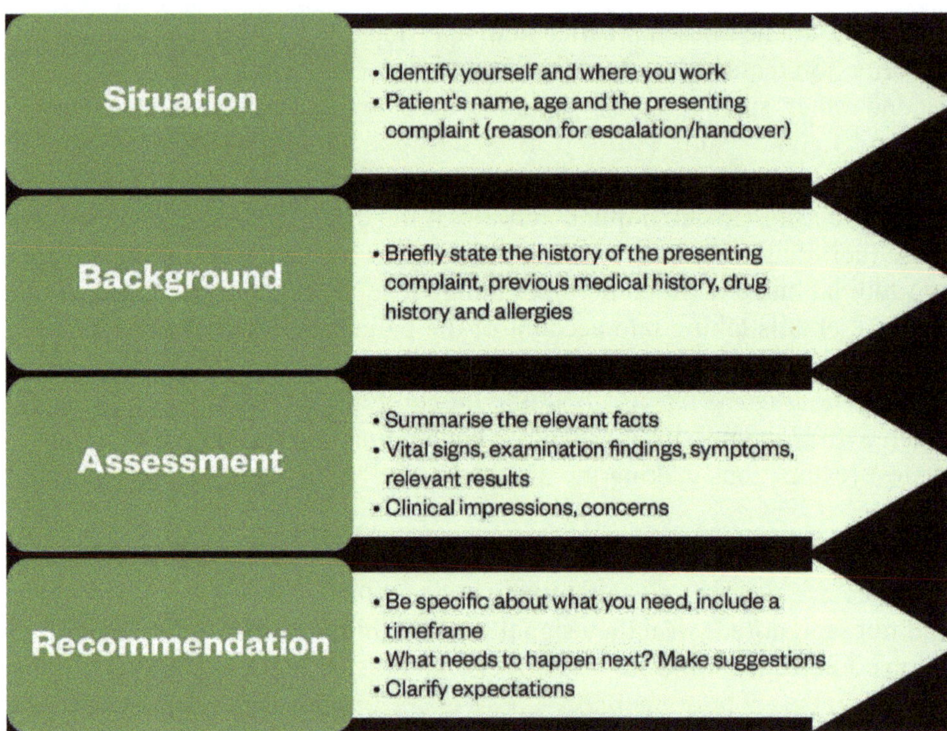

Figure 459 SBAR (situation, background, assessment, recommendation) tool

Further, there is safety-netting which should be used, this will require the patient to be given information on what the consultation will entail or what is expected from the consultation and also when next to seek medical help. This prompts the author to discuss the importance of note-taking in particular by pharmacists and safety netting when providing consultation. With regard to this, recognizing red-flag symptoms, and referring the patient immediately, pharmacists can enhance patient outcomes and the quality of healthcare systems

14.2 Pharmacokinetics and Pharmacodynamics

14.2.1 What is Pharmacokinetics?

The study of pharmacokinetics investigates drug and substance responses in the body following their absorption phase. **The drug's movement through the human body integrates three aspects: its distribution inside specific areas, body metabolic processes and elimination mechanisms.** Drug efficiency enhancement through Pharmacokinetic study represents its essential framework for establishing the rates of absorption and distribution as well as metabolism, and excretion to generate safer drug therapy outcomes. Pharmacokinetics contains four main processes alongside evaluation criteria, as shown in the figure below, also known as ADME (Absorption, Desorption, Metabolism, Excretion)

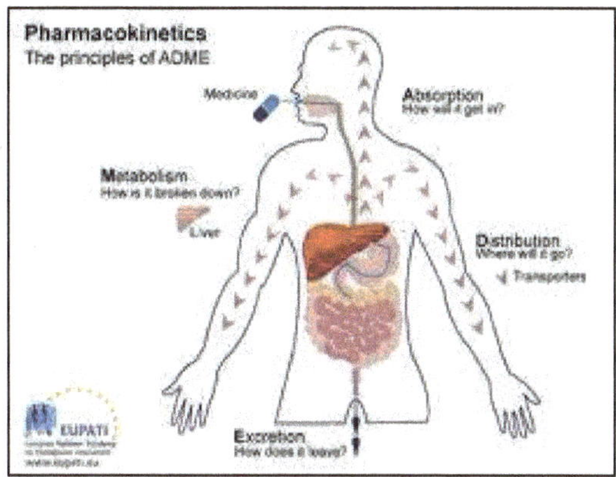

Figure 460 Pharmacokinetics

Absorption refers to the process by which drugs travel from their administration areas into the bloodstream. The drug enters the bloodstream through different methods, from oral delivery to intravenous injections and subcutaneous routes and inhalation methods. **Stereochemical properties of a drug, together with its designated administration method and any coexisting food or medicines in the digestive tract, determine the drug's absorption level. After blood absorption, the drug travels across the body until it reaches its targeted location.** The drug's ability to disperse throughout the body depends on aspects such as drug dimensions and form, its solubility in bloodstreams, combined with its binding affinity to bloodstream proteins. Drugs have the ability to penetrate through the blood-brain barrier, leading to critical effects on both their medical benefits and potential side effects.

Metabolism indicates how a drug transforms into smaller water-soluble molecules within the body, permitting their removal as waste. Enzymes located in the liver activate the drug breakdown process, which modifies both the drug's therapeutic value and toxicity levels. Several medications are transformed through metabolic processes in the kidneys and the intestinal system.

The body removes medications through Excretion, which is the process of drug removal from the body. A drug will exit the body through different routes, including the kidneys, liver, and lungs. Drug excretion depends on three main elements, which include the drug's chemical makeup, functional organ condition, and other medications that might interfere with elimination systems.

Systemic circulation experiences a fraction of the delivered dosage as bioavailability. Drugs' low availability produces inadequate circulating concentrations, which decreases therapeutic effectiveness. Developers working on new drugs should choose optimal routes and formulations along with proper dosages to enhance drug bioavailability.

The speed of drug elimination from the body is defined as clearance. **Drug half-life represents the period needed for drug concentration reduction to one-half of its initial value thus affecting the required duration between drug doses for maintaining therapeutic concentrations.** Short half-life drugs need frequent doses in comparison to drugs which have long half-life characteristics. The essential nature of drug discovery requires knowing drug pharmacokinetic properties since these properties aid in establishing proper dosing methods and selecting delivery methods, and deciding how long drugs should stay in the body for therapeutic success.

The plot demonstrates the relationship between drug concentrations in blood plasma or tissue samples throughout time while showing how the drug effects correlate with its blood plasma concentration. The drug starts to enter the bloodstream producing elevated plasma quantities. During the progression of time the drug concentration reaches its highest level that matches the peak intensity of its therapeutic results. The drug concentration reduces after reaching its highest value until complete detoxification takes place. **The therapeutic duration of a drug matches the period when drug concentration stays higher than minimum therapeutic thresholds thereby preserving its effectiveness level**. The length of time needed for a drug effect to start is revealed by the graph because it demonstrates when drug concentration reaches a therapeutic level that induces measurable results. Dosing strategies depend on the essential understanding of this drug relationship.

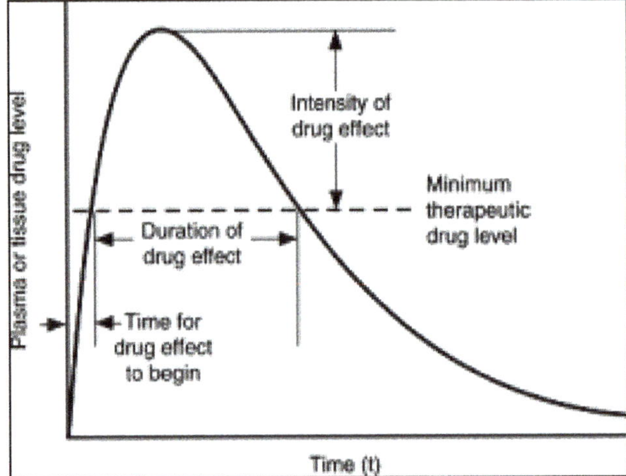

Figure 461 relationship between drug concentrations in blood plasma or tissue samples

14.2.2 Drug Absorption

The initial stage of pharmacokinetics starts with absorption that lets drugs cross from their administration site into bloodstream circulation. The given method of drug administration affects how much and how quickly a drug gets present in the bloodstream during its absorption phase. Different drug administration methods exist with separate absorption characteristics and specific hurdles available for each route. **A major limitation to effective drug absorption appears as the First-Pass Effect. Most oral and enteral medications undergo the First-Pass Effect because drugs pass from the gastrointestinal tract into systemic circulation through the liver as a primary step. During its liver processing some drug substance undergoes metabolic breakdown which decreases the amount of active medication that reaches bloodstream circulation.** The drug activity level diminishes throughout this process before achieving target sites. Medical practitioners need to either enhance their drug prescriptions or explore different delivery paths because the first-pass effect leads to substantial liver drug metabolism.

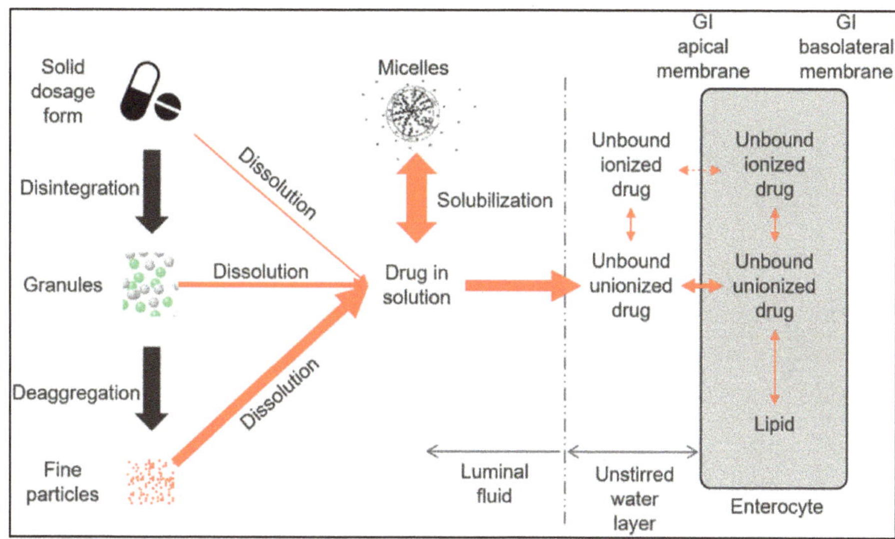

Figure 462 Process of Drug Absorption

14.2.2.1 Alternate Routes of Administration

Drugs can be affected by the first-pass effect by receiving administration through IV routes or through inhalation and SC, and IM methods, and transdermal procedures. Drugs administered through alternate routes can directly enter bloodstream circulation or other perfusion paths, such as respiratory or skin absorption, before initial liver metabolism occurs. **The bloodstream direct access of drugs through intravenous (IV) administration leads to total drug absorption, which makes this method best suited for urgent medical situations and complete availability needs**. The following table outlines the different routes of drug administration, highlighting their advantages, disadvantages, and specific considerations that healthcare providers must account for when selecting a method for medication delivery.

Table 261 Routes of Drug Administration

Route of Administration	Advantages	Disadvantages	Considerations
Oral (PO)	Convenient; solid/liquid formulations available; self-administered	First-pass effect can reduce bioavailability; slower onset of action	Affected by GI conditions, food intake, and gastric emptying
Enteral (NGT, GT, OGT)	Useful for patients who cannot swallow, continuous administration	Potential for irritation; absorption may be inconsistent	Ensure tube placement is correct and patent
Rectal	Avoids first-pass effect to some extent; useful in vomiting patients	Inconvenient for patients; absorption may be erratic	Variability in absorption depending on rectal conditions
Intravenous (IV)	Immediate effect; 100% bioavailability; fast action	Requires sterile technique; can cause pain and local reactions	Risk of infection and toxicity, must monitor closely

Intramuscular (IM)	Fast action; no first-pass effect	Painful; risk of local reactions such as swelling, bleeding	Absorption varies depending on muscle size and blood flow
Subcutaneous (SC)	Convenient for self-administration; avoids first-pass effect	Painful; may cause irritation or swelling at injection site	Site rotation and monitoring of site reactions needed
Transdermal	Steady drug delivery over time; avoids first-pass effect	Limited to small molecules; slow onset; skin reactions possible	Not suitable for all medications; affected by skin conditions
Inhalation	Rapid absorption; bypasses liver	Requires proper technique; may irritate airways	Particle size and inhalation technique crucial

The same rapid delivery of IV and inhalation administration involves complications that require sterile procedures and the potential development of local side effects. The drug delivery system of transdermal patches provides continuous drug administration across time, which helps drugs that need sustained effects. The technique restricts applicable medications since skin absorption requires small drug molecules to function. The following table provides detailed considerations for each route, focusing on how they impact drug

Table 262 Route-Specific Considerations

Route of Administration	Considerations	Bioavailability Impact
Oral (PO)	Gastric pH, food intake, and GI motility affect absorption. First-pass effect reduces bioavailability.	Lower bioavailability due to first-pass metabolism in the liver.
Enteral (NGT, GT, OGT)	Tube placement must be correct and secure. Medications must be liquid or crushable.	Similar to oral; potential inconsistent absorption.
Rectal	Absorption can be variable; bypasses some liver metabolism.	Variable bioavailability depending on rectal blood flow.
Intravenous (IV)	Complete bioavailability; direct into bloodstream.	100% bioavailability; no first-pass metabolism.
Intramuscular (IM)	Drug absorbed via muscle tissue; affected by blood flow.	Rapid bioavailability with steady absorption.
Subcutaneous (SC)	Absorption slower than IM; injected into fatty tissue.	Steady, predictable absorption unless blood flow is compromised.
Transdermal	Slow, continuous delivery; suitable for prolonged release drugs.	Avoids first-pass metabolism; slow, steady drug concentration.
Inhalation	Rapid absorption through lungs; requires effective technique.	High bioavailability; bypasses liver; fast action.

14.2.2.2 Life Span Considerations

Drugs are absorbed by the body depending on a person's age during treatment. The absorption rates for drugs differ in neonates and paediatrics because their developing stomach acid production and slow gastric emptying cause changes in bioavailability. **The liver of young patients does not function at full maturity, so first-pass metabolism performs poorly, resulting in elevated drug amounts in their bloodstream.** Older adults may experience slowed drug absorption through reduced gastrointestinal blood flow together with altered gastric acidity that decreases the speed of drug absorption. The drug absorption through transdermal patches becomes compromised when elderly patients have less subcutaneous fat tissue. Subcutaneous and intramuscular drugs experience delayed absorption through altered peripheral blood flow as a result of aging.

14.2.3 Distribution

A drug follows the distribution pathway to spread throughout the circulating blood while dissolving in body tissues post entry into systemic circulation. This vital pharmacokinetic stage establishes how much drug concentration reaches multiple target tissues and functions as the main factor in drug therapeutic outcomes. **Once absorbed or administered directly the drug transfers from blood vessels into the tissues before binding to receptors for producing chosen effects. The use of drugs results in unintended actions that produce unwanted effects because drugs may attach to inappropriate receptor sites.** The pain-relieving properties of ibuprofen generate stomach irritation which acts as one of its known side effects. The manner in which a drug distributes across the body depends upon blood circulation patterns, together with tissue composition and protein site occupation and obstruction by the blood-brain barrier and placental barrier.

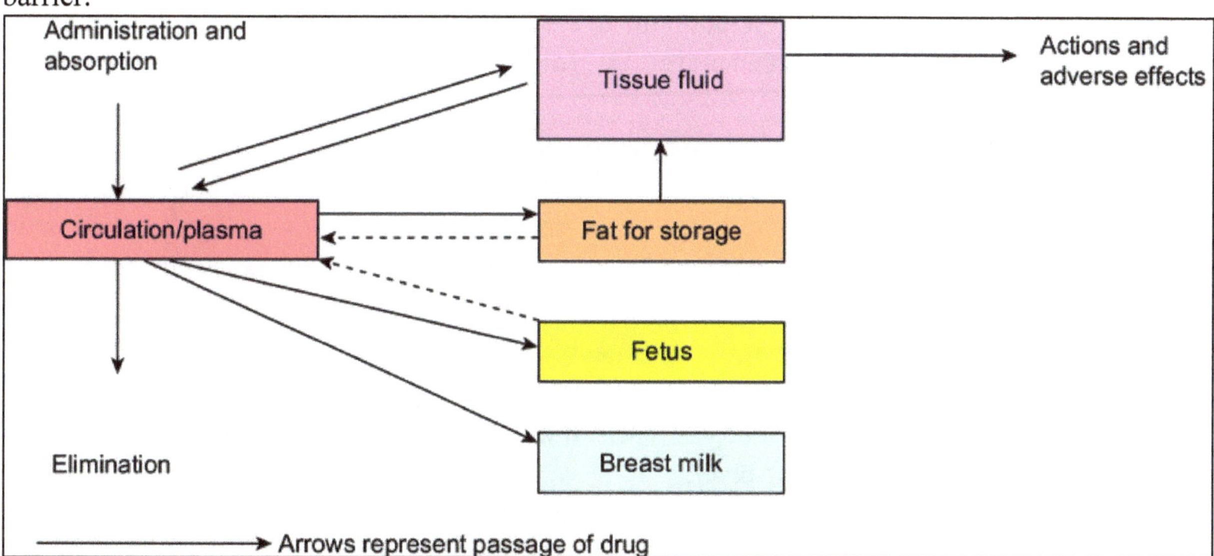

Figure 463 Drug Distribution

14.2.3.1 Blood Flow and Tissue Differences in Drug Distribution

Multiple factors control how drugs travel through the human body because the circulatory system determines their overall distribution throughout the body. **A drug delivery to its target tissue gets affected when blood circulation is reduced through dehydration and atherosclerosis or hypertension and heart failure conditions.** The liver along with kidneys and brain tissues receive medications swiftly but fat tissue only absorbs these drugs at a reduced rate because of differences in blood flow density. The fat-dissolving property of lipophilic drugs leads to their active accumulation within adipose tissue and especially affects those who are overweight.

14.2.3.2 Protein-Binding and Drug Distribution

The molecules within bloodstream do not completely remain unbound for circulation once a drug enters. Most drug molecules in the bloodstream connect to plasma albumin and other proteins. Pharmacologically active drug molecules exist as free agents because they have broken their bond with proteins thus enabling them to transport to target tissues for their effects. The bound drug exists inactive state until being progressively released. **Some drugs demonstrate such extensive protein binding that their action becomes extended by allowing minute drug amounts to detach over time reaching 95-98% of drug binding.** Drugs competing for plasma binding sites affect the actual drug efficacy that reaches the target tissues. When aspirin and warfarin both target the same plasma protein site their unbound quantities increase to cause stronger drug effects alongside greater possibilities of adverse outcomes like bleeding.

Table 263 Factors Affecting Drug Distribution

Factor	Description	Impact on Drug Distribution
Blood Flow	Blood flow varies across different tissues. High blood flow to organs like the liver, kidneys, and brain allows for rapid drug delivery.	Decreased blood flow (e.g., atherosclerosis, heart failure) can reduce drug delivery to tissues.
Tissue Characteristics	Tissues with higher vascularity (e.g., liver, kidneys) receive drugs faster. Lipophilic drugs tend to accumulate in fat tissues.	Distribution into fat tissue is slower for hydrophilic drugs, but lipophilic drugs may accumulate in adipose tissue.
Protein-Binding	Drugs bind to plasma proteins (e.g., albumin). Only unbound drugs are active and able to reach target tissues.	The percentage of bound drug affects the amount of free drug available for action. Drugs that are highly protein-bound require careful monitoring.
Blood-Brain Barrier	A selectively permeable barrier between the blood and brain tissue that restricts the entry of most drugs.	Only lipophilic drugs or those with specific carriers can cross the blood-brain barrier. This limits the types of drugs that can act on the CNS.
Placental Barrier	The placental barrier regulates the transfer of substances between the maternal and fetal circulation.	Some drugs can cross the placenta, potentially affecting fetal development. Certain medications may be harmful to the fetus.

14.2.3.3 Life Span Consideratin in Drug Distribution

Table 264 Drug Distribution among Neeonates and Adults

Age Group	Characteristics	Impact on Drug Distribution

Neonate & Pediatric	Lower body fat and higher total body water; immature blood-brain barrier; lower protein-binding capacity.	Decreased protein-binding capacity leads to higher free drug concentrations, increasing the risk of toxicity. The immature blood-brain barrier allows more drugs to affect the CNS.
Older Adults	Higher body fat; decreased albumin levels; decreased lean muscle mass and body water.	Increased body fat can cause prolonged drug action for lipophilic drugs. Decreased albumin means more free drug circulating, which may increase drug effects and potential toxicity.

14.2.3.4 Blood-Brain Barrier and Placental Barrier

Through the blood-brain barrier the protective mechanism inhibits various substances from reaching the brain tissue which protects the central nervous system (CNS) against toxins and outside pathogens. **Lipid-soluble medications and drugs with particular active transport pathways represent the sole options to penetrate the BBB.** The combination drug Sinemet® contains carbidopa along with levodopa to let levodopa penetrate the blood-brain barrier thus treating Parkinson's disease. Diphenhydramine (an antihistamine) together with other certain drugs cross the blood-brain barrier to reach the central nervous system resulting in CNS side effects particularly drowsiness. **The placental barrier functions similarly to a protective barrier that controls transfers between maternal and fetal substances.** Several drugs can penetrate the placenta to impact fetal development yet several drugs remain inaccessible to it. Multiple medications specifically anticonvulsants and antibiotics threaten both the development of the fetus and its functional health during maternal use in pregnancy. Medical professionals need to analyze the fetal consequences of medications when providing prescriptions to pregnant and breastfeeding individuals.

14.2.4 Metabolism

Metabolism Overview Building upon drug consumption, the body uses metabolic processes to create easier-to-excrete compounds, which are known as metabolites. Drugs that reach body tissues spread to every part of the body, undergo chemical conversion primarily in liver cells, enabled by enzyme action. The biotransformation processes modify drug molecules to convert inactive compounds into active drugs or to increase the water-solubility of active compounds for elimination from the body. **The metabolism process consists of three stages, which are modification (Phase I), followed by conjugation (Phase II), and further modification and excretion that can occur (Phase III).** The modification of drugs relies heavily on liver enzymes, particularly cytochrome P450. Drug metabolism rate, along with effectiveness, depends on depot binding strength and the influence of enzyme activity, and the available enzyme binding areas within the body. Knowledge about drug metabolism enables practitioners to modify treatment dosage and prevent adverse effects as well as handle drug-to-drug reactions.

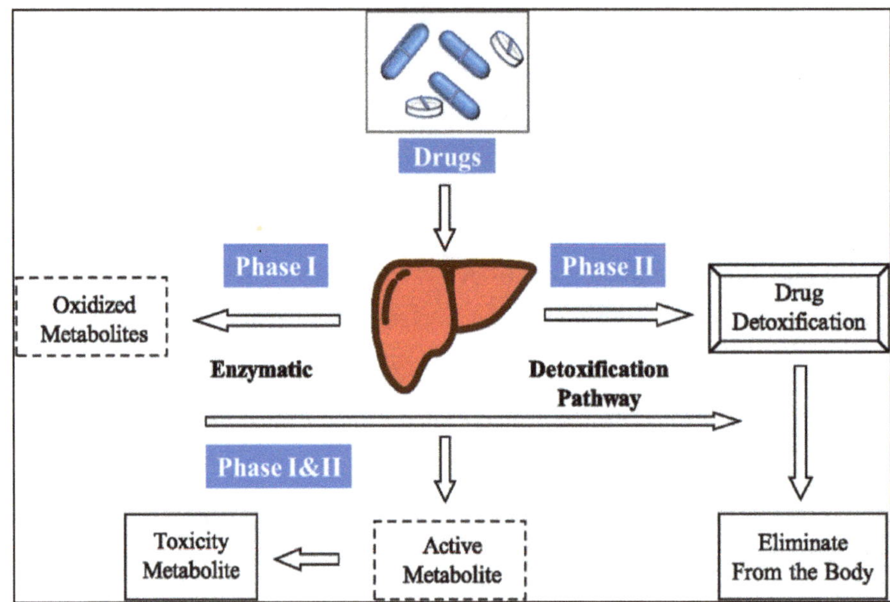

Figure 464 General Pathway of Drug Metabolism

14.2.5 Biotransformation Phases: Phase I and Phase II

The Biotransformation process has two distinct stages named Phase I and Phase II The drug molecule undergoes Phase I chemical transformations, which usually take place through oxidation, reduction, or hydrolysis instances. **The metabolic process produces transformation products of drugs, which demonstrate lower activity levels than the starting drug substance.** Some inactive drugs become active prodrugs through Phase I modifications to increase therapeutic benefit. Physical inactivity remains associated with sulfasalazine until the liver performs its metabolic function, which activates the medication for rheumatoid arthritis treatment. **During Phase II metabolism, drugs or their initial metabolites become attached to other molecules through conjugation reactions to create water-soluble, excretable forms**. During this stage, the drug becomes clinically inactive due to the biological inactivation process. As an active metabolite of diazepam, oxazepam becomes ready for elimination because it combines with glucuronide during Phase II metabolism.

Table 265: Biotransformation Phases and Their Mechanisms

Phase	Mechanism	Outcome	Example
Phase I	Modifies the chemical structure of the drug (oxidation, reduction, hydrolysis).	Converts drugs into metabolites that are often less active than the parent drug.	Diazepam metabolized into desmethyldiazepam and oxazepam.
Phase II	Conjugation: coupling the drug or its metabolites with another molecule (e.g., glucuronide).	Makes drugs more water-soluble and easier to excrete, often inactivating the drug.	Oxazepam conjugated with glucuronide for easier excretion.
Phase III	Additional modification and excretion from cells.	Facilitates the final elimination of conjugated drugs from cells.	Involves the final transport of metabolites into bile or urine.

14.2.5.1 Factors Affecting Metabolism

Drug metabolism is influenced by several factors, including enzyme activity, depot binding, and interactions with other drugs. **The most important enzymes for drug metabolism are monoamine oxidase (MAO) and cytochrome P450.** Enzyme induction, where repeated drug use increases enzyme production, can lead to tolerance, requiring higher drug doses to achieve the same effect. Conversely, enzyme inhibition, where one drug inhibits the activity of a metabolic enzyme, can lead to increased drug levels and potential toxicity. Depot binding is another factor that can affect metabolism. When drugs bind to inactive sites in fatty tissues, they are not available for metabolism, which can delay drug breakdown and excretion. **For example, tetrahydrocannabinol (THC), the psychoactive component of marijuana, binds to adipose tissue, leading to delayed metabolism and prolonged detection in urine.** Drugs that share the same metabolic pathway can compete for enzyme binding sites, affecting their metabolism. For example, alcohol and sedatives both use the cytochrome P450 enzyme, so taking both can result in slower metabolism of the sedative, increasing the risk of overdose.

Factor	Description	Impact on Drug Metabolism
Enzyme Activity	Liver enzymes (e.g., cytochrome P450, monoamine oxidase) are essential for drug breakdown.	Enzyme induction leads to faster metabolism; enzyme inhibition can lead to slower metabolism and toxicity.
Depot Binding	Drug molecules may bind to fat tissues, slowing their availability for metabolism.	Slows the breakdown of the drug and may extend its effects (e.g., THC).
Enzyme Induction	Repeated drug use increases enzyme production, leading to faster drug metabolism.	Leads to tolerance and requires higher doses to achieve the same effect.
Enzyme Inhibition	Some drugs inhibit the enzymes responsible for metabolizing other drugs, increasing their effects.	Increases the concentration of the inhibited drug, increasing the risk of side effects or toxicity (e.g., MAOIs and certain antidepressants).
Drug Interactions	Drugs that share metabolic pathways can compete for the same enzymes.	Reduces the efficiency of drug metabolism and can lead to adverse effects (e.g., alcohol and sedatives).

14.2.5.2 Clinical Significance of Metabolism

Understanding drug metabolism is essential for optimizing dosing regimens, particularly in patients with liver or kidney impairment. **The half-life of a drug, which refers to the time it takes for the drug's plasma concentration to reduce by half, is influenced by metabolism.** Drugs with short half-lives require more frequent dosing, while drugs with longer half-lives may only need a single dose per day. Patients with liver or kidney disease may require dose adjustments to prevent toxic buildup of the drug or its metabolites. Healthcare professionals must monitor drug levels, especially for drugs with narrow therapeutic windows, such as warfarin and some antibiotics.

14.2.5.3 Half-Life and Its Clinical Relevance

The duration it takes for a drug to decrease to half its initial concentration determines the necessary frequency with which health professionals need to administer it. **The length of time furosemide stays in the body amounts to about two hours as a result of its two-hour half-life. Some antidepressants, along with other drugs, show prolonged half-life that allows healthcare providers to prescribe treatment at decreased frequency.** Healthcare providers need a thorough understanding of drug half-life for managing medication planning and dosage adjustments because it affects treatment schedules of patients with liver or kidney impairment.

14.2.5.4 Life Span Considerations in Drug Metabolism

Neonatal and Pediatric patients possess liver enzymes which are underdeveloped so their drug metabolism occurs slower. Liver enzyme maturation occurs in children with age which provides them an enhanced metabolism rate requiring medication adjustments. **Drug metabolism performance in adults ages sixty and above decreases with advancing years thus elongating many pharmaceutical substances' half-lives.** Drug intake sensitivity becomes higher among elderly patients that requires healthcare providers to adjust their medication amounts to reduce possible toxic effects. Effective drug utilization depends on complete knowledge about medication breakdown mechanisms to provide safe medical treatment for all patient demographics. Healthcare providers achieve better therapeutic results with decreased adverse reactions through comprehensive assessments of enzyme activities combined with depot binding characteristics and drug compatibility studies and individual patient characteristics.

14.2.6 Elimination/Excretion

Drug metabolism ends with excretion as the body removes drugs and their reaction products from the system through this process. When distributing drugs throughout the body the remaining parent components alongside metabolites need to leave the system in order to avoid buildup and possible toxic effects. **The body uses kidneys, liver and lungs as its primary channels to eliminate drugs from the body.** When the kidneys perform filtration they capture several drug byproducts from blood circulation which may return to circulation through reabsorption or leave the body in urine. The liver releases medication byproducts as bile while alcohol together with anesthetic gases leave the body through the lungs. **Efficient drug excretion helps establish appropriate body drug levels and protect the patient from harmful outcomes.**

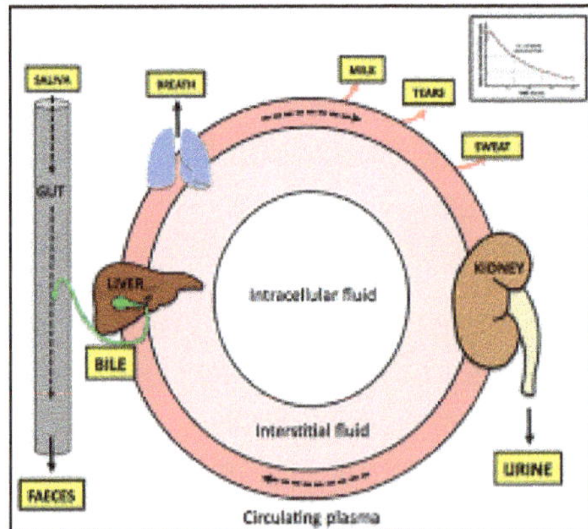

Figure 465 Drug Excretion

14.2.6.1 Routes of Excretion

1. **Kidneys**

The main excretory role of the kidneys involves blood filtration, which results in waste removal along with drug metabolites from the body. A person's age combined with their weight as well as their sex status alongside their kidney function determines how quickly medications leave their bodies. **Medical tests that evaluate kidney function include laboratory evaluations measuring serum creatinine, together with glomerular filtration rate (GFR)** and creatinine clearance tests. The elimination of drugs becomes impaired when kidney function declines in patients who have chronic kidney disease or heart failure so practitioners need to adjust drug doses.

2. **Liver**

Pharmacological substances move through the liver because this organ filters drug substances together with their metabolites into bile for excretion. The liver produces metabolites that travel through the gallbladder until reaching the small intestine before some products return to bloodstream circulation and the remaining parts are eliminated through feces. **Bronchogenic carcinomas provide information regarding liver function using ALT and AST enzymes which direct medication adjustments when liver health deteriorates.** Blood circulation difficulties affecting the liver will decrease its capacity to efficiently eliminate drugs from the body.

3. **Other Routes of Excretion**

Through various body routes drugs are **eliminated from the bloodstream by finding their way into sweat and tears as well as reproductive fluids including semen as well as breast milk**. Drugs enter the body through various routes that specifically endanger young infants and other susceptible groups by allowing drug substances to transfer into breast milk. Both healthcare providers and breastfeeding mothers need assessment of medication safety for their breasts while consulting drug references and medical professionals if required.

Table 266 Routes of Excretion

Route	Description	Excretion Mechanism	Considerations
Kidneys	Primary route of drug elimination. Blood is filtered, and byproducts are excreted in urine.	Filtration, reabsorption, and secretion via renal pathways.	Kidney function (e.g., GFR, serum creatinine) must be monitored to adjust drug doses.
Liver	Filters blood and excretes drugs into bile. Some drugs may be reabsorbed by the intestines.	Metabolism to metabolites, secretion into bile.	Liver function (ALT, AST) must be assessed, and dosages adjusted in cases of hepatic impairment.
Lungs	Excrete volatile substances like alcohol and anesthetic gases.	Exhalation of gaseous drugs.	Can lead to exposure risks; monitoring may be required.
Sweat, Tears, Reproductive Fluids, Breast Milk	Minor excretion routes, especially for small molecules.	Excretion via sweat, tears, seminal fluid, or milk.	Risk of drug exposure in infants via breast milk; consult drug references for safety.

14.2.6.2 Life Span Considerations in Excretion

Newborns and small children possess underdeveloped renal systems that negatively affect glomerular filtration rate alongside tubular secretion and reabsorption abilities. **These patients show reduced ability to eliminate medications through their body**. The prescribed doses for pediatric patients depend on their body weight due to the slower pace at which they eliminate drugs so smaller amounts receive lower doses. Regular assessment must occur to avoid drug side effects since young patients could develop higher levels of active medication substances in their blood. Drugs tend to remain in the bloodstream longer and present higher hazards for toxic effects during the aging process because older adults frequently experience decreased function in both their kidneys and liver. **Physicians recommend "start low and go slow" to older adults as an approach that begins with minimal dosing and requires adjustments according to treatment responses for avoiding adverse effects.** Medical staff should monitor kidney and liver function carefully because drug excretion becomes less efficient.

14.2.6.3 Clinical Significance of Excretion

Proper drug concentration levels in the human body depend heavily on the excretion process. An ineffective elimination process for drugs together with their metabolites risks accumulating toxins which affects patients with impaired renal or hepatic function particularly. Nurses need to adjust drug amounts and carefully observe patient toxicity symptoms because vulnerable groups such as **elderly adults neonates as well as children need special attention.** Healthcare providers need to notice drug interaction effects on excretion because drugs that affect kidney function alongside drugs that share metabolic pathways in the liver. The clinical understanding of drug excretion mechanisms enables healthcare professionals to manage appropriate drug dosages for therapeutic purposes along with adverse outcome reduction

14.2.7 What is Pharmacodynamics?

Pharmacodynamics (PD) examines drug-body interactions. Pharmacokinetics studies drug bodily movements but PD examines the molecular and physiological and biochemical drug effects on human systems. **Drug concentration and body effects constitute the main scope of PD analysis which includes descriptions of drug action methods as well as dose-response relations and duration of effects alongside adverse events.** Drug binding onto its body receptors constitutes a fundamental PD parameter. The drug chemical structure, along with the receptor nature, together with other binding possible molecules, impact this bond interaction. The pharmaceutical group known as agonists works by activating receptors, while the antagonists disrupt receptor action to generate their therapeutic benefits. Drugs classified as antagonists will occupy receptor binding sites to stop the receptor from activating thus inhibiting its activity. The nature of receptor concentration alongside its present state determines whether particular drugs will exhibit agonist and antagonist effects. **A drug demonstrates its ability to achieve the intended therapeutic outcome through efficacy, while potency describes how much substance it needs to reach this outcome**. The required concentration of drug needed to achieve a specific target effect is what defines potency. These two concepts typically correlate yet they do not need to affect each other. High potency does not guarantee high efficacy since the drug fails to generate meaningful effects at its target location. The safety levels of medications depend on the therapeutic index value. The therapeutic index expresses the safety measurement as the gap between minimum therapeutic dosage and the amount needed to cause harmful effects. **An agent classified as safe exhibits a high therapeutic index yet medications having a low therapeutic index tend to pose** significant risks to patients. The selectivity of medication involves its ability to communicate with specific targets yet avoid creating damage at alternative targets so scientists express this quality as the selectivity ratio. The way to express drug selectivity shows the relationship between main-target activating doses and secondary-target activating doses.

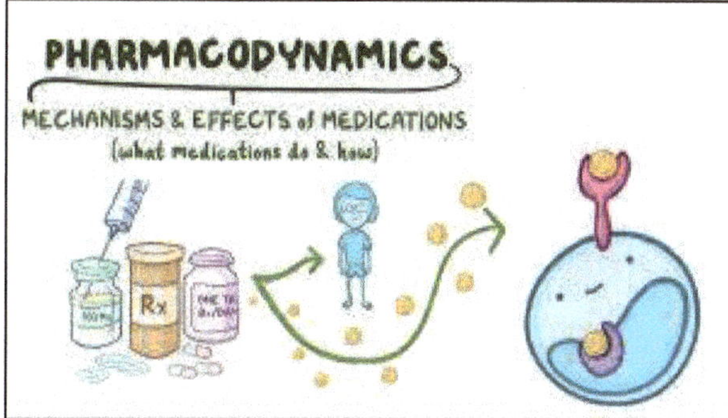

Figure 466 Pharmacodynamics

14.2.8 Mechanism of Action: Agonists and Antagonists

The mechanism of action describes the exact molecular-level processes which drugs use to create their therapeutic effects. **Drugs primarily function through receptor binding interactions on the cell surface yet diverse drugs also have direct effects on enzymes and cellular mechanisms.** The biochemical effect of agonists occurs when they combine with receptors to induce receptor activation and produce corresponding physiological effects. Drugs that function as agonists copy existing body chemicals like neurotransmitters and hormones during their action. The opioid analgesic morphine activates opioid receptors located in the brain to prevent pain signals and generate pain relief. These substances connect with receptors yet fail to start receptor activation. **These receptors only receive agonist blockade alongside naturally occurring substance inhibition to prevent typical binding activities.** The heart medicine atenolol functions as an antagonist which blocks beta-adrenergic receptors inside the heart so it can prevent adrenaline from working and lower blood pressure and heart rate. Understanding medications operates from the core principle of understanding agonist actions versus antagonist inhibitory functions.

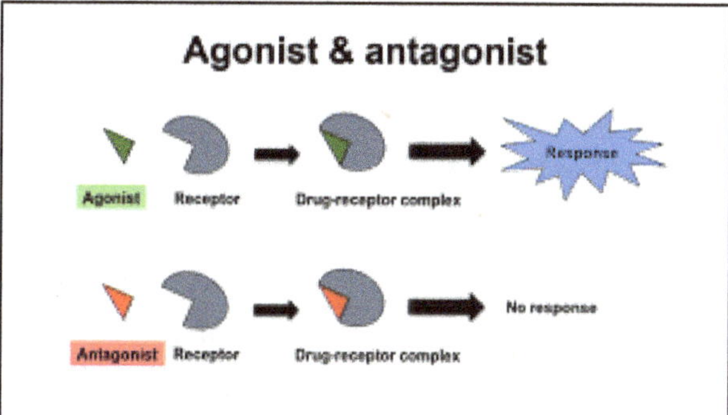

Figure 467 Mechanism of Agonist and Antagonist

14.2.9 Critical Thinking Activity Example: Atenolol

Atenolol (Tenormin) is a beta-blocker that acts as an antagonist at beta-adrenergic receptors in the heart. As an antagonist, atenolol competes with adrenaline and prevents it from binding to these receptors. The desired action of atenolol is to block the increase in heart rate and blood pressure typically caused by sympathetic stimulation. **Therefore, nurses should anticipate that atenolol will block the effects of beta receptors, specifically reducing the workload on the heart and managing conditions like hypertension and arrhythmias.** By understanding its antagonistic action, the nurse can predict its effect on the client's cardiovascular system.

14.2.10 Types of Medications

Pharmacodynamics focuses on different medication types separated into **prescription medications and over-the-counter (OTC) medications and herbal supplements.** Patients need to follow prescription medications because medical professionals issue these drugs under FDA oversight for both safety and effectiveness. These drugs act for defined therapeutic uses and doctors usually customize their prescriptions to match patients' medical needs. OTC medications can be obtained without medical prescription because patients typically use them to treat headaches along with colds and allergy symptoms. **Most individuals find OTC medications safe for correct usage but a client's use of these products merits attention from healthcare providers because they might impact other medications and preexisting medical issues.** Multiple people select herbal supplements alongside complementary and alternative medicines (CAM) yet these products remain exempt from FDA oversight and lack the extensive prescription drug testing protocol. Herbal remedies that might help with treatment can contain ingredients which negatively affect prescription medications thereby producing unwanted side effects and toxic effects. **The responsibility exists for nursing professionals to both explain complications of herbal supplements to patients and investigate how these supplements influence their prescribed medications.**

Table 267 Common Classes of Medications, Examples, Suffixes, and Roots

Class of Medication	Example	Common Suffixes	Common Roots
Analgesics	lidocaine	-caine	-morph, -morphe, -morphic
Antacids	omeprazole	-azole	-tidine
Antibiotics	levofloxacin	-mycin, -floxacin	bacter-, vir-, -cidal
Anticoagulants	warfarin	-arin	coagul-
Antidepressants	fluoxetine	-oxetine, -ipramine	serotonin, norepinephrine
Antihistamines	diphenhydramine	-dine, -mine	hist-
Anti-inflammatory	cortisone	-one	-corti-, -flam-, -prost-
Antipsychotics	olanzapine	-azine, -apine	dopa-, sero-, -plegia
Beta-blockers	metoprolol	-olol	adrenergic, beta-
Bronchodilators	albuterol	-terol	bronch-, -pnea
Corticosteroids	prednisone	-sone or -solone	
Diuretics	furosemide	-semide, -thiazide	-uret-, -osm-
Hypoglycemics	glipizide	-ide	gluc-, insulin-
Statins	atorvastatin	-statin	cholesterol, lipid-

14.3 Pharmacologic Agents: Commonly Used Drugs

14.3.1 Drug classes: antibiotics, antihypertensives, antidepressants.

14.3.1.1 Antibiotics

The visual representation demonstrates how different antibiotic categories work along with their operational methods towards controlling bacterial infections in a methodical approach. The different antibiotic classes attack bacterial cellular processes from different angles in order to stop bacterial reproduction and growth. **Protein synthesis becomes a target for antibiotic action by Aminoglycosides together with Macrolides and Lincomycins and Tetracyclines.** These antibiotics stop bacteria from making necessary proteins by connecting to the bacterial ribosome which causes essential survival and replication proteins to fail to be synthesized. The treatment method effectively targets Gram-positive and Gram-negative bacteria due to its broad applicability in treating different infections. **These antibiotics including Cephalosporins, Penicillins, Carbapenems and Glycopeptides disrupt bacterial cell wall synthesis.** Through blocking bacterial cell wall synthesis these antibiotics enable the microorganism to burst apart from osmotic pressure and perish. As a result these antibiotics exhibit strong effectiveness against the Gram-positive bacteria Streptococcus and **Staphylococcus species** although carbapenems show similar antibiotic activity on Gram-negative pathogens. Therapeutic actions of sulfonamides obstruct folate synthesis thus affecting essential bacterial DNA and nucleotide production pathways. The drugs destroy folate metabolic processes in bacteria thus blocking bacterial growth and replication. The medical benefit of this active substance extends to treating Gram-positive and Gram-negative bacterial infections including Escherichia coli and Staphylococcus aureus bacteria. The DNA replication process becomes blocked through Fluoroquinolones because these drugs attack DNA gyrase along with other essential bacterial enzymes. The proper replication of genetic material becomes impossible for bacteria when treated with these antibiotics which blocks cell survival and cell division therefore making this antibiotic effective against various bacteria in respiratory and urinary tract infections. **Healthcare providers can use their knowledge of bacterial growth mechanisms to pick appropriate antibiotics because it helps them determine which antibiotics will effectively halt microbial multiplication** while considering both the infection characteristics and bacterial types. Optimal treatment success and reduced development of antibiotic resistance become possible with this method.

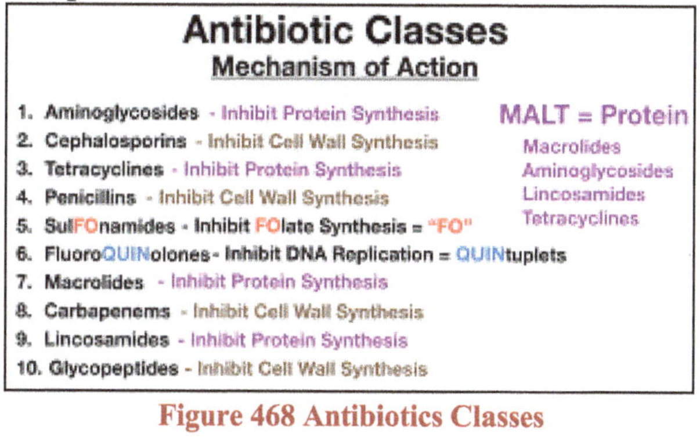

Antibiotic Classes
Mechanism of Action
1. Aminoglycosides - Inhibit Protein Synthesis
2. Cephalosporins - Inhibit Cell Wall Synthesis
3. Tetracyclines - Inhibit Protein Synthesis
4. Penicillins - Inhibit Cell Wall Synthesis
5. SulFOnamides - Inhibit FOlate Synthesis = "FO"
6. FluoroQUINolones - Inhibit DNA Replication = QUINtuplets
7. Macrolides - Inhibit Protein Synthesis
8. Carbapenems - Inhibit Cell Wall Synthesis
9. Lincosamides - Inhibit Protein Synthesis
10. Glycopeptides - Inhibit Cell Wall Synthesis
MALT = Protein
Macrolides
Aminoglycosides
Lincosamides
Tetracyclines

Figure 468 Antibiotics Classes

14.3.1.2 Antihypertensive

These images present in-depth information about antihypertensive drugs through their therapeutic classifications and mechanism-based divisions. **Antihypertensive medications are sorted into three categories displayed within the first chart: Diuretics, Renin-Angiotensin System Inhibitors and Sympathetic Inhibitors.** Among diuretics we find three main subtypes: Thiazides with Hydrochlorothiazide as an example while High Ceiling diuretics include Furosemide and

Potassium-sparing diuretics use Spironolactone as their representative drug. The medications produce their blood pressure lowering effects by encouraging fluid excretion and influencing kidney operations. **Medical intervention through the Renin-Angiotensin System Inhibitors contains three components including two classes of ACE inhibitors (Captopril and Enalapril amongst others) and ARBs (Losartan and Valsartan among others) as well as the Direct Renin Inhibitor Aliskiren.** Through their mechanism of renin-angiotensin pathway inhibition these medications stop angiotensin II from causing blood vessel constriction thus lowering blood pressure. The two classes of Sympathetic Inhibitors include β-adrenergic blockers such as Propranolol and Metoprolol as well as α-adrenergic blockers such as Prazosin and Terazosin that lower sympathetic nervous system activity and prevent heart rate increases and vascular resistance increases. **The Central Sympatholytics concentrate on controlling blood pressure through their action on the central nervous system by utilizing Clonidine as an example.** The second chart delves into Calcium Channel Blockers and Vasodilators. In smooth muscle cells calcium ion entry causes vasodilation and lower blood pressure through the mechanism of action of three types of calcium channel blockers: Phenylalkylamines (Verapamil) along with Benzothiazepines (Diltiazem) and Dihydropyridines (Amlodipine). **The first class of vasodilators known as Arteriolar Dilators uses Hydralazine as an example drug and includes direct blood vessel expansion to decrease systemic vascular resistance.** The distinct treatments groups of antihypertensive drugs enable medical providers to select personalized treatments that match the needs of individual patients while managing drug effectiveness alongside potential side effects.

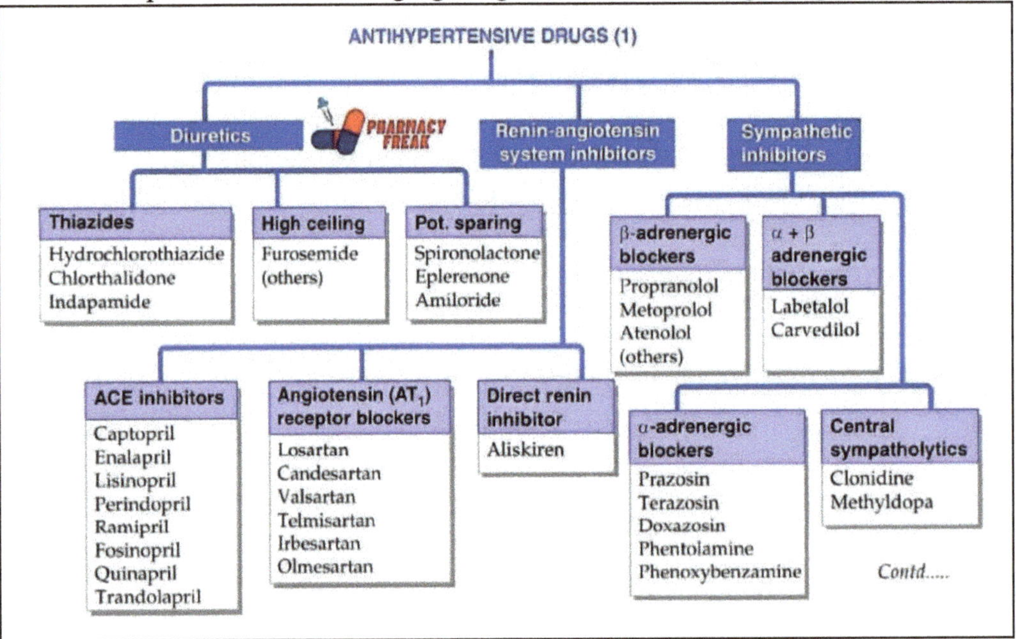

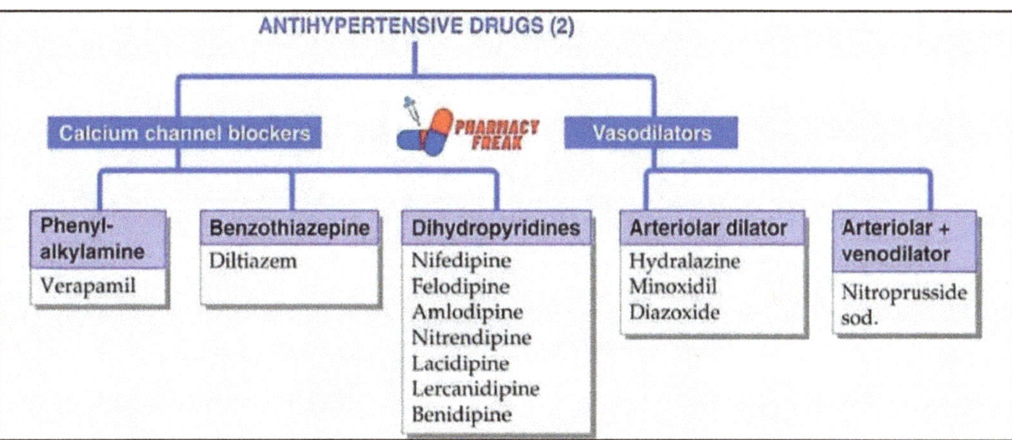

Figure 469 Classification of ANtihypertensive Drugs

14.3.1.3 Antsuppressants

This image demonstrates five antidepressant categories according to their action methods which include **Reversible Inhibitors of Monoamine Oxidase A (RIMAs), Selective Serotonin Reuptake Inhibitors (SSRIs), Tricyclic Antidepressants (TCAs), Atypical Antidepressants, and Serotonin and Noradrenaline Reuptake Inhibitors (SNRIs).** When patients take RIMA medications Moclobemide or Clorgyline their brain levels of serotonin norepinephrine and dopamine rise because these drugs stop the enzyme monoamine oxidase A from destroying these neurotransmitters. The medical effect of this mechanism makes symptoms of depression less severe. **The depressive symptoms decrease after the selective inhibition of serotonin reuptake by SSRIs including Fluoxetine and Sertraline and Paroxetine because their action leads to increased serotonin presence in the synaptic space for better mood regulation.** Both Imipramine and Amitriptyline as TCA medications work by blocking reuptake of serotonin and norepinephrine in the brain while producing more side effects because they affect multiple receptors. Three contemporary antidepressants Trazodone and Mirtazapine as well as Bupropion function through different pathways because **Bupropion primarily affects dopamine and norepinephrine and Mirtazapine increases serotonin and norepinephrine levels within the synapses.** SSRIs and TCAs are reserved for cases where patients do not respond well to these medicines. The dual-action mechanism of SNRIs including Venlafaxine and Duloxetine treats depression and anxiety simultaneously because they stop both serotonin and norepinephrine reuptake. Clinicians need this classification method to find the best antidepressant for each patient according to their individual symptoms and reaction to treatment along with their personal needs.

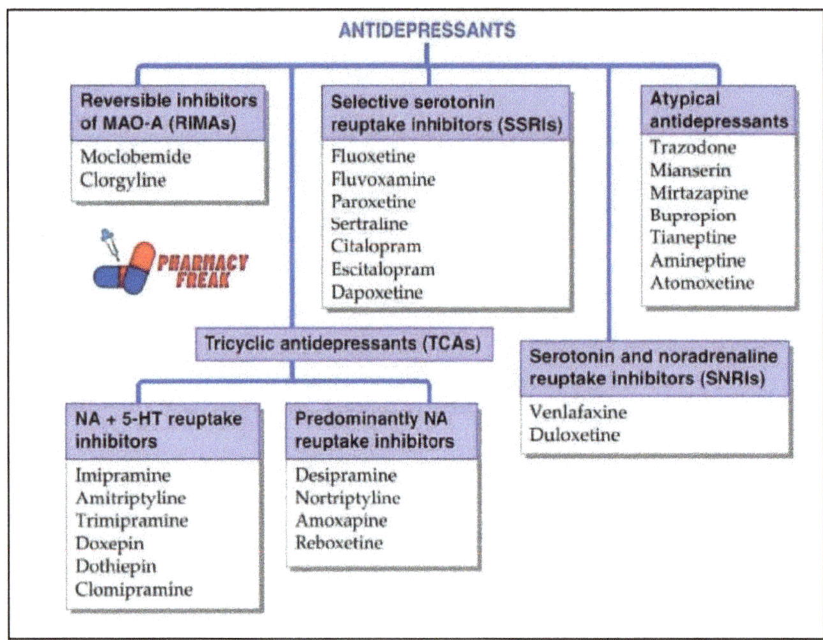

Figure 470 Classification of Antidepressants

14.3.2 Safe Prescribing Practices and Medication Errors

The implementation of proper medication prescribing techniques remains essential for error reduction because errors from medication prescription represent a major healthcare avoidable harm source. **The fundamental basis for generating preventive strategies for medication errors resides in fully understanding all stages of medication processing and their underlying causes together with all resulting error types and their consequences.**

14.3.2.1 Prescribing Medication Safely

During prescription medication steps several errors may happen especially when healthcare providers choose the wrong medication or set improper amounts or use improper delivery methods and neglect essential patient characteristics including allergic histories and existing conditions and organ health status. Safe medication prescribing requires both selecting the appropriate drug and documenting both dosage amount and administration route and schedule. A prevention of medical errors depends on direct communication exchanges between prescribers as well as pharmacists and nurses. The following list contains essential approaches for maintaining safe medication prescribing:

Accurate medication prescriptions and scheduling rates prevent major medical issues from occurring because of wrong amounts administered. Medical prescriptions need to comprise explicit information including the drug amount with the pill count together with dosage timing specifications. **Treatment instructions should exclude ambiguous terminology such as "take as directed" and "prn" (as needed) when add the concrete details about their implementation**. Electronic health records (EHRs) in combination with computerized physician order entry (CPOE) systems reduces prescribing errors in healthcare practice. Embedded within the system are multiple built-in features which confirm proper medicine dosage and drug interaction details while alerting healthcare providers about existing allergies or treatment restrictions to prevent various medication-related errors. **The process of prescribing medication requires practitioners to collect all essential information about patients together with their treatment plan data.** The physician must gather complete patient information by reviewing medical records alongside current medications alongside allergies together with kidney and liver functioning status. The information enables healthcare providers to select suitable medications while minimizing risks of adverse drug interactions or any contraindications.

Healthcare faces an ongoing challenge regarding prescription clarity since doctors often struggle to make their medical notes easy to read. The insufficient legible quality of prescriptions frequently induces significant medication errors so the Institute of Safe Medication Practices suggests prohibiting all handwritten drug prescriptions. Prescriptions written on computers or as electronic orders reduce the occurrence of medication errors that stem from poor handwriting. The practice of using abbreviations remains one of the leading sources that leads to medication prescription errors. **A medication prescription containing "QD" as an abbreviation could mistakenly be understood as "QID" by the reader due to the similar appearance between these medical terms**. The recommendation for safe prescribing practice includes complete avoidance of abbreviations in all medication orders.

14.3.2.2 Common Types of Medication Errors in Prescribing

Medication errors in the prescribing stage are varied and can occur due to human error, system failures, or miscommunication. Some common types include:

Table 268 Common Types of Errors

Type of Error	Description
Omission	Failure to prescribe a drug that is necessary for the patient's condition.
Wrong time	Medications prescribed at incorrect intervals or schedules.
Unauthorized medication	Prescribing a medication that has not been approved for a particular patient.
Improper dose	Incorrect dosage, either higher or lower than required.
Wrong route	Prescribing a drug via the wrong route (e.g., oral instead of intravenous).
Incorrect drug	Mistaking one drug for another with similar names or appearances.
Drug interactions	Prescribing medications that have adverse interactions with other prescribed drugs.

These errors can often be reduced through the use of **decision support tools** integrated into electronic prescribing systems, which provide warnings for contraindications, allergies, and drug-drug interactions.

14.3.2.3 Key Strategies for Preventing Medication Errors

The main approaches which eliminate medication errors include

1. **Improving Interprofessional Communication:**

The link between prescribers and nurses along with pharmacists needs to stay connected to reduce medication errors. During medication reconciliation a nurse must verify patient prescriptions with the person while properly recording all updated information. **Adults presenting medication orders with poor communication suffer from misinterpretation that produces harmful treatment effects**.

2. **Use of Medication Reconciliation**

The practice of medication reconciliation guarantees that complete details regarding patients' medicines will transmit safely across healthcare transition areas particularly from hospital admissions to discharges. T**hrough this process healthcare professionals can avoid several types of medication errors** including omitting prescriptions and treatment by incorrect dosage.

3. **Automated Medication Systems:**

Nursing practice becomes more secure when automated drug dispensing systems work together with barcoding to safely deliver medications to correct patients at precise timing. The systems determine both patient identity and medicine dose before delivery which minimizes prescription blunders.

4. **Regular Education and Training:**

Nursing personnel should participate in sustained educational programs to understand medication error origins and develop precise record keeping practices. Educational modules focused on safe prescribing methods that teach clinicians about medication reaction analysis and treatment complications will enhance their medical prescription ability.

5. **Promoting Error Reporting:**

The development of a work environment that enables healthcare personnel to report errors safely represents a fundamental requirement. The reporting of medical errors by healthcare providers produces analysis opportunities that unveil root **causes to establish organizational preventive measures for future errors including near-miss occurrences.**

14.3.2.4 Clinical Significance and Impact of Medication Errors

The direct impact on patients from medication errors creates consequences which affect patient safety across an extensive network. **The errors extend patients' hospitalization periods while driving up healthcare expenses also leading to fatal results at times**. Healthcare providers encounter negative effects from medication errors including feelings of guilt together with the erosion of trust and exposure to possible legal consequences**. High healthcare expenses arise from medication errors due to their substantial cost burden on the healthcare system.** Elderly patients along with patients who have multiple health conditions or consume several medications face an elevated risk for medication administration mistakes. Which requires extra attention because these patients exhibit modified drug breakdown and higher vulnerability toward medication side effects.

14.4 Clinical Guidelines for Drug Prescription

14.4.1 Managing drug interactions and contraindications

Patient safety alongside optimal treatment benefits are achieved through the essential management of drug interactions and contraindications in drug prescription clinical guidelines. **Containing two substances in a given system produces drug interactions because one compound alters the impact of the second substance either positively or negatively.** The interactions between various substances include both prescription drugs and over-the-counter drugs and food items to herbal supplements. The multiple drug interactions provide reasons why healthcare professionals must actively search for potential risks which demand strategic techniques to protect patients from harm.

14.4.1.1 Mechanisms of Drug Interactions

Drug interactions exist between pharmacodynamic and pharmacokinetic effects. Two or more drugs create pharmacodynamic interactions that result in either increased additive effects or **opposing effects or synergistic effects on the body functions.** An example of drug interaction occurs when opioids are combined with sedatives since the combined sedation effects enhance respiratory depression. Anti-diabetic drug efficacy decreases when patients take corticosteroids so healthcare providers **need to modify medication doses for effective blood glucose regulation. The absorption and metabolism of drugs together with their distribution and excretion processes (ADME)** are modified due to therapeutic agent pairing. Ketoconazole absorption becomes decreased through the influence of proton pump inhibitors because the drug needs acid **conditions to properly absorb. Metabolism processes become affected by rifampicin which stimulates cytochrome P450 enzymes to increase break down of digoxin leading to reduced drug efficacy.** Tobacco smoke exposure promotes drug metabolism reactions which potentially decreases the effectiveness of various medications.

14.4.1.2 Significance of Drug Interactions

Medical professionals should recognize many different levels of significance behind drug interaction outcomes. They can be:

These drug combinations represent danger zones which doctors should strictly avoid because they are completely contraindicated. **The simultaneous use of LMWHs with DOACs leads to dangerous bleeding complications which make such drug combinations medically inappropriate for patients**.

Drug interactions requiring intervention include those which present limited risk in typical use conditions yet need proper monitoring or adjustment of medication doses. **Medical professionals need to carefully adjust doses when combining antihypertensive drugs because it helps decrease blood pressure but produces side effects of hypotension.**

Healthcare professionals should treat those drug interactions which produce no meaningful impact on treatment results while avoiding intervention. **Each drug-drug interaction needs proper documentation even if it does not require immediate changes to therapy**. Medical professionals should keep an eye on such cases for additional developments. Some drug combinations create synergistic effects by giving more therapeutic benefits than the medication effects do individually such as using antihypertensives with antihypertensive drugs to decrease blood pressure or pairing ACE inhibitors with calcium channel blockers to treat ankle edema.

14.4.1.3 The Practicing Nurse Must Handle Drug Interactions and Contraindications Efficiently

Several important strategies must be followed to properly manage drug interactions.

Doctors must collect extensive medical details about their patients together with information about all their medications including **non-prescription treatments and herbal-based products and dietary supplements to detect possible drug interactions.** Academic providers must double-check all medical records before medication prescribing to prevent dangerous medication interactions.

Doctors can lower dangerous interactions through their decision support tools including clinical decision support systems and automated alerts functioning within electronic health records. Safe patient care **benefits from these technology tools which alert practitioners about present drug** interaction possibilities between medications and dietary substances and botanical treatments.

The evaluation process requires strict patient observation due to known interaction risks of prescribed medications. Medical professionals should conduct regular checks of blood pressure levels along with renal function checks and electrolyte assessments as this helps identify potential early adverse reactions. **Clinical follow-up checks provide physicians with the opportunity to modify medication amounts, to switch treatment or to remove harmful drugs from patient care plans.**

14.4.1.4 Managing Contraindications

Medicines should be avoided in patients if their use represents excessive health risks to patients. The drug must usually fall into two categories; absolute contraindications where it needs to avoid selection altogether and relative contraindications requiring careful consideration for usage. **Patients with either renal failure or gastric ulcers should not receive NSAIDs because these**

medications have negative effects on such conditions. Anticoagulant Warfarin should be carefully managed between absolute contraindications of pregnancy because it poses a risk of fetal bleeding complications and another relative contraindication exists.

14.4.2 Safe Medication Management for Chronic Conditions

Medication safety is important when it comes to the administration of medication since most patients take medications for a long time especially when they have chronic diseases. Several points to consider entail proper prescription of the drugs, proper checkups, educating the patients, and record keeping on the medications. It is meant to reduce the incidence of prescribing errors, maximize the chances of positive drug effects, and enhance patient's safety of those with chronic diseases. **Medication safety management relates to the action of using medications that are prescribed, dispensed and administered to patient in a safe manner with the least harm to the patient.** This is especially the case with patient with chronic illness who may be on treatment that may take years to complete. Some of the effects of substandard medication safety include wrong medication dosage, negative evidence of interaction and adverse effects that may cause more harm to the patient who will be admitted to the hospital.

Medication safety also supports the NHS Patient Safety Strategy of preventing harm to patients while doing their healthcare. **The CQC rates the healthcare organizations concerning the safety of medications administered in the system and, therefore, is a critical area for enhancement of practices among clinicians.** Medication management can enhance medication safety, polypharmacy and can also assist in limiting the prescription of multiple medications to an individual.

Key elements of Medication Safely Additionally, some of the other factors that are considered when discussing medication safely are as follows;

1. **Clinical competencies:** Professional performers in the clinical area must have adequate knowledge in the national and local guidelines on prescribing, the interactions, and contraindications of drugs. The prescriber should always consult other resources like **National Institute for Health and Care Excellence guidelines, BNF, up-to-date knowledge of Medicines and Healthcare products Regulatory Agency' safety alerts**. Brief training sessions, the process of prescribing audits, and general knowledge about the usage of the QOF for prescribing indicators should be regular.
2. **Patient Education and Information:** This is important for patients with such diseases as Asthma, Diabetes, and other chronic diseases, where they must be well informed about the drugs to be taken, their side effects, dosage and regarding the importance of compliance with the recommended regimen. **Information should be provided to the patient on the potentials of risks related to intake of prescribed and over counter drugs and products such as herbal that may cause a reaction with the prescribed drugs**. Patients should be engaged and assisted to disclose all the medicines they take, even those bought over the counter and make them understand how such drugs may influence their treatment.
3. **Records**: In particular, documentation of medication for a patient is of crucial importance since it avoids the mistakes that can be fatal for a patient and provides continuity of his/her medical treatment. **Additional required documentation points to all medications** that was prescribed, including dosage, frequency, and any changes made in a patient's treatment plan. This also encompasses recording of counter substances, natural products and any known allergies or **other untoward effects of drugs.** This must be done especially after any modification in the patient's prescription like during hospital discharge or consultations.

4. **Prescription Refills:** In the modern world, most diseases are chronic, and therefore, patients need repeat prescriptions. These prescriptions can be reviewed periodically, a date assigned to this and proper monitoring of the progress of the patient should be accomplished. Organized medication screenings should be done to determine whether the treatments that were prescribed should be continued or not and if any of the dosages should be changed. **With eRD, it is possible to optimize thempharmacological care** process while also tracking the prescribed medicines more effectively. Patient mediations can be **reviewed by other HCPCPs, including clinical pharmacists**, to detect factors like potential medication interaction or the use of medications in a patient with multiple diseases.
5. **Prescribing and Dispensing Systems:** It has been claimed that electronic prescribing and management of medicines will cut medication errors because of ways such **as increasing prescription orderliness, improving the stock control, and facilitating overall prescription reviews.** Prescribing systems need to undergo a constant evaluation to determine its efficiency and that the prescribers are knowledgeable about the proper functioning of the system. It is important to pay attention to the NHS Smartcard system when writing prescriptions for concomitant illness to be able to safely retrieve patient data and merge local information with the data on the NHS database.

14.4.2.1 Risks and Issues in Safe Medication Management

There are several risks associated with medication administration to the patient with chronic diseases. Some of these include:

1. **Lack of supervision:** This is one of the major causes of over-prescription or under prescription because there is no frequent check on the results. **A system by which long-term prescriptions can be continuously monitored for safety issues is of great significance**. A patient with a chronic disease may be prescribed several medications as part of his/her treatment. **Polypharmacy therefore simply refers to the careful regulation of medications that are consumed with a view to avoiding absolute toxicity that might result when two or more drugs react** together, or to make sure that the metabolism of the drugs is maintained hence intact for the benefit of the patient's condition.
2. **Telehealth and remote consultation:** The use of telehealth and more specifically telepharmacy subsequently creates new safety concerns as to prescribing medications. The lack of **actual confrontation with patients and the lack of possibility to check personal histories enhance the rate of medication errors**. To mitigate such a risk, it is helpful to have a set of recommendations for the best practices for remote consultations.
3. **Digital divide:** some patients may cannot, for whatever reason, or may not want to access technologies such as the **NHS app or electronic prescriptions.** It is proper to foster for all patients, including the ones who may be digitally marginalised, to receive all the support and information they require.

14.5 Moh Golden Points and Summary Question Answers

14.5.1 Moh Golden Points

Clinical decision-making must be informed by a patient-centered approach, ensuring decisions are tailored to individual patient needs, preferences, and values.

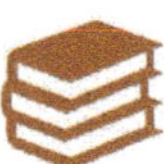
Evidence-based practice (EBP) and pharmacokinetics go hand-in-hand in providing accurate diagnoses and effective treatments. Pharmacokinetics is the science of how the body absorbs, distributes, metabolizes, and excretes drugs.

Recognizing red-flag symptoms such as unexplained weight loss, chest pain, or persistent fatigue is crucial. These symptoms may signal severe underlying conditions such as cancer or cardiovascular disease.

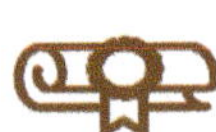
Pharmacodynamics focuses on how drugs interact with the body and receptors to produce their effects.

For patients with chronic conditions, regular medication reviews, careful monitoring, and clear communication are key.

Collaboration among healthcare teams is vital to improve patient outcomes. Effective communication—both within the healthcare team and with the patient—ensures that all relevant information is shared.

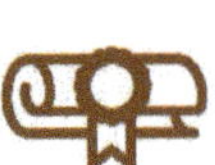
Healthcare professionals must continually engage in learning and reflective practice to enhance decision-making skills.

14.5.2 Summary Questions & Answers

1. What is the primary role of the pharmacist in identifying red-flag symptoms?
A. To diagnose the condition
B. To escalate the patient to the appropriate healthcare provide
C. To administer immediate treatment
D. To provide over-the-counter remedies

2. Which of the following is a pharmacokinetic interaction?
A. Two drugs enhancing each other's therapeutic effects
B. One drug affecting the absorption or metabolism of another drug
C. One drug blocking a receptor in the body
D. Two drugs causing an opposing effect on the body's systems

3. What does the term 'pharmacodynamics' refer to?
A. How the body absorbs, distributes, metabolizes, and excretes a drug
B. How drugs interact with body receptors to produce their effects
C. How drugs are chemically altered in the liver
D. How a drug passes through the blood-brain barrier

4. Which red-flag symptom is indicative of a potential myocardial infarction (heart attack)?
A. Right-sided chest pain after exercise
B. Central, crushing chest pain radiating to the back and jaw
C. Left-sided chest pain after a stressful event
D. Pain after eating fatty foods

5. Which of the following would be considered a red-flag symptom related to cancer?
A. Chronic cough lasting more than 3 weeks with unexplained weight loss
B. Headache with mild fever
C. Abdominal discomfort after eating
D. Shortness of breath after exercise

6. Which is a key factor in ensuring safe medication management for chronic conditions?
A. Avoiding all prescription medications
B. Monitoring the patient's medication use and revising prescriptions as needed
C. Prescribing the maximum dose to achieve quick relief
D. Limiting patient communication with healthcare providers

7. What should a healthcare provider do if they identify a red-flag symptom during a patient consultation?
A. Treat the symptom based on their own experience
B. Refer the patient to the appropriate healthcare provider or specialist
C. Ignore the symptom if it seems mild
D. Prescribe over-the-counter medication for immediate relief

8. Which of the following is an example of a safety-netting strategy after identifying a red-flag symptom?
A. Providing a follow-up plan and informing the patient about when to seek further medical attention
B. Discharging the patient immediately after providing medication
C. Giving the patient over-the-counter medication for immediate relief
D. Informing the patient to rest and wait for the symptom to resolve

9. What is the significance of pharmacokinetic interactions in drug therapy?

A. They can change the efficacy of one drug by altering the absorption, metabolism, or excretion of another drug.
B. They lead to immediate side effects, requiring urgent treatment.
C. They only affect the dosage form of a drug, not its pharmacological effect.
D. They occur when two drugs with similar actions are combined.

10. In clinical decision-making, what is the primary function of critical thinking?
A. To follow pre-established protocols without questioning
B. To apply intuition and personal bias to make decisions quickly
C. To evaluate evidence, recognize assumptions, and ensure the decision is evidence-based
D. To rely on gut feelings and past experiences to make quick judgments

14.5.3 Rationales

1. **Answer: B) To escalate the patient to the appropriate healthcare provider**

Rationale: The pharmacist's role in identifying red-flag symptoms is to escalate the patient to the appropriate healthcare provider for further investigation. Pharmacists can identify potential serious conditions but are not the primary diagnosticians.

2. **Answer: B) One drug affecting the absorption or metabolism of another drug**

Rationale: Pharmacokinetic interactions occur when one drug affects the absorption, distribution, metabolism, or excretion of another drug, altering its efficacy or safety profile.

3. **Answer: B) How drugs interact with body receptor to produce their effects**

Rationale: Pharmacodynamics refers to how drugs interact with receptors in the body to produce their therapeutic or adverse effects, distinguishing it from pharmacokinetics.

4. **Answer: B) Central, crushing chest pain radiating to the back and jaw**

Rationale: Central, crushing chest pain radiating to the back and jaw is a classic red-flag symptom of a myocardial infarction (heart attack), requiring immediate referral for urgent care.

5. **Answer: A) Chronic cough lasting more than 3 weeks with unexplained weight loss**

Rationale: A chronic cough lasting more than 3 weeks combined with unexplained weight loss is a red-flag symptom suggesting a potential serious condition, such as cancer, often requiring further diagnostic testing.

6. **Answer: B) Monitoring the patient's medication use and revising prescriptions as needed**

Rationale: Safe medication management in chronic conditions requires regular medication reviews and revisions to ensure that the treatment is still effective, appropriate, and minimizing harm.

7. **Answer: B) Refer the patient to the appropriate healthcare provider or specialist**

Rationale: The provider should refer the patient to the appropriate healthcare provider or specialist for further investigation, ensuring that any serious condition is promptly addressed.

8. **Answer: A) Providing a follow-up plan and informing the patient about when to seek further medical attention**

Rationale: Safety-netting involves providing the patient with a clear follow-up plan and instructions on when to seek further medical attention if symptoms worsen or do not improve.

9. **Answer: A) They can change the efficacy of one drug by altering the absorption, metabolism, or excretion of another drug**

Rationale: Pharmacokinetic interactions can alter the bioavailability of a drug, thereby changing its efficacy or risk profile, which is crucial for ensuring patient safety.

10. **Answer: C) To evaluate evidence, recognize assumptions, and ensure the decision is evidence-based**

Rationale: Critical thinking involves evaluating evidence, challenging assumptions, and ensuring that clinical decisions are made based on the best available information, not just intuition or bias.

15 Chapter 15: Family Nurse Practitioner's Role in Disease Prevention, Health Promotion, and Advanced Clinical Skills

15.1 Health Promotion and Disease Prevention

15.1.1 Nutrition, Physical Activity, and Lifestyle Modifications

Health promotion strategies are known to reduce nutrient deficiencies, diseases of inactivity like obesity, diabetes, and cardiovascular diseases through nutrition, physical activity, and appropriate change of lifestyle. **There is an opportunity for nurses to support patient decisions on what changes in dietary habits, choosing whole foods on the negative impact of processed food and high fat food products in the long run.** Also, it is important to encourage people to exercise to avoid obesity, reduce risks of heart diseases, and boosting energy levels. **The goal of moderate exercise should be achieved and include 150 minutes of aerobic activity in a week to lower the risks of chronic diseases.** It goes without saying that physical changes do not only include but are not limited to the restriction of certain foods and types of food, regular exercising, an important aspect of lifestyle alterations is stress, sleep, cessation of smoking and moderate use of alcohol. According to the stipulations by the ANA, FNPs play a central role of educating the patient on the implications of such changes, assisting him or her in outlining realistic goals, and then providing support towards achieving those goals in the future. Thus, collaborating with patients, FNPs can develop precise strategies based on change objective and realistic and catering to a patient's needs for improving her well-being and quality of life.

15.1.2 Vaccination Schedules and Preventative Measures

Vaccination has been described as one of the most effective tools and widespread in disease prevention. The necessity of vaccinations and following the strict vaccination schedule is one of the topics that **Family Nurse Practitioners should explain to the patient.** Vaccination is also important for the welfare of any human being and for developing the herd immunity which curb spread of pathogens in society. Some of the vaccination schedules provided by CDC include the child and adolescent vaccination, adult medical immunization recommendations, and vaccines for the special concern including flu, measles, chickenpox, hepatitis, and pneumonia among others. Thus, **FNPs have to ensure that patients know concerning the correct time for the relevant vaccinations to be administered.** Besides immunizations, enacted approach to reduction in the rates of diseases includes otherwise healthy routine examinations, cancer health examinations, and check-ups for clients with chronic health conditions. Through providing such a service and enhancing the knowledge of the patients regarding the necessity of such services, **FNPs contribute to decreased health costs, principally by decreasing the likelihood of the developement of such diseases.**

15.1.3 Mental Health and Substance Use Counseling

Counseling in mental health and substance use is therefore critical components of preventive healthcare and health enhancement. **The situation indicates that Family Nurse Practitioners are in a unique position to notice signs of mental illness, including depression, anxiety and stress, and substance use disorders.** Mental health issues should not be overlooked because if the early symptoms are not addressed it would lead to emergence of severe mental disorders. FNPs can diagnose mental disorders by interviewing patients, offer brief therapy, and if necessary, refer them to psychiatrists or counselors. Moreover, they can prevent substance use issues by availing treatments such as counseling, and assist those who wish to cut down on substance abuse, use of alcohol, tobacco, and other drugs. **The care of the mind is as important as the body since without proper treatment of the mind, the health, and relationships are affected, and vice versa.** Additionally, integrating substance use counseling into a broader context of patients' well-being may help them improve their lifestyles. Since an FNP is a vital member of the patient-centered care team, FNPs deconstruct stigmatization, encourage dialogues regarding mental health, and facilitate patients' access to relevant care which enables them to demystify the process and assist in recovery.

15.2 Chronic Disease Management

15.2.1 Skills in Managing Chronic Conditions (Diabetes, Hypertension, Heart Diseases)

It must be noted that chronic disease management is a complex process that involves the assessment, diagnosis, and treatment of different diseases such as diabetes, hypertension, and heart diseases; **FNPs have an essential role to play in the management of these diseases. This includes assessment of the intensity of diabetes, blood glucose levels, treatment to proper diet and physical activity as well as medication regime, and several complications of diabetes, as neuropathy and retinopathy**. Hypertension management involves the anticipation of patient's compliance to antihypertensive medications, frequent checks of blood pressure, and providing a suggestive strategy of lifestyle alterations like diet, exercise and losing weight. Concerning heart issues, FNPs assess for chest pain, fatigue, shortness of breath and they prevent further advancement of the conditions with medications like statins and beta-blockers. **The comorbidities are also a factor that is sometimes managed by other specialists and therefore FNPs need to evaluate the patient's overall picture.** Through constant knowledge and implementation of the clinical standards, FNP enables patients diagnosed with these chronic diseases to receive proper care toward the enhancement of their health status.

15.2.2 Lifestyle Interventions and Pharmacological Support

It has been observed that implementing annual lifestyle changes can have a very positive impact on such chronic diseases as diabetes, hypertension, or heart disease. The major activities that Family Nurse Practitioners in the northeastern region engage in the process of working with patients include healthy diet pattern, exercise, and smoking cessation. For example in diabetes care, FNPs help in training diabetes self-management, involving aspects such as counting of carbohydrates, portion control as well as exercise on how it affects the blood sugar level. **Some diet related to hypertension consist of decreased sodium intake and increase potassium intake of food products which highly influence the blood pressure level**. However, medical treatment using drugs is usually needed for the effective treatment of these conditions. They order medicines to be given to patients such as insulin or oral hypoglycemics for diabetes, antihypertensive for high blood pressure and statins or anticoagulant for heart disease. **A major aspect of chronic diseases involves medication management and since FNPs are trained to be primary caregivers** they must ensure that the patient understand how to use a medication, any side effects that may occur, and why they have to strictly adhere to the given regimen. Incorporating lifestyle modifications in addition to the use of medications, FNPs allow their clients the best treatment for chronic diseases.

15.2.3 Monitoring and Educating Patients

Educational interventions, as part of patient center care, and constant follow-up are crucial in managing chronic conditions. It is necessary to report, that the Family Nurse Practitioners are involved in monitoring the patient's condition through follow-up visits, tests, and laboratory tests. The major services provided to patients with chronic disease include assessment of glucometry, blood pressure and cholesterol levels in diabetic, hypertensive and cardiovascular diseases respectively. Therefore, through constant examination during the follow-up visit, the FNPs will be able to recognize developing problems like diabetic foot ulcers or hypertensive crisis that may worsen if not addressed on timely basis. **Also, it is crucial to communicate and fan educate the patients so that they may have sole responsibility of their health.** From the aforementioned facts, it is evident that FNP patients are taught on self-management skills, management of symptoms and signs that indicate worsening of condition. These are important in enabling patients to make informed choices pertaining to their health, for instance the time to review the medications and seek a doctors attention. **Educating patients and being supportive enables the FNPs to provide the patients with key information which will enable them to take the necessary steps needed when it comes to their health.**

15.3 Cultural Competency in Family Care

15.3.1 Understanding and Addressing Diverse Patient Needs

Cultural competency plays a critical role in enhancing FNP's ability to provide care to culturally diverse patient populations. Knowledge of cultural, ethnic, and socioeconomic aspects is particularly useful, since **FNPs approach patients with focus on their cultural and ethnical background and their preferences and values.** People from different cultures may have different perceptions over health and diseases and different ways of seeking for cure. These needs may vary, and FNP need to take these in to consideration in order to avoid creating any discomfort to the patients. This entails attending to the patient, especially by using questions that cannot be answered **with a simple yes or no answer and recognizing the role and impact of cultures in patient's behaviors.** They also need to have adequate information on cultures when it comes to family matters, roles and responsibilities, decision-making and communication. **Thus, incorporating cultural competence into those aspects of FNP education and training will increase the chances of FNP's delivering culturally appropriate patient-centered care while improving patient satisfaction and trust in healthcare services.**

15.3.2 Patient-Centered Care

Patient-centered care is one of the core values in family care that seeks to capture the patient's interests, including their choice and values, in the medical treatment decision. One of the approaches that are employed by **FNP is patient-centered care where the interests of the client are valued, and they work together with the practitioner.** This approach also creates hope for patients meaning they are not only the receivers of care but they play an active role in their health plan. More importantly, FNPs practice patient-centered care to ensure that they know the goals, the issues of concern, and expected outcomes of their clients. **The physicians and specialist are understanding and patient while explaining illnesses, the available cures and explicit advantages and disadvantages of each potential solution.** It also includes psychological aspect, which include giving emotional support and consideration of other issues that may affect the client physically, mentally or socially. Thus, the positive patient attitudes towards FNPs can be assumed to result from the enhanced satisfaction with the healthcare service and increased focus on individual patients promoted by FNPs. This makes care to be holistic, responsive and to value the life situation of the patient.

15.3.3 Overcoming Healthcare Access Barriers

Getting to medical care can sometimes be difficult for some people especially those in the underprivileged or minority groups. **By understanding these barriers, it is easier for Family**

Nurse Practitioners to tackle and eliminate challenges that may include financial restraints, geographical locations, language barriers as well as lack of transportation. For instance, FNPs can support their patient by giving them details about the availability of affordable or even charitable healthcare services and helping them attempt to get insurance payments. Moreover, FNPs have an ability to alleviate the problem in terms of accessibility through the use of telecommunication technology to offer remote health services or partner with community-based agencies to enhance service delivery in rural areas. **Cultural differences can be handled through such approaches as the use of friendly language, using of an interpreter or providing materials which portray culture that is familiar to the patient.** FNPs can also inform themselves in the fight against racism by embracing equality in the care of black and other ethnic peoples and putting pressure oneри organizations to adopt policies that advance the cause of the black community and any other discriminated group. In this way, due to the fact that FNPs are always aware of obstacles specific to particular patients, they work to help everyone and contribute to improvement of health equity and results in incomparable for some individuals.

15.4 Advanced Clinical Skills

15.4.1 Advanced Diagnostic Techniques

Improved clinical competencies in assessment and diagnosis are crucial for the FNP to identify various physical health conditions. Several facets are seen to be due to the use of advanced **diagnostic tools that allows FNPs to assess a patient holistically and at an initial stage of the disease.** One of the main functions that outline the concept of advanced diagnostic competencies includes knowledge in the interpretation of result findings in laboratory, and radiological images. Blood tests are samples which can give information on **the metabolic activity of an individual, the efficiency of vital internal organs, and infections or diseases**. Examples of useful biomarkers include cholesterol, liver enzymes and kidney functions that can provide information on the condition of heart and kidneys respectively. Similarly, some areas in structure, tumors, broken bones, and other conditions that cannot be diagnosed through physical examination and observation can be identified through **medical imaging like X-ray, MRI or CT scans among others**. Moreover, the results have to be combined with the overall clinical picture presented by the patient to come up with the right diagnosis in the case of FNPs. It does not only involve technical workforce but also understanding on how to communicate health information to the patients in a way that patients understand so that they can participate in decision making.

15.4.2 Managing Complex Cases

The typical complex cases which require an enhancement and a stronger level of clinical competency include those cases that **present with co-morbidity, risk and symptom complexities. FNP's has major responsibility in managing a patient's care plan of clients within varying stages of treatment with chronic health conditions and diseases and comorbidities with multi-system presentations.** One of the important competencies, which can be related to case management, is information integration of patient history, physical examination, possible diagnostic tests, and consultation with the other practitioners. In performing their work, FNPs should be able to determine strategies for providing care, keeping in mind both the short-term as well as the long-term care plan for the patient. This may involve using drugs therapeutically with varying patient lifestyle changes, integrating with other physicians and health care workers, and providing extensive education to patients in understanding and accepting the medical regimens. Also, **the management of complicated instances involves assessing or looking for signs of deterioration or variation in the patients or changing the treatment plan accordingly and coordinating follow-ups.** It is also important that FNPs learn to solve various decision-making problems that pertain in health matters including dealing with ethical issues or patient's expectations especially in cases where the patient's condition is critically ill and chances of extending life are rare. Instead, the patient should receive comprehensive and evidence-based care that takes into consideration the variouscolourcoded aspects of his or her case.

15.4.3 Assessing Lab Results and Medical Imaging

Specialised procedures are essential for fast and accurate diagnosis in difficult situations. It is also essential for **Family Nurse Practitioners (FNPs) to be knowledgeable in the interpretation of laboratory results and medical imaging.** Basic tests include tests that determine the patient's metabolic status, infection, and general health: Lab tests include blood tests, urine test, and cultures. For instance, high blood glucose levels may point to diabetes whereas high or low lipid profile can be suggestive of cardiovascular disease. However, **FNPs need to consider such results in relation to the patient's signs and symptoms and overall history.** Diagnostic imaging like, x-ray, MRI and CT offer a clearer picture of internal human body organs and limbs. The FNP has to analyze these images to look for signs of fracture line, tumors, indications of chronic diseases such as osteoarthritis. **The understanding of these results put the FNPs in a position to make decisions as well as to begin interventions and observe changes or deterioration of patients**.

15.4.4 Interpreting Diagnostic Tests

Interpretation of diagnostic tests not only involves importance of clinical decision making but also includes critical caring thinking. Family Nurse Practitioners can specify the problem given the results from blood test, imaging and specific screenings. **For instance, a normal ECG of a patient may show the existence of some rhythm disturbances or heart diseases, and blood tests, thyroid function tests, help in diagnosing hypothyroidism or hyperthyroidism.** Other aspect that FNPs should note is the fallacy of affirming the consequent, they should always compare the test result with other symptoms, risk factors, and history of the patient. They should also undertake rigorous testing limits so as to avoid circumstances where false negative of positive results in conducting relevant tests. Besides, FNPs explain offers and results to the patients in terms that the latter can easily comprehend in order to facilitate their physical treatment. Such an approach greatly involves patients in their treatment process and care to enhance their adherence to the treatment plan.

15.5 Legal and Ethical Responsibilities of FNP

15.5.1 Professional Ethical Challenges

Ethical dilemmas arise when individuals struggling to make decision involving clients, employers, society, self and profession or legal requirements, **for FNPs some of the areas of practice include; Ethical issues can present themselves in the context of patient treatment**, which may include decisions made on whether or not to procure treatment for a patient where the patient is in a vegetative state or a persistent vegetative state or in terminally ill patients, consent to treatment by patients, privacy violation and cases where the patient's wishes do not align with the physician's recommended procedures. **For example, an FNP may come across a patient who refuses to take some treatments despite being alive since they have certain beliefs that go against the grounds of an FNP** or due to their culture they speak against a certain treatment, this makes the FNP to experience a dilemma of either respecting the wish of the patient or the rules and regulations of the practice and the ethical consideration of the health care profession. Further, an FNP should support the rights of such groups as Minors or individuals with mental health issues, and the aspect of capacity and consent may be an issue. There are also ethical dilemmas arising from specific patients' information, especially in the healthcare sector, where the practitioners must demonstrate **different levels of patient confidentiality regarding statutory guidelines**

including HIPAA. In such circumstances, the FNPs should apply some ethical principles, including beneficence, non-maleficence, and justice. They also need to be current with their state's codes of professional conduct and cooperation with other healthcare professionals and the ethical committees whenever need arise so as to ensure that the needs of the patients are met legally and ethically.

15.5.2 Supervision, Licensure, and Practice Requirements

The performance of FNP is regulated by licensure and supervision rules and regulation whereby every state or country has its policies to enhance the safety of their patients and over-see the FNPs to ensure the offer right services within their practice. **Typically, the requirements for the FNPs to practice include having a valid RN license, and an APRN license in the area that one specializes in, this requires one to undergo a master's or doctoral degree in nursing as well as passing the national certification examination.** Licensure shows that FNPs are qualified for practice and that they observe the right standard to offer protections to patients. In addition, FNPs are mandated by the governing bodies to continue with education to update their knowledge with the current practice of healthcare and recommendations. However, supervision is the other key determinant in FNP practice after one acquires a license. In some states of the United States, FNPs may require practicing under the supervision of a physician or even collaboration in the context of a supervisory model and especially for diagnosis and prescription of treatments. While some states provide full practice authority that enables FNPs to practice independently some restrict entailing the following. **These policies as pertain to regulation are intended to safeguard both the healthcare consumer and the professional nurse in the position of the FNP to conform to the required professional conduct and standards** as well as practice safe clinical procedure. It is important for the FNPs to understand the legal regulation of their practice regarding the supervisory mechanisms, the procedure for getting licensed and the scope of practice acts.

15.6 Documentation Tools

15.6.1 SOAP Notes Template

Table 269 SOAP Notes Template

Section	Details
S: Subjective	- **Patient Information:** 24-year-old non-smoking female, accountant - **Presenting Complaint:** Frequent unilateral headaches with vomiting, nausea, and light sensitivity for one year, worsening over the last 20 days. - **Pain Description:** Unilateral, throbbing, sharp pain, 8/10 intensity. Dark room and sleep help reduce pain. - **Frequency:** 2-3 times a week at different times. - **Medications:** Tylenol 500mg PO (ineffective). - **Associated Symptoms:** No blurred vision, fever, body aches, sinus pain, rhinorrhea, cough, or chest pain. - **Past Medical History:** Denies chronic diseases or recent weight changes. - **Allergies:** None reported.
O: Objective	- **Vital Signs:** - HR = 90 bpm, regular - RR = 20 bpm - Temperature = 36.6°C (oral) - BP = 125/80 mmHg - SPO2 = 98% on room air - **Physical Exam:** - Height: 171 cm, Weight: 78 kg, BMI: 26.7 - Skin: Intact, no rashes or lesions - HEENT: Normocephalic, equal hair distribution, no tenderness, clear conjunctivae, no redness or jaundice, PERRLA, 20/30 vision without correction, TM clear, no discharge - Neck: Supple, anterior cervical lymph

	tender - Cardiovascular: Normal S1, S2, no murmurs - Abdomen: Normal bowel sounds, non-tender, no organomegaly - Cranial nerves I-XII: Intact
A: Assessment	- **Primary Diagnosis:** Migraine headache with aura - **Supporting Signs:** Frequent unilateral throbbing pain, vomiting, nausea, light sensitivity, and relief with sleep.
P: Plan	- **Medications:** - Sumatriptan 25mg PO PRN (as needed) - Gravol 50mg PO Q6hr PRN - **Monitoring:** Blood pressure monitoring - **Instructions:** - Take Sumatriptan as prescribed and seek help if ineffective. - Start Sumatriptan at the onset of symptoms, don't wait until they worsen. - Rest in a dark room during episodes. - Drink 6-8 glasses of fluid daily. - **Tests:** Blood work (CBC, Lytes, INR, Vit D, LFT, KFT, ESR, C-reactive protein). - **Follow-up:** In one month - **Referral:** Neurologist referral given.

15.6.2 Case Study Template

S: This ___ yr old fe/male presents for ____

History of Present Illness symptoms:
Review Of Symptoms/Systems: (For problem-focused visit, document only pertinent information)
Past Medical History: (For problem-focused visit, document only pertinent information)
Current Medications:
Medication allergies:
Social History: (For problem-focused visit, document only pertinent information)
Family History: ((For problem-focused visit, document only pertinent information)
Genogram: 3 generations with health problems, causes of deaths, etc.
or
History of major health or genetic disorders in family, including early death, spontaneous abortions or stillbirths

O: (listed are the components of the all normal physical exam)

General: Well appearing, well nourished, in no distress. Oriented x 3, normal mood and affect . Ambulating without difficulty.
Skin: Good turgor, no rash, unusual bruising or prominent lesions
Hair: Normal texture and distribution.
Nails: Normal color, no deformities
HEENT:
Head: Normocephalic, atraumatic, no visible or palpable masses, depressions, or scaring.
Eyes: Visual acuity intact, conjunctiva clear, sclera non-icteric, EOM intact, PERRL, fundi have normal optic discs and vessels, no exudates or hemorrhages
Ears: EACs clear, TMs translucent & mobile, ossicles nl appearance, hearing intact.
Nose: No external lesions, mucosa non-inflamed, septum and turbinates normal
Mouth: Mucous membranes moist, no mucosal lesions.
Teeth/Gums: No obvious caries or periodontal disease. No gingival inflammation or significant resorption.
Pharynx: Mucosa non-inflamed, no tonsillar hypertrophy or exudate
Neck: Supple, without lesions, bruits, or adenopathy, thyroid non-enlarged and non-tender
Heart: No cardiomegaly or thrills; regular rate and rhythm, no murmur or gallop
Lungs: Clear to auscultation and percussion
Abdomen: Bowel sounds normal, no tenderness, organomegaly, masses, or hernia
Back: Spine normal without deformity or tenderness, no CVA tenderness
Rectal: Normal sphincter tone, no hemorrhoids or masses palpable
Extremities: No amputations or deformities, cyanosis, edema or varicosities, peripheral pulses intact
Musculoskeletal: Normal gait and station. No misalignment, asymmetry, crepitation, defects, tenderness, masses, effusions, decreased range of motion, instability, atrophy or abnormal strength or tone in the head, neck, spine, ribs, pelvis or extremities.
Neurologic: CN 2-12 normal. Sensation to pain, touch, and proprioception normal. DTRs normal in upper and lower extremities. No pathologic reflexes.
Psychiatric: Oriented X3, intact recent and remote memory, judgment and insight, normal mood and affect.
Pelvic: Vagina and cervix without lesions or discharge. Uterus and adnexa/parametria nontender without masses.

A:

Assessment:
Includes health status and need for lifestyle changes.
Diagnosis and differential diagnosis:

P:

Laboratory:
X-Rays:
Medications:
Patient Education:
Other:

Follow-up:

15.7 Moh Golden Points and Summary Question Answers

15.7.1 Moh Golden Points

FNPs play a crucial role in promoting health through education on nutrition, physical activity, and lifestyle changes to prevent chronic diseases such as diabetes, hypertension, and cardiovascular diseases.

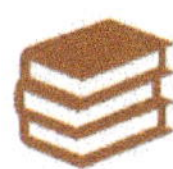

Being culturally competent fosters better communication, reduces misunderstandings, and promotes patient trust, which enhances treatment adherence and overall outcomes.

Managing chronic conditions such as diabetes, hypertension, and heart disease involves more than just prescribing medications.

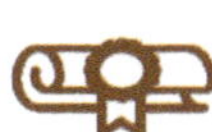

FNPs play a pivotal role in educating patients about vaccines and ensuring that individuals of all ages stay up to date with necessary immunization.

Family Nurse Practitioners need advanced skills in interpreting lab results, medical imaging, and diagnostic tests.

In a patient-centered approach, the FNP respects and incorporates the patient's preferences, values, and goals into the treatment plan.

FNPs work to eliminate these barriers by providing accessible care, advocating for resources, and ensuring that all patients receive timely medical attention regardless of their background or financial situation.

15.7.2 Summary Questions & Answers

1. Which of the following is a primary focus of Family Nurse Practitioners (FNPs) in chronic disease management? A) Prescribing medications only B) Focusing solely on acute care C) Providing patient education and lifestyle interventions D) Refer patients to specialists without providing care
2. What is the primary goal of cultural competency in family care? A) To eliminate cultural differences B) To tailor care based on a patient's cultural background C) To provide care without considering cultural factors D) To focus only on clinical symptoms
3. In managing diabetes, which of the following is a key lifestyle intervention that FNPs may recommend? A) Increasing sugar intake to boost energy B) Reducing physical activity to conserve energy C) Encouraging regular physical activity and balanced diet D) Limiting medication use as much as possible
4. Which of the following best describes patient-centered care? A) Focusing only on the physical aspects of patient health B) Prioritizing the doctor's preferences in care decisions C) Involving patients in their own treatment decisions and respecting their preferences D) Minimizing patient interaction with healthcare professionals
5. Which of the following is a key skill required for FNPs when managing complex cases? A) Avoiding interdisciplinary collaboration B) Simplifying patient care to treat only the primary condition C) Synthesizing information from various diagnostic tools and sources D) Ignoring patient preferences to focus on clinical data
6. What is the role of vaccinations in disease prevention? A) Vaccines only prevent minor illnesses B) Vaccines contribute to herd immunity and reduce disease transmission C) Vaccines are used to treat infections D) Vaccines have no role in prevention
7. Which of the following is a primary concern when interpreting lab results for chronic disease management? A) Relying only on one test to diagnose a condition B) Ignoring the patient's history and clinical presentation C) Integrating lab results with the patient's overall health status and symptoms D) Focusing solely on abnormal test results
8. A key aspect of overcoming healthcare access barriers is: A) Limiting access to healthcare for certain populations B) Providing care only in urban areas C) Addressing financial, social, and geographic barriers to care D) Ignoring patient concerns about healthcare access
9. In which of the following situations would an FNP be most likely to intervene with mental health counseling?

A) When a patient is experiencing physical symptoms only
B) When a patient shows signs of depression or anxiety
C) When a patient refuses all forms of treatment
D) When a patient has no history of mental health concerns

10. Which of the following is most important when managing patients with multiple chronic conditions?

A) Prescribing as many medications as possible
B) Focusing only on the primary condition
C) Coordinating care and monitoring all aspects of the patient's health
D) Avoiding any lifestyle changes to simplify care

15.7.3 Rationales

1. **Answer: C) Providing patient education and lifestyle interventions**

Rationale: FNPs take a holistic approach to chronic disease management, emphasizing the importance of patient education, lifestyle changes, and medication adherence to manage conditions such as diabetes, hypertension, and heart disease.

2. **Answer: B) To tailor care based on a patient's cultural background**

Rationale: Cultural competency allows FNPs to provide care that respects and integrates a patient's cultural beliefs, values, and preferences, leading to more effective and personalized care.

3. **Answer: C) Encouraging regular physical activity and balanced diet**

Rationale: Lifestyle interventions, including regular exercise and a healthy, balanced diet, are essential for managing blood sugar levels in diabetes and preventing complications.

4. **Answer: C) Involving patients in their own treatment decisions and respecting their preferences**

Rationale: Patient-centered care emphasizes collaboration between healthcare providers and patients, respecting the patient's values, needs, and desires to achieve the best outcomes.

5. **Answer: C) Synthesizing information from various diagnostic tools and sources**

Rationale: FNPs must integrate data from multiple sources, including diagnostic tests, patient history, and clinical presentation, to manage complex cases effectively.

6. **Answer: B) Vaccines contribute to herd immunity and reduce disease transmission**

Rationale: Vaccines help prevent the spread of infectious diseases, protect individuals from illness, and contribute to herd immunity, which decreases the overall transmission of disease in the community.

7. **Answer: C) Integrating lab results with the patient's overall health status and symptoms**

Rationale: Interpreting lab results in conjunction with the patient's medical history, physical exam, and symptoms allows FNPs to make accurate diagnoses and provide appropriate treatment.

8. **Answer: C) Addressing financial, social, and geographic barriers to care**

Rationale: FNPs work to ensure all patients have access to healthcare, regardless of their financial status, location, or other barriers that may prevent them from receiving care.

9. **Answer: B) When a patient shows signs of depression or anxiety**

Rationale: FNPs are trained to recognize the signs of mental health issues such as depression and anxiety and provide counseling or referrals to mental health professionals for further care.

10. **Answer: C) Coordinating care and monitoring all aspects of the patient's health**

Rationale: Managing patients with multiple chronic conditions requires a comprehensive approach that includes coordinated care, ongoing monitoring, and addressing all aspects of the patient's health, including lifestyle interventions and medication management.

16 Chapter 6: Golden Rules for Family Nurse Practitioners (FNPs)

16.1 Standard Screening Diseases

Table 270 Standard Screening Disease Consideration for Different Age Groups

Population	What the FNP Says	Clinical Note
Newborns	"I am assessing a newborn. As per standard neonatal screening, I will begin with congenital hearing assessment using OAE or AABR to evaluate cochlear and brainstem response."	→ Hearing screening completed using otoacoustic emissions or auditory brainstem response; recommended by the RUSP and AAP Joint Committee on Infant Hearing (JCIH).
	"Next, I will check oxygen saturation using pulse oximetry to rule out critical congenital heart disease."	→ Pulse oximetry completed; detects hypoxemia associated with congenital heart defects. Recommended as part of RUSP screenings.
	"Now to metabolic screening: a heel-prick blood sample is taken to test for heritable disorders such as PKU, hypothyroidism, sickle cell anemia, and cystic fibrosis."	→ Dried blood spot analysis pending/within normal limits; screens for 35 core conditions recommended by the RUSP to prevent disability or mortality.
	"If maternal Hepatitis B status is positive, I will administer HBIG and the first dose of the Hepatitis B vaccine within 12 hours of birth."	→ Timely administration reduces risk of chronic hepatitis B infection; CDC and AAP recommended protocol.
	"For infants with risk factors like NICU stay >5 days or ototoxic drug exposure, I will ensure follow-up diagnostic audiologic evaluation by 3 to 9 months."	→ As per JCIH guidelines, follow-up and ongoing surveillance needed for progressive or delayed-onset hearing loss.
	"For infants born to mothers with congenital infections such as CMV, Zika, or rubella, or with craniofacial anomalies, I will initiate early diagnostic hearing testing."	→ These infants are at higher risk for sensorineural hearing loss; recommendation based on JCIH 2019 and CDC surveillance strategies.

Infants/Children (0-18 yrs)	"I will now evaluate a toddler. Starting with vision—screening for strabismus and amblyopia at ages 3 to 5 is standard. I'll ask the child to identify shapes or letters."	→ Vision grossly intact; no deviation, corrected vision if required.
	"For hearing, I'll observe speech development and conduct otoacoustic testing if delays are noted."	→ Speech development age-appropriate; no red flags.
	"Developmental screening is next; I will assess for autism signs at 18 and 24 months using M-CHAT."	→ No repetitive behaviors or social deficits noted.
	"Lead exposure will be evaluated through blood test at 12-24 months if environmental risks are present."	→ No lead exposure risk; levels WNL if tested.
	"Iron deficiency anemia screening will be performed for at-risk children, especially those with poor diets."	→ Hgb checked, dietary counseling provided.
	"I will monitor BMI starting at age 2 and ensure all immunizations are up to date per CDC schedule."	→ BMI percentile documented; immunization schedule verified and updated.
Adolescents (18-21 yrs)	"This is an 18-year-old presenting for annual physical. I'll begin with blood pressure screening, ensuring measurements are within normative ranges."	→ BP 118/76, within normal limits.
	"Lipid screening will be ordered if patient is obese or has family history of heart disease."	→ Total cholesterol within range or pending results.
	"Now I will assess for STIs—HIV, gonorrhea, chlamydia—based on sexual activity and risk profile."	→ Chlamydia screening collected via urine NAAT; counseling provided.

	"Pap smear to be performed if sexually active and over age 21, per USPSTF guidelines."	→ Counseling given, test planned for next visit.
	"Next, I will conduct a mental health screening using PHQ-9 and assess suicide risk."	→ PHQ-9 score within mild range; no suicidal ideation.
	"Obesity screening will include BMI, diet recall, and physical activity evaluation."	→ BMI 28; nutrition and activity counseling provided.
Adults (22-39 yrs)	"I am assessing a 30-year-old adult for preventive care. Blood pressure will be measured and compared with past records."	→ BP remains stable; follow-up in 2 years if normal.
	"I will request lipid panel every five years or sooner if risks like smoking or diabetes are present."	→ Cholesterol results WNL, lifestyle reinforced.
	"STI screening is indicated based on risk profile; patient consents to annual testing."	→ Screening ordered, education provided.
	"If skin cancer risk is high due to sun exposure or family history, I will inspect nevi and advise dermatology follow-up."	→ Nevi symmetric and stable; patient advised self-monitoring.
	"Mental health screening and substance use history will be documented."	→ No depressive symptoms; alcohol use within moderate limits.
Adults (40-64 yrs)	"This patient is 50 years old. I begin with annual blood pressure check and lipid profile every 5 years."	→ BP elevated; lifestyle intervention discussed.
	"Diabetes screening using fasting glucose or HbA1c is indicated beginning at age 45."	→ HbA1c ordered, prior values elevated.
	"I will counsel patient on colorectal cancer screening. Colonoscopy recommended every 10 years starting at age 45."	→ Patient scheduled for colonoscopy; no prior history.
	"For women, mammography is recommended biennially from age 50 to 74."	→ Last mammogram 1 year ago, next due in 12 months.

	"Men with risk factors will be educated on prostate screening options and PSA."	→ Patient informed; decision deferred to next visit.
	"Osteoporosis risk evaluated in women ≥65 or earlier if fracture risk present."	→ DEXA scan ordered based on FRAX score.
	"Depression and substance use screenings repeated annually."	→ Negative screen, coping mechanisms reinforced.
Older Adults (65+ yrs)	"This is a 70-year-old patient. I will start with annual BP and cholesterol checks."	→ BP 134/78, lipid panel due in 6 months.
	"Colorectal cancer screening continues as long as patient has >10 years life expectancy."	→ Recent colonoscopy 3 years ago; within guideline.
	"Assessing vision and hearing for signs of presbyopia or presbycusis."	→ Mild hearing loss noted; audiology referral placed.
	"Osteoporosis screening performed for women and at-risk men using DEXA."	→ T-score -2.3; calcium/Vitamin D and weight-bearing exercise discussed.
	"Cognitive screening using Mini-Cog or MMSE for dementia and delirium signs."	→ Screening WNL; no signs of decline.
	"Immunization status reviewed: flu (annual), shingles, pneumonia, and Tdap updated."	→ Vaccines administered per CDC guideline.

16.2 Common Disease Screenings by Condition

16.2.1 A. Cardiovascular Disease (CVD) Screening

Table 271 Cardiovascular Screening Considerations

Condition	What the FNP Says	Clinical Note
Blood Pressure	"I will check your blood pressure today. For adults with normal readings, this should be repeated every 2 years, or yearly if previously elevated."	→ Adults ≥18 years should be screened every 2 years if BP <120/80 mmHg, and annually if ≥120/80 mmHg. Elevated BP may indicate risk for CVD and requires intervention. (USPSTF, ACC/AHA 2017)
Cholesterol	"We'll check your lipid panel, especially since you're over 20. High-risk patients may require more frequent screening."	→ Lipid screening every 4-6 years for low-risk adults ≥20; annually for those with diabetes, hypertension, or family history of premature heart disease. (ACC/AHA Guidelines)

Diabetes	"Since you're over 45, or have risk factors like obesity or hypertension, I recommend diabetes screening with fasting glucose or HbA1c."	→ Screen every 3 years starting at age 45, or earlier if risk factors are present. Tests include FPG, HbA1c, or OGTT. (USPSTF, ADA 2023)
Aortic Aneurysm	"You're a male between 65 and 75 with a smoking history; we'll order a one-time abdominal ultrasound to screen for aneurysm."	→ One-time abdominal ultrasound recommended for men 65-75 years who have ever smoked. Helps detect AAA before rupture. (USPSTF Grade B)

16.2.2 B. Cancer Screening

Table 272 Cancer Screening Considerations

Cancer Type	What the FNP Says	Clinical Note
Breast Cancer	"If you're between 50 and 74, a mammogram every 2 years is recommended. We'll consider earlier screening if you're high risk."	→ Biennial mammography for women 50-74; start earlier if BRCA mutation, family history, or high-risk factors are present. (USPSTF, ACS)
Cervical Cancer	"We'll do a Pap smear. If it's normal, repeat in 3 years. If combined with HPV test and both are negative, next in 5 years."	→ Women 21-65: Pap every 3 years or every 5 years with HPV co-testing. Early detection lowers cervical cancer mortality. (USPSTF, ACOG)
Colorectal Cancer	"Since you're over 45, it's time for colon cancer screening. Colonoscopy every 10 years or FIT annually are both options."	→ Adults ≥45 should begin screening with colonoscopy (every 10 yrs), FIT (annually), or sigmoidoscopy (every 5 yrs). (USPSTF, ACS 2021)
Lung Cancer	"Given your smoking history, a low-dose CT scan once a year is recommended."	→ Annual low-dose CT scan for adults 50-80 years with ≥20 pack-year smoking history, who currently smoke or quit within the past 15 years. (USPSTF 2021)

16.2.3 C. Infectious Disease Screening

Table 273 Infectious Disease Screening Considerations

Infection	What the FNP Says	Clinical Note
HIV	"As you're sexually active and in a high-risk group, I recommend an HIV test annually."	→ Annual HIV screening for high-risk individuals (MSM, IV drug users, sex workers, multiple partners). One-time test for all adults aged 15-65. (CDC, USPSTF)
Hepatitis B & C	"Due to your background and risk profile, we'll	→ One-time HCV screening for adults 18-79; periodic testing for high-risk populations. HBV testing for healthcare workers, individuals

	check for hepatitis B and C antibodies."	from endemic areas, and IV drug users. (CDC, USPSTF)
Tuberculosis (TB)	"Since you're a healthcare worker or recent immigrant, I'll perform a TB skin test or chest X-ray."	→ Annual or risk-based TB testing via TST or IGRA for high-risk groups like healthcare workers, immigrants, and immunocompromised individuals. (CDC, WHO)

16.3 Special Risk Groups and Screenings

16.3.1 Pregnant Women – Screening Recommendations

Table 274 Screening Considerations for Pregnant Women

Screening	What the FNP Says	Clinical Note
HIV	"At your first prenatal visit, we'll run a standard blood test for HIV to ensure early detection and treatment if needed."	→ Universal HIV screening recommended at first prenatal visit. Early treatment can prevent maternal-to-child transmission. (CDC, USPSTF, ACOG)
Syphilis	"We'll also screen for syphilis at this visit using a simple blood test."	→ Required during early pregnancy; repeated in the third trimester if high risk. Prevents congenital syphilis. (CDC, ACOG)
Gestational Diabetes	"Around 24 to 28 weeks, we'll perform a glucose tolerance test to check for gestational diabetes."	→ One-step or two-step glucose screening recommended at 24-28 weeks. Early management prevents fetal and maternal complications. (ADA, ACOG)
Hepatitis B	"We'll test for hepatitis B as part of your early prenatal labs."	→ All pregnant women should be screened for Hepatitis B during the first trimester to reduce perinatal transmission. (CDC, USPSTF)
Urinary Tract Infection	"We'll do a urine culture in your first trimester to check for any silent urinary infections."	→ Asymptomatic bacteriuria screening recommended early in pregnancy. Untreated cases can lead to pyelonephritis or preterm birth. (USPSTF, ACOG)

16.3.2 B. High-Risk Groups – Targeted Screenings

Table 275 Targetted Screening Considerations for High Risk Groups

High-Risk Group	What the FNP Says	Clinical Note
Obese Individuals	"Due to your BMI, we'll check your HbA1c and cholesterol levels to	→ Obesity is a risk factor for type 2 diabetes and dyslipidemia. Screen

	screen for diabetes and cardiovascular risk."	with HbA1c and lipid panel regularly. (ADA, ACC/AHA)
Smokers	"Because you currently smoke or have smoked heavily in the past, I'll order a low-dose CT for lung cancer screening and evaluate your cardiovascular risk factors."	→ Annual low-dose CT for individuals aged 50-80 with a 20+ pack-year history. Also, screen for hypertension, cholesterol, and peripheral artery disease. (USPSTF, ACC/AHA)

16.4 Vaccination Schedules & Preventative Measures (NHS/CDC Guidelines)

Table 276 Vaccination Schedules and Preventive Measures

Category	Age/Condition	Vaccines Recommended	Trade Names
Pediatric Immunization	8 weeks	6-in-1 (DTaP/IPV/Hib/HepB), Rotavirus, MenB	Infanrix hexa / Vaxelis, Rotarix, Bexsero
	12 weeks	6-in-1 (2nd dose), Rotavirus (2nd dose), Pneumococcal (PCV)	Infanrix hexa / Vaxelis, Rotarix, Prevenar 13
	16 weeks	6-in-1 (3rd dose), MenB (2nd dose)	Infanrix hexa / Vaxelis, Bexsero
	1 year	Hib/MenC, MMR (1st dose), Pneumococcal booster, MenB booster	Menitorix, MMRvaxPro / Priorix, Prevenar 13, Bexsero
	3 years 4 months	MMR (2nd dose), 4-in-1 booster	MMRvaxPro / Priorix, REPEVAX
	2-15 years (annual)	Flu vaccine	Fluenz (nasal spray)
Teenage Immunization	12-13 years	HPV vaccine	Gardasil 9
	14 years	Td/IPV booster, MenACWY	Revaxis, MenQuadfi
Adult Immunization	65 years	Flu (annual), Pneumococcal (PPV23), Shingles	Pneumovax 23, Shingrix
	70-79 years	Shingles vaccine	Zostavax / Shingrix
	75-79 years	RSV vaccine	Abrysvo
	75+ years (Spring/Winter)	COVID-19 vaccine (seasonal)	Various (seasonal update)

Pregnancy	Flu season	Inactivated flu vaccine	Various
	From 16 weeks gestation	Whooping cough (Tdap)	ADACEL
	From 28 weeks gestation	RSV vaccine	Abrysvo
Special Risk: Hep B-exposed Infants	At birth, 4 weeks, 12 months	Hepatitis B	Engerix B / HBvaxPRO
Special Risk: High TB Area Infants	Around 28 days	Tuberculosis	BCG
Clinical Risk: Asplenia/Splenic Dysfunction	All ages	MenACWY, MenB, PCV13, PPV23, Flu	Multiple
Clinical Risk: Cochlear Implants	All ages	PCV13 (≤10 years), PPV23 (≥2 years)	Prevenar 13, Pneumovax 23
Clinical Risk: Chronic Respiratory/ Cardiac Disease	All ages	PCV13, PPV23, Annual Flu	Multiple
Clinical Risk: Diabetes	All ages	PCV13, PPV23, Annual Flu	Multiple
Clinical Risk: Chronic Kidney Disease	Stage 3-5 CKD	PCV13, PPV23, Hep B, Annual Flu	Multiple
Clinical Risk: Chronic Liver Disease	All ages	PCV13, PPV23, Hep A, Hep B, Annual Flu	Multiple
Clinical Risk: Haemophilia	All ages	Hep A, Hep B	Multiple

Clinical Risk: Immunosuppression	All ages	PCV13, PPV23, Shingrix (if ≥50), Annual Flu	Multiple
Clinical Risk: Complement Disorders	All ages	MenACWY, MenB, PCV13, PPV23, Annual Flu	Multiple

16.4.1 Travel Vaccines (NHS/CDC)

Table 277 Travel Vaccine Schedule

Vaccine	Indication	Regions/Conditions	Doses	Notes
Cholera	For travellers to areas with poor sanitation and water hygiene	Africa, Asia, South America	2 doses, 1-6 weeks apart; booster dose if previously vaccinated	Given as a drink. A booster dose is recommended if previously vaccinated.
Dengue	For travellers with a history or risk of dengue	Tropical areas in Africa, Asia, Central/South America, the Caribbean, Pacific Islands	2 doses, 3 months apart	Administered via injection.
Diphtheria	Routine vaccination for polio, diphtheria, and tetanus protection	Africa, Central/Southeast Asia, South America, Haiti, Eastern Europe, Russia	Booster every 10 years if travelling	Additional booster required if more than 10 years since last dose.
Hepatitis A	For travellers to countries with poor sanitation and hygiene	Sub-Saharan and North Africa, Asia, Middle East, South and Central America, Eastern Europe	2 doses, 6-12 months apart	Initial dose at least 2 weeks before departure.
Hepatitis B	For travellers engaging in high-risk activities (e.g., sexual activity, injecting drugs, medical care)	Sub-Saharan Africa, Asia, Middle East, Southern/Eastern Europe, South America	3 doses, spread over 3-6 months	A combined hepatitis A/B vaccine is available.

Japanese Encephalitis	For long-term travellers to rural areas in endemic countries	Asia, including India, China, Japan, Thailand, Indonesia, Laos, Philippines, Cambodia, Vietnam	2 doses, 28 days apart	Ideal for those staying over a month in rural areas.
Meningococcal Meningitis (MenACWY)	For travellers to areas with a high risk of meningococcal disease	Africa, Saudi Arabia during Hajj, Umrah	1 dose, 2-3 weeks before travel	Mandatory for Hajj pilgrims. Babies under 1 year need 2 doses.
Measles, Mumps, Rubella (MMR)	For routine vaccination and travel to areas with endemic measles or mumps	Worldwide	2 doses, 1 month apart	Ensure full vaccination or immunity before travel.
Polio	For travellers to areas with polio risk	Pakistan, Afghanistan, parts of Africa	Booster every 10 years	Additional doses required if last dose was over 10 years ago.
Rabies	For travellers at risk of rabies exposure	Worldwide, especially areas where rabies is endemic and healthcare is inaccessible	3 doses over 28 days	Further treatment required if bitten by animals in rabies-endemic areas.
Tetanus	For routine protection or if last dose was over 10 years ago	Worldwide	Booster every 10 years	Given as part of the Td/IPV vaccine.
Tick-Borne Encephalitis	For travellers to areas with tick-borne encephalitis risk	Central, Eastern, Northern Europe, Eastern Russia, parts of East Asia (China, Japan)	3 doses, second dose 1-3 months after first	Booster every 3 years. Accelerated schedule available for those with time constraints.

Tuberculosis (BCG)	For travellers at high risk of TB exposure	Africa, parts of South and Southeast Asia	1 dose	Recommended for unvaccinated children or adults at risk of prolonged exposure to TB.
Typhoid	For travellers to areas with poor sanitation	Africa, South/Southeast Asia, South and Central America	1 dose injection or 3 oral doses	Booster every 3 years if risk continues.
Yellow Fever	For travellers to regions where yellow fever is endemic	Sub-Saharan Africa, parts of South America	1 dose, lifelong protection	Required for entry to some countries. Must be given at least 10 days before travel.

16.4.2 Special Population

Table 278 Vaccine Schedule for Special Population

Special Population	Vaccine Recommendations	Additional Notes
A. Pregnancy	**Recommended Vaccines**	
	Tdap (27-36 weeks of each pregnancy)	Protects against tetanus, diphtheria, and pertussis (whooping cough).
	Influenza (any trimester)	Ensure maternal and fetal protection against flu.
	COVID-19 (if not up-to-date)	Protects against COVID-19, especially for high-risk pregnant individuals.
	Avoid Live Vaccines	
	MMR (measles, mumps, rubella), Varicella	Live vaccines are contraindicated during pregnancy.
B. Immunocompromised Patients	**Avoid Live Vaccines**	
	MMR, Varicella, FluMist	Live vaccines can be harmful for immunocompromised individuals.
	Recommended Inactivated Vaccines	
	Pneumococcal	Protects against pneumonia.
	Hepatitis B	Provides protection against hepatitis B infection.

	Additional Doses	
	Immunocompromised individuals may need more frequent or additional doses of inactivated vaccines.	Consult healthcare provider for specific dosing schedules.
C. Healthcare Workers	Required Vaccines	
	Hepatitis B, MMR, Varicella, Influenza, Tdap, COVID-19	Ensure that healthcare workers are up-to-date on vaccines to protect themselves and patients.
	Regular Serologic Testing	Healthcare workers may need routine serologic testing to assess immunity levels, especially for Hepatitis B and MMR.

16.4.3 COVID-19 vaccination recommendations for moderately to severely immunocompromised individuals

Table 279 COVID-19 vaccination recommendations for moderately to severely immunocompromised individuals

Category	Age Group	Initial COVID-19 Vaccine	Booster Doses	Additional Doses	Notes
Already completed initial series	Children (6 months-4 years)	2 doses of 2024-2025 COVID-19 vaccine (same brand) spaced 6 months apart	2 doses, 6 months apart (same brand as initial series)	May get additional doses after 2 months from the last dose, consult healthcare provider	Follow the same vaccine brand for all doses, if possible.
	Children (5-11 years)	2 doses of 2024-2025 COVID-19 vaccine (either Moderna or Pfizer-BioNTech) spaced 6 months apart	2 doses, 6 months apart (either Moderna or Pfizer-BioNTech)	Additional doses can be considered after 2 months, after discussion with healthcare provider	

	People (12 years and older)	2 doses of 2024-2025 COVID-19 vaccine (any brand: Moderna, Pfizer-BioNTech, or Novavax) spaced 6 months apart	2 doses, 6 months apart (any brand)	May receive more doses, consult healthcare provider.	
Never received a COVID-19 vaccine	Children (6 months-4 years)	2 doses of 2024-2025 COVID-19 vaccine (same brand: Moderna or Pfizer-BioNTech)	1 dose, 6 months after initial series (same brand)	After 2 months, may get additional doses, depending on healthcare advice	
	Children (5-11 years)	2 doses of 2024-2025 COVID-19 vaccine (same brand: Moderna or Pfizer-BioNTech)	1 dose, 6 months after initial series (either brand)	Additional doses can be considered after 2 months, after discussion with healthcare provider	
	People (12 years and older)	2 doses of 2024-2025 COVID-19 vaccine (same brand: Moderna, Pfizer-BioNTech, or Novavax)	1 dose, 6 months after initial series (any brand)	Additional doses can be considered after 2 months from the last dose, based on consultation	
Started but did not complete initial series	Children (6 months-4 years)	Complete initial series with the same brand (Moderna or Pfizer-	1 dose of 2024-2025 COVID-19 vaccine, 6 months after completing	Additional doses can be given after 2 months from the last dose	

		BioNTech), then 1 more dose 6 months later	initial series (same brand)		
	Children (5-11 years)	Complete initial series with the same brand (Moderna or Pfizer-BioNTech), then 1 more dose 6 months later	1 dose of 2024-2025 COVID-19 vaccine, 6 months after completing initial series (either brand)	Additional doses after 2 months can be considered, after discussion with healthcare provider	
	People (12 years and older)	Complete initial series with the same brand (Moderna, Pfizer-BioNTech, or Novavax), then 1 more dose 6 months later	1 dose of 2024-2025 COVID-19 vaccine, 6 months after completing initial series (any brand)	May receive more doses after 2 months from the last dose, based on healthcare advice	
People who recently had COVID-19	All Ages	Can delay vaccine for 3 months after COVID-19 symptoms or positive test	Can receive vaccine 3 months after recovery	Delay getting the vaccine unless there is a personal risk for severe illness or other factors; consult healthcare provider	The delay is due to reduced likelihood of reinfection in the months following illness.

16.4.4 Non-Pharmaceutical Interventions (NPIs)

Non-pharmaceutical interventions (NPIs) are crucial for managing the transmission of contagious diseases when an epidemic is on the rise. They abstain from the use of drugs in combating the spread of the pathogen, but aim at preventing the transfer of disease-causing mechanisms to other people. The first and one of the most elementary steps includes hand hygiene, which helps to avoid pathogens that can be spread by touch. They include proper hand washing with soap and water, or when not possible, using hand sanitizer, can greatly minimize the chances of getting infected. **Masks are another essential NPI, particularly for respiratory diseases, because they**

minimize the spread of respiratory droplets, which have infectious particles in them. It is therefore advisable to use a physical space during epidemics to avoid touching and coming close to people to avoid spreading airborne diseases. Covering the mouth and nose when coughing or sneezing also plays a significant role in minimizing the spread of germs into the environment and on objects. Lastly, isolation and quarantine measures refer to the measures taken with the aim of preventing the spread of a disease by putting a distance between infected and susceptible individuals, **as in the case of COVID or TB.**

16.4.5 Preventative Screenings (Age-Appropriate)

Preventive care has remained a vital aspect of healthcare service delivery needed in curbing the spread of diseases. It is with regard to such screenings, depending on the age of the person and the diseases that are likely to cause harm to an individual. Such screening tests for children cover vision and hearing check-ups, anemia, lead level, and general physical growth. They also assist in the early identification of any complications that may occur with the child during development. That means women in the **age group of 21-65 should have a Pap smear at least once every three years, while those who wish to undergo HPV testing should go for it once every five years**. His maintenance includes colon cancer screening to show early symptoms of colorectal cancer in adults aged 45 years and above. **Individuals of 35 years or older, or those who have other risk factors, should pay attention to their lipid panel levels and diabetes screening.** The measurement of blood pressure, the assessment of the BMI, and the screening for depression, as well as alcohol and tobacco usage, should be conducted for every adult on a regular basis.

16.4.6 Vaccine Storage and Handling

Vaccines, like any other products that are stored and distributed to patients, come with certain rules that must be adhered to to maintain their effectiveness. Still, vaccines need to be stored under certain temperature conditions so that their effectiveness is not affected. **The routine vaccines are to be kept at 2°C–8°C, while frozen vaccines are to be stored at or below -15°C.** There is a need to check the temperature run constantly, and there should be alarms in the storage of vaccines to indicate a change in temperature. If it is required to reconstitute a vaccine, then the reconstitution should be done within the time span provided by the respective manufacturers in order to yield optimal results. Furthermore, every vaccine has its shelf life; in this regard, it is important to adhere to this limitation to avoid using expired vaccines.

16.4.7 Common Myths & Facts

The following are some of the myths and misconceptions of vaccines that have hampered the campaign: **Some of the common myths include that vaccines cause autism. Though this has been propagated in society, various research works have disputed this claim, and there is no substance to this.** The myths that are currently circulating include the claim that natural immunity is superior to the immunity that is derived from the vaccines. To the contrary, natural infections are usually more dangerous for individuals, and sometimes fatal, whereas vaccines offer a controlled form of protection against diseases. There is another myth that one can overwhelm the immune system if he or she takes too many vaccines. Meanwhile, the system also understands that the immune system is capable of processing thousands of **antigens every day. Further, a common myth is that the flu vaccine leads to flu illness and sickness.** The other is a flu shot, which is an inactivated virus, which means that it does not result in the flu, although you are likely to experience mild reactions like a sore throat or even a low-grade fever.

16.4.8 Key Considerations for Providers

Healthcare providers have a major contribution to make towards the achievement of successful vaccination programs. Immunization status should be checked in every patient Visit to determine who has received his or her immunizations. With the patients who have failed to access earlier time schedules, providers should provide new schedules that can take the patients through a recommended vaccination. Secondly, if possible, it is always preferred to use a combination vaccine, **for instance, DTaP-IPV-Hib, for the purpose of reducing the number of times an infant undergoes an injection.** This regulatory knowledge also refers to common side effects, such as fever or slight soreness of muscles, that the providers should inform the patients to make them understand that severe reactions like anaphylaxis are rare in occurrence. Lastly, healthcare providers need to report any reaction that occurs from vaccines in VAERS to ensure that the immunization program is safe and effective.

16.5 Pediatric Considerations

16.5.1 Principles of Growth and Development

Childhood development involves certain principles that explain the dynamics of growth as well as the different domains of physical, mental, and emotional development. **Cephalocaudal mode of development is the process that progresses from the head to the lower part of the body**, an aspect that is evidenced in the early stages of development when children are able to control their neck before sitting, crawling, or walking. This principle holds that the human body grows in a sequential way, starting with the head and upper limbs. **Analogously, proximodistal advancement touches upon the center-outward model of development in which the body's core muscles are acquired before the fine touch control over the limbs' extremities.** These developmental trends are developmental and correlated, with the majority of the children attaining the milestones like sitting, walking, and talking within a specified age bracket. However, it is true that there are slight differences in the growth process because a child grows depending on the specific rate at which he/she develops. **Development is a process that is associated with so many factors like genetic makeup, environment, health, and feeding; hence, all children are different.** Knowledge of these principles assists caregivers, educators, and teachers within health-related fields to enhance the general well-being of the learners.

16.5.2 Stages of Pediatric Development

Table 280 Stages of Pediatric Development

Stage	Age Range	Key Physical Changes	Developmental Focus	Clinical Considerations
Neonate	Birth-28 days	Reflexes (Moro, rooting), poor head control	Attachment, sensory stimulation	APGAR score, newborn screening
Infant	1-12 months	Rapid weight gain, motor milestones	Trust vs. Mistrust (Erikson), sensorimotor stage (Piaget), social smile	Growth monitoring, vaccinations
Toddler	1-3 years	Walking, potty training, speech emerges	Autonomy vs. Shame and Doubt, symbolic thought begins	Safety (accident prevention), toilet training guidance
Preschooler	3-5 years	Improved coordination, full sentences	Initiative vs. Guilt, imagination, role-playing	Vision/hearing screening, school readiness

School-Age	6-12 years	Steady growth, teeth changes, improved stamina	Industry vs. Inferiority, logical thought, peer interaction	Academic progress, mental health
Adolescent	13-18 years	Puberty, sexual maturity, growth spurts	Identity vs. Role Confusion, abstract thinking, independence	Sexual health education, emotional support, risk behavior counseling

16.5.3 Cognitive Development (Piaget)

Table 281 Cognitive Development

Age Range	Stage	Key Characteristics	Key Aspects
Infancy (0-2 years)	**Sensorimotor Stage**	Infants learn about the world through their senses and actions. Object permanence begins to develop.	Babies develop an understanding of their surroundings through sensory experiences and motor activities. Key developments include object permanence and early problem-solving.
Toddler/Preschool (2-7 years)	**Preoperational Stage**	Marked by egocentrism, magical thinking, and animism. Begin to engage in symbolic play and language development.	Children start to use words and images to represent objects and experiences. They struggle with understanding other viewpoints (egocentrism) and logical thinking.
School-age (7-12 years)	**Concrete Operational Stage**	Children	

16.5.4 Language Development

Table 282 Key Cosniderations for Language Development

Age Range	Developmental Milestone	Key Characteristics	Key Aspects
Infancy (0-12 months)	**Crying → Cooing → Babbling**	Crying as a primary communication, followed by cooing and babbling.	Early communication includes crying, cooing, and simple sounds. Babbling marks the first steps towards verbal communication.

Toddler (12-24 months)	First Words → Combining Words	Simple words emerge, leading to two-word phrases (e.g., "want cookie").	Vocabulary begins to expand. Two-word combinations mark the transition to more structured language use.
Preschool (2-5 years)	Expanding Vocabulary and Grammar	Use of sentences, increasing vocabulary, basic grammar structures.	Sentence complexity increases. Grammar usage becomes more sophisticated, and children begin to engage in storytelling.
School-age (6-12 years)	Refining Vocabulary and Literacy	Enhanced comprehension of language, use of complex sentence structures, and ability to read/write.	Increased exposure to formal and academic language. Children begin to read, write, and engage in more abstract language.
Adolescents (12+ years)	Complex Expression, Abstract Language	Mastery of sarcasm, abstract language, and figurative speech.	Adolescents become adept at using complex expressions, including irony, sarcasm, and metaphor. They can express abstract concepts and emotions.

16.5.5 Motor Development

Table 283 Key Considerations for Motor Development

Type of Motor Skill	Milestones	Key Aspects
Gross Motor	Rolling, sitting, crawling, walking, running, jumping	Gross motor skills involve large muscle groups and major body movements. These milestones follow a predictable sequence, with early motor control seen in neck and trunk stability before limb control.
Fine Motor	Grasping, drawing, dressing, writing	Fine motor skills require coordination of small muscle groups, such as hand-eye coordination for tasks like grasping objects, holding utensils, or writing.

16.5.6 Psychosocial Development (Erikson)

Table 284 Key Considerations for Psychosocial Development

Age Range	Stage	Key Tasks/Challenges	Key Aspects

Infancy (0-2 years)	Trust vs. Mistrust	Developing trust in caregivers and the world around them.	Infants learn to trust their caregivers to meet their basic needs. Successful resolution leads to feelings of safety and security.
Toddler (2-4 years)	Autonomy vs. Shame/Doubt	Developing independence and autonomy in actions and thoughts.	Toddlers strive for independence but may experience shame if they fail or are overly restricted.
Preschool (4-6 years)	Initiative vs. Guilt	Developing initiative to engage in activities and explore.	Preschoolers assert their power and control over the environment through directing play and other social interactions.
School-age (6-12 years)	Industry vs. Inferiority	Mastering skills and tasks, gaining self-confidence.	Children strive to achieve competence in academic, social, and athletic skills. Failure to succeed can lead to feelings of inferiority.
Adolescence (12-18 years)	Identity vs. Role Confusion	Establishing a personal identity and direction in life.	Adolescents explore their identity, careers, relationships, and values. Successful resolution leads to a solid sense of self.

16.5.7 Social/Emotional Development

Table 285 Social/Emotional Development Consideration

Age Range	Social/Emotional Milestone	Key Characteristics	Key Aspects
Infancy (0-2 years)	**Attachment to caregiver**	Infants form secure or insecure attachments based on caregiver response.	Early emotional bonds are critical for emotional regulation and future relationships.
Toddler (2-4 years)	**Parallel play, emotional expression**	Children begin to explore emotions and engage in independent play alongside others.	Children start recognizing their emotions and the emotions of others, though their play is often independent rather than cooperative.
Preschool (4-6 years)	**Cooperative play, gender identity**	Play becomes more interactive, and children begin	Preschoolers begin to form friendships and engage in more

		developing an understanding of gender roles.	cooperative play. Gender identity starts to emerge.
School-age (6-12 years)	**Peer influence, team play**	Peer relationships become more important, and children engage in team-based activities.	Children begin to understand social roles, group dynamics, and rules of play. Peer acceptance becomes a central concern.
Adolescents (12-18 years)	**Peer groups, romantic interests, self-image**	Adolescents explore group dynamics, develop romantic relationships, and form their identity.	Peer influence and relationships become central to the adolescent's development. Self-image and romantic relationships play a crucial role.

16.5.8 Influencing Factors

Table 286 Key Cosniderations for Influencing Factors

Factor	Impact on Development
Genetics	Genetic makeup influences growth potential, intelligence, and temperament.
Nutrition	Adequate nutrition is critical for brain and body development, impacting cognitive abilities and physical growth.
Health Conditions	Chronic illness, prematurity, and disability can delay or impair developmental milestones.
Environment	Home safety, quality of education, and exposure to language influence cognitive and emotional development.
Socioeconomic Status	Limited access to resources can result in deficits in cognitive stimulation, healthcare, and nutrition.
Cultural Practices	Cultural norms influence milestones, discipline, feeding practices, and overall expectations.

16.5.9 Clinical & Nursing Considerations

Table 287 Clinical and Nursing Consideration

Consideration	Description
Growth Charts	Track weight, height, and head circumference using WHO/CDC standards.

Developmental Screening Tools	Use tools like Denver II and ASQ to identify developmental delays early.
Anticipatory Guidance	Educate parents about developmental milestones and what to expect.
Immunization Schedules	Ensure vaccines are given on time according to national and international guidelines.
Parental Support	Provide guidance on responsive parenting and monitor for mental health concerns.
Adolescent Health	Focus on mental health, peer pressure, sexual behavior, and substance use prevention.

16.5.10 Major Growth and Development Theories in Pediatrics

Table 288 Major Growh and Development Theories in Pediatrics

Theory	Stage	Age Range	Key Concepts	Key Tasks / Positive Outcome	Clinical Relevance
Freud's Psychosexual Theory	**Oral**	Birth - 1 year	Mouth (feeding, sucking)	Trust, comfort	Understanding emotional responses like stress during toilet training or early sexual curiosity.
	Anal	1 - 3 years	Anus (toilet training)	Control, independence	Helps address issues like potty training stress or behavioral problems related to control.
	Phallic	3 - 6 years	Genitals (gender identity)	Oedipus/Electra complex	Addresses early sexual curiosity and gender identity.
	Latency	6 - 12 years	Dormant sexual feelings	Social skills, self-confidence	Focuses on developing social relationships and mastering new skills.

	Genital	12+ years	Maturation of sexual interests	Intimacy, independence	Supports interventions in adolescent identity formation and establishing intimate relationships.
Erikson's Psychosocial Theory	**Trust vs. Mistrust**	Birth – 1 year	Reliable caregiving	Trust in caregivers and the world	Essential for forming healthy bonds with caregivers and promoting trust.
	Autonomy vs. Shame/Doubt	1 – 3 years	Independence vs. overcontrol	Self-confidence, autonomy	Encourages independence, as seen in potty training and developing self-control.
	Initiative vs. Guilt	3 – 6 years	Exploration vs. reprimand	Initiative, purpose	Promotes exploration and taking the initiative, especially in social or learning environments.
	Industry vs. Inferiority	6 - 12 years	Competence vs. failure	Pride in achievements	Encourages pride in achievements, particularly in academic or social settings.
	Identity vs. Role Confusion	12 - 18 years	Self-definition	Stable sense of identity	Assists in guiding interventions in adolescence related to self-identity

					and independence.
Piaget's Cognitive Development	**Sensorimotor**	Birth - 2 years	Object permanence, cause-effect	Development of object permanence and early problem-solving skills	Helps in designing play therapy and early learning experiences for infants.
	Preoperational	2 - 7 years	Symbolic play, egocentrism, language explosion	Beginning of language and symbolic thinking	Shapes approaches to language development, play-based learning, and early literacy.
	Concrete Operational	7 - 11 years	Logical thinking, conservation, reversibility	Logical thought, understanding conservation	Guides educational strategies and problem-solving tasks.
	Formal Operational	12+ years	Abstract reasoning, hypothetical thinking	Ability to think about abstract ideas, future planning, and hypothetical reasoning	Vital for understanding and fostering abstract thought in adolescents.
Kohlberg's Moral Development	**Preconventional**	1-9 years	Obedience & punishment, individualism & exchange	Avoiding punishment, self-interest	Guides understanding of moral reasoning, especially in younger children.
	Conventional	9-15 years	Interpersonal relationships, law and order	Seeking approval, following rules for societal order	Crucial in understanding social rules, moral reasoning, and peer group influence.

	Postconventional	15+ years	Social contract, universal ethical principles	Justice, human rights, ethical principles	Essential for discussing ethics and moral dilemmas in adolescents.
Maslow's Hierarchy of Needs	**Physiological Needs**	All ages	Nutrition, sleep, safety	Meeting basic survival needs	Helps identify and address unmet physical needs that can impact development.
	Safety and Security	All ages	Stable home, predictable routines	Stable environment for development	Supports the creation of a secure environment for children to thrive.
	Love and Belonging	All ages	Parental bonding, peer relationships	Development of emotional bonds, peer relationships	Ensures healthy emotional connections with family, friends, and peers.
	Esteem	All ages	Encouragement, success in school	Achievement, recognition	Builds self-esteem through success and encouragement, particularly in academics.
	Self-actualization	All ages	Fulfillment of potential (creativity, problem-solving)	Reaching full potential, creativity, personal growth	Supports the growth of personal talents and aspirations.
Vygotsky's Sociocultural Theory	**Zone of Proximal Development (ZPD)**	All ages	Scaffolding, social dialogue	Learning through social interactions and support	Encourages guided learning through social interaction

					just beyond current ability	and cultural sensitivity.

16.5.11 Red Flags in Development

Red flags in development are signs that may alert one to the possibility that there may be a development problem or developmental concern. It is crucial for parents, caregivers, and anyone who comes in contact with children to become aware of these signs early enough so that the child can be aided accordingly. **Another indicator of developmental problems is the failure to engage in babbling and gesturing at the age of 12 months, as these are vital for communicating and interacting with other people.** Delay in the development of such simple gestures, such as pointing with an index finger or waving, at this age can signify language development and social skills delays. One of the other prominent signs is the absence of words at the age of 18 months. Generally, the time when children start speaking their first words is at the age of 12 months, and if a child does not talk at that age, a possible language or developmental issue could be present. Also, before 2 years of age, those children are expected to be able to speak simple phrases that **contain two words, such as 'want cookie' or 'go play'.** If this is not accomplished, it may be an indication of some delay in the child's expressive language.

Regression of skills at any age is also quite an alarming sign, which often speaks about a disease. Sometimes, with development, children may develop a disease, or there is a decrease in their abilities, for example, there are nervous system problems, walking, speaking, and training issues. **Last but not least, poor eye contact or lack of it when it is continuously maintained also may suggest social, emotional, or behavioural problems such as autism spectrum disorder.** Play and social skills are important in early childhood, and shyness, avoiding eye contact, and withdrawing from group activities may indicate further evaluation. Early identification of these signs can help caregivers to seek assistance and provide necessary intervention to ensure that children are given every chance to succeed in their development.

16.6 Obstetric Considerations

16.6.1 Preconception and Prenatal Care

Table 289 Key Considerations for Preconception and Prenatal Care

Category		Details
1. Preconception Care		
	Health Assessment	A thorough health assessment should be conducted to review chronic diseases (e.g., diabetes, hypertension), current medications, infections (e.g., TORCH infections), and mental health status. Any existing medical conditions should be managed before conception.
	Folic Acid	Folic acid supplementation (400-800 mcg/day) is recommended to prevent neural tube defects. This should begin at least 1 month before conception and continue during the first trimester.
	Immunizations	Immunizations should be updated, including MMR (Measles, Mumps, Rubella), Varicella (chickenpox), hepatitis B, Tdap (tetanus, diphtheria, pertussis), and flu. Women should

		ensure their immunization status is up to date before conception.
	Genetic Counseling	Couples with a family history of inherited disorders (e.g., cystic fibrosis, sickle cell disease) or those who are carriers of genetic conditions should undergo genetic counseling to assess risks and consider carrier screening.
	Lifestyle Advice	Health promotion strategies include smoking and alcohol cessation, achieving a healthy BMI (body mass index), adopting a balanced diet with proper nutrients, and starting a fitness regimen to prepare for pregnancy.
2. First Prenatal Visit		
	Pregnancy Confirmation	Pregnancy is confirmed using a β-hCG blood test. A urine test may also be used for home testing.
	Estimated Date of Delivery	The Estimated Date of Delivery (EDD) is determined using the last menstrual period (LMP) or an early ultrasound. Early ultrasounds are more accurate for determining the due date.
	Physical Exam & History	Complete a physical exam including vital signs (blood pressure, weight, height) and a comprehensive health history to identify any pre-existing health issues.
	Initial Labs	Initial labs include a complete blood count (CBC), blood type & Rh factor, rubella titer (to check immunity to rubella), hepatitis B/C, HIV, syphilis (RPR), urinalysis, and urine culture. A Pap smear should be done if indicated.
	Genetic Screening Options	Depending on the individual's risk factors, options for genetic screening may include tests for chromosomal abnormalities (e.g., Down syndrome), and other inherited conditions (e.g., cystic fibrosis, Tay-Sachs).
3. Antenatal Care		
	Routine Prenatal Visit Schedule	Visits are typically scheduled every 4 weeks until 28 weeks, every 2 weeks until 36 weeks, and weekly after 36 weeks. The frequency of visits may vary depending on individual health and risk factors.
	Monitoring and Screening	Routine monitoring includes tracking blood pressure and weight gain, measuring fundal height (from 20 weeks onward), and listening to fetal heart tones with a Doppler (~10–12 weeks). These measures ensure healthy pregnancy progression.
	Ultrasounds	A dating ultrasound is performed between 8-12 weeks to confirm the pregnancy dating. An anatomy scan, which

		checks fetal development and structure, is typically performed between 18-22 weeks.
	Gestational Diabetes Screening	All pregnant women should be screened for gestational diabetes between 24-28 weeks of pregnancy via a glucose tolerance test. Early screening may be needed for high-risk women (e.g., those with obesity or a family history of diabetes).
	Group B Strep Screening	Screening for Group B Streptococcus is recommended between 35-37 weeks to prevent neonatal infection during labor. Positive results typically require IV antibiotics during labor.
	Fetal Movements	Fetal movement typically begins to be noticeable by the mother around 18-20 weeks. Regular movement is monitored as an indicator of fetal well-being.

16.7 Comprehensive Maternal & Fetal Care in Pregnancy, Labor, and Postpartum

16.7.1 High-Risk Pregnancy Considerations

Table 290 Key Considerations for High-Risk Pregnancy

Condition	Description	Management/Monitoring
Preeclampsia/Eclampsia	Characterized by hypertension, proteinuria, and seizures (eclampsia in severe cases). Can lead to maternal and fetal complications like placental abruption or IUGR.	Monitor blood pressure, urine protein levels, assess for symptoms of seizures, magnesium sulfate for seizure prevention.
Gestational Diabetes	Insulin resistance due to pregnancy hormones. Risks for macrosomia, shoulder dystocia, preterm birth, and cesarean delivery.	Screen at 24-28 weeks, manage with diet and exercise, insulin if necessary, frequent fetal monitoring.
Placenta Previa/Abruption	Placenta previa: Placenta covers or is near the cervix; placenta abruption: Premature separation of placenta from the uterine wall.	Monitor for vaginal bleeding, ultrasound to assess placenta position, plan for cesarean if previa is present.
Preterm Labor	Contractions and cervical changes before 37 weeks gestation, increasing risk	Monitor for contractions, cervical length assessment, consider tocolysis,

	of preterm birth and neonatal complications.	corticosteroids for fetal lung maturity.
Intrauterine Growth Restriction (IUGR)	Fetus is not growing at a normal rate. Risk factors include placental insufficiency, maternal hypertension, or infections.	Monitor fetal growth with serial ultrasounds, Doppler studies, and biophysical profile (BPP), plan for early delivery if necessary.
Multiple Gestation	Carrying more than one fetus (e.g., twins or higher-order multiples). Increased risk for preterm birth, preeclampsia, and gestational diabetes.	Monitor for fetal growth, gestational diabetes screening, preeclampsia management, more frequent prenatal visits.
Rh Incompatibility	Occurs when Rh-negative mother carries an Rh-positive fetus, risking hemolytic disease of the newborn.	Administer Rhogam at 28 weeks gestation and postpartum if the newborn is Rh-positive.

16.7.2 Labor and Delivery

Table 291 Key Considerations for Labor and Delivery

Stage of Labor	Description	Key Considerations
First Stage	Onset of contractions → full cervical dilation (10 cm).	*Latent phase:* 0-6 cm dilation, *Active phase:* 6-10 cm dilation. Monitoring of contractions and fetal well-being is essential.
Second Stage	Full dilation → delivery of baby.	Focus on maternal pushing efforts, continuous fetal heart rate monitoring, and guidance for delivery.
Third Stage	Delivery of baby → delivery of placenta.	Monitor for signs of hemorrhage, ensure placenta is delivered intact.
Fourth Stage	Immediate postpartum (first 1-2 hours).	Monitor for hemorrhage, assess uterine tone, and ensure maternal recovery from anesthesia (if used).

16.7.3 Monitoring During Labor

Table 292 Key Considerations for Monitoring During Labor

Monitor	Description	Key Actions
Fetal Heart Rate (FHR)	Continuous monitoring of fetal heart tones, which can provide insight into fetal distress or well-being.	Use of external or internal monitors, assess baseline rate, variability, and any decelerations or accelerations.
Maternal Vital Signs	Monitor blood pressure, heart rate, temperature, and oxygen saturation to assess maternal health during labor.	Frequent checks, especially during active labor and after interventions.
Uterine Contractions	Monitor frequency, intensity, and duration of uterine contractions. This helps assess the progression of labor.	Palpation or electronic monitoring of contractions (frequency and strength).
Cervical Exams	Regular assessments of cervical dilation, effacement, and fetal station (the position of the fetal head in relation to the pelvis).	Performed during labor to evaluate progress. Frequent assessment in active labor.

16.7.4 Pain Management

Table 293 Key Pain Management Consideration

Type	Description	Options
Non-pharmacologic	Techniques that focus on relaxation, support, and education to ease the experience of labor.	Breathing techniques, position changes, support persons, massage, and hydrotherapy (warm baths or showers).
Pharmacologic	Medications that help manage pain during labor, with options varying by stage and maternal preference.	Epidural analgesia, opioids (e.g., fentanyl), local anesthesia (e.g., for episiotomy repair), nitrous oxide.

16.7.5 Postpartum Considerations

Table 294 Key Postpartum Considerations

Stage	Description	Key Actions
Immediate Postpartum Care	Postpartum care during the first few hours following delivery ensures maternal stability and assesses bonding and breastfeeding.	Monitor for hemorrhage (check fundus firmness and lochia), assess emotional well-being, and support early breastfeeding.
Postpartum Follow-Up	The follow-up visit usually occurs at 6 weeks postpartum but can be scheduled earlier if the patient has high-risk conditions.	Screen for postpartum depression, provide contraceptive counseling, assess healing of vaginal or cesarean incisions.

16.7.6 Fetal and Neonatal Considerations

Table 295 Key Fetal and Neonatal Considerations

Consideration	Description	Key Actions
Fetal Well-being	Assessment of the fetus's health through various screening tests and monitoring methods.	Non-stress test (NST), biophysical profile (BPP), growth scans, and Doppler studies.
Neonatal Care	Immediate care is provided to newborns post-delivery, which includes stabilization and prophylactic treatments.	APGAR score assessment, vitamin K injection, eye prophylaxis (e.g., erythromycin drops), temperature stabilization.
Breastfeeding Support	Assistance with initiating and maintaining breastfeeding, focusing on proper latch and maternal comfort.	Provide lactation consultation, position guidance, and address any complications such as nipple pain or low milk supply.
Newborn Screening	Routine tests are conducted to identify conditions that can affect the newborn's health.	Metabolic screening (e.g., PKU), hearing screening, and congenital heart disease screening (e.g., pulse oximetry).

16.7.7 Documentation & Education

Table 296 Key Considerations for Documentation and Education

Aspect	Description	Key Actions
Documentation	Accurate record-keeping throughout the pregnancy and labor process, ensuring all medical information is available for decision-making.	Document vital signs, assessments, interventions, fetal status, and maternal recovery.
Patient Education	Essential education for the patient about self-care, warning signs, and infant care.	Educate on signs of labor and when to go to the hospital, warning signs of complications (e.g., bleeding, headache, decreased fetal movement), and infant care, including breastfeeding and sleep safety.

16.7.8 Key Prenatal Tests by Trimester

Table 297 Key Prenatal Tests by Trimester

Trimester	Tests/Screening	Key Points
First Trimester (11-13 weeks)	- Maternal blood test (measuring hCG and PAPP-A levels) - Ultrasound (measuring fluid behind the	- A combination of tests is offered to screen for heart birth defects and chromosomal disorders. - High or low levels of hCG and PAPP-A can indicate chromosomal disorders. - Ultrasound

	neck) - Genetic screening (NIPT)	checks for extra fluid behind the neck, which could suggest a chromosomal disorder or heart defect.
Second Trimester (15-20 weeks)	- Maternal serum screen (Triple or Quad Screen: AFP, hCG, estriol, inhibin-A) - Ultrasound (18-20 weeks, including anatomy scan) - Fetal echocardiogram	- Serum screen measures proteins in the mother's blood to assess risk for certain birth defects. - Ultrasound checks major body structures, and fetal echocardiogram evaluates the baby's heart in more detail. - A "triple screen" measures 3 proteins, and a "quad screen" measures 4 proteins.
Third Trimester (28-40 weeks)	- Rhogam (if Rh negative) - Group B Strep (GBS) screening - Repeat labs - Fetal monitoring	- Rhogam is administered at 28 weeks and postpartum if needed for Rh incompatibility. - GBS screening occurs between 35-37 weeks to assess for bacterial infection risks that could affect the baby during delivery. - Regular fetal monitoring ensures baby's well-being and tracks development.

16.8 Geriatric Considerations

16.8.1 Geriatric Care Overview

Table 298 Geriatric Care Considerations

Category	Key Points
General Principles of Geriatric Care	Holistic, patient-centered approach, focus on function over disease, multidisciplinary care, recognizing normal aging vs. disease, emphasis on quality of life and autonomy.
Physiological Changes with Aging	**Cardiovascular**: ↓ cardiac output, ↑ vascular stiffness (HTN, orthostatic hypotension). **Respiratory**: ↓ lung elasticity (↑ infection risk, ↓ exercise tolerance). **Renal**: ↓ GFR, altered drug clearance. **GI**: ↓ motility, malabsorption (B12/iron). **Musculoskeletal**: ↓ bone density, sarcopenia (↑ falls). **Neurological**: Slowed reflexes (risk of misdiagnosing dementia). **Sensory**: ↓ vision/hearing/taste (isolation, malnutrition). **Skin**: Thinner, ↓ elasticity (pressure ulcer risk). **Immune**: ↓ immune response (↑ infections).
Pharmacological Considerations	**Start low, go slow**; **Polypharmacy** (≥5 medications); **Increased sensitivity** to medications, especially CNS-acting drugs. Use **Beers Criteria** and **STOPP/START** criteria to assess medications. Risks: Sedation/falls (e.g., benzodiazepines), GI bleeding (NSAIDs), confusion (anticholinergics, opioids), renal impairment (NSAIDs, ACE inhibitors).

16.8.2 Cognitive, Mental Health, and Functional Assessment

Table 299 Cognitive, Mental Health, and Functional Assessment

Category	Details
Cognitive and Mental Health	**Dementia**: Gradual decline in memory/language. **Delirium**: Acute confusion, often reversible. **Depression**: Anhedonia, somatic symptoms. Tools: MMSE, MoCA, GDS.
Functional Assessment	Focus on independence in ADLs and IADLs. **ADLs (Basic)**: Bathing, dressing, feeding, mobility. **IADLs**: Managing meds, finances, cooking, shopping. Tools: Katz Index, Lawton IADL scale, Timed Up and Go (TUG).
Geriatric Syndromes	Multifactorial conditions: **Falls**, **Frailty**, **Incontinence**, **Delirium**, **Malnutrition**, **Polypharmacy**, **Pressure ulcers**, **Depression**, **Sleep disorders**. Requires interprofessional, preventive approaches.

16.8.3 Chronic Conditions, Mobility, and Social Considerations

Table 300 Chronic Conditions, Mobility, and Social Consideration

Category	Details
Common Chronic Conditions	**Hypertension**: Adjust targets based on frailty. **Diabetes**: Relaxed HbA1c goals. **Osteoporosis**: DEXA scan, fall prevention. **Heart Failure**: Monitor fluid status. **COPD**: Monitor for hypoxia, pulmonary rehab. **Arthritis**: Pain management. **Cancer**: Balance screening with life expectancy.
Mobility and Fall Prevention	Assess gait, balance, vision, and environment. Tools: TUG, Berg Balance Scale. Use **assistive devices**, home modifications, **Vitamin D** and **calcium** supplementation, **strength exercises** like Tai Chi.
Social and Environmental Considerations	Evaluate living situation, support systems, financial insecurity, and promote community engagement. Plan for end-of-life care (e.g., hospice, palliative care).

16.8.4 Key Considerations, Assessment Tools, and Summary Checklist

Table 301 Key Considerations for Getriatric Care

Category	Key Points/Assessment Tools
Communication and Ethical Considerations	Use clear, slow speech; avoid medical jargon; Involve caregivers/family; Respect autonomy and advance directives; Discuss goals of care and code status; Use shared decision-making for complex choices; Address elder abuse or neglect if suspected.
Social and Environmental Considerations	Evaluate living situation, support systems; Screen for financial, transportation, or food insecurity; Promote community engagement and mental stimulation; Plan for end-of-life care (e.g., hospice, palliative care).

Comprehensive Geriatric Assessment (CGA)	A multidimensional, interdisciplinary diagnostic process evaluating: Medical conditions, Functional ability, Cognitive status, Mental health, Social circumstances, Environmental safety.
Summary Checklist for Geriatric Assessment	**Cognitive**: MMSE, MoCA. **Mood**: GDS (Geriatric Depression Scale). **Function**: ADLs, IADLs, TUG. **Nutrition**: Mini Nutritional Assessment (MNA). **Medications**: Beers Criteria, medication review. **Social Support**: Social history, caregiver involvement. **Hearing/Vision**: Whisper test, Snellen chart. **Pain**: Numeric or Verbal Descriptor Scale. **Falls**: TUG, fall history.

16.9 Physical Examination

Table 302 Physical Examination

References (Ernstmeyer, K. and Christman, E. (2021). *Chapter 7 Head and Neck Assessment*. [online] www.ncbi.nlm.nih.gov. Available at: https://www.ncbi.nlm.nih.gov/books/NBK593205/. Head to Toe Assessment (Adult -Bedside). (n.d.). Available at: https://www.westand4health.com/blackboard/video_resources/Head_to_Toe_Assessment_Checklist_2020.pdf [Accessed 10 May 2025].)

Adult Head to Toe	
• Introduce self	I am Lindsey Beus Student Nurse Practitioner & will be performing a Head to Toe assessment
General Survey	
• **Mental status:** Alert, Oriented x3 (Person, Place, Time & Situation) • General appearance/presence of discomfort or distress • Dress, grooming & hygiene	Can you tell me your name? Do you know what time it is? Where are you and what you are doing here?, Pt is Alert & Oriented Does not appear to be in Distress or show signs of Discomfort Dressed appropriately for climate, appears well Groomed & personal Hygiene appears well kept → signs of poor hygiene, restlessness or signs of pain, further assessment would be indicated
Skin	
• **Skin:** Pigmentation, texture, moisture, temperature → Comment on skin throughout exam	Now I will assess your **Skin**, can you stand up & show me your back. Inspecting your back, arms & legs → Face forward, I will inspect your abdomen & legs. Now I'll assess your arms & hands. Skin color is normal for ethnicity with even Pigmentation, Texture is smooth, it's Dry & Warm → Skin color can indicate underlying condition; Jaundice suggests liver disease or excessive hemolysis of RBCs
• **Lesions:** (Presence or absence) if present describe characteristics/ distribution	Lesions-Multiple scattered 2–4-mm round brown macules (freckles), symmetrically pigmented, on back, bilateral upper extremities & chest
• **Nails:** Capillary refill, hygiene, shape, lesions	Well-groomed(Hygiene) Nails with regular shape no **clubbing or cyanosis** & absence of lesions; →Clubbing of the nails is seen in heart disease, lung disease or cancer I will press on your nail to assess the Capillary refill & there is a quick return I will assess Skin turgor slightly pinching the skin to assess for hydration; the skin returns quickly which is a sign of hydration
Head & Hair	
→ Part hair on scalp with finger w/ pt tilting head down	I will start by assessing your Head, having you tilt it down. I will part your hair with my fingers & will be touching your scalp, feeling for any **Lesions or Nodules**: None noted
→ Pt to look into the distance & shine bright light obliquely into each pupil • **Pupils:** size, shape, regularity, equality • **Pupillary response:** Direct (pupil constricts in the same eye) & consensual reaction to light (pupil constriction in the opposite eye); Accommodation	I am going to shine the light again to assess Pupils & the light response Pupils are __**mm** (size), are Equal, Round, & Reactive Direct response to light is the pupil that has light applied to it constricts, noted bilaterally Consensual response to light is the **opposite eye constricts** when light applied. This indicated that **CN 3 Oculomotor** is **intact. CN 3** transmits impulses to the *constrictor muscles of the iris* of each eye For Accommodation, I will have you to look at my finger, then at the wall behind me & then back at my finger; When looking at my **finger pupils constrict**, then at **wall dilate & constrict** again when returning focus to my finger
(EOMs) Extraocular Muscle function: Present/Intact; Nystagmus present/absent-CN 3, 4, 6	Now to assess Extraocular Muscle function w/ **Convergence** by using the **6 Cardinal Fields of Gaze**. I want you to follow my finger with your eyes & keep your head still → Traces "H" with finger, Right-Left, Up & down (bilateral), then in toward the nose I'm looking for beats of Nystagmus, none noted with Normal conjugate movements. **CN 3,4 &6 intact; CN 3** (Oculomotor) responsible for moving the **R** eye, **CN 4** (Trochlear) moves the **L** & **CN 6** (Abducens) is responsible for contracting the *lateral rectus muscle* to abduct-turning the eye **laterally** → If one of these muscles was paralyzed the eyes would deviate from its normal position in direct gaze & would no longer appear conjugate (parallel)
Visual Acuity: Handheld Snellen; CN 2	Visual Acuity by placing the Snellen chart 14in. from your face, Cover your **R** eye & read the

→ While facing the patient mimic same side eye covered, bring finger in from up & lower outer **Visual Fields**: CN2 Visual fields test	smallest line that you can read from L-R. Now the L eye. Now with Both eyes. Tested **CN 2** & is functioning **Visual Fields** by using the **Static finger wiggle test**. I am going to hold my hands 2 ft apart & to the side of you. When you see my fingers come into view, I want you to say "now". With **Both** eyes, I want you to look at my eyes Now again but **Covering one eye** at a time. With your uncovered eye look into my uncovered eye Tested the **CN 2** (**Optic nerve**) & is functioning →Visual field defects indicate Anterior pathway defects-Glaucoma & optic neuropathy; Posterior pathway defects-Stroke & tumors, Should be referred for evaluation

Ears

Auricles: inspect anterior & posterior **External canal:** inspect for lesions, drainage, cerumen (ear wax) → Palpate external ear & mastoid for tenderness	Now yours **Ears**, **Auricles** (visible outer ear), Inspecting **Anterior auricle** (front), **Posterior auricle** (back); Size & shape are uniform, w/ no lesions or deformities. Next palpating **External ear & Mastoid** for tenderness-No tenderness or edema. →Mastoiditis can indicate Otitis Media **External canal** shows no **Lesions, Drainage or Cerumen**
Tympanic membrane: inspect, comment on landmarks, cone of light	Now to assess your **Tympanic Membranes** (TM) w/ the **Otoscope**, placing the otoscope into your ear, **Pulling the auricle up & back** **Right:** Landmarks **Incus, Malleus & Cone of light** at **5 o'clock** **Left:** Landmarks **Incus, Malleus & Cone of light** at **7 o'clock** Both TMs are intact, pearly gray, no perforations. →In acute Otitis Externa canal is often swollen, narrowed, moist, pale, & tender Stapes / Incus / Malleus (Handle) / Cone of light
• **Hearing:** Test with **whispered voice** or watch tick –CN 8	Do you feel you have a hearing loss or difficulty hearing? I will be testing your **Hearing** & **CN 8** (Vestibulocochlear) By stand 2 ft. behind you, I will have you occlude the non-tested ear & rub the tragus in a circular motion. By using a **Whispered voice** saying a combination of letters & numbers, having you repeat it back to me. 1st the R ear "3-U-1" Can you repeat? Now the L "2-B-6" Can you repeat? **CN 8 intact**

Nose & Sinuses

External structure: skeleton	"I will touch your **external structure** of the **nose**", "No pain induced while palpating skeleton"
• **Sinuses:** frontal, maxillary: palpate for tenderness	"Now I will be touching your face to palpate the **Frontal sinuses**(under the bony brows)", "Pressing up for **Maxillary sinuses**", "No pain or tenderness noted throughout" "Tenderness, facial pain, pressure with purulent nasal drainage present for greater than 7 days suggests acute bacterial rhonosinusitis"
Internal structures: • **Septum:** inspect for deviation, perforation, lesions, mucosa • **Turbinates:** inspect for color, lesions, edema, discharge	Next I will be looking into your nose with the **Otoscope** by placing it into each nostril". "**Septum** shows no deviation, perforation, lesions, with pink mucosa on the **right** side and same on the **left** side", "In viral rhinitis the mucosa is red & swollen", "**Turbinates** are pink with no erythema, no edema, no lesion or discharge Middle turbinate / Nasal passage / Septum / Inferior turbinate

Nose & Sinuses

External structure: skeleton	"I will touch your **external structure** of the **nose**", "No pain induced while palpating skeleton"
• **Sinuses:** frontal, maxillary: palpate for tenderness	"Now I will be touching your face to palpate the **Frontal sinuses**(under the bony brows)", "Pressing up for **Maxillary sinuses**", "No pain or tenderness noted throughout" "Tenderness, facial pain, pressure with purulent nasal drainage present for greater than 7 days suggests acute bacterial rhonosinusitis"

Neck

• **Trachea:** midline	"Now I will assess your **neck**. Look for swelling", "None noted" "I will place my finger along one side of the **Trachea** & note distance from it & sternocleidomastoid, compare on each side", "Trachea is midline"
Thyroid: → Inspect for enlargement → Palpate for enlargement, nodules, tenderness	"Now to assess the **Thyroid**, by having you extend your neck & I will have you **take sips of water** holding it in your mouth until I tell you to swallow", "Swallow, I can see the **thyroid cartilage, the cricoid cartilage & the thyroid gland** all rise when swallowing & all return to resting position after", "While swallowing, if the lower border of thyroid gland rises & look less symmetric is an abnormal finding" "Next, I will **stand behind** you to palpate the thyroid gland while you flex your neck forward" "No enlargement, nodules or tenderness Thyroid cartilage / Cricoid cartilage / Thyroid gland

	noted bilaterally", "Enlargement can indicate a goiter"	
Carotids: → Palpate for presence/absence → Quality of pulsation → Auscultate for bruits (Use first two fingers to palpate carotid over lower 1/3 of neck--each side separately)	"Now **palpate carotid pulses** one side at time", "Present, 2+, & equal bilaterally" → "Next I will **listen to carotid arteries** with **bell of stethoscope for bruits**, take deep breath and hold", "bruits is a blowing sound from turbulent blood flow, can be caused by atherosclerosis", "No bruit heard bilateral", "A continuous bruit may be heard in *hyperthyroidism* from Grave's disease or toxic multinodular goiter"	
Heart		
• **Neck veins:** observe and measure at 30 degrees; observe with HOB over 30 degrees Jugular Venous Pressure (JVP) measures the highest oscillation point "meniscus" of the jugular venous pulsations, JVP reflects pressure in the right atrium, central venous pressure, providing info about volume status & cardiac function (carotid pulse not affected by pressure being applied)	"To assess **Jugular Venous Pressure (JVP),** reflects pressure in the **right atrium**, I will have you lay on your back to observe & measure at a 90° & at 30° using a pillow", "I will examine from the **right side**, identifying **right internal jugular** venous pulsation, ruling out carotid artery. I will place the ruler at the **sternal angle** and a card horizontally from the highest point of the internal jugular vein pulsation (measuring in cm) & adding 5cm as the distance from the *sternal angle to the right atrium*. "It was 1cm at 30° & at 90° 1 cm adding 5cm = 6cm". "Abnormal is 3-4cm above the sternal angle at 30° or more than 7-8cm in total distance above the right atrium", "JVP elevation is correlated with both acute & chronic heart failure"	
Precordium: → inspect precordium: heaves, lifts → palpate precordium: pulsations, thrills **Apical impulse:** → Location, amplitude → Identify rate & rhythm at apical impulse -referred to PMI, point of maximum impulse	"**At 30°**, I will inspect your chest, precordium for any **heaves or lifts** which may indicate a large heart", "At the 2nd intercostal space, I'll place my palm against the chest", "No heaves", "Placing the ball of my hand on the chest to assess lifts", "None noted" "Apical pulse is palpated at mid-clavicular line 4-5th intercostal space, amplitude normal, listening for 1 min-rate 80 bpm"	(S1=Closure of Mitral valve/ S2= Closure of Aortic valve)
Auscultation (use bell and diaphragm): Identify landmarks and auscultate using **diaphragm; Listen to all areas w/ bell** o Aortic area, identify S1, S2 o Pulmonic area, identify S1, S2 o Tricuspid area, identify S1, S2 o Mitral area, identify S1, S2	"Now I will listen to the heart using the **Diaphragm** & **Bell of the stethoscope**" → "**Aortic** at the right 2nd intercostal" → "**Pulmonic** at the left 2nd intercostal space" → "**Tricuspid** at the left sternal border" → "**Mitral** (Apex) at 5th intercostal, mid-clavicular line" "Rate is regular, S1 and S2 present throughout & no S3 or S4"	
→ Have patient turn to **left side**; listen at mitral area w/ bell for mitral murmur	"I will have you **turn to your left side** so I can listen to the **Mitral area** with the **Bell** of the stethoscope for **mitral murmur**", "Bell hears low pitched, S3 &4, murmur of **Mitral stenosis**" "No noted"	
→ Have patient sit up, lean forward, diaphragm in aortic area for aortic murmur	"Diaphragm hears high pitched & murmurs of aortic", "Now if you will **sit up & lean forward**, I will use the **Diaphragm** in **Aortic area**, 2nd right intercostal", "Can you **exhale and hold breath**?", "No murmur note- would indicate Aortic regurgitation"	
Peripheral Vascular		
→ Palpate & comment presence/absence, symmetry • Temporal • Radial • Femoral • Popliteal • Posterior tibial • Dorsalis pedis	"I will palpate pulses throughout body" "Starting with- o **Temporal pulses** (sides of head) o **Radial pulses** (wrist) o **Femoral** (inside thigh) o **Popliteal** (back of knee) o **Posterior tibial** (ankle) o **Dorsalis Pedis** (top of foot) "All pulses are present, equal & 2 + throughout"	Radial Popliteal Posterior tibial Dorsalis pedis
→ Inspect lower extremities for signs of arterial insufficiency → Inspect lower extremities for varicosities → Inspect/palpate lower extremities for edema	"Now to inspect lower extremities for signs of **Arterial insufficiency**", "No erythema or loss of hair" "No signs of **Varicosities** noted, such as varicose veins" "I will **inspect & palpate** for **edema**", "none noted"	

<table>
<tr><td colspan="2">

Respiratory & Gastrointestinal (GI) (Video #3)

</td></tr>
<tr><td colspan="2">

Thorax & Lungs (Sitting up)

</td></tr>
<tr><td>

Inspection:
- **AP to lateral diameter:** comment on ratio
- **Respiratory effort:** use of accessory muscles, retraction of interspaces
- **Respiratory rate**

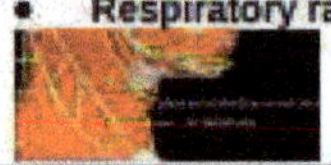

</td><td>

"To start I will compare the **Anteroposterior (AP) diameter to lateral diameter**", "I will observe your chest from the front & now the side", "The ratio appears to be 2:1; which is normal", "Now observing **respiratory effort**". "**Respiratory rate** is 16, skin color is appropriate for ethnicity, no audible sounds of breathing", "I will **inspect the neck *during inspiration*** for contraction of accessory muscles, Sternocleidomastoid (SCM) & Scalene muscles or supraclavicular retraction", "No contraction of the accessory muscles noted", "During ***expiration*** inspecting the intercostal or abdominal oblique muscles". "No intercostal retractions noted"

Supraclavicular

Intercostal

</td></tr>
<tr><td>

Percuss lung fields:
- **Posterior chest**
- **Location of diaphragm**

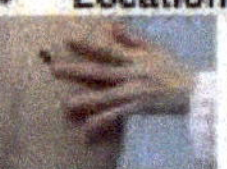 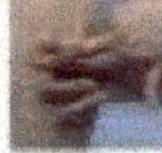 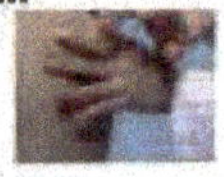

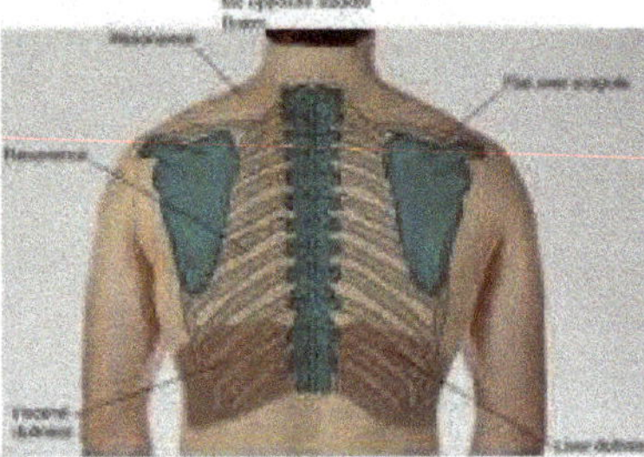

(Percussion helps you establish whether the underlying tissues are air-filled, fluid-filled, or consolidated)

</td><td>

"Now I will **percuss the lung fields of the posterior chest**; I will have you cross your arms in front of your chest", "I will hyperextend the middle finger of my L hand (pleximeter), with a quick sharp motion I will strike the pleximeter finger with the R pleximeter the R middle finger (plexor) hitting the distal interphalangeal joint using the same for each strike", "I will percuss one side of the chest & then the other in a ladder like pattern from medial scapular bone level to 10th rib", "Healthy lungs are **resonant**", "Abnormal is dullness replaces resonance when fluid or solid tissue replaces air-containing lungs or pleural space like a tumor, hemothorax"

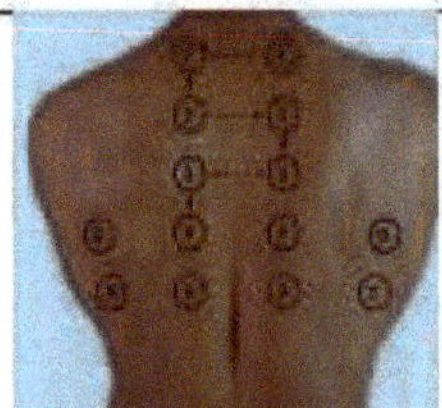

FIGURE 8-15. Percuss and auscultate in a "ladder" pattern.

→"Now to assess **location of the diaphragm** (descent of the diaphragm or) **diaphragmatic excursion**", "1st detect the level of diaphragmatic dullness during quiet respiration by holding the pleximeter finger (left middle) above & parallel to the expected level of dullness, percussing downward in progressive steps until dullness clearly replaces resonance comparing medially & laterally", "Now estimating the extent of diaphragmatic excursion by determining the distance between the *level of dullness* on *full expiration* & the *level of dullness* on *full inspiration*, normally about 3-5.5cm", "repeating it on other side". "Abnormally high level suggests pleural effusion or elevated hemidiaphragm from atelectasis or phrenic nerve paralysis"

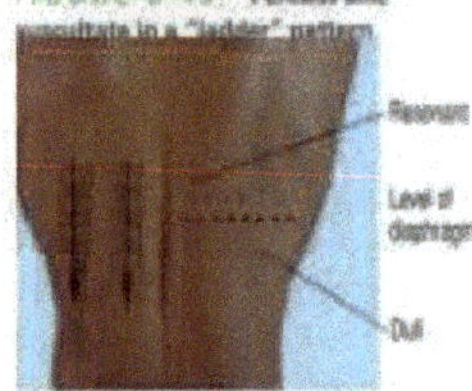

Identify the extent of diaphragmatic excursion.

</td></tr>
<tr><td>

Auscultate breath sounds:
- **Anterior:** Comment on findings /adventitious sounds
- **Posterior:** Comment on findings/ adventitious sounds

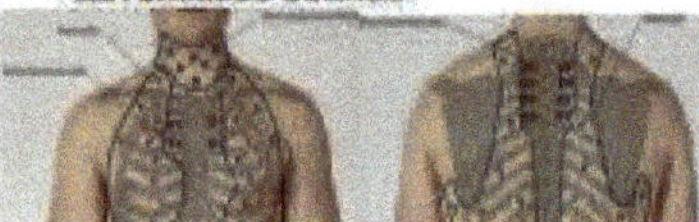

(Perform voice transmission tests (indicates consolidation) bronchophony, egophony, & whispered pectoriloquy; "Scooby doo" (bronchophony) or any change from "ee" sound to "ay" sound (egophony) or a clearer whispered voice (whispered pectoriloquy)

</td><td>

"Now I will **auscultate breath sounds** using diaphragm while you breathe deeply through an open mouth".

"1st **Anterior** lung sounds" "Vesicular lung sounds heard, with no adventitious sounds"

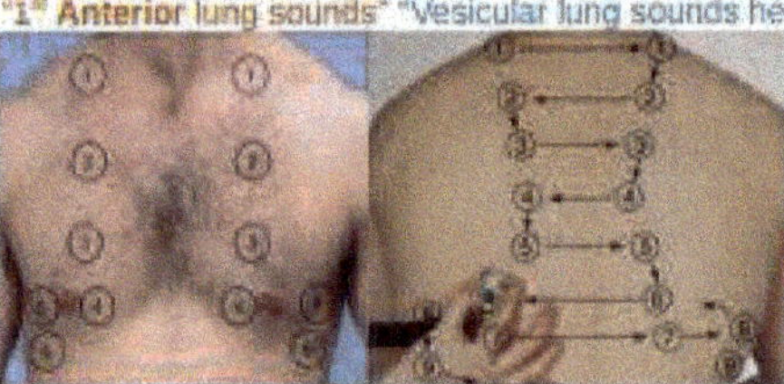

"2nd **Posterior** lung sounds". "Vesicular lung sounds heard, with no adventitious sounds"

"Example, Wheezes arise in the narrowed airways of asthma, COPD, and bronchitis"

</td></tr>
<tr><td>

Voice sounds: Egophony OR bronchophony

</td><td>

"Next to assess **Bronchophony**, I will have you say "**99**"

"I hear muffled & indistinct sound which is normal",

"Louder voice sounds are bronchophony which can indicate pneumonia"

</td></tr>
<tr><td colspan="2">

Abdomen (Lay down)

</td></tr>
<tr><td>

Inspect: Contour, masses, scars, skin

</td><td>

"Now, I will assess your **abdomen** starting with **inspection**"

"Contour is symmetrical appears rounded, no masses, scars or lesions"

</td></tr>
</table>

Auscultate: Bowel sounds in 4 quadrants 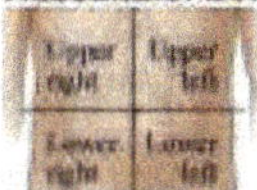 **Auscultate:** • Aorta • Renal arteries for bruits	"Next I will **auscultate** (listen) **to all 4 quadrants:** **Right Lower** • **Right Upper** • **Left Lower** • **Left Upper** "5-30 bowel sounds per minute in all 4 quadrants, normoactive" → **Auscultate** for **bruits over the aorta, iliac arteries & femoral arteries"** (using Bell) "No bruits heard", "Dull areas suggesting underlying mass or enlarged organ"	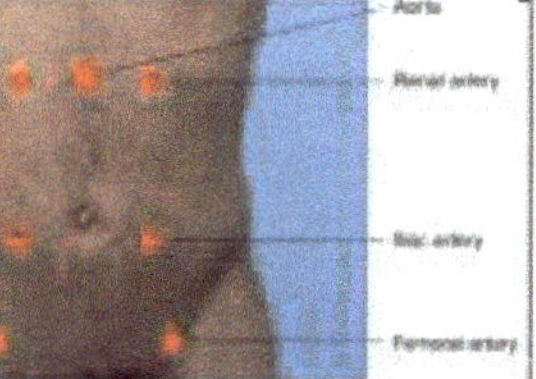 Auscultate for bruits
Percuss abdomen (Palpation 4 quadrants) • **Light palpation** 4 quadrants and flanks: Tenderness, masses • **Deep palpation** 4 quadrants and flanks: Tenderness, masses	"Next to **percuss** the abdomen in all 4 quadrants (RL, RU, LL, LU) & flanks" "1st **light palpation** by gently palpating to detect abdominal tenderness, muscular resistance & superficial organs or masses". "No tenderness or masses noted" "Then **deep palpation** is deeper depression of 2-3in", "No tenderness or masses noted" "Abdominal masses may be a pregnant uterus, diverticulitis, or distended bladder"	
Special Maneuvers: • **Percuss liver span** • **Palpate liver edge** • **Percuss for enlarged spleen along left costal margin** • **Palpate for enlarged spleen** • **Elicit rebound tenderness** • **Elicit CVA tenderness** • **Elicit Psoas sign/Obturator sign** • **Aortic span** 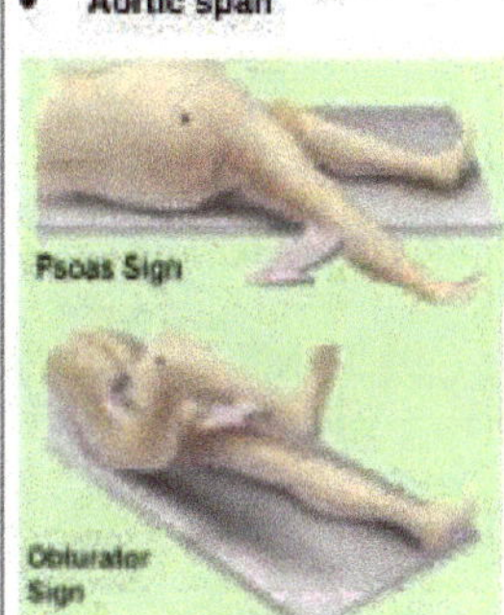 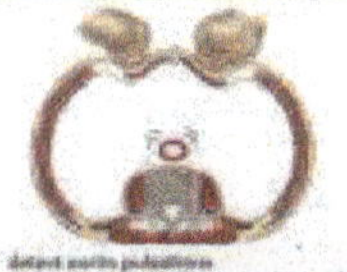 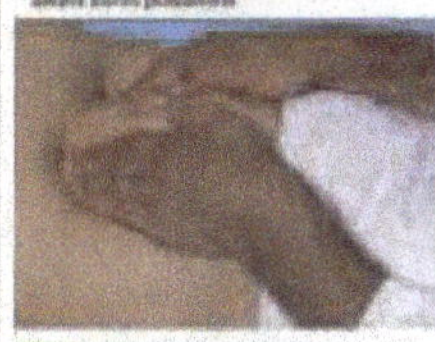	"Now to perform **Special Maneuvers:** →"**Percuss the Liver span** by starting RLQ moving up towards the liver, identify lower border of dullness midclavicular line, then identify the upper border liver dullness by starting at nipple line percussing downward until resonance shifts to liver dullness, normally measure 6-12cm", "Pt's measures 8cm", "Span of liver dullness is increased when the liver is enlarged". →"**Palpate Liver edge** by placing left hand behind pt parallel to the 11-12th rib, pushing up with left hand using right hand finger tips to palpate lower border of liver under costal margin (where ribs end)", "Take a deep breathe", "It is soft, sharp & regular with a smooth surface which is normal". "Sign of liver disease is firmness, blunt, rounding of its edge" →"**Percuss for enlarged Spleen along left costal margin** by percussing the left lower anterior chest wall from the border of cardiac dullness at the 6th rib to the anterior axillary line & down to the costal margin (Traube space) note the lateral extent of tympany", "Tympany is prominent" "Dullness on inspiration is a positive splenic percussion sign & is only moderately useful for detecting splenomegaly" →"**Palpate for enlarged spleen** with your right hand below the left costal margin pressing in toward the spleen", "take a deep breath?", "Begin palpation low, spleen tip is just palpable deep to the left costal margin", "Palpated high in the abdomen is a sign of Splenomegaly" →"**Elicit rebound tenderness** by pressing the RLQ to examine pain when released, assessing for peritoneal inflammation", "None noted" ------(Sit up)------ →"**Elicit CVA-Costovertebral angle tenderness** by having pt **sit up** percuss with the ulnar surface of your fist against hand. "No tenderness", "Pain with pressure or fist percussion supports →"**Elicit Psoas sign** 1st I will have you lift your right leg against my hand which is above your leg; Next I will have you turn onto your **left side**, extending the pt's right leg at the hip backwards. "No pain noted" "Increased abdominal pain either move is a positive sign, suggests irritation of the psoas muscle by an inflamed appendix" →"**Obturator sign** flexing the pt's right thigh at the hip, with the knee bent & rotate the leg internally", "No pain noted" "Right hypogastric pain is a positive obturator sign, from irritation of the obturator muscle by an inflamed appendix" →"**Aortic span** I will press firmly deep in the epigastrium, slightly to the left of the midline (above umbilicus), & identify the aortic pulsations", "pt's is 2.5cm" "Upper abdominal mass with expansile pulsations that is ≥3 cm in	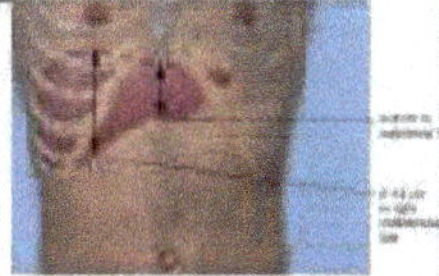 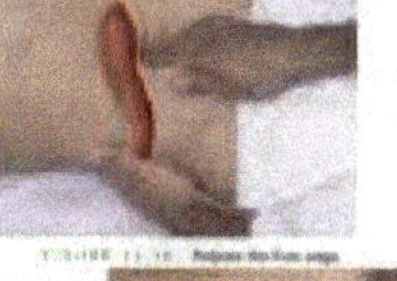 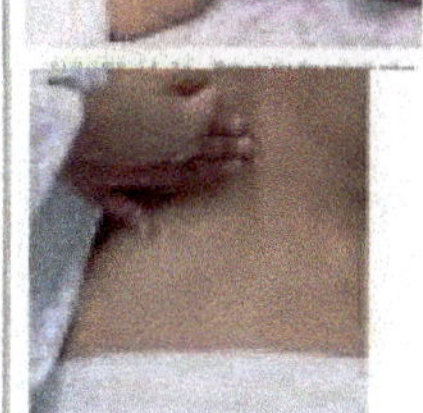 FIGURE 11-2? Percuss for costovertebral angle tenderness. (then Psoas sign→)

	diameter suggests an AAA (Abdominal Aortic Aneurysm)"

Breast (Verbalize only)	
"Inspection: Breast size, symmetry, contour, skin lesions/texture, nipples" "Redness suggests local infection or inflammatory carcinoma" →"Elicit **retractions or dimpling by 1st** having pt sit with **hands raised over head**; 2nd sitting with **hands pressed against hips while leaning forward** this brings out dimpling or retraction that otherwise may not be visible; inspecting the breast contours in each position "Breast dimpling or retraction is an sign of underlying cancer" **→"Palpate 4 quadrants each breast for tenderness, masses"** "**lateral portion** of the breast with the *patient turned to the side* with hand on forehead starting with the axilla palpating with 3 fingers with **concentric circles** moving closer to areola in a vertical strip pattern", "Then **medial portion** pt lays supine, placing her hand at her neck and lifting up her elbow until it is even with her shoulder", "Assessing bilaterally". "Hard irregular poorly circumscribed nodules, fixed to the skin or underlying tissues, strongly suggest cancer" **→"Palpate Areola/Nipples for tenderness, masses** (press or pinch lightly on nipple) **checking for discharge** • Instruct that assessment can be done at home monthly after period, since breasts less nodular **→"Palpate Axillary nodes: Lateral, Central, Subscapular & Pectoral** assessing for immobile, enlarged or tender nodes"	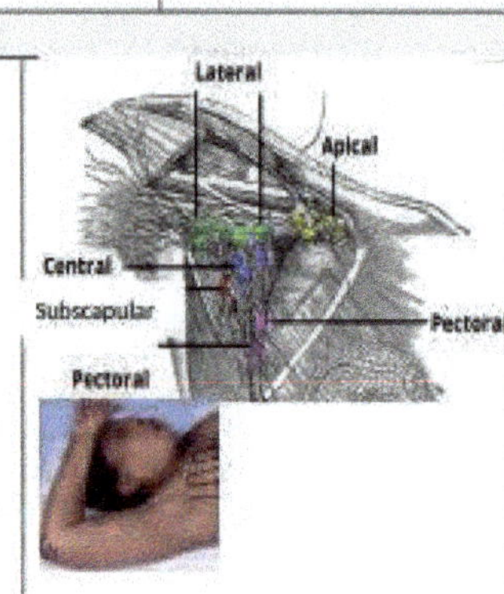

Video #4: MSK & Neuro Goal 10 minutes (Min 8 min/Maximum 15 min)		
• Wash hands (and apply gloves) • Introduce self	"I am Lindsey Beus Student Nurse Practitioner" "I have completed the general survey including vitals" "I will be assessing your **Musculoskeletal & Neurological** systems"	
Musculoskeletal		
Demonstrate: 1) Inspection 2) Palpation 3) Range of motion	I will 1st perform the **Musculoskeletal** exam; I will be **Inspecting, Palpating & performing Range of Motion** throughout the body; I will have you mimic my movement for ROM; Let me know if you have pain during ROM movements.	
TM joints: 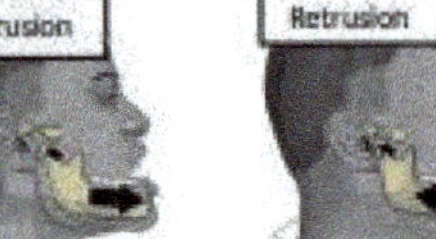 	**Temporomandibular joint (TMJ)** **Inspect** for swelling or redness-none noted **Palpating** joint by placing index finger in front of tragus of each ear & you will open your mouth, fingertips should drop into the joint spaces as the mouth opens-Which it does **ROM**, pt will open & close mouth. Protrusion moving lower jaw forward & Retrusion moving it inward- Moves smoothly; Swelling, tenderness, & decreased ROM sign of TMJ inflammation or arthritis	
Neck: • **Landmarks:** Cervical vertebrae, paravertebral muscles • **ROM:** Flexion, extension, lateral bending, rotation	Now to assess the **Neck** **Cervical vertebrae, paravertebral muscles** **Flexion** "Bring your chin to your chest" **Extension** "Look up at the ceiling" **Lateral bending** "Bring your ear to your shoulder" **Rotation** "Look over one shoulder, and then the	
Shoulder: • **Landmarks:** AC joint, bicipital groove, glenohumeral joint • **ROM:** Abduction, adduction, internal & external rotation, flexion, extension	Now assess the **Shoulder**; **Inspecting** skin or for swelling, deformity, muscle atrophy Starting from behind **Palpating** the **Acromioclavicular (AC) joint, bicipital groove, glenohumeral joint** **ROM:** **Flexion** "Raise your arms in front of you & overhead" (90°&180°) **Extension** "Extend your shoulder behind you" (60°) **Abduction** "Raise your arms out to the side & overhead" **Adduction** "Cross your arm in front of your body" (AC joint) **Internal rotation** "Place one hand behind your back and touch your shoulder blade."	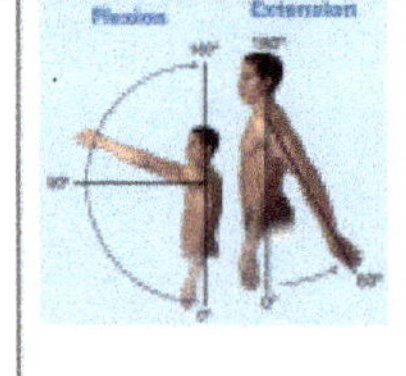

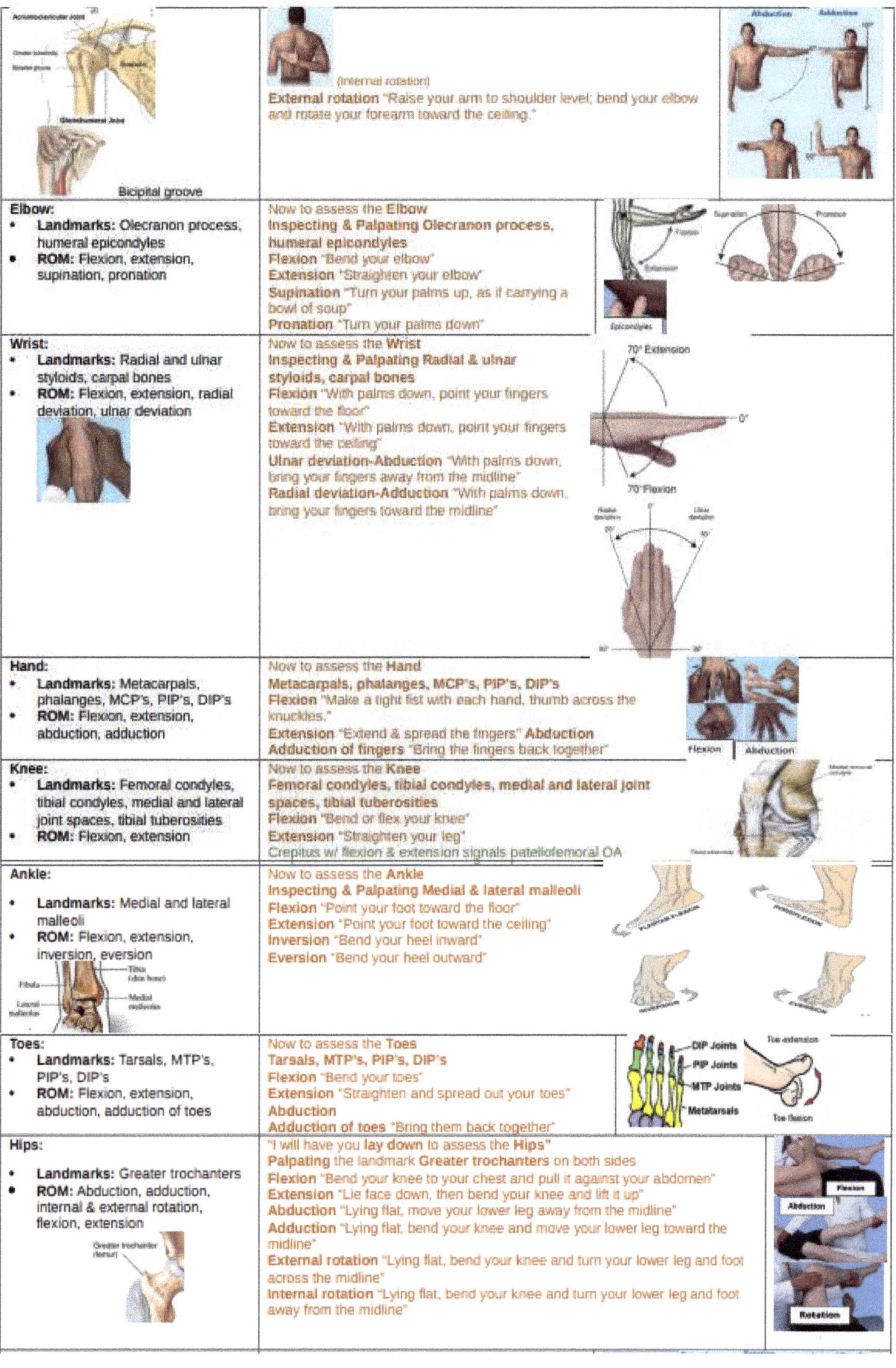

Bicipital groove	(internal rotation) **External rotation** "Raise your arm to shoulder level; bend your elbow and rotate your forearm toward the ceiling."
Elbow: • **Landmarks:** Olecranon process, humeral epicondyles • **ROM:** Flexion, extension, supination, pronation	Now to assess the **Elbow** **Inspecting & Palpating Olecranon process, humeral epicondyles** **Flexion** "Bend your elbow" **Extension** "Straighten your elbow" **Supination** "Turn your palms up, as if carrying a bowl of soup" **Pronation** "Turn your palms down"
Wrist: • **Landmarks:** Radial and ulnar styloids, carpal bones • **ROM:** Flexion, extension, radial deviation, ulnar deviation	Now to assess the **Wrist** **Inspecting & Palpating Radial & ulnar styloids, carpal bones** **Flexion** "With palms down, point your fingers toward the floor" **Extension** "With palms down, point your fingers toward the ceiling" **Ulnar deviation-Abduction** "With palms down, bring your fingers away from the midline" **Radial deviation-Adduction** "With palms down, bring your fingers toward the midline" 70° Extension 0° 70° Flexion
Hand: • **Landmarks:** Metacarpals, phalanges, MCP's, PIP's, DIP's • **ROM:** Flexion, extension, abduction, adduction	Now to assess the **Hand** **Metacarpals, phalanges, MCP's, PIP's, DIP's** **Flexion** "Make a tight fist with each hand, thumb across the knuckles." **Extension** "Extend & spread the fingers" **Abduction** **Adduction of fingers** "Bring the fingers back together" Flexion | Abduction
Knee: • **Landmarks:** Femoral condyles, tibial condyles, medial and lateral joint spaces, tibial tuberosities • **ROM:** Flexion, extension	Now to assess the **Knee** **Femoral condyles, tibial condyles, medial and lateral joint spaces, tibial tuberosities** **Flexion** "Bend or flex your knee" **Extension** "Straighten your leg" Crepitus w/ flexion & extension signals patellofemoral OA
Ankle: • **Landmarks:** Medial and lateral malleoli • **ROM:** Flexion, extension, inversion, eversion	Now to assess the **Ankle** **Inspecting & Palpating Medial & lateral malleoli** **Flexion** "Point your foot toward the floor" **Extension** "Point your foot toward the ceiling" **Inversion** "Bend your heel inward" **Eversion** "Bend your heel outward"
Toes: • **Landmarks:** Tarsals, MTP's, PIP's, DIP's • **ROM:** Flexion, extension, abduction, adduction of toes	Now to assess the **Toes** **Tarsals, MTP's, PIP's, DIP's** **Flexion** "Bend your toes" **Extension** "Straighten and spread out your toes" **Abduction** **Adduction of toes** "Bring them back together" DIP Joints PIP Joints MTP Joints Metatarsals
Hips: • **Landmarks:** Greater trochanters • **ROM:** Abduction, adduction, internal & external rotation, flexion, extension	"I will have you **lay down** to assess the **Hips**" **Palpating** the landmark **Greater trochanters** on both sides **Flexion** "Bend your knee to your chest and pull it against your abdomen" **Extension** "Lie face down, then bend your knee and lift it up" **Abduction** "Lying flat, move your lower leg away from the midline" **Adduction** "Lying flat, bend your knee and move your lower leg toward the midline" **External rotation** "Lying flat, bend your knee and turn your lower leg and foot across the midline" **Internal rotation** "Lying flat, bend your knee and turn your lower leg and foot away from the midline" Flexion Abduction Rotation

Spine: • **Landmarks:** Vertebrae, paravertebral muscles, sciatic notch • **ROM:** Flexion, extension, lateral bending, rotation	Now to assess the **Spine** **Vertebrae, paravertebral muscles, sciatic notch** **Flexion** "Bend forward and try to touch your toes" **Extension** "Bend back as far as possible" **Lateral bending** "Bend to the side from the waist" **Rotation** "Rotate from side to side" 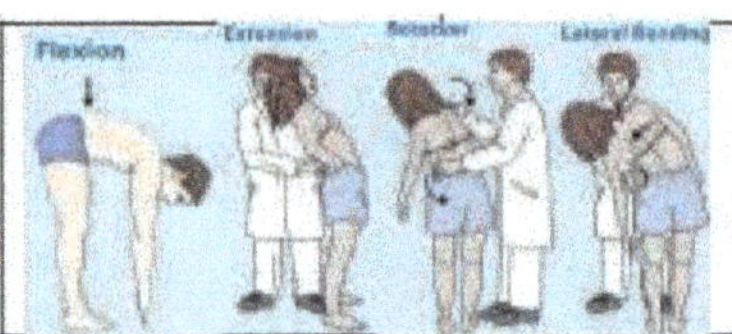
Neurological	
Mental Status: • **Cognitive function:** Pick **ONE** and demonstrate a technique to test: Serial 7's or 3's, memory, word comprehension, naming, reading, writing, or copying figures • **Higher intellectual function:** Pick **ONE** and demonstrate a technique to test: Information, vocabulary, abstract reasoning, or judgment	**Assess Mental Status** **Cognitive function:** Will you spell "WORLD" backwards. [D - L - R - O - W] **Higher intellectual function** through **Abstract reasoning:** What does "The squeaky wheel gets the grease" mean? What is the similarity between "An orange and an apple"?
Cranial Nerves: • **CN 2 Optic:** Visual acuity, visual fields • **CN 3 Oculomotor:** Pupil response, upper lid movement • **CN 4 Trochlear:** Look for EOMs with cardinal fields of gaze • **CN 5 Trigeminal sensory:** Light touch, pain to 3 facial dermatomes Trigeminal motor: Strength of temporal and masseter muscles • **CN 6 Abducens:** Observe lateral eye movement w/cardinal field of gaze • **CN 7 Facial motor:** Frown, smile & show teeth, wrinkle forehead • **CN 8 Acoustic:** Whispered voice (with ears) • **CN 9 & 10 Glossopharyngeal & Vagus motor:** symmetrical rising of palate, uvula, hoarseness (with *Mouth & Pharynx*) Sensory: Gag reflex, taste not required • **CN 11 Spinal accessory motor:** Turn head, shrug against resistance • **CN 12 Hypoglossal motor:** Tongue protrudes midline	Now to assess **Cranial Nerves:** **CN 2 Optic:** o **Visual acuity:** using the **Static finger wiggle test**. I am going to hold my hands 2 feet apart & to the side of you. When you see my fingers come into view, I want you to say "now". With **both** eyes, I want you to look at my eyes → Now we will do this again but **covering one eye** at a time. With your uncovered eye look into my uncovered eye o **Visual fields:** Placing the Snellen chart 14in. from your face, cover your **R** eye & read the smallest line that you can read from Left-Right, then **L**, **both** eyes **CN 3 Oculomotor:** o **Pupil response:** I will shine light was shown into your eye it *constricted* which is the **Direct response to light**- noted bilaterally; **Consensual response to light** is when the opposite eye constricts when the other eye had direct light applied. **CN 3 Oculomotor,** intact bilaterally o Upper lid movement **Cardinal field of gaze: Tests CN3, 4 & 6** **CN 4 Trochlear:** Look for EOMs **CN 6 Abducens:** Observe lateral eye movement → I want you to follow my finger with your eyes & keep your head still, looking for beats of **nystagmus.** Normal conjugate movements **CN 5 Trigeminal sensory:** o Light touch, pain to 3 facial dermatomes o Trigeminal motor: Strength of temporal and masseter muscles **CN 7 Facial motor:** Frown, smile & show teeth, wrinkle forehead
	CN 8 Acoustic: Whispered voice (with *ears*) → I will stand 2 ft. behind you, occlude the non-tested ear & rub the tragus in a circular motion. **Whisper test:** by **whispering a combination of letters & numbers** into each ear & have you repeat what I said back. 1st the Right ear "3-U-1" Can you repeat?, Now the Left ear "2-B-8" Can you repeat? **CN 9 & 10 Glossopharyngeal & Vagus motor:** → I will have you stick your tongue out and place the **tongue blade** onto it? "Say Ah...", Symmetrical rising of palate, uvula, hoarseness (w/ *Mouth & Pharynx*) **CN 12 Hypoglossal motor:** Tongue protrudes midline o Sensory: Gag reflex, taste not required **CN 11 Spinal accessory motor:** o Turn head o Shrug against resistance
Motor-Inspection: • Muscle bulk, tone • Unusual movements, tremors, fasciculation (Hold one hand w/ yours and, while supporting the elbow, flex & extend the pt's fingers, wrist, elbow, put the shoulder through a moderate ROM)	**Motor-Inspection:** • **Muscle Bulk:** Inspect the size & contours of muscles; Inspecting for signs of atrophy paying attention to hands, shoulders, thighs & legs. (No signs of atrophy) • **Muscle Tone:** I am going to hold your hand and move it through ROM, there is slight residual tension "muscle tone" • No **unusual movements, tremors, fasciculation**

Muscle Strength: • Test muscle strength against resistance in major muscle groups Grade muscle strength 0-5 • Upper extremities • Lower extremities • Shoulder girdle: Pronator drift - arms extended, palms up	• Now Test **Muscle strength** against resistance in major muscle groups: **Upper extremities:** o "Flex your arm, don't let me pull down" o "Don't let me push up" o "Now grasp my fingers" (Grips) Grade muscle strength **5** (Normal) **Lower extremities:** o "Lift your leg against my hand" o "Try to bring your legs together" o "Spread both legs against my hands" o "Straighten your leg" o "Dorsiflexion-pull foot up" o "Push foot down-plantar flexion" Grade muscle strength **5** (Normal) **Shoulder girdle:** o Pronator drift: "Extend your arms out with palms up"-No drifting of either hand or pronation Grade muscle strength **5** (Normal) 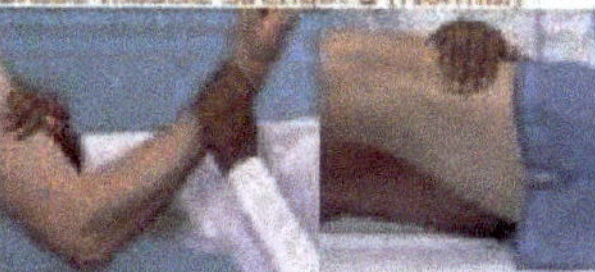
Sensory: Major dermatomes of extremities Test for light touch and pain separately: • Light touch (cotton) • Pain (broken tongue blade, paper clip) • Vibratory sense with 128 Hz tuning fork • Position sense great toe and index finger bilaterally	**Sensory:** Major dermatomes of extremities • **Light touch (cotton):** "Tell me when you feel the cotton against your skin?" Assessing bilateral upper extremities & lower extremities • **Pain (paper clip)** "I will be pressing an object against your skin", "Is this sharp or dull?" • **Vibratory sense with 128 Hz tuning fork** (Tap tuning fork & place it on distal interphalangeal joint of the pt's finger; then interphalangeal joint of the big toe) "I will be placing the tuning fork onto your hand & then foot, put your hands out & close your eyes, tell me when you feel the vibration stop"
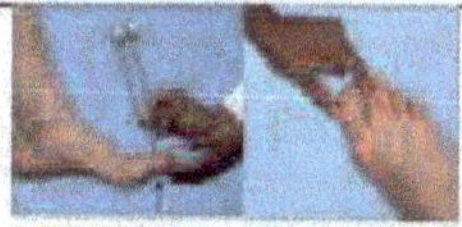	Assessing bilateral hands & feet • **Position sense great toe and index finger bilaterally** Proprioception (Joint Position Sense). Grasp the patient's big toe, holding it by its sides between your thumb & index finger, then pull it away from the other toes. Demonstrate "up" & "down" as you move the patient's toe clearly upward & downward. "I will be moving your index finger up & down, now close your eyes & say "up" or "down" when I move it" (bilateral) "Now with your big toe, close your eyes & say "up" or "down" when I move it" (bilateral)
Reflexes: **Deep tendon reflexes:** • Triceps • Biceps • Brachioradialis • Knee (Patellar) • Ankle (Achilles) • Plantar response (Normal or Babinski-abnormal) 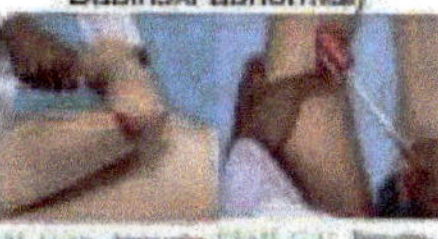 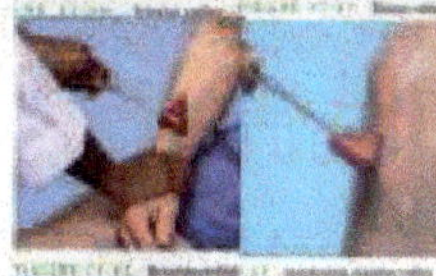 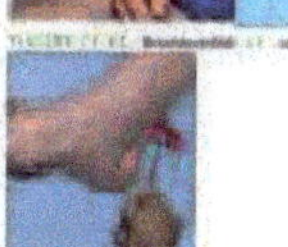	Now assessing **Reflexes:** **Deep tendon reflexes:** • **Triceps:** o "While sitting, flex your arm at the elbow with palm down, slightly crossing your chest" (Strike the triceps tendon with a direct blow directly behind and just above the elbow) o Contraction of the triceps muscle & extension at the elbow (Normal) o **Grade 2** (Avg. normal) • **Biceps:** (Place your thumb or finger firmly on the biceps tendon. Aim the strike with the reflex hammer directly through your digit toward the biceps tendon) o "I will be hitting my thumb toward bicep tendon with the hammer" o **Grade 2** (Avg. normal) • **Brachioradialis** o "Pt rests hand on lap, strike the radius with the flat edge above the wrist" o **Grade 2** (Avg. normal) Watch for flexion and supination of the forearm • **Knee (Patellar)** o "Sitting with knees flexed, I will briskly tap the patellar tendon" o **Grade 2** (Avg. normal) Note contraction of the quadriceps with extension at the knee • **Ankle (Achilles)** o "Point your foot and I will strike the Achilles tendon" o **Grade 2** (Avg. normal) Strike the Achilles tendon, & watch and feel for plantar flexion at the ankle • **Plantar response** (Normal or Babinski-abnormal) o "I am going to stroke the sole of your foot (heel – ball)" o Response is negative, toes did not fan out, which is normal for adult pt

Cerebellar Function: Equilibrium & Gait Gait • Heel to toe (tandem) walking • Romberg: feet together, eyes closed, arms at side for 20-30 seconds	**Cerebellar Function: Equilibrium & Gait** **Gait: Heel to toe (tandem) walking** • "Will you walk heel-to-toe in a straight line, walking on your toes & then heels" • tests plantar flexion & dorsi-flexion of the ankles as well as balance **Romberg:** feet together, eyes closed, arms at side for 20-30 seconds • "Will you stand with feet, arms at sides, together with eyes open for 20-30sec", "Now, with eyes closed" • Pt able to maintain upright posture and no swaying (or minimal-normal) noted
Coordination: Demonstrate **EITHER** rapid alternating movements **OR** point-to-point Upper extremities Lower extremities	**Coordination:** Point-to-Point Movements Arms—Finger-to-Nose Test "I will have you touch my index finger, then your nose, alternating 7x" (Move your finger so the patient has to change directions & extend the arm fully to reach your finger) "Accuracy & smoothness of movement is noted, no tremor" "Now we will repeat this but you will touch my finger (staying in 1 place) then raise your arm over your head, repeating it 7x". "Then with your eyes closed" "Now the other arm" "Pt was able to touch finger with eyes open or close (Normal), this test the position sense & fx of both the labyrinth of the inner ear & the cerebellum"

Pelvic Exam (Verbal only)

- "For the Pelvic exam, I am verbalizing the procedure only. Have pt empty bladder."
- Materials for procedure: Gloves, speculum, sponge forceps, cotton balls, brush, two glass slides, liquid medium, lubricant & Kleenex
- "I will raise the HOB, moving your bottom to the end of the exam table. Placing a sheet around your legs arranging it so that only perineum is visible. Now separate your legs & let them relax. I would palpate perineal tone.
- I would then instruct you to hold your breath & strain or push down looking for any urine or descent of the vagina wall.
- Are you having any loss of urine with coughing or sneezing?
- Using the speculum to examine the vagina & cervix for color, discharge and lesions
- Then perform an internal exam by inserting my fingers into the vagina & palpating for masses or tenderness.
- Then palpate & elevate the cervix, while palpating for the uterus with my other hand.
- I would then perform an internal pelvic exam.
- I would put on gloves and use my left hand to hold the speculum and right hand to palpate the uterus & ovaries between fingers and palpating hand flat on the lower abdomen.
- I would locate the cervix & note the size, mobility, position and consistency of the cervix.
- I would assess if there is pain with movement of the cervix.
- I would press downward with my abdominal hand palm up, put one finger on either side of the cervix and attempt to outline the uterus.

Opthalamoscopic exam → Dims light, positions patient appropriately → Turn on & set ophthalmoscope to "0" → Holds ophthalmoscope correctly (left eye for left eye, right for right eye) uses index finger to switch lens → Hold 15in away from pt at a 15° angle, then move closer to visualize • **Verbalizes major structures of eye** (cornea, vitreous, optic disc, vessels (vein/arteries) & macula)	"I am going to **dim the light** to perform the **Opthalamoscopic Exam**: I will assess your eyes with the **Opthalamscope.** I will move in close to view your eye Look up & over my shoulder as I shine the light into your eye 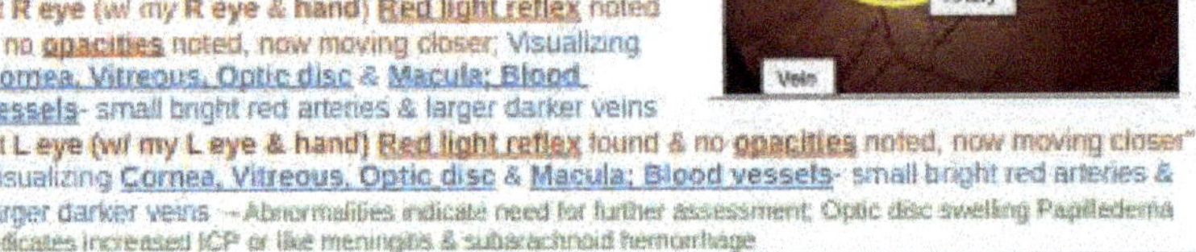 Pt **R eye** (w/ my **R eye & hand**) **Red light reflex** noted & no **opacities** noted, now moving closer; Visualizing **Cornea, Vitreous, Optic disc** & **Macula; Blood vessels**- small bright red arteries & larger darker veins Pt **L eye (w/ my L eye & hand) Red light reflex** found & no **opacities** noted, now moving closer", Visualizing **Cornea, Vitreous, Optic disc** & **Macula; Blood vessels**- small bright red arteries & larger darker veins →Abnormalities indicate need for further assessment; Optic disc swelling Papilledema indicates increased ICP or like meningitis & subarachnoid hemorrhage

• **Hearing:** Test with **whispered voice** or watch tick –CN 8 **Tuning fork test:** 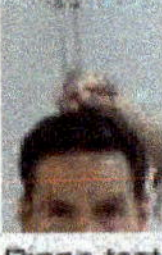 **Weber test** (lateralization) Rinne test (*Air conduction (AC): bone conduction (BC)*) 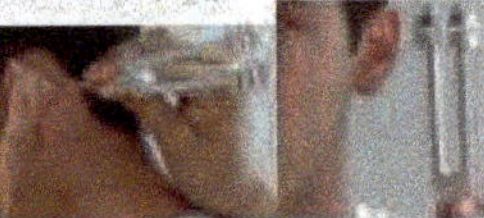	"Do you feel you have a hearing loss or difficulty hearing?", "Nest I will test you **hearing** and **Cranial Nerve 8, Vestibulocochlear nerve**, I will stand 2 ft. behind you", "I will have you occlude the non-tested ear and rub the tragus in a circular motion" "I will **whisper a combination of letters and numbers** into each ear and have you repeat what I said back", "I will exhale 1st to ensure a whispered voice", "1" the Right ear "3-U-1" Can you repeat?", "Now the Left ear "2-B-6" Can you repeat?"
	→"Next the **Weber test**, **testing Conductive vs. sensorineural hearing loss**", "We are in a quiet room and I am using a **tuning fork of 512 hertz**", "I will tap it against my forarm to start the vibration", "I will place **tuning fork** at middle of your ***head*** and tell me which ear the sound is best heard or if it is equal"-"In ***unilateral conductive hearing loss***, sound is heard in the impaired ear possibly from otitis media or perforation of the ear drum"/ "In unilateral ***sensorineural hearing loss***, sound is heard in the good ear" →"Now **Rinne test**, I will place the tuning fork 1st at the **Mastoid bone** (behind the ear) testing **Bone Conduction**", "Tell me when you no longer here the tuning fork", "Once no longer hearing the tuning fork I will immediately hold the tuning fork with U facing forward, **next to your ear** & do you hear the sound again?" (Yes) "this maximizes the sound transmission which is normal finding to have heard it longer in air conduction than bone conduction" "In ***conductive hearing loss*** sound is heard through bone as long or longer than through air" "In ***sensorineural hearing loss***, sound is heard longer through air"

16.10 Microbiology Considerations

16.10.1 Microbiology Foundation

Table 303 Microbiology Foundational Cosniderations

Category	Subcategory	Examples	Key Features	Clinical Implications/Diagnosis
Microorganism Classification	**Bacteria**	*E. coli, Staphylococcus aureus*	Prokaryotic, single-celled organisms, cell wall (Gram + or -), can be aerobic or anaerobic	Can cause infections like UTIs, skin infections, pneumonia, sepsis, depending on bacterial strain and environment
	Viruses	*HIV, Influenza, Hepatitis B*	Acellular, need host to replicate, composed of DNA or RNA and a protein coat (capsid)	Viruses require antiviral treatment (e.g., HIV) or vaccines (e.g., Hep B, Influenza)
	Fungi	*Candida albicans, Aspergillus*	Eukaryotic, can be single-celled or multicellular, can be pathogenic in immunocompromised individuals	Can lead to opportunistic infections, especially in immunocompromised patients like candidiasis, aspergillosis
	Parasites	*Plasmodium, Giardia, Tapeworms*	Eukaryotic, complex life cycles, often involving an intermediate host	Can cause gastrointestinal symptoms (Giardia), systemic effects (Plasmodium causing malaria), and other parasitic diseases
	Prions	*Creutzfeldt-Jakob disease*	Protein-only infectious agents, no nucleic acids	Can lead to neurodegenerative diseases, prion diseases are usually fatal with no cure
Laboratory Diagnostics	**Gram Stain**	-	Staining technique to	Helps in identifying bacterial species

			differentiate Gram-positive and Gram-negative bacteria based on cell wall structure	and choosing appropriate antibiotics
	Culture & Sensitivity (C&S)	-	Cultures grown on media to identify bacteria, followed by testing for antibiotic susceptibility	Critical for selecting the correct antibiotic therapy for bacterial infections
	PCR (Polymerase Chain Reaction)	-	Amplifies DNA/RNA sequences to detect specific pathogens (e.g., HIV, COVID-19, TB)	Useful for detecting pathogens that are difficult to culture or for viruses
	ELISA (Enzyme-Linked Immunosorbent Assay)	-	Tests for antibodies or antigens (e.g., for HIV, Hepatitis B)	Identifies past infections or current exposure to pathogens
	Serology	-	Blood tests to identify the immune response to infections through detection of specific antibodies (IgM, IgG)	Useful for identifying past infections and immune responses
	Blood Smear	-	A microscopic examination of blood to identify infections like malaria or parasitic organisms	Key for diagnosing malaria, parasitic infections like Babesia or Trypanosoma
Pathogenic Microorganisms and Diseases	**Staphylococcus aureus**	Skin infections, sepsis, endocarditis	Gram-positive cocci, facultative anaerobe, part of normal skin flora	Causes abscesses, pneumonia, bloodstream infections, and can

			but can cause severe infections when opportunistic	be resistant to antibiotics (e.g., MRSA)
	Streptococcus pyogenes	Strep throat, rheumatic fever	Gram-positive cocci, β-hemolytic, group A streptococcus	Causes pharyngitis, scarlet fever, and post-streptococcal complications like glomerulonephritis
	E. coli	UTIs, food poisoning	Gram-negative rod, facultative anaerobe, part of normal intestinal flora	Can cause UTIs, gastroenteritis, and bloodstream infections, some strains (e.g., E. coli O157:H7) can be highly virulent
	Mycobacterium tuberculosis	Tuberculosis	Slow-growing acid-fast bacilli	Causes pulmonary and extrapulmonary tuberculosis, requires prolonged antibiotic therapy
	Clostridium difficile	Antibiotic-associated diarrhea, colitis	Gram-positive, anaerobic, spore-forming bacteria	Often occurs after antibiotic therapy, causes colitis, may lead to life-threatening complications (e.g., toxic megacolon)
	Neisseria meningitidis	Meningitis	Gram-negative diplococcus, part of the normal nasopharyngeal flora	Causes bacterial meningitis, can be life-threatening and requires prompt treatment
Important Viruses	**Influenza virus**	Flu	RNA virus, enveloped, causes seasonal respiratory infections	Requires vaccines and antiviral treatment for

16.10.2 Antimicrobial Considerations and Resistance

Table 304 Antimicrobbial Considerations and Resistence

Category	Drug Class	Examples	Target Pathogens	Key Considerations
Antimicrobial Drug Classes	**Penicillins**	Amoxicillin, Penicillin G	Gram-positive bacteria	Effective for strep throat, skin infections; watch for penicillin allergies.
	Cephalosporins	Ceftriaxone, Cefazolin	Broad-spectrum	Treats pneumonia, UTIs; classified into generations based on activity spectrum.
	Macrolides	Azithromycin, Erythromycin	Respiratory infections	Commonly used for pneumonia, bronchitis; risk of QT prolongation in high doses.
	Aminoglycosides	Gentamicin	Gram-negative bacteria, serious infections	Used in severe infections, kidney toxicity, must monitor drug levels.
	Fluoroquinolones	Ciprofloxacin, Levofloxacin	UTIs, GI infections	Broad spectrum, risk of tendon rupture, avoid in children and pregnant women.
	Antivirals	Acyclovir, Oseltamivir	HSV, Influenza	Effective for HSV, flu; early administration is key for effectiveness.
	Antifungals	Fluconazole, Amphotericin B	Candida, systemic mycoses	Monitor for liver toxicity, particularly with long-term use.
	Antiparasitics	Metronidazole, Mebendazole	Giardia, intestinal worms	Treats parasitic infections, consider drug interactions

			and side effects like nausea.

16.10.3 Immunology, Transmission, Infection Control, and Antimicrobial Considerations

Table 305 Immunology, Transmission, Infection Control, and Antimicrobial Considerations

Category	Subcategory	Details	Clinical Implications
Immunology and Host Response	**Innate Immunity**	Immediate, nonspecific defense mechanisms such as physical barriers (skin, mucous membranes), phagocytes (neutrophils, macrophages), and natural killer (NK) cells. Activated as the first line of defense.	Provides immediate defense against pathogens, essential in the early stages of infection. Can lead to inflammation and fever.
	Adaptive Immunity	Specific, memory-based immunity involving B and T cells. B cells produce antibodies for pathogen recognition, while T cells directly attack infected cells. Involves primary (first exposure) and secondary (subsequent exposure) immune responses.	Offers long-term immunity and provides protection from future infections. Vaccination enhances adaptive immunity by priming the immune system.
	Antigens	Foreign substances, such as pathogens or toxins, that trigger an immune response. Typically, antigens are proteins or polysaccharides found on the surface of pathogens.	Key signals for immune activation. Targeted by antibodies to neutralize pathogens or mark them for destruction.
	Antibodies (IgG, IgM, etc.)	Proteins produced by B cells that bind to specific antigens. IgG provides long-term immunity, whereas IgM is the first to appear in acute infections.	Neutralize or mark pathogens for destruction. IgG is vital for immunological memory, while IgM helps in early-stage defense.

	Vaccination	Vaccines train the immune system by introducing a small, non-infectious part of a pathogen (antigen) to trigger an immune response, stimulating both B and T cells. Examples include MMR, DTaP, COVID-19, and HPV vaccines.	Primarily used to prevent infection. Stimulates long-term immunity and prepares the immune system to respond faster and more effectively to future infections.
Modes of Transmission	**Contact**	Spread through direct contact (e.g., skin-to-skin, mucous membranes) or indirect contact (e.g., contaminated surfaces). Pathogens like MRSA, C. difficile, and VRE are transmitted via contact.	Requires isolation of infected patients, use of gloves, gowns, and stringent hygiene practices to prevent cross-contamination.
	Droplet	Spread via respiratory droplets generated when an infected person coughs, sneezes, or talks. Pathogens include Influenza, pertussis, and SARS-CoV-2.	Masks are essential in protecting against droplet transmission. Infected individuals should be placed in isolation with appropriate precautions.
	Airborne	Pathogens are transmitted through tiny airborne particles that remain suspended in the air. TB, measles, and varicella are airborne diseases.	Requires use of N95 masks, isolation in negative pressure rooms, and strict infection control measures.
	Vector-borne	Transmission via insects or other organisms (vectors). Examples include Malaria (mosquitoes), Lyme disease (ticks).	Involves preventive measures such as the use of insect repellents, bed nets, and avoiding areas with high vector presence.
	Fecal-oral	Pathogens transmitted through contaminated food, water, or direct contact with fecal matter.	Hygiene practices, sanitation, clean water, and safe food handling

		Norovirus, cholera, and hepatitis A are classic examples.	are critical to prevent fecal-oral transmission.
	Bloodborne	Pathogens spread through blood or body fluids. HIV, Hepatitis B, and Hepatitis C are common bloodborne pathogens.	Requires use of proper PPE, sterilization of medical equipment, and safe handling of needles and sharps to prevent exposure.
Infection Control Measures	**Standard Precautions**	Basic infection control measures for all patients, including hand hygiene, gloves, and proper disposal of contaminated materials.	These are foundational to reducing the risk of transmission in healthcare settings. Ensures protection against all types of infections.
	Contact Precautions	Used for infections transmitted through direct or indirect contact with the patient or their environment. Pathogens include MRSA, VRE, and C. difficile.	Requires use of gowns, gloves, and appropriate cleaning/disinfection protocols. Isolate patients when necessary to prevent the spread of infection.
	Droplet Precautions	Used for infections transmitted by respiratory droplets. Includes diseases like influenza and pertussis.	Requires masks, patient isolation, and room ventilation. Masks must be worn when in close proximity to the patient.
	Airborne Precautions	Used for infections transmitted through airborne particles. Diseases include TB and measles.	Involves the use of N95 respirators, placement in negative pressure rooms, and restricting patient movement outside of their isolation area.
	Protective (Reverse) Precautions	Measures to protect immunocompromised or neutropenic patients from outside infections.	Requires strict isolation, use of high-efficiency filtration systems, and restriction of visitors or unnecessary contacts.
Antimicrobial Considerations	**Penicillins**	Amoxicillin, Penicillin G. Targets Gram-positive	Effective for common infections. Overuse can

		bacteria, used for treating pneumonia, strep throat, and skin infections.	lead to resistance. Requires allergy screening prior to administration.
	Cephalosporins	Ceftriaxone, cefazolin. Broad-spectrum antibiotics effective against both Gram-positive and Gram-negative organisms.	Commonly used in surgical prophylaxis and broad-spectrum infection treatment. Second- and third-generation cephalosporins target resistant bacteria.
	Macrolides	Azithromycin, erythromycin. Used primarily for respiratory infections (e.g., pneumonia, bronchitis) and sexually transmitted infections (e.g., chlamydia).	Effective for both Gram-positive and atypical pathogens. Careful use in elderly patients due to risk of QT interval prolongation.
	Aminoglycosides	Gentamicin. Targets Gram-negative bacteria, often used for severe infections like sepsis.	Requires monitoring for nephrotoxicity and ototoxicity. Typically used in combination with other antibiotics for synergistic effects.
	Fluoroquinolones	Ciprofloxacin, levofloxacin. Effective for UTIs, GI infections, and some respiratory infections.	Risk of tendon rupture in older adults. Prescribe with caution in those with renal impairment.
	Antivirals	Acyclovir, oseltamivir. Used for viral infections such as herpes simplex virus (HSV), influenza, and chickenpox.	Early initiation is key for efficacy. Some antivirals can cause kidney damage in long-term use or overdose.
	Antifungals	Fluconazole, amphotericin B. Used for Candida infections, systemic mycoses, and Aspergillus infections.	Often require monitoring for liver toxicity. Amphotericin B requires renal function monitoring due to nephrotoxicity.

	Antiparasitics	Metronidazole, mebendazole. Used for parasitic infections such as Giardia, amoebiasis, and helminths.	Treatment duration varies; side effects like GI distress and skin reactions are

16.10.4 Comprehensive Microbiology in Public Health and Epidemiology (WHO/CDC Guidelines)

Table 306 Comprehensive Considerations of Microbioogy in Public Health

Category	Subcategory	Details	Key Actions and Implications
Outbreak Investigations	**Foodborne Illness**	Common pathogens include *Salmonella*, *E. coli*, *Listeria*, and *Campylobacter*; often linked to contaminated food or water.	**Steps:** Identify source of infection (trace back food source), conduct culture and PCR testing, implement quarantine if necessary, conduct contact tracing, and inform the public.
	Influenza	Outbreaks occur seasonally, caused by influenza A and B viruses; requires identifying strains such as H1N1, H3N2, and variants.	**Steps:** Test patient specimens, identify virus type, monitor epidemiological trends, and activate emergency vaccination campaigns if necessary.
	Vector-borne Diseases	*Malaria*, *Dengue*, *Zika*, and *Yellow Fever* are spread by mosquitoes; *Plasmodium* species (malaria) and *Aedes* mosquitoes (Dengue, Zika).	**Steps:** Surveillance of mosquito populations, use of insecticide-treated nets (ITNs), vector control (indoor spraying), and emergency vaccination where needed.
	Zoonotic Diseases	Infections like *Hantavirus*, *Ebola*, *Rabies*, *Avian Influenza* (H5N1), and *Zika virus* which	**Steps:** One Health approach, collaboration across human, animal, and environmental health sectors, use of

		jump from animals to humans.	animal health surveillance, and risk communication to the public.
Surveillance of Emerging Infections	**Global Networks**	**Global Influenza Surveillance and Response System (GISRS)**, *Epidemic Intelligence Service (EIS)*, and other global systems track infectious diseases globally.	**Actions:** Real-time monitoring of infectious diseases, sharing data globally for timely interventions, and tracking new pathogen strains to inform public health guidelines.
	Zoonotic Infections	Diseases such as *Avian Influenza*, *Zika*, and *COVID-19* often have cross-species transmission (animal-to-human).	**Actions:** Surveillance systems integrate data from human, animal, and environmental health. Use genetic sequencing to track transmission routes of new diseases.
	Antimicrobial Resistance (AMR)	Resistance of pathogens like *MRSA* and *ESBL* to multiple antibiotics creates treatment challenges.	**Actions:** Promote antimicrobial stewardship, monitor antibiotic resistance patterns, improve infection control measures, and prevent unnecessary prescriptions.
Vaccination Programs	**Routine Immunization**	Vaccines for *Measles*, *Polio*, *Hepatitis B*, *Mumps*, *Rubella*, *Hib*, *Rotavirus* are given on a set schedule to prevent common diseases.	**Actions:** Ensure high vaccination coverage, particularly in vulnerable populations (e.g., children, elderly, healthcare workers). Collaborate internationally to

			address immunization gaps.
	Outbreak Response Vaccination	Emergency vaccination campaigns for diseases like *Yellow Fever*, *Cholera*, and *Meningitis* during an outbreak.	**Actions:** Swift deployment of vaccines, typically within 48 hours of outbreak detection. Utilize mass vaccination strategies in affected areas.
	Targeted Vaccination for High-Risk Groups	Focus on pregnant women, infants, the elderly, and immunocompromised individuals, who are at higher risk for severe disease.	**Actions:** Prioritize vaccines in clinical settings and during mass immunization efforts. Encourage targeted vaccination campaigns and monitoring of high-risk groups.
Key Public Health Initiatives	**Global Health Security**	Response to emerging diseases, pandemics, and biosecurity threats, including surveillance of new pathogens.	**Actions:** Strengthen national response mechanisms, ensure timely sharing of health data, coordinate international responses to prevent disease spread.
	Community Engagement	Active involvement of communities in health initiatives, including vaccination campaigns and hygiene awareness.	**Actions:** Implement community health education programs, engage local leaders in public health initiatives, and promote behavior change in disease prevention.
	Cross-Sector Collaboration	Collaboration across sectors such as education, agriculture,	**Actions:** Facilitate partnerships among public health, animal health, agriculture, and

		environment, and urban planning to tackle complex public health challenges.	environmental sectors for effective disease prevention and management.
Epidemiological Surveillance	**Disease Reporting**	Reporting of cases of infectious diseases to national and global health authorities such as the CDC, WHO, and local public health departments.	**Actions:** Develop and maintain real-time surveillance systems, provide accurate data for epidemic prediction and intervention, and utilize GIS mapping for disease hotspots.
	Rapid Response Teams	Mobilizing rapid response teams, including public health professionals, epidemiologists, and laboratory scientists, during disease outbreaks.	**Actions:** Quickly deploy teams to investigate, contain, and mitigate outbreaks using data-driven models. Develop rapid diagnostic tools and response protocols.
	Data Collection and Analysis	Collection and analysis of data to understand disease trends, track outbreaks, and predict future public health threats.	**Actions:** Use big data analytics, GIS mapping, and social media data for early detection of outbreaks, and guide decision-making in health interventions.
Infection Control Measures	**Hand Hygiene**	Preventing the transmission of pathogens by washing hands regularly with soap and water.	**Actions:** Promote global hygiene campaigns, ensure access to soap and water, and educate communities on proper handwashing techniques.

	Transmission-Based Precautions	Standard precautions and additional precautions for contact, droplet, and airborne transmission.	**Actions:** Isolate infected individuals, use personal protective equipment (PPE), and implement environmental controls in healthcare settings.
	Isolation/Quarantine	Isolate infected individuals to prevent disease spread, especially in cases of highly contagious diseases.	**Actions:** Establish quarantine zones for confirmed or suspected cases, monitor contacts, and maintain strong communication with public health officials.

16.11 Antibiotic Consideration

16.11.1 Antibiotic Overview

Bacteria are categorized based on their shape, such as **cocci** (spherical) and **bacilli** (rod-shaped), and their Gram stain properties, with **Gram-positive bacteria** staining violet and **Gram-negative bacteria** staining red. **Antibiotics like Penicillin target the bacterial cell wall, inhibiting its synthesis, while others like Aminoglycosides and Tetracyclines** interfere with protein synthesis by binding to bacterial ribosomes. The treatment of **pneumonia** is highlighted, particularly **Community-Acquired Pneumonia (CAP)** and **Healthcare-Associated Pneumonia (HCAP),** with recommended antibiotics including **Azithromycin**, **Vancomycin**, and **Ceftriaxone**. The importance of addressing **antibiotic resistance**, particularly **Methicillin-Resistant Staphylococcus Aureus (MRSA),** is emphasized, alongside the need for tailored antibiotic choices based on the type of bacteria and the infection being treated to ensure effective outcomes.

16.11.2 Principles of Antibiotics

Principles of antibiotic use are essential for effective patient care and combating antimicrobial resistance. **Empiric therapy** is the initial treatment provided based on the most likely pathogens causing an infection, often before culture results are available. This approach is critical in severe or life-threatening infections, where waiting for culture results could delay necessary treatment. **Definitive therapy** is initiated once culture and sensitivity results are obtained, allowing for a more targeted approach by selecting the most effective antibiotic for the identified pathogen. **Prophylactic use** refers to the preventive administration of antibiotics, often used in situations like surgical or dental procedures to prevent infections in patients at high risk. **Antibiotic stewardship** focuses on the rational use of antibiotics to maximize effectiveness while minimizing the risks of resistance and adverse effects. The primary goals of antibiotic therapy are to ensure the **right drug, right dose, right duration**, and **right route** of administration to optimize patient outcomes and reduce the emergence of resistant organisms.

16.11.3 Classification of Antibiotics

16.11.3.1 According to Mechanism of Action

Table 307 Table 1 Classification of Antibiotics According to the Mechanism of Action

S.No.	ANTIBIOTICS	MECHANISM OF ACTION
1	Beta-lactam antibiotics (Penicillin, Cephalosporin, Monobactams, Carbapenems) Cycloserin, Bacitracin, Vancomycin, Fosfomycin	Cell wall synthesis inhibitors.
2.	Polypeptides (Polymixins, Colistin, Tyrothricn) Polyenes (Amphoteracin-B, Nyststin, Hamycin), Azoles (Ketoconazole, Fluconazole, Itraconazole),	Drugs that affect cell membrane.
3.	Tetracyclines, Chloramphenicol, Erythromycin, Clindamycin, Linezolid,	Protein synthesis inhibitors.
4.	Aminoglycoside.	Alter protein synthesis by misreading of mRNA code.
5.	Acyclovir, Zidovudine.	DNA synthesis inhibitors.
6.	Rifampin, Metronidazole,	Drugs that affect DNA function.
7.	Nalidixic acid and Fluroquinolones,	DNA gyrase inhibitors.
8.	Ritoxavir.	RNA dependent RNA polymerase inhibitors.
9.	Rifamycin.	DNA dependent RNA polymerase inhibitors.
10.	Sulfonamide, Sulfones, PAS, Dapsone, Trimethoprim, pyrimethamine, Ethambutol.	Antimetabolites.

16.11.3.2 According to Spectrum

Table 308 Antibiotic Classification According to Spectrum

Type	Antibiotics	Target
Broad-Spectrum Antibiotics	Doxycycline, Minocycline, Aminoglycosides (except for streptomycin), Ampicillin, Amoxicillin/clavulanic acid (Augmentin), Azithromycin, Carbapenems (e.g., imipenem), Piperacillin/tazobactam, Quinolones (e.g., ciprofloxacin), Tetracycline-class drugs (except sarecycline), Chloramphenicol, Ticarcillin, Trimethoprim/sulfamethoxazole (Bactrim), Ofloxacin	Effective against both Gram-positive and Gram-negative bacteria
Extended-Spectrum Antibiotics	Ceftriaxone, Cefepime, Piperacillin-tazobactam, Meropenem, Ceftazidime	Target a broader range of Gram-negative bacteria, including resistant strains, along with Gram-positive bacteria

Narrow-Spectrum Antibiotics	Azithromycin, Clarithromycin, Erythromycin, Clindamycin	Target a specific group of bacteria, either Gram-positive or Gram-negative, but not both

16.11.3.3 According to Prophylactic Usage

Table 309 Classification According to Prophylatctic Usage

Surgery	Infective pathogen	Antibiotic	Alternative for Penicillin and/or Cephalosporin Allergy
Gastrointestinal			
ESOPHAGEAL, NON OBSTRUCTED GASTRODUODENAL AND JEJUNAL	gram negative bacilli, gram positive cocci	CEFAZOLIN	CLINDAMYCIN + GENTAMICIN
OBSTRUCTED GASTRODUODENAL AND JEJUNAL	gram negative bacilli, gram positive cocci and anaerobes	CEFAZOLIN + METRONIDAZOLE - - - - - - - - AMPI/SULBACTAM	CLINDAMYCIN + GENTAMICIN
UNCOMPLICATED APPENDECTOMY	gram negative bacilli and anaerobes	CEFAZOLIN + METRONIDAZOLE - - - - - - - - AMPI/SULBACTAM	CIPROFLOXACIN + METRONIDAZOLE
ILEAL AND COLORECTAL	gram negative bacilli, Enterococci and anerobes	CEFAZOLIN + METRONIDAZOLE	CIPROFLOXACIN + METRONIDAZOLE
Biliary tract			
OPEN AND LAPAROSCOPIC PROCEDURES	gram negative bacilli, gram positive cocci	CEFAZOLIN	CLINDAMYCIN + GENTAMICIN
BILIARY PROCEDURES WITH POSSIBLE MANIPULATION (PTC, ERCP)	gram negative bacilli, gram positive cocci, anaerobes	CEFAZOLIN + METRONIDAZOLE	CIPROFLOXACIN + METRONIDAZOLE
Head and Neck			
CLEAN		None	None
WITH PLACEMENT OF PROSTHESIS	gram negative bacilli, gram positive cocci	CEFAZOLIN	CLINDAMYCIN + GENTAMICIN
CLEAN-CONTAMINATED	gram negative bacilli, gram positive cocci	CEFAZOLIN	CLINDAMYCIN + GENTAMICIN
Urologic			
CYSTOURETHROSCOPY		Targeted therapy	Targeted therapy
OPEN SURGERIES OR LAPAROSCOPY (INCLUDING NEPHROSTOMY TUBE PLACEMENT IF INFECTED OR WITH STONES)	gram negative bacilli, gram positive cocci	CEFAZOLIN	CLINDAMYCIN + GENTAMICIN

16.11.4 Comprehensive Guide to Antibiotics, Resistance, and Stewardship Strategies

Table 310 Comprehensive Guide to Antibiotics, Resistance, and Stewardship Strategies

Category	Subcategory	Details	Examples	Clinical Implications/Notes
Common Pathogens & Antibiotics	***Streptococcus pneumoniae***	First-line antibiotics for common infections such as pneumonia, otitis media, and meningitis	Penicillin, amoxicillin, ceftriaxone	Amoxicillin effective for less severe cases, ceftriaxone for more severe cases

	Staphylococcus aureus (MSSA)	Common cause of skin and soft tissue infections, osteomyelitis, endocarditis	Dicloxacillin, cefazolin, nafcillin	Dicloxacillin is preferred for MSSA; cefazolin for surgical prophylaxis
	Staphylococcus aureus (MRSA)	More resistant strain requiring potent antibiotics for severe infections	Vancomycin, linezolid, doxycycline, clindamycin	Vancomycin is the first-line treatment, but linezolid is an alternative for oral treatment
	Escherichia coli	Common cause of UTIs, gastroenteritis, and sepsis	Nitrofurantoin (for UTIs), cephalexin, TMP-SMX	Nitrofurantoin is the drug of choice for uncomplicated UTIs
	Pseudomonas aeruginosa	Common in immunocompromised patients and associated with hospital-acquired infections	Piperacillin-tazobactam, cefepime, meropenem, ciprofloxacin	Requires broad-spectrum treatment with beta-lactams and fluoroquinolones for severe infections
	Clostridioides difficile	Cause of antibiotic-associated diarrhea and pseudomembranous colitis	Oral vancomycin, fidaxomicin	Oral vancomycin is the most effective for severe C. difficile infection
	Anaerobes (e.g., Bacteroides)	Common in intra-abdominal infections, abscesses, and chronic infections	Metronidazole, clindamycin	Metronidazole is preferred for anaerobic infections, clindamycin for severe cases
	Atypicals (Mycoplasma, Chlamydia, Legionella)	Causes atypical pneumonia and other respiratory infections	Azithromycin, doxycycline	Doxycycline for mild, azithromycin for outpatient care
	Enzymatic Inactivation	Bacteria produce enzymes that	β-lactamases, carbapenemases	Inhibits the antibiotic action,

Antibiotic Resistance Mechanisms		break down antibiotics like beta-lactams and carbapenems		leading to resistant strains such as MRSA, CRE
	Target Modification	Bacteria alter the binding sites of antibiotics, e.g., MRSA alters penicillin-binding proteins (PBP)	MRSA (modified PBPs), Streptococcus pneumoniae	MRSA alters its PBP to prevent penicillin binding, making it resistant to beta-lactams
	Efflux Pumps	Pump antibiotics out of bacterial cells before they can have an effect	Pseudomonas aeruginosa, Acinetobacter baumannii	Antibiotics are expelled from bacterial cells, reducing effectiveness of drugs like aminoglycosides
	Porin Mutations	Mutations in the porin channels that prevent antibiotics from entering the bacterial cell	Pseudomonas, Enterobacteriaceae	These mutations prevent beta-lactams and fluoroquinolones from entering the bacteria
	Biofilm Formation	Bacteria form protective layers that make them resistant to treatment	Chronic infections like CF, catheters, prosthetic infections	Biofilms protect bacteria in chronic infections, making them harder to treat
Adverse Effects & Monitoring	**Aminoglycosides**	Toxic effects due to accumulation in tissues such as the kidneys and ears	Nephrotoxicity, ototoxicity	Trough levels must be monitored to prevent toxicity, especially in renal and elderly patients
	Vancomycin	Can cause infusion-related reactions (Red Man Syndrome) and renal toxicity	"Red man syndrome", nephrotoxicity, monitor trough levels	Monitor blood levels (trough) to prevent nephrotoxicity; slow infusion to

			prevent red man syndrome
Tetracyclines	Common side effects include GI issues and photosensitivity	Tooth discoloration, photosensitivity, avoid in pregnancy	Avoid in children and pregnant women, may cause tooth discoloration in developing teeth
Fluoroquinolones	Serious adverse effects including tendon rupture, QT prolongation, and CNS issues	Tendon rupture, QT prolongation, CNS effects	Caution in elderly due to risk of tendon damage and CNS side effects
Macrolides	Can cause gastrointestinal upset, but also QT prolongation, especially with other QT-prolonging drugs	GI upset, QT prolongation	Monitor for QT prolongation, avoid in patients with a history of arrhythmias
Clindamycin	Commonly associated with Clostridioides difficile infection (C. difficile colitis)	High risk of C. difficile colitis	Monitor for diarrhea and stop immediately if C. diff symptoms occur
Sulfonamides	Severe allergic reactions, including Stevens-Johnson syndrome	Hypersensitivity, Stevens-Johnson syndrome, hyperkalemia	Monitor for skin rash, hypersensitivity reactions, and electrolyte imbalances
β-lactams (penicillin)	Commonly associated with allergies, GI upset, and occasionally hematological effects	Allergy, GI upset	Monitor for allergic reactions, especially anaphylaxis
Metronidazole	Can cause disulfiram-like	Disulfiram reaction with	Avoid alcohol during treatment

		reactions when taken with alcohol	alcohol, metallic taste	to prevent disulfiram-like reactions
Special Population Considerations	Pediatrics	Avoid tetracyclines (teeth and bone issues), fluoroquinolones (cartilage toxicity)	Weight-based dosing, avoid sulfonamides (kernicterus risk)	Careful with dosing, avoid nephrotoxic and hepatotoxic drugs
	Pregnancy and Lactation	Use safe antibiotics, avoid drugs that may harm fetus	Safe: Penicillins, cephalosporins, azithromycin	Avoid tetracyclines, fluoroquinolones, sulfonamides during pregnancy due to teratogenicity
	Geriatrics	Adjust dosing based on renal function, monitor for drug interactions	Monitor for drug interactions and CNS side effects	Renal function often decreases with age, so dose adjustment is critical
	Renal/Hepatic Impairment	Adjust for drugs primarily excreted by kidneys, avoid hepatotoxic agents	Adjust vancomycin, aminoglycosides, avoid hepatotoxic drugs like rifampin	Check creatinine clearance, adjust dosing for renal or liver dysfunction
Key Stewardship Strategies	**Strategy**	**Details**	**Examples**	**Clinical Implications**
	Avoid unnecessary antibiotics	Limit use of antibiotics for viral infections to prevent resistance	Avoid using antibiotics for common colds or viral URIs	Prevent unnecessary resistance development, educate on appropriate use
	Use culture-guided therapy	Start therapy based on cultures to target the pathogen specifically	Strep throat treated based on rapid strep test, UTI with culture results	Helps avoid broad-spectrum antibiotics, reduces

				resistance development
	De-escalate when possible	Once cultures are received, switch to more specific antibiotics	Switch from broad-spectrum to narrow-spectrum antibiotics (e.g., from pip/tazo to ceftriaxone)	Reduces unnecessary broad-spectrum use and minimizes resistance development
	Limit treatment duration	Follow evidence-based guidelines for appropriate duration to minimize resistance	5 days for uncomplicated pneumonia, 3 days for uncomplicated UTI	Shorter courses when appropriate reduce resistance risk and side effects
	Use local antibiograms	Use local antibiograms to determine regional resistance patterns	Review antibiogram for most effective empiric treatment	Ensures use of the most effective antibiotics for a specific region

16.11.5 Antibiogram and Local Resistance Pattern

An antibiogram is a report on the susceptibility of bacterial pathogens to radio antimicrobial agents, which is part of the regular working document of a clinical microbiology laboratory. It is used as a crucial weapon to direct empiric therapy and make a proper choice of antibiotics available in a certain region. **Antibiograms are generally created from bacteria identified in clinical contexts, including hospitals or clinics, where bacterial samples obtained from patients are tested against antibiotics.** Local resistance patterns are the rates of antibiotic resistance in a geographic region or within any particular healthcare facility. These can differ according to the world regions, the patient groups, and the infection control measures applied. Thereby, **the best informed decisions can be made about the antibiotics that should be prescribed in a particular region, in an attempt to prevent ineffective treatment and further spread of resistance.** Antibiograms are usually done frequently and are crucial for achieving the best outcomes, reducing the emergence of resistance, and promoting of antibiotic-wise use.

16.11.6 Antibiotics Flow Chart

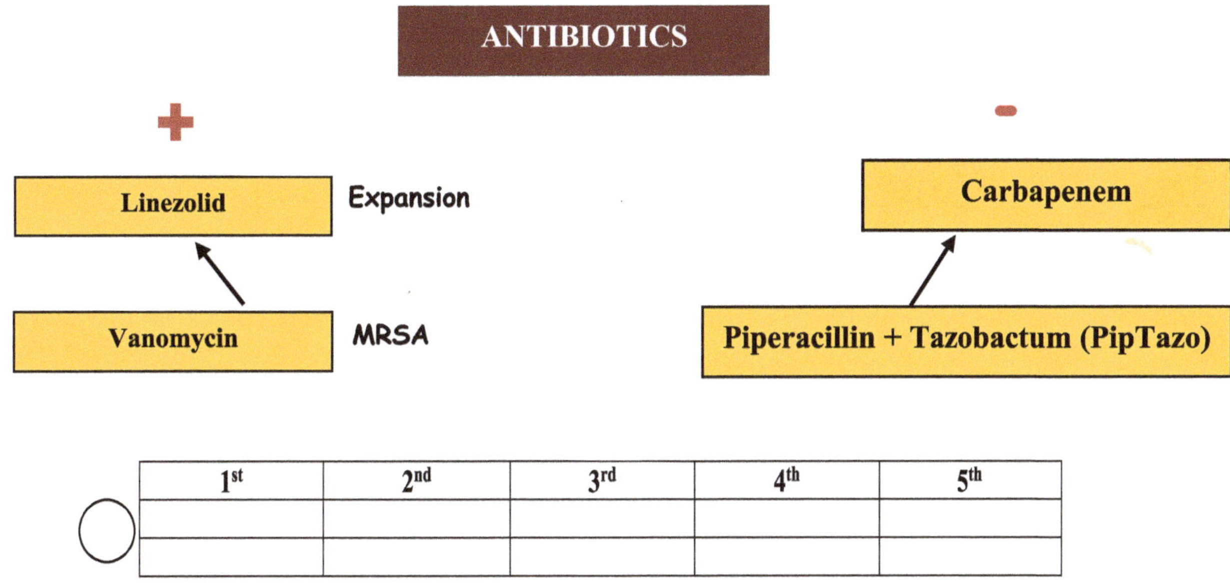

16.12Research, Quality Improvement Considerations

16.12.1 Definitions and Key Differences

Research, **Quality Improvement (QI), and Evidence-Based Practice (EBP)** each serve distinct yet interconnected purposes in healthcare, focusing on improving patient outcomes and healthcare delivery. Research aims to generate new knowledge that can be generalized across broader populations, often using systematic and rigorous methodologies, such as quantitative or qualitative studies. It typically requires **Institutional Review Board (IRB) approval when involving human subjects.** In contrast, QI focuses on improving **specific local processes or systems through cyclical, data-driven methodologies like the PDSA (Plan-Do-Study-Act) cycle. QI** efforts usually do not require IRB approval, though they may still undergo review to ensure ethical standards are met. EBP, on the other hand, integrates the best available research evidence with clinical expertise and patient values to inform clinical decision-making. While EBP does not necessitate IRB approval, it does involve a rigorous process of applying evidence within the clinical context, ensuring that the chosen interventions align with patient preferences and clinical judgment.

Table 311 Key Differences

Aspect	Research	Quality Improvement (QI)	Evidence-Based Practice (EBP)
Purpose	Generate new knowledge	Improve local processes/systems	Apply best evidence to clinical decision-making
Focus	Generalizable findings	Local problem-solving	Integration of evidence, expertise, and values
Methodology	Systematic, rigorous (quantitative/qualitative)	Cyclical, data-driven (PDSA)	Combines research, clinical judgment, and patient preference
IRB Required?	Yes (for human subjects)	Usually not, but may need review	No

16.12.2 Research Considerations

16.12.2.1 Research Methodology, Process, and Evidence Hierarchy

Table 312 Research Methodology, Process, and Evidence Hierarchy

Category	Details
Quantitative Research	*Randomized Controlled Trials (RCTs)*: Considered the gold standard in research for establishing causal relationships by randomly assigning participants to treatment or control groups. *Cohort Studies*: Observational studies where participants are followed over time to see how exposures affect outcomes.
Qualitative Research	*Phenomenology*: Focuses on exploring lived experiences of individuals to understand the essence of a phenomenon. *Grounded Theory*: Aims to develop theories grounded in data collected from participants. *Ethnography*: Involves in-depth study of cultures and communities through immersion.
Mixed Methods	Combines both qualitative and quantitative approaches to gather comprehensive data. This approach is used to validate and enhance findings by integrating numerical data and personal, contextual insights from individuals or communities.
Translational Research	Focuses on translating basic scientific research into practical applications that can improve healthcare and clinical practices. It includes T1 (bench to bedside), T2 (clinical trials), T3 (practice in communities), and T4 (population-level impact) phases.
Steps in the Research Process	1. *Identify a Research Problem*: Define the issue to be studied. 2. *Review Literature*: Conduct a thorough review of existing studies. 3. *Formulate Research Question/Hypothesis*: Develop a clear and testable hypothesis. 4. *Choose Design*: Select the appropriate research design (experimental, non-experimental). 5. *Obtain Ethical Approval (IRB)*: Ensure the study complies with ethical guidelines for human subjects. 6. *Collect and Analyze Data*: Gather and statistically or thematically analyze data. 7. *Interpret Results*: Draw conclusions based on data analysis. 8. *Disseminate Findings*: Publish or present findings to the broader scientific community.
Levels of Evidence	1. *Systematic Reviews/Meta-Analyses of RCTs*: Synthesize findings from multiple RCTs to provide high-level evidence. 2. *Randomized Controlled Trials (RCTs)*: High-quality evidence with controlled environments. 3. *Cohort Studies*: Observational, often used to examine the cause and effect in large groups over time. 4. *Case-Control Studies*: Compare individuals with a condition to those without to identify risk factors. 5. *Descriptive/Qualitative Studies*: Studies focusing on exploring patterns or experiences.

16.13 Sympathetic and Parasympathetic Considerations

Table 313 Fundamental considerations for both the sympathetic and parasympathetic nervous systems

System	Function	Clinical Relevance	Assessment	Treatment Considerations	General Considerations
Sympathetic Nervous System	Regulates "fight or flight" responses—increasing heart rate, blood pressure, redirecting blood flow to muscles, dilating bronchi, and releasing glucose.	**Overactivity**: Hypertension, tachycardia, anxiety, hyperhidrosis. **Underactivity**: Orthostatic hypotension, reduced sweating, impaired stress response.	Monitor vital signs (e.g., blood pressure, heart rate) and assess for signs of hyperactivity (sweating, rapid heartbeat).	**Adrenergic agents** (agonists or antagonists) to modify sympathetic tone. **Caution** with medications affecting sympathetic pathways, especially in hypertensive or cardiac patients.	**Balance**: Both sympathetic and parasympathetic systems work together to regulate bodily functions. **Autonomic Dysfunction**: Present in conditions like diabetic autonomic neuropathy, Parkinson's disease, or multiple system atrophy. **Medication Effects**: Many drugs influence these systems, such as beta-blockers, adrenergic agents. **Implications in Diagnosis**: Tests like tilt-table testing, HR

					variability, or sweat tests assess autonomic function.
Parasympathetic Nervous System	Regulates "rest and digest" activities—slowing heart rate, stimulating digestion, promoting saliva production, and conserving energy.	**Overactivity**: Bradycardia, hypotension. **Underactivity**: Impaired digestion, delayed gastric emptying, reduced saliva production.	Observe resting vagal tone (e.g., heart rate variability). Monitor symptoms like rapid heartbeat, dry mouth, or gastrointestinal disturbances.	**Cholinergic agonists** or **anticholinergics** to modify parasympathetic activity. **Caution** with medications that affect parasympathetic functions, especially in elderly or psoriasis patients.	**Balance**: Both systems must be balanced for optimal function. Autonomic dysfunction occurs when balance is disrupted, contributing to various clinical conditions. **Autonomic Dysfunction**: Found in diseases like Parkinson's or multiple system atrophy. **Medication Effects**: Many drugs, including anticholinergics, affect parasympathetic function.

16.14 Oncology Consideration

Table 314 Oncology Care Consideration

Category	Details
1. Patient Evaluation	**Histological and Staging Assessment**: Accurate tumor type, grade, and extent of spread (TNM system). **Performance Status**: Using

	scales like ECOG or Karnofsky to gauge the patient's ability to tolerate treatments. **Comorbidities**: Chronic illnesses (e.g., cardiovascular, respiratory, or renal diseases) affecting treatment choices.
2. Treatment Planning	**Multidisciplinary Approach**: Involving oncologists, surgeons, radiologists, and supportive care teams. **Personalized Therapy**: Including surgery, chemotherapy, radiation therapy, targeted therapy, and immunotherapy. **Goals of Care**: Curative, control, or palliative based on cancer stage and patient preferences.
3. Side Effect Management	**Proactively Manage Common Adverse Effects**: Cytopenias, nausea, mucositis, neuropathy. **Supportive Care Measures**: Growth factors, antiemetics, pain management, nutritional support.
4. Monitoring and Follow-up	**Regular Assessments**: For treatment response, toxicity, and disease progression. **Surveillance Imaging and Tumor Markers**: Regular imaging and testing to monitor disease status.
5. Psychosocial and Quality of Life Aspects	**Emotional, Psychological, and Social Impacts**: Address the emotional challenges of cancer diagnosis and treatment. **Palliative and End-of-Life Care**: Provide support if needed, focusing on comfort and symptom management.
6. Special Populations	**Elderly**: Adjust treatments considering frailty, comorbidities, and functional status. **Pregnancy**: Balancing maternal treatment and fetal safety. **Immunocompromised Patients**: Increased infection risk; chemotherapy and immunotherapy considerations.
7. Prevention and Screening	**Cancer Screenings**: Pap smear, mammography, colonoscopy, PSA, etc. **Lifestyle Modifications**: Smoking cessation, diet, and exercise to reduce cancer risk.
8. Genetic and Molecular Testing	**Molecular Profiling**: Used to guide targeted therapies. **Hereditary Cancer Syndromes**: Consider testing in familial cases to identify genetic predispositions.
9. Research and Clinical Trials	**Encourage Participation in Trials**: Provide access to emerging therapies and contribute to advancing oncology knowledge.

16.15Leadership and Management Considerations

16.15.1 Definitions and Distinctions

Leadership and management can be said to have some similarities, but are tied in different capacities or structures within an organization. Leadership is always future-focused and involves influencing people, creating change, and fostering innovation. It may establish operations, foster culture and values, and may be of either a formal or cultural nature. **Management, on the other hand, is more concerned with procedure and work-based or procedural stability and order**. Organizational leaders typically hold more specialized positions, **authoritatively bound to organizational regulations and regulation implementation processes.** While leadership fosters change and encourages the employees to follow the desired change, management imposes order, making sure that none of the available resources are wasted and that certain goals are met. Every organisation needs leadership to chart the course for change and innovation, and it also needs management to ensure business as usual.

16.15.2 Leadership Theories and Styles

Leadership theories and leadership styles give boundary conditions to describe how leaders work in a team and organization. The Trait Theory holds that leadership qualities are inherent, while the Behavioral Theory postulates that leadership is an adaptive process. **Situational Theory stresses that the level of leadership one takes has to correspond with the situation.** Transformational Leadership is all about achieving organizational change by appealing to the higher aims of the employees, whereas Transactional Leadership requires employees to perform their tasks through positive reinforcement. On the same note, Servant Leadership entails identifying the best ways to support the members of a team, and it is aimed at empowering them. **Leadership styles vary: autocratic leaders make decisions unilaterally, democratic leaders encourage everyone to participate, laissez-faire leaders do not interfere, while transactional leaders work towards the achievement of goals.** Tulsa defines servant leadership as a character that promotes trust and long-term orientation. Leadership means flexibility, E4, and any type is effective when appropriate for the specific company and circumstances.

16.15.3 Core Management Functions (Fayol's Principles)

Fayol introduced five functions of management as follows: these four are**; planning, organizing, staffing, directing, and controlling.** The orderly arrangement of activities that include establishing objectives and outlooks, and deciding on strategies, is known as planning. Managing entails the formation of teams, the acquisition and allocation of resources, and the definition of roles to achieve the set goals. Staffing deals with finding, selecting, and maintaining the right people in the organization to meet the human capital needs of the organization. **While managing is focused on organizing and controlling workers to ensure they achieve the objectives of the firm, directing involves leading workers towards the achievement of preset objectives.** Lastly, controlling is maintaining a check on the performance and making sure that all is going as planned, and rectifying if not. These functions also combine to facilitate performance in any organization. These functions are as follows: **SWOT analysis, Gantt charts, and Key Performance Indicators (KPIs)** also aid in the systematic performance of these functions since they allow for the collection of data and other crucial information regarding the organization's goals and general progress during tasks.

16.15.4 Communication and Conflict Resolution

Administrative communication is a vital determinant of leadership and management since it plays a crucial role in the dissemination of information**. Verbal, nonverbal, written, and electronic communication comprise the concept of business communication that is essential within an organization**. However, challenges like hierarchy, culture, and poor listening skills can hinder communication. Eye contact, postures and positions, summarizing, and clarifying are crucial tools in eliminating the barriers that hinder active listening. Another important competency that can be found in leaders and managers is conflict resolution, which can be performed with several methods: The five strategies are: managerial decision to avoid, managerial decision to accommodate, managerial decision to compete, managerial decision to compromise, and managerial decision to collaborate. Of these, collaboration is considered to be most effective because it aims to find a solution that will be beneficial to all parties involved. The SBAR model stands for **Situation, Background, Assessment, Recommendation, and is a framework that**

was designed to help maintain effective communication, particularly in emergencies, since there is much emphasis put on the transference of key information.

16.15.5 Change Management

Various models are available to help an organization implement change since change is critical when an organization faces fluctuating environments. According to Lewin's Change Model, the change process is divided into the following three stages: This addresses the preparatory work that has to be done before effecting change, the change process, and then the consolidation process that comes after the change. Kotter's 8 Step Model of Change can be seen clearly as follows: Create a Sense of Urgency, Set the Direction, Get the Support, Remove Obstacles, Build Coalitions, Generate Quick Wins, Work on Anchor New Approaches in the Corporate, as well as Sustainability. **The ADKAR Model Awareness, Desire, Knowledge, Ability, Reinforcement emphasizes that the change must be looked at from the organizational member's perspective, making sure that each organizational member has the awareness**, desire, knowledge, ability, and reinforcement in order to change. It also needs communication, coordination, and endorsement by all employees to embrace the change processes aimed at implementing any change process. Such a process also involves the comparison of the formulated strategies and the need to modify such strategies in the light of various organizational concerns in the long run.

16.15.6 Nursing Leadership and Management

The nurse leaders and managers have crucial responsibilities of guaranteeing that the patients receive proper care in a timely and effective manner. Nursing leaders balance the interests and advocate for both the patient and the employees, making safety and quality care achievable. Staff development is crucial in enhancing quality delivery in healthcare facilities, and nursing managers need to employ strategies for hiring, training, and retaining human capital. It is important to talk about delegation and supervision because they play crucial roles within the area of nursing management, directing tasks and their completion. There may be a traditional divide between various care professions; **however, it is essential to promote interprofessional cooperation among healthcare managers.** Also, the patient safety concerns are further advanced by the nursing leaders through quality improvement programs to avoid or minimize on errors in the provision of healthcare services. Measures like pressure ulcers, falls, and healthcare-acquired infections are some of the outcome-level nursing markers used to monitor the quality of the care that is delivered to patients, and should always be nursing sensitive.

16.15.7 Strategic Planning and Decision Making

Strategic planning is the first step in developing an overall structure for an organization so that its current and future goals will reflect the mission, vision, and values of the organization. It involves setting specific goals and objectives that must be measurable, achievable, relevant to the goal, and time-bound. The rational model is a well-known approach to decision-making, in addition to the intuition model of decision-making, where the decisions made are based on intuition and instinct. While decentralization of decision-making means that **many individuals have an opportunity to directly contribute, it entails that the decision-making process involves the participation of many people.** Evidence-based decision making involves the process of basing decisions on facts and research, rather than guessing and assuming that such a course of action is best. By incorporating these strategies, leaders can be certain that decisions are consistent with the goals of the organization and are not only sensitive to a specific condition.

16.15.8 Delegation and Supervision

Another set of important management functions in healthcare and almost any other field involves delegation and supervision to address the distribution of tasks as well as to monitor the activities of subordinates. **The five rights of delegation: The following rights ensure that delegation is done effectively: right task, right circumstance, right person, right direction/communication, right supervision/evaluation**. The right task involves ensuring that a task is suitable for delegation, while the right circumstance involves making sure that the circumstances in which delegation is exercised are correct. **Right person can be defined as recruiting and selecting the most capable candidate for the given work, while right direction/communication is aimed at providing accurate directions or information when offering instructions**. , therefore, the last step in management is supervision and evaluation where they check if the work is on track, offer correction if needed, and make sure the work is done rightly. Delegation is a solution to increase productivity, to increase the capacity of employees, and in an organization to ensure that all tasks are handled with efficiency, resulting to improvement in team performance.

16.15.9 Risk, Quality, and Safety Management

The general understanding of risk, quality, and safety management is of paramount importance, more so within the healthcare industry. It is the process of identifying, evaluating, and minimizing threats, including adverse events, patient injury, or loss in financial terms. Measures such as incident reporting, liability assessment, as well as adverse event evaluation are crucial and helpful in managing and mitigating risks. Quality improvement or QI aims at achieving goal-oriented changes by following processes that are supported by facts and data. Tools for pacing include: **PDSA cycles, Lean, and Six-Sigma aim at identifying the problems and finding the methods that can be applied to improve these areas after applying a change. One of the cornerstones of QI is patient safety**, which involves employing methods such as **RCA and FMEA** to understand and avoid mistakes. Benchmarking entails the comparisons made of the organisation against national or accreditation standards in a bid to assess its performance and progress in its drive for optimality and improved success in patient care.

16.15.10 Team Building and Motivation

Organisation effectiveness relies heavily on one's ability to build a team, develop motivation, and ensure that the group achieves its set goals and objectives. The passage also highlights that leaders should establish trust, respect, and psychological safety for employees to have a positive employee experience. Rewarding the efforts increases the morale of the employees, and innovating and valuing diverse ideas fosters stronger teamwork. There are numerous theories that are used to explain motivation in leadership practice: **According to the Maslow's Hierarchy of Needs,** people work to achieve higher-order needs; while, according to Herzberg's Two-Factor Theory, motivators and hygiene factors of workers have their different effect; McGregor differentiated between **Theory X and Theory Y that assumed employees lack of responsibility; and finally, perspectives of Self-Determination Theory in terms of autonomy, competence and relatedness.** These theories will help the leaders to improve the levels of engagement, satisfaction, and performance of the team to ensure it is on par with the set organizational goals.

16.15.11 Legal and Ethical Considerations

In this unit, I will outline some of the organisational and legal issues that are fundamental to leaders and managers of healthcare facilities. It refers to a legal requirement whereby patients must be made comprehensively aware of the consequences of some treatments and procedures in order for them to give their consent. It becomes a legal and ethical requirement to maintain a patient's identity and his/her information confidential, especially where the facility is operating under HIPAA regulations. Supervisors also need to stick to the scope of practice criteria to guarantee that particular tasks are accomplished by competent workers. The ethical theories embedded in organizational and practical contexts are autonomy, beneficence, nonmaleficence, justice, and fidelity. Some frameworks in ethical decision-making are the **MORAL model, which stands for Massage the dilemma, Outline the options, Review the criteria, Affirm the position, Look back.** Whistle-blowing and advocacy are also realistic elements since they enable individuals to raise concerns about unethical practices while also championing patient advocacy and the public's welfare. These aspects guarantee ethical practice in healthcare systems so that the hospitals offer the finest services to their clients

16.15.12 Cultural Competence and Diversity

Cultural competence and Diversity are very important in ensuring that quality and fair health care is offered to people. Political parties involved in the healthcare delivery systems should appreciate and incorporate the culture of their people in order to be responsive to the cultural beliefs of their patients. **The use of interpreters and having accommodating policies will ensure that there are no barriers in terms of language or culture between the patient and the health care provider.** Cultural safety, where patient's cultural values and beliefs are considered, ensures trust and ultimately results in better patient care. All managers must embrace equality in the workplace by ensuring that the working environment is fair to everyone. This entails eradicating prejudice from the unconscious mind, conducting diversity practice and making the workforce diverse as the population of the community. Cultural competence can improve patient satisfaction and health through effective patient care, organizational functioning, and multiculturalism.

16.15.13 Budgeting and Resource Management

The allocation of funds and resources is essential to ensure that these organizations work economically and effectively in the long run. **The operating budget, capital budget, and personnel budget assist various organisations in allocating resources to optimum resource utility.** Recurrent budgets provide for working expenses and operating expenses, while capital budgets are reserved for large investments in a project. The personnel budgets are very important in the administration to make sure that there is an adequate health workforce to meet the increasing health needs. It is a way of making optimum use of its resources and at the same time minimizing the expenses incurred in its operation. **Average factors, such as HPPD, help to understand how effective or efficient the staffing has been, as well as the effective utilization of the resources.** Cost-benefit analysis is an effective means of the financially justified evaluation of a range of projects, and its significance is explained by the need to achieve better results and growth within an organization. Budgeting facilitates the appropriate utilization of resources, hence enhancing the efficiency of service production and delivery.

16.16 Evidence-Based Practice (EBP) Considerations

16.16.1 Definition

Evidence-Based Practice (EBP) is the conscientious integration of the best available research evidence, clinical expertise, and patient preferences in the decision-making process to improve patient care. It seeks to use current best practices, grounded in solid scientific research, to guide healthcare professionals in their clinical decisions. **Researchers define EBP as the "conscientious use of current best evidence in making decisions about patient care."** The primary goal of EBP is to provide the most effective care for patients, utilizing practices that are scientifically validated and tailored to the individual needs of the patient.

16.16.2 EBP Components (3-legged stool)

Table 315 Table 5 EBP Components

Component	Description	Purpose
Best Research Evidence	Refers to the current, high-quality scientific studies and clinical trials that provide data and conclusions to inform clinical practice.	To ensure that clinical decisions are based on the most reliable and up-to-date evidence available.
Clinical Expertise	The healthcare provider's personal experience, skills, and expertise, including their ability to interpret evidence and apply it in patient care.	To enhance the application of evidence, ensuring it aligns with the clinical context and the provider's expertise.
Patient Values and Preferences	Incorporating the patient's individual needs, preferences, and values into the clinical decision-making process.	To ensure that patient-centered care is delivered and that decisions reflect the patient's choices and values.

16.17 Steps in the EBP Process (The 7 A's)

Table 316: Steps in the EBP Process

Step	Action	Explanation
Ask	Formulate a clinical question using the PICO format.	PICO stands for Patient, Intervention, Comparison, and Outcome. It helps in defining the focus of the question.
Acquire	Search for the best available evidence to answer the question.	Use databases like PubMed, Cochrane, or Google Scholar to find relevant studies, clinical trials, and reviews.
Appraise	Critically evaluate the quality and applicability of the evidence.	Assess the study's methodology, sample size, and findings to determine if it is relevant to your clinical practice.
Apply	Integrate the evidence into clinical practice while considering patient values.	Apply the research findings in a way that is relevant to the patient's condition, preferences, and context.
Assess	Evaluate the outcomes of the intervention or decision.	Measure the effectiveness of the applied intervention by monitoring patient outcomes and satisfaction.
Adjust	Modify the approach based on the evaluation and emerging evidence.	If the outcomes are not as expected, adjust the intervention and approach as new evidence becomes available.
Advocate	Promote and share the findings and outcomes of EBP in the healthcare environment.	Disseminate results to improve practice by informing colleagues and ensuring that improvements are sustained.

16.18PICO Format (Clinical Questions)

Table 317 PICO Format

Element	Explanation	Example
P (Patient/Population/Problem)	Describes the patient group or clinical issue being addressed.	P: Elderly patients with hypertension
I (Intervention)	The intervention being tested or implemented.	I: Yoga
C (Comparison)	The comparison intervention or treatment, if applicable.	C: Standard exercise
O (Outcome)	The desired result or effect of the intervention.	O: Lowering of blood pressure (systolic and diastolic)
Example Question	Combines all components into a structured clinical question.	**In elderly patients with hypertension (P), is yoga (I) more effective than standard exercise (C) in lowering blood pressure (O)?**

16.18.1 Quality Improvement (QI)

16.18.1.1 Definition

Quality Improvement (QI) refers to the systematic, data-guided efforts to improve the quality of healthcare services and outcomes. QI aims to enhance healthcare delivery by focusing on immediate, impactful improvements in specific settings. By using scientific methodologies and real-time data, QI seeks to optimize processes and care for better patient outcomes. The primary goal is to increase efficiency, reduce errors, and improve patient satisfaction.

16.18.1.2 QI Methodologies

Several methodologies guide QI efforts, including:

- **PDSA Cycle**: A simple iterative model (Plan-Do-Study-Act) for testing and refining improvements.
- **Six Sigma (DMAIC)**: A structured approach focused on eliminating defects (Define, Measure, Analyze, Improve, Control).
- **Lean**: Focuses on eliminating waste and maximizing value.
- **Root Cause Analysis (RCA)**: Retrospective analysis to identify causes of adverse events.
- **Failure Mode & Effects Analysis (FMEA)**: A proactive approach to predict potential errors and their impacts.

16.18.1.3 Common QI Focus Areas

QI initiatives often target key areas such as:

- Reducing falls and healthcare-associated infections (HAIs)
- Minimizing medication errors
- Improving hand hygiene compliance
- Enhancing discharge processes and pain control
- Boosting patient satisfaction and staff communication

16.18.1.4 Tools Used in QI

QI projects utilize several tools for data collection, analysis, and visualization:

- **Flowcharts**: Map out processes and identify inefficiencies.
- **Run Charts/Control Charts**: Track data over time to monitor improvements.
- **Fishbone Diagram**: Identify root causes of problems.
- **Pareto Chart**: Highlight major issues based on frequency or impact.
- **Checklists**: Ensure key actions and standards are met.

16.18.2 Ethical and Regulatory Considerations

16.18.2.1 Informed Consent

Informed consent is crucial for all clinical research involving human subjects. It ensures participants are fully aware of the risks, benefits, and procedures involved in a study. In the context of **QI or EBP, informed consent is generally not required as these activities do not involve direct patient intervention** in the same way that clinical trials do. However, transparency with patients about data collection and interventions remains essential.

16.18.2.2 Privacy & HIPAA

Protecting patient privacy is paramount. **HIPAA (Health Insurance Portability and Accountability Act) mandates the secure handling of patient data**. Both research and clinical practice must adhere to privacy laws to prevent unauthorized access to sensitive health information.

16.18.2.3 IRB Approval

The Institutional Review Board (IRB) is responsible for ensuring that any clinical research involving human participants adheres to ethical standards and federal regulations. While IRB approval is required for research involving direct patient interventions, it is typically not required for QI initiatives, although institutional policies may vary.

16.18.2.4 Conflict of Interest

Conflicts of interest must be disclosed in **research and EBP projects.** Any potential bias, whether financial, personal, or professional, should be transparent to maintain the integrity of the findings and ensure patient safety.

16.18.3 Data Collection & Analysis

16.18.3.1 Quantitative Methods

Quantitative data are essential for measuring outcomes in QI, EBP, and research. This data often comes from structured sources such as surveys, metrics, and Electronic Health Records (EHR). Common statistical tools for analyzing quantitative data include **SPSS, SAS, R, and Excel. These tools help to interpret the data, identify patterns, and evaluate interventions.**

16.18.3.2 Qualitative Methods

Qualitative data collection involves more subjective information, **such as patient interviews, focus groups, and open-ended surveys.** These methods are useful for understanding patient experiences, healthcare provider insights, and complex social factors. Tools like NVivo are commonly used for qualitative data analysis, enabling themes and patterns to be identified within unstructured data.

16.18.3.3 Data Analysis in QI

In QI, baseline data is often compared with benchmarks to measure improvement. **This allows healthcare professionals to determine whether changes** in practice have led to measurable improvements in patient outcomes.

16.18.4 Dissemination of Findings

16.18.4.1 Research

Disseminating research findings is vital for advancing knowledge in healthcare. Research findings are often shared through **peer-reviewed journals (e.g., *JAMA*, *AJN*), academic conferences, or dissertations**. This ensures that evidence-based practices are shared widely with the medical community.

16.18.4.2 QI Projects

For QI projects, dissemination occurs **through internal reports, dashboards, and QI presentations within the institution.** These presentations help staff understand the impact of the improvements and the next steps for continued progress.

16.18.4.3 EBP Projects

EBP findings are typically shared through **clinical protocols, updated guidelines, posters, and internal reports.** These materials help inform clinical practice by integrating the latest research evidence with patient care.

16.18.5 Interrelationship: Research, QI, and EBP

16.18.5.1 Research generates evidence → informs EBP

Research plays a pivotal role in **generating high-quality evidence that directly informs EBP decisions**. By identifying the most effective interventions and practices, research provides the foundation for clinical guidelines.

16.18.5.2 QI identifies local problems → may prompt EBP implementation or new research

QI activities help identify specific issues or inefficiencies within a healthcare setting, which can then prompt new research or the application of EBP strategies to address these challenges.

16.18.5.3 EBP uses research to solve clinical problems → evaluated through QI metrics

EBP integrates research evidence **with clinical expertise to solve real-world problems**. The effectiveness of EBP interventions is evaluated through QI metrics, allowing healthcare providers to measure the impact of changes in practice.

16.19150 Practice Questions with Answers

1. Which of the following is the primary route of drug elimination in the body? A. Liver B. Kidneys C. Lungs D. Sweat
2. What is the first-pass effect in drug absorption? A. Drug breakdown in the stomach B. The effect of drugs passing through the liver before reaching systemic circulation C. The speed of drug absorption D. The influence of blood flow on drug distribution
3. Which organ primarily metabolizes drugs in the body? A. Heart B. Kidneys C. Liver D. Lungs
4. Which type of drug interaction can occur if two drugs share metabolic pathways in the liver? A. Potentiation B. Drug toxicity C. Synergy D. Bioavailability enhancement
5. Which of the following factors can affect drug distribution in the body? A. Blood flow B. Tissue composition C. Protein-binding capacity D. All of the above
6. What is the mechanism of action for an agonist drug? A. It prevents receptor activation B. It binds to a receptor and activates it C. It inhibits enzyme activity D. It directly binds to DNA
7. Which class of medication includes drugs like fluoxetine and sertraline? A. Beta-blockers B. SSRIs (Selective Serotonin Reuptake Inhibitors) C. Antihypertensives D. Antipsychotics
8. Which of the following medications is used to treat alcohol use disorder (AUD)? A. Disulfiram B. Lorazepam C. Amoxicillin D. Sildenafil
9. What is the main cause of serotonin syndrome? A. Overdose of antipsychotic drugs B. Excessive serotonin levels caused by drugs that increase serotonin

C. Kidney failure D. Drug interactions in the liver
10. Which clinical sign is characteristic of serotonin syndrome? A. Bradycardia B. Hypothermia C. Hyperreflexia D. Decreased muscle tone
11. What is the first-line treatment for serotonin syndrome? A. Cyproheptadine B. Ibuprofen C. Dantrolene D. Amoxicillin
12. What class of medication does atenolol belong to? A. Calcium channel blockers B. Beta-blockers C. Antipsychotics D. Opioid analgesics
13. What is the therapeutic goal of a beta-blocker like atenolol? A. To activate beta-adrenergic receptors B. To block beta-adrenergic receptors and reduce heart rate C. To increase sympathetic nervous system activity D. To dilate blood vessels
14. Which medication is commonly prescribed for the management of hypertension? A. Levothyroxine B. Enalapril C. Metoprolol D. Amoxicillin
15. What is the main function of a diuretic in hypertension treatment? A. To block the renin-angiotensin system B. To increase the elimination of sodium and water C. To block beta-adrenergic receptors D. To decrease the heart rate=
16. Which medication can cause serotonin toxicity if combined with other serotonergic drugs? A. Prednisone B. Fluoxetine C. Propranolol D. Hydralazine
17. What is the most important factor in determining drug dosage in elderly patients? A. Age B. Body mass C. Kidney and liver function D. Gender
18. Which of the following best describes the role of pharmacodynamics? A. The study of how drugs are absorbed, metabolized, and excreted B. The study of the body's effects on drugs

C. The study of drug interactions D. The study of drug effects on the body
19. What is the primary site for drug metabolism? A. Kidneys B. Liver C. Lungs D. Small intestine
20. Which class of drug is used to reduce inflammation? A. Antihistamines B. Analgesics C. Anti-inflammatory drugs D. Beta-blockers
21. What is the most common side effect of opioids? A. Tachycardia B. Constipation C. Hypertension D. Hyperglycemia
22. Which type of medication would be used for a patient suffering from generalized anxiety disorder (GAD)? A. SSRIs B. Antibiotics C. Antidiuretics D. Corticosteroids
23. What condition is commonly associated with the use of tetracycline antibiotics? A. Diarrhea B. Photosensitivity C. Edema D. Hyperglycemia
24. Which of the following is a common symptom of peritonsillar abscess? A. Fever and sore throat B. Yellowish exudate in the mouth C. Painless swollen lymph nodes D. Severe headache
25. What is the most likely cause of an avulsed tooth? A. Tooth decay B. Trauma or injury C. Poor oral hygiene D. Gum disease
26. What type of drug is cyproheptadine used to treat? A. Antihypertensive B. Serotonin syndrome C. Anxiety disorders D. Pain management
27. What is the primary function of selective serotonin reuptake inhibitors (SSRIs)? A. To block dopamine receptors B. To inhibit serotonin reuptake and increase serotonin levels

C. To increase norepinephrine levels D. To block histamine receptors
28. Which of the following is a side effect of high-dose corticosteroids? A. Hypoglycemia B. Osteoporosis C. Hyperkalemia D. Bradycardia
29. What is the correct treatment for a patient diagnosed with strep throat? A. Antiviral medication B. Antibiotics (e.g., penicillin or amoxicillin) C. Analgesics for pain relief only D. Surgery
30. Which of the following is the most important factor in prescribing antibiotics for infection? A. Cost of the drug B. The type of bacteria causing the infection C. The patient's preference D. The patient's ability to swallow the medication
31. What is the primary cause of auricular hematoma? A) Viral infection B) Trauma C) Bacterial infection D) Aging
32. Which imaging method is used to diagnose acoustic neuroma? A) MRI B) X-ray C) CT scan D) Ultrasound
33. What is the first-line treatment for acute otitis media? A) Steroid injections B) Antibiotics C) Surgical drainage D) Pain relievers
34. What condition is indicated by the presence of dendritic ulcers on the cornea during a slit-lamp examination? A) Acute angle-closure glaucoma B) Herpes keratitis C) Retinal detachment D) Pterygium
35. Which medication is commonly used to reduce intraocular pressure in acute angle-closure glaucoma? A) Acetazolamide B) Metronidazole C) Clindamycin D) Fluconazole
36. What is a common risk factor for developing polycystic ovary syndrome (PCOS)?

A) Increased caffeine consumption B) Insulin resistance C) High levels of estrogen D) Smoking
37. What is the primary cause of atrophic vaginitis? A) Bacterial infection B) Low estrogen levels C) Fungal infection D) Trauma
38. Which of the following is a treatment option for bacterial vaginosis? A) Oral metronidazole B) Oral fluconazole C) Topical clindamycin D) Oral acyclovir
39. Which test is recommended for diagnosing retinopathy in patients with autoimmune disease? A) Slit-lamp examination B) Optical coherence tomography (OCT) C) Tonometry D) Visual field testing
40. What is the common symptom of Sjogren's syndrome? A) Dry eyes and mouth B) Weight loss C) Swelling in the legs D) Abdominal pain
41. What is the definitive treatment for orbital cellulitis? A) Topical antibiotics B) Intravenous antibiotics C) Surgical drainage D) Steroid therapy
42. Which of the following is a common complication of untreated endometritis? A) Sepsis B) Ovarian cysts C) Menstrual irregularities D) Uterine fibroids
43. What is the initial management step for acute angle-closure glaucoma? A) Laser iridotomy B) Oral antibiotics C) Topical corticosteroids D) Medications to lower intraocular pressure
44. What is a common sign of myometritis? A) Painful urination B) Abdominal tenderness C) Decreased menstrual flow D) Hot flashes
45. Which imaging method is used to confirm orbital cellulitis?

A) X-ray B) CT scan C) MRI D) Slit-lamp examination
46. Which of the following treatments is recommended for age-related macular degeneration (AMD)? A) Anti-VEGF injections B) Antibiotics C) Corticosteroid eye drops D) Surgical removal of the macula
47. What is the most common cause of contact-lens related keratitis? A) Fungal infection B) Poor contact lens hygiene C) Bacterial infection D) Viral infection
48. What is the primary diagnostic method for diagnosing pterygium? A) Fundoscopy B) Physical examination C) Slit-lamp examination D) MRI
49. Which type of vaginal infection is treated with oral fluconazole? A) Trichomoniasis B) Yeast infection C) Bacterial vaginosis D) Herpes simplex
50. What is the primary symptom of retinal detachment? A) Redness of the eye B) Sudden vision loss C) Blurred vision D) Painful eye movement
51. What condition is commonly associated with optic neuritis? A) Multiple sclerosis B) Glaucoma C) Cataract D) Retinal detachment
52. What is a key sign of vulvovaginitis caused by bacterial vaginosis? A) Yellowish vaginal discharge B) Fishy odor to vaginal discharge C) Painful urination D) Redness in the vaginal area
53. What treatment is recommended for vulvovaginitis caused by trichomoniasis? A) Antifungal creams B) Antibiotics such as metronidazole C) Topical corticosteroids D) Oral fluconazole

54. Which condition is indicated by an enlarged optic disc and visual field loss? A) Glaucoma B) Retinal detachment C) Age-related macular degeneration D) Conjunctivitis
55. What is the typical treatment for atrophic vaginitis in postmenopausal women? A) Antibiotics B) Vaginal estrogen therapy C) Surgical removal of the uterus D) Oral contraceptives
56. What condition is associated with the presence of drusen in the macula? A) Retinal detachment B) Glaucoma C) Age-related macular degeneration D) Conjunctivitis
57. What is a common complication of untreated PCOS? A) Infertility B) Endometriosis C) Cervical cancer D) Uterine fibroids
58. What is the primary symptom of entropion? A) Eye dryness B) Tearing and irritation from eyelashes rubbing the cornea C) Double vision D) Glare sensitivity
59. What is the most effective treatment for endometritis after miscarriage? A) Hormonal therapy B) IV antibiotics C) Surgical removal of fibroids D) Oral contraceptives
60. Which infection causes a thick white or creamy discharge in women? A) Trichomoniasis B) Bacterial vaginosis C) Yeast infection D) Gonorrhea
61. What is the primary treatment for polycystic ovary syndrome (PCOS)? A) Antibiotics B) Birth control pills C) Insulin therapy D) Surgery
62. What is the common symptom of atrophic vaginitis? A) Increased menstrual bleeding B) Vaginal dryness and discomfort C) Pelvic pain D) Fever and chills
63. Which of the following is an effective non-hormonal method of contraception?

A) Copper IUD B) Oral contraceptives C) Contraceptive patch
64. What is the most common cause of secondary amenorrhea? A) Pregnancy B) Stress C) Polycystic ovary syndrome D) Excessive exercise
65. What is the primary treatment for Bell's Palsy? A) Antiviral medications B) Corticosteroids C) Pain relievers D) Surgery
66. Which of the following is a classic sign of giant cell arteritis (GCA)? A) Jaw claudication B) Severe headaches without nausea C) Facial drooping D) Muscle weakness
67. What is the most common causative organism of acute bacterial meningitis in adults? A) Haemophilus influenzae B) Neisseria meningitidis C) Streptococcus pneumoniae D) Listeria monocytogenes
68. Which symptom is typically seen in a patient with a transient ischemic attack (TIA)? A) Sudden, severe headache B) Sudden numbness or weakness on one side of the body C) Long-lasting confusion D) Decreased vision in both eyes
69. What is a key treatment for subarachnoid hemorrhage (SAH)? A) IV antibiotics B) Immediate surgical intervention C) Corticosteroids D) Blood pressure management
70. What is the first-line treatment for carpal tunnel syndrome (CTS)? A) Surgery B) NSAIDs for pain relief C) Corticosteroid injections D) Wrist splints and ergonomic adjustments
71. What is the typical first-line pharmacological treatment for acute bacterial meningitis? A) Antiviral medications B) IV antibiotics (e.g., ceftriaxone, vancomycin) C) NSAIDs D) Corticosteroids

72. What is the initial symptom commonly reported by patients with trigeminal neuralgia? A) Sharp, stabbing facial pain B) Severe headache C) Blurred vision D) Muscle weakness
73. Which of the following is a classic symptom of multiple sclerosis (MS)? A) Unilateral facial paralysis B) Fluctuating neurological symptoms such as weakness and visual changes C) Severe, continuous headaches D) Unilateral vision loss
74. What is the most effective treatment for polycystic ovary syndrome (PCOS) related acne? A) Birth control pills B) Insulin therapy C) Anti-androgens (e.g., spironolactone) D) Metformin
75. What is a common complication of untreated giant cell arteritis (GCA)? A) Stroke B) Vision loss C) Diabetes D) Ovarian cysts
76. What diagnostic test is typically used to confirm a diagnosis of subarachnoid hemorrhage? A) MRI B) CT scan of the head C) Blood tests D) Lumbar puncture
77. What is the most common cause of TIA in older adults? A) Diabetes B) Hypertension C) Atherosclerosis D) Hyperlipidemia
78. What condition is typically treated with riluzole and edaravone? A) Multiple sclerosis B) Bell's palsy C) Amyotrophic lateral sclerosis (ALS) D) Trigeminal neuralgia
79. Which treatment option is most effective for acute bacterial meningitis caused by Streptococcus pneumoniae? A) Ceftriaxone with dexamethasone B) Intravenous fluids C) Acetaminophen D) Pain relief only
80. Which of the following is a hallmark sign of Bell's palsy? A) Unilateral facial paralysis B) Severe headaches with photophobia C) Severe neck stiffness D) Visual disturbances

81. Which of the following can be a long-term complication of untreated acute bacterial meningitis?
A) Hearing loss
B) Paralysis
C) Memory loss
D) Depression

82. What condition is characterized by sharp, electric shock-like facial pain triggered by activities such as chewing or brushing teeth?
A) Tension headaches
B) Trigeminal neuralgia
C) Bell's palsy
D) Acute bacterial meningitis

83. Which condition is associated with sudden, severe headaches and positive Brudzinski's sign and Kernig's sign?
A) Tension-type headache
B) Subarachnoid hemorrhage
C) Acute bacterial meningitis
D) Multiple sclerosis

84. What is the first-line treatment for Bell's Palsy?
A) Antiviral therapy
B) Corticosteroids
C) Physical therapy
D) Surgery

85. What is the most common cause of subdural hematoma in elderly patients?
A) Trauma
B) Tumors
C) Chronic hypertension
D) Infection

86. Which of the following conditions causes significant facial weakness and difficulty swallowing due to upper and lower motor neuron degeneration?
A) ALS
B) Bell's Palsy
C) Multiple sclerosis
D) Carpal tunnel syndrome

87. Which treatment is recommended for acute bacterial meningitis caused by Neisseria meningitidis?
A) Antibiotics and antivirals
B) Intravenous antibiotics
C) Pain relievers only
D) Hydration and rest

88. What is a common sign of acute bacterial meningitis in infants?
A) Bulging fontanelle
B) Seizures
C) Fever and vomiting
D) Excessive crying

89. Which of the following is a common complication of subarachnoid hemorrhage?

A) Seizures B) Stroke C) Chronic headaches D) Hearing loss
90. What is the primary pharmacological treatment for carpal tunnel syndrome (CTS)? A) NSAIDs B) Corticosteroids C) Antiviral medication D) Antibiotics
91. What is the primary treatment for sciatica caused by a herniated disc? A) Surgery B) NSAIDs and physical therapy C) Muscle relaxants only D) Immediate steroid injections
92. What is the hallmark sign of Systemic Lupus Erythematosus (SLE)? A) Butterfly-shaped rash B) Night sweats C) Joint stiffness in the morning D) Fever with sore throat
93. Which of the following is NOT a common symptom of sciatica? A) Radiating pain from lower back to leg B) Numbness and tingling in the foot C) Worsening pain when bending D) Difficulty swallowing
94. Which condition is associated with a positive Brudzinski's sign? A) Stroke B) Meningitis C) Trigeminal neuralgia D) Multiple sclerosis
95. What is the primary pharmacological treatment for rotator cuff tendinitis? A) NSAIDs B) Corticosteroids C) Muscle relaxants D) Antibiotics
96. What is the first-line treatment for Carpal Tunnel Syndrome (CTS)? A) Surgery B) Wrist splints C) Corticosteroid injections D) Physical therapy only
97. Which of the following is a characteristic of a comminuted fracture? A) A clean break with no displacement B) Bone fragments are displaced into several pieces C) Fracture through the skin D) Fracture is limited to the bone surface
98. What diagnostic tool is used to confirm the diagnosis of a subarachnoid hemorrhage?

A) X-ray
B) MRI
C) CT scan
D) Lumbar puncture

99. Which of the following is an indication for surgical intervention in fractures?
A) Non-displaced fractures
B) Comminuted fractures with displacement
C) Stable fractures with minor swelling
D) Fractures without deformity

100. What is a common symptom of a traumatic brain injury (TBI)?
A) Sudden onset of joint pain
B) Loss of consciousness
C) Swelling in the leg
D) Difficulty swallowing

101. What is the first step in managing a sprained ankle?
A) Immediate surgery
B) Rest, Ice, Compression, Elevation (R.I.C.E.)
C) Apply heat to the injury
D) Massage the affected area

102. Which type of fracture occurs when the bone is exposed through the skin?
A) Closed fracture
B) Compound fracture
C) Greenstick fracture
D) Transverse fracture

103. Which test is used to diagnose carpal tunnel syndrome (CTS)?
A) X-ray
B) MRI
C) Nerve conduction studies
D) Blood tests

104. What type of fracture is common in children due to their softer bones?
A) Comminuted fracture
B) Greenstick fracture
C) Oblique fracture
D) Transverse fracture

105. Which condition involves inflammation of the bursa in joints, often caused by repetitive motions?
A) Gout
B) Bursitis
C) Tendinitis
D) Arthritis

106. What is a common treatment for osteomyelitis?
A) Topical antibiotics
B) Surgery to remove necrotic bone tissue
C) Physical therapy
D) NSAIDs only

107. What is the role of acetylcholine in the nervous system?

A) It controls muscle relaxation
B) It regulates mood and appetite
C) It helps with learning and memory
D) It inhibits neurotransmission

108. Which neurotransmitter is known as the "pleasure hormone"?
A) Serotonin
B) Dopamine
C) Glutamate
D) Epinephrine

109. What is the most common cause of fractures in adults?
A) Osteoporosis
B) Trauma
C) Infections
D) Genetic disorders

110. Which of the following is a common treatment for a herniated disc causing sciatica?
A) Surgery
B) NSAIDs and physical therapy
C) Antidepressants
D) Ice and rest

111. What is a hallmark symptom of Achilles tendonitis?
A) Pain in the shoulder
B) Pain in the wrist
C) Pain in the posterior aspect of the ankle
D) Pain in the elbow

112. What is a common complication of a compound fracture?
A) Infection
B) Swelling
C) Bruising
D) Displacement

113. What is the primary diagnostic tool for evaluating fractures?
A) MRI
B) X-ray
C) CT scan
D) Physical examination

114. What condition is characterized by progressive muscle weakness and difficulty speaking and swallowing?
A) Amyotrophic Lateral Sclerosis
B) Multiple sclerosis
C) Carpal Tunnel Syndrome
D) Bell's palsy

115. What is a positive finding in the Romberg test suggestive of?
A) Proprioceptive or cerebellar disorder
B) Stroke
C) Spinal cord injury
D) Bell's palsy

116. What is the purpose of GABA as a neurotransmitter?

<table>
<tr><td>A) To increase muscle contraction
B) To decrease neuronal excitability
C) To stimulate the release of adrenaline
D) To regulate mood and appetite</td></tr>
<tr><td>117. Which of the following is a diagnostic test for meningitis?
A) MRI
B) Lumbar puncture (CSF analysis)
C) X-ray
D) Nerve conduction studies</td></tr>
<tr><td>118. What condition is associated with the "worst headache of your life"?
A) Tension headache
B) Subarachnoid hemorrhage
C) Cluster headache
D) Acute bacterial meningitis</td></tr>
<tr><td>119. What is the main neurotransmitter involved in muscle contraction?
A) GABA
B) Acetylcholine
C) Dopamine
D) Glutamate</td></tr>
<tr><td>120. Which of the following is a common cause of traumatic brain injury (TBI)?
A) Stroke
B) Sports-related injuries
C) Autoimmune diseases
D) Poor posture</td></tr>
<tr><td>121. Which of the following is NOT typically used to treat tendonitis?
A) Ice therapy
B) Steroid injections
C) Surgery
D) Physical therapy</td></tr>
<tr><td>122. What is the typical first step in managing a muscle strain?
A) Immediate surgery
B) Rest, Ice, Compression, Elevation (R.I.C.E.)
C) Massage
D) Heat therapy</td></tr>
<tr><td>123. What is the main function of the peripheral nervous system (PNS)?
A) To process information
B) To control voluntary movement
C) To transmit sensory and motor signals between the body and the brain
D) To maintain balance</td></tr>
<tr><td>124. What is a common consequence of untreated acute bacterial meningitis?
A) Hearing loss
B) Nausea and vomiting
C) Memory loss
D) Personality changes</td></tr>
<tr><td>125. What is the most common treatment for Giant Cell Arteritis (GCA)?</td></tr>
</table>

A) NSAIDs
B) Corticosteroids
C) Surgery
D) Physical therapy

126. What diagnostic tool is commonly used for diagnosing multiple sclerosis (MS)?
A) MRI
B) X-ray
C) CT scan
D) Blood test

127. What is the primary function of the somatic motor division of the PNS?
A) To regulate involuntary functions
B) To carry sensory impulses to the brain
C) To send motor signals from the CNS to muscles
D) To control heart rate

128. What condition is associated with facial drooping and inability to close the eye?
A) Bell's palsy
B) Trigeminal neuralgia
C) Stroke
D) Myasthenia gravis

129. Which of the following medications is commonly used to treat sciatica?
A) Antidepressants
B) Muscle relaxants
C) Antiplatelet drugs
D) Insulin

130. What is the primary cause of osteomyelitis?
A) Viral infection
B) Bacterial infection
C) Fungal infection
D) Autoimmune disease

131. Which neurotransmitter is involved in the body's "fight or flight" response?
A) Serotonin
B) Epinephrine
C) GABA
D) Acetylcholine

132. What is the main characteristic of a Grade 2 muscle strain?
A) Complete muscle rupture
B) Mild muscle discomfort
C) Moderate muscle tear with swelling and pain
D) Mild stretching of the muscle

133. What is the first-line treatment for a sprained ankle?
A) Surgery
B) Rest, Ice, Compression, Elevation (R.I.C.E.)
C) Ice only
D) Heat therapy

134. What is the primary goal of physical therapy for a sprained ankle?

A) To increase flexibility
B) To strengthen muscles and improve stability
C) To reduce inflammation
D) To immobilize the ankle

135. What is the purpose of the straight leg raise test in sciatica evaluation?
A) To assess knee function
B) To evaluate lumbar range of motion
C) To check for nerve root irritation
D) To test for muscle weakness

136. Which of the following is a major risk factor for osteoporosis?
A) High calcium intake
B) Smoking
C) Regular exercise
D) Low body weight

137. What is a common symptom of patellar tendinitis (jumper's knee)?
A) Swelling and pain in the shoulder
B) Pain around the kneecap, especially during jumping
C) Pain in the heel
D) Pain in the wrist

138. What is a common cause of tendinitis?
A) Poor posture
B) Sedentary lifestyle
C) Repetitive movements and overuse
D) Low-calcium diet

139. What is a common sign of carpal tunnel syndrome?
A) Shoulder pain
B) Numbness and tingling in the fingers
C) Pain in the knee
D) Muscle weakness in the legs

140. What is the primary cause of a subdural hematoma?
A) Chronic alcohol use
B) Head trauma
C) Infections
D) Bone fractures

141. What is the hallmark symptom of fibromyalgia?
A) Muscle weakness
B) Widespread musculoskeletal pain
C) Joint swelling
D) Radiating pain down the legs

142. Which of the following is a common symptom of fibromyalgia?
A) Numbness in the hands
B) "Fibro fog" and difficulty concentrating
C) Swelling of the joints
D) Sharp, stabbing pain in the lower back

143. What is the primary treatment for fibromyalgia?

A) Steroid injections B) Antidepressants and pain relievers C) Surgery D) Physical therapy only
144. Which of the following is NOT a cause of bursitis? A) Repetitive motion B) Trauma or injury C) Gout or rheumatoid arthritis D) Genetic predisposition
145. Which test is used to diagnose carpal tunnel syndrome? A) MRI B) Tinel's sign and Phalen's test C) X-ray D) Complete blood count
146. What is the first-line treatment for acute gout attacks? A) Surgery B) NSAIDs, colchicine, or corticosteroids C) Antidepressants D) Muscle relaxants
147. Which joint is most commonly affected during a gout attack? A) Knee B) Wrist C) First metatarsophalangeal joint of the great toe D) Elbow
148. What is the potential consequence of untreated chronic gout? A) Heart failure B) Chronic tophaceous gout causing joint deformation C) Arthritis in the wrists D) Muscle atrophy
149. Which of the following is a typical sign of carpal tunnel syndrome? A) Pain radiating down the arm B) Numbness and tingling in the fingers, especially at night C) Swelling around the wrist D) Sharp pain in the wrist after trauma
150. What is a common risk factor for developing gout? A) High intake of low-purine foods B) Increased alcohol consumption C) Low blood pressure D) Excessive physical activity

1.	• **B. Kidneys** – The kidneys are the primary organs responsible for excreting most drugs and their metabolites through urine.
2.	• **B. The effect of drugs passing through the liver before reaching systemic circulation** – The first-pass effect refers to the metabolism of drugs in the liver before they reach the bloodstream, reducing their active concentration.
3.	• **C. Liver** – The liver is the primary site for drug metabolism, where many drugs are processed by liver enzymes.
4.	• **B. Drug toxicity** – If two drugs share metabolic pathways in the liver, they may compete for the same enzymes, increasing the risk of drug toxicity due to altered metabolism.
5.	• **D. All of the above** – Blood flow, tissue composition, and protein-binding capacity all influence the distribution of drugs throughout the body.
6.	• **B. It binds to a receptor and activates it** – An agonist drug binds to a receptor and activates it, mimicking the action of the body's natural ligands.
7.	• **B. SSRIs (Selective Serotonin Reuptake Inhibitors)** – SSRIs, such as fluoxetine and sertraline, increase serotonin levels by inhibiting its reuptake in the brain.
8.	• **A. Disulfiram** – Disulfiram is used to treat alcohol use disorder by causing a severe reaction when alcohol is consumed, discouraging alcohol intake.
9.	• **B. Excessive serotonin levels caused by drugs that increase serotonin** – Serotonin syndrome is caused by an excess of serotonin, often due to drug interactions or overdose of serotonergic drugs.
10.	• **C. Hyperreflexia** – Hyperreflexia, or increased reflex responses, is a characteristic clinical sign of serotonin syndrome.
11.	• **A. Cyproheptadine** – Cyproheptadine is an antihistamine that can block serotonin receptors and is used as the first-line treatment for serotonin syndrome.
12.	• **B. Beta-blockers** – Atenolol is a beta-blocker, which works by blocking beta-adrenergic receptors to reduce heart rate and blood pressure.
13.	• **B. To block beta-adrenergic receptors and reduce heart rate** – Beta-blockers like atenolol block beta receptors, which reduces heart rate and lowers blood pressure.
14.	• **B. Enalapril** – Enalapril is an ACE inhibitor commonly prescribed for hypertension because it relaxes blood vessels and reduces blood pressure.
15.	• **B. To increase the elimination of sodium and water** – Diuretics work by helping the kidneys eliminate excess sodium and water, which reduces blood volume and lowers blood pressure.
16.	• **B. Fluoxetine** – Fluoxetine is an SSRI, and when combined with other serotonergic drugs, it can cause serotonin toxicity by increasing serotonin levels in the body.
17.	• **C. Kidney and liver function** – In elderly patients, kidney and liver function are crucial in determining drug dosage, as these organs process and eliminate medications.
18.	• **D. The study of drug effects on the body** – Pharmacodynamics is the study of how drugs affect the body, including their mechanisms of action and therapeutic effects.
19.	• **B. Liver** – The liver is the primary site of drug metabolism, where most drugs undergo chemical changes through enzymes like cytochrome P450.
20.	• **C. Anti-inflammatory drugs** – Anti-inflammatory drugs, such as NSAIDs, reduce inflammation and are used to treat conditions like arthritis.

21.	• **B. Constipation** – Constipation is a common side effect of opioid drugs because they reduce gastrointestinal motility.
22.	• **A. SSRIs** – SSRIs are commonly prescribed for generalized anxiety disorder (GAD) to regulate serotonin levels and improve mood and anxiety.
23.	• **B. Photosensitivity** – Tetracycline antibiotics can cause photosensitivity, increasing the risk of sunburn when exposed to sunlight.
24.	• **A. Fever and sore throat** – Peritonsillar abscess is characterized by fever and severe sore throat, often with difficulty swallowing.
25.	• **B. Trauma or injury** – An avulsed tooth is commonly caused by trauma or injury, such as a blow to the mouth.
26.	• **B. Serotonin syndrome** – Cyproheptadine is used to treat serotonin syndrome by blocking serotonin receptors and reversing symptoms.
27.	• **B. To inhibit serotonin reuptake and increase serotonin levels** – SSRIs inhibit the reuptake of serotonin, leading to increased serotonin levels in the brain.
28.	• **B. Osteoporosis** – High-dose corticosteroids can lead to osteoporosis by reducing calcium absorption and increasing bone resorption.
29.	• **B. Antibiotics (e.g., penicillin or amoxicillin)** – Strep throat is caused by a bacterial infection, and antibiotics like penicillin are used to treat it.
30.	• **B. The type of bacteria causing the infection** – The specific bacteria causing an infection determines which antibiotic should be prescribed for treatment.
31.	• **B) Trauma** – Auricular hematoma is caused by trauma to the ear, leading to blood accumulation between the cartilage and skin.
32.	• **A) MRI** – MRI is the preferred imaging method for diagnosing acoustic neuroma because it provides detailed images of the brain and inner ear.
33.	• **B) Antibiotics** – Antibiotics are the first-line treatment for acute otitis media to address the bacterial infection causing the condition.
34.	• **B) Herpes keratitis** – Dendritic ulcers on the cornea observed during a slit-lamp examination are a hallmark sign of herpes keratitis caused by the herpes simplex virus.
35.	• **A) Acetazolamide** – Acetazolamide is used to reduce intraocular pressure in acute angle-closure glaucoma by inhibiting the production of aqueous humor.
36.	• **B) Insulin resistance** – Insulin resistance is a common risk factor for polycystic ovary syndrome (PCOS) and is linked to hormonal imbalances in the body.
37.	• **B) Low estrogen levels** – Atrophic vaginitis is primarily caused by low estrogen levels, especially in postmenopausal women, leading to vaginal dryness and discomfort.
38.	• **A) Oral metronidazole** – Oral metronidazole is the first-line treatment for bacterial vaginosis caused by anaerobic bacterial overgrowth.
39.	• **B) Optical coherence tomography (OCT)** – OCT is a non-invasive imaging method commonly used to diagnose and monitor retinopathy, especially in patients with autoimmune diseases.
40.	• **A) Dry eyes and mouth** – Sjogren's syndrome is an autoimmune disorder characterized by dry eyes and mouth due to damage to exocrine glands, such as the salivary and lacrimal glands.

41. • B. Intravenous antibiotics – Orbital cellulitis is a severe infection requiring intravenous antibiotics to prevent further complications like abscess formation or vision loss.
42. • A. Sepsis – Untreated endometritis can lead to sepsis, a systemic infection that can be life-threatening if not treated promptly.
43. • D. Medications to lower intraocular pressure – Acute angle-closure glaucoma requires immediate lowering of intraocular pressure with medications to prevent optic nerve damage.
44. • B. Abdominal tenderness – Myometritis causes abdominal tenderness due to inflammation of the uterine muscles, often following childbirth or infection.
45. • B. CT scan – A CT scan is used to confirm orbital cellulitis, allowing the identification of abscesses or other complications associated with the infection.
46. • A. Anti-VEGF injections – Anti-VEGF injections are used to treat age-related macular degeneration (AMD) by inhibiting abnormal blood vessel growth in the retina.
47. • B. Poor contact lens hygiene – Poor hygiene and improper care of contact lenses increase the risk of keratitis, a serious eye infection.
48. • B. Physical examination – Pterygium is diagnosed through a physical examination, where the growth of tissue from the conjunctiva onto the cornea is visible.
49. • B. Yeast infection – Oral fluconazole is used to treat yeast infections caused by *Candida* species, leading to symptoms like thick white discharge.
50. • B. Sudden vision loss – Retinal detachment often presents with sudden vision loss or the sensation of a shadow or curtain in the field of vision.
51. • A. Multiple sclerosis – Optic neuritis, characterized by inflammation of the optic nerve, is commonly associated with multiple sclerosis, an autoimmune disease affecting the central nervous system.
52. • B. Fishy odor to vaginal discharge – A fishy odor is characteristic of bacterial vaginosis, caused by an imbalance in vaginal flora, particularly *Gardnerella* bacteria.
53. • B. Antibiotics such as metronidazole – Metronidazole is the first-line treatment for trichomoniasis, a sexually transmitted infection caused by *Trichomonas vaginalis*.
54. • A. Glaucoma – An enlarged optic disc and visual field loss are classic signs of glaucoma, a condition that causes optic nerve damage due to increased intraocular pressure.
55. • B. Vaginal estrogen therapy – Vaginal estrogen therapy is the most effective treatment for atrophic vaginitis, especially in postmenopausal women, to restore vaginal health.
56. • C. Age-related macular degeneration – Drusen in the macula are a hallmark feature of age-related macular degeneration (AMD), which can lead to vision loss.
57. • A. Infertility – Untreated PCOS commonly leads to infertility due to irregular ovulation and hormonal imbalances that disrupt fertility.
58. • B. Tearing and irritation from eyelashes rubbing the cornea – Entropion causes the eyelid to turn inward, leading to irritation and damage to the cornea from the eyelashes.
59. • B. IV antibiotics – The primary treatment for endometritis after a miscarriage is IV antibiotics to prevent or treat infection in the uterus.

60. • **C. Yeast infection** – A thick, white, creamy discharge is typical of a vaginal yeast infection caused by *Candida* species.
61. • **B. Birth control pills** – Birth control pills are commonly prescribed to manage the hormonal imbalance in PCOS, which can help regulate menstrual cycles and improve acne.
62. • **B. Vaginal dryness and discomfort** – Atrophic vaginitis, commonly occurring in postmenopausal women, is characterized by vaginal dryness, discomfort, and thinning of vaginal tissues due to low estrogen levels.
63. • **A. Copper IUD** – The copper intrauterine device (IUD) is a non-hormonal, long-term contraceptive method that prevents pregnancy by creating an unfavorable environment for sperm.
64. • **A. Pregnancy** – Pregnancy is the most common cause of secondary amenorrhea (absence of menstruation), leading to missed periods.
65. • **B. Corticosteroids** – Corticosteroids are the first-line treatment for Bell's palsy to reduce inflammation and promote recovery of the facial nerve.
66. • **A. Jaw claudication** – Jaw claudication, or pain when chewing, is a classic symptom of giant cell arteritis (GCA), which involves inflammation of the temporal arteries.
67. • **C. Streptococcus pneumoniae** – Streptococcus pneumoniae is the most common causative organism of acute bacterial meningitis in adults, requiring immediate antibiotic treatment.
68. • **B. Sudden numbness or weakness on one side of the body** – Sudden numbness or weakness on one side of the body is a hallmark symptom of a transient ischemic attack (TIA), which is a mini-stroke.
69. • **D. Blood pressure management** – The key treatment for subarachnoid hemorrhage (SAH) is blood pressure management to prevent further bleeding or complications.
70. • **D. Wrist splints and ergonomic adjustments** – Wrist splints and ergonomic adjustments are the first-line non-surgical treatments for carpal tunnel syndrome to alleviate pressure on the median nerve.
71. • **B. IV antibiotics (e.g., ceftriaxone, vancomycin)** – IV antibiotics are the standard treatment for acute bacterial meningitis, especially in cases caused by *Streptococcus pneumoniae* or *Neisseria meningitidis*.
72. • **A. Sharp, stabbing facial pain** – Trigeminal neuralgia is characterized by sharp, stabbing facial pain that occurs suddenly and is triggered by activities such as chewing or brushing teeth.
73. • **B. Fluctuating neurological symptoms such as weakness and visual changes** – Multiple sclerosis is characterized by fluctuating neurological symptoms like weakness, numbness, and visual disturbances.
74. • **C. Anti-androgens (e.g., spironolactone)** – Anti-androgens like spironolactone are used to treat acne associated with PCOS by blocking the effects of excess androgen hormones.
75. • **B. Vision loss** – A common complication of untreated giant cell arteritis (GCA) is vision loss due to inflammation and occlusion of the arteries supplying the eyes.
76. • **B) CT scan of the head** – A CT scan of the head is typically used to confirm the diagnosis of subarachnoid hemorrhage, which is visible on imaging as blood in the brain.

77. • C) Atherosclerosis – Atherosclerosis, or the buildup of plaque in arteries, is the most common cause of TIAs in older adults and can restrict blood flow to the brain.
78. • C) Amyotrophic lateral sclerosis (ALS) – Riluzole and edaravone are used to treat amyotrophic lateral sclerosis (ALS), a neurodegenerative disease that affects motor neurons.
79. • A) Ceftriaxone with dexamethasone – Ceftriaxone with dexamethasone is the treatment of choice for bacterial meningitis caused by *Streptococcus pneumoniae* to address both the infection and inflammation.
80. • A) Unilateral facial paralysis – Bell's palsy is characterized by sudden, unilateral facial paralysis, which often prevents the person from closing one eye or smiling on one side of the face.
81. • A) Hearing loss – Hearing loss is a common long-term complication of untreated acute bacterial meningitis, especially when the infection affects the auditory pathways.
82. • B) Trigeminal neuralgia – Trigeminal neuralgia presents with sharp, electric shock-like facial pain triggered by touch or chewing.
83. • C) Acute bacterial meningitis – Acute bacterial meningitis is characterized by sudden severe headache, fever, and signs like positive Brudzinski's and Kernig's signs.
84. • B) Corticosteroids – Corticosteroids are used as the primary treatment for Bell's palsy to reduce inflammation and improve recovery of the facial nerve.
85. • A) Trauma – Trauma is the most common cause of subdural hematomas in elderly patients, often resulting from a fall or minor head injury.
86. • A) ALS – ALS (Amyotrophic Lateral Sclerosis) causes muscle weakness, difficulty swallowing, and other symptoms due to the degeneration of both upper and lower motor neurons.
87. • B) Intravenous antibiotics – Intravenous antibiotics are recommended for Neisseria meningitidis infections causing bacterial meningitis to treat the infection effectively.
88. • A) Bulging fontanelle – A bulging fontanelle is a common sign of increased intracranial pressure due to infection, such as in acute bacterial meningitis, in infants.
89. • B) Stroke – Stroke is a common complication of subarachnoid hemorrhage due to disrupted blood flow and subsequent brain damage.
90. • B) Corticosteroids – Corticosteroids are used to reduce inflammation and manage symptoms in carpal tunnel syndrome (CTS).
91. • B) NSAIDs and physical therapy – NSAIDs and physical therapy are effective in treating sciatica caused by a herniated disc by reducing inflammation and improving mobility.
92. • A) Butterfly-shaped rash – A butterfly-shaped rash across the cheeks and nose is a classic symptom of Systemic Lupus Erythematosus (SLE), an autoimmune disease.
93. • D) Difficulty swallowing – Sciatica typically presents with radiating pain and numbness in the legs, not difficulty swallowing.
94. • B) Meningitis – A positive Brudzinski's sign is indicative of meningitis, an infection of the meninges that causes neck stiffness and irritation.
95. • A) NSAIDs – NSAIDs are the primary pharmacological treatment for rotator cuff tendinitis, as they help reduce inflammation and manage pain.
96. • B) Wrist splints – Wrist splints are the first-line non-surgical treatment for car

97. • B) Bone fragments are displaced into several pieces – A comminuted fracture involves the bone breaking into several pieces, which may require surgery for realignment.
98. • C) CT scan – A CT scan is used to confirm the diagnosis of a subarachnoid hemorrhage, as it can detect blood in the brain.
99. • B) Comminuted fractures with displacement – Comminuted fractures with displacement typically require surgical intervention to align and stabilize the bone.
100. B) Loss of consciousness – A common symptom of traumatic brain injury (TBI) is loss of consciousness, often due to a direct blow to the head.
101. • B. Rest, Ice, Compression, Elevation (R.I.C.E.) – The R.I.C.E. method is the initial treatment for a sprained ankle, helping reduce swelling and promoting healing.
102. • B. Compound fracture – A compound fracture occurs when the bone is exposed through the skin, increasing the risk of infection.
103. • C. Nerve conduction studies – Nerve conduction studies are the primary diagnostic tool for carpal tunnel syndrome (CTS), as they measure the speed of nerve impulses.
104. • B. Greenstick fracture – Greenstick fractures are common in children due to their softer bones, resulting in a partial break without complete separation.
105. • B. Bursitis – Bursitis is the inflammation of the bursa, often due to repetitive motions or overuse of joints, causing pain and swelling.
106. • B. Surgery to remove necrotic bone tissue – Osteomyelitis may require surgery to remove necrotic tissue in severe cases, along with antibiotic treatment.
107. • C. It helps with learning and memory – Acetylcholine is a neurotransmitter crucial for memory and learning, as well as muscle function.
108. • B. Dopamine – Dopamine is known as the "pleasure hormone," involved in reward, motivation, and mood regulation.
109. • B. Trauma – Trauma, such as falls or accidents, is the most common cause of fractures in adults, particularly in those with osteoporosis.
110. • B. NSAIDs and physical therapy – For a herniated disc causing sciatica, NSAIDs reduce inflammation, and physical therapy helps with mobility and pain management.
111. • C. Pain in the posterior aspect of the ankle – Achilles tendonitis presents with pain at the back of the ankle, especially during activities like running or jumping.
112. • A. Infection – A common complication of a compound fracture is infection due to the exposure of bone to the environment.
113. • B. X-ray – X-rays are the primary diagnostic tool for evaluating fractures, allowing visualization of the bone structure and any breaks.
114. • A. Amyotrophic Lateral Sclerosis – Amyotrophic lateral sclerosis (ALS) is characterized by progressive muscle weakness and difficulty speaking and swallowing due to the degeneration of motor neurons.
115. • A. Proprioceptive or cerebellar disorder – A positive Romberg test suggests a problem with proprioception or cerebellar function, often indicating neurological issues.

116.	• **B. To decrease neuronal excitability** – GABA (gamma-aminobutyric acid) is the main inhibitory neurotransmitter in the brain, helping to reduce neuronal excitability and prevent overstimulation.
117.	• **B. Lumbar puncture (CSF analysis)** – A lumbar puncture, or CSF analysis, is the primary diagnostic test for meningitis, as it checks for abnormal white blood cell counts or pathogens in the cerebrospinal fluid.
118.	• **B. Subarachnoid hemorrhage** – The "worst headache of your life" is a hallmark symptom of a subarachnoid hemorrhage, which can result in a brain bleed.
119.	• **B. Acetylcholine** – Acetylcholine is the neurotransmitter that plays a key role in muscle contraction by transmitting signals from nerve endings to muscle fibers.
120.	• **B. Sports-related injuries** – Traumatic brain injury (TBI) is most commonly caused by sports-related injuries, such as concussions from impacts or falls.
121.	• **C. Surgery** – Surgery is generally not used to treat tendonitis unless other treatments (such as rest and physical therapy) fail to resolve the condition.
122.	• **B. Rest, Ice, Compression, Elevation (R.I.C.E.)** – R.I.C.E. is the standard first step in managing a muscle strain, as it helps reduce swelling and supports healing.
123.	• **C. To transmit sensory and motor signals between the body and the brain** – The peripheral nervous system (PNS) is responsible for carrying sensory and motor signals to and from the brain and spinal cord.
124.	• **A. Hearing loss** – A common consequence of untreated acute bacterial meningitis is hearing loss, which may result from damage to the auditory pathways.
125.	• **B. Corticosteroids** – The primary treatment for Giant Cell Arteritis (GCA) is corticosteroids, which help reduce inflammation and prevent vision loss.
126.	• **A. MRI** – MRI is commonly used to diagnose multiple sclerosis (MS) by detecting plaques or lesions in the brain and spinal cord caused by demyelination.
127.	• **C. To send motor signals from the CNS to muscles** – The somatic motor division of the PNS is responsible for sending voluntary motor signals from the central nervous system (CNS) to skeletal muscles.
128.	• **A. Bell's palsy** – Bell's palsy is associated with facial drooping and an inability to close one eye, due to damage to the facial nerve (cranial nerve VII).
129.	• **B. Muscle relaxants** – Muscle relaxants are commonly prescribed for sciatica to relieve muscle spasms associated with nerve compression from a herniated disc.
130.	• **B. Bacterial infection** – Osteomyelitis is primarily caused by a bacterial infection, often *Staphylococcus aureus*, which spreads to the bones from the bloodstream or nearby tissues.
131.	• **B. Epinephrine** – Epinephrine is the primary neurotransmitter involved in the "fight or flight" response, preparing the body for rapid action by increasing heart rate and blood flow to muscles.
132.	• **C. Moderate muscle tear with swelling and pain** – A Grade 2 muscle strain is characterized by a moderate muscle tear, causing swelling, pain, and some loss of function.
133.	• **B. Rest, Ice, Compression, Elevation (R.I.C.E.)** – The first-line treatment for a sprained ankle is R.I.C.E. to reduce swelling and promote recovery.

134.	• **B. To strengthen muscles and improve stability** – The primary goal of physical therapy for a sprained ankle is to strengthen muscles, improve stability, and prevent re-injury.
135.	• **C. To check for nerve root irritation** – The straight leg raise test is used to assess nerve root irritation, particularly in cases of sciatica caused by a herniated disc.
136.	• **B. Smoking** – Smoking is a major risk factor for osteoporosis as it inhibits bone formation and increases the rate of bone loss.
137.	• **B. Pain around the kneecap, especially during jumping** – Patellar tendinitis, or jumper's knee, causes pain around the kneecap, especially during activities like jumping or running.
138.	• **C. Repetitive movements and overuse** – Tendinitis is commonly caused by repetitive movements or overuse of a particular joint or tendon, leading to inflammation.
139.	• **B. Numbness and tingling in the fingers** – Carpal tunnel syndrome is characterized by numbness and tingling in the fingers, especially at night, due to compression of the median nerve.
140.	• **B. Head trauma** – Subdural hematomas are often caused by head trauma, especially in elderly individuals with fragile blood vessels.
141.	• **B. Widespread musculoskeletal pain** – Fibromyalgia is characterized by widespread musculoskeletal pain, often accompanied by fatigue and sleep disturbances.
142.	• **B. "Fibro fog" and difficulty concentrating** – Fibromyalgia often involves "fibro fog," which includes difficulty concentrating, memory issues, and cognitive dysfunction.
143.	• **B. Antidepressants and pain relievers** – The primary treatment for fibromyalgia includes antidepressants and pain relievers to manage symptoms and improve quality of life.
144.	• **D. Genetic predisposition** – Bursitis is usually caused by repetitive motion or injury, not genetic predisposition, which makes option D incorrect.
145.	• **B. Tinel's sign and Phalen's test** – Tinel's sign and Phalen's test are commonly used to diagnose carpal tunnel syndrome by provoking symptoms of nerve compression in the wrist.
146.	• **B. NSAIDs, colchicine, or corticosteroids** – The first-line treatment for acute gout attacks includes NSAIDs, colchicine, or corticosteroids to reduce inflammation and pain.
147.	• **C. First metatarsophalangeal joint of the great toe** – Gout typically affects the first metatarsophalangeal joint, causing severe pain and swelling in the big toe.
148.	• **B. Chronic tophaceous gout causing joint deformation** – Untreated chronic gout can lead to the formation of tophi, which are deposits of uric acid crystals that deform joints.
149.	• **B. Numbness and tingling in the fingers, especially at night** – Carpal tunnel syndrome is characterized by numbness and tingling in the fingers, often worse at night due to median nerve compression.
150.	• **B. Increased alcohol consumption** – Increased alcohol consumption is a common risk factor for developing gout, as it increases uric acid levels in the body.

References

Amegadzie, J.E., 2021. *Pharmaco-epidemiological study of cardiorespiratory safety of β2-agonists for the treatment and management of asthma, chronic obstructive pulmonary disease (DOPD) and asthma-COPD overlap* (Doctoral dissertation, Memorial University of Newfoundland).

Stamm, B., Royan, R., Cui, J., Long, D.L., Lineback, C.M., Akinyelure, O.P., Plante, T.B., Levine, D.A., Howard, V.J., Howard, G. and Gorelick, P.B., 2024. Trends in Black-White Differences of Antihypertensive Treatment in Individuals With and Without History of Stroke. *Stroke*, *55*(8), pp.2034-2044.

Sehgal, A.R., 2004. Overlap between whites and blacks in response to antihypertensive drugs. *Hypertension*, *43*(3), pp.566-572.

Augnito., n.d.. *Accurate clinical documentation with SOAP notes.* Augnito. Retrieved February 17, 2025, from https://augnito.ai/resources/accurate-clinical-documentation-with-soap-notes/

Berglund, C., 2019. *Nursing Staff Development for Novice Nurse Practitioners in Acute Care* (Doctoral dissertation, Walden University).

Celermajer, D.S., Chow, C.K., Marijon, E., Anstey, N.M. and Woo, K.S., 2012. Cardiovascular disease in the developing world: prevalences, patterns, and the potential of early disease detection. *Journal of the American College of Cardiology*, *60*(14), pp.1207-1216.

Centers for Disease Control and Prevention., 2024. *Evidence-based practice: What it is and why it matters.* CDC. Retrieved February 17, 2025, from https://www.cdc.gov/genomics/media/pdfs/2024/04/Evidence-Based_Practice_508.pdf

Chipps, B.E., Albers, F.C., Reilly, L., Johnsson, E., Cappelletti, C. and Papi, A., 2021. Efficacy and safety of as-needed albuterol/budesonide versus albuterol in adults and children aged≥ 4 years with moderate-to-severe asthma: rationale and design of the randomised, double-blind, active-controlled MANDALA study. *BMJ Open Respiratory Research*, *8*(1), p.e001077.

Connor, L., Dean, J., McNett, M., Tydings, D.M., Shrout, A., Gorsuch, P.F., Hole, A., Moore, L., Brown, R., Melnyk, B.M. and Gallagher-Ford, L., 2023. Evidence-based practice improves patient outcomes and healthcare system return on investment: Findings from a scoping review. *Worldviews on Evidence-Based Nursing*, *20*(1), pp.6-15.

Cooper, C.P. and Saraiya, M., 2018. Cervical cancer screening intervals preferred by US women. *American journal of preventive medicine*, *55*(3), pp.389-394.

Dlamini, C.P., Khumalo, T., Nkwanyana, N., Mathunjwa-Dlamini, T.R., Macera, L., Nsibandze, B.S., Kaplan, L. and Stuart-Shor, E.M., 2020. Developing and implementing the family nurse practitioner role in Eswatini: implications for education, practice, and policy. *Annals of Global Health*, *86*(1).

Donohoe, J., 2015. *Implementing an education programme and SOAP Notes framework to improve nursing documentation* (Doctoral dissertation, Royal College of Surgeons in Ireland).

Dumic, I., Nordin, T., Jecmenica, M., Stojkovic Lalosevic, M., Milosavljevic, T. and Milovanovic, T., 2019. Gastrointestinal tract disorders in older age. *Canadian Journal of Gastroenterology and Hepatology*, *2019*(1), p.6757524.

Fenstermacher, K. and Hudson, B., 2019. *Practice Guidelines for Family Nurse Practitioners E-Book: Practice Guidelines for Family Nurse Practitioners E-Book.* Elsevier Health Sciences.

Fraze, T.K., Briggs, A.D., Whitcomb, E.K., Peck, K.A. and Meara, E., 2020. Role of nurse practitioners in caring for patients with complex health needs. *Medical care*, *58*(10), pp.853-860.

Gilbert, C., Earleywine, M. and Altman, B.R., 2021. Perceptions of cognitive behavioral therapy, aerobic exercise, and their combination for depression. *Professional Psychology: Research and Practice*, *52*(6), p.551.

Godshall, M. and Cannon, J., 2023. ADRENAL INSUFFICIENCY. *Pediatric CCRN® Certification Review: Comprehensive Review, PLUS 300 Questions Based on the Latest Exam Blueprint*, p.121.

Gubala, V., Harris, L.F., Ricco, A.J., Tan, M.X. and Williams, D.E., 2012. Point of care diagnostics: status and future. *Analytical chemistry*, *84*(2), pp.487-515.

Haghdoost, F. and Togha, M., 2022. Migraine management: Non-pharmacological points for patients and health care professionals. *Open Medicine*, *17*(1), pp.1869-1882.

Holtzman, M.J., 2012. Asthma as a chronic disease of the innate and adaptive immune systems responding to viruses and allergens. *The Journal of clinical investigation*, *122*(8), pp.2741-2748.

Hughes, K. and Eastman, C., 2021. Thyroid disease: Long-term management of hyperthyroidism and hypothyroidism. *Australian journal of general practice*, *50*(1/2), pp.36-42.

Kekii, E.B., 2014. *A Motivational Interviewing Approach to Improve Self-Care in Older Adults with Congestive Heart Failure* (Doctoral dissertation, Walden University).

Lin, C.T., McKenzie, M., Pell, J. and Caplan, L., 2013. Health care provider satisfaction with a new electronic progress note format: SOAP vs APSO format. *JAMA internal medicine*, *173*(2), pp.160-162.

Lin, Y.J., Anzaghe, M. and Schülke, S., 2020. Update on the pathomechanism, diagnosis, and treatment options for rheumatoid arthritis. *Cells*, *9*(4), p.880.

Martin, Z., Spry, G., Hoult, J., Maimone, I.R., Tang, X., Crichton, M. and Marshall, S., 2022. What is the efficacy of dietary, nutraceutical, and probiotic interventions for the management of gastroesophageal reflux disease symptoms? A systematic literature review and meta-analysis. *Clinical Nutrition ESPEN*, *52*, pp.340-352.

Melo, M.D.M., Silva, I.P.D., Freitas, L.S., Mesquita, S.K.D.C., Sonenberg, A. and Costa, I.K.F., 2023. Family Nurse Practitioners: an exploratory study. *Revista da Escola de Enfermagem da USP*, *57*, p.e20220362.

Nowaczyk, A., Szwedowski, D., Dallo, I. and Nowaczyk, J., 2022. Overview of first-line and second-line pharmacotherapies for osteoarthritis with special focus on intra-articular treatment. *International Journal of Molecular Sciences*, *23*(3), p.1566.

Olalekan, R.M., Raimi, A.A. and Adias, T.C., 2021. Silent Pandemic': Evidence-Based Environmental and Public Health Practices to Respond to the Covid-19 Crisis. *Science-Based Approaches to Respond to COVID and Other Public Health Threats*, *103*.

Pearce, P.F., Ferguson, L.A., George, G.S. and Langford, C.A., 2016. The essential SOAP note in an EHR age. *The Nurse Practitioner*, *41*(2), pp.29-36.

Podder, V., Lew, V. and Ghassemzadeh, S., 2020. SOAP notes [Internet]. *StatPearls. Treasure Island (FL): StatPearls Publishing.*

Porreca, A., D'Agostino, D., Romagnoli, D., Del Giudice, F., Maggi, M., Palmer, K., Falabella, R., De Berardinis, E., Sciarra, A., Ferro, M. and Artibani, W., 2021. The clinical efficacy of nitrofurantoin for treating uncomplicated urinary tract infection in adults: a systematic review of randomized control trials. *Urologia Internationalis*, *105*(7-8), pp.531-540.

Prosser, T. and Bollmeier, S.G., 2017. Asthma and COPD. *Pulmonary and Emergency Medicine. American College of Clinical Pharmacy*.

Sackett, D.L., 1998. Evidence-based medicine. *Spine*, *23*(10), pp.1085-1086.

Senno, A.T. and Brannon, R.K., 2022. Respiratory Diseases: Asthma, Pneumonia, Influenza, Tuberculosis, and COVID-19. In *Maternal-Fetal Evidence Based Guidelines* (pp. 269-296). CRC Press.

Solomons, N.M. and Spross, J.A., 2011. Evidence-based practice barriers and facilitators from a continuous quality improvement perspective: an integrative review. *Journal of nursing management*, *19*(1), pp.109-120.

Sung, J.J., Luk, A.K., Ng, S.S., Ng, A.C., Chiu, P.K., Chan, E.Y., Cheung, P.S., Chu, W.C., Wong, S.H., Lam, T.Y. and Wong, S.Y., 2021. Effectiveness of one-stop screening for colorectal, breast, and prostate cancers: A population-based feasibility study. *Frontiers in Oncology*, *11*, p.631666.

Wilcox, T., De Block, C., Schwartzbard, A.Z. and Newman, J.D., 2020. Diabetic agents, from metformin to SGLT2 inhibitors and GLP1 receptor agonists: JACC focus seminar. *Journal of the American College of Cardiology*, *75*(16), pp.1956-1974.

World Health Organization, 2023. *Global report on hypertension: the race against a silent killer*. World Health Organization.

Yin, H.L., Yin, S.Q., Lin, Q.Y., Xu, Y., Xu, H.W. and Liu, T., 2017. Prevalence of comorbidities in chronic obstructive pulmonary disease patients: a meta-analysis. *Medicine*, *96*(19), p.e6836.

Zheng, Y., Ley, S.H. and Hu, F.B., 2018. Global aetiology and epidemiology of type 2 diabetes mellitus and its complications. *Nature reviews endocrinology*, *14*(2), pp.8

www.ingramcontent.com/pod-product-compliance
Lightning Source LLC
Chambersburg PA
CBHW052339210326
41597CB00037B/6195

9781967349609